Care of childbearing women and neonates demands a nurse's best s[...] Give your students the cle[...] instruction they need to s[...]

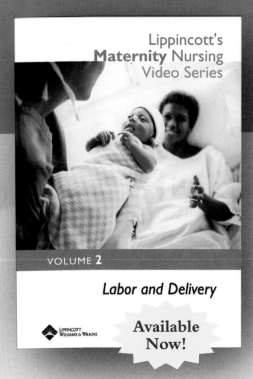

Lippincott's
Maternity Nursing
Video Series

VOLUME **2**

Labor and Delivery

LIPPINCOTT
WILLIAMS & WILKINS

Available Now!

Lippincott's Maternity Nursing
Video Series

Created with today's visual learners in mind, each of these documentary-style videos guides users through a specific phase of maternity nursing—from prenatal care, through labor and delivery, to postpartum care—while broadening their clinical expertise and enhancing their decision-making ability.

Begin your students' journey to understanding...

- **Several scenarios** address a range of pregnancy experiences, types of labors and deliveries, and postpartum experiences to prepare students for any challenge.
- **Nurse, patient, and family interviews** help users maximize their communication skills and establish therapeutic relationships.
- **A range of formats**—VHS, DVD, or Streaming Video—lets you choose the one that's best for you.

They'll build skill and confidence each step of the way...

- **Volume 1: Prenatal Care** addresses family adaptations to pregnancy, ways to promote a healthy pregnancy, and nursing management of at-risk pregnancies.
  VHS: ISBN: 0-7817-8250-3 • DVD: ISBN: 0-7817-9778-0
- **Volume 2: Labor and Delivery** begins from the moment of admission and addresses the nurse's role in assessment, monitoring, pain management, emotional support, stabilization of the newborn, and maternal-neonatal bonding.
  VHS: ISBN: 0-7817-7590-6 • DVD: ISBN: 0-7817-9547-8
- **Volume 3: Cesarean Delivery** covers several labor scenarios, including nursing care during an emergency C-section, and planned C-section.
  VHS: ISBN: 0-7817-9532-X • DVD: ISBN: 0-7817-6599-4
- **Volume 4: Postpartum Care** presents three normal range cases, from 12 hours to 6 weeks postpartum, with emphasis on maternal and newborn assessment, pain management, and family teaching.
  VHS: ISBN: 0-7817-7511-6 • DVD: ISBN: 0-7817-6545-5

2006 • Set of 4 VHS tapes: ISBN: 0-7817-6071-2 • Set of 4 DVDs: ISBN: 0-7817-8626-6

Add these skill-building videos to your curriculum...
ORDER TODAY!
Call TOLL FREE 1-800-638-3030
Visit us on the Web at **LWW.com/nursing** or **nursingcenter.com**
Or visit your local health science bookstore

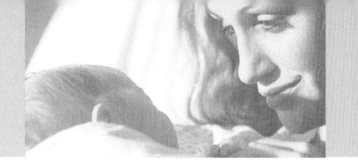

Essentials *of* Maternity, Newborn, *and* Women's Health Nursing

Susan Scott Ricci, ARNP, MSN, MEd
Nursing Faculty
University of Central Florida
Orlando, Florida
Former Nursing Program Director and Faculty
Lake Sumter Community College
Leesburg, Florida

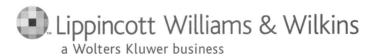
Lippincott Williams & Wilkins
a Wolters Kluwer business
Philadelphia · Baltimore · New York · London
Buenos Aires · Hong Kong · Sydney · Tokyo

Acquisitions Editor: Elizabeth Nieginski
Development Editor: Danielle DiPalma
Senior Production Editor: Tom Gibbons
Director of Nursing Production: Helen Ewan
Senior Managing Editor/Production: Erika Kors
Art Director: Joan Wendt
Senior Manufacturing Manager: William Alberti
Indexer: Victoria Boyle
Compositor: Circle Graphics
Printer: R. R. Donnelley

9 8 7 6 5 4 3 2 1

Library of Congress Cataloging-in-Publication Data

Ricci, Susan Scott.
   Essentials of maternity, newborn and women's health nursing / Susan Scott Ricci.
      p. ; cm.
   Includes bibliographical references and index.
   ISBN 0-7817-5220-5 (pbk. : alk. paper)
   1. Maternity nursing. 2. Gynecologic nursing. I. Title.
   [DNLM: 1. Maternal-Child Nursing. 2. Obstetrical Nursing. 3. Pregnancy Complications—nursing. WY 157.3 R491e 2007]
RG951.R53 2007
618.1'0231—dc22

                                                                    2005031006

LWW.com

This book is dedicated to our Heavenly Father and to my loving family: my husband Glenn, my daughter Jennifer, my son Brian and my sister Patty. Words cannot express my appreciation for their unfailing patience, their wholehearted support and encouragement during this endeavor.

SUSAN SCOTT RICCI

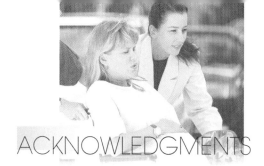

ACKNOWLEDGMENTS

To author a textbook is both an exciting and a challenging experience. It will be a privilege to contribute to the knowledge base of the next generation of nursing students. Words can't express my appreciation to Elizabeth Nieginski for believing in my vision and working tirelessly to bring this work to fruition. I would like to especially thank Danielle DiPalma for her editorial expertise and for keeping the project moving. She has been my anchor in the storm of chapter drafts and revisions. In addition, I would like to thank Maryann Foley for her professional collaboration and attention to detail within the chapters.

I would like to thank photographer Gus Freedman and photo producer Amy Geller for their dedicated work on the photo shoot. I would like to thank the following institutions for their help in getting the photos for this book:

UMass Memorial Health Care
The Birthplace at Wellesley
Brigham and Women's Hospital
Newton-Wellesley Hospital

Also thanks to the many nurses, midwives, doctors, and families for their participation in this book, especially Debbie Turner, Paula McGarr, Susan Martinson, Grace Jackson, and Marianne Cummings. I'm sure I have left out several other people who played a role in the development of this textbook, so a global appreciation is extended to the Lippincott Williams & Wilkins staff.

S.S.R.

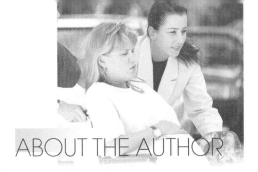

ABOUT THE AUTHOR

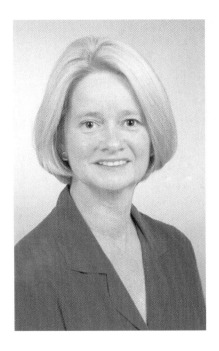

Susan Scott Ricci has a diploma from Washington Hospital Center School of Nursing, with a BSN, MSN, from Catholic University of America in Washington D.C., an M.Ed. in Counseling from the University of Southern Mississippi, and an ARNP in Women's Health from the University of Florida. She has worked in numerous women's health care settings including labor and delivery, postpartum, prenatal, and family planning ambulatory care clinics. Susan is a women's health care nurse practitioner, who has spent 30+ years in nursing education teaching in LPN, ADN, and BSN programs. She is involved in several professional nursing organizations and holds memberships in Sigma Theta Tau International Honor Society of Nursing, National Association of Ob/Gyn Nurses, Who's Who in Professional Nursing, American Nurses Association, and the Florida Council of Maternal-Child Nurses.

With Susan Scott Ricci's wealth of practical and educational experience, she has decided to concentrate on the "essential facts" of nursing instruction and reduce the amount of "nice to know" information that is presented to students. As an educator, she recognized the tendency for nursing educators to want to "cover the world" when teaching rather than focusing on "the facts" that students need to know to practice nursing. With this thought, Susan has directed her energy to the *birth* of this essentials textbook.

She recognizes that instructional time is shrinking as the world of health care is expanding exponentially. Therefore, with the valuable instructional time allotted, she has recognized the urgent need to present pertinent facts as concisely as possible to promote application of knowledge within nursing practice.

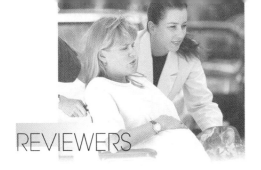

REVIEWERS

Marjorie L. Archer, MS, RN
Vocational Nursing Coordinator/Faculty
North Central Texas College
Gainesville, Texas

Linda Barren, MS, RNC
Division Head of Health Services; Assistant Professor
Oklahoma State University—Oklahoma City
Oklahoma City, Oklahoma

Cheryl Becker, RN, MN
Chair, Health Sciences
Tenured Teaching Faculty
Bellevue Community College
Kirkland, Washington

Betty Bertrand, RNC
Instructor, LVN Program
Texarkana College
Texarkana, Texas

Nancy Bingaman, MSN
Instructor, Nursing
Monterey Peninsula College
Monterey, California

Beverly Bradley, MSN
Coordinator, Nursing
Trident Technical College
Charleston, South Carolina

Vera C. Brancato
Associate Professor of Nursing
Kutztown University
Spring City, Pennsylvania

Patricia Burkard, MSN
Associate Professor, Nursing
Moorpark College
Moorpark, California

Deborah Campagna, RN, BSN, MSN, LCCE, FACCE
Associate Professor, Nursing
Hudson Valley Community College
Troy, New York

Diane Campbell, MSN, RN
Clinical Assistant Professor
Purdue University—West Lafayette
West Lafayette, Indiana

Annie M. Carson, RN, BScN
Teaching Master, Professor
Cambrian College of Applied Arts and Technology
Sudbury, Ontario

Connie Daily, MSN, RN
Nursing Instructor
Shawnee Community College
Ullin, Illinois

Shelly Daily, MSNc, RN, APN
Assistant Professor
Arkansas Technical University
Russelville, Arkansas

London Draper, MSN, RN
Assistant Professor
Weber State University
Ogden, Utah

Pat Durham-Taylor, PhD
Professor, Nursing
Truckee Meadows Community College
Reno, Nevada

Cathy Emeis, PhD
Clinical Instructor
Beth-El College of Nursing & Health Sciences,
    University of Colorado
Colorado Springs, Colorado

Teri Fernandez, MSN
Instructor
Yavapai College
Prescott, Arizona

Rhonda Ferrell, MSN, RN
Department Head, Health Education
James Sprunt Community College
Kenansville, North Carolina

Gay Goss, PhD, RN
Associate Professor of Nursing
California State University, Dominguez Hills
Carson, California

Pamela Gwin, RNC
Director, Vocational Nursing Program
Brazosport College
Lake Jackson, Texas

Anna Hefner, MSN, CPNP
Director, Academic Support and Nursing
    Computer Center; Associate Professor
Azusa Pacific University
Azusa, California

Mary F. King, RN, MS
Level III and Level IV Course Coordinator;
    Nursing Instructor
Phillips Community College of the University
    of Arkansas
Helena, Arkansas

Diana Kunce, MS, RN
Instructor
Tarleton State University
Stephenville, Texas

Kay LaCount, BSN, MSN
Chair, Nursing
Bay De Noc Community College
Escanaba, Michigan

Kelli Lewis, BSN, MSN
Practical Nursing Instructor/Allied Health Division
Rend Lake College
Ina, Illinois

Jeanne Linhart, MS, RN
Associate Professor of Nursing
Rockland Community College
Suffern, New York

Susan Lloyd, PhD, RN, CNS
MSN Program Director
California State University—Los Angeles
Los Angeles, California

Barbara Manning, MS, RN
Nursing Instructor
Northwest Mississippi Community College
Senatobia, Mississippi

Rhonda Martin, MS, RN
Clinical Instructor in Nursing
University of Tulsa
Tulsa, Oklahoma

Eva Mauldin, MA, BSN, RN
Associate Professor II
Odessa College
Odessa, Texas

Susan Mayer, MS, CS, RNC
Nursing Faculty
Glendale Community College
Glendale, Arizona

Kay McKinley, BS, RN
Nursing Instructor
Victor Valley College
Victorville, California

Beth Mogle, MSN, WHNP, RN
Nursing Instructor
Kirtland Community College
Roscommon, Michigan

Linda Pasto, BSN, MSN
Nursing Professor
Tompkins Cortland Community College
Dryden, New York

Sarah Plunkett, BS, MS
Instructor of Nursing
Tulsa Community College
Tulsa, Oklahoma

Shana Ruggenberg, RN, MSN
Assistant Professor of Nursing
Pacific Union College
Angwin, California

Lorna Shletzbaum, RN, MN
Nursing Instructor
Tacoma Community College
Tacoma, Washington

Faye Sigman, RN, BSN, MSN
Associate Professor and Dean of Nursing and Allied
    Health
Dyersburg State Community College
Dyersburg, Tennessee

Brenda Y. Smith, RN, EdD, MN, BSN, CNM, ICCE
Chairperson
East Arkansas Community College
Forrest City, Arkansas

Janet Somlyay, MSN, RN, CSN, CPNP
Assistant Lecturer
University of Wyoming
Laramie, Wyoming

Barbara Stoner, BS, MS
Clinical Nurse Coordinator
Arapahoe Community College
Littleton, Colorado

Linda J. Tucker, RNC
Nurse Manager
Medical Careers Development Center
Southfield, Michigan

Bobbie Walker, RN, MSN, IBCLC
Full-Time Nursing Faculty
Montgomery College – Takoma Park
Takoma Park, Maryland

Darlyn Weikel, RN, MS
Associate Professor, Practical Nursing
North Central Technical College
Wausau, Wisconsin

Julie Wells, BS
Instructor, Health Services
Mohawk Valley Community College
Utica, New York

Barbara Wilford, MS
Professor
Lorain County Community College
Elyria, Ohio

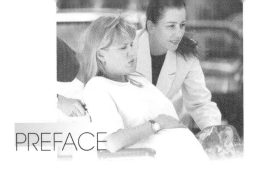

PREFACE

The principle of going from simple to complex concepts in nursing education is well established, and yet many textbooks bombard their students with "nice to know" concepts rather than "need to know" ones. With time in nursing curricula shrinking and the world of health knowledge expanding, where does one find the happy medium to accomplish both challenges?

This textbook was written on the premise that students need to know the "facts" and not necessarily the whole world of knowledge surrounding that one fact. It is my hope that the essential facts will be imparted to nursing students, which will empower them to guide individuals and communities toward higher levels of wellness throughout the life cycle. In addition, they will strive to look beyond the moment to anticipate, to identify, and to address common problems that would allow timely, evidence-based interventions to reduce long-term sequelae. This will validate their unique and valued role in health care.

This textbook is designed as a practical approach to understanding the health of women and newborns. Women in our society are becoming empowered to make informed and responsible choices regarding their health, but to do so they need the advocacy and support of nurses who care for them. This textbook focuses on women throughout their lifespan and arms the student or practicing nurse with essential information to care for women and their families, to assist them to make the right choices safely, intelligently and with confidence.

Organization

Each chapter of this textbook reviews an important dimension of a woman's general health throughout her life cycle and addresses risk factors, lifestyle choices that influence her well-being, appropriate interventions, and nursing education topics to preserve her health and that of her newborn.

The text is divided into 8 units:

Unit 1: Introduction to Maternity, Newborn, and Women's Health Nursing

Unit 1 helps build a foundation for the student beginning the study of maternal-newborn and women's health nursing by exploring contemporary issues and trends and community-based nursing.

Unit 2: Women's Health Throughout the Lifespan

Unit 2 introduces the student to select women's health topics, including structure and function of the reproductive system, common reproductive concerns, sexually transmitted infections, problems of the breast, and benign disorders and cancers of the female reproductive tract. This unit encourages students to assist women in maintaining their quality of life, reducing their risk of disease, and becoming active partners with their health care professional.

Unit 3: Pregnancy

Unit 3 addresses topics related to normal pregnancy, including fetal development, genetics, and maternal adaptation to pregnancy. Nursing management during normal pregnancy is presented in a separate chapter encouraging application of basic knowledge to nursing practice. This nursing care chapter covers maternal and fetal assessment throughout pregnancy; interventions to promote self-care and minimize common discomforts, and patient education.

Unit 4: Labor and Birth

Unit 4 begins with a chapter on the normal labor and birth process, including maternal and fetal adaptations. This is followed by a chapter discussing the nurse's role during normal labor and birth, which includes maternal and fetal assessment, pharmacologic and non-pharmacologic comfort measures and pain management, and specific nursing interventions during each stage of labor and birth.

Unit 5: Postpartum Period

Unit 5 focuses on maternal adaptation during the normal postpartum period. Both physiologic and psychological aspects are explored. Paternal adaptation is also considered. This unit also focuses on related nursing management, including assessment of physical and emotional status, promoting comfort, assisting with elimination, counseling about sexuality and contraception, promoting nutrition, promoting family adaptation, and preparing for discharge.

Unit 6: The Newborn

Unit 6 covers physiologic and behavioral adaptations of the normal newborn. It also delves into nursing management of the normal newborn to include immediate assessment and specific interventions, as well as ongoing assessment, physical examination, and specific interventions during the early newborn period.

Unit 7: Childbearing at Risk

Unit 7 shifts the focus to at-risk pregnancy, childbirth, and postpartum care. Pre-existing conditions of the woman, pregnancy-related complications, at-risk labor, emergencies associated with labor and birth, and medical conditions and complications affecting the postpartum woman are all covered. Treatment and nursing management are presented for each medical condition. This organization allows the student to build on a solid foundation of normal material when studying the at-risk content.

Unit 8: The Newborn at Risk

Unit 8 continues to focus on at-risk content. Issues of the newborn with birth weight variations, gestational age variations, congenital conditions, and acquired disorders are explored. Treatment and nursing management are presented for each medical condition. This organization helps cement the student's understanding of the material.

Recurring Features

In order to provide the instructor and student with an exciting and user-friendly text, a number of recurring features have been developed.

Key Terms

A list of terms that are considered essential to the chapter's understanding is presented at the beginning of each chapter. Each key term appears in boldface, with the definition included in the text. Key terms can also be found in the glossary at the end of the text.

Learning Objectives

Learning Objectives included at the beginning of each chapter guide the student in understanding what is important and why. These valuable learning tools also provide opportunities for self-testing or instructor evaluation of student knowledge and ability.

WOW

Each chapter opens with inspiring Words of Wisdom, which offer helpful, timely, or interesting thoughts. These WOW statements set the stage for each chapter and give students valuable insight into nursing care of women and newborns.

Healthy People 2010

Throughout the textbook, relevant Healthy People 2010 objectives are outlined in recurring boxes. These serve as a roadmap for improving the health of women, mothers, and their newborns.

Teaching Guidelines

An important tool for achieving health promotion and disease prevention is health education. Throughout the textbook, Teaching Guidelines are aimed at raising awareness and providing nursing students with simple, clear information to impart to their patients.

Nursing Care Plans

Nursing Care Plans provide concrete examples of each step of the nursing process within numerous chapters. These Nursing Care Plans illustrate common health problems of women and newborns that are managed in a variety of settings. To make the Nursing Care Plans more meaningful, a scenario is presented at the beginning of each one.

Nursing Procedures

Step-by-step Nursing Procedures are presented in a clear, concise format to facilitate competent performance of relevant procedures.

Drug Guides

These tables include medication, action, indication, and nursing implications. An understanding of drugs used in the care of pregnant women and newborns is essential to protect and promote the health of this special population.

Consider This!

In every chapter students are asked to *Consider This!* These first-person narratives engage students in real-life scenarios experienced by their patients. These personal accounts evoke empathy and help students perfect their caregiving skills. Each box ends with an opportunity for further contemplation, encouraging students to think critically about the scenario.

Tables, Boxes, Drawings, and Photographs

Abundant tables and boxes summarize key content throughout the book. Additionally, beautiful drawings and photographs help students visualize the content presented. These important aspects of the text allow for quick, easy access of material.

Key Points

At the end of each chapter, Key Points provide a quick review of essential chapter elements. These bulleted lists help students focus on the important aspects of the chapter.

References and Helpful Informational Resources

References and Helpful Informational Resources, which were used to develop chapter content, enable students to further explore topics of interest. Many on-line resources are provided. These resources can be shared with women and their families to enhance patient education and support.

Chapter Worksheets

Chapter worksheets are placed at the end of each chapter to assist the student in reviewing the essentials. Chapter worksheets include:

- **Multiple Choice Questions**—These review questions are written to test the students' ability to apply chapter material. Questions cover maternal-newborn and women's health content that students might encounter on their national licensing exam (NCLEX). The questions are straightforward and factual in nature to rule out regional/cultural variations.
- **Critical Thinking Exercises**—These exercises challenge students to apply new knowledge and experiences to real-life situations. Questions encourage students to think critically, problem solve, and consider their own perspective on given topics.
- **Study Activities**—These interactive activities promote student participation in the learning process. This section includes many on-line and community-based exercises.

Teaching-Learning Package

Instructor's Resource CD-ROM

This valuable resource for instructors is compatible with WebCT and Blackboard, and includes all the materials you need to teach your Maternity Nursing course:

- Test Generator, featuring hundreds of questions within a powerful tool to help you create your quizzes and tests

- PowerPoint presentations, corresponding to every chapter and serving as a supplement for your overheads, for your handouts, or for you to post on-line
- Image Bank, giving you access to photographs and illustrations from the text in a convenient, searchable format
- Lecture Outlines, for organizing your classroom instruction
- Sample syllabi, for setting up your course
- Assignments and reading comprehension quizzes, for testing your students' understanding

Front-of-Book CD-ROM

This free front-of–book CD-ROM features 25 minutes of video clips highlighting the following topics:

- Developmental Stages of Pregnancy
- Vaginal Labor and Delivery
- Scheduled Cesarean Section
- Assisting the Client with Breastfeeding

The CD-ROM also includes 275 NCLEX-style questions for student review, including traditional and alternate-format questions.

Free Connection Web Site

Visit http://thePoint.lww.com for on-line versions of the text's powerful teaching/learning tools, as well as additional supplements and information about the book.

Electronic Study Guide to Accompany Essentials of Maternity, Newborn, and Women's Health Nursing

This exciting new resource, built for your WebCT or Blackboard Learning Management System, provides review questions to help students apply and retain the key information from each chapter. Featuring NCLEX-style practice questions and other thought-provoking exercises, the Electronic Study Guide provides you with a great new tool for assessing your students' mastery of information and for tracking their proficiency within the world of maternity nursing.

Contact your sales representative or visit www.LWW.com/Nursing for more details.

SUSAN SCOTT RICCI

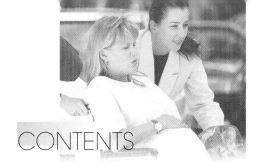

CONTENTS

Unit 3
Pregnancy 209

Unit 4
Labor and Birth 305

Unit 8

The Newborn at Risk 635

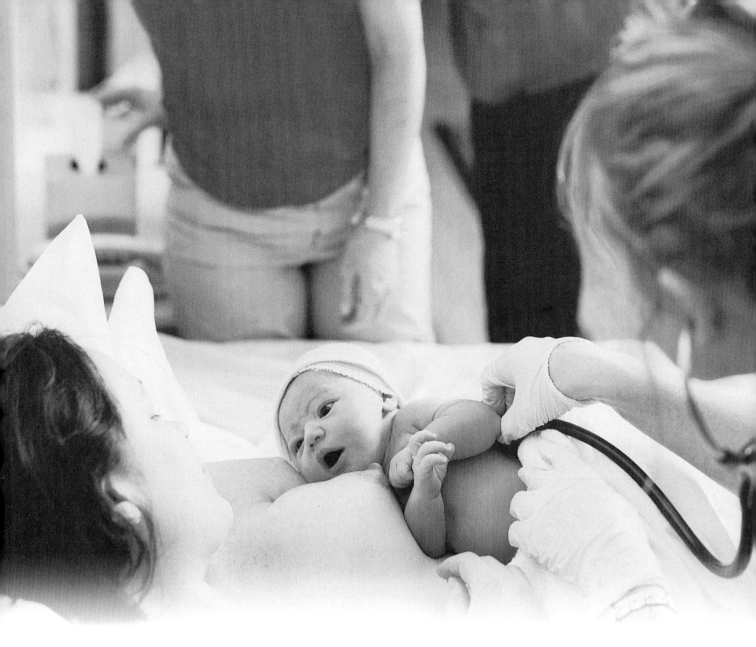

Introduction to Maternity, Newborn, and Women's Health Nursing

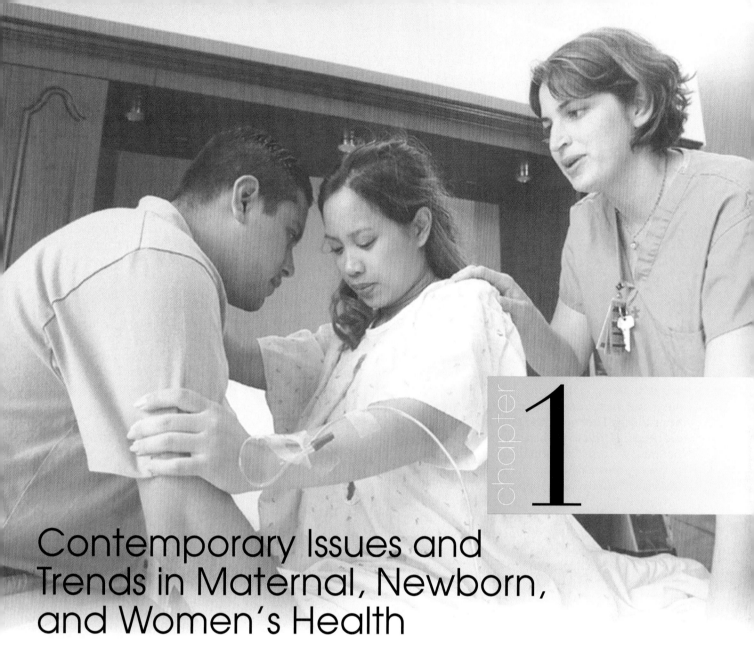

chapter 1

Contemporary Issues and Trends in Maternal, Newborn, and Women's Health

KeyTERMS

abortion
certified nurse midwife
   (CNM)
doula
empowerment
ethics
family-centered care
health indicators
infant mortality rate
intrauterine fetal surgery
maternal mortality rate
nurse practice acts

LearningOBJECTIVES

After studying the chapter content, the student should be able to accomplish the following:

1. Define the key terms.
2. Identify the current trends in health care that affect women.
3. Outline the barriers that women have in accessing health care.
4. List three women's health care indicators and how they are being addressed.
5. Describe the nursing implications of current trends in women's health care.
6. Discuss the role of the nurse throughout the life cycle continuum.

WOW

Being pregnant and giving birth are like crossing a narrow bridge. People can accompany you to the bridge. They can greet you on the other side. But you walk that bridge alone. . . .

A person's ability to lead a fulfilling life and to participate fully in society depends largely on his or her health status. This is especially true for women, who often shoulder the combined burden of child rearing, family health care, and career building. To fulfill her responsibility to her loved ones, a woman must first care for her own personal health.

Now more than ever, nearly every health care experience involves the contribution of a nurse. From birth to death, and every health care emergency in between, will likely involve the presence of a nurse. A knowledgeable, supportive, comforting nurse often results in a superior health care experience. Skilled nursing practice depends on a solid base of knowledge and clinical expertise delivered in a caring, holistic manner. It is imperative that nurses use their knowledge and passion to reach out to their patients. They must help meet every woman's health care needs regardless of where a woman is in her life cycle continuum. Nurses can help their patients to live healthier lives by providing emotional support, comfort, information, advice, advocacy, support, and family counseling.

This chapter presents a general overview of issues and trends in health care with which nurses often grapple in caring for families with children. Nurses must know how to approach these issues in a knowledgeable and systematic way to reduce conflict and to provide professional care.

Maternal and Women's Health Care Perspectives

Past Trends

Centuries ago, granny midwives handled the normal birthing process for most women. Their training was obtained through an apprenticeship with a more experienced midwife. Most doctors only participated in childbirth in the most extreme cases of difficulty. All births took place in the home setting.

Childbirth in colonial America was a difficult and sometimes dangerous experience. During the 17th and 18th centuries, women giving birth died as a result of exhaustion, dehydration, infection, hemorrhage, or seizures (Lehrman, 2003). In addition to her anxieties about pregnancy, an expectant mother was filled with apprehensions about the death of her newborn child. The death of a child during infancy was far more common than it is today. Approximately 50% of all children died before the age of five (Lehrman, 2003). This can be compared with the 0.07% **infant mortality rate** of today, which is a dramatic improvement (World Factbook, 2003).

During the early 1900s, physicians attended about half the births in the United States. Midwives often cared for women who could not afford a doctor. Most women were attracted to hospitals because these institutions offered pain management that was not available in home births. Natural childbirth practices advocating birth without medication and focusing on relaxation techniques were introduced in the 1950s. These techniques opened the door to childbirth education classes and helped bring the father back into the picture. Both partners were participating in the whole family experience by taking an active role in pregnancy, childbirth, and parenting (Fig. 1-1).

During the 1960s, consumer organizations formed and advocated for family-centered maternity care (FCMC). The International Childbirth Education Association

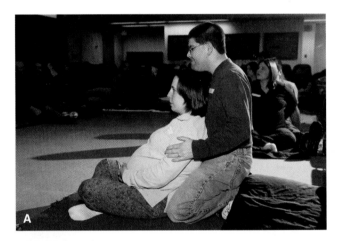

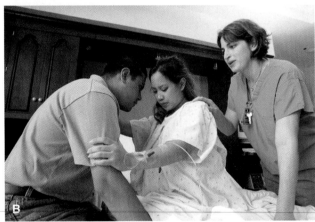

● Figure 1-1 Today, fathers and partners are welcome to take an active role in the pregnancy and childbirth experience. (**A**) Couples can participate together in childbirth education classes. (Photo by Gus Freedman.) (**B**) Fathers and partners can assist the woman throughout her labor and delivery. (Photo by Joe Mitchell.)

(ICEA), the American Society for Psychoprophylaxis in Obstetrics (ASPO), and the National Association of Parents and Professionals for Safe Alternatives in Childbirth (NAPSAC) all stressed a strong commitment to family values and responsibility in childbearing. In the 1970s, female consumers and women health professionals challenged many assumptions of the obstetric system and demanded new models of care delivery. From the 1980s to the present, increased access to care for all women (regardless of their ability to pay) and new hospital redesigns (labor, delivery, and recovery [LDR] rooms; and labor, delivery, recovery, and postpartum [LDRP] spaces) to keep "families together" during the childbirth experience breathed new life into FCMC (Fig. 1-2).

Family-centered care is the delivery of safe, satisfying, quality health care that focuses on and adapts to the physical and psychosocial needs of the family. It is a cooperative effort of families and other caregivers that

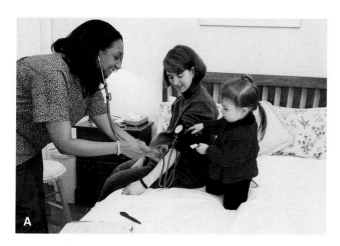

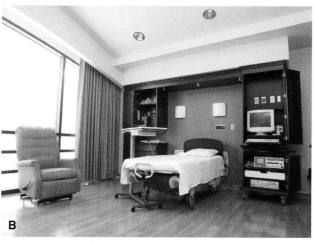

● Figure 1-2 Many different settings are available for prenatal care, labor, and delivery. (**A**) Birthing centers and (**B**) labor, delivery and recovery (LDR) rooms have inviting, home-like atmospheres and encourage family-centered care. (A, Photo by Gus Freedman; B, photo by Joe Mitchell.)

recognizes the strength and integrity of the family. The basic principles of family-centered care are as follows:

• Childbirth is considered a normal, healthy event in the life of a family.
• Childbirth affects the entire family and relationships will change.
• Families are capable of making decisions about their own care if given adequate information and professional support (Murray et al., 2002).

FCMC is based on the premise that the family is the constant. Family members support one another well beyond the health care provider's brief time with them during the childbearing process. FCMC views birth as a normal life event, rather than a medical procedure. The core values of FCMC that need to be integrated into all nursing care provided to families include mutual respect and trust of all parties, "informed choice" used by the family, **empowerment** of the family unit, collaboration in all decision making, and flexibility, quality, and individualized care for all family members (Phillips, 2003).

In many ways, childbirth practices in the United States have come full circle, as we see the return of nurse midwives and doulas. **Certified nurse midwives (CNMs)** have postgraduate training in the care of normal pregnancy and delivery, and are certified by the American College of Nurse Midwives (ACNM). A **doula** is a birth assistant who provides quality emotional, physical, and educational support to the woman and family during childbirth and the postpartum period. Childbirth choices are often based on what works best for the mother, child, and family. Box 1-1 summarizes a time line of childbirth in America.

Current Trends

Modern women are often faced with multiple responsibilities that compete for their time and attention, including the health of their parents, their children, and their partner. These responsibilities may decrease a woman's ability to tend to her own mental and physical health (nutrition, exercise, leisure activities, and so forth). A woman who neglects her health may have to deal with the consequences for the remainder of her life.

Today women are part of an evolving health care delivery system. The cost of health care is soaring and the federal government, insurance agencies, hospitals, and health care providers are joining together in an attempt to bring it under control. Several changes in the health care arena have resulted, many of which have brought about an increasingly complex health care system. Many people feel "lost in the maze."

Health care functions within the parameters of a market setting, offering goods and services that carry cost to health care consumers and patients. If a woman is pregnant, diabetic, and needs to go to an endocrinologist, she

---

BOX 1-1

CHILDBIRTH IN AMERICA: A TIME LINE

1700s	Men did not attend births, because it was considered indecent.
	Women faced birth, not with joy and ecstasy, but with fear of death.
	Female midwives attended the majority of all births at home.
1800s	There is a shift from using midwives to doctors among middle class women.
	The word *obstetrician* was formed from the Latin, meaning "to stand before."
	Puerperal (childbed) fever was occurring in epidemic proportions.
	Louis Pasteur demonstrated that streptococci were the major cause of puerperal fever that was killing mothers after delivery.
	The first cesarean section was performed in Boston in 1894.
	The x-ray was developed in 1895 and was used to asses pelvic size for birthing purposes (Feldhusen 2003).
1900s	Twilight sleep (a heavy dose of narcotics and amnesiacs) was used on women during childbirth in the United States.
	The United States was 17th out of 20 nations in infant mortality rates.
	Fifty to 75% of all women gave birth in hospitals by 1940.
	Nurseries were started because moms could not care for their baby for several days after receiving chloroform gas.
	Dr. Grantley Dick–Reed (1933) wrote a book entitled *Childbirth Without Fear* that reduced the "fear–tension–pain" cycle women experienced during labor and birth.

Dr. Fernand Lamaze (1984) wrote a book entitled *Painless Childbirth: The Lamaze Method* that advocated distraction and relaxation techniques to minimize the perception of pain.

Amniocentesis is first performed to assess fetal growth in 1966.

In the 1970s the cesarean section rate was about 5%. By 1990 it rose to 24%, where it stands currently (Martin, 2002).

The 1970s and 1980s see a growing trend to return birthing back to the basics—nonmedicated, nonintervening childbirth.

In the late 1900s, freestanding birthing centers—LDRPs—were designed, and the number of home births began to increase.

2000s One in four women undergo a surgical birth (cesarean).

CNMs once again assist couples at home, in hospitals, or in freestanding facilities with natural childbirths. Research shows that midwives are the safest birth attendants for most women, with lower infant mortality and maternal rates, and fewer invasive interventions such as episiotomies and cesareans (Keefe 2003).

Childbirth classes of every flavor abound in most communities.

According to the latest available data, the United States ranks 21st in the world in maternal deaths. The maternal mortality rate is approximately 7 in 1000 live births.

According to the latest available data, the United States ranks 27th in the world in infant mortality rates. The infant mortality rate is approximately 7 in 1000 live births (United Nations, 2003).

---

has very little choice except to purchase the services needed or go without care. In the managed care environment of health care today, the woman will need to go through her "primary health care professional" or "gatekeeper" to receive a referral to a specialist. Often she must trust her primary provider to make that choice for her, instead of making that decision on her own.

The best managed care principles value a comprehensive approach with a focus on prevention, early intervention, and continuity of care. The goal is to consider the merit of services, procedures, and treatments in view of the resources available, thus the gatekeeper role, which ensures that care is timely and necessary. In a perfect world, all women would receive necessary quality care throughout their lives, but we don't live in the perfect managed care world. With cost-cutting strategies, there are many implications for women:

• Decreased length of hospital stay for newborns and high-risk neonates, which is often met by increased at-home care given by women as caretakers
• Loss of continuity of care and an establishment of a trusting relationship with her health care provider when the insurance plan does not cover the same provider she may have been receiving care from for years
• Potential prohibition of OB/GYN physicians from making referrals for specialists if they are not classified as primary physicians (gatekeepers)
• Restricting clinical judgment that impacts quality and individualization of care, which may potentially increase mother and infant morbidity by dictating length of stay in the hospital when more observation and nursing care are needed
• Restricting the number and type of diagnostic studies ordered by the health care provider, which may jeopar-

dize the health and well-being of the newborn and mother, and precludes the parents from making decisions about future pregnancy events (Youngkin & Davis, 2004)

Other trends in the health care system include

- Changing demographics—an aging population
- Economic forces that affect resources
- Profound growth of technology and information
- Proliferation of unlicensed assistive personnel providing health care
- Communications and cultural issues associated with the increasingly diverse needs of multicultural patients
- Shortages of trained health care professionals
- Movement of health care away from acute settings into the community

Currently, the problem surmounting all health care considerations is cost. Although cost containment is important to restrain spiraling health care spending, costs and efforts to contain them should not affect the quality or safety of care delivered. The old saying that "an ounce of prevention is worth a pound of cure" has been shown to lower costs significantly. Mammograms, cervical cancer screenings, prenatal care, and smoking cessation programs are a few examples that yield positive outcomes and reduce overall health care costs. Using technologic advances to diagnose and treat breast cancer early positively saves lives as well as fiscal resources.

Nurses can be leaders in providing quality care within a limited-resource environment by stressing to the women for whom they care the importance of making healthy lifestyle and food choices, seeking early interventions for minor problems before they become major ones, and educating themselves about health-related issues that affect them so they can select the best option for themselves and their families. Prevention services and health education are the cornerstones of delivering quality women's health care.

These are just a few of the changes in the health care system that consumers face when they need services. These dramatic changes present a significant opportunity for the nursing profession. Nurses who clearly articulate their role in this changing environment will be able to help their patients to navigate this increasingly complicated health care system.

Future Trends/Needs for Women's Health

Based on our changing demographics concerning age, ethnic background, education, workforce participation, and booming childbearing statistics, the future trend for women's health will need to

- Broaden the focus on women's health, not just during pregnancy, but throughout the entire life cycle
- Integrate women's and perinatal health services to compensate for poor coordination of services by increasing

numbers of OB/GYNs being designated primary care providers
- Expand comprehensive, integrated programs and services addressing women's unique needs across their life span
- Offer better provider education about the consequences of chronic health problems as well as enlighten all women about better lifestyle choices to prevent the progression of chronic conditions
- Promote social policies that ensure economic security and health care insurance coverage for women
- Recognize sociocultural differences that affect women's caregiving roles, domestic violence, access to health information, lifestyle preferences, autonomy to make health decisions, and learning/motivation for health prevention and promotion activities
- Focus scientific research for more specific drug treatments for breast cancer, osteoporosis, autoimmune diseases, and menopause
- Develop better diagnostic procedures for heart disease, diabetes, arthritis, lupus, inflammatory diseases, and detection of genetic disorders earlier
- Support health care educational programs to increase entry of diverse-culture students to provide a broad range of women's health services

Health Care Indicators

Health indicators are used to measure the health of the nation. They are global in nature and provide each country with guidelines to assess their own health status. General global health indicators include infant mortality rate, at-risk birth weight, potential years of life lost, life expectancy, disability-free life expectancy, and self-rated health status (Osei et al., 2003). The *leading health indicators* reflect the major health concerns in the United States at the beginning of the 21st century. These indicators were selected on the basis of their ability to motivate action, the availability of data to measure progress, and their importance as public health issues (Healthy People 2010). The current leading health indicators include

- Physical activity
- Overweight and obesity
- Tobacco use
- Substance abuse
- Responsible sexual behavior
- Mental health
- Injury and violence
- Environmental quality
- Immunization
- Access to health care (Healthy People 2010)

The objectives of Healthy People 2010 are categorized according to the health indicators. Healthy People 2010 is a broad-based, collaborative federal and state initiative that has set national disease prevention and health promotion objectives to be achieved by the end of the decade. The initiative has two goals: to increase the quality and years of healthy life and to eliminate health disparities among Americans. An example of health disparity exists in people with disabilities. Just because these individuals were born with an impairing condition or have experienced a disability or injury that has long-term consequences does not negate their need for health promotion and disease prevention. In fact, their need for health-promoting behaviors is accentuated. Many women with disabling conditions such as lupus, rheumatoid arthritis, multiple sclerosis, or osteoporosis do not view themselves as disabled, despite immense physical limitations. Nurses need to remember that wellness is the lens of their self-perception. The accompanying Healthy People 2010 box highlights national health goals for maternal and infant health.

HEALTHY PEOPLE *2010*

National Health Goals—Maternal and Infant Health

✓ **Goal:** Reduce fetal and infant deaths.

✓ **Goal:** Reduce maternal deaths.

✓ **Goal:** Reduce maternal illness and complications resulting from pregnancy.

✓ **Goal:** Increase the proportion of pregnant women who receive early and adequate prenatal care.

✓ **Goal:** Increase the proportion of pregnant women who attend a series of prepared childbirth classes.

✓ **Goal:** Increase the proportion of very low-birth weight (VLBW) infants born at level III hospitals or subspecialty perinatal centers.

✓ **Goal:** Reduce cesarean births among low-risk (full-term, singleton, vertex presentation) women.

✓ **Goal:** Reduce low birth weight (LBW) and VLBW.

✓ **Goal:** Reduce preterm births.

✓ **Goal:** Increase the proportion of mothers who achieve a recommended weight gain during their pregnancies.

✓ **Goal:** Increase the percentage of healthy, full-term infants who are laid down to sleep on their backs.

✓ **Goal:** Reduce the occurrence of developmental disabilities.

✓ **Goal:** Reduce the occurrence of spina bifida and other neural tube defects (NTDs).

✓ **Goal:** Increase the proportion of pregnancies begun with an optimum folic acid level.

✓ **Goal:** Increase abstinence from alcohol, cigarettes, and illicit drugs among pregnant women.

✓ **Goal:** Reduce the occurrence of fetal alcohol syndrome (FAS).

✓ **Goal:** Increase the proportion of mothers who breast-feed their babies.

✓ **Goal:** Ensure appropriate newborn bloodspot screening, follow-up testing, and referral to services.

Mortality Rates

The federal government has pledged to improve maternal–child care outcomes and thus reduce the statistics of mortality rates for both women and children. The **maternal mortality rate** counts the number of deaths from any cause during the pregnancy cycle per 100,000 live births. In the United States, the maternal mortality rate is 7.5. The infant mortality rate counts the number of deaths of infants younger than one year of age per 1000 live births. In the United States, the infant mortality rate is 7.0 (Centers for Disease Control and Prevention [CDC], 2004, National Center for Health Statistics [NCHS], 2005).

During the past several decades, mortality and morbidity have dramatically decreased as a result of an increased emphasis on hygiene, good nutrition, exercise, and prenatal care for all women. However, women and infants are still experiencing complications at significant rates. The United States is one of the most medically and technologically advanced nations and has the highest per-capita spending on health care in the world, yet current mortality rates in the United States indicate the need for continued improvement.

A few facts might help present a clearer picture:

- The current maternal mortality rate is approximately 7.5 maternal deaths per 100,000 live births (CDC, 2004).
- The current infant mortality rate is approximately 7.0 infant deaths per 100,000 live births (CDC, 2004; NCHS, 2005).
- Two to three women die in the United States every day from pregnancy complications, and more than 30% of pregnant women (1.2 million women annually) experience some type of illness or injury during childbirth (CDC, 2004).
- The United States ranks 21st (below 20 other countries) in rates of maternal deaths (deaths per 100,000 live births).
- The United States ranks 27th (below 26 other countries with a population of at least 2.5 million) in rates of infant deaths (deaths per 100,000 live births; United Nations, 2003). One reason cited for the high infant mortality rate in the United States is the high rate of very-low-birth-weight births in the country relative to other developed countries (NCHS, 2005).
- Most pregnancy-related complications are preventable. The most common are ectopic pregnancy, preterm labor, hemorrhage, emboli, hypertension, infection, stroke, diabetes, and heart disease.
- The leading causes of pregnancy-related mortality for the years 1991 to 1999 (the last years for which data are available) are embolism (20%), hemorrhage (17%), pregnancy-related hypertension (16%), and infection (13%; CDC, 2003).
- More than half of all infant deaths in 2002 were attributable to five leading causes: congenital malformations (20%), disorders relating to short gestation and unspeci-

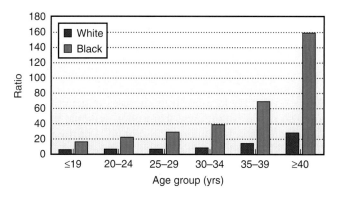

* Deaths per 100,000 live births.

● Figure 1-3 Pregnancy-related mortality ratios by race and age, United States, 1991–1999. (Retrieved May 2005 from http://www.cdc.gov/mmwr/preview/mmwrhtml/ss5202a1.htm.)

fied LBW (17%), sudden infant death syndrome (SIDS; 8%), newborns affected by maternal complications of pregnancy (6%), and newborns affected by complications of placenta, cord, and membranes (4%) (Martin et al., 2005).

- The maternal mortality and morbidity rates for African-American women have been three to four times higher than for whites (Chang, 2003; Fig. 1-3).

- Infant mortality rates are higher for African-American, Latin-American, and Native American babies. The rate for African-American babies is twice that of white babies (Keefe, 2003; Fig. 1-4).

Why is there such disparity within the United States? The problem is multifaceted, but lack of care during pregnancy is a major contributing factor to a poor outcome. Prenatal care is well known to prevent complications of pregnancy and to support the birth of healthy infants. Unfortunately, not all women are able to receive the same quality and quantity of health care during a pregnancy. More than 40% of African-American, Native American, and Latino women do not obtain prenatal care during their first trimester of pregnancy (Condon, 2004).

Several of the risk factors that contribute to high mortality rates can be lessened or prevented with good preconception and prenatal care. First, preconception screening and counseling offer an opportunity to identify maternal risk factors before pregnancy begins. Examples include daily folic acid consumption (a protective factor) and alcohol use (a risk factor). During preconception counseling, health care providers can also refer women for medical and psychosocial or support services for any risk factors identified. Counseling should be culturally appropriate and linguistically proficient.

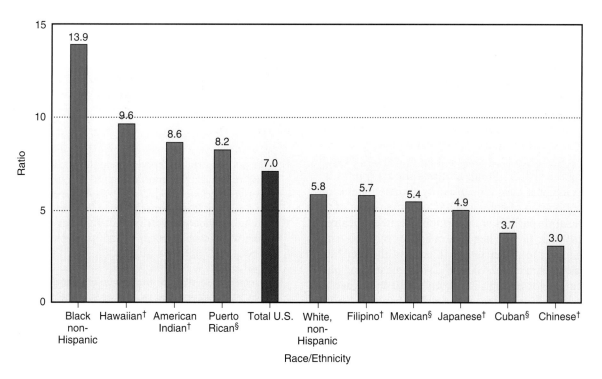

* Per 1,000 live births.
† Can include persons of Hispanic and non-Hispanic origin.
§ Persons of Hispanic origin may be of any race.

● Figure 1-4 Infant mortality rates by selected racial/ethnic populations—United States, 2002. (Retrieved May 2005 from http://www.cdc.gov/mmwr/preview/mmwrhtml/mm5405a5.htm.)

Prenatal visits offer an opportunity to provide information about the adverse effects of substance use and serve as a vehicle for referrals to treatment services. The use of timely, high-quality prenatal care can help to prevent poor birth outcomes and improve maternal health by identifying women who are at particularly high risk, and then can be used to take steps to reduce risks, such as the risk of high blood pressure or diabetes. Interventions targeted at prevention and cessation of substance use during pregnancy may be helpful in further reducing the rate of preterm delivery and LBW. Continued promotion of folic acid intake can help to reduce the rate of NTDs.

In addition, providing access to quality prenatal care for all pregnant women without ability to pay will help reduce the mortality rates tremendously. Access to family planning services can also play a major role in preventing maternal deaths by reducing health risks associated with unplanned pregnancy.

Maternal mortality rates are nearly four times higher for women of color than for white women (Keefe, 2003). Researchers do not entirely understand what accounts for these disparities, but some suspected causes of higher maternal mortality rates for minority women include low socioeconomic status, limited or no insurance coverage, bias among health care providers (which may foster distrust), and quality of care available in the community. Language and legal barriers may also add to the various reasons why some immigrant women do not receive good prenatal care.

After birth, other health promotion strategies can significantly improve an infant's health and chances of survival. Breast-feeding has been shown to reduce rates of infection in infants and to improve long-term maternal health. Emphasizing to mothers that they should place their infants on their backs to sleep will help reduce the incidence of SIDS. Encouraging mothers to join support groups to prevent postpartum depression and gain assistance with sound child-rearing practices will help toward improving the health of both mothers and their infants.

The CDC has called the disparity in maternal mortality rates in women of color and white women "one of the largest racial disparities among public health indicators" (CDC, 1999, p. 493). They have called for more research and monitoring to understand and address the racial disparities, along with increased funding for prenatal and postpartum care. Not enough is known about the causes of racial disparities in maternal and infant health, so additional research is needed to identify causes and design initiatives to reduce these disparities. In addition, the CDC is calling on Congress to expand programs to provide preconception and prenatal care to underserved women to address the racial disparities.

The Health Resources and Services Administration (HRSA)'s Maternal and Child Health Bureau (MCHB) has primary federal responsibility for improving the health of mothers and children in the United States. More than 27 million infants, children, and pregnant women are served by an MCHB program annually (Dyck et al., 2003).

A few of their programs and initiatives to improve the health of mothers, infants, and children and to reduce mortality rates are described in Box 1-2.

The Report Card on Women's Health

Women of today face not only diseases of genetic origin but also diseases that arise from poor personal habits as well. Even though women represent 51% of the population, only recently have researchers and the medical community focused attention on the special health needs of women. One significant study that was published in August 2000 assessed the overall health of women at the state and national level. It identified an urgent need to improve women's access to health insurance and health care services, place a stronger emphasis on prevention, and invest in more research on women's health (National Women's Law Center [NWLC] et al., 2000).

The study identified several health care indicators that measure women's access to health care services. It measured the degree to which women receive preventive health care and engage in health-promoting activities (Box 1-3).

The report card gave the nation an overall grade of "unsatisfactory," and not a single state received a grade of "satisfactory." Among the other substandard findings were the following:

- No state has focused enough attention on preventive measures, such as smoking cessation, exercise, nutrition, and screening for diseases.

BOX 1-2

MCHB PROGRAMS AND INITIATIVES

- *Healthy Start*—through community outreach, home visitation, and a network of support services, targets the poorest neighborhoods where the likelihood of maternal and infant mortality and LBW is highest.
- *Health and Human Services (HHS) Interagency Council on Low Birth Weight*—has been established to promote multidisciplinary research on LBW and preterm births, scientific exchange, policy initiatives, and collaboration among HHS agencies.
- *Food fortification*—along with the national campaign to educate women about the preventive benefits of taking folic acid, has resulted in decreases in the prevalence of spina bifida and anencephaly.
- *Increased research*—concerning genetic, environmental, and behavioral factors that have an influence on pregnancy outcomes for mother and infant is being undertaken.
- *CDC's Pregnancy Risk Assessment Monitoring System (PRAMS)*—is an ongoing, state-specific surveillance system designed to identify and monitor select maternal behaviors and experiences before, during, and after pregnancy. PRAMS surveillance now covers approximately two thirds of all US births (Dyck et al., 2003).

- Too many women lack health insurance coverage. Nationally, nearly one in seven women (14%) have no health insurance.
- No state has adequately addressed women's health needs in the areas of reproductive health, mental health, and violence against women.
- Limited research has been done on health conditions that primarily affect women and that affect women differently than men (NWLC et al., 2000).

Cardiovascular Disease (CVD)

Poor health habits affect all women. Smoking, drug abuse, high cholesterol, and obesity lead to high mortality and morbidity rates in our nation. CVD is the number one cause of death of women, regardless of racial or ethnic group. Approximately 500,000 women die annually in the United States of CVD, equaling a rate of about one death per minute (Alexander et al., 2004) Women who endure a heart attack are more likely than men to die and oftentimes are more difficult to diagnose than men because of their vague and varied symptoms. Heart disease is still thought of as a "man's disease" and thus is not considered as a diagnosis when a woman presents to the emergency room.

The common perception held by many nurses that CVD is a man's disease could cost women their lives. Many nurses believe erroneously that only men need to worry about heart attacks and stroke, but CVD is an equal-opportunity killer. Consider these *myths:*

- Breast cancer kills more women than CVD.
- CVD is more deadly in men.
- Men and women experience the same symptoms.

Now examine the *facts* about CVD:

- CVD is the number one killer of women and stroke is number three.
- One in 10 women age 45 to 64 has some form of CVD.
- CVD is more challenging to diagnose in women than men.
- One of two American women dies of CVD, whereas 1 in 30 dies of breast cancer.
- Approximately 35% of heart attacks in women go unnoticed or unreported.
- Health care professionals do not take CVD symptoms seriously in women.
- Heart attack is twice as deadly in women as men (American Heart Association [AHA], 2004).

Nurses need to take heed and look beyond the obvious "crushing chest pain" textbook symptom that heralds a heart attack in men, because women present much differently and the diagnosis is missed if CVD is not on their radar screen of possibilities. Look for the following risk factors in women:

- Cigarette smoking
- Smoking and use of oral contraceptives or hormone replacement therapy
- Obesity
- Consuming a diet high in saturated fats
- Stress
- Sedentary lifestyle
- Hypertension
- Hyperlipidemia
- Strong family history
- Diabetes mellitus
- Postmenopausal

Figure 1-5 presents a sample *health risk assessor* to help nurses and patients assess the patient's risk of heart attack.

Consider CVD as a possibility in women who present with any of the following clinical symptoms: chest discomfort in the center of the chest that goes away and comes back (can be described as pressure, squeezing, or feeling of fullness); discomfort in one or both arms or shoulders, the back, neck, jaw, or stomach; shortness of breath; nausea; lightheadedness; breaking out in a cold sweat; paleness; atypical abdominal pain; and unexplained fatigue (AHA, 2004).

Prevention efforts to reduce the number victims of CVD in women include

- A low-cholesterol, low-fat diet
- Aspirin therapy and treatment of hypertension
- Daily exercise
- Achieving an ideal weight
- Smoking cessation measures
- Cholesterol-lowering agents
- Stress management (Condon, 2004)

Heart Risk Assessor — Women

Below are some easy-to-complete questions about your health and lifestyle that will help you assess your risk of a heart attack. The questions are designed to encourage discussion with your healthcare professional. Circle your points for each risk factor. Add them up and place your total points in the box. Then use the graph below to determine your risk.

1. HOW OLD ARE YOU?

Age	Points
35 – 39	–4
40 – 44	0
45 – 49	3
50 – 54	6
55 – 59	7
60 – 64	8
65 – 69	8
70 and over	8

2. DO YOU SMOKE?

	Points
Yes	2
No	0

3. DO YOU HAVE DIABETES?

	Points
Yes	4
No	0

Score (Total Points) [ ]

Now determine your risk. To do this, use the graph. Find your score on the left, run your finger across the line to match your age, and place an X at this point.

4. WHAT IS YOUR BLOOD PRESSURE?

Look up your points on the table below. Your systolic pressure (higher number) is on the left and your diastolic pressure (the lower number) is along the top.

Systolic	Diastolic 79 or less	80 – 84	85 – 89	90 – 99	100 or more
Less than 120	–3	0	0	2	3
120 – 129	0	0	0	2	3
130 – 139	0	0	0	2	3
140 – 159	2	2	2	2	3
160 or more	3	3	3	3	3

Don't know, but I have been told it is:	
Low	–3
Normal	0
High	2

5. WHAT IS YOUR TOTAL CHOLESTEROL LEVEL?

Total cholesterol (mg/dL)	Points
Less than 160	–2
160 – 199	0
200 – 239	1
240 – 279	1
280 and over	3

Don't know, but I have been told it is:	
Low	–2
Average	1
High	3

6. WHAT IS YOUR HDL (GOOD) CHOLESTEROL LEVEL?

HDL (good) cholesterol (mg/dL)	Points
Less than 35	5
35 – 44	2
45 – 49	1
50 – 59	0
60 and over	–3

Don't know, but I have been told it is:	
High	–3
Average	1
Low	5

Use the Heart Risk Assessor as a general guide. **If you have already had a heart attack or have heart disease, your heart attack risk is significantly higher. Only your healthcare professional can evaluate your risk and recommend treatment plans to reduce your risk.** If you don't know your cholesterol level or blood pressure, ask your healthcare professional if your levels should be checked.

Heart Attack Risk Groups, Women Age 35 and Older

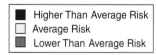

Heart Attack Risk*

- ■ Higher Than Average Risk
- □ Average Risk
- ■ Lower Than Average Risk

The **red** zone indicates a higher than average risk for a heart attack. The **yellow** zone indicates an average risk for a heart attack. It is desirable for you to be in the lower or **green** zone, which indicates a lower than average risk of a heart attack.

If you have already had a heart attack or have heart disease, your heart attack risk is significantly higher. Only your healthcare professional can evaluate your risk and recommend treatment plans to reduce your risk.

* Risk estimates were derived from the results of the Framingham Heart Study
Provided as an educational service from

 Bristol-Myers Squibb Company

D3-F091-7-99
© 1999 Bristol-Myers Squibb Company, Princeton NJ 08543

● Figure 1-5 Sample Health Risk Assessor form to help detect the risk for heart attack in women. (Used with permission from Bristol-Myers-Squibb Company.)

Cancer

Cancer falls as the second leading cause of death among women (Grantham, 2002). Women have a one in three lifetime risk of developing cancer, and one out of every four deaths is from cancer (Alexander et al., 2004). Although much attention is focused on cancer of the reproductive system, lung cancer is the number one killer of women. This is largely the result of the higher rates of smoking by women as well as the effects of second-hand smoke. Lung cancer has no early symptoms, making early detection almost impossible. Because of this, lung cancer has the lowest survival rate of any cancer. More than 90% of people who get lung cancer die of the disease (Breslin & Lucas, 2003).

Breast cancer occurs in one in every eight women in a lifetime, with more than 183,000 women diagnosed annually in the United States. It is the most common malignancy in women, and second only to lung cancer as a cause of cancer mortality in women (American Cancer Society [ACS], 2004). Although a positive family history of breast cancer, aging, and irregularities in the menstrual cycle at an early age are major risk factors, others include excess weight, not having children, oral contraceptive use, excessive alcohol consumption, a high-fat diet, and long-term use of hormone replacement therapy (ACS, 2003). Early detection and treatment appear to be the best chance for a cure, and reducing the risk of cancer by decreasing avoidable risks continues to be the best preventive plan.

Improving Women's Health

What can we do as a nation to improve the health of women? There is no single answer to address the multitude of issues that were identified in the state-to-state study. Women's health is a complex issue, and no single policy is going to change the overall dismal state ratings. Some policies may include

- Expand health care to the uninsured
- Overcome barriers to accessing care
- Address the issue of violence toward women
- Focus on wellness and prevention education programs

Although progress in science and technology have helped reduce the incidence and improve survival rates in several diseases, women's health issues continue to have an impact on our society. By eliminating or decreasing some of the risk factors and causes for prevalent diseases and illnesses, society and science could solve certain chronic health problems. By focusing on the causes and effects of particular illnesses, many women's health issues of today could be resolved.

Social Issues

Many social issues influence health care, including poverty, limited access to health care (especially prenatal care), and violence against women. These issues and possible interventions as they relate to nursing care are discussed next.

Poverty and Women

Despite many global economic gains during the last century, poverty continues to grow, and the gap between rich and poor is widening. Major gaps continue between the economic opportunities and status afforded to women and those offered to men. A disproportionate share of the burden of poverty rests on women's shoulders and undermines their health. For example:

- 70% of the 1.2 billion people living in poverty are female.
- Iron deficiency anemia, which is a direct result of malnutrition and poverty, affects twice the number of women compared with men.
- Half a million women die needlessly from pregnancy-related complications annually, the causes of which are exacerbated by issues of poverty and geographic remoteness.
- On average, women are paid 30% to 40% less than men for comparable work (World Health Organization [WHO], 2000).

Poverty, particularly for women, is more than monetary deficiency. Women continue to lag behind men in control of cash, credit, and collateral. Other forms of impoverishment may include deficiencies in literacy, education, skills, employment opportunities, mobility, and political representation, as well as pressures on their available time and energy linked to their role responsibilities. These poverty factors may diminish a woman's development and affect her health status (WHO, 2000).

Barriers to Accessing Health Care

Women are the major consumers of health care services, in many cases negotiating not only their own care, but also that of their family members. Compared with men, women have a greater rate of health problems, longer life spans, and more significant reproductive health needs. Their access to care is often complicated by their disproportionately lower incomes and greater responsibilities, juggling work and family concerns.

The Kaiser Women's Health Study (Salganicoff et al., 2002) surveyed approximately 4000 women between the ages of 18 to 64 and found that their health care needs were not being met, especially for women of color, those who are poor, and those who are uninsured.

For many, affordability of care is a major concern. A significant portion of women cannot afford to go to the doctor and fill their drug prescriptions, even when they have insurance coverage. Many health insurance plans do not include prescription coverage and thus the person must pay "out of pocket" (Box 1-4).

According to the Kaiser Women's Health Study (Salganicoff et al., 2002), women also have issues about

---

BOX 1-4

THE KAISER WOMEN'S HEALTH STUDY HIGHLIGHTS

- Low-income women were twice as likely (23%) as those with higher incomes (10%) to have fair or poor health status.
- Low-income women 45 to 64 years old reported
  49% had arthritis
  41% had hypertension
  32% had anxiety or depression
- Latinos were the most likely to report poor health (29%).
- African-American women were most likely to report activity limitations (16%).
- African-American women (45–64 years old) reported hypertension (57%) and arthritis (40%).
- One in six Latino and African-American women (45–64 years old) were diagnosed with diabetes during the past five years.
- One in three low-income women have no health insurance.
- Fifty-seven percent of uninsured women work either full- or part-time.
- Thirty-seven percent of Latino women are without insurance coverage.
- One in seven women reported their insurance plans did not provide adequate coverage to meet their health care needs

- One half of low-income women delayed or never received treatment because of lack of approval for treatment or tests.
- Seventeen percent of women did not have a regular health provider; 46% of uninsured women did not have a regular provider; and 31% of Latinos and 24% of low-income women lacked a regular provider.
- Seventeen percent of women of color reported they had difficulty communicating with their provider and left the office.
- Latino (31%) and uninsured (24%) women experienced access problems and barriers to care, and were least likely to have had a doctor visit within the past year.
- Women on Medicaid (40%), Latino women (38%), and African-American women (27%) were more likely to rely on hospital clinics and health centers for health care.
- Uninsured women were consistently less likely than women with private coverage to obtain any recommended preventive screening tests (Salganicoff et al., 2002).

---

the quality of care they receive. More than one in five women (22%) expressed concerns about the quality of care compared with 17% of men. This issue was a particular problem for women in fair or poor health (40%). Almost one in five women (18%) changed providers within the past five years because of dissatisfaction with care and concerns over quality—twice the rate of men (Salganicoff et al., 2002). Because access to health care is often unstable, relationships with health care providers are often short lived, resulting in care that can be spotty and disjointed (Salganicoff et al., 2002).

The value of prenatal care has been extensively documented in the literature as being equated with better pregnancy outcomes. The proportion of women beginning prenatal care during the first trimester of pregnancy remained stable at 83.2% in 2000 (US Department of Health and Human Services, 2002). However, finances, transportation, language and/or cultural barriers, clinic hours, and poor attitudes of the health care workers often limit women's access to prenatal care.

Financial Barriers

Financial barriers are one of the most important factors that limit care. Many women have limited or no health care and simply cannot afford the insurance. Although Medicaid covers prenatal care in most states, the paperwork and enrollment process is so burdensome that many women do not register.

Transportation

Transportation to and from appointments can be challenging for patients who do not drive or own a car or cannot use public transportation. The frequency of prenatal health care visits can be quite burdensome, compounding the transportation issue. The transportation issue becomes even more difficult if the woman has small children that she must take along with her. These challenges can prevent the pregnant patient from making her scheduled appointments.

Consider THIS!

I was a 17-year-old pregnant migrant worker needing prenatal care. Although my English wasn't good, I was able to show the receptionist my "big belly" and ask for services. All the receptionist seemed interested in was a social security number and health insurance—neither of which I had. She proceeded to ask me personal questions concerning who the father was and commented on how young I looked. The receptionist then "ordered" me in a loud voice to sit down and wait for an answer by someone in the back, but never contacted anyone that I could see. It seemed to me like all eyes were on me while I found an empty seat in the waiting room. After sitting there quietly for over an hour without any attention or answer, I left.

Thoughts: Why did she leave before receiving any health care service? What must she have been feeling during her wait? Would you come back to this clinic again? Why or why not?

Language Barriers

Language is how people communicate with each other to increase their understanding or knowledge base. If a health care worker cannot speak the same language as the client or does not have a trained interpreter available, a barrier is created. This language barrier might prevent the client from accessing prenatal care that could increase the chances affecting the pregnancy outcome. Frequently, communication between people who speak the same language can be misinterpreted.

Cultural Barriers

Culture is the sum of the beliefs and values that are learned, shared, and transmitted from generation to generation by a particular group. Cultural beliefs and values vary among different groups, and nurses must be aware, understand, and respect cultural beliefs different from their own. Nurses who feel their cultural values and pattern of behavior are superior (ethnocentrism) frequently set up barriers that inhibit diverse cultures from receiving prenatal health care.

Clinic Hours

Clinic hours must meet the needs of the patients, not the health care providers who work there. Evening and/or weekend service hours might be needed to meet the working client's schedule. It is important to evaluate the availability and accessibility of the offered service.

Poor Attitudes of Health Care Workers

Some health care workers exhibit negative attitudes toward poor and/or culturally diverse families, which could prohibit women from seeking health care. Long delays, hurried examinations, and rude comments by staff might increase a patient's level of discomfort with the health care team and may discourage return appointments.

Violence and Women

Violence against women is a major health concern—one that costs the health care system millions of dollars and thousands of lives. Violence affects women of all ages, ethnic backgrounds, races, educational levels, socioeconomic levels, and all walks of life. Nurses often come in contact with abused women, but fail to identify, acknowledge, or report the abuse. Pregnancy is often a time when physical abuse starts or escalates, resulting in poorer outcomes for the mother and the baby. Assessing for abuse carries the responsibility of listening for and following up on a possible incidence of abuse. Nurses serve their clients best by not trying to rescue them, but by helping them build on their strengths, providing support, and thereby empowering them to help themselves. All nurses need to include "RADAR" in every client visit (Box 1-5). For a thorough discussion of violence and women, see Chapter 9.

BOX 1-5
RADAR

R–Routinely screen every patient for abuse.
A–Ask direct, supportive, and nonjudgmental questions.
D–Document all findings.
A–Assess your client's safety.
R–Review options and provide referrals.

Legal and Ethical Issues

Law and **ethics** are interrelated and affect the entire nursing practice. Professional nurses must understand the limits in their scope of practice, standards of care, institutional or agency policies, and state laws. Every nurse is responsible for knowing current information regarding ethics and laws related to their practice. Three sources of rules and regulations provide guidelines for safe and legal nursing practice:

1. State **Nurse Practice Acts**
2. Standards of Care set by the American Nurses Association (ANA)
3. Policies and procedures set by the employer

Ethics provide rules and principles that can be used for resolving ethical dilemmas. The ANA recently revised their code of ethics (ANA, 2001), which should guide nurses in their ethical practice. Ethical decisions in maternal health frequently involve maternal–fetal conflict, in which the status of the fetus as a person is still being debated. In maternity care, the ethical assumption is made that the pregnant woman's decision regarding medical intervention will be beneficial to both the expectant mother and her fetus. This is not always the case when the mother's needs or wishes may injure the fetus. Abortion, substance abuse, and fetal therapy are examples that might bring about ethical conflict to all involved in the decisions that influence that family unit.

Throughout the world, effects of violence, abuse, as well as rape confront nurses daily in their practice settings. Women are the primary victims of these "human crimes." Clearly, these acts harm women, and nurses need to look to the ethical principle of nonmaleficence to justify action.

The principle of nonmaleficence asserts an obligation not to inflict harm on others. It is usually translated as, "First, do no harm." Once nurses are convinced that these abusive acts violate the principle of nonmaleficence, they can turn to their own ANA code of ethics for guidance (ANA, 2001).

According to the ANA code of ethics, nurses have an ethical duty to respect the dignity and human rights of other persons and to treat them with compassion regardless of health condition, ethnicity, or life style (ANA, 2001, p. 7). In addition, the nurse is to "promote, advocate, and strive to protect the health and safety of the patient" (ANA, 2001, p. 12). Ethical codes demand action and mandate nurses do something about violation of human rights, not only for the abused women by reporting it, but also on the professional, local, and national levels.

Human abuse, wherever it occurs, diminishes every human being. The challenge to all nurses is what they can do to make a difference in abused women's lives and to reduce its incidence. The right ethical choice is to move beyond ethical beliefs to ethical action (Silva & Ludwick, 2002).

Abortion

Abortion was a volatile legal, social, and political issue even before the *Roe v. Wade* decision to legalize abortion by the Supreme Court in 1973. The term **abortion** describes the willful or purposeful termination of a pregnancy, usually within the first three months. Each year, an estimated 46 million abortions occur worldwide. In 2000, 1.3 million abortions took place in the United States. Forty-nine percent of pregnancies among American women are unintended, and 50% of them are terminated by abortion (Alan Guttmacher Institute, 2004). The highest percentages of reported abortions in 2000 were for women who were younger than 25 years of age (52%), white (57%), and unmarried (81%). In 2000, the racial characteristics of women obtaining abortions were 57% white, 46% black, and 7% other (Whitcomb, 2004). Abortion is one of the most common procedures performed in the United States. It has become a hotly debated political issue that separates people into two camps: pro-choice and pro-life. The pro-choice group supports the right of any woman to make decisions about her reproductive functions on the basis or her own moral and ethical beliefs. The pro-life group feels strongly that abortion is killing and deprives the fetus of the basic right to life. Both sides will continue to deliberate this very emotional issue for years to come.

Today there are several modalities available to terminate a pregnancy: dilation and curettage, vacuum extraction, or medical termination by ingesting the medications methotrexate/misoprostol (Cytotec) or mifepristone (RU 486). When a woman chooses to terminate her pregnancy, she now has options, depending on how far the pregnancy has developed. For a surgical intervention she has up to 14 weeks' gestation; for a medical intervention she has up to 9 weeks' gestation (Goss, 2002). Regardless of the method a woman chooses, all procedures require that women have emotional support, a stable environment in which to recover, and nonjudgmental care throughout.

Abortion is a complex issue, and the controversy lies not only in the public arena, but many nurses struggle with the conflict between their personal convictions and their professional duty. Nurses are taught to be supportive patient advocates and interact with a nonjudgmental attitude under all circumstances, but nurses are not immune to having their own personal and political views, and they may be very different from the patients'. Nurses need to clarify their own personal values and beliefs on this issue and be able to provide nonbiased care before assuming responsibility for clients who might be in a position to consider abortion. Their decision to care for or refuse to care for the patient affects staff unity, influences staffing decisions, and challenges the ethical concept of duty (Marek, 2004).

The ANA's *Code of Ethics for Nurses* upholds the nurse's right to refuse to care for a patient undergoing an abortion if the nurse ethically opposes the procedure (ANA, 2001). Nurses need to make their values and beliefs known to their managers before the situation occurs so alternate staffing arrangements can be made. Open communication and acceptance of personal beliefs of one another can promote a comfortable working environment.

Substance Abuse

Substance abuse can cause fetal injury and thus has legal and ethical implications. In some instances, courts have issued jail sentences when pregnant women caused harm to their fetuses. Many state laws require reporting evidence of prenatal drug exposure and might charge pregnant women with negligence and endangerment of a child. The punitive approach to fetal injury raises the question of how much government control is appropriate and how much should be allowed in the interest of child safety (Box 1-6).

Fetal Therapy

Intrauterine fetal surgery is a procedure that involves opening the uterus during pregnancy, performing a surgery, and replacing the fetus in the uterus. The risks to the fetus and the mother are both great, but may be used to correct anatomic lesions (London et al., 2003). Some argue that medical technology should not interfere with nature and thus this intervention should not take place. Others would vote for the better quality of life for the child made possible with the surgical intervention. For many people, these are ethical debates and intellectual discussions. For nurses, these procedures may be part of a daily routine.

Nurses do play an important supportive role in caring and advocating for their patients and their families. As medical science expands the use of technology, frequent ethical situations will surface that test a nurse's belief system. Encouraging open discussions to address potential emotional issues and differences in opinion among staff members is healthy and opens the door for increasing tolerance of differing points of view. In caring for patients undergoing ethically sensitive procedures, the nurse can

- Offer objective information to the woman and her family
- Recognize and validate the woman's myriad feelings
- Project a nonjudgmental attitude
- Respect the decision made by the family
- Assess the family's emotional support system
- Ask questions using reflection to ascertain feelings
- Use appropriate touch to demonstrate support
- Make appropriate referrals for continuity of care

BOX 1-6
PREGNANT, HOOKED, AND BOOKED

In 1992, a South Carolina court sent Cornelia Whitner, 34, who had used cocaine while pregnant, to jail for eight years because she violated state laws regarding child abuse and neglect. According to the court, she should have known that cocaine use would result in the birth of a damaged baby; therefore, she had to be punished (Lester 1999). Ms. Whitner is an African-American woman who was born and raised in South Carolina. When her youngest son was born she was arrested. A test indicated that he had been exposed to cocaine during her pregnancy. Ms. Whitner was never counseled about her substance abuse problem during her pregnancy and was never offered treatment as a way to avoid arrest. When she was indicted, there was not a single inpatient residential drug treatment program in the entire state designed to treat pregnant drug users (Anderson 2000).

Based on the advice of her court-appointed attorney, Ms. Whitner pled guilty to the charge of child abuse. At her guilty plea and sentencing hearing, Ms. Whitner admitted that she was chemically dependent and requested help. Although Ms. Whitner and her attorney emphasized both the need and the desire for treatment, the court sentenced her to eight years in prison.

Author's Note: The public's concern for the welfare of the child is often expressed as anger at the mother. As a result, policy makers tend to punish these women with jail sentences or removal of their children from their custody. Research shows that treatment for drug addictions is effective. The federal government spends millions annually on services for drug-exposed children in school. If that were spent on early intervention, we could prevent the children's deficits from occurring. But to do this, we must first accept that substance abuse by pregnant women is similar to other treatable health problems. We must remove the societal stigma associated with drug use and advocate treatment for these women. Substance abuse should be viewed as a sickness, not a crime.

Nursing Management

The health care system is intricately woven into the political and social structure of society. Nurses who understand social, legal, and ethical health care issues can play an active role in meeting the health care needs of women. Nurses striving to address these complex concerns might want to consider the following suggestions:

1. Be aware of your own beliefs, attitudes, and misconceptions.
2. Examine and debate your feelings to validate or change them.
3. Stay current about the impact of social/legal/ethical issues on the family.
4. Be sensitive to different beliefs and values from your own.

5. Stay knowledgeable about community resources for all issues.
6. Offer your expertise on these issues to community groups.
7. Become a client advocate by ensuring clients know all their options.
8. Maintain your expertise in clinical practice to avoid litigation.
9. Speak to your legislators about your opinion regarding political action.

It is imperative that nurses take a proactive role in advocating and empowering their clients. Nurses need to enable women to increase control over the determinants of health to help improve their health status. A woman may become empowered when she develops skills not only to cope with her environment, but also when she works to change it. Nurses can take on that mentoring role with women and their families, and help improve their health outcome.

KEY CONCEPTS

- Nurses need to evoke empowerment in their patients by enabling, permitting, and investing them with the power of knowledge.
- Family-centered care is the delivery of safe, satisfying, quality health care that focuses on and adapts to the physical and psychosocial needs of the family.
- Child-birthing practices evolved from female attendants at home to male physicians delivering babies in hospitals with the use of analgesia by the early 1900s.
- Today, freestanding birthing centers, LDRP units, and home births are the norm.
- Changing demographics, economics, growth of technology and information, an increasing multicultural patient base, and a shortage of health care workforce to meet demands have made the health care system difficult to navigate.
- Women with health problems, who need health care services the most, often have the hardest time getting care because of plan coverage policies, affordability concerns, and limited transportation to access that service.
- Healthy People 2010 is a broad-based collaborative federal and state initiative that has set national disease prevention and health promotion objectives to be achieved by the end of the decade.
- All states need to address disease prevention and health promotion to make a difference in the health status of our nation.
- Some of the social issues affecting women's health care include poverty, access to health care (especially prenatal care), and violence.
- Every nurse is responsible for knowing current information regarding ethics and laws related to their practice.

● State nurse practice acts, standards of care, and agency policies and procedures are three categories of safeguards that determine the law's view of nursing practice. The recently revised *Code of Ethics for Nurses* by the ANA should act as an ethical guide for the practice of nursing.

● The nurse's role in advocating for women's health must encompass local, state, and national issues that influence access to care and research.

References

Alexander, L. L., LaRosa, J. H., Bader, H., Garfield, S. (2004). *New dimensions in women's health* (3rd ed.). Sudbury, MA: Jones and Bartlett Publishers.

American Cancer Society. (2004). *Breast cancer facts and figures.* [Online] Available at www.cancer.org/docroot/STT/stt_0.asp.

American Cancer Society. (2005). What are the risk factors for breast cancer? *Cancer Reference Information.* [Online] Available at www.cancer.org/docroot/CRI/content/CRI_2_4_2X_What_are_the_risk_factors_for_breast_cancer_5.asp?sitearea=.

American Heart Association. (2005). *Cardiovascular disease and women.* [Online] Available at www.americanheart.org.

American Nurses Association. (2001). *Code of ethics for nurses with interpretive statements.* Washington, DC: American Nurses Publishing.

Anderson, W. (2000). *Letter to President and CEO of NAACP.* South Carolina Advocates for Pregnant Women (SCAPW). [Online] Available at http://scapw.org/NAACPltr.htm.

Breslin, E. T., & Lucas, V. A. (2003). *Women's health nursing: toward evidence-based practice.* St. Louis, MO: WB Saunders.

Centers for Disease Control and Prevention. (2004). *Safe motherhood: promoting health for women before, during and after pregnancy.* Atlanta: CDC, Division of Reproductive Health.

Centers for Disease Control and Prevention. (2003). *Fact sheet: pregnancy-related mortality surveillance—United States, 1991–1993.* [Online] Available at www.cdc.gov/od/oc/media/pressrel/fs030220.htm. Accessed May 2005.

Centers for Disease Control and Prevention. (1999). State-specific maternal mortality among black and white women—United States, 1987–1996. *MMWR, 48,* 492–496. Also available at www.cdc.gov/epo/mmwr/preview/mmwrhtm/mm4823a3.htm.

Chang, J., et al. (2003). Pregnancy-related mortality surveillance—United States, 1991–1999. *MMWR, 52* (SS02), 1–8.

Condon, M. C. (2004). *Women's health: an integrated approach to wellness and illness.* Upper Saddle River, NJ: Prentice Hall.

Dick–Read, G. (1933). *Childbirth without fear.*

Dyck, P. V., Lackritz, E., & Cordero, J. (2003). *Progress review on maternal, infant, and child health.* Washington, DC: US Department of Health and Human Services, Public Health Service. Also available at www.cdc.gov/nchs/about/otheract/hpdata2010/fa16/mich.htm.

Family Health International, Inc. (2005). *Maternal mortality and morbidity.* [Online] Available at www.fhi.org/en/Topics/maternalmort.htm.

Feldhusen, A. E. (2003). *The history of midwifery and childbirth in America.* [Online] Available at www.midwiferytoday.com/articles/timeline.asp.

Goss, G. L. (2002). Pregnancy termination: understanding and supporting women who undergo medical abortion. *AWHONN Lifelines, 6,* 46–50.

Grantham, C. (2002). *Women's issues then and now.* [Online] Available at www.cwrl.utexas.edu/~ulrich/femhist/medicine.shtml.

Keefe, C. (2003). *Overview of maternity care in the US.* [Online] Available at www.cfmidwifery.org/pdf/OverviewofMatCareApr2003.pdf.

Lamaze, F. (1984). *Painless childbirth: the Lamaze method.* Lincolnwood, IL: NTC Publishers.

Lehrman, G. (2003). *Childbirth in early America.* [Online] Available at www.gliah.uh.edu/historyonline/childbirth.cfm.

Lester, B. (1999). *Drug-abusing moms and babies—victims of stigma.* Brown University News Service. [Online] Available at www.brown.edu/Administration/News_Bureau/Op-Eds/Lester.html.

London, M. L., Ladewig, P. W., Ball, J. W., & Bindler, R. C. (2003). *Maternal–newborn & child nursing: family-centered care.* Upper Saddle River, NJ: Prentice Hall.

Marek, M. J. (2004). Nurses' attitudes toward pregnancy termination in the labor and delivery setting. *JOGNN, 33,* 472–479.

Martin, J., et al. (2002). Births final data for 2001. *National Vital Statistics Reports, 49*(5),16.

Martin, J. A., Kochanek, K. D., Strobino, D. M., Guyer, B., & MacDorman, M. F. (2005). Annual summary of vital statistics—2003. *Pediatrics, 115,* 619–634.

Maternal Child Health Bureau. (2001). *Child health USA.* Rockville, MD: Maternal Child Health Bureau, Health Resources and Services Administration, US Department of Health & Human Services.

Murray, S. S., McKinney, E. S., & Gorrie, T. M. (2006). *Foundations of maternal–newborn nursing* (4th ed.). Philadelphia: WB Saunders.

National Center for Health Statistics. (2005). More babies born at very low birthweight: linked to rise in infant mortality in 2002. In *NCHS news release fact sheets.* [Online] Available at www.cdc.gov/nchs/pressroom/05news/lowbirthwt.htm.

National Women's Law Center, FOCUS/University of Pennsylvania, and the Lewin Group. (2000). *Making the grade on women's health: a national state-by-state report card.* Washington, DC: National Women's Law Center.

Osei, W., Jackson, M., & Miller, S. (2003). *Global health indicators for regional health authorities.* Epidemiology, research and evaluation unit. [Online] Available at www.health.gov.sk.ca/ph_ph_ere_ghi.pdf.

Phillips, C. R. (2003). *Family-centered maternity care.* Sudbury, MA: Jones and Bartlett Publishers.

Salganicoff, A., Beckerman, J. Z., Wyn, R., & Ojeda, V. D. (2002). *Women's health in the United States: health coverage and access to care.* Report no. 6027. Menlo Park, CA: The Henry J. Kaiser Family Foundation.

Save the Children. (2005). *State of the world's mothers* (6th ed., pp. 1–52). Westport, CT: David and Lucille Packard Foundation.

Silva, M., & Ludwick, R. (2002). Ethic column: domestic violence, nurses and ethics: what are the links? *Online Journal of Issues in Nursing.* [Online] Available at www.nursingworld.org/ojin/ethicol/ethics_8.htm.

The Alan Guttmacher Institute. (2004). *Facts in brief: induced abortion.* [Online] Available at www.agi-usa.org/pubs/fb_induced_abortion.html.

United Nations. (2003). *United Nations demographic yearbook.* New York: United Nations.

U.S. Department of Health and Human Services. (2000). *Healthy people 2010* (2nd ed.). Washington, D.C.: U.S. Government Printing Office.

U.S. Department of Health and Human Services. (2002). *Women's health USA 2002.* Rockville, MD: US Department of Health and Human Services, Health Resources and Services Administration, Maternal and Child Health Bureau. Also available at http://mchb.hrsa.gov/data/women.htm.

Whitcomb, D. J. (2004). Abortion surveillance: trends, characteristics and the necessity of the data collection. *AWHONN Lifelines, 8,* 112–114.

World Factbook. (2005). *Infant mortality rate.* Washington, DC: Central Intelligence Agency.

World Health Organization. (2005). *Gender, health and poverty fact sheet.* [Online] Available at www.who.int/inf-fs/en/fact251.html.

Youngkin, E. Q., & Davis, M. S. (2004). *Women's health: a primary care clinical guide.* Upper Saddle River, NJ: Pearson Prentice Hall.

Web Resources

American Dietetic Association, **www.eatingright.org**

American Heart Association National Center, **www.americanheart.org**

Association of Reproductive Health Professionals, **www.arhp.org**

CancerNet, **www.cancernet.nci.nih.gov**

Centers for Disease Control and Prevention, **www.cdc.gov**

Initiative to Eliminate Racial and Ethnic Disparities in Health, **http://raceandhealth.hhs.gov**

National Abortion Federation, **www.naf.org**

National Coalition for Women with Heart Disease, **www.womenheart.org**

Office of Minority Health, **www.omhrc.gov**

Planned Parenthood Federation of America, **www.ppfa.org**

Public Health Service, **www.ahcpr.gov**

The Alan Guttmacher Institute, **www.agi-usa.org**

ChapterWORKSHEET

● MULTIPLE CHOICE QUESTIONS

1. Most women in the 1900s were attracted to hospitals for their child-birthing needs because they

    a. Felt the sterile environment of a hospital would reduce infections

    b. Wanted analgesia to reduce the discomfort of their labors

    c. Needed to have privacy, which was not afforded in the home

    d. Sought a male physician with more experience to deliver them

2. The maternal mortality rate differs from the infant mortality rate in its measurement of

    a. The deaths-per-live births comparison

    b. How the statistics were gathered

    c. The time frame in which the data were formulated

    d. The health index for the various countries

3. The number one cause of mortality for women in the United States is

    a. Breast cancer

    b. Childbirth complications

    c. Injury resulting from violence

    d. Heart disease

4. Research reports that women receiving prenatal care have better pregnancy outcomes. Why are many women in the United States not receiving this valuable service?

    a. They don't feel it is necessary for a normal pregnancy

    b. Many use denial to cope with their pregnancy

    c. No health insurance to cover the expense of care

    d. Some do not trust traditional medical practices

● CRITICAL THINKING EXERCISE

1. As a nurse working in a federally funded low-income clinic offering women's health services, you are becoming increasing frustrated with the number of "no-shows" or appointments missed in your maternity clinic. Some clients come for their initial prenatal intake appointment and never come back. You realize that some just forget their appointments, but most don't even call to notify you. Many of the clients are high risk and thus are jeopardizing their health and the health of their future child.

    a. What changes in the clinic service hours might address this situation?

    b. Outline what you might say at your next staff meeting to address the issue of clients making one clinic visit and then never returning.

    c. What strategies might you use to improve attendance and notification?

    b. Describe what cultural and customer service techniques might be needed.

● STUDY ACTIVITIES

1. Within your clinical group discussion, debate the following statement: Should access to health care be a right or a privilege?

2. List three reasons why one in four women is not receiving prenatal care in the United States.

3. Choose an Internet website from the ones listed here pertaining to women's health and select an article from that site to discuss in your clinical group.

    www.4woman.gov/
    www.healthywomen.org
    www.ivillage.com

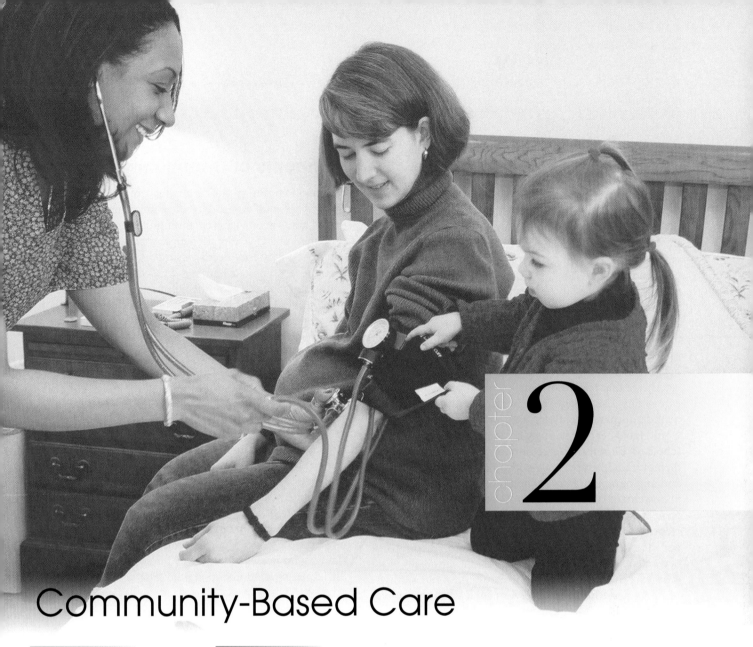

Community-Based Care

KeyTERMS

community
community-based nursing
complementary and
    alternative medicine
cultural competence
cultural encounter
cultural self-awareness
cultural skill
epidemiology
home visits
outpatient clinics
primary prevention
secondary prevention
telephone consultation
    services
tertiary prevention

LearningOBJECTIVES

After studying the chapter content, the student should be able to accomplish the following:

1. Define the key terms.
2. Differentiate community-based nursing practice from acute care settings.
3. Describe nursing roles in community-based health care.
4. Explain the difference between primary, secondary, and tertiary health care and give an example of how each may be provided in the community.
5. Identify at least three barriers to cultural competence.
6. Outline strategies for integrating elements of alternative/complementary therapies and scientific health care practice.

Nursing in the United States began as **community-based nursing.** Self-trained women cared for the sick and dying, assisted women in laboring and birthing, and provided health education to those without access to it. Community-based nursing is the application of the nursing process in caring for individuals and families in **community** settings. The focus of community-based nursing is illness-oriented care of individuals and families throughout their life cycle. Its goal is to help people manage acute or chronic health conditions in community and home settings. It emphasizes all levels of prevention (i.e., primary, secondary, and tertiary), but focuses more on secondary and tertiary levels. Secondary health care typically refers to relatively serious or complicated care that has historically been provided in the acute care setting. Examples of community-based secondary care include outpatient surgery for complex procedures that would have been previously done in the hospital setting (cholecystectomy, hysterectomy, appendectomy), chemotherapy, radiotherapy, magnetic resonance imaging (MRI), and angiography. Tertiary health care encompasses the management of chronic, complicated, long-term health problems that is now delivered in the community setting. Centers for cardiac rehabilitation, home health care for bed-bound elderly people, home care for respiratory-dependent people, and hospice care for the terminally ill are a few examples of tertiary health care community settings.

Preventive health care serves people of all ages and at all levels of health. Improving access to health care means bringing health services that support a continuum of care to people where they live.

Nurses are essential in each of these community-based settings and for each level of care described. Nursing practice in the community is similar to that within the acute care setting because assessing, performing procedures, administering medications, coordinating care services and equipment, counseling patients and their families, and teaching clients and their families regarding their care are all part of the care administered by nurses in the community.

During the past several years, the health care delivery system has changed dramatically. The health care business is focused on controlling costs, sometimes at the expense of patient care. To control costs, people are spending less time in the hospital. Patients are being discharged "sicker and quicker" from their hospital beds. The health care system has moved from reactive treatment strategies in hospitals to a proactive approach in the community. This has resulted in an increasing emphasis on health promotion and illness prevention within the community.

Concepts of Community

Because community-based nursing care is part of the continuum of health care services, it is important for nurses to understand the concepts of community. Often community is defined as a collection of people sharing common characteristics, interests, needs, resources, and environments that interact with one another. The common features of a community may be common rights and privileges as members of a designated city or common ties of identity, values, norms, culture, language, or social support. Women are caregivers to children, parents, spouses, and neighbors, and provide important social support in these roles. A person can be a part of many communities during the course of daily life. Examples would be area of residence (home, apartment, shelter), gender, place of employment (organization or home), language spoken (Spanish, Chinese, English), educational background or college student status, culture (Italian, African-American, Indian), career (nurse, business woman, housewife), place of worship (church or synagogue), and community memberships (Women's Garden Club, YMCA, Women's Support Group, school PTA). In community-based nursing, the community is the unit of service. In community-based settings, the providers of care are concerned not only with the clients who present themselves for service, but also with the larger population of potential or at-risk clients.

Community-Based Nursing

The health needs of society and consumer demand brought about community-based and community-focused services. The movement from an illness-oriented "cure" perspective in hospitals to a focus on health promotion and primary health care in community-based settings has dramatically changed employment opportunities for today's nurses. This shift to emphasizing primary care, and outpatient treatment and management will very likely continue. As a result, employment growth in a variety of community-based settings can be expected for properly trained nurses.

The 2000 National Sample Survey of Registered Nurses (USDHHS/DON 2001) found the following trends in registered nurse (RN) employment settings:

- The percent of RNs working outside the hospital setting is 40.1%.
- RNs employed in community-based settings showed a 36% increase between 1992 and 2000, which was largely the result of an increase in nurses working in home health care and managed care organizations.

Community-based settings include ambulatory care, home health care, occupational health, school health, and hospice settings (Table 2-1). Clinical practice within the community may also include case management, research, quality improvement, and discharge planning. Nurses with advanced practice and experience may be employed in areas of staff development, program development, and community education.

Nurses must be educationally and experientially prepared to provide care in very diverse settings. The goals of Healthy People 2010 to increase quality and years of healthy life and to eliminate health disparities are attainable through community-based health care activities and interventions. The focus of health initiatives today shifts the emphasis of health care to the people themselves and their needs, reinforcing and strengthening their capacity to shape their own lives. This shift of emphasis away from dependence on health professionals toward personal involvement and patient responsibility gives nurses the opportunity to interact with individuals in a variety of self-help roles.

Table 2-1 Community-Based Practice Settings

Setting	Description
Ambulatory care settings	Doctor's offices Health maintenance organizations (HMOs) Day surgery centers Freestanding urgent care centers Family planning clinics Mobile mammography centers
Home health care services	High-risk pregnancy/neonate care Maternal/child newborn care Skilled nursing care Hospice care
Health Department services	Maternal/child health clinics Family planning clinics Sexually transmitted infection programs Immunization clinics Substance abuse programs Jails and prisons
Long-term care	Skilled nursing facilities Nursing homes Hospices Assisted living
Other community-based settings	Parish nursing programs Summer camps Childbirth education programs School health programs Occupational health programs

Nurses in the community-based arena are well positioned to be the primary force in identifying the challenges and implementing changes in women's health for the future.

Community-Based Nursing Roles

Many nurses find the shift from acute care to community settings a challenge. However, nurses working in community-based settings share many of the same roles and responsibilities as their colleagues in acute care settings. For example, nursing assessment and interventions are practiced in a variety of community settings. As nurses build their experiences in community-based settings, they will also develop their roles in case management, patient education, collaborative practice, counseling, research, and advocacy for individuals and families. See Table 2-2 for examples of these roles. The nurse who implements these roles in the community demonstrates a caring and comprehensive client-centered nursing practice.

Community-Based Nursing Interventions

Nursing interventions involve any treatment that the nurse performs to enhance the client's outcome. Although certain nursing interventions are universal in most settings, the ones described in Box 2-1 are particularly prevalent in community-based practice.

Community-Based Nursing Challenges

Despite the positive benefits achieved by caring for families within their own home environments and community, challenges also exist. Clients are being discharged from acute care facilities very early in their recovery course and present with more health care needs than in the past. As a result, nursing care and procedures in the home and community are more complex and time-consuming for the nurse. An example of this would be a high-risk woman discharged from the hospital after childbirth by cesarean with a systemic infection, pelvic abscesses, deep vein thrombosis in her leg, and anorexia. The home health nurse would be making **home visits** to administer heparin and antibiotics intravenously rather than to spend time educating her about child care and follow-up appointments. In the past, this woman would have remained hospitalized for this therapy, but home infusion therapy is now cheaper and allows the client to be discharged sooner.

This demand on the nurse's time may limit the amount of time spent on prevention measures, education, and addressing the family's psychosocial issues. Families may need more time with the nurse to meet all their issues and concerns. With large client caseloads, nurses may feel stretched to spend the time needed and still meet the time restrictions dictated by their health care agencies. To maximize a home care visit, the nurse should plan the tasks to be accomplished (Box 2-2).

Table 2-2 Community-Based Nursing Roles

Role	Example
Direct care provider	Involves the direct delivery of care including client assessment, taking vital signs, medication administration, and changing dressings—for example, a nurse working in an OB/GYN office practice completing prenatal assessment of pregnant client
Educator	Teaches individuals, families, and groups about health maintenance, threats to health, and relevant lifestyle choices that impact health—for example, a home health nurse instructing parents how to care for their high-risk newborn after discharge
Case manager	Coordinates support services for the elderly, assists with insurance issues, arranges transportation for the disabled, and coordinates home visits to high-risk pregnant clients—for example, a home health nurse coordinating home care with several community services
Collaborator	Works with family, teachers, physicians, and social workers for clients with complex or chronic health problems to deliver the most comprehensive, effective, cost-conscious care—for example, a community health nurse partnering with various disciplines to bring care to a preterm infant with multiple health care needs
Advocate	Acts on behalf of the client to ensure they receive necessary care and services—for example, a clinic nurse advocating on behalf of a substance-abusing pregnant woman to receive appropriate treatment for her addiction
Counselor	Assists clients to use problem-solving techniques to decide on the most appropriate course of action for them by listening objectively, clarifying, and offering guidance—for example, a nurse working with couples in a genetic counseling clinic
Researcher	Shares current research findings with new mothers—for example, a school nurse working in community education who shares research findings about the importance of vaccinations for public health in the local high school teenage pregnancy program

---

BOX 2-1

COMMUNITY-BASED NURSING INTERVENTIONS

- *Health screening*—detects unrecognized or preclinical illness among individuals so they can be referred for definitive diagnosis and treatment (e.g., mammogram or Pap smear)
- *Health education programs*—assisting clients in making health-related decisions about self-care, use of health resources, and societal health issues such as smoking bans and motorcycle helmet laws (e.g., childbirth education or breast self-examination)
- *Medication administration*—preparing, giving, and evaluating the effectiveness of prescription and over-the-counter drugs (e.g., hormone replacement therapy in menopausal women)
- *Telephone consultation*—identifying the problem to be addressed; listening and providing support, information, or instruction; documenting advice/instructions given to concerns raised by caller (e.g., consultation for a new mother with a newborn with colic)

- *Health system referral*—facilitating the location, services offered, and telephone number for contacting that agency (e.g., referring a woman for breast prosthesis after a mastectomy)
- *Instructional*—teaching an individual or a group about a medication, disease process, lifestyle changes, community resources, or latest research findings concerning their environment (e.g., childbirth education class)
- *Nutritional counseling*—demonstrating the direct relationship between nutrition and illness while focusing on need for diet modification to promote wellness (e.g., Women, Infants, and Children [WIC], counselor interviewing an anemic pregnant client)
- *Risk identification*—recognize personal or group characteristics that predispose one to develop a specific health problem and modify or eliminate them (McCloskey & Bulechek, 2000; e.g., genetic counseling of 42-year-old pregnant woman at risk for a Down syndrome infant)

BOX 2-2

HOME CARE VISITATION PLANNING

- Review previous interventions to eliminate unsuccessful ones.
  - Check previous home visit narrative to validate interventions.
  - Communicate with previous nurse to ask questions and clarify.
  - Formulate plan of interventions based on data received (e.g., client preference of intravenous (IV) placement or order of fluids).
- Prioritize client needs based on their potential to threaten the client's health status.
  - Use Maslow's hierarchy of needs to set forth a plan of care.
  - Address life-threatening physiologic issues first (e.g., an infectious process would take precedence over anorexia).
- Develop goals that reflect primary, secondary, and tertiary prevention levels.
  - *Primary prevention*—Have the patient consume adequate fluid intake to prevent dehydration.
  - *Secondary prevention*—Administer drug therapy as prescribed to contain and treat an existing infectious process.
  - *Tertiary prevention*—Instruct the client on good hand-washing technique to prevent spread and future secondary infections.
- Bear in mind the client's readiness to accept intervention and education.
  - Ascertain the client's focus and how they see their needs.
  - Address minor client issues that might interfere with intervention (e.g., if the client is in pain, attempting to teach her about her care will be lost; her pain must be addressed first before she is ready to learn).
- Consider the timing of the visit to prevent interfering with other client activities.

- Preschedule all visits at convenient times per client if possible.
- Reschedule a home visit if a client event comes up suddenly (e.g., if the client has a favorite soap opera to watch, attempt to schedule around that event if at all possible).
- Outline nursing activities to be completed during the scheduled visit.
  - Know the health care agency's policy and procedures for home visits.
  - Consider the time line and other visits scheduled that day.
  - Research evidence-based best practices to use in the home (e.g., if the client is fatigued, be able to be flexible to accommodate her needs and allow for periods of rest so that she may conserve her energy).
- Obtain necessary materials/supplies before making the visit.
  - Assemble all equipment needed for any procedure in advance.
  - Secure any equipment that might be needed if a problem occurs (e.g., bring additional IV tubing and a catheter to make sure the procedure can be carried out without delay).
- Determine criteria to be used to evaluate the effectiveness of the home visit.
  - Revisit outcome goals to determine the effectiveness of the intervention.
  - Assess the client's health status to validate improvement.
  - Monitor changes in the client's behavior toward health promotion activities and disease prevention (e.g., verify/observe that the client demonstrates correct hand-washing technique after instruction and reinforcement during the home care visit).

Nurses making home care and community visits have fewer resources available to them when compared with the acute care setting. Intervention decisions have to be made in isolation at times. The nurse must possess excellent assessment skills and the ability to communicate effectively with the family to be successful in carrying out the appropriate plan of care needed.

Nurses interested in working in community-based settings must be able to apply the nursing process in a less structured or controlled environment compared with the hospital. Nurses must be able to assimilate information well beyond the immediate physical and psychosocial needs of the client in a controlled acute care setting, and deal with environmental threats, lifestyle choices, family issues, different cultural patterns, financial burdens, transportation problems, employment hazards, communication barriers, limited resources, and client acceptance and compliance.

Although opportunities for employment in community-based settings are plentiful, a baccalaureate degree may be required for many positions. Many public health departments will hire only nurses with a bachelor of science in nursing (BSN) degree. Previous medical/surgical experience in an acute care setting is typically sought by home health agencies before hiring a nurse, because they must function fairly independently within the home environment.

The nurse must also be familiar with and respectful of many different cultures and socioeconomic levels when visiting clients in their homes. The nurse must remain objective in dealing with such diversity and demonstrate an understanding and appreciation for cultural differences. Home-based interventions must be individualized to address the cultural, social, and economic diversity among clients within their own environment (Littleton & Engebretson, 2005).

Community-Based Nursing Care for Women and Infants

A woman's reproductive years span half her lifetime, on average. This is not a static period, but rather one that encompasses several significant stages. As her reproductive goals change, so do a woman's health care needs. Because of these changing needs, comprehensive community-centered care is critical. These services should include

- Contraceptive services
- Abortion services
- Infertility services
- Screening for sexually transmitted infections and cancer of the reproductive system
- Preconceptional risk assessment and care
- Maternity care (including prenatal, birth, and post-partum/newborn care)

Prenatal Care

Early, adequate prenatal care has long been associated with improved pregnancy outcomes (March of Dimes, 2005). Adequate prenatal care is a comprehensive process in which problems associated with pregnancy are identified and treated. Basic components of prenatal care are early and continuing risk assessment, health promotion and medical and psychosocial interventions, and follow-up. Within the community setting, several services are available to provide health care for pregnant women. These are highlighted in Box 2-3.

Although many families living in affluent neighborhoods have access to private prenatal care, some are unaware of the various community resources available to them within their communities. Most public health services are available for consultation, local hospitals have "hotlines" for questions, and public libraries have pregnancy-related resources as well as Internet access. Nurses can be a very helpful "link" between needs and resources for all women regardless of their economic status.

Technologically advanced care for high-risk pregnancies has proved to improve maternal child outcomes. Between 1980 and 2000, the LBW infant mortality rate declined from 694 per 1000 to 422 per 1000, and by 2000 declined to approximately 250 per 1000 live births (Iyasu et al., 2002). Widespread use of better high-technology care has been credited with this decline. The idea of regionalized high-risk care was promulgated by the American Academy of Pediatrics in the late 1970s. The goal was to promote uniformity nationwide, covering the prenatal care of high-risk pregnancies and high-risk new-borns. Advanced technology found in level III perinatal regional centers along with community-based prenatal surveillance programs has resulted in better risk-adjusted mortality rates (Mackey & Alexander, 2003; Schwartz et

---

BOX 2-3

MATERNAL AND INFANT COMMUNITY HEALTH CARE SERVICES

- State public health prenatal clinics provide access to care based on a sliding scale payment schedule or have services paid for by Medicaid.
- Federally funded community clinics typically offer a variety of services, which may include prenatal, pediatric, adult health, and dental services. A sliding scale payment schedule or Medicaid may cover costs.
- Hospital outpatient health care services offer maternal–child health services. Frequently they are associated with a teaching hospital in which medical school students, interns, and OB/GYN residents rotate through the clinic services to care for patients during their education process.
- Private OB/GYN offices are available for women with health insurance seeking care during their pregnancies. Some physicians in private practice will accept Medicaid patients as well as private patients.
- Community free clinics offer maternal–child services in some communities for women with limited economic resources (homeless, unemployed).
- Freestanding birth centers offer prenatal care for low-risk mothers as well as childbirth classes to educate couples regarding the birthing process. Most centers accept private insurance and Medicaid for reimbursement services.

- Midwifery services are available in many communities where midwives provide women's health services. They usually accept a multitude of payment plans from private pay to health insurance to Medicaid for reimbursement purposes.
- WIC provides food, nutrition counseling, and access to health services for low-income women, infants, and children. WIC is a federally funded program and is administered by each state. All persons receiving Aid to Families with Dependent Children (AFDC), food stamps, or Medicaid are automatically eligible for WIC. An estimated 45% of the infants born in the United States are served by WIC (USDA Food and Nutrition Service, 2004; Fig. 2-1).
- Childbirth classes offer pregnant women and their partners a series of educational classes on childbirth preparation. Women attend them during their last trimester of pregnancy. Some classes are free and some have a fee.
- Local La Leche League groups provide mother-to-mother support for breast-feeding, nutrition, and infant care problem-solving strategies. All women who have an interest in breast-feeding are welcome to participate in the meetings, which are typically held in the home of a La Leche member.

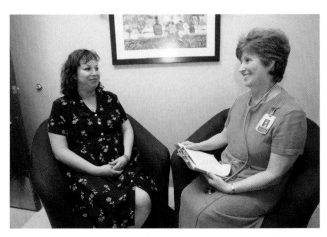

● Figure 2-1 A trained registered nurse screens a pregnant woman at a WIC clinic. If the woman meets income and nutritional eligibility requirements, she may receive vouchers to purchase nutritious foods. (Photo by Joe Mitchell.)

al., 2000). For example, fetal monitoring and ultrasound technology have traditionally been used within acute care settings to monitor the progress of many high-risk pregnancies. However, with the increased cost of hospital stays, many services were moved to outpatient facilities and into the home. The intent was to reduce health care costs and to monitor women with complications of pregnancy in the home rather than in the hospital. Home-versus-hospital care has the potential to produce cost savings. Such services offered in the home setting might include

- Infusion therapy to treat infections or combat hydration
- Hypertension monitoring for women with pregnancy-induced hypertension
- Uterine monitoring for mothers who are high risk for preterm labor
- Fetal monitoring to evaluate fetal well-being
- Portable ultrasound to perform a biophysical profile to assess fetal well-being

Care During Labor and Delivery

The nine months of pregnancy are all about choices: cloth or disposable diapers, breast-feed or bottle feed, doctor or midwife, where to give birth—at a birthing center, at home, or at a hospital. Deciding where a woman chooses to give birth depends on her pregnancy risk status. For the pregnant women identified as high risk as a result of medical or social risk factors, the hospital is the safest place for her to give birth. Potential complications can be addressed because medical technology, skilled professionals, and neonatal services are available. For low-risk women, a freestanding birthing center or a home birth is an option.

Birthing Center

A *birthing center* is a cross between a home birth and a hospital. Birthing centers offer a "homelike" setting but with close proximity to a hospital facility in case of com-

plications. Midwives often are the sole care providers in freestanding birthing centers, with obstetricians as backups in case of emergencies. Birthing centers usually have fewer restrictions and guidelines for families to follow and allow for more freedom in making laboring decisions. The cost and the cesarean section rate are much lower when compared with a hospital (Ramsey, 2004). The normal discharge time after birth is normally measured in hours (4–24 hours), not days.

Birthing centers provide an alternative to parents who are not comfortable with a home birth, yet who do not want to give birth in a hospital. Advantages of birthing centers include nonintervening obstetric care, freedom to eat and move around during labor, ability to give birth in any position, and the right to have any number of family and friends attend the birth. Disadvantages are that some centers have rigid screening criteria, which may eliminate healthy mothers from using birth centers; many have rigid rules concerning transporting the mother to the hospital (e.g., prolonged labor, ruptured membranes); and many have no pediatrician on staff if the newborn has special needs after birth (Cooper, 2004).

Birthing centers aim to provide a relaxing home environment and promote a culture of normality. Birth is viewed as a normal physiologic process, and most centers use a nonintervening view of labor and birth. The range of services for the expectant family often includes prenatal care, childbirth education, intrapartum care, and postpartum care, including home follow-up and family planning (Fig. 2-2). One of the hallmarks of the freestanding birthing center is that it has the ability to provide truly family-centered care by approaching pregnancy and birth as a normal family event and encouraging participation of all family members. Education is often provided by centers, encouraging families to become informed and self-reliant in the care of themselves and their families (ICEA, 2001).

Home Birth

For centuries women have been having babies in their home. Many feel more comfortable and relaxed when giving birth in their own environment. Home births are recommended for women with low-risk pregnancies and no labor complications. Many women who want no medical interventions and a very family-centered birth choose to have a home birth. Advantages of home birth include

- Incurring the lowest cost
- Laboring and delivering in the privacy, comfort, and familiarity of home while surrounded by loved ones
- Maintaining control over every aspect affecting the woman's labor (e.g., positions, attire, support people)
- Allowing labor to progress normally, without interference and unnecessary interventions
- Having continuous one-on-one care given by the midwife throughout the childbirth process
- Establishing a trusting relationship with the nurse midwife (APA, 2003)

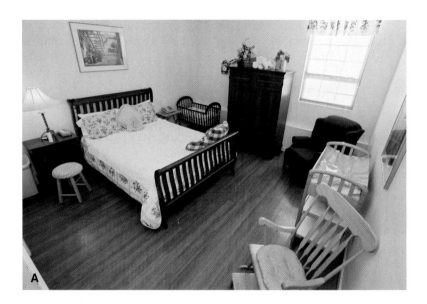

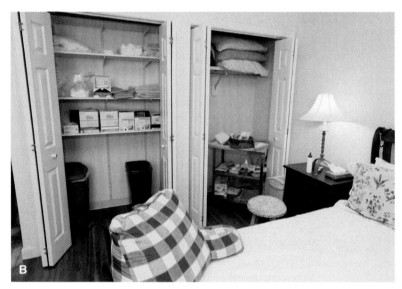

● Figure 2-2 Birth centers aim to provide a relaxing home environment and promote a culture of normality, while offering a full range of health care services to expectant family. (Photos by Gus Freedman.)

Disadvantages of having a home birth include

- Limited anesthetic pain medication
- Danger to mother and baby if an unanticipated emergency arises (placenta abruptio, uterine rupture, cord prolapse, or a distressed fetus). The time it takes to get to the hospital could be detrimental.
- The necessity of an emergency backup plan for a doctor on standby and a nearby hospital should an emergency occur (Ramsey, 2004)

Nursing Management

The choice between a birthing center, home birth, and hospital depends widely on the woman's personal preferences, her risk status, and her distance from a hospital (30 minutes away). Some women choose an all-natural birth with no medications and no medical intervention, whereas others would feel more comfortable in a setting in which medications and a trained staff are available if needed. Presenting the facts (pros and cons) to women and allowing them to choose in collaboration with their health care provider is the nurse's role. Safety for the low-risk childbearing woman is paramount, but at the same time nurses must protect the right to choose birth options and continue to promote family-centered care in all maternity settings.

Postpartum and Newborn Care

Recent reforms in health care financing have reduced the hospital stays significantly for women after giving birth. Community-based nursing is part of an effort that extends care beyond the hospital setting. When new mothers are discharged from the hospital, most are still experiencing perineal discomfort, incisional pain, and uterine cramping. Furthermore, they are fatigued, constipated, and unsure about their feeding and caring for their newborn without consultation. These new mothers need to be made aware of available community resources, which might include telephone consultation by nurses, **outpatient clinics,** and home visits.

Telephone Consultation

Many hospitals offer **telephone consultation services** by their maternity nurses. The discharged mother is given the phone number of the nursing unit on the day of discharge and is instructed to call if she has any questions or concerns. Because the nurses on the unit are familiar with her birth history and the newborn, they are in a good position to assist her in adjusting to her new role. Although this service is usually free, not all families recognize a problem early or use this valuable informational resource.

Outpatient Clinics

Outpatient clinics offer another community-based site for the childbearing family to access services. Usually the mother has received prenatal care before her birthing experience and thus has established some rapport with the nursing staff there. The clinic staff is usually willing to answer any questions or concerns she may have concerning the health of herself or her newborn. Appointments usually include an examination of the mother and newborn, and instructions about umbilical cord, care, and nutritional issues for both mother and infant.

Home Visits

Home visits offer similar services as a scheduled clinic visit, but in addition provide the nurse an opportunity to assess the family's adaptation/dynamics and the home environment. During the last decade, hospital stays averaged 24 to 48 hours or less for vaginal births and 72 to 96 hours for cesarean births (CDC, 2004). Federal legislation went into effect in 1998 that prohibited insurers from restricting hospital stays for mothers and newborns to less than 2 days for vaginal births or 4 days for cesarean births (CDC, 2004). These shortened stays have reduced the educational opportunities for new mothers to learn to care for themselves and their newborns.

Postpartum care in the home environment should include

- Monitoring the physical and emotional well-being of the family members
- Identifying potential or developing complications for the mother and newborn
- Bridging the gap between discharge and ambulatory follow-up for mothers and their newborns (Lynch et al., 2001)

Because hospital stays are reduced, high-risk newborns are also being cared for in community settings. High-tech care once was reserved exclusively for the hospital. Now, however, the increasing cost of complex care and the preva-

lence of managed care have forced high-technology equipment into the living rooms of high-risk infant's homes. Families have become "health care systems" by providing physical, emotional, social, and developmental home care for their technology-dependent infants. A few conditions that would persist or continue after discharge might include

- Preterm infants with ongoing oxygen dependency, strictures and bowel obstructions, or retinopathy
- LBW infants needing nutritional or hypercaloric formulas and adjunct feeding devices (e.g., tube feeding or gastrostomy)
- Hydrocephalus
- Cerebral palsy

Examples of home technology equipment may include

- Renal dialysis
- Mechanical ventilation for bronchopulmonary dysplasia
- Electronic apnea monitoring for preterm infants
- Home oxygen equipment
- IV infusions for antibiotics
- Hyperalimentation
- Respiratory nebulizer
- Phototherapy
- Suction equipment

All family members must work together to provide 24-hour care. Family members must negotiate with insurers for reimbursement of durable medical equipment, to troubleshoot equipment problems, and to make sure they manage inventories of supplies and equipment. In addition, the parents or caretakers must be able to assess the infant for signs of illness; determine the problem; decide when to call nurses, pharmacists, and physical therapists; and interpret and implement physician prescriptions. Technology in the home requires nurses to focus on the family "home care system" to provide total care to the infant.

Nurses can play a key role in assisting families with successful adaptation by guiding preparedness and increasing their confidence in caring for their infants at home. This adaptation begins with the hospital discharge nurse. This nurse can help prepare the family to care for their infant by providing instruction and hands-on experience within a supportive environment until their confidence increases. Family members should be active participants in the transition-to-home plan. Recognition of parental needs and addressing each area in the discharge plan will ease the transition home.

The home health nurse can further assess the family's preparedness through several brief questions:

How well prepared are you to take care of your infant's physical, emotional, and technologic equipment needs?

How well prepared are you obtain the home services you need for your infant?

How well prepared are you manage the stress of home care?

These simple questions convey the nurse's concern for the infant and family while obtaining a thorough assessment of the family learning needs.

Once preparedness has been assessed, the nurse can intervene as necessary. For example, if the caretakers do not judge themselves to be prepared to maintain machinery, technology, medication, or developmental therapy, then the nurse can demonstrate the care to the family. The nurse can also assist the family to anticipate the common problems that might occur, such as running out of supplies, having enough medication or special formula mixture to last throughout the weekend, and keeping backup batteries for powering machines or portable oxygen. The outcome of the preparedness assessment and intervention is that safety of the infant is established and maintained.

Nursing of families who are using complex home care equipment requires caring for the infant and their family members' physical and emotional well-being as well as providing effective solutions to problems they may encounter. Home health nurses need to identify, mobilize, and adapt a myriad of community resources to support the family in giving the best possible care in the home setting. Preparing families for high-technology care before hospital discharge, with home health nurses continuing and reinforcing that focus, will help ease the burden of managing high-technology equipment in the home.

Women's Health Care

Community-based women's health services have received increased emphasis during the last few decades simply because of economics. Women use more health care services than men, make as much as 90% of health care decisions, and are the majority of the population (CDC, 2001). Women spend 66 cents of every health care dollar, and 7 of the 10 most frequently performed surgeries in the United States are specific to women (Breslin & Lucas, 2003). Examples of community-based women's health care services that can be freestanding or hospital-based include

- *Screening centers* that offer mammograms, Pap smears, bone density assessments, genetic counseling, ultrasound, breast examinations, complete health risk appraisals, laboratory studies (complete blood count, cholesterol testing, thyroid testing, glucose testing for diabetes, follicle-stimulating hormone [FSH] levels), and electrocardiograms
- *Educational centers* that provide childbirth education, preconception classes, women's health lectures, sibling preparation classes, instruction on breast self-examinations, breast-feeding, and computers for research
- *Counseling centers* that offer various support groups: genetics, psychotherapy, substance abuse, sexual assault, and domestic violence
- *Surgical centers* that provide plastic surgery, urologic and gynecologic surgeries, abortion, liposuction, and loop electrode excision

- *Wellness centers* that make available stress reduction techniques, massage therapy, guided imagery, hypnosis, smoking cessation, weight reduction, tai chi, yoga, and women's fitness/exercise classes
- *Alternative/wholeness healing centers* that provide acupuncture, aroma therapy, biofeedback, therapeutic touch, facials, reflexology, and herbal remedies
- *Retail centers* that offer breast pump rental and purchase, baby scales, nursing clothes and supplies, breast prostheses, and lactation consultants

Women have multiple selections regarding services and settings, and have many choices regarding health care providers. In the past, most women received health care services from physicians such as obstetricians, gynecologists, and family physicians. Today, nurse midwives and nurse practitioners are becoming more prevalent in providing well-women care.

Nurses who work in community-based settings need to be familiar with the many health issues commonly encountered by women within their communities. All nurses who work with women of any age in community-based settings, including the workplace, schools, practitioner offices, and clinics, should possess a thorough understanding of the scope of women's health care and be prepared to intervene appropriately to prevent problems and to promote health.

Levels of Prevention in Community-Based Nursing

The concept of prevention is a key focus of community-based nursing practice. Prevention means to ward off an event before it occurs. The emphasis on health care delivery in community-based settings has moved beyond primary preventive health care (e.g., well-child checkups, routine physical examinations, prenatal care, and treatment of common acute illnesses) and now encompasses secondary and tertiary care.

Primary Prevention

The concept of **primary prevention** involves preventing the disease or condition before it occurs through health promotion activities. It encompasses a vast array of areas, including nutrition, good hygiene, sanitation, immunization, adequate shelter, smoking cessation, family planning, and the use of seat belts (Matteson, 2001). Primary preventive interventions for women are directed by four goals. These goals include

1. Maintaining balance, perspective, and priorities in life to improve ability to cope with life stress in effective ways and to handle multiple roles
2. Developing and maintaining healthy relationships to prevent abuse
3. Developing and maintaining a healthy sense of self to deal effectively with the role changes of the life cycle

4. Developing and maintaining physical health and preventing illness by eating a balanced diet, using safety precautions, practicing safe sex, preventing osteoporosis, and not smoking or drinking (Clark, 2003)

Prevention of NTDs, which include anencephaly and spina bifida, is an example of primary prevention. NTDs arise from improper development of the neural tube during embryogenesis. Anencephaly is incompatible with life. Spina bifida can range from mild to severe with associated morbidity, which may include paraplegia, bladder and bowel incontinence, and mental impairment. The worldwide incidence of fetal NTDs ranges from 1 to 8 per 1000 live births and varies considerably geographically. In the United States, approximately 2500 babies are born each year with NTDs, about 6 in every 10,000 live births (Wald, 2004). Primary prevention of NTDs by all pregnant women taking folic acid supplementation between 0.4 to 0.8 mg daily 3 months before and 3 months after conception reduces the risk of first occurrence of NTD by 50% or more (Wald, 2004). All women of childbearing age should be advised to take 4 mg folic acid daily as soon as they plan to become pregnant and continue throughout the pregnancy to prevent this devastating condition.

Secondary Prevention

Secondary prevention is the early detection and treatment of adverse health conditions. Pregnancy testing, blood pressure readings, cholesterol levels, fecal occult blood, breast examinations, mammography screening, hearing and vision examinations, and Pap smears to detect cancer or sexually transmitted infections are examples of this level of prevention. Such interventions do not prevent the start of the health problem but are intended to detect it and start treatment early to prevent further complications (Anderson & McFarlane, 2000).

Consider the benefits of secondary prevention related to HIV infection. Without intervention, an estimated one in four HIV-positive women in the United States will transmit HIV perinatally. This means approximately 1750 HIV-positive infants would be born each year, with lifetime estimated medical costs of $282 million. The estimated cost of secondary prevention (counseling, testing, and AZT) is $68 million. This represents a savings of $114 million in health care costs. This estimate excludes lifetime productivity savings and quality-of-life improvements related to HIV infections averted (CDC, 1999).

Tertiary Prevention

Tertiary prevention is designed to reduce or limit the progression of a disease or disability after an injury. The purpose of tertiary prevention is to rehabilitate or restore individuals to their maximum potential (Sorrell & Redmond, 2002). Tertiary prevention measures are supportive and restorative. Two areas in which tertiary prevention are particularly warranted for women include sexually transmitted infections and abuse. Tertiary prevention efforts would focus on minimizing and managing the effects of chronic sexually transmitted infections such as herpes, HIV infection, and untreated syphilis. With regard to abuse, tertiary prevention would involve working with women who have suffered long-term consequences of violence. The focus of the nurse would be to maximize the woman's strengths, to heal from the trauma and loss, and to build support systems. These examples represent the essence of the tertiary level of prevention.

The Nurse's Role in Community-Based Preventive Care

Women's health needs are many and varied. All health professionals have a special role in health promotion, health protection, and disease prevention. Community-based nurses provide health care for women at all three levels of prevention. This care often involves advocacy for services to meet the particular needs of women.

Much of community nursing involves prevention, early identification, and prompt treatment of health problems, and monitoring for emerging threats that might lead to health problems. For example, a nurse could help reduce the incidence of AIDS by taking the following steps:

- *Primary*—educating clients on the practice of "safe sex"
- *Secondary*—urging testing and counseling for clients who practice "unprotected sex," as well as providing referrals and follow-up for clients who test positive for HIV
- *Tertiary*—providing care and support, advocacy, case management, and other therapeutic interventions to slow disease progression and keep viral counts down

Nurses who work with clients in community settings are frequently in a position to assist in identification, management, treatment, and prevention of health problems. As a result, these nurses need a general understanding of the basic principles and concepts of **epidemiology.** Using an epidemiologic approach can provide nurses with the language to describe and analyze health concerns in population-based care. Epidemiology is the study of factors that influence the frequency and distribution of disease, injury, or other health-related events, and their causes, for the purpose of establishing programs of prevention and control (O'Toole, 2003). Its ultimate goal is to identify the underlying causes of a disease, then apply findings to disease prevention and health promotion. Epidemiology uses research and statistical data collection to find answers to the following questions:

Who in the population is affected by the disease, disorder, or injury?

What is the occurrence of this health problem in the community?

Can the causative factors and risk factors contributing to the problem be determined? (Hitchcock et al., 1999)

Healthy People 2010 (US Department of Health and Human Services, 2000a) was written based on epidemiologic principles. This report presents health statistics and data, describes health threats, discusses interventions, and sets goals and objectives directed toward prevention and management (McEwen, 2002). A few examples of objectives demonstrating epidemiologic concepts that address women's health needs are presented in the accompanying box "Healthy People 2010."

Cultural Issues in Community-Based Care

The population in the United States has a mix of cultural groups, highlighted by ever-increasing diversity. The Center for Immigration Studies (2004) reports that the US immigration population has reached 33 million, with people arriving from every corner of the world. One million immigrants come to the United States each year, and more than half are of childbearing age. Latin America accounts for more than 50% of immigrants to the United States. By the year 2050, people of African, Asian, and Latino backgrounds will make up one half our population (Hawke, 2004).

The nursing population in the United States does not begin to approximate the diversity in the general population. According to the US Department of Health and Human Services (2000b), 12% (or 324,000) of the 2.7 million RNs in the United States identify themselves as being from racial/ethnic minority backgrounds. This stands in contrast to 30% of the general population, which describes themselves as being from a racial or ethnic minority (Mattson, 2003).

This growing diversity has strong implications for the provision of health care. For years nurses have struggled with the issues of providing optimal health care that meets the needs of women and their families from varied cultures and ethnic groups. In addition to displaying competence in technical skills, nurses must also become competent in caring for clients from ethnic and racial backgrounds. Adapting to different cultural beliefs and practices requires flexibility and accepting others' viewpoints. Nurses must really listen to clients and learn about their beliefs of health and wellness. To provide culturally appropriate care to diverse populations, nurses need to know, understand, and respect culturally influenced health behaviors. Table 2-3 lists selected beliefs and behaviors from various cultures that may help nurses understand their childbearing patients.

Characteristics of Culture

Culture is complex and not easily dissected. It can be thought of as a fabric with many interwoven colored threads. Each colored thread represents one aspect of culture—values, worldview, time orientation, personal–space orientation, language, touch, and family organization. Understanding one's values is key to understanding their behavior, because behavior generally reflects values. A culture's worldview helps its peoples understand how life fits into the "big picture" and allows them to make sense of that which is knowable (e.g., evil, disease, natural disaster).

It is very important for nurses to research and understand cultural characteristics, values, and beliefs of the various people to whom they deliver care so that false assumptions and stereotyping do not lead to insensitive care. Table 2-4 provides a comparison of common cultural characteristics, values, and beliefs. Time orientation, personal space, family orientation, and language are discussed in the following paragraphs.

Time Orientation

The strict concept of time that organizes American health care service is not shared by many other cultures around the world, where a more relaxed attitude toward time prevails. Time measures productivity in many health care settings and nurses can get angry or frustrated when women from different cultures arrive late for appointments and do not seem to be concerned about their "lateness."

Personal Space

Personal space, which is an appropriate distance between conversing people, varies widely between cultural groups. Overall, this distance is generally closer between people of the same gender and wider when the interaction involves people of the opposite sex. Touch is incorporated in cultures with close distance zones (Hispanic, Mediterranean, Eastern Indian, Middle Eastern) and is not used in cultures

---

HEALTHY PEOPLE *2010*

Objectives for Women's Health Needs

✓ **Goal:** Reduce pregnancies among adolescents from 72 pregnancies to 46 pregnancies per 1000

✓ **Goal:** Reduce AIDS among adolescents and adults (incidence) from 19.5 new cases to 1 new case per 100,000

✓ **Goal:** Reduce fetal and infant deaths during the perinatal period from 7.5% to 4.5% per 1000 live births

✓ **Goal:** Increase the proportion of women with health insurance from 87% to 100%

✓ **Goal:** Reduce the percentage of cases of osteoporosis from 10% to 8%

✓ **Goal:** Reduce cervical cancer deaths per 100,000 women from 3 to 2

✓ **Goal:** Reduce lung cancer deaths per 100,000 women from 45 to 41

✓ **Goal:** Reduce pregnancy complications per 100 deliveries from 32 to 20

Source of data: US Department of Health and Human Services. (2000). *Healthy people 2010* (conference ed.). Washington, DC: Government Printing Office.

Table 2-3 Selected Cultural Beliefs and Behaviors during the Childbearing Period

Topic	Belief or Behavior
Pregnancy	A pregnant woman is considered ill or weak. (Latino) Pregnancy is a "hot" condition, so meat should be avoided and sodium intake increased. (African-American) Drinking milk during pregnancy may result in a large baby and hard labor. (Asian) "Cold" foods, including vegetables, should be avoided during pregnancy. (Chinese) A pregnant woman's workload should be reduced. (Native American) Planning for the infant prior to delivery defies God's will. (Arab)
Birth	Pain speeds delivery so pain relief should be avoided. (African-American) Emotional expression during labor is expected. (Arab and Italian) Labor can be stimulated by the use of herbal preparations. (Latino) Changes in the moon's phase may trigger labor. (African-American) Delivery should take place in a squatting position. (Asian) The pregnant woman's mother-in-law should attend her during delivery. (Chinese) Women will want to wear their headscarves during labor and birth. (Muslim)
Conception	Pregnancy is more apt to happen during monthly menses. (African-American) Infertility is perceived as failure to fulfill family role expectations. (Chinese) Herbs can be used to "heat" the womb to increase the chances of conception. (Latino) Islam forbids exposing a developing fetus to alcohol and drugs. (Muslim)
Contraception	Pregnancy should be avoided by abstinence. (Chinese, Filipino, Latino, Catholic) A wife who asks her husband to use a condom marks herself as a prostitute. (Latino) Charms and ceremonies may prevent conception. (Native American) An ice water and vinegar douche slows sperm and kills them. (African-American) Islam forbids permanent sterilization for both men and women. (Muslim)
Menstruation	Menstruation opens one up to infection. (African-American) One must avoid sex during menstruation and wear shoes to prevent poisons from entering the body. (African-American) Avoiding hot, spicy food can alleviate menstrual cramping. (Latino) Exposure of an infant to a menstruating woman may cause an umbilical hernia. (African-American, Latino)
Postpartum	Bathing should be avoided after delivery. (Mexican) Outside visitors should be discouraged after delivery. (Korean) Drinking cold water after delivery should be avoided. (Asian) Beef and seafood cause itching at the episiotomy site. (Asian)

Modified from Clark (2003) and Moore and Moos (2003).

with more distanced personal space (North American, Muslims, Native Americans) (Moore & Moos, 2003).

Family Orientation

Families may be patriarchal (male/father centered), matriarchal (female/mother centered), or egalitarian (equal). Patriarchal family orientation is most common throughout the world. Health care workers need to know which type of family organization is present to be able to relate to family dynamics and to understand who will be making health care decisions for all family members (Fig. 2-3).

Language

Language barriers can complicate communication between nurses and patients from different cultures. There are more than 6000 languages and dialects spoken around the world today. Types of language barriers that impede communication include foreign languages; different dialects and regionalisms; and the use of idioms, slang, and street talk (Munoz & Luckmann, 2005). A skilled interpreter can assist nurses to overcome the anxiety and frustration produced by language barriers. In addition, Box 2-4 provides guidelines to help nurses establish a therapeutic relationship with people of different cultures speaking a different language.

Culturally Competent Nursing Care

Cultural competence is defined as the knowledge, willingness, and ability to adapt health care to enhance its acceptability to and effectiveness with patients from diverse cultures (Clark, 2003). Cultural competence is a dynamic

Table 2-4 Comparison of Common Cultural Characteristics, Values, and Beliefs

American Characteristics (Anglo-European)	Other Contrasting Cultures' Characteristics
Individualism	Family focus (Asian)
Independent	Interdependence (Hmong)
Obsession with personal hygiene	Not concerned with body odors or frequent bathing (Zimbabwe)
Emphasis on youth	Value of elders (Japanese)
Health care decisions made by women	Decisions made by elders (Indian)
Time is precise	Time is flexible (Northern Europe)
Technology oriented	Confidence in natural systems (Latinos)
Direct eye contact valued	Direct eye contact violates privacy (Navajos)
Reliance on biomedical remedies	Traditional healers, folk medicine (Chinese)
Active participation of fathers at birth	Taboo against presence of father (Africa)
Childbearing cycle can be hazardous	Childbirth is normal, natural (Cherokee)
Disbelief in supernatural phenomena	Strong belief in "evil spirits" (Hispanics)
Independent during postpartum	Dependent for 40 days (Mexican)

Sources: Steefel (2003), Levine et al. (2004), and Moore and Moos (2003).

process during which nurses obtain cultural information and then apply that knowledge. Nurses must look at patients through their own eyes and the eyes of patients and family members. Nurses must develop nonjudgmental acceptance of cultural differences in clients, using diversity as a strength that empowers them to achieve mutually acceptable health care goals (Kersey–Matusiak, 2000). This cultural awareness allows nurses to see the entire picture and improves the quality of care and health outcomes.

Cultural Self-Awareness

The first step of the journey toward cultural competence is **cultural self-awareness.** Nurses need to become aware of, appreciate, and become sensitive to the values, beliefs, customs, and behaviors that have shaped their own culture. It is only through this self-exploration that they can then look beyond their own culture and "see" patients from different cultures. During this process, nurses should examine their own biases and prejudices toward other cultures. Without being aware of the influence of their own cultural values, nurses may have a tendency to impose their own beliefs, values, and patterns of behavior on other cultures. The goal of self-cultural awareness is to help nurses become aware of how their background and their clients' backgrounds differ (Habel, 2001).

An example of the first step in achieving cultural awareness is to explore your "preunderstandings" of diverse cultures based on your history and culture, and know this is how you form your prejudices. It is important to be aware that in many cultures pregnancy and childbirth are primarily taken care of within a woman's domain in the home setting. Expecting a husband to help or support his wife during labor is contrary to the traditions of some cultures. Awareness that this cultural norm is different from the nurse's own frame of reference prevents the "labeling" of culturally diverse husbands as disinterested in the childbirth process and prevents you from forming prejudices.

Cultural Knowledge

The second step is gaining cultural knowledge about various worldviews of different cultures. Some of the ways nurses can acquire knowledge are by reading about different cultures, attending continuing education courses on different cultures, accessing Web sites, and attending cultural diversity conferences. The goal of cultural knowledge is to become familiar with culturally/ethnically diverse groups, worldviews, beliefs, practices, lifestyles, and problem-solving strategies.

An example of the second step in gaining cultural knowledge is to know that touch is not welcome by many cultures. For example, Hmong women are not comfortable with vaginal examinations, which traditionally are not performed in their culture. The genitals are considered to be a private area of the body, with the only exposure occurring during the sexual act with one's husband (Levine et al., 2004). For nurses working with Hmong women, cloth covering and positioning to promote privacy are needed to demonstrate understanding of their culture.

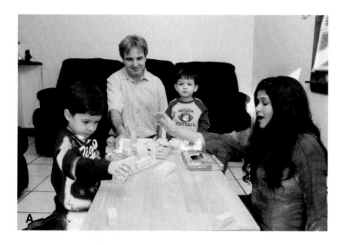

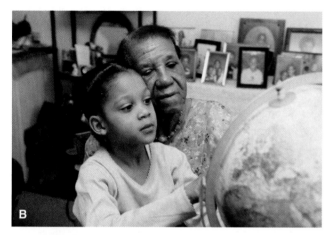

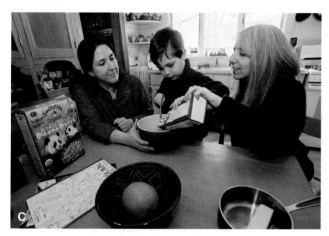

● Figure 2-3 It is important for nurses to recognize family dynamics when providing health care to patients. Many different family structures exist and influence patient needs. (**A**) The traditional nuclear family, which is composed of two parents and their biological or adopted children. (**B**) The extended family, which includes the nuclear family, plus other family members such as grandparents, aunts, uncles, and cousins. (**C**) Gay and lesbian families comprise two people of the same sex sharing in a committed relationship, with or without children. (Photos by Gus Freedman.)

BOX 2-4
GUIDELINES FOR COMMUNICATING WITH CLIENTS

- Convey empathy by experiencing what that person is experiencing. Example: If that client has just been told she has breast cancer, mentally place yourself into "her shoes" and "feel" her feelings at that time.
- Show respect by valuing that person and viewing them as special. Example: Address all patients with a formal title to retain their individuality and demonstrate personal respectfulness.
- Build trust by having confidence or faith in that person. Example: Be honest about what can be done to "fix" the problem and do not promise anything more to patients than you can deliver.
- Establish a rapport by initiating social, friendly conversation first. Example: Ask questions about the client's homeland, about how long she has lived in the United States, and about family before asking health-related questions.
- Listen actively by giving verbal and body language clues that you are interested in that person and her problem. Example: Use eye contact, an open posture, and sit at the same level to promote open communication between parties.
- Demonstrate genuine interest by using words of concern and demonstrating a caring attitude that shows you are interested in their total well-being. Example: Using a "concerned facial expression" when listening to a patient's problems conveys interest in that patient as an individual (Munoz & Luckmann, 2005).

Cultural Skills

The third step toward becoming culturally competent is acquiring **cultural skills.** This step involves learning how to do a competent cultural assessment. Nurses who have achieved cultural skills can individually assess each client's unique cultural values, beliefs, and practices without depending solely on written facts about specific cultural groups. Principles of cultural assessment include the following:

- View all cultures in the context they were developed.
- Examine underlying premises for cultural beliefs and behaviors.
- Interpret behavior within the context of the particular culture.
- Recognize the potential for intracultural variation (Bowers, 2000).

An example of the third step in acquiring cultural skills can be demonstrated in asking all postpartum women what they would like to drink, rather than bringing them cold juice or water. Many cultures (Latinos and Asians) that prescribe to the theory of cold (yin) and hot (yang) consider cold drinks harmful after birth—a cold state. These mothers need to restore balance by taking warm drinks. To add confusion to nurses, hot and cold actually refer to the property rather than the temperature of a substance, which is all the more reason to ask rather than assume what women want to drink after birth (Steefel, 2003).

Cultural Encounter

The final step in the journey to becoming culturally competent is a **cultural encounter.** This involves participating in cross-cultural interactions with people from culturally diverse backgrounds. Cultural encounters may include attending religious services or ceremonies and participating in important family events. Although nurses may have several friends in different cultural groups, they are not necessarily knowledgeable about the group as a whole. In fact, the values, beliefs, and practices of the few people nurses encounter on a social basis may not represent that specific cultural group for which they provide care. Thus, it is important to have as many cultural encounters as possible to avoid cultural stereotyping (Salimbene & Gerace, 2003; Fig. 2-4).

An example of the final step (cultural encounter) in achieving cultural competence would be to participate in a culturally diverse group discussion to work on changing policies and procedures within the health care unit. Invite several cultural brokers that represent diverse cultures to discuss specific childbirth practices that affect the childbearing health care setting. A cultural broker is someone who is fluent in the language and is knowledgeable about the value systems, customs, mores, and daily living experiences of the population served. The ultimate goal is to facilitate a more positive experience for all cultures.

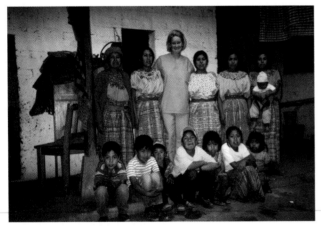

● Figure 2-4 Cultural encounters help nurses develop an understanding and appreciation for people from culturally diverse backgrounds. Caring for women and children in Guatemala provided rich opportunities for a group of American nurses to develop cultural competence.

Consider THIS!

Our medical mission took a team of nurse practitioners into the rural mountains of Guatemala to offer medical services to people who had never had any. One day, a distraught mother brought her 10-year-old daughter to the mission clinic, asking me if there was anything I could do about her daughter's right wrist. She had sustained a fracture a year ago and it had not healed properly. As I looked at the girl's malformed wrist, I asked if it had been splinted to help with alignment, knowing what the answer was going to be. The interpreter enlightened me by saying that this young girl would never marry and have children because of this injury. I appeared puzzled at the interpreter's prediction of this girl's future. It was later explained to me that if the girl couldn't make tortes from corn meal for her husband because of her wrist disability, she would not be worthy of becoming someone's wife and thus would probably live with her parents the rest of her life.

I reminded myself during the week of the medical mission not to impose my cultural values on the women for whom I was caring and to accept their cultural mores without judgment. These silent self-reminders served me well throughout the week, for I was open to learning about their lifestyles and customs.

Thoughts: What must the young girl be feeling at the age of 10, being rejected for a disability that wasn't her fault? What might have happened if I had imposed my value system on this patient? How effective would I have been in helping her if she didn't feel accepted? This incident ripped my heart out, for this young girl will be deprived of a fulfilling family life based on a wrist disability. This is just another example of female suppression that happens all over the world—such a tragedy—and yet a part of their culture, on which nurses should not pass judgment.

Barriers to Cultural Competence

Barriers to cultural competence can be grouped into two categories: those related to providers and those related to systems (Mazanec & Tyler, 2003). When health care providers lack knowledge of their patients' cultural practices and beliefs or when the provider's beliefs are different than those of the client, the provider may be unprepared to respond when the patient expresses unexpected health care decisions. System-related barriers occur when most agencies have not been designed for cultural diversity, want everyone to conform to the established rules and regulations, and attempt to fit everyone into the same mold.

If nurses are to meet the needs of all their patients and families, they must understand that cultural competence does not mean substituting one's own cultural identity with another, ignoring the variability within cultural groups, or even appreciating the cultures being served. Instead, a respect for difference, an eagerness to learn, and a willingness to accept that there are many ways of viewing the world will distinguish nurses who integrate cultural competence into their daily practice from those who give "lip service" to it (Gonzalez et al., 2000).

Complementary and Alternative Medicine

The use of **complementary and alternative medicine** (CAM) is not unique to ethnic culture groups. Interest in CAM therapies continues to grow nationwide and will affect care of the childbearing and child-rearing families. CAM use spans people from all walks of life. Overall, CAM use is seen more in women than men, and in people with higher educational levels. Prayer specifically for health reasons was the most commonly used CAM therapy (NCCAM, 2004a). Research indicates that more than 42% of adults use some form of alternative practice, and one in three pregnant women use CAM therapies, some of which may be potentially harmful (Ranzini et al., 2001).

Types of Complementary and Alternative Medicine

CAM includes diverse practices, products, and health care systems that are not currently considered to be part of conventional medicine (NCCAM, 2004b). Complementary medicine is used *together with* conventional medicine, such as using aromatherapy to reduce discomfort after surgery. Alternative medicine is used *in place of* conventional medicine, such as eating a special natural diet to treat cancer instead of undergoing surgery, chemotherapy, or radiation that has been recommended by a conventional doctor.

Integrative medicine combines mainstream medical therapies and CAM therapies for which there is some scientific evidence of safety and effectiveness (NCCAM, 2004b). These include acupuncture, reflexology, therapeutic touch, meditation, yoga, herbal therapies, nutritional supplements, homeopathy, naturopathic medicine, and many more used for the promotion of health and well-being (Youngkin & Davis, 2004). See Table 2-5 for selected CAM therapies and treatments.

The theoretic underpinnings of alternative health propose that health and illness are complex interactions of the mind, body, and spirit. It is then surmised that many aspects of patients' health experiences are not subject to traditional scientific methods. This field does not lend itself readily to scientific study or to investigation, and therefore is not easily embraced by many hard-core scientists (Sorrell & Redmond, 2002). Much of what we consider to be alternative medicine comes from the Eastern world, folk medicine, and religious and spiritual practices. There is no unifying basic theory for the numerous treatments or modalities, except (as noted previously) that health and illness are considered to be complex interactions among the body, mind, and spirit.

Nursing Management

Because of heightened interest in complementary treatments and their widening use, anecdotal efficacy, and growing supporting research evidence, nurses need to be sensitive to and knowledgeable enough to answer many of the questions patients ask and to guide them in a safe, objective way (Tryens et al., 2004). Traditional remedies need to be integrated with mainstream medicine

Table 2-5 Selected Complementary and Alternative Therapies

Therapy	Description
Aromatherapy	Use of essential oils to stimulate the sense of smell for balancing mind, body, and spirit
Homeopathy	Based on the theory of "like treats like"; helps restore the body's natural balance
Acupressure	Restores balance by pressing an appropriate point so self-healing capacities can take over
Feng Shui (pronounced fung shway)	The Chinese art of placement. Objects are positioned in the environment to induce harmony with chi.
Guided imagery	Uses consciously chosen positive and healing images, along with deep relaxation to reduce stress and to help people cope
Reflexology	Uses deep massage on identified points on the foot or hand to scan and rebalance body parts that correspond with each point
Therapeutic touch	Includes balancing energy by centering, invoking an intention to heal, and moving the hands from the head to the feet several inches from the skin
Herbal medicine	The therapeutic use of plants for healing and treating disease and conditions
Spiritual healing	Praying, chanting, presence, laying on of hands, rituals, and meditation to assist in the healing process

Adapted from Littleton and Engebretson (2002).

when patients are taking modern drugs. Many patients who use complementary or alternative therapies do not reveal this fact to their health care provider. One of the nurse's most important roles during the *assessment* phase of the nursing process is to encourage clients to communicate their use of these therapies to eliminate the possibility of harmful interactions and contraindications with current medical therapies. When assessing clients, it is important to ask specific questions about any nonprescription medications they may be taking, including vitamins, minerals, or herbs. Clients should also be questioned about any therapies they are taking that have not been ordered by their primary health care provider.

A few common *nursing diagnoses* that might be applicable for clients using CAM are as follows:

- Deficient knowledge regarding the benefits of CAM
- Deficient knowledge regarding the potential risks linked with CAM
- Ineffective health maintenance related to traditional medicine

Nurses who treat patients who practice CAM may want to consider some of the following tips:

- Be culturally sensitive to nontraditional treatments.
- Acknowledge and respect different beliefs, attitudes, and lifestyles.
- Keep an open mind; standard medical treatments do not work for all women.
- Accept CAM and integrate it if it brings comfort without harm.
- Provide accurate information, not unsubstantiated opinions.
- Advise clients how they can best monitor their condition using CAM.
- Discourage practices only if they are harmful to the client's health.
- Instruct the client to weigh the risks and benefits of CAM use.
- Avoid confrontation when asking clients about CAM.
- Be reflective, nonjudgmental, and open-minded about CAM.

The nurse can offer clients the following guidelines:

- Do not take for granted that because a substance is a natural herb or plant product, it is beneficial or harmless.
- Seek medical care when ill.
- Always inform the provider if herbs are being used.
- Avoid taking herbal remedies if you are pregnant or lactating.
- Be sure that any product package contains a list of all ingredients and amounts of each.
- Frequent or continual use of large doses of a given CAM preparation is not advisable.
- Possible harm may result if therapies are mixed (e.g., vitamin E, garlic, and aspirin all have anticoagulant properties).

- Research CAM through resources such as books, Web sites, and articles (Clark et al., 2003).

Nurses need to remember that when they provide guidance to women concerning CAM therapies, stress to them that they check with their health care provider before taking any "natural" substance. The use of complementary therapies is widespread, especially by women desiring to alleviate the nausea and vomiting of early pregnancy. Ginger tea, sea-bands, and vitamin B_6 are typically used to treat morning sickness (Gaffney & Smith, 2004). Although these may not cause any ill effects during the pregnancy, the fact that most substances ingested cross the placenta and have the potential to reach the growing embryo, it is imperative to emphasize to all pregnant women that it is better to be safe than sorry. Women at risk for osteoporosis are seeking alternative therapies to hormone replacement since the release of data from the Women's Health Initiative (WHI) study placed doubt on estrogen. Some of the alternative therapies for osteoporosis include soy isoflavones, progesterone cream, magnet therapy, tai chi, and hip protectors (Kessenich, 2004). In addition, menopausal women seek CAM therapies to reduce the incidence of hot flashes. Once again, despite many "natural herbs" claims, most of the therapies have not undergone scientific inquiry and thus could place the woman at risk if mixed with traditional medicines.

A large increase in the use of CAM has occurred during the past decade. This situation has precipitated many issues, including the safety and true value of many of the therapies. Nurses must educate themselves about the pros and cons of CAM and be prepared to discuss and help their patients make sense of it all. Expanding our consciousness by understanding and respecting diverse cultures and CAM will enable nurses to provide the best potential treatment for patients and their families entrusted to our delivery of community-based care.

KEY CONCEPTS

- Community-based nursing uses the nursing process in caring for patients within community settings and applies primary, secondary, and tertiary prevention levels.
- Health care delivery has moved from acute care settings out into the community, with an emphasis on health promotion and illness prevention.
- Nurses have a variety of job opportunities in ambulatory care settings, home health care, occupational health, school health, hospice, and others.
- The goals of Healthy People 2010 to increase quality and years of healthy life and to eliminate health disparities are attainable through community-based health care activities and interventions.
- Nursing interventions in community-based settings include those of health screening, education, medication administration, telephone consultation,

nutritional counseling, and acting as referral agent, counselor, and researcher.

- The goal of epidemiology is to identify the underlying causes of a disease, then apply findings to disease prevention and health promotion.
- Cultural competence is a dynamic process during which nurses obtain cultural information and then apply that knowledge.
- Steps to gaining cultural competence include cultural self-awareness, cultural knowledge, cultural skills, and cultural encounters.
- The field of complementary and alternative health and medicine is almost entirely community based.
- Nurses must educate themselves about complimentary/alternative therapies to be able to advise patients in community-based settings who use them.

References

American Pregnancy Association (APA). (2003). *Birthing choices: care providers and labor locations.* [Online] Available at www.american-pregnancy.org/planningandpeparing/birthingchoices.html.

Anderson, E. T., & McFarlane, J. (2000). *Community as partner* (3rd ed.). Philadelphia: Lippincott Williams & Wilkins.

Bowers, P. (2000). *Cultural perspectives in childbearing.* [Online] Available at http://nsweb.nursingspectrum.com/ce/ce263.htm.

Breslin, E. T., & Lucas, V. A. (2003). *Women's health nursing: toward evidence-based practice.* St. Louis, MO: Saunders.

CDC. (2004). *Longer hospital stays for childbirth.* National Center for Health Statistics. [Online] Available at www.cdc.gov/nchs/products/pubs/pubd/hestats/hospbirth.htm.

CDC. (2001). *New study profiles women's use of health care.* [Online] Available at www.cdc.gov/od/oc/media/pressrel/r010725.htm.

CDC. (1999). *Status of perinatal HIV prevention: US declines continue.* Division of HIV/AIDS Prevention. [Online] Available at www.cdc.gov/hiv/pubs/facts/perinatl.htm.

Center for Immigration Studies. (2004). *Current numbers.* [Online] Available at www.cis.org/topics/currentnumbers.html.

Clark, C. C., Colbath, J. D., & Reitz, S. E. (2003). *A complementary potpourri.* [Online] Available at http://nsweb.nursingspectrum.com/ce/ce199.htm.

Clark, M. J. (2003). *Community health nursing: caring for populations* (4th ed.). Upper Saddle River, NJ: Prentice Hall.

Cooper, T. (2004). Changing the culture: normalizing birth. *British Journal of Midwifery, 12,* 45–50.

Gaffney, L., & Smith, C. A. (2004). Use of complementary therapies in pregnancy: the perceptions of obstetricians and midwives in South Australia. *Australia and New Zealand Journal of Obstetrics and Gynecology, 44,* 24–29.

Gonzalez, R. I., Gooden, M. B., & Porter, C. P. (2000). Eliminating racial and ethnic disparities in health care. *American Journal of Nursing, 100,* 56–58.

Habel, M. (2001) *Putting patient teaching into practice.* [Online] Available at www.cyberchalk.com/nurse/courses/nurseweek/nw0650/c6/references.htm.

Hawke, M. (2004). Mosaic of diversity. *Nursing Spectrum.* [Online] Available at http://community.nursingspectrum.com/MagazineArticles/article.cfm?AID=11786.

Hitchcock, J. E., Schubert, P. E., & Thomas, S. A. (1999). *Community health nursing: caring in action.* New York: Delmar Publishers.

ICEA. (2001). ICEA position statement and review: the birth place. *International Journal of Child Education, 17,* 36–41.

Iyasu, S., Tomashek, K., & Barfield, W. (2002). Infant mortality and low birth weight among black and white infants—United States, 1980–2000. *MMWR, 51*(27), 589–592.

Kersey–Matusiak, G. (2000). An action plan for cultural competence. *Nursing Spectrum.* [Online] Available at http://nsweb.nursingspectrum.com/ce/ce255.htm.

Kessenich, C. R. (2004). Alternative therapies in osteoporosis. *Nursing Spectrum.* [Online] Available at http://nsweb.nursingspectrum.com/ce/ce282.htm.

Levine, M. A., Anderson, L., & McCullough, N. (2004). Hmong birthing: bridging the cultural gap in a rural community in northern California. *AWHONN Lifelines, 8,* 147–149.

Littleton, L. Y., & Engebretson, J. C. (2002). *Maternal, neonatal, and women's health nursing.* New York: Delmar.

Lynch, A. M., Kordish, R. A., & Williams, L. R. (2001). Maternal–child nursing: postpartum home care. In Rice, R. (Ed.), *Home health nursing: concepts and application* (3rd ed., pp. 379–398). St. Louis: Mosby.

Mackey, M. C., & Alexander, J. W. (2003). Program management of high risk pregnancy: outcomes and costs. *Disease Management Health Outcomes, 11,* 1–6.

March of Dimes. (2005). *Why prenatal care?* March of Dimes Birth Defect Prevention Foundation. [Online] Available at www.modimes.org.

Matteson, P. S. (2001). *Women's health during the childbearing years: a community-based approach.* St. Louis: Mosby.

Mattson, S. (2003). Cultural diversity in the workplace. *AWHONN Lifelines, 7,* 154–158.

Mazanec, P., & Tyler, M. K. (2003). Cultural considerations in end-of-life care. *American Journal of Nursing, 103,* 50–58.

McCloskey, J. C., & Bulechek, G. M. (2000). *Nursing interventions classification (NIC)* (3rd ed.). St. Louis: Mosby.

McEwen, M. (2002). *Community-based nursing: an introduction* (2nd ed.). St. Louis: Saunders.

Moore, M. L., Moos, M. K. (2003). *Cultural competence in the care of childbearing families.* March of Dimes nursing module. White Plains, NY: Educational Services of March of Dimes.

Munoz, C. C., & Luckmann, J. (2005). *Transcultural communication in nursing* (2nd ed.). Clifton Park, NY: Delmar Learning.

National Center for Complementary and Alternative Medicine (NCCAM). (2004a). *The use of complementary and alternative medicine in the United States.* [Online] Available at http://nccam.nih.gov.

National Center for Complementary and Alternative Medicine (NCCAM). (2004b). *What is complementary and alternative medicine (CAM)?* [Online] Available at http://nccam.nih.gov.

O'Toole, M. T. (2003). *Encyclopedia & dictionary of medicine, nursing & allied health* (7th ed.). Philadelphia: Saunders.

Ramsey, L. (2004). Birthing options: birthing center, home, and hospitals. *PageWise.* [Online] Available at http://ncnc.essortment.com/birthingoptions_rikm.htm.

Ranzini, A., Allen, A., & Lai, Y. (2001). Use of complementary medicine and alternative therapies among obstetric patients. *Obstetrics and Gynecology, 4*(Suppl. 1), S46.

Salimbene, S., & Gerace, L. M. (2003). *Cultural competence for today's nurses—culture and women's health.* [Online] Available at http://nsweb.nursingspectrum.com/ce/m29a-1.htm.

Schwartz, R. M., Muri, J. H., Overpeck, M. D., Pezzullo, J. C., & Kogan, M. D. (2000). Use of high-technology care among women with high-risk pregnancies in the United States. *Maternal Child Health Journal, 4,* 7–18.

Sorrell, J. M., & Redmond, G. M. (2002). *Community-based nursing practice: learning through student's stories.* Philadelphia: FA Davis.

Steefel, L. (2003). No cookie cutter approach to postpartum culture care. *Nursing Spectrum.* [Online] Available at http://community.nursingspectrum.com/MagazineArticles/article.cfm?AID=9717.

Tryens, E., Coulston, L., & Tlush, E. (2004). *Understanding the complexities of herbal medicine.* [Online] Available at http://nsweb.nursingspectrum.com/ce/ce290.htm.

Turnock, B. J. (2001). *Public health: what it is and how it works* (2nd ed.). Gaithersburg, MD: Aspen Publishers.

USDA Food and Nutrition Service. (2004). *WIC: the special supplemental nutrition program for women, infants and children.* [Online] Available at www.fns.usda.gov/wic/aboutwic.

US Department of Health and Human Services. (2000a). *Healthy people 2010.* [Online] Available at www.healthypeople.gov.

US Department of Health and Human Services, Health Resources and Services Administration, Bureau of Health Professions. (2000b). *National sample survey of RNs final report.* [Online] Available at www.hrsa.gov.

US Department of Health and Human Services, Division of Nursing, Bureau of Health Professions (USDHHS/DON). (2001). *The registered nurse population: national sample survey of registered nurses, March 2000.* Washington, DC: Government Printing Office.

Wald, N. J. (2004). Folic acid and the prevention of neural-tube defects. *New England Journal of Medicine, 350,* 101–103.

Youngkin, E. Q., & Davis, M. S. (2004). *Women's health: a primary care clinical guide* (3rd ed.). Upper Saddle River, NJ: Prentice Hall.

Web Resources

Acupuncture, **www.acupuncture.com**
Alliance for Hispanic Health, **www.hispanichealth.org**
American Botanical Council, **www.herbalgram.org**
American Holistic Nurses Association, **www.ahna.org**
American Nurses Association, **www.nursingworld.org**
Association for Women's Health, Obstetrics, and Neonatal Nursing, **www.ahonn.org**
Center for Immigration Studies, **www.cis.org**
Centers for Disease Control and Prevention, **www.cdc.gov/mmwr**
Cross-Cultural Health Care Program, **www.xculture.org**
DiversityRx, **www.diversityrx.org**
Herb Research Foundation, **www.herbs.org**
National Center for Homeopathy, **www.homeopathic.org**
NIH Complementary and Alternative Medicine, **www.altmed.od.nih.gov/oam**
Office of Minority Health, **www.omhrc.gov**
The Holistic Health Center, **www.forholistichealth.com**
Transcultural Nursing Society, **www.tcns.org**

ChapterWORKSHEET

● MULTIPLE-CHOICE QUESTIONS

1. A nurse with cultural competence is one who is

   a. Well versed in the customs and beliefs of his or her own culture

   b. Open to the values and beliefs of other cultures

   c. Knowledgeable about various cultures and able to apply it in treatment settings

   d. Active in establishing policies to address care for diverse cultures

2. Which prevention level includes early diagnosis, screening, and treatment?

   a. Primary prevention

   b. Secondary prevention

   c. Tertiary prevention

   d. Community prevention

3. The Anglo-European culture in the United States tends to emphasize

   a. Youth, technology, time as precise

   b. Value of elders, spiritual phenomena, belief in fate

   c. Flexible time, confidence in natural systems, family focus

   d. Independence, extended family, folk medicine

4. A pregnant client asks the nurse about taking an herb to boost her energy levels. An appropriate response by the nurse would be to

   a. Discourage it because she is pregnant and it might be harmful

   b. Encourage her taking it because she will probably feel better

   c. Make no comment because it might be culturally oriented

   d. Tell her to double her prenatal vitamins to improve her energy

5. When talking about CAM therapies with a patient, which of the following would be a nonjudgmental question to ask?

   a. "Are you practicing alternative medicine?"

   b. "You're not taking anything that we don't know about, are you?"

   c. "What activities are you doing to promote wellness for yourself?"

   d. "Are you playing it safe and staying away from herbs?"

● CRITICAL THINKING EXERCISE

1. As a nurse working in a women's health clinic serving a culturally diverse population, you are concerned that many of the client's cultural beliefs are not being addressed, and thus the clients are not keeping their scheduled appointments. Many of the nurses that work there seem to feel that the clients should adopt Western cultural values and beliefs, and leave their own cultural beliefs behind now that they live in the United States. You are planning to address this concern at the next staff meeting.

   a. What resources would you use to research this topic before the meeting?

   b. What information will you present to address the nursing staff's attitudes toward their culturally diverse clientele?

   c. What steps would you take to help the nursing staff to become culturally competent?

● STUDY ACTIVITIES

1. Form a panel discussion group representing at least three different cultures. Ask each panel member to describe predominant health care practices based on their cultural background and compare them with those of the United States.

2. Accepting cultural differences with an open mind and heart, expressing a willingness to work with others from different cultures, and keeping a flexible attitude describes _____.

3. Select one of the Helpful Informational Resources websites to explore cultural diversity. After reviewing the website, answer the following questions: Would this resource be helpful for nurses to learn about the various cultures with which they interact in their practice? Why or why not?

4. Arrange for a visit to a community health center that offers services to various cultural immigrants. Interview the staff concerning strategies used to overcome communication barriers and different health care practices.

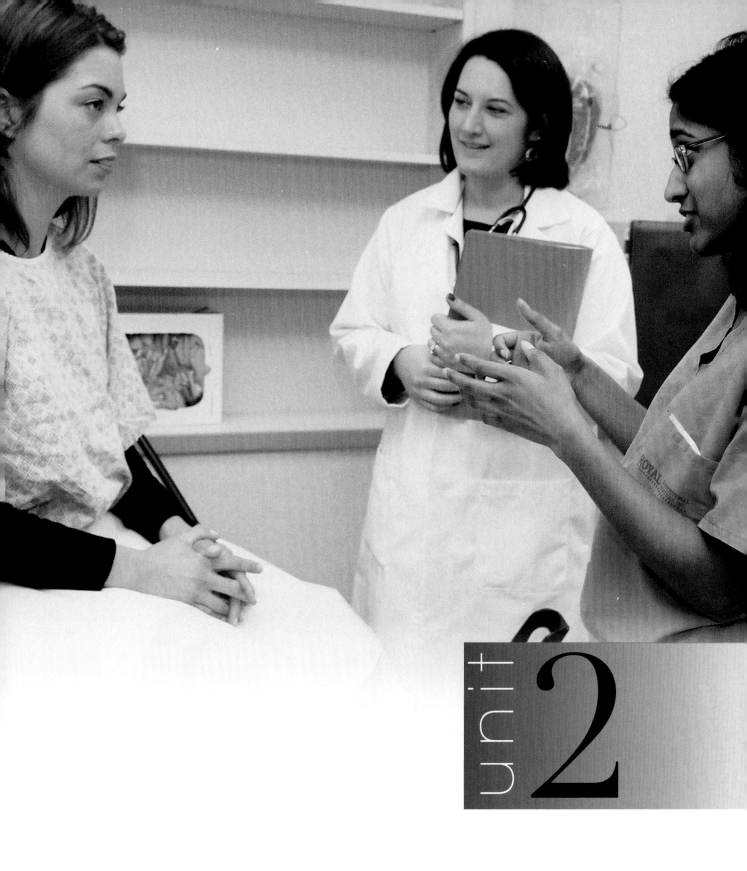

Women's Health
Throughout the Lifespan

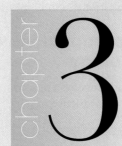

chapter 3

Anatomy and Physiology of the Reproductive System

KeyTERMS

breasts
cervix
endometrium
estrogen
fallopian tubes
follicle-stimulating
   hormone (FSH)
luteinizing hormone (LH)
menstruation
ovaries
ovulation
penis
progesterone
testes
uterus
vagina
vulva

LearningOBJECTIVES

After studying the chapter content, the student should be able to accomplish the following:

1. Define the key terms.
2. Discuss the structure and function of the major external and internal female genital organs.
3. Outline the phases of the menstrual cycle, dominant hormones involved, and changes taking place in each phase.
4. Identify external and internal male reproductive structures and the function of each in hormonal regulation.

The reproductive system consists of organs that function in the production of offspring. In humans and other mammals, the female reproductive system produces the female reproductive cells (the eggs, or ova) and contains an organ (uterus) in which development of the fetus takes place; the male reproductive system produces the male reproductive cells (the sperm) and contains an organ (penis) that deposits the sperm within the female. Nurses need to have a thorough understanding of anatomy and physiology of the male and female reproductive systems to be able to care for them and the conditions that might affect their reproductive organs. This chapter will review the female and male reproductive systems and the menstrual cycle as it relates to reproduction.

Female Reproductive Anatomy and Physiology

The female reproductive system is composed of both internal and external reproductive organs.

Internal Female Reproductive Organs

The internal female reproductive organs consist of the vagina, the uterus, the fallopian tubes, and the ovaries. These structures develop and function according to the specific hormone influences that affect fertility and childbearing (Fig. 3-1).

Vagina

The **vagina** is a highly distensible musculomembranous canal situated in front of the rectum and behind the bladder. It is a tubular, fibromuscular organ lined with mucous membrane that lies in a series of transverse folds called rugae. The rugae allow for extreme dilatation of the canal during labor and birth. The vagina is a canal that connects the external genitals to the uterus. It receives the penis and the sperm ejaculated during sexual intercourse, and it serves as an exit passageway for menstrual blood and for the fetus during childbirth. The front and back walls normally touch each other so that there is no space in the vagina except when it is opened (e.g., during a pelvic examination or intercourse). In the adult, the vaginal cavity is 3 to 4 inches long. Muscles that control its diameter surround the lower third of the vagina. The upper two thirds of the vagina lies above these muscles and can be easily stretched. During a woman's reproductive years, the mucosal lining of the vagina has a corrugated appearance and is resistant to bacterial colonization. Before puberty and after menopause (if the woman is not taking estrogen), the mucosa is smooth secondary to lower levels of estrogen (Venes, 2005).

Uterus

The **uterus** is a pear-shaped muscular organ at the top of the vagina. It lies behind the bladder and in front of the rectum and is anchored in position by eight ligaments. It is not firmly attached or adherent to any part of the skeleton. A full bladder tilts it backward; a distended rectum, forward. It alters its position by gravity or with change of posture. It is the size and shape of an inverted pear. It is the site of menstruation, implantation of a fertilized ovum, development of the fetus during pregnancy, and labor. Before the first pregnancy, it measures approximately 3 inches long, 2 inches wide, and 1 inch thick. After a pregnancy, the uterus remains larger than before the pregnancy. After menopause, it becomes smaller and atrophies.

The uterine wall is relatively thick and composed of three layers: the endometrium (innermost layer), the myometrium (muscular middle layer), and the perimetrium (outer serosal layer that covers the body of the uterus). The **endometrium** is the mucosal layer that lines the uterine cavity in nonpregnant women. It varies in thickness from 0.5 mm to 5 mm and has an abundant supply of glands and blood vessels (Cunningham et al., 2004). The myometrium makes up the major portion of the uterus and is composed of smooth muscle linked by connective tissue with numerous elastic fibers. During pregnancy, the upper myometrium undergoes marked hypertrophy, but there is limited change in the cervical muscle content.

Anatomic subdivisions of the uterus include the convex portion above the uterine tubes (the fundus); the central portion (the corpus or body) between the fundus and the cervix; and the cervix, or neck, which opens into the vagina.

Cervix

The **cervix,** the lower part of the uterus, opens into the vagina and has a channel that allows sperm to enter the uterus and menstrual discharge to exit. It is composed of fibrous connective tissue. During a pelvic examination, the part of the cervix that protrudes into the upper end of the vagina can be visualized. Like the vagina, this part of the cervix is covered by mucosa, which is smooth, firm, and doughnut-shaped, with a visible central opening called the external os (Fig. 3-2). Before childbirth, the external cervical os is a small, regular, oval opening. After childbirth, the opening is converted into a transverse slit that resembles lips (Fig. 3-3). Except during menstruation or ovulation, the cervix is usually a good barrier against bacteria.

The canal or channel of the cervix is lined with mucus-secreting glands. This mucus is thick and impenetrable to sperm until just before the ovaries release an egg

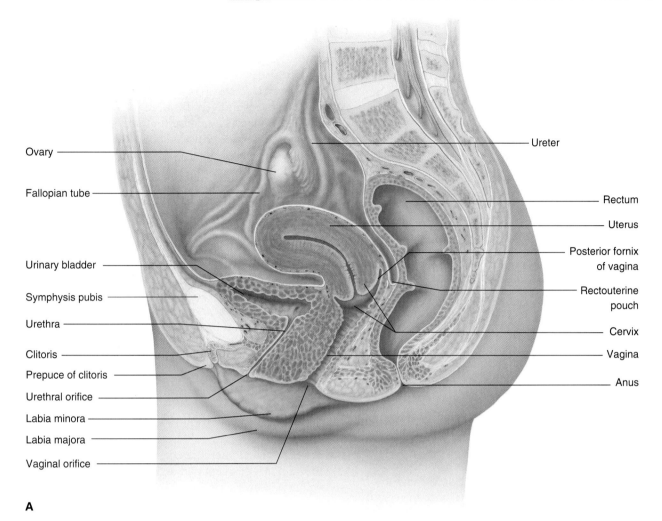

Ovary

Fallopian tube

Urinary bladder

Symphysis pubis

Urethra

Clitoris

Prepuce of clitoris

Urethral orifice

Labia minora

Labia majora

Vaginal orifice

Ureter

Rectum

Uterus

Posterior fornix of vagina

Rectouterine pouch

Cervix

Vagina

Anus

A

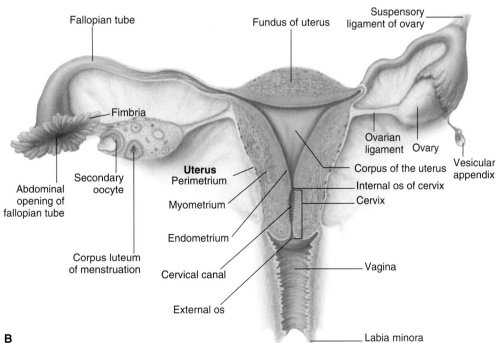

Fallopian tube

Fundus of uterus

Suspensory ligament of ovary

Fimbria

Abdominal opening of fallopian tube

Secondary oocyte

Corpus luteum of menstruation

Uterus
Perimetrium

Myometrium

Endometrium

Cervical canal

External os

Ovarian ligament   Ovary

Vesicular appendix

Corpus of the uterus

Internal os of cervix

Cervix

Vagina

Labia minora

B

● Figure 3-1 The internal female reproductive organs. (**A**) Lateral view. (**B**) Anterior view. (Source: The Anatomical Chart Company [2001]. *Atlas of human anatomy.* Springhouse, PA: Springhouse.)

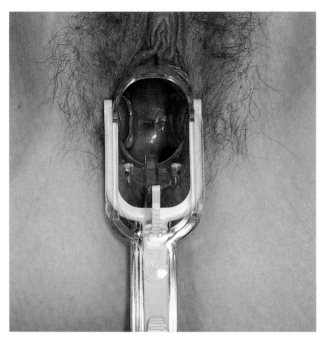

● Figure 3-2 Appearance of normal cervix. Note: This is the cervix of a multipara female. (Photo by B. Proud.)

(**ovulation**). At ovulation, the consistency of the mucus changes so that sperm can swim through it, allowing fertilization. At the same time, the mucus-secreting glands of the cervix actually become able to store live sperm for 2 or 3 days. These sperm can later move up through the corpus and into the fallopian tubes to fertilize the egg; thus, intercourse 1 or 2 days before ovulation can lead to pregnancy. Because some women do not ovulate consistently, pregnancy can occur at varying times after the last menstrual period. The channel in the cervix is narrow, too narrow for the fetus to pass through during pregnancy, but during labor it stretches to let the newborn through.

Corpus

The corpus, or the main body of the uterus, is a highly muscular organ that enlarges to hold the fetus during pregnancy. The inner lining of the corpus (endometrium) undergoes cyclic changes as a result of the changing lev-

els of hormones secreted by the ovaries: it is thickest during the part of the menstrual cycle in which a fertilized egg would be expected to enter the uterus and is thinnest just after menstruation. If fertilization does not take place during this cycle, most of the endometrium is shed and bleeding occurs, resulting in the monthly period. If fertilization does take place, the embryo attaches to the wall of the uterus, where it becomes embedded in the endometrium (about 1 week after fertilization); this process is called implantation (Condon, 2004). Menstruation then ceases during the 40 weeks (280 days) of pregnancy. During labor, the muscular walls of the corpus contract to push the baby through the cervix and into the vagina.

Fallopian Tubes

The **fallopian tubes** are hollow, cylindrical structures that extend 2 to 3 inches from the upper edges of the uterus toward the ovaries. Each tube is about 7 to 10 cm long (4 inches) and approximately 0.7 cm in diameter. The end of each tube flares into a funnel shape, providing a large opening for the egg to fall into when it is released from the ovary. Cilia (beating, hair-like extensions on cells) line the fallopian tube and the muscles in the tube's wall. The fallopian tubes convey the ovum from the ovary to the uterus and sperm from the uterus toward the ovary. This movement is accomplished via ciliary action and peristalsis. If sperm is present in the fallopian tube as a result of sexual intercourse or artificial insemination, fertilization of the ovum can occur. If the egg is fertilized, it will divide over a period of 4 days while it moves slowly down the fallopian tube and into the uterus.

Ovaries

The **ovaries** are a set of paired glands resembling unshelled almonds set in the pelvic cavity below and to either side of the umbilicus. They are usually pearl-colored and oblong. They are homologous to the testes. Each ovary weighs from 2 to 5 grams and is about 4 cm long, 2 cm wide, and 1 cm thick (Speroff & Fritz, 2005). Several ligaments help hold each ovary in position. The ovaries link the reproductive system to the body's system of endocrine glands, as they produce the ova (eggs) and secrete, in cyclic fashion, the female sex hormones **estrogen** and **progesterone.** After an ovum matures, it passes into the fallopian tubes. The ovaries are not attached to the fallopian tubes but are suspended nearby from a ligament.

External Female Reproductive Organs

The external female reproductive organs collectively are called the **vulva** (which means "covering" in Latin). The vulva serves to protect the urethral and vaginal openings and is highly sensitive to touch to increase the female's pleasure during sexual arousal (Sloane, 2002). The structures that make up the vulva include the mons pubis, the labia majora and minora, the clitoris, the structures within the vestibule, and the perineum (Fig. 3-4).

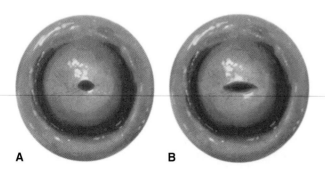

A   **B**

● Figure 3-3 (**A**) Nulliparous cervical os. (**B**) Parous cervical os.

Mons pubis

Symphysis pubis

Clitoris
Prepuce
Body
Urethral orifice
Glans

Hymen
Labia majora
Vaginal orifice
Labia minora
Perineal
membrane

Anus

External anal
sphincter

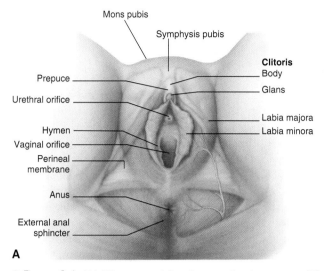

A

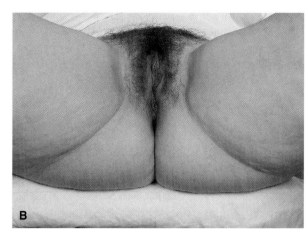

B

● Figure 3-4 (**A**) The external female reproductive organs. (**B**) Normal appearance of external structures. (Photo by B. Proud.)

Mons Pubis

The mons pubis is the elevated, rounded fleshy prominence over the symphysis pubis. This fatty tissue and skin is covered with pubic hair after puberty. It protects the symphysis pubis during sexual intercourse.

Labia

The labia majora (large lips), which are relatively large and fleshy, are comparable to the scrotum in males. The labia majora contain sweat and sebaceous (oil-secreting) glands; after puberty, they are covered with hair. Its function is to protect the vaginal opening. The labia minora (small lips) are the delicate hairless inner folds of skin that can be very small or up to 2 inches wide. They lie just inside the labia majora and surround the openings to the vagina and urethra. The labia minora grow down from the anterior inner part of the labia majora on each side. They are highly vascular and abundant in nerve supply. They lubricate the vulva, swell in response to stimulation, and are highly sensitive.

Clitoris and Prepuce

The clitoris is a small, cylindrical mass of erectile tissue and nerves. It is located at the anterior junction of the labia minora. There are folds above and below the clitoris. The joining of the folds above the clitoris forms the prepuce, a hood-like covering over the clitoris; the junction below the clitoris forms the frenulum. A rich supply of blood vessels gives it a pink color. The clitoris, like the penis, is very sensitive to touch, stimulation, and temperature and can become erect. The word "clitoris" is from the Greek word for key, which in ancient times was thought to be the key to a woman's sexuality. For its small size, it has a generous blood and nerve supply. There are more free nerve endings of sensory reception located on the clitoris than on any other part of the body, and it is, unsurprisingly, the most

erotically sensitive part of the genitalia for most females. Its function is sexual stimulation (Mattson & Smith, 2004).

Vestibule

The vestibule is an oval area enclosed by the labia minora laterally. It extends from the clitoris to the fourchette and is perforated by six openings. Opening into the vestibule are the urethra from the urinary bladder, the vagina, and two sets of glands. The opening to the vagina is called the introitus, and the half-moon-shaped area behind the opening is called the fourchette. Through tiny ducts beside the introitus, Bartholin's glands, when stimulated, secrete mucus that supplies lubrication for intercourse. Skene's glands are located on either side of the opening to the urethra. They secrete a small amount of mucus to keep the opening moist and lubricated for the passage of urine (Olds et al., 2004).

The vaginal opening is surrounded by the hymen (maidenhead). The hymen is a tough, elastic, perforated, mucosa-covered tissue across the vaginal introitus. In a virgin, the hymen may completely cover the opening, but it usually encircles the opening like a tight ring. Because the degree of tightness varies among women, the hymen may tear at the first attempt at intercourse, or it may be so soft and pliable that no tearing occurs. In a woman who is not a virgin, the hymen usually appears as small tags of tissue surrounding the vaginal opening, but the presence or absence of the hymen can neither confirm nor rule out sexual experience (Mattson & Smith, 2004).

Perineum

The perineum is the most posterior part of the external female reproductive organs. This external region is located between the vulva and the anus. It is made up of skin, muscle, and fascia. The perineum can become lacerated or incised during childbirth and needs to be repaired with sutures. Incising the perineum area to provide more space for the presenting part is called an episiotomy. Although still a common obstetric procedure, the use of episiotomy has decreased over the past 25 years. The procedure should be applied selectively rather than routinely. An episiotomy can add to postpartum discomfort, perineal trauma, and potential fecal incontinence (Cunningham et al., 2004).

Erection, Lubrication, and Orgasm

With sexual stimulation, tissues in the clitoris, in the breasts, and around the vaginal orifice fill with blood and the erectile tissues swell. At the same time, the vagina begins to expand and elongate to accommodate the penis. As part of the whole vasocongestive reaction, the labia majora and minor swell and darken in color. As sexual stimulation intensifies, the vestibular glands secrete mucus to moisten and lubricate the tissues to facilitate insertion of the penis.

The zenith of intense stimulation is orgasm, the spasmodic and involuntary contractions of the muscles in the region of the vulva, the uterus, and the vagina that produce a pleasurable sensation to the woman. Typically the woman feels warm and relaxed after an orgasm. Within a short time after orgasm, the two physiologic mechanisms that created the sexual response, vasocongestion and muscle contraction, rapidly dissipate.

Breasts

The two mammary glands, or **breasts,** are accessory organs of the female reproductive system that are specialized to secrete milk following pregnancy. They overlie the pectoralis major muscles and extend from the second to the sixth ribs and from the sternum to the axilla. Each breast has a nipple located near the tip, which is surrounded by a circular area of pigmented skin called the areola. Each breast is composed of 15 to 20 lobes, which contain glands (alveolar) and a duct (lactiferous) that leads to the nipple and opens to the outside (Fig. 3-5). The lobes are separated by dense connective and adipose tissues, which also help support the weight of the breasts.

During pregnancy, placental estrogen and progesterone stimulate the development of the mammary glands. Because of this hormonal activity, the breasts may double in size during pregnancy. At the same time, glandular tissue replaces the adipose tissue of the breasts.

Following childbirth and the expulsion of the placenta, levels of placental hormones (progesterone and lactogen) fall rapidly, and the action of prolactin (milk-producing hormone) is no longer inhibited. Prolactin stimulates the production of milk within a few days after childbirth, but in the interim, a deep yellow fluid called colostrum is secreted. Colostrum contains more minerals and protein but less sugar and fat than mature breast milk. Colostrum secretion may continue for approximately a week after childbirth, with gradual conversion to mature milk. Colostrum is rich in maternal antibodies, especially immunoglobulin A (IgA), which offers protection for the newborn against enteric pathogens.

The Female Reproductive Cycle

The female reproductive cycle is a complex process that encompasses an intricate series of chemical secretions and reactions to produce the ultimate potential for fertility and birth. The female reproductive cycle is a general term encompassing the ovarian cycle, the endometrial cycle, the hormonal changes that regulate them, and the cyclical changes in the breasts. The endometrium, ovaries, pituitary gland, and hypothalamus are all involved in the cyclic changes that help to prepare the body for fertilization. Absence of fertilization results in **menstruation,** the monthly shedding of the uterine lining. Menstruation marks the beginning and end of each menstrual cycle.

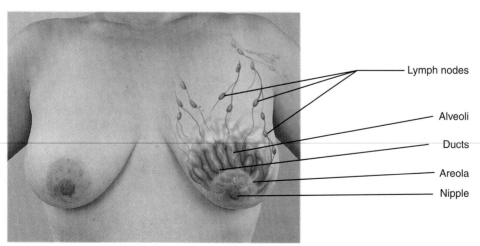

Lymph nodes

Alveoli

Ducts

Areola

Nipple

● Figure 3-5 Anatomy of the breasts. (Photo by B. Proud.)

In the United States, the average age at menarche is 12.8 years, with a range between 8 and 18. Most women will experience 300 to 400 menstrual cycles within their lifetime (Youngkin & Davis, 2004). Events preceding the first menses have an orderly progression: *thelarche,* the development of breast buds; *adrenarche,* the appearance of pubic and then axillary hair, followed by a growth spurt; and *menarche,* a girl's first menses. Cycles vary in frequency from 21 to 36 days, bleeding lasts 3 to 8 days, and blood loss averages 20 to 80 mL (Mattson & Smith, 2004). The average cycle is 28 days long. Irregular menses can be associated with irregular ovulation, stress, disease, and hormonal imbalances (Cunningham et al., 2004).

Menopause refers to the cessation of regular menstrual cycles. It is the end of menstruation and childbearing capacity. It is usually marked by atrophy of the breasts, uterus, tubes, and ovaries (Bachmann, 2004). Many women pass through menopause without untoward symptoms. These women remain active and in good health with little interruption of their daily routines. Other women experience vasomotor symptoms, which give rise to sensations of heat, cold, sweating, headache, insomnia, and irritability (Kessenich, 2004). The average age of natural menopause—defined as 1 year without a menstrual period—is 51 (Alexander et al., 2004). (See Chapter 4 for more information.)

Although menstruation is a normal process, the various world cultures have taken a wide variety of attitudes toward it, seeing it as everything from a sacred time to an unclean time. In a society where menstruation is viewed negatively, nurses can help women develop a more positive image of this natural physiologic process.

The female reproductive cycle involves two cycles that occur simultaneously: the ovarian cycle, during which ovulation occurs, and the endometrial cycle, during which menstruation occurs. Ovulation divides these two cycles at midcycle. Ovulation occurs when the ovum is released from its follicle; after leaving the ovary, the ovum enters the fallopian tube and journeys toward the uterus. If sperm fertilizes the ovum during its journey, pregnancy occurs. Figure 3-6 summarizes the menstrual cycle.

Ovarian Cycle

The ovarian cycle is the series of events associated with a developing oocyte (ovum or egg) within the ovaries. While men manufacture sperm daily, often into advanced age, women are born with a single lifetime supply of ova that are released from the ovaries gradually throughout the childbearing years. In the female ovary, 2 million oocytes are present at birth, and about 400,000 follicles are still present at puberty. The excess follicles are depleted during the childbearing years, with only 400 follicles ovulated during the reproductive period (Speroff & Fritz, 2005).

The ovarian cycle begins when the follicular cells (ovum and surrounding cells) swell and the maturation process starts. The maturing follicle at this stage is called a graafian follicle. The ovary raises many follicles monthly, but usually only one follicle matures to reach ovulation. The ovarian cycle consists of three phases: the follicular phase, ovulation, and the luteal phase.

Follicular Phase

This phase is so named because it is when the follicles in the ovary grow and form a mature egg. This phase starts on day 1 of the menstrual cycle and continues until ovulation, approximately 10 to 14 days. The follicular phase is not consistent in duration because of the time variations in follicular development. These variations account for the differences in menstrual cycle lengths (Breslin and Lucas, 2003). The hypothalamus is the initiator of this phase. Increasing levels of estrogen secreted from the maturing follicular cells and the continued growth of the dominant follicle cell induce proliferation of the endometrium and myometrium. This thickening of the uterine lining supports an implanted ovum if pregnancy occurs.

Prompted by the hypothalamus, the pituitary gland releases **follicle-stimulating hormone (FSH),** which stimulates the ovary to produce 5 to 20 immature follicles. Each follicle houses an immature oocyte or egg. The follicle that is targeted to mature fully will soon rupture and expel a mature oocyte in the process of ovulation. A surge in **luteinizing hormone (LH)** from the anterior pituitary gland is actually responsible for affecting the final development and subsequent rupture of the mature follicle.

Ovulation

At ovulation, a mature follicle ruptures in response to a surge of LH, releasing a mature oocyte (ovum). This usually occurs on day 14 in a 28-day cycle. When ovulation occurs, there is a drop in estrogen. Typically ovulation takes place approximately 10 to 12 hours after the LH peak and 24 to 36 hours after estrogen levels peak (Speroff and Fritz, 2005). The distal ends of the fallopian tubes become active near the time of ovulation and create currents that help carry the ovum into the uterus. The lifespan of the ovum is only about 24 hours; unless it meets a sperm on its journey within that time, it will die.

During ovulation, the cervix produces thin, clear, stretchy, slippery mucus that is designed to help the sperm travel up through the cervix to meet the ovum for fertilization. Some women can feel a pain on one side of the abdomen around the time the egg is released. This is known as *mittelschmerz,* a German word meaning "middle pain." The one constant, whether a women's cycle is 28 days or 120 days, is that ovulation takes place 14 days before menstruation (Mattson & Smith, 2004).

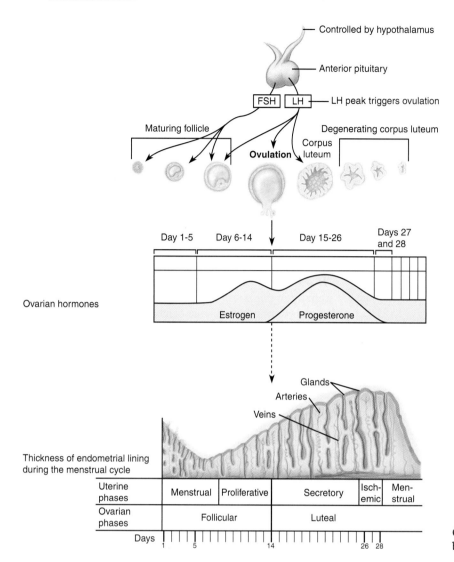

Figure 3-6 Menstrual cycle summary based on a 28-day (average) menstrual cycle.

I had been married 2 years when my husband and I decided to start a family. I began thinking back to my high-school biology class and tried to remember about ovulation and what to look for. I also used the Internet to find the answers I was seeking. As I was reading, it all started to come into place. During ovulation, a woman's cervical mucus increases and she experiences a 'wet sensation' for several days midcycle. The mucus also becomes stretchable during this time. In addition, her temperature rises slightly and then falls if no conception takes place. Armed with this knowledge, I began to check my temperature daily before arising and checking the consistency of my mucus. I figured that if these signs could help prevent pregnancy by warning of the unsafe time, they could help me discover the best time to conceive. Within 3 months I became pregnant using my body's natural signals.

Thoughts: How does knowledge of the reproductive system help nurses take care of couples who are trying to become pregnant?

Luteal Phase

The luteal phase begins at ovulation and lasts until the menstrual phase of the next cycle. After the follicle ruptures as it releases the egg, it closes and forms a corpus luteum. The corpus luteum secretes increasing amounts of the hormone progesterone, which interacts with the endometrium to prepare it for implantation. At the beginning of the luteal phase, progesterone induces the endometrial glands to secrete glycogen, mucus, and other substances. These glands become tortuous and have large lumens due to increased secretory activity. The progesterone secreted by the corpus luteum causes the temperature of the body to rise slightly until the start of the next period. A significant increase in temperature, usually 0.5 to 1 degrees Fahrenheit, is generally seen within a day or two after ovulation has occurred; the temperature remains elevated for 12 to 16 days, until menstruation begins (Youngkin & Davis, 2004). This rise in temperature can be plotted on a graph and gives an indication of when ovulation has occurred. In the absence of fertilization, the corpus luteum begins to degenerate, and consequently ovarian hormone levels decrease. As estrogen and progesterone levels decrease, the endometrium undergoes involution. In a 28-day cycle, menstruation then begins approximately 14 days after ovulation in the absence of pregnancy. FSH and LH are generally at their lowest levels during the luteal phase and highest during the follicular phase.

Endometrial Cycle

The endometrial cycle occurs in response to cyclic hormonal changes. The three phases of the endometrial cycle are the proliferative phase, the secretory phase, and the menstrual phase.

Proliferative Phase

The proliferative phase starts with enlargement of the endometrial glands in response to increasing amounts of estrogen. The blood vessels become dilated and the endometrium increases in thickness dramatically. It lasts from about day 5 of the menstrual cycle to the time of ovulation. This phase depends on estrogen stimulation resulting from ovarian follicles.

Secretory Phase

The secretory phase follows ovulation to about 3 days before the next menstrual period. Under the influence of progesterone, the endometrium becomes thickened and more vascular (growth of the spiral arteries) and glandular (secreting more glycogen and lipids). These dramatic changes are all in preparation for implantation, if it were to occur. Estrogen levels drop sharply during this phase as progesterone dominates.

Menstrual Phase

The menstrual phase begins as the spiral arteries rupture secondary to ischemia, releasing blood into the uterus, and the endometrium is sloughed off. If fertilization does not take place, the corpus luteum degenerates. As a result, both estrogen and progesterone levels fall and the thickened endometrial lining sloughs away from the uterine wall and passes out via the vagina. The beginning of the menstrual flow marks the end of one menstrual cycle and the start of a new one. Most women report bleeding for an average of 3 to 5 days (Mattson & Smith, 2004).

Menstrual Cycle Hormones

The menstrual cycle involves a complex interaction of hormones. The predominant hormones include gonadotropin-releasing hormone (GnRH), FSH, LH, estrogen, progesterone, and prostaglandins. Box 3-1 summarizes menstrual cycle hormones.

Gonadotropin-Releasing Hormone (GnRH)

Gonadotropin-releasing hormone (GnRH) is secreted from the hypothalamus in a pulsatile manner throughout

---

BOX 3-1

SUMMARY OF MENSTRUAL CYCLE HORMONES

- Luteinizing hormone (LH) rises and stimulates the follicle to produce estrogen.
- As estrogen is produced by the follicle, estrogen levels rise, inhibiting the output of LH.
- Ovulation occurs after an LH surge damages the estrogen-producing cells, resulting in a decline in estrogen.
- The LH surge results in establishment of the corpus luteum, which produces estrogen and progesterone.
- Estrogen and progesterone levels rise, suppressing LH output.
- Lack of LH promotes degeneration of the corpus luteum.
- Cessation of the corpus luteum means a decline in estrogen and progesterone output.
- The decline of the ovarian hormones ends their negative effect on the secretion of LH.
- LH is secreted, and the menstrual cycle begins again.

---

the reproductive cycle. It pulsates slowly during the follicular phase and increases during the luteal phase. GnRH induces the release of FSH and LH to assist with ovulation.

Follicle-Stimulating Hormone (FSH)

FSH is secreted by the anterior pituitary gland and is primarily responsible for the maturation of the ovarian follicle. FSH secretion is highest and most critical during the first week of the follicular phase of the reproductive cycle.

Luteinizing Hormone (LH)

LH is secreted by the anterior pituitary gland and is required for both the final maturation of preovulatory follicles and luteinization of the ruptured follicle. As a result, estrogen production declines and progesterone secretion continues. Thus, estrogen levels fall a day before ovulation, and progesterone levels begin to rise.

Estrogen

Estrogen is secreted by the ovaries and is crucial for the development and maturation of the follicle. Estrogen is predominant at the end of the follicular phase, directly preceding ovulation. After ovulation, estrogen levels drop sharply as progesterone dominates. In the endometrial cycle, estrogen induces proliferation of the endometrial glands. Estrogen also causes the uterus to increase in size and weight because of increased glycogen, amino acids, electrolytes, and water. Blood supply is expanded as well. Estrogen inhibits FSH production and stimulates LH production.

Progesterone

Progesterone is secreted by the corpus luteum. Progesterone levels increase just before ovulation and peak 5 to

7 days after ovulation. During the luteal phase, progesterone induces swelling and increased secretion of the endometrium. This hormone is often called the hormone of pregnancy because of its calming effect (reduces uterine contractions) on the uterus, allowing pregnancy to be maintained.

Prostaglandins

Prostaglandins are a closely related group of oxygenated fatty acids that are produced by the endometrium, with a variety of effects throughout the body. Although they have regulatory effects and are sometimes called hormones, prostaglandins are not technically hormones because they are produced by all tissues rather than by special glands (Sloane, 2002). Prostaglandins increase during follicular maturation and play a key role in ovulation by freeing the ovum inside the graafian follicle. Large amounts of prostaglandins are found in menstrual blood. Research is ongoing as to the various roles prostaglandins have on the menstrual cycle (Cunningham et al., 2004).

Male Reproductive System

The male reproductive system, like that of the female, consists of those organs functioning to produce a new individual. The male organs are specialized to produce and maintain the male sex cells, or sperm; to transport them, along with supporting fluids, to the female reproductive system; and to secrete the male hormone testosterone. The organs of the male reproductive system include the two testes (where sperm cells and testosterone are made), the penis, the scrotum, and the accessory organs (epididymis, vas deferens, seminal vesicles, ejaculatory duct, urethra, bulbourethral glands, and prostate gland).

Internal Male Reproductive Organs

The internal structures include the testes, the ductal system, and accessory glands (Fig. 3-7).

Testes

The **testes** are oval bodies the size of large olives that lie in the scrotum; usually the left testis hangs a little lower than the right one. The testes have two functions: producing sperm and synthesizing testosterone (the primary male sex hormone). Sperm is produced in the seminiferous tubules of the testes. The testes also produce the male hormone testosterone and a portion of the seminal fluid, the liquid in which sperm are carried. The epididymis, which lies against the testes, is a coiled tube almost 20 feet long. It collects sperm from the testes and provides the space and environment for sperm to mature (Fig. 3-8).

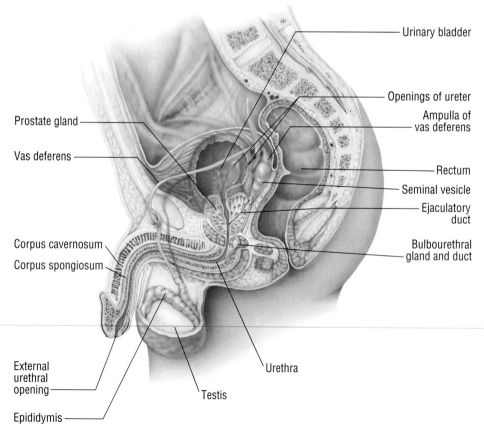

● Figure 3-7 Lateral view of the internal male reproductive organs. (Source: The Anatomical Chart Company. [2001]. *Atlas of human anatomy*. Springhouse, PA: Springhouse.)

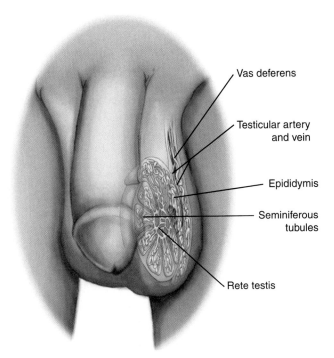

● Figure 3-8 Internal structures of a testis.

Labels on figure: Vas deferens, Testicular artery and vein, Epididymis, Seminiferous tubules, Rete testis

The Ductal System

The vas deferens is a cordlike duct that transports sperm from the epididymis. One such duct travels from each testis up to the back of the prostate and enters the urethra to form the ejaculatory ducts. Other structures, such as blood vessels and nerves, also travel along with each vas deferens and together form the spermatic cord. The urethra is the terminal duct of the reproductive and urinary systems, serving as a passageway for semen (fluid containing sperm) and urine. It passes through the prostate gland and the penis and opens to the outside.

Accessory Glands

The seminal vesicles, which produce nutrient seminal fluid, and the prostate gland, which produces alkaline prostatic fluid, are both connected to the ejaculatory duct leading into the urethra. The paired seminal vesicles are convoluted pouchlike structures lying posterior to and at the base of the urinary bladder in front of the rectum. They secrete an alkaline fluid that contains fructose and prostaglandins. The fructose supplies energy to the sperm on its journey to meet the ovum, and the prostaglandins assist in sperm mobility.

The prostate gland lies just under the bladder in the pelvis and surrounds the middle portion of the urethra. Usually the size of a walnut, this gland enlarges with age. The prostate and the seminal vesicles above it produce fluid that nourishes the sperm. This fluid provides most of the volume of semen, the secretion in which the sperm is expelled during ejaculation. Other fluid that makes up

the semen comes from the vas deferens and from mucous glands in the head of the penis.

The bulbourethral glands (Cowper's glands) are two small structures about the size of peas, located inferior to the prostate gland. They are composed of several tubes whose epithelial linings secrete a mucuslike fluid. It is released in response to sexual stimulation and lubricates the head of the penis in preparation for sexual intercourse. Their existence is said to be constant, but they gradually diminish in size with advancing age.

External Male Reproductive Organs

The penis and the scrotum form the external genitalia in the male (Fig. 3-9).

Penis

The **penis** is the organ for copulation and serves as the outlet for both sperm and urine. The skin of the penis is thin, with no hairs. The prepuce (foreskin) is a circular fold of skin that extends over the glans unless it is removed by circumcision shortly after birth. The urinary meatus, located at the tip of the penis, serves as the external opening to the urethra (Fig. 3-10). The penis is composed mostly of erectile tissue. Most of the body of the penis consists of three cylindrical spaces (sinuses) of erectile tissue. The two larger ones, the corpora cavernosa, are side by side. The third sinus, the corpus spongiosum, surrounds the urethra. Erection results when nerve impulses from the autonomic nervous system dilate the arteries of the penis, allowing arterial blood to flow into the erectile tissues of the organ.

Scrotum

The scrotum is the thin-skinned sac that surrounds and protects the testes. The scrotum also acts as a climate-control system for the testes, because they need to be slightly cooler than body temperature to allow normal

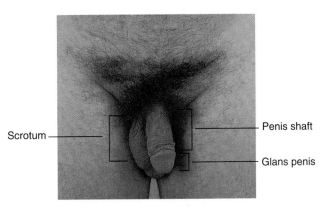

Labels on figure: Scrotum, Penis shaft, Glans penis

● Figure 3-9 The external male reproductive organs. (Photo by B. Proud.)

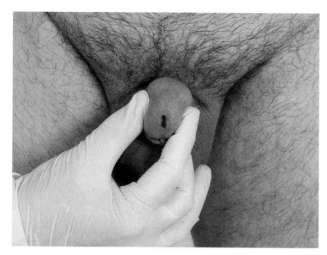

● Figure 3-10 The urinary meatus. (Photo by B. Proud.)

sperm development. The cremaster muscles in the scrotal wall relax or contract to allow the testes to hang farther from the body to cool or to be pulled closer to the body for warmth or protection (Sloane, 2002). A medial septum divides the scrotum into two chambers, each of which encloses a testis.

Erection, Orgasm, and Ejaculation

With sexual stimulation, the arteries leading to the penis dilate and increase blood flow into erectile tissues. At the same time, the erectile tissue compresses the veins of the penis, reducing blood flow away from the penis. Blood accumulates, causing the penis to swell and elongate and producing an erection. As in women, the culmination of sexual stimulation is an orgasm, a pleasurable feeling of physiologic and psychological release.

Orgasm is accompanied by emission (movement of sperm from the testes and fluids from the accessory glands) into the urethra, where it is mixed to form semen. As the urethra fills with semen, the base of the erect penis contracts, which increases pressure and forces the semen through the urethra to the outside (ejaculation). During ejaculation, the ducts of the testes, epididymis, and vas deferens contract, causing expulsion of sperm into the urethra, where the sperm mixes with the seminal and prostatic fluids. These substances, together with mucus secreted by accessory glands, form the semen, which is discharged from the urethra.

KEY CONCEPTS

● The female reproductive system produces the female reproductive cells (the eggs, or ova) and contains an organ (uterus) where the fetus develops. The male reproductive system produces the male reproductive

cells (the sperm) and contains an organ (penis) that deposits the sperm within the female.

● The internal female reproductive organs consist of the vagina, the uterus, the fallopian tubes, and the ovaries. The external female reproductive organs make up the vulva. These include the mons pubis, the labia majora and minora, the clitoris, structures within the vestibule, and the perineum.

● The breasts are accessory organs of the female reproductive system that are specialized to secrete milk following pregnancy.

● The main function of the reproductive cycle is to stimulate growth of a follicle to release an egg and prepare a site for implantation if fertilization occurs.

● Menstruation, the monthly shedding of the uterine lining, marks the beginning and end of the cycle if fertilization does not occur.

● The ovarian cycle is the series of events associated with a developing oocyte (ovum or egg) within the ovaries.

● At ovulation, a mature follicle ruptures in response to a surge of LH, releasing a mature oocyte (ovum).

● The endometrial cycle is divided into three phases: the follicular or proliferative phase, the luteal or secretory phase, and the menstrual phase.

● The menstrual cycle involves a complex interaction of hormones. The predominant hormones are gonadotropin-releasing hormone (GnRH), follicle-stimulating hormone (FSH), luteinizing hormone (LH), estrogen, progesterone, and prostaglandins.

● The organs of the male reproductive system include the two testes (where sperm cells and testosterone are made), penis, scrotum, and accessory organs (epididymis, vas deferens, seminal vesicles, ejaculatory ducts, urethra, bulbourethral glands, and prostate gland).

References

Alexander, L. L., LaRosa, J. H., Bader, H., & Garfield, S. (2004). *New dimensions in women's health* (3rd ed.). Boston: Jones and Bartlett.

Bachmann, G. (2004), Menopause. *eMedicine*. [Online] Available: http://www.emedicine.com/med/topic3289.htm.

Breslin, E. T., & Lucas, V. A. (2003). *Women's health nursing: toward evidence-based practice*. St. Louis, MO: Saunders.

Condon, M. C. (2004). *Women's health: an integrated approach to wellness and illness*. Upper Saddle River, NJ: Prentice Hall.

Cunningham, F. G., Leveno, K. J., Bloom, S. L., et al. (2004). *Williams obstetrics* (22nd ed.). New York: McGraw-Hill.

Kessenich, C. R. (2004). Inevitable menopause. *Nursing Spectrum*. [Online] Available: http://nsweb.nursingspectrum.com/ce/ce232.htm.

Mattson, S., & Smith, J. E. (2004). *Core curriculum for maternal-newborn nursing* (3rd ed.). St. Louis, MO: Elsevier Saunders.

Olds, S. B., London, M. L., Ladewig, P. W., & Davidson, M. R. (2004). *Maternal-newborn nursing and women's health* (7th ed.). Upper Saddle River, NJ: Pearson Prentice Hall.

Sloane, E. (2002). *Biology of women* (4th ed.). New York: Delmar.

Speroff, L., & Fritz, M. A. (2005). *Clinical gynecologic endocrinology and infertility* (7th ed.). Philadelphia: Lippincott Williams & Wilkins.

Venes, D. (2005) *Taber's cyclopedia medical dictionary* (20th ed.). Philadelphia: F. A. Davis.

Writing Group for the Women's Health Initiative Investigators. (2002). Risks and benefits of estrogen plus progestin in healthy postmenopausal women: principal results from the Women's Health Initiative randomized controlled trial. *JAMA, 288*(3), 321–333.

Youngkin, E. Q., & Davis, M. S. (2004) *Women's health: A primary care clinical guide* (3rd ed.). Upper Saddle River, NJ: Prentice Hall.

Web Resources

Alan Guttmacher Institute: **www.agi-usa.org**
American Society for Reproductive Medicine: **www.asrm.com**
Kinsey Institution: **www.indiana.edu/~kinsey/index.html**
Sexuality Information of the United States: **www.siecus.org**
National Women's Health Information Center: **www.4woman.gov**
National Women's Health Resource Center: **www.healthywomen.org**
Society for Women's Health Research: **www.womens-health.org**

ChapterWORKSHEET

● MULTIPLE CHOICE QUESTIONS

1. The predominant anterior pituitary hormones that orchestrate the menstrual cycle include:

   a. Thyroid-stimulating hormone (TSH)

   b. Follicle-stimulating hormone (FSH)

   c. Corticotropin-releasing hormone (CRH)

   d. Gonadotropin-releasing hormone (GnRH)

2. Which glands are located on either side of the female urethra and secrete mucus to keep the opening moist and lubricated for urination?

   a. Cowper's

   b. Bartholin's

   c. Skene's

   d. Seminal

3. The ovarian cycle comprises all of the following phases *except:*

   a. Secretory

   b. Follicular

   c. Ovulation

   d. Luteal

4. Which hormone is produced in high levels to prepare the endometrium for implantation just after ovulation by the corpus luteum?

   a. Estrogen

   b. Prostaglandins

   c. Prolactin

   d. Progesterone

5. Sperm maturation and storage in the male reproductive system occurs in the:

   a. Testes

   b. Vas deferens

   c. Epididymis

   d. Seminal vesicles

● CRITICAL THINKING EXERCISE

1. The school health nurse was asked to speak to the 10th-grade biology class in the local high school about menstruation. The teachers felt that the students misunderstood this monthly event and wanted to dispel some myths about it. After explaining the factors influencing the monthly menses, one girl asks, "Could someone get pregnant if she had sex during her period?"

   a. How should the nurse respond to this question?

   b. What factor regarding the menstrual cycle was not clarified?

   c. What additional topics might this question lead into that might be discussed?

● STUDY ACTIVITIES

1. Select a website under *Web Resources* to explore to find information concerning a topic of interest regarding women's health. Be prepared to discuss it in class.

2. List the predominant hormones and their function in the menstrual cycle.

3. The ovarian cycle describes the series of events associated with the development of the _____ within the ovaries.

4. Sperm cells and the male hormone testosterone are made in which of the following structures? Select all that apply:

   a. Vas deferens

   b. Penis

   c. Scrotum

   d. Ejaculatory ducts

   e. Prostate gland

   f. Testes

   g. Seminiferous tubules

   h. Bulbourethral glands

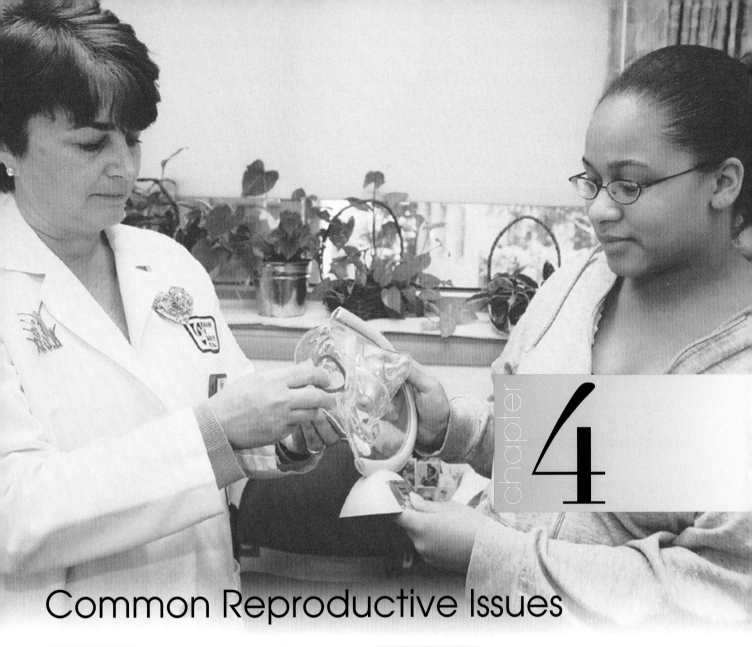

Common Reproductive Issues

chapter 4

KeyTERMS

abortion
abstinence
amenorrhea
basal body temperature
   (BBT)
cervical cap
cervical mucus ovulation
   method
coitus interruptus
condoms
contraception
contraceptive sponge
Depo-Provera
diaphragm
dysmenorrhea
dysfunctional uterine
   bleeding (DUB)
emergency contraception
   (EC)

endometriosis
fertility awareness
infertility
lactational amenorrhea
   method (LAM)
Lunelle injection
menopause
Norplant
oral contraceptives
premenstrual syndrome
   (PMS)
Standard Days Method
   (SDM)
sterilization
symptothermal method
transdermal patch
tubal ligation
vaginal ring
vasectomy

LearningOBJECTIVES

*After studying the chapter content, the student
should be able to accomplish the following:*

1. Define the key terms.
2. Describe common reproductive concerns in terms of
   symptoms, diagnostic tests, and appropriate
   interventions.
3. Identify risk factors and outline appropriate client
   education needed in common reproductive
   disorders.
4. Compare and contrast the various contraceptive
   methods available and their overall effectiveness.
5. Discuss the physiologic and psychological aspects of
   menopause.
6. Delineate the nursing management needed for
   women experiencing common reproductive
   disorders.

Good health throughout the life cycle begins with the individual. Women today can expect to live well into their 80s and need to be proactive in maintaining their own quality of life. Women need to take steps to reduce their risk of disease and need to become active partners with their healthcare professional to identify problems early, when treatment may be most successful (Teaching Guidelines 4-1). Nurses can assist women to maintain their quality of life by helping them to become more attuned to their body and its clues and can use the assessment period as an opportunity for teaching and counseling.

Common reproductive issues addressed in this chapter that nurses might encounter in caring for women include menstrual disorders, infertility, contraception, abortion, and menopause.

Menstrual Disorders

Many women sail through their monthly menstrual cycles with little or no concern. With few symptoms to worry about, their menses are like clockwork, starting and stopping at nearly the same time every month. For others, the menstrual cycle causes physical and emotional symptoms that initiate visits to their healthcare provider for consultation. The following menstruation-related conditions will be discussed in this chapter: amenorrhea, dysmenorrhea, dysfunctional uterine bleeding (DUB), premenstrual syndrome (PMS), premenstrual dysphoric disorder (PMDD), and endometriosis.

 TEACHING GUIDELINES 4-1

Tips for Being an Active Partner in Managing Your Health

- Become an informed consumer. Read, ask, and search.
- Know your family history and know factors that put you at high risk.
- Maintain a healthy lifestyle and let moderation be your guide.
- Schedule regular medical checkups and screenings for early detection.
- Ask your healthcare professional for a full explanation of any treatment.
- Seek a second medical opinion if you feel you need more information.
- Know when to seek medical care by being aware of disease symptoms.

To gain an understanding of menstrual disorders, it is important to know the terms used in describing them (Box 4-1).

Amenorrhea

Amenorrhea is the absence of menses during the reproductive years. Amenorrhea is a normal feature in prepubertal, pregnant, and postmenopausal females. The two categories of amenorrhea are *primary* and *secondary* amenorrhea. Primary amenorrhea is defined as either (1) absence of menses by age 14, with absence of growth and development of secondary sexual characteristics, or (2) absence of menses by age 16, with normal development of secondary sexual characteristics (Bielak, 2002). Ninety-eight percent of American girls menstruate by age 16 (Minjarez & Carr, 2002). Secondary amenorrhea is the absence of menses for three cycles or 6 months in women who have previously menstruated regularly.

Etiology

There are multiple causes of primary amenorrhea:

- Extreme weight gain or loss
- Congenital abnormalities of the reproductive system
- Stress from a major life event
- Excessive exercise
- Eating disorders (anorexia nervosa or bulimia)
- Cushing's disease
- Polycystic ovarian syndrome
- Hypothyroidism
- Turner syndrome
- Imperforate hymen
- Chronic illness
- Pregnancy
- Cystic fibrosis
- Congenital heart disease (cyanotic)
- Ovarian or adrenal tumors (Thompson, 2004)

BOX 4-1

MENSTRUAL DISORDER VOCABULARY

- Meno = menstrual-related
- Metro = time
- Oligo = few
- A = without, none or lack of
- Rhagia = excess or abnormal
- Dys = not or pain
- Rhea = flow

Causes of secondary amenorrhea might include:

- Pregnancy
- Breastfeeding
- Emotional stress
- Pituitary, ovarian, or adrenal tumors
- Depression
- Hyperthyroid or hypothyroid
- Malnutrition
- Hyperprolactinemia
- Rapid weight gain or loss
- Chemotherapy or radiation therapy to the pelvic area
- Vigorous exercise, such as long-distance running
- Kidney failure
- Colitis
- Use of tranquilizers or antidepressants
- Postpartum pituitary necrosis (Sheehan syndrome)
- Early menopause (Nelson & Bakalov, 2004)

Assessment

A thorough history and physical examination is needed to determine the etiology. The history should include questions about the women's menstrual history; past illnesses; hospitalizations and surgeries; obstetric history; use of prescription and over-the-counter drugs; recent or past lifestyle changes; and history of present illness, with an assessment of any bodily changes.

The physical examination should begin with an overall assessment of the woman's nutritional status and general health. Height and weight should be taken, along with vital signs. Hypothermia, bradycardia, hypotension, and reduced subcutaneous fat may be observed in women with anorexia nervosa. Facial hair and acne might be evidence of androgen excess secondary to a tumor. The presence or absence of axillary and pubic hair may indicate adrenal and ovarian hyposecretion or delayed puberty. A general physical examination may uncover unexpected findings that are indirectly related to amenorrhea. For example, hepatosplenomegaly, which may suggest a chronic systemic disease or an enlarged thyroid gland, might point to a thyroid disorder as well as a reason for amenorrhea (Nelson & Bakalov, 2004).

Common laboratory tests that might be ordered to determine the cause of amenorrhea include:

- Karyotype (might be positive for Turner syndrome)
- Ultrasound to detect ovarian cysts
- Pregnancy test to rule out pregnancy
- Thyroid function studies to determine thyroid disorder
- Prolactin level (an elevated level might indicate a pituitary tumor)
- Follicle-stimulating hormone (FSH) level (an elevated level might indicate ovarian failure)
- Luteinizing hormone (LH) level (an elevated level might indicate gonadal dysfunction)
- 17-ketosteroids (an elevated level might indicate an adrenal tumor)
- Laparoscopy to detect polycystic ovary syndrome
- CT scan of head if a pituitary tumor is suspected (Cavanaugh, 2003)

Treatment

Therapeutic intervention depends on the cause of the amenorrhea. The treatment of primary amenorrhea involves the correction of any underlying disorders and estrogen replacement therapy to stimulate the development of secondary sexual characteristics. If a pituitary tumor is the cause, it might be treated with drug therapy, surgical resection, or radiation therapy. Surgery might be needed to correct any structural abnormalities of the genital tract. Therapeutic interventions for secondary amenorrhea may include:

- Cyclic progesterone, when the cause is anovulation, or oral contraceptives
- Bromocriptine to treat hyperprolactinemia
- Gonadotropin-releasing hormone (GnRH), when the cause is hypothalamic failure
- Thyroid hormone replacement, when the cause is hypothyroidism (Littleton & Engebretson, 2002)

Nursing Management

Counseling and education are primary interventions and appropriate nursing roles. The nurse should address the diverse causes of amenorrhea, the relationship to sexual identity, possible infertility, and the possibility of a tumor or a life-threatening disease. In addition, the nurse should inform the woman about the purpose of each diagnostic test, how it is performed, and when the results will be available to discuss with her. Sensitive listening, interviewing, and presenting treatment options are paramount to gain the woman's cooperation and understanding.

Nutritional counseling is also vital in managing this disorder, especially if the woman has findings suggestive of an eating disorder. Although not all causes can be addressed by making lifestyle changes, the nurse can still emphasize maintaining a healthy lifestyle (Teaching Guidelines 4-2).

Dysmenorrhea

Dysmenorrhea refers to painful menstruation. The term is derived from the Greek words dys, meaning difficult/painful/abnormal, and rrhea, meaning flow. It may affect more than half of menstruating women (Alzubaidi & Calis, 2004). Uterine contractions occur during all periods, but in some women these cramps can be frequent and very intense. Dysmenorrhea is categorized as primary or secondary.

Etiology

Primary dysmenorrhea is caused by increased prostaglandin production by the endometrium in an ovulatory cycle. This hormone causes contraction of the uterus, and levels tend

T E A C H I N G   G U I D E L I N E S   4 - 2

Tips for Maintaining a Healthy Lifestyle

- Balance energy expenditure with energy intake.
- Modify diet to maintain ideal weight.
- Avoid excessive use of alcohol and mood-altering or sedative drugs.
- Avoid cigarette smoking.
- Identify areas of emotional stress and seek assistance to resolve them.
- Balance work, recreation, and rest.
- Maintain a positive outlook regarding the diagnosis and prognosis.
- Participate in ongoing care to monitor replacement therapy or associated conditions.
- Maintain bone density through:
  - Calcium intake (1,200–1,500 mg daily)
  - Weight-bearing exercise (30 minutes or more daily)
  - Hormone replacement therapy (Nelson & Bakalov, 2004)

to be higher in women with severe menstrual pain than women who experience mild or no menstrual pain. These levels are highest during the first 2 days of menses, when symptoms peak (Hart, 2005). This results in increased rhythmic uterine contractions from vasoconstriction of the small vessels of the uterine wall. This condition usually begins within a few years of the onset of ovulatory cycles at menarche.

Secondary dysmenorrhea is painful menstruation due to pelvic or uterine pathology. It may be caused by endometriosis, adenomyosis, fibroids, pelvic infection, an intrauterine device, cervical stenosis, or congenital uterine or vaginal abnormalities. Adenomyosis involves the ingrowth of the endometrium into the uterine musculature. Endometriosis involves ectopic implantation of endometrial tissue in other parts of the pelvis (Youngkin & Davis, 2004). It occurs most commonly in the third or fourth decades of life. Endometriosis is the most common cause of secondary dysmenorrhea and is associated with pain beyond menstruation, dyspareunia, and infertility (Speroff & Fritz, 2005). Treatment is directed toward removing the underlying pathology.

Clinical Manifestations

Affected women experience sharp, intermittent spasms of pain, usually in the suprapubic area. Pain may radiate to the back of the legs or the lower back. Systemic symptoms of nausea, vomiting, diarrhea, fatigue, fever, headache, or dizziness are fairly common. Pain usually develops within hours of the start of menstruation and peaks as the flow becomes heaviest during the first day or two of the cycle (Clark & Steele, 2004).

Assessment

As with any gynecologic complaint, a thorough focused history and physical examination is needed to make the diagnosis of primary or secondary dysmenorrhea. In primary dysmenorrhea, the history usually reveals the typical cramping pain with menstruation, and the physical examination is completely normal. In secondary dysmenorrhea, the history discloses cramping pain starting after 25 years old with a pelvic abnormality, a history of infertility, heavy menstrual flow, irregular cycles, and little response to nonsteroidal anti-inflammatory drugs (NSAIDs), oral contraceptives, or both (Alzubaidi & Calis, 2004).

During the initial interview, the nurse might ask some of the following questions to assess the woman's symptoms:

- "At what age did you start your menstrual cycles?"
- "Have your cycles always been painful, or did the pain start recently?"
- "When in your cycle do you experience the pain?"
- "How would you describe the pain you feel?"
- "Are you sexually active?"
- "What impact does your cycle have on your physical and social activity?"
- "When was the first day of your last menstrual cycle?"
- "Was the flow of your last menstrual cycle a normal amount for you?"
- "Do your cycles tend to be heavy or last longer than 5 days?"
- "Are your cycles generally regular and predictable?"
- "What have you done to relieve your discomfort? Is it effective?"
- "Has there been a progression of symptom severity?"
- "Do you have any other symptoms?"

A detailed sexual history is essential to assess for inflammation and scarring (adhesions) secondary to pelvic inflammatory disease (PID). Women with a previous history of PID, sexually transmitted infections (STIs), multiple sexual partners, or unprotected sex are at increased risk.

The physical examination performed by the healthcare provider centers on the bimanual pelvic examination. This examination is done during the nonmenstrual phase of the cycle. The nurse needs to offer an explanation to the woman about how it is to be performed, especially if is her first pelvic examination. The nurse should prepare the woman for it in the examining room by offering her a cover gown to put on and covering her lap with a privacy sheet on the examination table. The nurse will remain in the examining room throughout the examination to assist the healthcare provider with any procedures or specimens and offer the woman reassurance.

Common laboratory tests that may be ordered to determine the cause of dysmenorrhea might include:

- Complete blood count to rule out anemia
- Urinalysis to rule out a bladder infection
- Pregnancy test to rule out pregnancy

- Cervical culture to exclude STI
- Erythrocyte sedimentation rate to detect an inflammatory process
- Stool guaiac to exclude gastrointestinal bleeding or disorders
- Pelvic and/or vaginal ultrasound to detect pelvic masses or cysts
- Diagnostic laparoscopy and/or laparotomy to visualize pathology that may account for the symptoms

Treatment

Therapeutic intervention is directed toward pain relief and building coping strategies that will promote a productive lifestyle. Treatment measures usually include treating infections if present; suppressing the endometrium if endometriosis is suspected by administering low-dose oral contraceptives; administering prostaglandin inhibitors to reduce the pain; administering Depo-Provera; and initiating lifestyle changes. Table 4-1 lists selected treatment options for dysmenorrhea.

Nursing Management

Educating the client about the normal events of the menstrual cycle and the etiology of her pain is paramount in achieving a successful outcome. Explaining the normal menstrual cycle will teach the woman the correct terms so she can communicate her symptoms more accurately and will help dispel myths. Provide the woman with monthly graphs or charts to record menses, the onset of pain, the timing of medication, relief afforded, and coping strategies used. This involves the woman in her care and provides objective information so that therapy can be modified if necessary.

The nurse should explain in detail the dosing regimen and the side effects of the medication therapy selected. Commonly prescribed drugs include NSAIDs such as ibuprofen (Motrin), naproxen (Naprosyn), and Advil. They alleviate dysmenorrhea symptoms by decreasing intrauterine pressure and inhibiting prostaglandin synthesis, thus reducing pain (Skidmore-Roth, 2005). COX-2 inhibitors such as Vioxx or Bextra are also used, but they

Table 4-1 Treatment Options for Dysmenorrhea

Therapy Options	Dosage	Comments
Nonsteroidal Anti-inflammatory Agents (NSAIDs)		
Ibuprofen (Ibuprin, Advil, Motrin)	400–800 mg TID	Take with meals. Don't take with aspirin. Avoid alcohol. Watch for signs of GI bleeding.
Naproxen (Anaprox, Naprelan, Naprosyn, Aleve)	250–500 mg TID	Same as above
Cyclooxygenase-2 Inhibitors (COX-2)		
Valdecoxib (Bextra)	20 mg BID	More costly than NSAIDs, but decreased risk of GI bleeding
Rofecoxib (Vioxx)	50 mg QD	Same as above
Celecoxib (Celebrex)	200 mg BID	Same as above
Hormonal Contraceptives		
Low-dose oral contraceptives	Taken daily (42/7 days; 63/7 or 84/7)	Take active pills for an extended time to reduce number of monthly cycles (Policar, 2002).
Depo-medroxyprogesterone (DMPA), Depo-Provera	150 mg IM every 12 wks	Within 9–12 months of DMPA therapy, 75% of women will be amenorrheic (Homes & Laden, 2002).
Lifestyle Changes Daily exercise Limit salty foods Weight loss Smoking cessation Relaxation techniques		Gives sense of control over life

are more costly than NSAIDs. If pain relief is not achieved in two to four cycles, a low-dose combination oral contraceptive may be initiated. Client teaching and counseling should include information about how to take pills, side effects, and danger signs to watch for.

Additional information includes lifestyle changes that the woman can make to restore some sense of control and active participation in her care (Teaching Guidelines 4-3).

Dysfunctional Uterine Bleeding

Dysfunctional uterine bleeding (DUB) is a disorder that occurs most frequently in women at the beginning and end of their reproductive years. It is defined as irregular, abnormal bleeding that is not caused by pregnancy, a tumor, or an infection (Bradley, 2005). It is frequently associated with anovulatory cycles, which are common for the first year after menarche and later in life as women approach menopause.

The pathophysiology of DUB is related to a hormone disturbance. With anovulation, estrogen levels rise as usual in the early phase of the menstrual cycle. In the absence of ovulation, a corpus luteum never forms and progesterone is not produced. The endometrium moves into a hyperproliferative state, ultimately outgrowing its estrogen supply. This leads to irregular sloughing of the endometrium and excessive bleeding (Aeby & Frattarelli, 2002). If the bleeding is heavy enough and frequent enough, anemia can result.

DUB is similar to several other types of uterine bleeding disorders and sometimes overlaps these conditions. They include:

- Menorrhagia (abnormally long, heavy periods)
- Oligomenorrhea (bleeding occurs at intervals of more than 35 days)

- Metrorrhagia (bleeding between periods)
- Menometrorrhagia (bleeding occurs at irregular intervals with heavy flow lasting more than 7 days)
- Polymenorrhea (too frequent periods)

Etiology

The possible causes of DUB may include:

- Adenomyosis
- Pregnancy
- Hormonal imbalance
- Fibroid tumors (see Chapter 7)
- Endometrial polyps or cancer
- Endometriosis
- Intrauterine device (IUD)
- Polycystic ovary syndrome
- Morbid obesity
- Steroid therapy
- Hypothyroidism
- Blood dyscrasias/clotting disorder

Clinical Manifestations

The common symptoms associated with DUB include vaginal bleeding between periods, irregular menstrual cycles (usually less than 28 days between cycles), infertility, mood swings, hot flashes, vaginal tenderness, variable menstrual flow ranging from scanty to profuse, obesity, acne, and diabetes. Signs of polycystic ovary syndrome might be present, since it is associated with unopposed estrogen stimulation, elevated androgen levels, and insulin resistance and is a common cause of anovulation (Albers, Hull, & Wesley, 2004).

Assessment

A thorough history should be taken to differentiate between DUB and other conditions that might cause vaginal bleeding, such as pregnancy and pregnancy-related conditions (abruptio placentae, ectopic pregnancy, abortion, or placenta previa); systemic conditions such as Cushing's disease, blood dyscrasias, liver disease, renal disease, or thyroid disease; and genital tract pathology such as infections, tumors, or trauma (Queenan & Whitman, 2004). The healthcare provider, with the nurse assisting, performs a pelvic examination to identify any structural abnormalities.

Common laboratory tests that may be ordered to determine the cause of DUB include:

- Complete blood count, which is useful to reveal anemia
- Prothrombin time (PT) to detect blood dyscrasias
- Pregnancy test to rule out a spontaneous abortion or ectopic pregnancy
- Thyroid-stimulating hormone (TSH) level to screen for hypothyroidism
- Transvaginal ultrasound to measure endometrium
- Pelvic ultrasound to view any structural abnormalities
- Endometrial biopsy to check for intrauterine pathology
- Dilation and curettage (D&C) for diagnostic evaluation

 TEACHING GUIDELINES 4-3

Tips to Manage Dysmenorrhea

- Exercise increases endorphins and suppresses prostaglandin release.
- Limit salty foods to prevent fluid retention.
- Increase water consumption to serve as a natural diuretic.
- Increase fiber intake with fruits and vegetables to prevent constipation.
- Use heating pads or warm baths to increase comfort.
- Take warm showers to promote relaxation.
- Sip on warm beverages, such as decaffeinated green tea.
- Keep legs elevated while lying down or lie on side with knees bent.
- Use stress management techniques to reduce emotional stress.
- Practice relaxation techniques to enhance ability to cope with pain.
- Stop smoking and decrease alcohol use (Hart, 2004).

Treatment

Treatment of DUB depends on the cause of the bleeding and the age of the client. When known, the underlying cause of the disorder is treated. Otherwise, the goal of treatment is to relieve the symptoms so that uterine bleeding does not interfere with a woman's normal activities or cause anemia (Dodds & Sinert, 2005).

Management of DUB might include medical care with pharmacotherapy or insertion of an IUD. Oral contraceptives are used for cycle regulation as well as contraception. They help prevent the risks associated with prolonged unopposed estrogen stimulation of the endometrium. NSAIDs and the levonorgestrel-releasing IUD (Mirena) decrease menstrual blood loss significantly (Lethaby, Cooke, & Rees, 2003).

If the client does not respond to medical therapy, surgical intervention might include D&C, endometrial ablation, or hysterectomy. Endometrial ablation is an alternative to hysterectomy. A thermal balloon is used to ablate the tissue, and improvement is found in 90% of women (Speroff & Fritz, 2005).

The drug categories used in the treatment of DUB are:

- *Estrogens:* cause vasospasm of the uterine arteries to decrease bleeding
- *Progestins:* used to stabilize an estrogen-primed endometrium
- *Oral contraceptives:* regulate the cycle and suppress the endometrium
- *NSAIDs:* inhibit prostaglandins
- *Levonorgestrel-20 Intrauterine System:* suppresses endometrial growth
- *Iron salts:* replenish iron stores lost during heavy bleeding

Nursing Management

Educate the client about normal menstrual cycles and the possible reasons for her abnormal pattern. Inform the woman about treatment options. Instruct her about any prescribed medications and potential side effects. Do not simply encourage the woman to "live with it": complications such as infertility can result from lack of ovulation, severe anemia can occur secondary to prolonged or heavy menses, and endometrial cancer can occur associated with prolonged buildup of the endometrial lining without menstrual bleeding (Debernardo, 2004). Adequate follow-up and evaluation for women who do not respond to medical management is essential.

See Nursing Care Plan 4-1: Overview of a Woman With Dysfunctional Uterine Bleeding (DUB).

Premenstrual Syndrome

Premenstrual syndrome (PMS) describes a wide range of recurrent symptoms that occur during the last half of the menstrual cycle and resolve with the onset of menstruation (Braverman & Neinstein, 2002). A woman experiencing PMS may have a wide variety of seemingly unrelated symptoms; for that reason, it is difficult to define and more challenging to diagnose. PMS affects millions of women during their reproductive years: up to 85% of menstruating women report having one or more premenstrual symptoms, and up to 10% report disabling, incapacitating symptoms (Dickerson, Mazyck, & Hunter, 2003).

Etiology

The exact cause of PMS is not known. It is thought to be related to the interaction between hormonal events and neurotransmitter function, specifically serotonin. Not all women respond to serotonin reuptake inhibitors (SSRIs), however, which implies that other mechanisms may be involved (Braverman & Neinstein, 2002).

Clinical Manifestations

Although little consensus exists in the medical literature and among researchers about what constitutes PMS, the physical and psychological symptoms are very real. The extent to which the symptoms debilitate or incapacitate a woman is highly variable.

There are more than 200 symptoms assigned to PMS, but irritability, tension, and dysphoria are the most prominent and consistently described (Dickerson et al., 2003). Diagnostic criteria for PMS consists of having a least one of the following affective and somatic symptoms during the 5 days before menses in each of the three previous cycles:

- Affective symptoms: depression, angry outbursts, irritability, anxiety
- Somatic symptoms: breast tenderness, abdominal bloating, edema, headache
- Symptoms relieved from days 4 to 13 of the menstrual cycle (ACOG, 2000)

There are two different syndromes recognized: PMS and *premenstrual dysphoric disorder* (PMDD). As defined by the American Psychological Association, PMDD is a more severe variant of PMS. Experts equate the difference between PMS and PMDD to the difference between a mild tension headache and a migraine (Healthy Women, 2005). PMDD markedly interferes with work and school, or with social activities and relationships with others. In PMDD, the main symptoms are mood disorders such as depression, anxiety, tension, and persistent anger or irritability. Physical symptoms such as headache, joint and muscle pain, lack of energy, bloating, and breast tenderness are also present.

According to the American Psychiatric Association, a woman must have at least five of the typical symptoms to be diagnosed with PMDD (Lowdermilk & Perry, 2004). These must occur during the week before and a few days after the onset of menstruation and must include one or more of the first four symptoms:

1. Affective lability: sadness, tearfulness, irritability
2. Anxiety and tension
3. Persistent or marked anger or irritability

Nursing Care Plan 4-1

Overview of a Woman With Dysfunctional Uterine Bleeding (DUB)

Stacy, a 52-year-old obese woman, comes to her gynecologist with the complaint of heavy erratic bleeding. Her periods were fairly regular until about 4 months ago, and since that time they have been unpredictable, excessive, and prolonged. Stacy reports she is tired all the time, can't sleep, and feels "out of sorts" and anxious. She is fearful she has cancer.

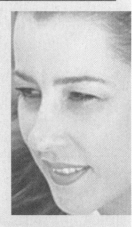

Nursing Diagnosis: Fear related to current signs and symptoms possibly indicating a life-threatening condition

Outcome Identification and *evaluation*	Interventions with *rationales*
The client will acknowledge her fears as *evidenced by statements made that fear and anxiety have been lessened after explanation of diagnosis.*	Distinguish between anxiety and fear to *determine appropriate interventions.* Check complete blood count and assess for possible anemia secondary to excessive bleeding to *determine if fatigue is contributing to anxiety and fears. Fatigue occurs because the oxygen-carrying capacity of the blood is reduced.* Reassure client that symptoms can be managed *to help address her current concerns.* Provide client with factual information and explain what to expect *to assist client with identifying fears and help in her coping with her condition.* Provide symptom management *to reduce concerns associated with the cause of bleeding.* Teach client about early manifestations of fear and anxiety *to aid in prompt recognition and minimize escalation of anxiety.* Assess client's use of coping strategies in the past and reinforce use of effective ones *to help control anxiety and fear.* Instruct client in relaxation methods, such as deep-breathing exercises and imagery *to provide her with additional methods for controlling anxiety and fear.*

Nursing Diagnosis: Deficient knowledge related to perimenopause and its management

Client will demonstrate understanding of her symptoms *as evidenced by making health-promoting lifestyle choices, verbalizing appropriate health care practices, and adhering to measures to comply with therapy.*	Assess client's understanding of perimenopause and its treatment *to provide a baseline for teaching and developing a plan of care.*

(continued)

Overview of a Woman With Dysfunctional Uterine Bleeding (DUB) (continued)

Outcome Identification and *evaluation*	Interventions with *rationales*
	Review instructions about prescribed procedures and recommendations for self-care, frequently obtaining feedback from the client *to validate adequate understanding of information.*
	Outline link between anovulatory cycles and excessive buildup of uterine lining in perimenopausal women *to assist client in understanding the etiology of her bleeding.*
	Provide written material with pictures *to promote learning and help client visualize what is occurring to her body during perimenopause.*
	Inform client about the availability of community resources and make appropriate referrals as needed *to provide additional education and support.*
	Document details of teaching and learning *to allow for continuity of care and further education, if needed.*

4. Depressed mood, feelings of hopelessness
5. Difficulty concentrating
6. Sleep difficulties
7. Increased or decreased appetite
8. Increased or decreased sexual desire
9. Chronic fatigue
10. Headache
11. Constipation or diarrhea
12. Breast swelling and tenderness (Hendrick, 2005)

Assessment

To establish the diagnosis of PMS, the nurse interviewing the woman needs to elicit a description of cyclic symptoms occurring before the woman's menstrual period. The woman should chart her symptoms daily for two cycles. These data will help demonstrate symptoms clustering around the luteal phase of ovulation, with resolution after bleeding starts. Ask the woman to bring her list of symptoms to the next appointment. Symptoms can be categorized using the following:

- A: anxiety: difficulty sleeping, tenseness, mood swings, clumsiness
- C: craving: headache, cravings for sweets, salty foods, chocolate
- D: depression: feelings of low self-esteem, anger, easily upset
- H: hydration: weight gain, abdominal bloating, breast tenderness
- O: other: hot flashes or cold sweats, nausea, change in bowel habits, aches or pains, dysmenorrhea, acne breakout (Clark, 2004)

Treatment

Treatment of PMS is often frustrating for both patients and healthcare providers. Clinical outcomes can be expected to improve as a result of recent consensus on the diagnostic criteria for PMS and PMDD, data from clinical trials, and the availability of evidence-based clinical guidelines (Dickerson et al., 2003).

Therapeutic interventions for PMS and PMDD address the symptoms because the exact cause of this condition is still unknown. Treatments may include vitamin supplements, diet changes, exercise, lifestyle changes, and medications (Box 4-2).

The management of PMS or PMDD requires a multidimensional approach because these conditions are not likely to have a single cause, and they appear to affect multiple systems within a woman's body; therefore, they are not likely to be amenable to treatment with a single therapy. Because there are no diagnostic tests that can reliably determine the existence of PMS or PMDD, it is the woman herself who must decide that she needs help during this time of the month. The woman must embrace multiple therapies and become an active participant in her treatment plan to find the best level of symptom relief.

Nursing Management

Educate the client about the management of PMS or PMDD. Advise her that lifestyle changes often result in significant symptom improvement without pharmacotherapy. Explain the relationship between cyclic estrogen fluctuation and changes in serotonin levels and how the different management strategies help maintain serotonin

BOX 4-2

TREATMENT OPTIONS FOR PMS AND PMDD

○ Lifestyle changes
  ▪ Reduce stress.
  ▪ Exercise three to five times each week.
  ▪ Eat a balanced diet and increase water intake.
  ▪ Decrease caffeine intake.
  ▪ Stop smoking.
  ▪ Limit intake of alcohol.
  ▪ Attend a PMS/women's support group.
○ Vitamin and mineral supplements
  ▪ Multivitamin daily
  ▪ Vitamin E, 400 units daily
  ▪ Calcium, 1,200 mg daily
  ▪ Magnesium, 200–400 mg daily
○ Medications
  ▪ NSAIDs taken a week prior to menses
  ▪ Oral contraceptives (low dose)
  ▪ Antidepressants (SSRIs)
  ▪ Anxiolytics (taken during luteal phase)
  ▪ Diuretics to remove excess fluid

levels, thus improving symptoms. It is important to rule out other conditions that might cause erratic or dysphoric behavior. If the initial treatment regimen does not work, the woman should return for further testing. Behavioral counseling and stress management might help women regain control during these stressful periods. Reassuring the woman that support and help are available through many community resources/support groups can be instrumental in her acceptance of this monthly disorder. Nurses can be a very calming force for many women experiencing PMS or PMDD.

Endometriosis

Endometriosis is one of the most common gynecologic diseases, affecting more than 5.5 million women in the United States. In this condition, bits of functioning endometrial tissue are located outside of their normal site, the uterine cavity. This endometrial tissue is commonly found attached to the ovaries, fallopian tubes, the outer surface of the uterus, the bowels, the area between the vagina and the rectum (rectovaginal septum), and the pelvic side wall (Fig. 4-1). The places where the tissue attaches are called implants, or lesions. Endometrial tissue found outside the uterus responds to hormones released during the menstrual cycle in the same way as endometrial lining within the uterus.

At the beginning of the menstrual cycle, when the lining of the uterus is shed and menstrual bleeding begins, these abnormally located implants swell and bleed also. In short, the woman with endometriosis experiences several "mini-periods" throughout her abdomen, wherever this endometrial tissue exists.

Etiology and Risk Factors

It is not currently known why endometrial tissue becomes transplanted and grows in other parts of the body. Several theories exist, but to date none has scientifically proven the true etiology of this condition. However, several factors

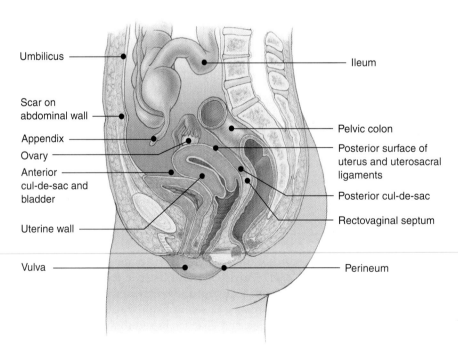

● Figure 4-1 Common sites of endometriosis formation.

that increase a woman's risk of developing endometriosis have been identified:

- Increasing age
- Family history of endometriosis in a first-degree relative
- Short menstrual cycle (less than 28 days)
- Long menstrual flow (more than 1 week)
- Young age of menarche (younger than 12)
- Few (one or two) or no pregnancies (Speroff & Fritz, 2005)

Clinical Manifestations

Endometriosis is chronic and progressive. Symptoms include:

- Infertility (Kapoor & Davila, 2004)
- Pain before and during menstrual periods
- Pain during or after sexual intercourse
- Painful urination
- Depression
- Fatigue
- Painful bowel movements
- Chronic pelvic pain
- Hypermenorrhea (heavy menses)
- Pelvic adhesions
- Irregular and more frequent menses
- Premenstrual vaginal spotting

The two most common symptoms are infertility and pain. Endometriosis occurs in 38% of infertile women and in 71% to 87% of women with chronic pelvic pain (Youngkin & Davis, 2004). About 30% to 40% of women with this condition are infertile, making it one of the top three causes of female infertility (NICHD, 2002).

Assessment

Nurses encounter women with endometriosis in a variety of settings: community health settings, schools, clinics, day surgical centers, and hospitals. Healthcare professionals must not trivialize or dismiss the concerns of these women, because early recognition is essential to preserve fertility. Elicit a description of signs and symptoms and obtain a health history to determine risk factors.

The pelvic examination typically correlates with the extent of the endometriosis. The usual finding is non-specific pelvic tenderness. The hallmark finding is the presence of tender nodular masses on the uterosacral ligaments, the posterior uterus, or the posterior cul-de-sac (Hsu, 2004).

After a thorough history and a pelvic examination, the health care practitioner may suspect endometriosis, but the only certain method of diagnosing it is by seeing it. This can be done through laparoscopy, the direct visualization of the internal organs with a lighted instrument inserted through an abdominal incision. A tissue biopsy of the suspected implant taken at the same time and examined microscopically can confirm the diagnosis.

Nurses can play a role in offering a thorough explanation of the condition and why tests are needed to diagnose endometriosis. The nurse can set up appointments for imaging studies, such as a pelvic or transvaginal ultrasound to assess pelvic organ structures, although a laparoscopy is needed for a definitive diagnosis.

Treatment

Therapeutic management of the client with endometriosis needs to take into consideration the following factors: severity of symptoms, desire for fertility, degree of disease, and the client's therapy goals. The aim of therapy is to suppress levels of estrogen and progesterone, which cause the endometrium to grow. Treatment can include surgery or medication (Table 4-2).

Nursing Management

In addition to the interventions outlined above, the nurse should encourage the client to adopt healthy lifestyle habits with respect to diet, exercise, sleep, and stress management. Referrals to support groups and Internet resources can help the woman to understand this condition and to cope with chronic pain. A number of organizations provide information about the diagnosis and treatment of endometriosis and offer support to women and their families (Box 4-3).

Infertility

Infertility is defined as the inability to conceive a child after 1 year of regular sexual intercourse unprotected by contraception, or to carry a pregnancy to term (DeMasters, 2004). *Secondary infertility* is the inability to conceive after a previous pregnancy. Many people take the ability to conceive and produce a child for granted, but infertility affects about 6.1 million Americans, or 10% of the reproductive-age population, according to the American Society for Reproductive Medicine (2002). Infertility is a widespread problem that has an emotional, social, and economic impact on couples. Nurses must recognize infertility and understand its causes and treatment options so that they can help couples understand the possibilities as well as the limitations of current therapies for infertility. The caring aspect of professional nursing is an essential component of meeting the special needs of these couples (Brucker & McKenry, 2004). Prevention of infertility through education should also be incorporated into any client–nurse interaction.

Etiology and Risk Factors

Multiple known and unknown factors affect fertility. Female-factor infertility is detected in about 40% of cases, male-factor infertility in about 40% of cases. The remaining 20% fall into a category of combined (both male and female factors) or unexplained infertility (Gray

Table 4-2 Treatment Options for Endometriosis

Therapy Options	Comment
Surgical Intervention	
Conservative surgery	Removal of implants/lesions using laser, cautery, or small surgical instruments. This intervention will reduce pain and allows pregnancy to occur in the future.
Definitive surgery	Abdominal hysterectomy, with or without bilateral salpingo-oophorectomy. Will eliminate pain but will leave a woman unable to become pregnant in the future.
Medication Therapy	
NSAIDs	First-line treatment to reduce pain; taken early when premenstrual symptoms are first felt
Oral contraceptives	Suppresses cyclic hormonal response of the endometrial tissue
Progestogens	Used to cast off the endometrial cells and thus destroy them
Antiestrogens	Suppresses a woman's production of estrogen, thus stopping the menstrual cycle and preventing further growth of endometrium
Gonadotropin-releasing hormone analogues (GnRH-a)	Suppresses endometriosis by creating a temporary pseudomenopause

et al., 2004). In women, ovarian dysfunction (40%) and tubal/pelvic pathology (40%) are the primary contributing factors to infertility.

Risk factors for infertility include:

- *For women:*
  - Overweight or underweight (can disrupt hormone function)
  - Hormonal imbalances leading to irregular ovulation
  - Fibroids
  - Tubal blockages

- Chronic illnesses such as diabetes, thyroid disease, asthma
  - STIs
  - Age older than 27
  - Endometriosis
  - History of PID
  - Smoking and alcohol consumption
  - Multiple miscarriages
  - Psychological stress
- *For men:*
  - Exposure to toxic substances (lead, mercury, x-rays)
  - Cigarette or marijuana smoke
  - Heavy alcohol consumption
  - Use of prescription drugs for ulcers or psoriasis
  - Exposure of the genitals to high temperatures (hot tubs or saunas)
  - Hernia repair
  - Frequent long-distance cycling
  - STI
  - Undescended testicles (cryptorchidism)
  - Mumps after puberty (Women's Health Guide, 2004)

BOX 4-3

ORGANIZATIONS AND WEB RESOURCES TO ASSIST THE CLIENT WITH ENDOMETRIOSIS

- American College of Obstetricians and Gynecologists (ACOG): www.acog.org or e-mail at resources@acog.org
- American Society of Reproductive Medicine: www.asrm.org or e-mail at asrm@asrm.org
- Center for Endometriosis Care: http://www.centerforendo.com/
- Endometriosis Association: www.endometriosisassn.org or www.KillerCramps.org
- Endometriosis Association support groups: e-mail at support@endometriosisassn.org
- NICHD Information Resource Center: www.nichd.nih.gov or e-mail at NICHDClearinghouse@mail.nih.gov
- National Women's Health Information Center (Dept. of Health and Human Services): http://www.4women.gov

Assessment

Infertile couples are under tremendous pressure and can be by nature secretive, considering their problem to be very personal. The couple is often beset by feelings of inadequacy and guilt, and many are subjected to pressures from both family and friends. As their problem becomes more chronic, they may begin to blame one another, with consequent martial discord. Seeking help is often a very difficult step for them, and it may take a lot of courage to discuss something about which they feel deeply embarrassed or upset. The nurse working in this specialty setting must be aware of the conflict and problems couples present with and must be very sensitive to their needs.

A full medical history should be taken from both partners, along with a physical examination. The data needed for the infertility evaluation are very sensitive and of a personal nature, so the nurse must use very professional interviewing skills.

There are numerous causes of and contributing factors to infertility, so it is important to use the process of elimination, determining what problems don't exist in order to better comprehend the problems that do exist. At the first visit, a plan of investigation is outlined and a complete health history is taken. This first visit forces many couples to confront the reality that their desired pregnancy may not occur naturally. The nurse can alleviate some of the anxiety associated with diagnostic testing by offering explanations as to the timing and reasons for each test.

Male Factors

The initial screening evaluation for the male partner should include a reproductive history and a semen analysis. From the male perspective, three things must happen for conception to take place: there must be an adequate number of sperm; those sperm must be healthy and mature; and the sperm must be able to penetrate and fertilize the egg. Semen analysis is the most important indicator of male fertility. The man should abstain from sexual activity for 24 to 48 hours before giving the sample. For a semen examination, the man is asked to produce a specimen by ejaculating into a specimen container and delivering it to the laboratory for analysis within 1 to 2 hours. When the specimen is brought to the laboratory, it is analyzed for volume, viscosity, number of sperm, sperm viability, motility, and sperm shape. If semen parameters are normal, no further male evaluation is necessary (Youngkin & Davis, 2004).

The physical examination routinely includes:

- Assessment for the presence of appropriate male sexual characteristics, such as body hair distribution, development of the Adam's apple and muscle development
- Examination of the penis, scrotum, testicles, epididymis, and vas deferens for abnormalities (e.g., nodules, irregularities, varicocele)
- Assessment for normal development of external genitalia (small testicles)
- Performance of a digital internal examination of the prostate to check for tenderness or swelling (DeMasters, 2004).

Female Factors

The initial assessment of the woman should include a thorough history of factors associated with ovulation and the pelvic organs. Diagnostic tests to determine female infertility may include:

- Assessment of ovarian function
  - Menstrual history: regularity of cycles
  - Ovulation predictor kits used midcycle
  - Urinary LH level
  - Clomiphene citrate challenge test
  - Endometrial biopsy to document luteal phase
- Assessment of pelvic organs
  - Papanicolaou (Pap) smear to rule out cervical cancer or inflammation
  - Cervical culture to rule out *Chlamydia* infection
  - Postcoital testing to evaluate sperm–cervical mucus interaction
  - Hysterosalpingogram (HSG) to assess tubal patency
  - Ultrasound to assess pelvic structures
  - Hysterosalpingography to visualize structural defects
  - Laparoscopy to visualize pelvic structures and diagnose endometriosis

Home Ovulation Predictor Kits

Home ovulation predictor kits contain monoclonal antibodies specific for LH and use the ELISA test to determine the amount of LH present in the urine. A significant color change from baseline indicates the LH surge and presumably the most fertile day of the month for the woman.

Clomiphene Citrate Challenge Test

The clomiphene citrate challenge test is used to assess a woman's ovarian reserve (capability of her eggs to become fertilized). FSH levels are drawn on cycle day 3 and on cycle day 10 after the woman has taken 100 mg clomiphene citrate on cycle days 5 through 9. If the FSH level is greater than 15, the test is considered abnormal and the likelihood of conception with her own eggs is very low (Youngkin & Davis, 2004).

Endometrial Biopsy

Another assessment of ovulation that indicates whether the secretion of progesterone is adequate is an endometrial biopsy. A strip of endometrial tissue is removed just before menstruation. Histologic documentation of secretory endometrial development implies that ovulation has taken place. An endometrium that does not conform to the normal histologic pattern indicates a defect in the luteal phase.

Postcoital Testing

Postcoital testing is done to assess the receptivity of the cervical mucus to sperm. Cervical mucus from the woman is examined 2 to 8 hours after intercourse during the expected time of ovulation, and the number of live, motile sperm present is assessed. Cervical mucus is also evaluated for stretchability (spinnbarkeit) and consistency (Marchiano, 2004). The results are described in Table 4-3.

Hysterosalpingogram

In a hysterosalpingogram, 3 to 10 mL of an opaque contrast medium is slowly injected through a catheter into the endocervical canal so that the uterus and tubes can be visualized during fluoroscopy and radiography. If the

Table 4-3 Postcoital Test Results

Normal: Normal amounts of sperm are seen in the
          sample.
          Sperm are moving forward through the
          cervical mucus.
          The mucus stretches at least 2 in (5 cm).
          The mucus dries in a fernlike pattern.

Abnormal: Mucus cannot stretch 2 in (5 cm).
          Mucus does not dry in a fernlike pattern.
          No sperm or a large percentage of dead
          sperm are seen in the sample.
          Sperm are clumped.

Nissi, J. (2004). Postcoital test. *WebMD*. (Online) Available at:
http://my.webmd.com/hw/infertility_reproduction/ux1259.asp

fallopian tubes are patent, the dye will ascend upward to distend the uterus and the tubes and spill out into the peritoneal cavity (Fig. 4-2).

Laparoscopy

A laparoscopy is usually performed early in the menstrual cycle. During the procedure, an endoscope is inserted through a small incision in the anterior abdominal wall. Visualization of the peritoneal cavity in an infertile woman may reveal endometriosis, pelvic adhesions, tubal occlusion, fibroids, or polycystic ovaries (Lowdermilk & Perry, 2004).

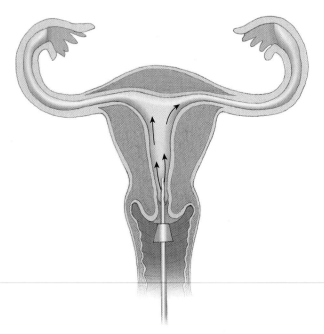

● Figure 4-2 Insertion of a dye for a hysterosalpingogram. The contrast dye outlines the uterus and fallopian tubes on x-ray to demonstrate patency.

Treatment

The test results are presented to the couple and different treatment options are suggested. The majority of infertility cases are treated with drugs or surgery. Various ovulation-enhancement drugs and timed intercourse might be used for the woman with ovulation problems. The woman should understand the drug's benefits and side effects before consenting to take them. Depending on the type of drug used and the dosage, some women may experience multiple births. If the woman's reproductive organs are damaged, surgery can be done to repair them. Still other couples might opt for the high-tech approaches of artificial insemination (Fig. 4-3), in vitro fertilization (IVF; Fig. 4-4), and egg donation or contract for a gestational carrier or surrogate (Brucker & McKenry, 2004). Table 4-4 lists selected infertility options.

Nursing Management

Consider THIS!

We had been married for 3 years and wanted to start a family, but much to our dismay nothing happened after a year of trying. I had some irregular periods and was finally diagnosed with endometriosis and put on Clomid. After 3 years of taking Clomid on and off, I went to a fertility expert. The doctor lasered the endometriosis tissue, sent air through my tubes to make sure they were patent, and put me back on Clomid, but still with no luck. Finally 2 years later we were put on an IVF waiting list and prayed we would have the money for the procedure when we were chosen. By then I felt a failure as a woman. We then decided that it was more important for us to be parents than it was for me to be pregnant, so we considered adoption. We tried for another year without any results.

We went to the adoption agency to fill out the paperwork for the process to begin. Our blood was taken and we waited for an hour, wondering the whole time why it was taking so long for the results. The nurse finally appeared and handed a piece of paper to me with the word "positive" written on it. I started to cry tears of joy, for a pregnancy had started and our long journey of infertility was finally ending.

Thoughts: For many women the dream of having a child is not easily realized. Unwanted infertility can affect self-esteem, disrupt relationships, and result in depression. This couple experienced many years of frustration in trying to have a family. What help can be offered to couples during this time? What can be said to comfort the woman who feels she is a failure?

Nurses play an important role in the care of infertile couples. The nurse is most effective when he or she offers care and treatment in a professional manner and regards the couple as valued and respected individuals. The nurse's focus must encompass the whole person, not just the

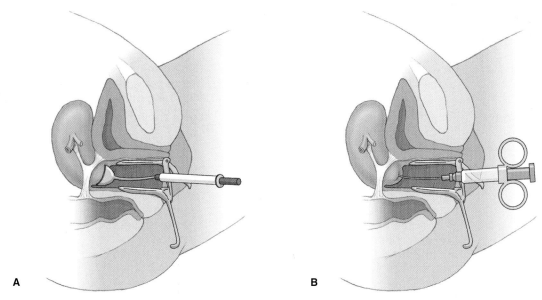

● Figure 4-3 Artificial insemination. Sperm are deposited next to the cervix (**A**) or injected directly into the uterine cavity (**B**).

results of the various infertility studies. Throughout the entire process, the nurse's role is to provide information, anticipatory guidance, stress management, and counseling. The couple's emotional distress is usually very high, and the nurse must be able to recognize that anxiety and provide emotional support. The nurse may need to refer couples to a reproductive endocrinologist or surgeon, depending on the problem identified.

There is no absolute way to prevent infertility per se because so many factors are involved in conception. Nurses can be instrumental in educating men and women about the factors that contribute to infertility.

The nurse can also outline the risks and benefits of treatments so that the couple can make an informed decision.

With advances in genetics and reproductive medicine also come a myriad of ethical, social, and cultural issues that will affect the couple's decisions. With this in mind, nurses must provide an opportunity for the couple to make informed decisions in a nondirective, nonjudgmental environment. Through the use of advocacy and anticipatory guidance, nurses can assist and support couples through the diagnosis and treatment of infertility (Jones, 2004).

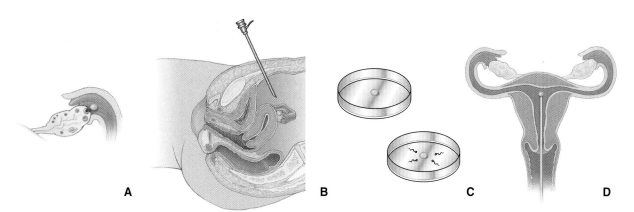

● Figure 4-4 Steps involved in in vitro fertilization. (**A**) Ovulation. (**B**) Capture of the ova (done here intra-abdominally). (**C**) Fertilization of ova and growth in culture medium. (**D**) Insertion of fertilized ova into uterus.

Table 4-4 Selected Treatment Options for Infertility

Procedure	Comments	Nursing Considerations
Fertility Drugs		
Clomiphene citrate (Clomid)	A nonsteroidal synthetic antiestrogen used to induce ovulation	Nurse can advise the couple to have intercourse every other day for 1 week starting after day 5 of medication.
Human menopausal gonadotropin (HMG); Pergonal	Induces ovulation by direct stimulation of ovarian follicle	Same as above
Artificial Insemination		
	The insertion of a prepared semen sample into the cervical os or intrauterine cavity	Nurse needs to advise couple that the procedure might need to be repeated if not successful the first time.
	Enables sperm to be deposited closer to improve chances of conception	
	Husband or donor sperm can be used	
Assisted Reproductive Technologies*		
In vitro fertilization (IVF)	Oocytes are fertilized in the lab and transferred to the uterus.	Nurse advises woman to take medication to stimulate ovulation so the mature ovum can be retrieved by needle aspiration.
	Usually indicated for tubal obstruction, endometriosis, pelvic adhesions, and low sperm counts	
Gamete intrafallopian transfer (GIFT)	Oocytes and sperm are combined and immediately placed in the fallopian tube so fertilization can occur naturally.	Nurse needs to inform couple of risks and have consent signed.
	Requires laparoscopy and general anesthesia, which increases risk	
Intracytoplasmic sperm injection (ICSI)	One sperm is injected into the cytoplasm of the oocyte to fertilize it.	Nurse needs to inform the male that sperm will be aspirated by a needle through the skin into the epididymis.
	Indicated for male factor infertility	
Donor oocytes or sperm	Eggs or sperm are retrieved from a donor and the eggs are inseminated; resulting embryos are transferred via IVF.	Nurse needs to support couple in their ethical/religious discussions prior to deciding.
	Recommended for women > 40 and those with poor-quality eggs	
Gestational carrier (surrogacy)	Laboratory fertilization takes place and embryos are transferred to the uterus of another woman, who will carry the pregnancy.	Nurse should encourage an open discussion regarding implications of this method with the couple.
	Medical-legal issues have resulted over the "true ownership" of the resulting infant.	

*When other options have been exhausted, these are considered.

Finances and insurance coverage often dictate the choice of treatment. Nurses can help couples decipher their insurance coverage and can help them weigh the costs of various procedures by explaining what each will provide in terms of information about their infertility problems.

Assisting them to make a priority list of diagnostic tests and potential treatment options will help the couple plan their financial strategy.

Many infertile couples are not prepared for the emotional roller-coaster of grief and loss during infertility treatments. Financial concerns and coping as a couple are two major areas of stress when treatment is undertaken. During the course of what may be months, or even years, of infertility care, it is essential to develop a holistic approach to nursing care. Stress management and anxiety reduction need to be addressed, and referral to a peer support group such as Resolve might be in order (Box 4-4).

Contraception

In the United States, there are approximately 60 million women in their childbearing years, ages 15 to 44. Overall, 64% of those 60 million women use contraception, but still more than 3 million unintended pregnancies occur every year (U.S. Bureau of the Census, 2003). Although numerous fertility-control methods are available, the United States continues to have the highest unintended pregnancy rate when compared to other Western countries. Every minute of every day, 10 people become infected with HIV, most through heterosexual contact; 190 women conceive an unwanted pregnancy; 1 woman dies from a pregnancy-related cause; and 40 women undergo unsafe abortions, as outlined in the UNFPA State of the World Population 2000 Report. Much of this suffering could be prevented by access to safe, efficient, appropriate, modern contraception for everyone who wants it (UNFPA, 2000).

Contraception is any method that prevents conception or childbirth. A woman's reproductive life spans almost 40 years, and throughout those years, a variety of contraceptive methods may be used. Oral contraceptives, sterilization of the female, and the male condom are the most popular methods in the United States (Alan Guttmacher Institute, 2004a,b).

Couples must decide which method is appropriate for them to meet their changing contraceptive needs throughout their life cycles. Nurses can educate and assist couples during this selection process. This part of chapter will outline the most common birth control methods available.

In an era when many women wish to delay pregnancy and at the same time face potential STIs, choices are difficult. There are numerous methods available today, and many more will be offered in the near future. The ideal contraceptive method for many women would have to have the following characteristics: ease of use, safety, effectiveness, minimal side effects, "naturalness," non-hormonal method, and immediate reversibility (Burkman, 2002). Currently, no one contraceptive method offers everything. Box 4-5 outlines the contraceptive methods

---

BOX 4-4

ORGANIZATIONS AND WEB RESOURCES TO ASSIST THE CLIENT WITH INFERTILITY

- Resolve: A nationwide network of chapters dedicated to providing education, advocacy, and support for men and women facing the crisis of infertility. They provide a helpline, medical referral services, member-to-member contact system. (http://www.resolve.org)
- American Society of Reproductive Medicine (ASRM): Provides fact sheets and other resources on infertility, treatments, insurance, and other issues (http://www.asrm.org)
- International Counsel on Infertility (INCIID): Provides information about infertility, support forums, and a directory of infertility specialists (http://www.inciid.org)
- American Fertility Association: Offers education, referrals, research, support, and advocacy for couples dealing with infertility (http://www.americaninfertility.org)
- Bertarelli Foundation: The Human Face of Infertility: Aims to promote and improve understanding of infertility by offering resources (http://www.bertarelli.edu)
- International Consumer Support for Infertility: An international network engaged in advocacy on behalf of infertile couples via fact sheets and information (http://www.icsi.ws)

BOX 4-5

OUTLINE OF CONTRACEPTIVE METHODS

Reversible Methods
Behavioral
- Abstinence
- Fertility awareness
- Withdrawal (coitus interuptus)
- Lactational amenorrhea method (LAM)

Barrier
- Condom (male and female)
- Diaphragm
- Cervical cap
- Sponge

Hormonal
- Oral contraceptives
- Injectable contraceptive
- Transdermal patches
- Vaginal ring
- Implantable contraceptives
- Intrauterine devices
- Emergency contraceptives

Abortion
Permanent Methods
- Tubal ligation for women
- Vasectomy for men

available today. Table 4-5 provides a detailed summary of each type, including information on failure rates, advantages, disadvantages, STI protection, and danger signs.

Contraceptives methods can be divided into three types: behavioral methods, barrier methods, and hormonal methods.

Behavioral Methods

Behavioral methods refer to any natural contraceptive method that does not require hormones, pharmaceutical compounds, physical barriers, or surgery to prevent pregnancy. These methods require couples to take an active role in preventing pregnancy through their sexual behaviors.

Abstinence

Abstinence (not having vaginal or anal intercourse) is one of the least expensive forms of contraception and has been used for thousands of years. Basically, pregnancy cannot occur if sperm is kept out of the vagina. It also reduces the risk of contracting HIV/AIDS and other STIs, unless body fluids are exchanged through oral sex; however, some infections, like herpes and HPV, can be passed by skin-to-skin contact. There are many pleasurable alternatives for sex play without intercourse ("outercourse"), such as kissing, masturbation, erotic massage, sexual fantasy, sex toys such as vibrators, and oral sex.

Many people have strong feelings about abstinence based on religious and moral beliefs. There are many good and personal reasons to choose abstinence. For some it is a way of life, while for others it is a temporary choice. Some people choose abstinence because they want to:

• Wait until they are older
• Wait for a long-term relationship
• Avoid pregnancy or STIs
• Follow religious or cultural expectations

Fertility Awareness

Fertility awareness is a natural method of contraception in which no contraceptive devices are used; instead, certain observations, techniques, and calculations are used to determine the "fertile" and the "safe" periods in a monthly menstrual cycle. There are normal physiologic changes caused by hormonal fluctuations during the menstrual cycle that can be observed and charted. This information can be used to avoid a pregnancy or encourage one. Fertility awareness methods rely upon the following assumptions:

• A single ovum is released from the ovary 14 days before the next menstrual period. It lives approximately 24 hours.
• Sperm can live up to 5 days after intercourse. The "unsafe period" during the menstrual cycle is thus approximately 6 days: 3 days before and 3 days after ovulation. Since

(text continues on page 82)

Table 4-5 Summary of Contraceptive Methods

Type	Description	Failure Rate	Pros	Cons	STI Protection	Danger Signs	Comments
Abstinence	Refrain from sexual activity	None	Costs nothing	Difficult to maintain	100%	None	Must be joint couple decision
Fertility awareness	Refrain from sex during fertile period	27%	No side effects; acceptable to most religious groups	High failure rate with incorrect use	None	None	Requires high level of couple commitment
Withdrawal (coitus interruptus)	Man withdraws before ejaculation	19%	Involves no devices and is always available	Requires considerable self-control by the man	None	None	Places woman in trusting and dependent role

Method	Description	Failure rate	Advantages	Disadvantages		Contraindications	Nursing considerations
Lactational amenorrhea method (LAM)	Uses lactational infertility for protection from pregnancy	1–2% chance of pregnancy in first 6 months	No cost Not coitus-linked	Temporary method; effective for only 6 months after giving birth	None	None	Mother must breastfeed infant on demand without supplementation for 6 months
Male condom	Thin sheath placed over an erect penis, blocking sperm	14%	Widely available; low cost; physiologically safe	Decreased sensation for man; interferes with sexual spontaneity; breakage	Provides protection against STIs	Latex allergy	Couple must be instructed on proper use of condom
Female condom	Polyurethane sheath inserted vaginally to block sperm	21%	Use controlled by woman; eliminates postcoital drainage of semen	Expensive for frequent use; cumbersome; noisy during sex act; for single use only	Provides protection against STIs	Allergy to polyurethane	Couple must be instructed on proper use of condom
Diaphragm with spermicide	Shallow latex cup with spring mechanism in its rim to hold it in place in the vagina	20%	Does not use hormones; considered medically safe; provides some protection against cervical cancer	Requires accurate fitting by healthcare professional; increase in UTIs	None	Allergy to latex, rubber, polyurethane, or spermicide Report symptoms of toxic shock syndrome; change size if excessive weight gain or loss	Woman must be taught to insert and remove diaphragm correctly.
Cervical cap with spermicide	Soft cup-shaped latex device that fits over base of cervix	17%	No use of hormones; provides continuous protection while in place	Requires accurate fitting by healthcare professional; odor may occur if left in too long	None	Irritation, allergic reaction; abnormal Pap test; risk of toxic shock syndrome	Instructions on insertion and removal must be understood by client.

(continued)

Table 4-5 Summary of Contraceptive Methods (continued)

Type	Description	Failure Rate	Pros	Cons	STI Protection	Danger Signs	Comments
Sponge with spermicide	Disk-shaped polyurethane device containing a spermicide that is activated by wetting it with water	14–28%	Offers immediate and continuous protection for 24 hours; OTC	Can fall out of vagina with voiding; is not form-fitting in the vagina	None	Irritation, allergic reactions; toxic shock syndrome can occur if sponge left in too long	Caution woman not to leave sponge in beyond 24 hours.
Oral contra-ceptives (combina-tion)	A pill that suppresses ovulation by combined action of estrogen and progestin	1%	Easy to use; high rate of effectiveness; protection against ovarian and endometrial cancer	User must remember to take pill daily; user may experience undesirable side effects; high cost for some women; prescription needed	None	Dizziness, nausea, mood changes, high blood pressure, blood clots, heart attacks, strokes	Each woman must be assessed thoroughly to make sure she is not a smoker and does not have a history of thrombo-embolic disease.
Oral contra-ceptives (progestin-only minipills)	A pill containing only progestin that thickens cervical mucus to prevent sperm from penetrating	2%	No estrogen-related side effects; may be used by lactating women; may be used by women with history of thrombo-phlebitis	Must be taken with meticulous accuracy; may cause irregular bleeding; less effective than combination pills	None	Irregular bleeding, weight gain, increased incidence of ectopic pregnancy	Women should be screened for history of functional ovarian cysts, previous ectopic pregnancy, hyperlipi-demia prior to giving prescription

Method	Description	Failure rate	Advantages	Disadvantages	Contraindications	Side effects	Nursing considerations
Lunelle injectable	An injectable form of progestin and estrogen given monthly	<1%	Woman will regain fertility 2–3 months after last injection; no need for daily pill taking	Must make arrangements for monthly injection; possible weight gain	None	Irregular spotting; similar to oral combination pills	Screen potential candidate's ability to schedule monthly appointment for injection
The patch (Ortho Evra)	Transdermal patch that releases estrogen and progestin into circulation	1%	Easy system to remember; very effective	May cause skin irritation where it is placed; may fall off and not be noticed and thus provide no protection	None	Less effective in women weighing > 200 pound	Instruct woman to apply patch every week for 3 weeks and then not to wear one during week 4
The ring (NuvaRing)	Vaginal contraceptive ring about 2 inches in diameter that is inserted into the vagina; releases estrogen and progestin	1%	Easy system to remember; very effective	May cause a vaginal discharge; can be expelled without noticing and not offer protection	None	Similar to oral contraceptives	Instruct woman to use a backup method if ring is expelled and remains out for > 3 hours
Depo-Provera injection	An injectable progestin that inhibits ovulation	<1%	Long duration of action (3 months); highly effective; estrogen-free; may be used by smokers; can be used by lactating women	Menstrual irregularities; return visit needed every 12 weeks; weight gain, headaches, depression; return to fertility delayed up to 12 months	None	If depression is a problem, this method may increase the depression.	Inform woman that fertility is delayed after stopping the injections.

(continued)

Table 4–5 Summary of Contraceptive Methods (continued)

Type	Description	Failure Rate	Pros	Cons	STI Protection	Danger Signs	Comments
Implant (Norplant) As of 2003, the manufacturer decided not to continue to market this device.	A time-release implant (matchstick rods) of levonorgestrel for 5 years	<1%	Long duration of action; low dose of hormones; reversible; estrogen-free	Irregular bleeding; weight gain; breast tenderness; headaches; difficulty in removal	None	If bleeding is heavy, anemia may occur.	Before insertion, assess woman to make sure she is aware that this method will produce about 5 years of infertility
Intrauterine devices (IUDs)	A T-shaped device inserted into the uterus that releases copper or progesterone or levonorgestrel	<1%	Is immediately and highly effective; allows for sexual spontaneity; can be used during lactation; return to fertility not impaired; requires no motivation by the user after insertion	Insertion requires a skilled professional; menstrual irregularities; prolonged amenorrhea; can be unknowingly expelled; may increase the risk of pelvic infection; user must regularly check string for placement; no protection against STIs; delay of fertility after discontinuing for possibly 6 to 12 months	None	Cramps, bleeding, pelvic inflammatory disease; infertility; perforation of the uterus	Instruct woman how to locate string to check monthly for placement

Postcoital emergency contraceptives (ECs)	Combination or progestin-only pills taken within 72 hours after unprotected intercourse	80%	Provides a last chance to prevent a pregnancy	Risk of ectopic pregnancy if EC fails	None	Nausea, vomiting, abdominal pain, fatigue, headache	Inform woman that ECs do not interrupt an established pregnancy, and the sooner they are taken, the more effective they are.
Permanent sterilization Male	Sealing, tying, or cutting the vas deferens	<1%	One-time decision provides permanent sterility; short recovery time; low long-term risks	Procedures are difficult to reverse; initial cost may be high; chance of regret; some pain/discomfort after procedures	None for both	Post operative complications—pain, bleeding, infection	Counsel both as to permanence of procedure and urge them to think it through prior to signing consent
Female	Fallopian tubes are blocked to prevent conception	<1%					

Sources: Samra, 2003; FDA, 2002; Youngkin & Davis, 2004; Hatcher, 2004; and Sloane, 2002.

bodily changes start to occur before ovulation, the woman can become aware of them and not have intercourse on these days or use another method to prevent pregnancy.

• The exact time of ovulation cannot be determined, so 2 to 3 days are added to the beginning and end to avoid pregnancy

Techniques used to determine fertility include the cervical mucus ovulation method, the basal body temperature (BBT) method, and the symptothermal method (Hatcher et al., 2004).

Fertility awareness methods are moderately effective but are very unforgiving if not carried out as prescribed: not following the guidelines might cause a 27% failure or pregnancy rate per cycle (Youngkin & Davis, 2004). Fertility awareness can be used in combination with coital abstinence or barrier methods during fertile days if pregnancy is not desired.

Cervical Mucus Ovulation Method

The **cervical mucus ovulation method** is used to assess the character of the cervical mucus. Cervical mucus changes consistency during the menstrual cycle and plays a vital role in fertilization of the egg. In the days preceding ovulation, fertile cervical mucus helps draw sperm up and into the fallopian tubes, where fertilization usually takes place. It also helps maintain the survival of sperm. As ovulation approaches, the mucus becomes more abundant, clear, slippery, and smooth; it can be stretched between two fingers without breaking. Under the influence of estrogen, this mucus looks like egg whites. It is called spinnbarkeit mucus (Fig. 4-5). After ovulation, the cervical mucus becomes thick and dry under the influence of progesterone.

The cervical position can also be assessed to confirm changes in the cervical mucus at ovulation. Near ovulation, the cervix feels soft and is high/deep in the vagina, the os is slightly open, and the cervical mucus is copious and slippery (Hatcher et al., 2002).

This method works because the woman becomes aware of her body changes that accompany ovulation. When she notices them, she abstains from sexual intercourse or uses another method to prevent pregnancy. Each woman is an individual, so each woman's unsafe time of the month is unique. In using this method, one size doesn't fit all.

Basal Body Temperature

The **basal body temperature (BBT)** refers to the lowest temperature reached upon wakening. The woman takes her temperature orally before rising and records it on a chart. Preovulation temperatures are suppressed by estrogen, whereas postovulation temperatures are increased under the influence of heat-inducing progesterone. Temperatures typically rise within a day or two after ovulation and remain elevated for approximately 2 weeks (at which point bleeding usually begins). If using this method by itself, the woman should avoid unprotected intercourse until the BBT has been elevated for 3 days.

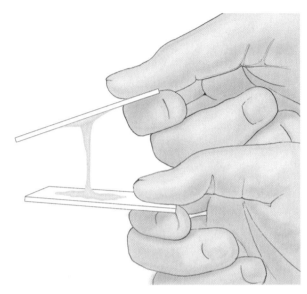

● Figure 4-5 Spinnbarkeit is the property of cervical mucus to stretch a distance before breaking.

Other fertility awareness methods should be used along with BBT for better results (Fig. 4-6).

Symptothermal Method

The **symptothermal method** relies on a combination of techniques to recognize ovulation, including BBT, cervical mucus changes, alterations in the position and firmness of the cervix, and other symptoms of ovulation, such as increased libido, mittelschmerz, pelvic fullness or tenderness, and breast tenderness (Sloane, 2002). Combining all these predictors increases awareness of when ovulation occurs and increases the effectiveness of this method. A home predictor test for ovulation is also available in most pharmacies. It measures LH levels to pinpoint the day before or the day of ovulation. These are widely used for fertility and infertility regimens.

The Standard Days Method

The **Standard Days Method (SDM)** is a new natural method of contraception developed by Georgetown University Medical Center's Institute for Reproductive Health. Women with menstrual cycles between 26 and 32 days long can use the SDM to prevent pregnancy by avoiding unprotected intercourse on days 8 through 19 of their cycles. An international clinical trial of the SDM showed that the method is more than 95% effective when used correctly (Arevalo & Sinai, 2003). SDM identifies the 12-day "fertile window" of a woman's menstrual cycle. These 12 days takes into account the lifespan of the women's egg (about 24 hours) and the viability of the sperm (about 5 days) as well as the variation in the actual timing of ovulation from one cycle to another.

To help women keep track of the days on which they should avoid unprotected intercourse, a string of 32 color-

Basal body temperature

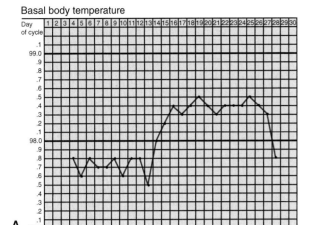

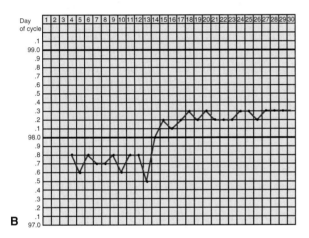

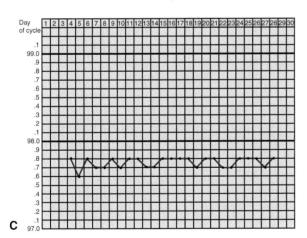

● Figure 4-6 Basal body temperature graph. (**A**) The woman's temperature dips slightly at midpoint in the menstrual cycle, then rises sharply, an indication of ovulation. Toward the end of the cycle (the 24th day), her temperature begins to decline, indicating that progesterone levels are falling and that she did not conceive. (**B**) The woman's temperature rises at the midpoint in the cycle and remains at that elevated level past the time of her normal menstrual flow, suggesting that pregnancy has occurred. (**C**) There is no preovulatory dip, and no rise of temperature anywhere during the cycle. This is the typical pattern of a woman who does not ovulate.

coded beads (CycleBeads) is used, with each bead representing a day of the menstrual cycle. Starting with the red bead, which represents the first day of her menstrual period, the woman moves a small rubber ring one bead each day. The brown beads are the days when pregnancy is unlikely, and the white beads represent her fertile days (Arevalo, 2003). This method has been used in underdeveloped countries for women with limited educational resources (Fig. 4-7).

Withdrawal (Coitus Interruptus)

In withdrawal, or **coitus interruptus,** a man controls his ejaculation during sexual intercourse and ejaculates outside the vagina. It is better known colloquially as "pulling out in time" or "being careful." It is one of the oldest and most widely used means of preventing pregnancy in the world (Sloane, 2002). The problem with this method is that the first few drops of the true ejaculate contain the greatest concentration of sperm, and if some pre-ejaculatory fluid escapes from the urethra before orgasm, conception may result. This method requires that the woman rely solely on the cooperation and judgment of the man.

Lactational Amenorrhea Method

The **lactational amenorrhea method (LAM)** is an effective temporary method of contraception used by breastfeeding mothers. Continuous breastfeeding can postpone ovulation and thus prevent pregnancy. Breastfeeding stimulates the hormone prolactin, which is necessary for milk production and also inhibits the release of another hormone, gonadotropin, which is necessary for ovulation.

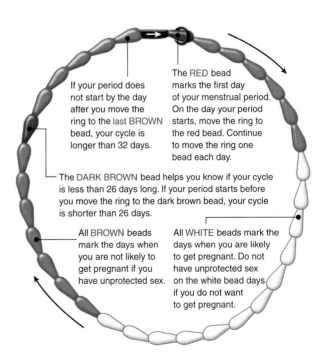

● Figure 4-7 CycleBeads help women use the Standard Days Method.

Breastfeeding as a contraceptive method can be effective for 6 months after delivery only if a woman:

- Has not had a period since she gave birth
- Breastfeeds her baby at least six times daily on both breasts
- Breastfeeds her baby "on demand" at least every 4 hours
- Does not substitute other foods for a breast-milk meal
- Provides nighttime feedings at least every 6 hours
- Does not rely on this method after 6 months (Planned Parenthood, 2005)

Barrier Methods

Barrier contraceptives are forms of birth control that prevent pregnancy by preventing the sperm from reaching the ovum. Mechanical barriers include condoms, diaphragms, cervical caps, and sponges. These devices are placed over the penis or cervix to prevent passage of sperm. They physically obstruct the passage of sperm through the cervix. Chemical barriers called spermicides may be used along with mechanical barrier devices. They come in creams, jellies, foam, suppositories, and vaginal films. They chemically destroy the sperm in the vagina.

These contraceptives are called barrier methods because they not only provide a physical barrier for sperm, but also protect against STIs. Since the HIV/AIDS epidemic started in the early 1980s, these methods have become extremely popular.

Many of these barrier methods contain latex. Allergy to latex was first recognized in the late 1970s, and since then it has become a major health concern, with increasing numbers of people affected. According to the American Academy of Allergy, Asthma and Immunology (2004), 6% of the general population, 10% of healthcare workers, and 50% of spina bifida patients are sensitive to natural rubber latex. Since the late 1980s, with the establishment of policies dictating barrier requirements resulting from the HIV/AIDS epidemic, there has been an exponential increase in the use of latex gloves and condoms (Lenehan, 2004). Teaching Guidelines 4-4 provides tips for individuals with latex allergy.

Condoms

Condoms are made for both males and females. The male condom is made from latex or polyurethane or natural membrane and may be coated with spermicide. Male condoms are available in many colors, textures, sizes, shapes, and thicknesses. When used correctly, the male condom is put on over an erect penis before it enters the vagina and is worn throughout sexual intercourse (Fig. 4-8).

The female condom is a polyurethane pouch inserted into the vagina. It consists of an outer and inner ring that is inserted vaginally and held in place by the pubic bone. Some women complain that the female condom is cumbersome to use and makes noise during intercourse. Female condoms are readily available, are inexpensive, and can be carried inconspicuously by the woman. The female

TEACHING GUIDELINES 4-4

Tips for Individuals Allergic to Latex

- Symptoms of latex allergy include:
  ○ Skin rash, itching, hives
  ○ Itching or burning eyes
  ○ Swollen mucous membranes in the genitals
  ○ Shortness of breath, difficulty breathing, wheezing
  ○ Anaphylactic shock (OSHA, 2003)
- Use of or contact with latex condoms, cervical caps, and diaphragms is contraindicated for men and women with a latex allergy.
- If the female partner is allergic to latex, have the male partner apply a natural condom over the latex one.
- If the male partner experiences penile irritation after condom use, try different brands or place the latex condom over a natural condom.
- Use polyurethane condoms rather than latex ones.
- Use female condoms; they are made out of polyurethane.
- Switch to another birth control method that isn't made with latex, such as oral contraceptives, IUDs, Depo-Provera, fertility awareness, and other non-barrier methods. However, these methods do not protect against sexually transmitted infections.

condom is the first contraceptive device to protect women against STIs under her control.

Diaphragm

The **diaphragm** is a soft latex dome surrounded by a metal spring. Used in conjunction with a spermicidal jelly or cream, it is inserted into the vagina to cover the cervix (Fig. 4-9). The diaphragm may be inserted up to 4 hours before intercourse but must be left in place for at least 6 hours afterwards. Diaphragms are available in a range of sizes and styles. The diaphragm is available only by prescription and must be professionally fitted by a healthcare professional. The device should be replaced every 2 years and may need to be refitted after weight loss or gain or term birth (Hatcher et al., 2004). The woman also needs to receive thorough instruction about its use and should practice putting it in and taking it out before she leaves the medical office (Fig. 4-10). This contraceptive is not effective unless it is used correctly.

Cervical Cap

The **cervical cap** is smaller than the diaphragm and covers only the cervix; it is held there by suction. Caps are made from rubber and are used with spermicide the same way diaphragms are (Fig. 4-11). The cap may be inserted up to 12 hours before intercourse and provides protection for 48 hours. The dome of the cap is filled about one-third

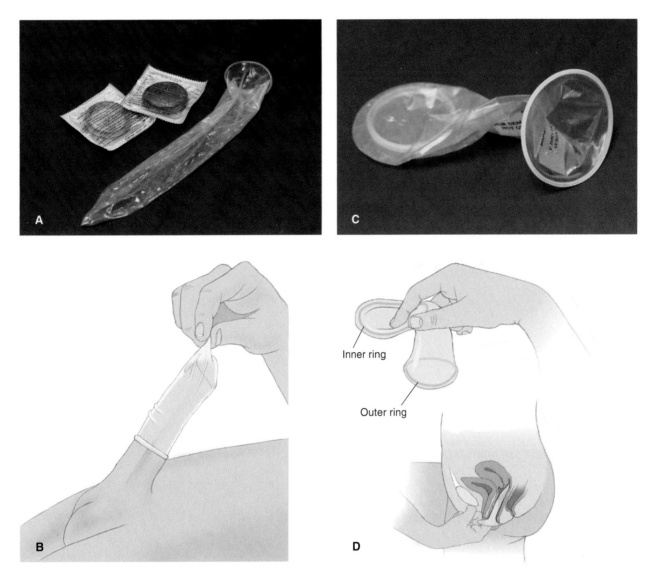

● Figure 4-8 (**A**) Male condom. (**B**) Applying a male condom. Being certain that space is left at the tip helps to ensure the condom will not break with ejaculation. (**C**) The female condom. (**D**) Insertion technique.

full with spermicide. Spermicide should not be applied to the rim because it might interfere with the seal that must form around the cervix. The cap is available only by prescription and must be fitted by a healthcare professional.

Contraceptive Sponge

After being removed from the market in 1995, the **contraceptive sponge** is once again being marketed to women after receiving approval from the U.S. Food and Drug Administration (FDA). It should be available in summer 2005 (Weise, 2005). At one time, it was a very popular nonprescription birth control device for women, but a decade ago Wyeth stopped making it rather than upgrade its manufacturing plant after the FDA found deficiencies there, even though the device's effectiveness and safety were never questioned.

The contraceptive sponge is a soft concave device that prevents pregnancy by covering the cervix and releasing spermicide. While it was less effective than several other methods and does not offer protection against STIs, the sponge achieved a wide following among women who appreciated the spontaneity with which it could be used and its easy availability.

Hormonal Methods

Several options are available to women who want long-term but not permanent protection against pregnancy. These methods of contraception work by altering the hormones within a woman's body. They rely on estrogen and progestin or progestin alone to prevent ovulation. When used consistently, these methods are a most reliable way

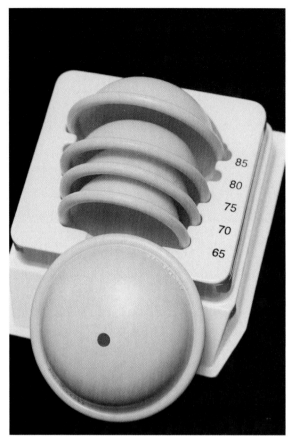

● Figure 4-9 Diaphragm.

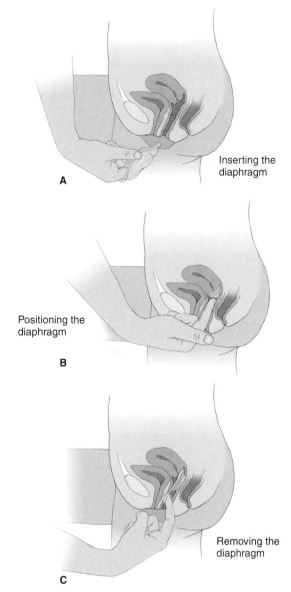

● Figure 4-10 Application of a diaphragm. (**A**) To insert, fold the diaphragm in half, separate the labia with one hand, then insert upwards and back into the vagina. (**B**) To position, make certain the diaphragm securely covers the cervix. (**C**) To remove, hook a finger over the top of the rim and bring the diaphragm down and out.

to prevent pregnancy. Hormonal methods include oral contraceptives, injectables, implants, vaginal rings, and transdermal patches.

Oral Contraceptives

As early as 1937, scientists recognized that the injection of progesterone inhibited ovulation in rabbits and provided contraception. Breakthrough bleeding was reported in early clinical trials in women, and the role of estrogen in cycle control was launched. This established the rationale for modern combination **oral contraceptives** (OCs) that contain both estrogen and progesterone (Wysocki et al., 2002). In 1960 the FDA approved the first combination OC, Enovid-10 (150 mcg estrogen and 9 mg progesterone) for use in the United States.

Today, nearly 50 combination OCs are available in the United States. The most notable change in over 40 years of OC improvement has been the lowering of the estrogen dose to as low as 20 mcg and the introduction of new progestins. Oral contraceptives are the most popular method of nonsurgical contraception, used by approximately 18 million women in the United States (Wysocki et al., 2002) (Fig. 4-12).

Unlike the original OCs that women took decades ago, the new low-dose forms have fewer health risks attached to them. OCs, while most commonly prescribed

for contraception, have long been used in the management of a wide range of conditions and have many health benefits, such as:

- Reduced incidence of ovarian and endometrial cancer
- Prevention and treatment of endometriosis
- Decreased incidence of acne and hirsutism
- Decreased incidence of ectopic pregnancy
- Decreased incidence of acute PID
- Reduced incidence of fibrocystic breast disease
- Decreased perimenopausal symptoms
- Increased menstrual cycle regularity

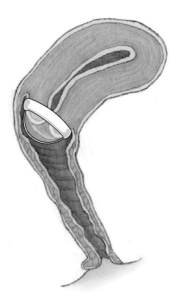

● Figure 4-11 A cervical cap is placed over the cervix and used with a spermicidal jelly the same as a diaphragm.

• Protection against colorectal cancer
• Reduced iron-deficiency anemia by treating menorrhagia
• Reduced incidence of dysmenorrhea (Zieman, 2002)

OCs work primarily by suppressing ovulation by adding estrogen and progesterone to a woman's body, thus mimicking pregnancy. This hormonal level stifles gonadotropin-releasing hormone (GnRH), which in turn suppresses FSH and LH and thus inhibits ovulation. Cervical mucus also thickens, which hinders sperm transport into the uterus. Implantation is inhibited by suppression of the maturation of the endometrium and alterations of uterine secretions (Trussell, 2003).

The combination pills are prescribed as monophasic pills, which deliver fixed dosages of estrogen and progestin, or as multiphasic ones. Multiphasic pills (e.g., biphasic and triphasic OCs) alter the amount of progestin and estrogen within each cycle. To maintain adequate hormonal levels

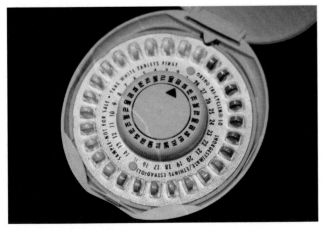

● Figure 4-12 Oral contraceptive.

for contraception and enhance compliance, OCs should be taken at the same time daily (Lowdermilk & Perry, 2004).

OCs that contain progestin only are called *minipills.* They are prescribed for women who cannot take estrogen. They work primarily by thickening the cervical mucus to prevent penetration of the sperm and make the endometrium unfavorable for implantation. Progestin-only pills must be taken at a certain time every 24 hours. Breakthrough bleeding and a higher risk of pregnancy have made these OCs less popular than combination OCs (Murray et al., 2006).

Extended OC regimens have been used for the management of menstrual disorders and endometriosis for years but now are attracting wider attention. Surveys asking women about their willingness to reduce their menstrual cycles from 12 to 4 annually were returned with a resounding "yes!" (Sulak et al., 2002). Recent studies have shown that the extended use of active OC pills carries the same safety profile as the conventional 28-day regimens (Wysocki et al., 2002). The extended regimen consists of 84 consecutive days of active combination pills, followed by 7 days of placebo. The woman has four withdrawal-bleeding episodes a year. Seasonale, a combination OC, is on the market for women who choose to reduce the number of periods that they have.

The balance between the benefits and the risks of OCs must be determined for each woman when she is being assessed for this type of contraceptive. It is a highly effective contraceptive when taken properly but can aggravate many medical conditions, especially in women who smoke. Table 4-6 lists advantages and disadvantages of OCs. A thorough history and pelvic examination, including a Pap smear, must be completed before the medication is prescribed and yearly thereafter.

Nurses need to provide OC users with a great deal of education before they leave the health care facility. They need to be able to identify early signs and symptoms that might indicate a problem. The mnemonic "ACHES" can help women remember the early warning signs that necessitate a return to the health care provider (Box 4-6).

Injectable Contraceptives

The **Lunelle injection** is a long-term reversible contraceptive for women. It contains the same hormones as the combination OCs. It is administered once every 28 to 33 days by intramuscular injection. It provides immediate, very effective contraception if given within 5 days after the last normal menses. Its mechanism of action, contraindications, and side effects are similar to those of oral contraceptives (Hatcher et al., 2004).

Depo-Provera is the trade name for an injectable contraceptive that delivers progesterone every 12 weeks. Depo-Provera works by suppressing ovulation and the production of FSH and LH by the pituitary gland. A single injection of 150 mg into the buttocks acts like other

Table 4-6 Advantages and Disadvantages of Oral Contraceptives

Advantages	Disadvantages
Regulate and shorten menstrual cycle	Offer no protection against STIs
Decrease severe cramping and bleeding	Pose slightly increased risk of breast cancer
Reduce anemia	Modest risk for vein thrombosis and pulmonary emboli
Reduce ovarian and colorectal cancer risk	Increased risk for migraine headaches
Decrease benign breast disease	Increased risk for myocardial infarction, stroke, and hypertension for women who smoke
Reduce risk of endometrial cancer	
Improve acne	May increase risk of depression
Minimize perimenopausal symptoms	User must remember to take pill daily
Decrease incidence of rheumatoid arthritis	High cost for some women (Dickey, 2002)
Improve PMS symptoms	
Protection against loss of bone density	

progestin-only products to prevent pregnancy for 3 months at a time (Fig. 4-13).

Transdermal Patches

A **transdermal patch,** Ortho Evra, is also available. The patch is applied weekly for 3 weeks, followed by a patch-free week during which withdrawal bleeding occurs. The patch delivers continuous levels of progesterone and estrogen. Recommended application sites include the upper arm, buttocks, and lower abdomen. Compliance with combination contraceptive patch use has been shown to be significantly greater than compliance with OCs (Herndon & Zieman, 2004). The patch provides combination hormone therapy with a side effect profile similar to that of OCs. The manufacturer is currently evaluating extended regimens for the patch (Youngkin & Davis, 2004) (Fig. 4-14).

Vaginal Rings

The contraceptive **vaginal ring,** NuvaRing, is a flexible, soft, transparent ring that is inserted by the user for a

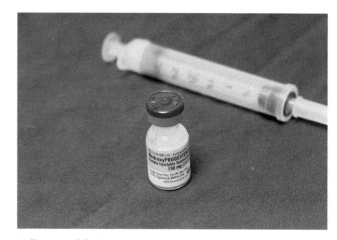

● Figure 4-13 Injectable contraceptive.

BOX 4-6

EARLY SIGNS OF COMPLICATIONS FOR OC USERS

A Abdominal pain may indicate liver or gallbladder problems.

C Chest pain or shortness of breath may indicate a pulmonary embolus.

H Headaches may indicate hypertension or impending stroke.

E Eye problems might indicate hypertension or a attack.

S Severe leg pain may indicate a thromboembolic event (Lowdermilk & Perry, 2004).

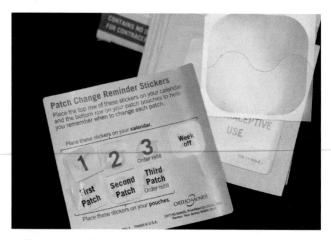

● Figure 4-14 Transdermal patch.

3-week period of continuous use followed by a ring-free week to allow withdrawal bleeding (Fig. 4-15). The ring can be inserted by the woman and does not have to be fitted. The woman compresses the ring and inserts it into the vagina, behind the pubic bone, as far back as possible, but precise placement is not critical. The hormones are absorbed through the vaginal mucosa. It is left in place for 3 weeks and then removed and discarded. Effectiveness and adverse events are similar to those seen with combination OCs. Clients need to be counseled regarding timely insertion of the ring and what to do in case of accidental expulsion. This device is also being tested for extended regimens to reduce menstrual bleeding.

Implantable Contraceptives

Norplant is a subdermal time-release implant that delivers synthetic progestin, levonorgestrel. Once in place, it delivers 5 years of continuous, highly effective contraception. The original system consists of six Silastic capsules that are implanted in a fanlike pattern through a small incision, usually on the inside of a woman's upper arm. A one- and two-capsule Norplant system has been approved by the FDA but has not been marketed yet in the United States (Hatcher et al., 2002). Norplant, like progestin-only pills, acts by thickening cervical mucus so sperm cannot penetrate. The side effects are also similar to progestin-only pills: irregular bleeding, headaches, weight gain, breast tenderness, and depression. Fertility is restored quickly after it is removed. Norplant requires a minor surgical procedure for both insertion and removal. It is not currently available in the United States.

Intrauterine Devices (IUDs)

Intrauterine devices (IUDs) are small plastic T-shaped objects that are placed inside the uterus to provide contraception (Fig. 4-16). They prevent pregnancy by making the endometrium of the uterus hostile to implantation of a fertilized ovum by causing a nonspecific inflammatory reaction (Sloane, 2002). They may contain copper or progesterone to enhance their effectiveness. One or two attached strings protrude into the vagina so that the user can check for placement.

Currently there are three IUDs available in the United States: the copper ParaGard-T-380A; Progestasert, a progesterone device; and the levonorgestrel intrauterine system (LNG-IUS) Mirena, a levonorgestrel-releasing device. The ParaGard-T-380A is approved for 10 years of use. The Progestasert may stay in place 1 year, then must be removed and replaced. Mirena provides intrauterine conception for up to 5 years (Wysocki et al., 2002). Box 4-7 highlights warning signs of potential complications.

Emergency Contraception

Emergency contraception (EC) reduces the risk of pregnancy after unprotected intercourse or contraceptive failure such as condom breakage (Sloane, 2002). It is used within 72 hours of unprotected intercourse to prevent pregnancy. The sooner ECs are taken, the more effective they are. They reduce the risk of pregnancy for a single act of unprotected sex by almost 80% (Weismiller, 2004). The four methods available in the United States are progestin-only OCs, combination OCs, EC kits (Preven or Plan B; Fig. 4-17), and preemptive endometrial aspiration. Table 4-7 lists recommended oral medication and intrauterine regimens.

Contrary to popular belief, ECs do not induce abortion and are not related to Mifepristone or RU-486, the so-called abortion pill approved by the FDA in 2000. Mifepristone chemically induces abortion by blocking the body's progesterone receptors, which are necessary for pregnancy maintenance. ECs simply prevent embryo creation and uterine implantation from occurring in the first place. There is no evidence that ECs have any effect on an already implanted ovum. The side effects are nausea and vomiting.

Abortion

Abortion is defined as the expulsion of an embryo or fetus before it is viable (Alexander et al., 2004). Abortion can be a medical or surgical procedure. The purpose of abortion is to terminate a pregnancy. Surgical abortion is the most common procedure performed in the United States, approximately 1.6 million annually, and might be the most common surgical procedure in the world (Speroff & Fritz, 2005). Both medical and surgical abortions are safe and legal in the United States; an abortion is considered a woman's constitutional right based on the fundamental right to privacy (Sloane, 2002).

Since the landmark U.S. Supreme Court decision *Roe v. Wade* legalized abortion in 1973, debate has continued over how and when abortions are provided. Every state has laws regulating some aspects of the provision of abortion, and many have passed restrictions such as parental consent or notification requirements, mandated counseling and waiting periods, and limits on funding for abortion.

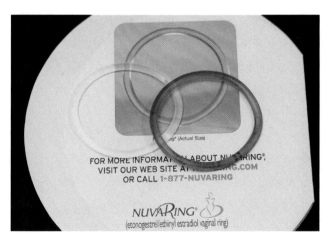

● Figure 4-15 Vaginal ring.

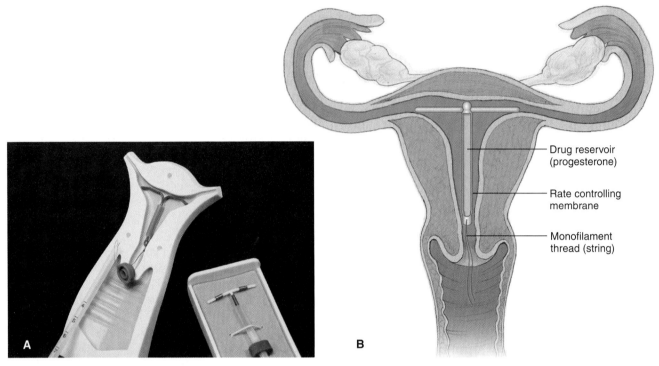

Drug reservoir
(progesterone)

Rate controlling
membrane

Monofilament
thread (string)

● Figure 4-16 (**A**) Intrauterine device. (**B**) An IUD in place in the uterus.

Each state addresses these matters independently, and the laws that are passed or enforced are a legislative decision and a function of the political system. Although opponents of abortion continue to be very much a part of the current debates, recently they have refocused their attention on "regulation legislation" to reduce the number of abortions not medically necessary. For this continuing emotional debate, we will all have to stay tuned to see what the future holds within the political arena.

Surgical Abortion

Surgical abortion is usually carried out by vacuum aspiration or suction curettage. It is an ambulatory procedure done under local anesthesia. The cervix is dilated prior to surgery and then the products of conception are removed by suction evacuation. The uterus may gently be scraped by curettage to make sure that the uterus is empty. The entire procedure lasts about 10 minutes.

Medical Abortion

In a *medical abortion,* the woman takes certain medications to induce a miscarriage to remove the products of conception. There are two methods currently used to terminate a pregnancy during the first trimester. The first method uses methotrexate (an antineoplastic agent) followed by misoprostol (a prostaglandin agent) given as a vaginal suppository or in oral form 3 to 7 days later. Methotrexate induces abortion because of its toxicity to trophoblastic tissue, the growing embryo. Misoprostol works by causing uterine contractions, which helps to expel the products of conception. This method is 90% to 98% successful in completing an abortion (Hatcher et al., 2004).

BOX 4-7

WARNINGS FOR IUD USERS OF POTENTIAL COMPLICATIONS

P Period late, pregnancy, abnormal spotting or bleeding
A Abdominal pain, pain with intercourse
I Infection exposure, abnormal vaginal discharge
N Not feeling well, fever, chills
S String length shorter or longer or missing
(Hatcher et al., 2002)

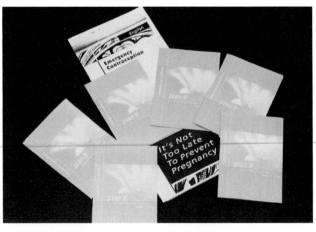

● Figure 4-17 Emergency contraceptive kit.

Table 4-7 Emergency Contraception (EC) Options

Product	First Dose (Within 72 Hours)	Second Dose (Taken 12 Hours Later)
Combined OCs Preven Ovral	2 tablets	2 tablets
Lo/Ovral, Nordette Levlen, TriLevlen Triphasil	4 tablets	4 tablets
Progestin-Only OCs Ovrette	20 tablets	20 tablets
Plan B	1 tablet	1 tablet
Intrauterine Devices Copper-containing IUD such as Paragard-T-380A	Inserted within 7 days after unprotected sexual episode	Can be left in for long-term contraception

The second method used to induce first-trimester abortions involves using mifepristone (a progesterone antagonist) followed 48 hours later by misoprostol (a prostaglandin agent), which causes contractions of the uterus and expulsion of the uterine contents. Mifepristone, the generic name for RU-486, is sold under the brand names Mifeprex and Early Option. Mifepristone is a potent oral anti-progestogen; it blocks the action of progesterone that prepares the endometrium for implantation and then maintains the pregnancy. This method is 95% effective when used within 49 days after the last menstrual cycle (Hatcher et al., 2004).

Sterilization

Sterilization is an attractive method of contraception for those who are certain they do not want any or more children. Sterilization refers to surgical procedures intended to render the person infertile (Lowdermilk & Perry, 2004). Sterilization is among the most popular method of contraception in the United States and worldwide (Youngkin & Davis, 2004). More women than men undergo surgical sterilization. According to the U.S. Centers for Disease Control & Prevention (CDC), approximately 18% of women undergo female sterilization in comparison to 7% of men in the United States (CDC, 2004). Sterilization should be considered a permanent end to fertility because reversal surgery is difficult, expensive, and not highly successful.

Tubal Ligation

Tubal ligation, the sterilization procedure for women, can be performed postpartum, after an abortion, or as an interval procedure unrelated to pregnancy. A laparoscope is inserted through a small subumbilical incision to provide a view of the fallopian tubes. They are grasped and sealed with a cauterizing instrument or with rings, bands, or clips or cut, and tied (Fig. 4-18).

A new approach used to visualize the fallopian tubes is through the cervix instead of the abdominal incision. This procedure, called transcervical sterilization, offers several advantages over conventional tubal ligation: general anesthesia and incisions are not needed, thereby increasing safety, lowering costs, and improving access to sterilization. A tiny coil is introduced and released into the fallopian tubes through the cervix. The coil promotes tissue growth in the fallopian tubes, and over a period of 3 months, this growth blocks the tubes (Schwartz & Gabelnick, 2002). This new technique has become increasingly popular.

Vasectomy

Male sterilization is accomplished with a surgical procedure known as a **vasectomy.** It is usually performed under local anesthesia in an urologist's office, and most men can return to work and normal activities in a day or two. The procedure involves making a small incision into the scrotum and cutting the vas deferens, which carries sperm from the testes to the penis (Fig. 4-19). After vasectomy, semen no longer contains sperm. This is not immediate, though, and the man must submit semen specimens for analysis until two specimens show that no sperm is present (Murray & McKinney, 2006).

Nursing Management

The choice of a contraceptive method is a very personal one involving many factors. What makes a woman choose

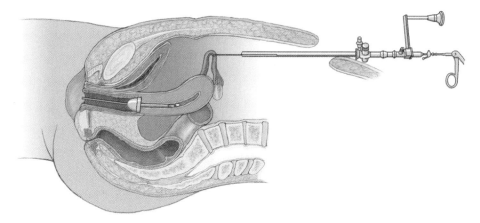

● Figure 4-18 Laparoscopy for tubal sterilization.

one contraceptive method over another? In making contraceptive choices, couples must balance their sexual lives, their reproductive goals, and each partner's health and safety. The search for a choice that satisfies all three objectives is challenging. A method that works for a sexually active teenage girl may not meet her needs later in life. Several considerations influence a person's choice of contraceptives:

- Motivation
- Cost
- Cultural and religious beliefs (Box 4-8)
- Convenience
- Effectiveness
- Side effects
- Desire for children in the future
- Safety of the method
- Comfort level with sexuality
- Protection from STIs
- Interference with spontaneity

If a contraceptive is to be effective, the woman must understand how it works, must be able to use it correctly and consistently, and must be comfortable and confident with it.

A nurse can provide clients with facts to help them decide which contraceptive method is right for them. The nurse can educate clients about which methods are available and their advantages and disadvantages, efficacy, cost, and safety.

Assessment

When assessing which contraceptive method might meet the client's needs, the nurse might ask:

- Do your religious beliefs interfere with any methods?
- Will this method interfere with your sexual pleasure?
- Are you aware of the various methods currently available?
- Is cost a major consideration, or does your insurance cover it?
- Does your partner influence which method you choose?
- Have you heard anything troubling about any of the methods?
- How comfortable are you touching your own body?
- What are your future plans for having children?

Counseling can help the woman choose a contraceptive method that is efficacious and fits her personal preferences and lifestyle. Although deciding on a contraceptive is a very personal decision between a woman and her

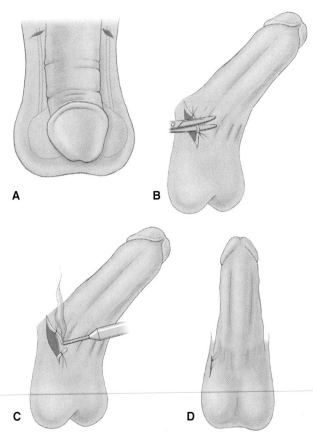

● Figure 4-19 Vasectomy. (**A**) Site of vasectomy incisions. (**B**) The vas deferens being cut with surgical scissors. (**C**) Cut ends of the vas deferens are cauterized to completely ensure blockage of the passage of sperm. (**D**) Final skin suture.

A **B** **C** **D**

SELECTED RELIGIOUS CHOICES FOR FAMILY PLANNING AND ABORTION

- Roman Catholic—Abstinence and natural family planning; no abortion
- Judaism—Yes for family planning and abortion in first trimester
- Islam—Family planning accepted; abortion only for serious reasons
- Protestant Christianity—Firmly in favor of family planning; mixed on abortion
- Buddhism—Long experience with family planning and abortion
- Hinduism—Accept both family planning and abortion
- Native American religions—Accept both family planning and abortion
- Chinese religions—Taoism and Confucianism accept both (Maguire, 2004)

partner, nurses can assist in this process by assessing the following areas:

- Medical history: smoking status, cancer of reproductive tract, diabetes mellitus, migraines, hypertension, thromboembolic disorder, allergies, risk factors for cardiovascular disease
- Family history: cancer, cardiovascular disease, hypertension, stroke, diabetes
- OB/GYN history: menstrual disorders, current contraceptive, previous STIs, PID, vaginitis, sexual activity
- Personal history: use of tampons and female hygiene products, plans for childbearing, comfort with touching herself, number of sexual partners and their involvement in the decision
- Diagnostic testing: urinalysis, complete blood count, Pap smear, wet mount to check for STIs, HIV/AIDS tests, lipid profile, glucose level
- Physical examination: height, weight, blood pressure, breast examination, thyroid palpation, pelvic examination

Figure 4-20 shows a Family Planning flow record to be used during the assessment. After collecting the assessment data above, consider the medical factors to help decide if she is a candidate for all methods or whether some should be eliminated. For example, if she reports she has multiple sex partners and has a lengthy history of various pelvic infections, she would not be a good candidate for an IUD, based on her infection history. Barrier methods (male or female condoms) of contraception might be recommended to this client to offer protection against STIs.

Nursing Diagnoses

A few nursing diagnoses that might be appropriate based on the nurse's assessment during the decision-making process might be:

- Deficient knowledge related to:
  - methods available
  - side effects/safety
  - correct use of method chosen
  - previous myths believed
- Risk for infection related to:
  - unprotected sexual intercourse
  - past history of STIs
  - methods offering protection

Nursing diagnoses applicable to the contraceptive would be:

- Health-seeking behaviors related to:
  - perceived need for limiting number of children
  - overall health relative to contraceptives
- Risk for ineffective health maintenance related to:
  - not being familiar with the various contraceptive methods
  - being unaware of high-risk sexual behavior leading to STIs
- Fear related to:
  - not understanding the correct procedure to use
  - unintended pregnancy occurring if not used correctly
  - general health concerning the long-term side effects

Nursing Interventions

It is important for the nurse to establish a trusting relationship with the client. The following guidelines are helpful in counseling and educating the client or couple about contraceptives:

- Encourage the client/couple to participate in choosing a method.
- Provide client education. The client/couple must be informed users before the method is agreed upon. Education should be targeted to the client's level so it is understood. Provide step-by-step teaching and an opportunity for practice for certain methods (cervical caps, diaphragms, vaginal rings, and condoms). See Teaching Guidelines 4-5 and Figure 4-21.
- Obtain written informed consents, which are needed for IUDs, implants, abortion, or sterilization. Informed consent implies that the client is making a knowledgeable, voluntary choice; has received complete information about the method, including the risks; and is free to change her mind before using the method or having the procedure (Youngkin & Davis, 2004).
- Discuss contraindications for all selected contraceptives.
- Consider the client's cultural and religious beliefs when providing care.
- Address myths and misperceptions about the methods under consideration in your initial discussion of contraceptives. Clearing up misconceptions will permit new learning to take hold and a better client response to whichever methods are explored and ultimately selected. Some common ones include:
  - Breastfeeding protects against pregnancy.

FAMILY PLANNING FLOW (VISIT) RECORD

Name:_____

ID #:_____

Date of Birth:_____

	Date:			Date:	
Current Method					
Reason for Visit					
LMP					
SUBJECTIVE DATA	**Pt.**	**Comments**		**Pt.**	**Comments**
Severe headaches					
Depression					
Visual abnormalities					
Dyspnea/chest pain					
Breast changes					
SBE					
Abdominal pain					
Nausea and vomiting					
Dysuria/frequency					
Menstrual irregularities					
Vaginal discharge/infections					
Leg pain					
Surgery, injury, infections, or serious illness since last visit					
Allergic reaction					
Pregnancy plans					
Other					
OBJECTIVE DATA	**Weight**	**B.P.**		**Weight**	**B.P.**
Other					
Lab					
ASSESSMENT					
Check here if assessment continues on progress notes	O			O	
PLAN					
Type of contraceptive given					
COUNSELING/EDUCATION					
Next appointment					
SIGNATURE/TITLE					
SIGNATURE/TITLE					

O = normal   ✓ = abnormal

● Figure 4-20 Family planning flow (visit) record.

T E A C H I N G   G U I D E L I N E S   4 - 5

Tips for Cervical Caps, Diaphragms, Vaginal Rings, and Condoms

Cervical cap insertion/removal technique:
- It is important to be involved in the fitting process.
- To insert the cap, pinch the sides together, compress the cap dome, insert into the vagina, and place over the cervix.
- Use one finger to feel around the entire circumference to make sure there are no gaps between the cap rim and the cervix.
- After a minute or two, pinch the dome and tug gently to check for evidence of suction. The cap should resist the tug and not slide off easily.
- To remove the cap, press the index finger against the rim and tip the cap slightly to break the suction, and gently pull out the cap.
- The woman should practice inserting and removing the cervical cap three times to validate her proficiency with this device.

Client teaching and counseling regarding the cervical cap:
- Fill the dome of the cap up about 1/3 full with spermicide cream or jelly. Do not apply spermicide to the rim, since it may interfere with the seal.
- Wait approximately 30 minutes after insertion before engaging in sexual intercourse to be sure that a seal has formed between the rim and the cervix.
- Leave the cervical cap in place for a minimum of six hours after sexual intercourse. It can be left in place for up to 48 hours without additional spermicide being added.
- Do not use during menses due to the potential for toxic shock syndrome. Use an alternative method such as condoms during this time.
- Inspect the cervical cap prior to insertion for cracks, holes, or tears.
- After using the cervical cap, wash it with soap and water, dry thoroughly, and store in its container.

Diaphragm insertion/removal technique:
- Always empty the bladder prior to inserting the diaphragm.
- Inspect diaphragm for holes or tears by holding it up to a light source, or fill it with water and check for a leak.
- Place approximately a tablespoon of spermicidal jelly or cream in the dome and around the rim of the diaphragm.
- The diaphragm can be inserted up to 6 hours prior to intercourse.
- Select the position that is most comfortable for insertion:
  ○ Squatting
  ○ Leg up, raising the nondominant leg up on a low stool
  ○ Reclining position, lying on her back in bed
  ○ Chair method, sitting forward on the edge of a chair

- Hold the diaphragm between the thumb and fingers and compress it to form a "figure-eight" shape.
- Insert the diaphragm into the vagina, directing it downward as far as it will go.
- Tuck the front rim of the diaphragm behind the pubic bone so that the rubber hugs the front wall of the vagina.
- Feel for the cervix through the diaphragm to make sure it is properly placed.
- To remove the diaphragm, insert the finger up and over the top side and move slightly to the side, breaking the suction.
- Pull the diaphragm down and out of the vagina.

Client teaching and counseling regarding the diaphragm:
- Avoid the use of oil-based products such as baby oil, since this may weaken the rubber.
- Wash the diaphragm with soap and water after use and dry thoroughly.
- Place the diaphragm back into the storage case.
- The diaphragm may need to be refitted after weight loss or gain or childbirth.
- Diaphragms should not be used by women with latex allergies.

Vaginal ring insertion/removal technique and counseling:
- Each ring is used for one menstrual cycle, which consists of 3 weeks of continuous use followed by a ring-free week to allow for menses.
- No fitting is necessary—one size fits all.
- The ring is compressed and inserted into the vagina, behind the pubic bone, as far back as possible.
- Precision placement is not essential.
- Backup contraception is needed for 7 days if the ring is expelled for more than 3 hours during the three-week period of continuous use.
- The vaginal ring is left in place for 3 weeks, then removed and discarded.
- The vaginal ring is not recommended for women with uterine prolapse or lack of vaginal muscle tone (Youngkin & Davis, 2004).

Male condom insertion/removal technique and counseling:
- Always keep the condom in its original package until ready to use.
- Store in a cool, dry place.
- Spermicidal condoms should be used if available.
- Check expiration date before using.
- Use a new condom for each sexual act.
- Condom is placed over the erect penis prior to insertion.
- Place condom on the head of the penis and unroll it down the shaft.

(continued)

TEACHING GUIDELINES 4-5

Tips for Cervical Caps, Diaphragms, Vaginal Rings, and Condoms (continued)

- Leave a half-inch of empty space at the end to collect ejaculate.
- Avoid use of oil-based products, because they may cause breakage.
- After intercourse, remove the condom while the penis is still erect.
- Discard condom after use.

Female condom insertion/removal technique and counseling:
- Practice wearing and inserting prior to first use with sexual intercourse.
- Condom can be inserted up to 8 hours before intercourse.

- Condom is intended for one-time use.
- It can be purchased over the counter—one size fits all.
- Avoid wearing rings to prevent tears; long fingernails can also cause tears.
- Spermicidal lubricant can be used if desired.
- Insert the inner ring high in the vagina, against the cervix.
- Place the outer ring on the outside of the vagina.
- Make sure the erect penis is placed inside the female condom.
- Remove the condom after intercourse. Avoid spilling the ejaculate.

○ Pregnancy can be avoided if the male partner "pulls out" before he ejaculates.
○ Pregnancy can't occur during menses.
○ Douching after sex will prevent pregnancy.
○ Pregnancy won't happen on the first sexual experience.
○ Taking birth control pills protects against STIs.
○ The woman is too old to get pregnant.
○ Irregular menstruation prevents pregnancy.
- Focus on the following specific information for each method outlined:
  ○ How this particular method works to prevent pregnancy
  ○ How effective it is under normal circumstances of use
  ○ Noncontraceptive benefits to overall health
  ○ Advantages and disadvantages of all methods
  ○ Cost involved
  ○ Danger signs that need to be reported to healthcare provider
  ○ Frequency of office visits needed
- Outline factors that place the client at risk for method failure. There are several reasons why there are contra-

ceptive failures. A few that nurses could help to educate their clients about are outlined in Table 4-8.
- Help clients who have chosen abstinence or fertility awareness methods to define what sexual activities they want and don't want. This helps them set sexual limits or boundaries. Help them to develop communication and negotiation skills that will allow them to be successful. Supporting, encouraging, and respecting a couple's choice of abstinence is vital for nurses.
- Emphasize that a second method to use as a backup is always needed.
- Provide both oral and written instructions on the method chosen.
- Discuss the need for STI protection if not using a barrier method.
- Inform the client about the availability of ECs.
- Abortion is a very emotional, deeply personal issue. Give support and accurate information. If for personal, religious, or ethical reasons you feel unable to actively participate in the care of a woman undergoing an abortion, you still have the professional responsibility to ensure that the woman receives the nursing care and help she requires. This may necessitate a transfer to another area or a staffing reassignment.

Contraception is an important issue for all couples, and the method used should be decided by the woman and her partner jointly. The nurse can facilitate this process by providing unbiased, accurate information about all methods available. As a nurse you need to reflect honestly on your feelings towards contraceptives while allowing the client's feelings to be central. Nurses should be aware of the practical issues involved in contraceptive use and must be determined to avoid making assumptions, making decisions on the woman's behalf, and making judgments about her and her situation. To do so, the nurse must keep up to date on the latest methods available and convey this information to clients. Nurses can encourage female clients to take control of

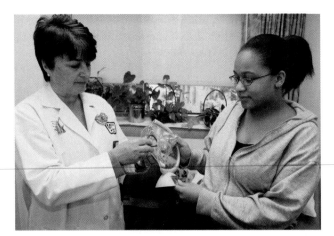

● Figure 4-21 The nurse demonstrates insertion of a vaginal ring during client teaching.

Table 4-8 Contraceptive Problems and Educational Needs

Contraceptive Failure Problem	Client Education Needed
Not following instructions for use of contraceptive correctly	Take pill the same time every day. Use condoms properly and check condition before using. Make sure diaphragm or cervical cap covers cervix completely. Check IUD for placement monthly.
Inconsistent use of contraceptive	Contraceptives must be used regularly to achieve maximum effectiveness. All it takes is one unprotected act of sexual intercourse to become pregnant.
Condom broke during sex	2% to 5% will break or tear during use. Check expiration date. Store condoms properly. Use only a water-based lubricant. Watch for tears caused by long fingernails. Use spermicides to decrease possibility of pregnancy if failure occurs.
Use of antibiotics or other herbs taken with OCs	Use alternative methods during the antibiotic therapy, plus 7 additional days. Implement on day 1 of taking antibiotics.
Belief that you can't get pregnant during menses or that it is safe "just this one time."	It may be possible to become pregnant on almost any day of the menstrual cycle.

Source: Herndon & Zieman, 2004.

their lives by sharing information that allows them to plan their futures.

Menopause

The change of life. The end of fertility. The beginning of freedom. Whatever people call it, menopause is a unique and personal experience for every woman. **Menopause** refers to the cessation of regular menstrual cycles. It is the end of menstruation and childbearing capacity. The average age of natural menopause—defined as 1 year without a menstrual period—is 51 years old (Alexander et al., 2004). With current female life expectancy at 80, this event comes in the middle of women's adult life. Interestingly, humans are virtually the only species to outlive their reproductive capacities.

Menopause signals the end of an era for many women. It concludes their ability to reproduce, and some women find advancing age, altered roles, and these physiologic changes to be overwhelming events that may precipitate depression and anxiety (Kessenich, 2004).

Why or how does this happen? A woman is born with approximately 500,000 ova, but only 300 to 400 ever mature fully to be released during the menstrual cycle. The absolute number of ova in the ovary is a major determinant of fertility. Over the course of her premenopausal life there is a steady decline in the number of immature ova. No one understands this depletion, but it does not occur in isolation. Maturing ova are surrounded by follicles that produce two major hormones: estrogen, in the form of estradiol, and progesterone. The cyclic maturation of the ovum is directed by the hypothalamus. The hypothalamus triggers a cascade of neurohormones, which act through the pituitary and the ovaries as a pulse generator for reproduction.

This hypothalamic-pituitary-ovarian axis begins to break down long before there is any sign that menopause is imminent. Some scientists believe that the pulse generator in the hypothalamus simply degenerates; others speculate that the ovary becomes more resistant to the pituitary hormone FSH and simply shuts down (Sloane, 2002). The final act in this well-orchestrated process is amenorrhea.

As menopause approaches, more and more of the menstrual cycles become anovulatory. This period of time, usually 2 to 8 years, before cessation of menstruation is termed *perimenopause* (Shoupe, 2002). In perimenopause, the ovary begins to sputter, producing irregular and missed periods and an occasional hot flash. When menopause finally appears, viable ova are gone. Estrogen levels plummet by 90%, and estrone, produced in fat cells, replaces estradiol as the body's main form of estrogen. The major hormone produced by the ovaries during the reproductive years is estradiol; the estrogen found in postmenopausal women is estrone. Estradiol is much more biologically active than estrone (Sloane, 2002). In addition, testosterone levels decrease with menopause.

Menopause, with a dramatic decline in estrogen, affects not only the reproductive organs, but also other bodily systems:

• Brain: hot flashes, disturbed sleep, mood and memory problems

- Cardiovascular: lower levels of HDL and increase in risk of cardiovascular disease
- Skeletal: rapid loss of bone density increases the risk of osteoporosis
- Breasts: duct and glandular tissues are replaced by fat
- Genitourinary: vaginal dryness, stress incontinence, cystitis
- Gastrointestinal: less calcium is absorbed from food, increasing the risk for fractures
- Integumentary: skin becomes dry and thin, and collagen levels decrease
- Body shape: more abdominal fat; waist size swells relative to hips

Assessment

Menopause is a universal and irreversible part of the overall aging process involving a woman's reproductive system. While not a disease state, menopause does place women at greater risk for the development of many conditions of aging. Proactive disease prevention can help the woman become aware of her risk for postmenopausal diseases, as well as strategies to prevent them. The nurse can be instrumental in assessing risk factors and planning interventions in collaboration with the client. These might include:

- Screening for osteoporosis, cardiovascular disease, and cancer risk
  - Assessment of blood pressure to identify hypertension
  - Blood cholesterol to identify hyperlipidemia risk
  - Mammogram to find a cancerous lesion
  - Pap smear to identify cervical cancer
  - Pelvic examination to identify endometrial cancer or masses
  - Digital rectal examination to assess for colon cancer
  - Bone density testing as a baseline at menopause to identify osteopenia (low bone mass), which might lead to osteoporosis
- Assessing lifestyle to plan strategies to prevent chronic conditions:
  - Dietary intake of fat, cholesterol, and sodium
  - Weight management
  - Calcium intake
  - Use of tobacco, alcohol, and caffeine
  - Performance of breast self-examinations

Treatment

Menopause should be managed individually. In the past, despite the wide diversity of symptoms and risks, the traditional reaction was to reach for the one-size-fits-all therapy: hormone therapy. Today the medical community is changing its thinking in light of the Women's Health Initiative study, which reported that long-term hormone replacement therapy (HRT) increased the risks of heart attacks, strokes, and breast cancer; in short, the overall health risks of HRT exceeded the benefits (Writing Group 2002, p. 321). As expected, the fallout from this study and others forced practitioners to reevaluate their usual ther-

apies and tailor treatment to each client's history, needs, and risk factors.

There is a universe of treatment options out there, but factors in the client's history should be the driving force when determining therapy. Women need to educate themselves about the latest research findings and collaborate with their healthcare provider on the right menopause therapy. The following factors should be considered in management:

- HRT is not indicated to treat or prevent cardiovascular disease, according to Women's Health Initiative study. Instead, consider lipid-lowering agents and lifestyle changes if risk or disease is present.
- HRT should not be taken for more than 5 years for vasomotor symptoms. Use the lowest dose possible for any hormone therapy.
- Consider nonhormonal therapies such as bisphosphonates and selective estrogen receptor modulators (SERMs).
- Consider weight-bearing exercises, calcium, vitamin D, smoking cessation, and avoidance of alcohol to treat or prevent osteoporosis.
- Annual breast examinations and mammograms are essential.
- Local estrogen creams can be used for vaginal atrophy.
- Consider herbal therapies for symptoms (Kaunitz, 2005).

Although numerous symptoms have been attributed to menopause (Box 4-9), some of them are more closely related to the aging process than to estrogen deficiency. A few of the more common menopausal conditions and their management will be discussed.

Hot Flashes and Night Sweats

Hot flashes and night sweats are classic signs of estrogen deficiency and the predominant complaint of perimenopausal women. A *hot flash* is a transient and sudden sen-

---

BOX 4-9

COMMON SYMPTOMS OF MENOPAUSE

- Hot flashes or flushes of the head and neck
- Dryness in the eyes and vagina
- Personality changes
- Anxiety and/or depression
- Loss of libido
- Weight gain and water retention
- Night sweats
- Fatigue
- Irritability
- Insomnia
- Stress incontinence
- Heart palpitations (Ernst, 2003)

sation of warmth that spreads over the body, particularly the neck, face, and chest. Hot flashes are caused by vasomotor instability. Nearly 85% of menopausal women experience them (Alexander et al., 2003). Hot flashes are an early and acute sign of estrogen deficiency. These flashes can be mild or extreme and can last from 2 to 30 minutes (Shoupe, 2002).

There are many options for treating hot flashes. Treatment must be based on symptom severity, the client's medical history, and the client's values and concerns. Although the gold standard in the treatment of hot flashes is estrogen, this is not recommended for all women. The following are suggestions for the management of hot flashes:

- Pharmacologic options
  - Estrogen replacement therapy (ERT) unless contra-indicated
  - Androgen therapy (potentiates estrogen)
  - Progestin therapy (Depo-Provera injection every 3 months)
  - Clonidine (central alpha-adrenergic agonist) weekly patch
  - Propranolol (beta-adrenergic blocker)
  - Gabapentin (Neurontin): antiseizure drug
  - Vitamin E, 100 mg daily
  - SSRIs
- Lifestyle changes
  - Lower room temperature; use fans.
  - Wear clothing in layers for easy removal.
  - Limit caffeine and alcohol intake.
  - Drink 8 to 10 glasses of water daily.
  - Stop smoking or cut back.
  - Avoid hot drinks and spicy food.
  - Take calcium (1,200–1,500 mg) and vitamin D (400–600 IU).
  - Try relaxation techniques, deep breathing, and meditation.
  - Exercise daily, but not just before bedtime.
  - Maintain a healthy weight.
  - Identify stressors and learn to manage them.
  - Keep a diary to identify triggers of hot flashes.
- Alternative therapies
  - Soy: daily intake of 25 to 50 grams
  - Black cohosh: helps control hormone surges
  - Chamomile: mild sedative to alleviate insomnia
  - Chaste berry (Vitex): balances progesterone and estrogen
  - Dong quai: acts as a form of phytoestrogen
  - Ginseng: helps improve memory and balances hormones
  - St. John's wort: reduces depression and fatigue
  - Valerian root: induces sleep and relaxation (McKee & Warber, 2005)

Although scientific evidence for many of these alternative remedies might be lacking, their use has skyrock-eted. While there might indeed be some benefits to their use, evidence of the efficacy of alternative products in menopause is largely anecdotal. Small, preliminary clinical trials might demonstrate the safety of some of the nonpharmacologic products, but longitudinal, randomized, placebo-controlled clinical trials that demonstrate their efficacy have yet to be conducted. Nurses should be aware of the purported action of these agents, as well as any potential adverse effects or drug interactions that women may experience.

Urogenital Changes

Menopause can be a physically and emotionally challenging time for women. In additional to the psychological burden of leaving behind the reproductive phase of life and the stigma of an "aging" body, sexual difficulties due to urogenital changes plague most women but are frequently not addressed.

Vaginal atrophy occurs during menopause because of declining estrogen levels. These changes include thinning of the vaginal walls, an increase in pH, irritation, increased susceptibility to infection, dyspareunia, loss of lubrication with intercourse, and a decrease in sexual desire related to the changes (Lowry et al., 2003).

Management of these changes might include the use of estrogen vaginal tablets (Vagifem) or Premarin cream; Estring, an estrogen-releasing vaginal ring that lasts for 3 months; testosterone patches; and over-the-counter moisturizers and lubricants (Astroglide). A positive outlook on sexuality and a supportive partner are also needed to make the sexual experience enjoyable and fulfilling (Bachmann, 2002).

Osteoporosis

Women are greatly affected by osteoporosis after menopause. Osteoporosis is a condition in which bone mass declines to such an extent that fractures occur with minimal trauma. Bone loss begins in the third or fourth decade of a woman's life and accelerates rapidly after menopause. It affects 8 million women, with millions more at high risk for developing it. This translates to 1 in 2 women over the age of 50 having an osteoporosis-related fracture in their lifetime (Alexander et al., 2003). This condition puts many women into long-term care, with a resulting loss of independence. Figure 4-22 shows the skeletal changes associated with osteoporosis.

Most women with osteoporosis don't know they have the disease until they sustain a fracture, usually of the wrist or hip. Risk factors include:

- Increasing age
- Postmenopausal status without hormone replacement
- Small frame, thin-boned
- Caucasian or Asian
- Impaired eyesight
- Rheumatoid arthritis
- Family history of osteoporosis

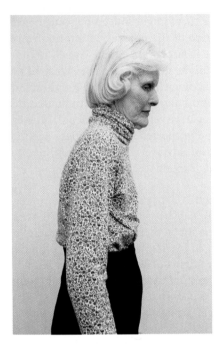

● Figure 4-22 Skeletal changes associated with osteoporosis.

- Sedentary lifestyle
- History of treatment with:
  ○ Antacids with aluminum
  ○ Heparin
  ○ Steroids
  ○ Thyroid replacement drugs
- Smoking and consuming alcohol
- Low calcium and vitamin D intake
- Excessive amounts of caffeine
- Anorexia nervosa or bulimia (Colyar, 2004)

Screening tests to measure bone density are not good predictors for young women who might be at risk for developing this condition. Dual-energy x-ray absorptiometry (DXA or DEXA) is a screening test that calculates the mineral content of the bone at the spine and hip. It is highly accurate, fast, and relatively inexpensive (Sloane, 2002).

The best management for this painful, crippling, and potentially fatal disease is prevention. Women can modify many risk factors by engaging in daily weight-bearing exercise, such as walking; increasing calcium and vitamin D intake; quitting smoking; and reducing their intake of alcohol and caffeine.

Medications that can help in preventing and managing osteoporosis include:

- ERT (Premarin)
- SERMs (Evista)
- Calcium and vitamin D supplements (Tums)
- Bisphosphonates (Actonel or Fosamax)
- Calcitonin (Miacalcin) (Bachmann, 2002)

Cardiovascular Disease

Although cardiovascular disease is still thought of as a "man's disease," it is the major killer of postmenopausal women 50 to 75 years of age (Sloane, 2002). Half a million women die annually in the United States of cardiovascular disease, with strokes accounting for about 20% of the deaths (Alexander et al., 2004).

For the first half of a woman's life, estrogen seems to be a protective substance for the cardiovascular system by smoothing, relaxing, and dilating blood vessels. It even helps boost HDL and lower LDL levels, helping to keep the arteries clean from plaque accumulation. But when estrogen levels plummet as women age and experience menopause, the incidence of cardiovascular disease increases dramatically.

Menopause is not the only factor that increases a woman's risk for cardiovascular disease. Lifestyle and medical history factors such as the following play a major role:

- Smoking
- Obesity
- High-fat diet
- Sedentary lifestyle
- High cholesterol levels
- Family history of cardiovascular disease
- Hypertension
- Apple-shaped body
- Diabetes

Nursing Management

There is no "magic bullet" in managing menopause. Nurses can counsel women about their risks and help them to prevent disease and debilitating conditions with specific health-maintenance education. Women should make their own decisions, but the nurse should make sure they are armed with the facts to do so intelligently. Nurses can offer a thorough explanation of the menopausal process, including the latest research findings, to help women understand and make decisions about this inevitable event.

Nurses should also promote "tried-and-true" tips for healthy living by encouraging women to:

- Participate actively in maintaining their health
- Exercise regularly
- Take supplemental calcium and eat appropriately to prevent osteoporosis
- Stop smoking to prevent lung and heart disease
- Reduce caffeine and alcohol intake to prevent osteoporosis
- Reduce dietary intake of fat, cholesterol, and sodium to prevent cardiovascular disease
- Maintain a health weight for body frame
- Control stress
- Perform breast self-examinations to detect breast lesions

These life approaches may be low-tech, but they can stave off menopause-related complications such as cardiovascular disease, osteoporosis, and depression. These tips for healthy living work well, but the client needs to be motivated and stick with it.

Summary

Sexual health is a concept that means different things to different people. In a global sense, it includes reproductive concerns in a woman's life from menarche through menopause, as this chapter has addressed. Nurses should aim to have a holistic approach to the sexual health of women and focus on health-promotion advice that will assist them to adapt to their changing bodies and needs throughout the life cycle. There will be incredible advances in all areas of women's health in the near future, and nurses must keep current in terms of new therapies to meet women's needs.

KEY CONCEPTS

- Establishing good health habits and avoiding risky behaviors early in life will prevent chronic conditions later on.
- There are more than 100 symptoms of PMS, and at least two different syndromes have been recognized: PMS and premenstrual dysphoric disorder (PMDD).
- Endometriosis is a condition in which bits of functioning endometrial tissue are located outside of their normal site, the uterine cavity.
- Infertility is a widespread problem that has an emotional, social, and economic impact on couples.
- More than half (53%) of all unintended pregnancies occur in women who report using some method of birth control during the month of conception.
- Hormonal methods include oral contraceptives, injectables, implants, vaginal rings, and transdermal patches.
- Recent studies have shown that the extension of active oral contraceptive pills carries the same safety profile as the conventional 28-day regimens.
- Currently there are three IUDs available in the United States: the copper ParaGard-T-380A; Progestasert, a progesterone device; and the levonorgestrel intrauterine system (LNG-IUS) Mirena, a levonorgestrel-releasing device.
- Sterilization is the most popular method of contraception in the United States and worldwide.
- Menopause, with a dramatic decline in estrogen levels, affects not only the reproductive organs but also other bodily systems.
- Most women with osteoporosis don't know they have the disease until they sustain a fracture, usually of the wrist or hip.

- Half a million women die annually in the United States of cardiovascular diseases, with strokes accounting for about 20% of the deaths.
- Nurses should aim to have a holistic approach to the sexual health of women from menarche through menopause.

References

ACOG Practice Bulletin (2000). Clinical management guidelines for obstetricians-gynecologists, number 15: premenstrual syndrome. *Obstetrics & Gynecology, 95,* 1–9.

Aeby, T. C., & Frattarelli, L. C. (2002) Dysfunctional uterine bleeding. *eMedicine Journal* [Online]. Available at: http://author.emedicine.com/ped/topic628.htm

Albers, J. R., Hull, S. K., & Wesley, R. M. (2004). Abnormal uterine bleeding. *American Family Physician, 69*(8), 1915–1926.

Alan Guttmacher Institute (2004a). Contraceptive use. [Online] Available at: http://www.agi-usa.org/pubs/fb_contr_use.html

Alan Guttmacher Institute (2004b). Contraceptive use in the United States. [Online] Available at: http://www.guttmacher.org/in-the-know/prevention.html

Alexander, L. L., LaRosa, J. H., & Bader, H. (2004). *New dimensions in women's health,* (3rd ed.). Boston: Jones and Bartlett.

Alzubaidi, N., & Calis, K. A. (2004). Dysmenorrhea. *EMedicine.* [Online] Available at: http://www.emedicine.com/med/topic606.htm

American Academy of Allergy, Asthma, and Immunology (2004). *Tips to remember: latex allergy.* [Online] Available at: http://www.aaaai.org/patients/publicedmat/tips/latexallergy.stm

American Society for Reproductive Medicine. (2002). *Frequently asked questions about infertility.* [Online]. Available at: http://www.asrm.org/Patients/faqs.html

Arevalo, M. (2003). CycleBeads: easy, effective natural family planning. [Online] Available at: http://www.cyclebeads.com

Arevalo, M., & Sinai, I. (2003) *The Standard Days Method: a new effective method of family planning. Field Notes.* Washington DC: Georgetown University Institute for Reproductive Health.

Bachmann, G. (2002). Menopause. *eMedicine.* [Online] Available at: http://www.emedicine.com/med/topic3289.htm

Bielak, K. M. (2002). Amenorrhea. [Online] Available at: http://www.emedicine.com/ped/topic2779.htm

Bradley, L. D. (2005). Abnormal uterine bleeding. *Nurse Practitioner, 30*(10), 38–51.

Braverman, P. K., & Neinstein, L. S. (2002). Dysmenorrhea and premenstrual syndrome. In L. S. Neinstein (Ed.), *Adolescent health care, a practical guide* (4th ed., pp. 952–965). Philadelphia: Lippincott Williams & Wilkins.

Brevet, D. B., & Wiggins, M. (2002). Preventing and treating STDs. *Advance for Nurses, 3*(23), 15–18.

Brucker, P. S., & McKenry, P. C. (2004). Support from health care providers and the psychological adjustment of individuals experiencing infertility. *JOGNN, 33*(5), 597–603.

Burkman, R. T. (2002). Patterns in contraception. *The Female Patient Supplement.* New Jersey: Quadrant HealthCom Inc.

Burstein, G. R., Lowry, R., Klein, J. D., & Santelli, J. S. (2003). Missed opportunities for sexually transmitted diseases, human immunodeficiency virus, and pregnancy prevention services during adolescent health supervision visits. *Pediatrics, 111*(5), 996–1001.

Carey, J. C., & Rayburn, W. F. (2002). *Obstetrics and gynecology* (4th ed.). Philadelphia: Lippincott Williams & Wilkins.

Cavanaugh, B. M. (2003). *Nurse's manual of laboratory and diagnostic tests* (4th ed.). Philadelphia: F. A. Davis.

Centers for Disease Control and Prevention (CDC) (2002). Sexually transmitted diseases treatment guidelines. *MMWR, 51*(RR-6), 1–77.

Centers for Disease Control and Prevention (CDC) (2003). Advancing HIV prevention: new strategies for a changing epidemic—United States. *MMWR, 52*(15), 329.

Centers for Disease Control and Prevention (CDC) (2004). Contraceptive use. *National Center for Health Statistics.* [Online] Available at: http://www.cdc.gov/nchs/fastats/usecontr/htm

Clark, A. D., & Steele, T. (2005). Dysmenorrhea. *eMedicine.* [Online] Available at: http://www.emedicine.com/emerg/topic156.htm

Clark, L. R. (2004). Premenstrual syndrome. *eMedicine.* [Online] Available at: http://www.emedicine.com/ped/topic1890.htm

Colyar, M. (2004). Bone density testing. *Advance for Nurse Practitioners, 12*(7), 24–25.

Crandall, C. J. (2004). Sexually transmitted infections (STIs) in women. *Medicine Net.* [Online]. Available at: http://www.medicinenet.com/script/main/art.asp?articlekey=482&pf=3&track=qpa482

Debernardo, R. L. (2004). Dysfunctional uterine bleeding. *Medline Plus* [Online]. Available at: http://www.nlm.nih.gov/medlineplus/print/ency/article/000903.htm

DeMasters, J. (2004). Male infertility. *Advance for Nurses, 6*(1), 19–25.

Dickerson, L. M., Mazyck, P. J., & Hunter, M. H. (2003). Premenstrual syndrome. *American Family Physician, 67*(8), 1743–1752.

Dodds, N., & Sinert, R. (2005). Dysfunctional uterine bleeding. *eMedicine* [Online]. Available at: http://www.emedicine.com/emerg/topic155.htm

Gray, D. E., Guinn, C., Norwood, B., & Ch'ien, A. (2004). The quest for conception: An overview of the NP's role in fertility care. *Advance for Nurse Practitioners, 12*(6), 55–60.

Hart, J. A. (2005). Painful menstrual periods. *Medline Plus* [Online]. Available at http://www.nlm.nih.gov/medlineplus/ency/article/003150.htm

Hatcher, R. A., et al. (2004). *Contraceptive technology* (18th ed.). New York: Ardent Media, Inc.

Healthy Women. (2005). Menstrual disorders. National Women's Health Resource Center [Online]. Available at: http://www.healthywomen.org/content.cfm?L1=3&L2=53.0

Hendrick, V. (2005). Premenstrual syndrome. *National Women's Health Information Center* [Online]. Available at: http://www.4women.gov/faq/pms.htm

Herndon, E. J., & Zieman, M. (2004). New contraceptive options. *American Family Physician* [Online]. Available at: http://wwwaafp.org/afp/20040215/853.html

Hsu, K. (2004). Endometriosis. *eMedicine* [Online]. Available at: http://www.emedicine.com/EMERG/topic165.htm

Jones, S. L. (2004). The confluence of two clinical specialties: genetics and assisted reproductive technologies. *MEDSURG Nursing, 13*(2), 114–121.

Kapoor, D., & Davila, W. (2004). Endometriosis. *eMedicine.* [Online] Available at: http://www.emedicine.com/med/topic3419.htm

Kaunitz, A. M. (2005). Beyond the pill: New data and options in hormonal and intrauterine contraception. *American Journal of Obstetrics and Gynecology, 192*, 998–1004.

Kessenich, C. R. (2004). Inevitable menopause. *Nursing Spectrum.* [Online] Available: http://nsweb.nursingspectrum.com/ce/ce232.htm

Lenehan, G. P. (2004). Latex allergy: separating fact from fiction. *Travel Nursing*, pp. 12–17.

Lethaby, A., Cooke, I., & Rees, M. (2003). Progesterone/progestogen releasing intrauterine systems verses either placebo or any other medication for heavy menstrual bleeding. *Cochrane Database Systematic Review* (4), CD002126.

Littleton, L. Y., & Engebretson, J. C. (2002). *Maternal, neonatal, and women's health nursing.* New York: Delmar.

Lowdermilk, D. L., & Perry, S. E. (2004). *Maternity & women's health care* (8th ed.). St. Louis: Mosby, Inc.

Lowry, S. L., Olesh, R. C., Mobasser, S., & Wool, E. N. (2003). Loss of libido during menopause. *Hormone Replacement Therapy: Issues in Patient Management.* New Jersey: MPE Communications, Inc.

Marchiano, D. (2004). Infertility. *Medline Plus.* [Online] Available at: http://www.nlm.nih.gov/medlineplus/ency/article/001191.htm

Matteson, P. S. (2001) *Women's health during the childbearing years: a community-based approach.* St. Louis: Mosby, Inc.

McKee, J., & Warber, S. L. (2005). Integrative therapies for menopause. *Southern Medical Journal, 98*(3), 319–326.

Minjarez, D. A., & Carr, B. R. (2002). Amenorrhea. In R. E. Rakel & E. T. Bope (Eds.), *Conn's current therapy* (pp. 1072–1075). Philadelphia: W. B. Saunders.

Mitan, L. A. P., & Slap, G. B. (2002) Dysfunctional uterine bleeding. In L. S. Neinstein (Ed.), *Adolescent health care: A practical guide* (4th ed., pp. 966–972). Philadelphia: Lippincott Williams & Wilkins.

Moreo, K. (2003). HIV/AIDS and HIV nephropathy. *Nephrology Nursing Journal, 30*(1), 64–68.

Morris, R. T. (2002). Human papillomavirus and genital neoplasia. In S. B. Ransom, M. P. Dombrowski, M. I. Evans, & K. A. Ginsburg (Eds.), *Contemporary therapy in obstetrics and gynecology.* Philadelphia: W. B. Saunders.

Murray, S. S. & McKinney, E. S. (2006). *Foundations of maternal-newborn nursing* (4th ed.). Philadelphia: W. B. Saunders.

myDr Women's Health Center (2003). Menstruation [online]. Available: http://www.mydr.com.au/default.asp?article=3041

National Institute of Child Health and Human Development (NICHD) (2002). *Endometriosis.* NICHD Information Resource Center, NIH Pub. No. 02-2413 [Online] Available at: www.nichd.nih.gov

Nelson, L. M., & Bakalov, V. (2004). Amenorrhea. *eMedicine.* [Online] Available at: http://www.emedicine.com/med/topic117.htm

OSHA (2003). *Latex allergy.* U.S. Department of Labor, Occupational Safety & Health Administration. [Online] Available at: http://www.osha.gov/SLTC/latexallergy

Planned Parenthood (2005). Facts about birth control [Online]. Available at: http://www.plannedparenthood.org/bc/bcfacts4.html

Policar, M. (2002, March). Extended OC regimens: practical applications. In *Contraceptive technology.* Conference by Contemporary Forums, Washington DC.

Queenan, J. T., & Whitman, G. F. (2004). Dysfunctional uterine bleeding. *eMedicine.* [Online] Available at: http://www.emedicine.com/med/topic2353.htm

Samra, O. M. (2003). Birth control overview. *eMedicine.* [Online] Available at: http://www.emedicinehealth.com/fulltext/35411.htm

Schwartz, J. L., & Gabelnick, H. L. (2002). Current contraceptive research. *Perspectives on Sexual and Reproductive Health, 34*(6), 310–315.

Shoupe, D. (2002). Practical strategies for treating hot flashes. *Women's Health (Gynecology Edition), 2*(1), 49–55.

Skidmore-Roth, L. (2005). *Mosby's drug guide for nurses* (6th ed.). St. Louis, MO: Elsevier Mosby.

Sloane, E. (2002). *Biology of women* (4th ed.). New York: Delmar.

Speroff, L., & Fritz, M. A. (2005). *Clinical gynecologic endocrinology and fertility,* (7th ed.). Philadelphia: Lippincott Williams & Wilkins.

Strine, T. W., Chapman, D. P., & Ahluwalia, I. B. (2005). Menstrual-related problems and psychological distress among women in the United States. *Journal of Women's Health, 14*(4), 316–323.

Sulak, P. J., Kuehl, T. J., Ortiz, M., & Shull, B. L. (2002). Acceptance of altering the standard 21-day/7-day oral contraceptive regimen to delay menses and reduce hormone withdrawal symptoms. *American Journal of Obstetrics & Gynecology, 186*(6), 1142–1149.

Theroux, R., & Taylor, K. (2003). Women's decision making about the use of hormonal and nonhormonal remedies for the menopausal transition. *JOGNN, 32*(6), 712–724.

Thompson, S. R. (2004). Primary amenorrhea. *Medline Plus.* [Online] Available at: http://www.nlm.nih.gov/medlineplus/ency/article/001218.htm

Trussell, J. (2003). Contraceptive efficacy. In R. Hatcher et al. (Eds.), *Contraceptive technology* (18th rev. ed.). New York: Ardent Media, Inc.

Trussel, J., & Vaughan, B. (1999). Contraceptive failure, method-related discontinuation and resumption of use: results from the 1995 national survey of family growth. *Family Planning Perspectives, 31*(2), 64–72.

UNFPA (2000). *The state of the world population 2000 report.* [Online] Available at: http://www.unfpa.org/swp/swpmain.htm

United Nations (2003). United Nations Population Information Network [Online] Available at: http://www.un.org/popin/data.html

U.S. Bureau of the Census (2003). *National population estimates-characteristics.* [Online] Available at: http://eire.census.gov/popest/data/national/tables/asro/NA-EST2002-ASRO-01.php

Weise, E. (2005). Contraceptive sponge is back, but why did it leave? *USA Today,* [Online] Available at: http://www.usatoday.com/news/health/2005-04-24-today-sponge_x.htm

Weismiller, D. G. (2004). Emergency contraceptive. *American Family Physician, 70*(4), 707–718.

Williams, J. K. (2002). Unintended pregnancy: incidence and consequences. *The Female Patient Supplement,* December.

Women's Health Guide (2004). *Infertility risk factors.* University of Maryland Medicine. [Online]. Available at: http://www.umm.edu/women/infrisk.htm

Workowski, K., Levine, W., & Wasserheit, J. (2002). U.S. Centers for Disease Control and Prevention guidelines for the treatment of sexually transmitted diseases: an opportunity to unify clinical and public health practice. *Annals of Internal Medicine, 137*(4), 255–262.

Workowski, K. A., & Berman, S. M. (2002). CDC sexually transmitted disease treatment guidelines. *Clinical Infectious Diseases, 35*(Suppl 2), S135–137.

Writing Group for the Women's Health Initiative Investigators. (2002). Risks and benefits of estrogen plus progestin in healthy postmenopausal women: principal results from the Women's Health Initiative randomized controlled trial. *JAMA, 288*(3), 321–333.

Wysocki, S., Dominguez, L., & Schnare, S. (2002). Hormonal contraceptives: extending the benefits. *American Journal of Nurse Practitioners, 6*(12), 19–29.

Youngkin, E. Q., & Davis, M. S. (2004). *Women's health: a primary care clinical guide* (3rd ed.). New Jersey: Prentice Hall.

Zieman, M. (2002). Benefits beyond contraception. *The Female Patient Supplement.* New Jersey: Quadrant HealthCom Inc.

Web Resources

American College of Obstetricians and Gynecologists (ACOG): (202) 863-2518, **http://www.acog.org**

American Psychiatric Association: (202) 682-6000, **http://psych.org**

American Society for Reproductive Medicine: (205) 978-5000, **http://www.asrm.org**

Centers for Disease Control and Prevention: (202) 329-1819, **http://www.cdc.gov**

Emergency Contraception Hotline: (888) 668-2528, **http://www.not-2-late.com**

Endometriosis Association: (414) 355-2200, **http://www.ovf.com/endohtml.html**

Hormone Foundation: (800) 467-6663, **http://hormone.org**

International Counsel on Infertility Information Dissemination: (703) 379-9178, **http://www.inciid.org**

National Institute of Mental Health: (301) 443-4513, **http://www.nimh.nih.gov**

National Women's Health Resource Center: (877) 986-9472, **http://www.healthywomen.org**

National Women's Information Center (NWHIC): (800) 994-9662, **http://www.4women.gov**

North American Menopause Society: http://www.menopause.org

Planned Parenthood Federation of America, Inc.: (800) 669-0156, **http://www.plannedparenthood.org**

Premenstrual Institute: (248) 624-3366, **http://www.pmsinst.com**

Resolve, The National Infertility Association: (617) 623-0744, **http://www.resolve.org**

ChapterWORKSHEET

● MULTIPLE CHOICE QUESTIONS

1. A couple is considered infertile after how many months of trying to conceive?

   a. 6 months

   b. 12 months

   c. 18 months

   d. 24 months

2. A couple reports that their condom broke while they were having sexual intercourse last night. What would you advise to prevent pregnancy?

   a. Inject a spermicidal agent into her vagina immediately.

   b. Obtain emergency contraceptives from their doctor.

   c. Douche with a solution of vinegar and hot water tonight.

   d. Take a strong laxative now and again at bedtime.

3. Which of the following combination contraceptives has been approved for extended continuous use?

   a. Seasonale

   b. NuvaRing

   c. Ortho Evra

   d. Mirena

4. Which of the following measures helps *prevent* osteoporosis?

   a. Iron supplementation

   b. Sleeping 8 hours nightly

   c. Eating lean meats only

   d. Walking 3 miles daily

5. Which of the following activities will *increase* a woman's risk of cardiovascular disease if she is taking oral contraceptives?

   a. Eating a high-fiber diet

   b. Smoking cigarettes

   c. Taking daily multivitamins

   d. Drinking alcohol

6. Hormone replacement therapy (HRT) taken by menopausal women reduces:

   a. Weight gain

   b. Bone density

   c. Hot flashes

   d. Heart disease

7. Throughout life, a woman's most proactive activity to promote health would be to engage in:

   a. Consistent exercise

   b. Socialization with friends

   c. Quality quiet time with herself

   d. Consuming water

● CRITICAL THINKING EXERCISE

1. Ms. London, 25, comes to your family planning clinic requesting to have an intrauterine device (IUD) inserted because "birth control pills give you cancer." In reviewing her history, you note she has been into the STI clinic three times in the past year with vaginal infections and was hospitalized for pelvic inflammatory disease (PID) last month. In questioning her about her sexual history, she reports having sex with multiple partners and not always using protection.

   a. Is an IUD the most appropriate method for her? Why or why not?

   b. What myths/misperceptions will you address in your counseling session?

   c. Outline the safer sex discussion you plan to have with her.

● STUDY ACTIVITIES

1. Arrange to shadow a nurse working in family planning for the morning. Observe the following: What questions does the nurse ask to ascertain the kind of family planning method that is right for this woman? What teaching goes along with each method? What follow-up care is needed? Share your findings with your classmates during a clinical conference.

2. Surf the Internet and locate three resources for infertile couples to consult that provide support and resources.

3. Sterilization is the most prevalent method of contraception used by married couples in the United States. Contact a local urologist and gynecologist to learn the procedure involved and the cost of a male and female sterilization. Which procedure poses less risk to the person and costs less?

4. Take a field trip to a local drugstore to check out the variety and costs of male and female condoms. How many different brands did you find? What was the range of costs?

5. Noncontraceptive benefits of combined oral contraceptives include which of the following? Select all that apply.

   a. Protection against ovarian cancer

   b. Protection against endometrial cancer

   c. Protection against breast cancer

   d. Reduction in incidence of ectopic pregnancy

   e. Prevention of functional ovarian cysts

   f. Reduction in deep venous thrombosis

   g. Reduction in the risk of colorectal cancer

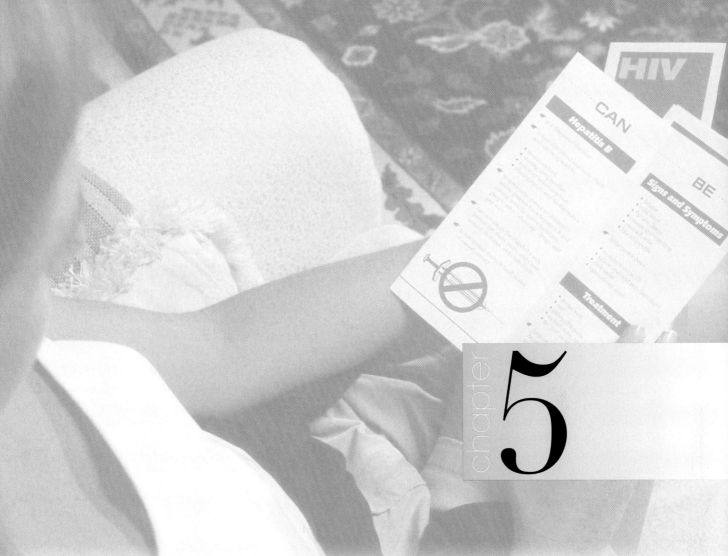

chapter 5

Sexually Transmitted Infections

KeyTERMS

bacterial vaginosis
gonorrhea
pelvic inflammatory
  disease (PID)
sexually transmitted
  infection (STI)
syphilis
trichomoniasis
vulvovaginal candidiasis

LearningOBJECTIVES

*After studying the chapter content, the student should be able to
accomplish the following:*

1. Define the key terms.
2. Describe the spread and control of sexually transmitted infections.
3. Identify risk factors and outline appropriate client education needed in common
   sexually transmitted infections.
4. Discuss how contraceptives can play a role in the prevention of sexually
   transmitted infections.
5. Discuss the physiologic and psychological aspects of sexually transmitted
   infections.
6. Delineate the nursing management needed for women with sexually
   transmitted infections.

Sexually transmitted infections (STIs) are infections of the reproductive tract caused by microorganisms transmitted through vaginal, anal, or oral sexual intercourse (CDC, 2002). STIs pose a serious threat not only to women's sexual health but also to the general health and well-being of millions of people worldwide. STIs constitute an epidemic of tremendous magnitude. An estimated 65 million people live with an incurable STI, and another 15 million are infected each year (CDC, 2004).

STIs are biologically sexist, presenting greater risk and causing more complications among women than among men. STIs may contribute to cervical cancer, low birthweight, fetal wastage (abortions and death) and vertical transmission (maternal-to-fetal transmission while in utero), infertility, ectopic pregnancy, chronic pelvic pain, and death. STIs know no class, racial, ethnic, or social barriers—all individuals are vulnerable if exposed to the infectious organism. The problem of STIs has still not been tackled adequately on a global scale and until this is done, numbers worldwide will continue to increase.

Biological and behavioral factors place teenagers at high risk. An estimated two thirds of all infections occur among persons under the age of 25 (Burstein et al., 2003). The incidence of STIs continues to rise in the United States.

Education about safer sex practices—and the resulting increase in the use of condoms—can play a vital role in reducing STI rates all over the world. Clearly, knowledge and prevention are the best defenses against STIs. The prevention and control of STIs is based on the following concepts (CDC, 2002):

1. Education and counseling of persons at risk about safer sexual behavior
2. Identification of asymptomatically infected individuals and of symptomatic individuals unlikely to seek diagnosis and treatment
3. Effective diagnosis and treatment of infected individuals
4. Evaluation, treatment, and counseling of sex partners of people who are infected with an STI
5. Preexposure vaccination of people at risk for vaccine-preventable STIs

Nurses play an integral role in identifying and preventing STIs. They have a unique opportunity to educate the public about this serious public health issue by communicating the methods of transmission, symptoms associated with each condition, tracking the updated CDC treatment guidelines, and offering clients strategic preventive measures to reduce the spread of STIs.

Discussion of STIs can be categorized in many fashions. We will use the CDC framework, which groups STIs according to the major symptom manifested (Box 5-1).

Infections Characterized by Vaginal Discharge

Vaginitis is a generic term that means inflammation and infection of the vagina. There can be hundreds of causes for vaginitis, but more often then not the cause is infection by one of three organisms:

- *Candida,* a fungus
- *Gardnerella,* a bacterium
- *Trichomonas,* a protozoan

The complex balance of microbiological organisms in the vagina is recognized as a key element in the maintenance of health. Subtle shifts in the vaginal environment may allow organisms with pathologic potential to proliferate, causing infectious symptoms.

Vulvovaginal Candidiasis

Vulvovaginal candidiasis is one of the most common causes of vaginal discharge. It is also referred to as yeast, monilia, and a fungal infection. It is not considered an

---

BOX 5-1

CDC CLASSIFICATIONS OF SEXUALLY TRANSMITTED INFECTIONS

- Infections characterized by vaginal discharge
- Vulvovaginal candidiasis
  ○ Trichomoniasis
  ○ Bacterial vaginosis
- Infections characterized by cervicitis
  ○ Chlamydia
  ○ Gonorrhea
- Infections characterized by genital ulcers
  ○ Genital herpes simplex
  ○ Syphilis
- Pelvic inflammatory disease (PID)
- Human immunodeficiency virus (HIV)
- Human papillomavirus infection (HPV)
- Vaccine-preventable STIs
  ○ Hepatitis A
  ○ Hepatitis B
- Ectoparasitic infections
  ○ Pediculosis pubis
  ○ Scabies

STI because *Candida* is a normal constituent in the vagina and becomes pathologic only when the vaginal environment becomes altered. An estimated 75% of women will have at least one episode of vulvovaginal candidiasis, and 40% to 50% will have two or more episodes in their lifetime (CDC, 2002).

Clinical Manifestations

Typical symptoms, which can worsen just before menses, include:

- Pruritus
- Vaginal discharge (thick, white, curd-like)
- Vaginal soreness
- Vulvar burning
- Erythema in the vulvovaginal area
- Dyspareunia
- External dysuria

Predisposing factors for candidiasis include:

- Pregnancy
- Use of oral contraceptives with a high estrogen content
- Use of broad-spectrum antibiotics
- Diabetes mellitus
- Use of steroid and immunosuppressive drugs
- HIV infection
- Wearing tight, restrictive clothes and nylon underpants
- Trauma to vaginal mucosa from chemical irritants or douching

Figure 5-1 shows the typical appearance of vulvovaginal candidiasis.

Diagnosis

The diagnosis of candidiasis is based on the history of symptoms and a pelvic examination. The speculum examination will reveal white plaques on the vaginal walls. The definitive diagnosis is made by a wet smear, which reveals the filamentous hyphae and spores characteristic of a fungus when viewed under a microscope.

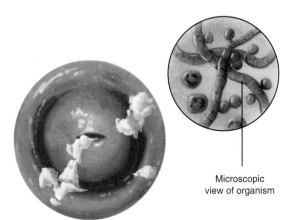

Microscopic view of organism

● Figure 5-1 Vulvovaginal candidiasis. (Source: The Anatomical Chart Company. [2002]. *Atlas of pathophysiology*. Springhouse, PA: Springhouse.)

Treatment

Treatment of candidiasis includes one of the following medications:

- Miconazole cream or suppository
- Clotrimazole tablet
- Terconazole cream or suppository
- Fluconazole oral tablet (CDC, 2002, p. 46)

Most of the above medications are used intravaginally in the form of a cream, tablet, or suppositories used for 3 to 7 days. If fluconazole (Diflucan) is prescribed, a 160-mg oral tablet is taken as a single dose.

Topical azole preparations are effective in the treatment of vulvovaginal candidiasis, relieving symptoms and producing negative cultures in 80% to 90% of women who complete therapy (CDC, 2002). If vulvovaginal candidiasis is not treated effectively during pregnancy, the newborn can develop an oral infection known as thrush during the birth process; that infection must be treated with a local azole preparation after birth.

Preventive measures for women with frequent vulvovaginal candidiasis infections include:

- Reducing the dietary intake of simple sugars and soda
- Wearing white, 100% cotton underpants
- Avoiding wearing tight pants
- Showering rather than taking tub baths
- Washing with a mild, unscented soap and drying the genitals gently
- Avoiding the use of bubble baths or scented bath products
- Washing underwear in unscented laundry detergent and hot water
- Drying underwear in a hot dryer to kill the yeast that cling to the fabric
- Removing wet bathing suits promptly
- Practicing good body hygiene
- Avoiding vaginal sprays/deodorants
- Avoiding wearing pantyhose (or cut out the crotch to allow air circulation)
- Using white, unscented toilet paper and wiping from front to back
- Avoiding douching (which washes away protective vaginal mucus)
- Avoiding the use of superabsorbent tampons (use pads instead)

Trichomoniasis

Trichomoniasis is another common vaginal infection that causes a discharge. The woman may be markedly symptomatic or asymptomatic. Men are asymptomatic carriers. Although this infection is localized, there is increasing evidence of preterm birth and postpartum endometritis in women with this vaginitis (CDC, 2002). *Trichomonas vaginalis* is a ovoid, single-cell protozoan parasite that can be observed under the microscope making a jerky swaying motion.

Clinical Manifestations

Typical symptoms include:

- A heavy yellow/green or gray frothy or bubbly discharge
- Vaginal pruritus and vulvar soreness
- Dyspareunia
- Dysuria
- Colpitis macularis ("strawberry" look on cervix)

Figure 5-2 shows the typical appearance of trichomoniasis.

Diagnosis

The diagnosis is confirmed when a motile flagellated trichomonad is visualized under the microscope.

Treatment

A single dose of oral metronidazole for both partners is a common treatment for this infection. Sex partners of women with trichomoniasis should be treated. Clients should be instructed to avoid sex until they and their sex partners are cured (i.e., when therapy has been completed and both partners are symptom-free) (CDC, 2002). People taking metronidazole should be counseled to avoid alcohol because mixing the two causes severe nausea and vomiting (Sloane, 2002).

Bacterial Vaginosis

A third common infection of the vagina is **bacterial vaginosis,** caused by the gram-negative bacillus *Gardnerella vaginalis.* It is the most prevalent cause of vaginal discharge or malodor, but up to 50% of women are asymptomatic. Bacterial vaginosis is a sexually associated infection characterized by alterations in vaginal flora in which *Lactobacilli* in the vagina are replaced with high concentrations of anaerobic bacteria. The cause of the microbial alteration is not fully understood but is associated with having multiple sex partners, douching, and lack of vaginal lactobacilli (CDC, 2002). Research suggests that bacterial vaginosis is associated with preterm labor, chorioamnionitis, postpartum endometritis, and pelvic inflammatory disease (CDC, 2002).

Clinical Manifestations

The primary symptoms of bacterial vaginosis are a thin, white homogeneous vaginal discharge and a characteristic "stale fish" odor. Figure 5-3 shows the typical appearance of bacterial vaginosis.

Diagnosis

To diagnose BV, three of the four criteria must be met:

- Thin, white homogeneous vaginal discharge
- pH > 4.5
- Positive "whiff test" (secretion is mixed with a drop of 10% potassium hydroxide on a slide, producing a characteristic stale fishy odor)
- The presence of clue cells on wet-mount examination (CDC, 2002)

Treatment

Treatment for bacterial vaginosis includes oral metronidazole or clindamycin cream. Treatment of the male partner has not been beneficial in preventing recurrence (CDC, 2002, p. 43).

Nursing Management

The nurse's role is one of primary prevention and education to limit recurrences of these infections. Primary prevention begins with changing the sexual behaviors that place women at risk for infection. In addition to assessing women for the common signs and symptoms and risk

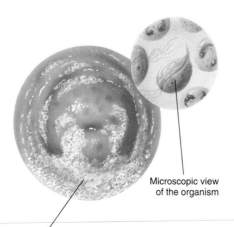

Microscopic view
of the organism

Greenish-gray cervical
discharge

● Figure 5-2 Trichomoniasis. (Source:
The Anatomical Chart Company.
[2002]. *Atlas of pathophysiology.*
Springhouse, PA: Springhouse.)

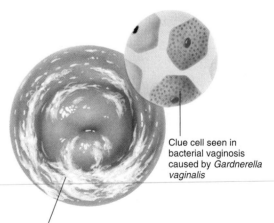

Clue cell seen in
bacterial vaginosis
caused by *Gardnerella
vaginalis*

Discharge with fishy odor

● Figure 5-3 Bacterial vaginosis. (Source: The
Anatomical Chart Company. [2002]. *Atlas of
pathophysiology.* Springhouse, PA: Springhouse.)

factors, the nurse can help women to avoid vaginitis or to prevent a recurrence by teaching them to take the precautions highlighted in Teaching Guidelines 5-1.

Infections Characterized by Cervicitis

Chlamydia

Chlamydia is the most common bacterial STI in the United States. The CDC estimates that there are 4 million new cases each year; the highest predictor for the infection is age. Chlamydia causes half of the 1 million recognized cases of pelvic inflammatory disease (PID) in the United States each year, and treatment costs run over $1 billion yearly. The highest rates of infection are among those ages 15 to 19, regardless of demographics or location (CDC, 2002). Asymptomatic infection is common among both men and women. Men primarily develop urethritis. In women, chlamydia is linked with cervicitis, acute urethral syndrome, salpingitis, PID, and infertility (Youngkin & Davis, 2004).

Chlamydia trachomatis is the bacterium that causes chlamydia. It is an intracellular parasite that cannot produce its own energy and depends on the host for survival. It is often difficult to detect, and this can pose problems for women due to the long-term consequences of untreated infection. Moreover, lack of treatment provides more opportunity for the infection to be transmitted to sexual partners. Newborns delivered to infected mothers may develop conjunctivitis or pneumonitis and have a 50% to 70% risk of acquiring the infection (Sloane, 2002).

Clinical Manifestations

The majority of women (70% to 80%) are asymptomatic (CDC, 2002). If the client is symptomatic, clinical manifestations include:

- Mucopurulent vaginal discharge
- Urethritis

 T E A C H I N G   G U I D E L I N E S   5 - 1

Preventing Vaginitis

- Avoid douching to prevent altering the vaginal environment.
- Use condoms to avoid spreading the organism.
- Avoid tights, nylon underpants, and tight clothes.
- Wipe from front to back after using the toilet.
- Avoid powders, bubble baths, and perfumed vaginal sprays.
- Wear clean cotton underpants.
- Change out of wet bathing suits as soon as possible.
- Become familiar with the signs and symptoms of vaginitis.
- Choose to lead a healthy lifestyle.

- Bartholinitis
- Endometritis
- Salpingitis
- Dysfunctional uterine bleeding

Significant risk factors for chlamydia include:

- Being an adolescent
- Having multiple sex partners
- Having a new sex partner
- Engaging in sex without using a barrier contraceptive (condom)
- Using oral contraceptive
- Being pregnant
- Having a history of another STI (Grella, 2005).

Diagnosis

The diagnosis can be made with nucleic acid amplification methods by polymerase chain reaction or ligase chain reaction (DNA probe, such as GenProbe or Pace2). These are highly sensitive and specific when used on urethral and cervicovaginal swabs. They can also be used with good sensitivity and specificity on first-void urine specimens (Brevet & Wiggins, 2002). Several other diagnostic tests exist, including culture, nucleic acid probes, and enzyme-linked immunoassays. The chain reaction tests are the most sensitive and cost effective. The CDC strongly recommends screening of asymptomatic women at high risk in whom infection would otherwise go undetected (CDC, 2002).

Treatment

Antibiotics are usually used in treating this STI. The CDC treatment options for chlamydia include doxycycline or azithromycin. Because of the common coinfection of chlamydia and gonorrhea, a combination regimen of ceftriaxone with doxycycline or azithromycin is frequently prescribed (CDC, 2002, p. 33). Additional CDC guidelines for patient management include annual screening of all sexually active women aged 20 to 25 years old; screening of all high-risk people; and treatment with antibiotics effective against both gonorrhea and chlamydia for anyone diagnosed with a gonococcal infection (CDC, 2002).

Gonorrhea

Gonorrhea is a serious and potentially very severe bacterial infection. It is one of the oldest STIs: reference is made to the condition in the Old Testament of the Bible. It is rapidly becoming more and more resistant to cure. In the United States, an estimated 600,000 new gonorrhea infections occur annually (CDC, 2002). In common with all other STIs, it is an equal-opportunity infection—no one is immune to it, regardless of race, creed, sex, or sexual preference.

The cause of gonorrhea is a gram-negative diplococcus, *Neisseria gonorrhoeae*. The site of infection is the columnar epithelium of the endocervix. Gonorrhea is almost exclusively transmitted by sexual activity. In pregnant women, gonorrhea is associated with chorioamnionitis, premature labor, premature rupture of membranes, and postpartum endometritis (Gibbs et al., 2004). It can also be transmitted to the newborn in the form of ophthalmia neonatorum during birth by direct contact with gonococcal organisms in the cervix. Ophthalmia neonatorum is highly contagious and if untreated leads to blindness of the newborn.

Clinical Manifestations

Between 50% and 90% of women infected with gonorrhea are totally symptom-free (Sloane, 2002). Because women are so frequently asymptomatic, they are regarded as the real "problem" in the spread of gonorrhea. If symptoms are present, they might include:

- Abnormal vaginal discharge
- Dysuria
- Cervicitis
- Abnormal vaginal bleeding
- Bartholin's abscess
- PID
- Neonatal conjunctivitis in newborns
- Mild sore throat (for pharyngeal gonorrhea)
- Rectal infection (asymptomatic)
- Perihepatitis (King, 2004)

Risk factors include low socioeconomic status, living in an urban area, single status, inconsistent use of barrier contraceptives, and multiple sex partners.

Sometimes a local gonorrhea infection is self-limiting (there is no further spread), but usually the organism ascends upward through the endocervical canal to the endometrium of the uterus, further on to the fallopian tubes, and out into the peritoneal cavity. When the peritoneum and the ovaries become involved, the condition is known as *pelvic inflammatory disease* (PID). The scarring to the fallopian tubes is permanent. This damage is a major cause of infertility and is a possible contributing factor in ectopic pregnancy (Sloane, 2002).

If gonorrhea remains untreated, it can enter the bloodstream and produce a disseminated gonococcal infection. This severe form of infection can invade the joints (arthritis), the heart (endocarditis), the brain (meningitis), and the liver (toxic hepatitis). Figure 5-4 shows the typical appearance of gonorrhea.

Diagnosis

The CDC recommends screening for all women at risk for gonorrhea. Pregnant women should be screened at the first prenatal visit and again at 36 weeks of gestation. Nucleic acid hybridization tests (GenProbe) are used for diagnosis. Any woman suspected of having gonorrhea should be tested for chlamydia also because coinfection (45%) is extremely common (Lowdermilk & Perry, 2004).

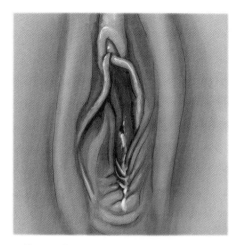

● Figure 5-4 Gonorrhea.

Treatment

The treatment of choice for uncomplicated gonococcal infections is cefixime orally or ceftriaxone intramuscularly. Azithromycin orally or doxycycline should accompany all gonococcal treatment regimens if chlamydial infection is not ruled out (CDC, 2002). Pregnant women should not be treated with quinolones or tetracyclines. Cephalosporins or a single 2-g intramuscular dose of spectinomycin should be used during pregnancy (CDC, 2002). To prevent gonococcal ophthalmia neonatorum, a prophylactic agent should be instilled into the eyes of all newborns; this procedure is required by law in most states. Erythromycin or tetracycline ophthalmic ointment in a single application is recommended (CDC, 2002).

Nursing Management

The prevalence of chlamydia and gonorrhea is increasing dramatically, and these infections can have long-term effects on people's lives. Sexual health is an important part of a person's physical and mental health, and nurses have a professional obligation to address it. Nurses need to be particularly sensitive when addressing STIs because women are often embarrassed or feel guilty. There is still a social stigma attached to STIs, so women need to be reassured about confidentiality.

The nurse's level of knowledge about chlamydia and gonorrhea should include treatment strategies, referral sources, and preventive measures. The nurse should be skilled at education and counseling and should be comfortable with women diagnosed with these infections.

High-risk groups include single women, women younger than 25 years, African-American women, women with a history of STIs, those with new or multiple sex partners, those with inconsistent use of barrier contraception, and women living in communities with high infection rates (Kirkham et al., 2005). Assessment involves taking a health history that includes a comprehensive sexual history. Questions about the number of sex partners and the use of safer sex practices are appropriate. Previous and current symptoms should be reviewed. Seeking treatment and informing sex partners should be emphasized.

The four-level P-LI-SS-IT model (Box 5-2) can be used to determine interventions for various women because it can be adapted to the nurse's level of knowledge, skill, and experience. Of utmost importance is the willingness to listen and show interest and respect in a nonjudgmental manner.

In addition to meeting the health needs of women with chlamydia and gonorrhea, the nurse is responsible for educating the public about the increasing incidence of these infections. This information should include high-risk behaviors associated with these infections, signs and symptoms, and the treatment modalities available. The nurse should stress that both of these STIs can lead to infertility and long-term sequelae. Safer sex practices need to be taught to people in non-monogamous relationships.

The nurse must know the physical and psychosocial responses to these STIs to prevent transmission and the disabling consequences. If this epidemic is to be halted, nurses must take a major front-line role now.

Infections Characterized by Genital Ulcers

Genital Herpes Simplex

Genital herpes is a recurrent, life-long viral infection. The CDC estimates that 50 million Americans have *genital herpes simplex* (HSV) infection, with a half million new cases annually (CDC, 2002). Two serotypes of HSV have been identified: HSV-1 and HSV-2. Today, approximately 10% of genital herpes infections are thought to be caused by HSV-1 and 90% by HSV-2 (Sloane, 2002). HSV-1 causes the familiar fever blisters or cold sores on the lips, eyes, and face. HSV-2 invades the mucous membranes of the geni-

tal tract and is known as herpes genitalis. Most persons infected with HSV-2 have not been diagnosed.

The herpes simplex virus is transmitted by contact of mucous membranes or breaks in the skin with visible or nonvisible lesions. Most genital herpes infections are transmitted by individuals unaware that they have an infection. Many have mild or unrecognized infections but still shed the herpes virus intermittently. HSV is transmitted primarily by direct contact with an infected individual who is shedding the virus. Kissing, sexual contact, and vaginal delivery are means of transmission.

Along with the increase in the incidence of genital herpes has been an increase in neonatal herpes simplex viral infections, which are associated with a high incidence of mortality and morbidity. The risk of neonatal infection with a primary maternal outbreak is between 30% to 50%; it is less than 1% with a recurrent maternal infection (CDC, 2002).

Clinical Manifestations

The clinical manifestations of HSV can be divided into the primary episode and recurrent infections. The first or *primary episode* is usually the most severe, with a prolonged period of viral shedding. Primary HSV is a systemic disease characterized by multiple painful vesicular lesions, mucopurulent discharge, superinfection with *Candida,* fever, chills, malaise, dysuria, headache, genital irritation, inguinal tenderness, and lymphadenopathy. The lesions in the primary herpes episode are frequently located on the vulva, vagina, and perineal areas. The vesicles will open and weep and finally crust over, dry, and disappear without scar formation (Fig. 5-5). This viral shedding process usually takes up to 2 weeks to complete. The virus remains dormant in the nerve cells for life, resulting in periodic outbreaks. Having sex with an infected partner places the individual at risk for contracting HSV.

Recurrent infection episodes are usually much milder and shorter in duration than the primary one. Tingling, itching, pain, unilateral genital lesions, and a more rapid resolution of lesions are characteristics of recurrent infections. Recurrent herpes is a localized disease characterized by typical HSV lesions at the site of initial viral

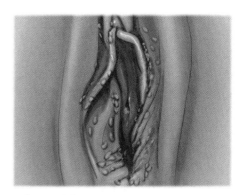

● Figure 5-5 Genital herpes simplex.

BOX 5-2

THE P-LI-SS-IT MODEL

P Permission—gives the woman permission to talk about her experience

LI Limited Information—information given to the woman about STIs
   • Factual information to dispel myths about STIs
   • Specific measures to prevent transmission
   • Ways to reveal information to her partners
   • Physical consequences if the infections are untreated

SS Specific Suggestions—an attempt to help women change their behavior to prevent recurrence and prevent further transmission of the STI

IT Intensive Therapy—involves referring the woman or couple for appropriate treatment elsewhere based on their life circumstances

entry. Recurrent herpes lesions are fewer in number and less painful and resolve more rapidly (Youngkin & Davis, 2004).

Recurrent genital herpes outbreaks are triggered by precipitating factors such as emotional stress, menses, and sexual intercourse, but more than half of recurrences occur without a precipitating cause. Immunocompromised women have more frequent and more severe recurrent outbreaks than normal hosts (King, 2004).

Living with genital herpes can be difficult due to the erratic, recurrent nature of the infection, the location of the lesions, the unknown causes of the recurrences, and the lack of a cure. Further, the stigma associated with this infection may affect the individual's feelings about herself and her interaction with partners. Potential psychosocial consequences may include emotional distress, isolation, fear of rejection by a partner, fear of transmission of the disease, loss of confidence, and altered interpersonal relationships (White & Mortensen, 2003).

Diagnosis

Diagnosis of HSV is often based on clinical signs and symptoms and confirmed by viral culture of fluid from the vesicle. Papanicolaou (Pap) smears are an insensitive and nonspecific diagnostic test for herpes simplex virus infection and should not be relied on for diagnosis.

Treatment

No cure exists, but antiviral drug therapy helps to reduce or suppress symptoms, shedding, and recurrent episodes. Advances in treatment with acyclovir, famciclovir, and valacyclovir have resulted in improved quality of life for those infected with HSV. However, these drugs neither eradicate latent virus nor affect the risk, frequency, or severity of recurrences after the drug is discontinued (CDC, 2002). Suppressive therapy is recommended for individuals with six or more recurrences per year. The natural course of the disease is for recurrences to be less frequent over time.

The management of genital herpes includes antiviral therapy. The safety of antiviral therapy has not been established during pregnancy. Therapeutic management also includes counseling regarding the natural history of the disease, the risk of sexual and perinatal transmission, and the use of methods to prevent further spread. Nurses must also address the psychosocial aspects of this STI with women by discussing appropriate coping skills, acceptance of the life-long nature of the condition, and options for treatment and rehabilitation.

Syphilis

Syphilis is a complex curable bacterial infection caused by the spirochete *Treponema pallidum*. It is a serious systemic disease that can lead to disability and death if untreated. Rates of syphilis in the United States are currently declin-

ing, but they remain high among young adult African-Americans in urban areas and in the south (CDC, 2002). It continues to be one of the most important STIs both because of its biological effect on HIV acquisition and transmission and because of its impact on infant health (Workowski & Berman, 2002).

The syphilis spirochete can cross the placenta at any time during pregnancy. One out of every 10,000 infants born in the United States has congenital syphilis (CDC, 2002). Maternal infection consequences include spontaneous abortion, prematurity, stillbirth, and multisystem failure of the heart, lungs, spleen, liver, and pancreas, as well as structural bone damage and nervous system involvement and mental retardation (Gilbert & Harmon, 2003).

Clinical Manifestations

Syphilis is divided into four stages: primary, secondary, latency, and tertiary. *Primary syphilis* is characterized by a chancre (painless ulcer) at the site of bacterial entry that will disappear within 1 to 6 weeks without intervention (Fig. 5-6). Motile spirochetes are present on darkfield examination of ulcer exudate. In addition, painless bilateral adenopathy is present during this highly infectious period. *Secondary syphilis* appears 2 to 6 months after the initial exposure and is manifested by flulike symptoms and a maculopapular rash of the trunk, palms, and soles. Alopecia and adenopathy are both common during this stage. The secondary stage of syphilis lasts about 2 years. Once the secondary stage subsides, the *latency* period begins. This stage is characterized by the absence of any clinical manifestations of disease, although the serology is positive. This stage can last as long as 20 years. If not treated, *tertiary* or late syphilis occurs, with life-threatening heart disease and neurologic disease that slowly destroys the heart, eyes, brain, central nervous system, and skin.

Diagnosis

Darkfield microscopic examinations and direct fluorescent antibody tests of lesion exudate or tissue are the definitive

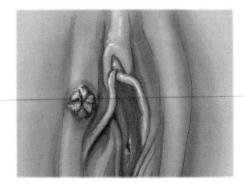

● Figure 5-6 Chancre of primary syphilis.

methods for diagnosing early syphilis. A presumptive diagnosis can be made by using two serologic tests:

- Nontreponemal tests (Venereal Disease Research Laboratory [VDRL] and rapid plasma reagin [RPR])
- Treponemal tests (fluorescent treponemal antibody absorbed [FTA-ABS] and *T. pallidum* particle agglutination [TP-PA]) (CDC, 2002).

Treatment

Fortunately, there is effective treatment for syphilis. Penicillin G, administered by either the intramuscular or intravenous route, is the preferred drug for all stages of syphilis. For pregnant or nonpregnant women with syphilis of less than 1 year's duration, the CDC recommends 2.4 million units of benzathine penicillin G intramuscularly in a single dose. If the syphilis is of longer duration (>1 year) or of unknown duration, 2.4 million units of benzathine penicillin G is given intramuscularly once a week for 3 weeks. The preparations used, the dosage, and the length of treatment depends on the stage and clinical manifestations of disease (CDC, 2002). Other medications, such as doxycycline, are available if the client is allergic to penicillin.

Women should be re-evaluated at 6 and 12 months after treatment for primary or secondary syphilis with additional serologic testing. Women with latent syphilis should be followed clinically and serologically at 6, 12, and 24 months (King, 2004).

Nursing Management

Genital ulcers from either herpes or syphilis can be devastating to women, and the nurse can be instrumental in helping her through this difficult time. Referral to a support group may be helpful. Teaching Guidelines 5-2 highlights appropriate teaching points for the patient with genital ulcers.

 TEACHING GUIDELINES 5-2

Caring for Genital Ulcers

- Abstain from intercourse during the prodromal period and when lesions are present.
- Wash hands with soap and water after touching lesions to avoid autoinoculation.
- Use comfort measures such as wearing nonconstricting clothes, wearing cotton underwear, urinating in water if urination is painful, taking lukewarm sitz baths, and air drying lesions with a hair dryer on low heat.
- Avoid extremes of temperature such as ice packs or hot pads to the genital area as well as application of steroid creams, sprays, or gels.
- Use condoms with all new or noninfected partners.
- Inform healthcare professionals of your condition.

Pelvic Inflammatory Disease

Pelvic inflammatory disease is an ascending infection of the upper female reproductive tract, most often caused by untreated chlamydia or gonorrhea (Fig. 5-7). An estimated 1 million cases are diagnosed annually, resulting in 250,000 hospitalizations (CDC, 2005). It is a serious health problem in the United States, costing an estimated $10 billion annually in terms of hospitalizations and surgical procedures (Murray et al., 2002). Complications include ectopic pregnancy, pelvic abscess, infertility, recurrent or chronic episodes of the disease, chronic abdominal pain, pelvic adhesions, and depression (Youngkin & Davis, 2004). Because of the seriousness of the complications of PID, an accurate diagnosis is critical.

Clinical Manifestations and Diagnosis

Because of the wide variety of clinical manifestations of PID, clinical diagnosis can be challenging. To reduce the risk of missed diagnosis, the CDC has established criteria to establish the diagnosis of PID. Minimal criteria (all must be present) are lower abdominal tenderness, adnexal tenderness, and cervical motion tenderness. Additional supportive criteria that support a diagnosis of PID are:

- Abnormal cervical or vaginal mucopurulent discharge
- Oral temperature above 101°F
- Elevated erythrocyte sedimentation rate
- Elevated C-reactive protein level
- *N. gonorrhoeae* or *C. trachomatis* infection documented
- White blood cells on saline vaginal smear (CDC, 2002)

The only way to definitively diagnose PID is through an endometrial biopsy, transvaginal ultrasound, or laparoscopic examination.

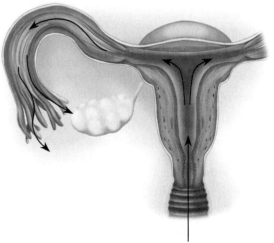

Spread of gonorrhea or chlamydia

● Figure 5-7 Pelvic inflammatory disease. Chlamydia or gonorrhea spreads up the vagina into the uterus and then to the fallopian tubes and ovaries.

Risk factors for PID include:

- Adolescence or young adulthood
- Nonwhite female
- Having multiple sex partners
- Early onset of sexual activity
- History of PID or STI
- Having intercourse with a partner who has untreated urethritis
- Recent insertion of an intrauterine device (IUD)
- Nulliparity
- Cigarette smoking
- Engaging in sex during menses (Youngkin & Davis, 2004)

Treatment

Treatment of PID must include empiric, broad-spectrum antibiotic coverage of likely pathogens. The client is treated on an ambulatory basis with oral antibiotics or is hospitalized and given antibiotics intravenously. The decision to hospitalize a woman is based on clinical judgment and the severity of her symptoms. Frequently, oral antibiotics are initiated, and if no improvement is seen within 72 hours, the woman is admitted to the hospital. Treatment then includes intravenous antibiotics, increased oral fluids to improve hydration, bed rest, and pain management. Follow-up is needed to validate that the infectious process is gone to prevent the development of chronic pelvic pain.

Nursing Management

Depending on the clinical setting (hospital or community clinic) where the nurse encounters the woman diagnosed with PID, a risk assessment should be done to ascertain what interventions are appropriate to prevent a recurrence. Explaining the various diagnostic tests needed to the woman is important to gain her cooperation. The nurse needs to discuss with the woman the implications of PID and the risk factors for the infection; her sexual partner should be included if possible. Sexual counseling should include practicing safer sex, limiting the number of sexual partners, using barrier contraceptives consistently, avoiding vaginal douching, considering another contraceptive method if she has an IUD and has multiple sexual partners, and completing the course of antibiotics prescribed (Abbuhl & Reyes, 2004). Review the serious sequelae that may occur if the condition is not treated or if the woman does not comply with the treatment plan. Ask the woman to have her partner go for evaluation and treatment to prevent a repeat infection. Provide nonjudgmental support while stressing the importance of barrier contraceptive methods and follow-up care.

Human Immunodeficiency Virus (HIV)

An estimated 900,000 people currently live with HIV, and an estimated 40,000 new HIV infections have occurred annually in the United States (CDC, 2003). Men who have sex with men represent the largest proportion of new infections, followed by men and women infected through heterosexual sex and injection drug use (CDC, 2004). The number of women with HIV infection and AIDS has been increasing steadily worldwide. The World Health Organization (WHO) estimates that over 19 million women are living with HIV/AIDS worldwide, accounting for approximately 50% of the 40 million adults living with HIV/AIDS (NIAID, 2004). HIV disproportionately affects African-American and Hispanic women: together they represent less than 25% of all U.S. women, yet they account for more than 82% of AIDS cases in women (CDC, 2003). Worldwide, more than 90% of all HIV infections have resulted from heterosexual intercourse. Women are particularly vulnerable to heterosexual transmission of HIV due to substantial mucosal exposure to seminal fluids. This biological fact amplifies the risk of HIV transmission when coupled with the high prevalence of nonconsensual sex, sex without condoms, and the unknown and/or high-risk behaviors of their partners (NIAID, 2004).

Therefore, the face of HIV/AIDS is becoming the face of young women. That shift will ultimately exacerbate the incidence of HIV because women spread it not only through sex, but also through nursing and childbirth.

Acquired immunodeficiency syndrome (AIDS) is a breakdown in the immune function caused by HIV, a retrovirus. The infected person develops opportunistic infections or malignancies that become fatal (Murray & McKinney, 2006).

Twenty years have passed since HIV/AIDS began to affect our society. Since then 40 million people have been infected by the virus, with AIDS being the fourth leading cause of death globally (CDC, 2004). The morbidity and mortality of HIV continues to hold the attention of the medical community. While there has been a dramatic improvement in both morbidity and mortality with the use of highly active antiretroviral therapy (HAART), the incidence of HIV infection continues to rise. More than 90% of individuals infected with HIV worldwide do not know they are infected (CDC, 2004).

The fetal and neonatal effects of acquiring HIV through perinatal transmission are devastating and eventually fatal. An infected mother can transmit HIV infection to her newborn before or during birth and through breastfeeding. Most cases of mother-to-child HIV transmission, the cause of more than 90% of pediatric-acquired infections worldwide, occur late in pregnancy or during delivery. Transmission rates vary from 25% in untreated non-breastfeeding populations in industrialized countries to about 40% among untreated breastfeeding populations in developing countries (NIAID, 2004).

Despite the dramatic reduction in perinatal transmission, hundreds of infants will be born infected with HIV.

In terms of epidemiology, fatality rate, and its social, legal, ethical, and political aspects, HIV/AIDS has become a public health crisis and has generated more concern than any other infectious disease in modern medical history (Sloane, 2002). To date, there is no cure for this fatal viral infection.

Clinical Manifestations

The HIV virus is transmitted by intimate sexual contact, by sharing needles for intravenous drug use, from mother to fetus during pregnancy, or by transfusion of blood or blood products. When a person is initially infected with HIV, he or she goes through an acute primary infection period for about 3 weeks. The HIV viral load drops rapidly because the host's immune system works well to fight this initial infection. The onset of the acute primary infection occurs 2 to 6 weeks after exposure. Symptoms include fever, pharyngitis, rash, and myalgia. Most people do not associate this flulike condition with HIV infection. After initial exposure, there is a period of 3 to 12 months before seroconversion. The person is considered infectious during this time.

After the acute phase, the infected person becomes asymptomatic, but the HIV virus begins to replicate. Even though there are no symptoms, the immune system runs down. A normal person has a CD4 T-cell count of 450 to 1,200 cells per microliter. When the CD4 T-cell count reaches 200 or less, the person has reached the stage of AIDS. The immune system begins a constant battle to fight this viral invasion, but over time it falls behind. A viral reservoir occurs in T cells that can store various stages of the virus. The onset and severity of the disease correlate directly with the viral load; the more HIV virus that is present, the worse the person will feel.

As profound immunosuppression begins to occur, an opportunistic infection will occur, qualifying the person for the diagnosis of AIDS. The diagnosis is finally confirmed when the CD4 count is below 200. As of now, AIDS will eventually develop in everyone who is HIV positive.

Because the HIV virus over time depletes the CD4 cell population, infected people become more susceptible to opportunistic infections. Currently, the AIDS virus and response to treatment are tracked based on CD4 count rather than viral load. Untreated HIV will progress to AIDS in about 10 years, but this progression can be delayed by antiretroviral therapy (Moreo, 2003).

Diagnosis

Newly approved quick tests for HIV produce results in 20 minutes and also lower the healthcare worker's risk of occupational exposure by eliminating the need to draw blood. The CDC's Advancing HIV Prevention initiative, launched in 2003, has made increased testing a national priority. The initiative calls for testing to be incorporated into routine medical care and to be delivered in more nontraditional settings.

Fewer than half of adults aged 18 to 64 have ever had an HIV test, according to the CDC. The agency estimates that one fourth of the 900,000 HIV-infected people in the United States do not know they are infected. This means they are not receiving treatment that can prolong their lives, and they may be unknowingly infecting others. In addition, even when people do get tested, one in three failed to return to the testing site to learn their results when there was a 2-week wait. The CDC hopes that the new "one-stop" approach to HIV testing changes that pattern. About 40,000 new HIV cases are reported each year in the United States, and that number has held steady for the past few years despite massive efforts in prevention education (CDC, 2002).

The OraQuick Rapid HIV-1 Antibody Test detects the HIV antibody in a blood sample taken with a finger-stick or from an oral fluid sample. Both can produce results in as little as 20 minutes with more than 99% accuracy (Hemmila, 2004). The FDA has approved two other rapid blood tests: Reveal Rapid HIV-1 Antibody Test and the Uni-Gold Recombigen HIV Test.

Testing for HIV should be offered to anyone seeking evaluation and treatment for STIs. Counseling before and after testing is an integral part of the testing procedure. Informed consent must be obtained before an HIV test is performed. HIV infection is diagnosed by tests for antibodies against HIV-1 and HIV-2 (HIV-1/2). Antibody testing begins with a sensitive screening test (e.g., the enzyme immunoassay [ELISA]). This is a specific test for antibodies to HIV that is used to determine whether the person has been exposed to the HIV retrovirus. Reactive screening tests must be confirmed by a more specific test (e.g., the Western blot [WB]) or an immunofluorescence assay (IFA). This is a highly specific test that is used to validate a positive ELISA test finding. If the supplemental test (WB or IFA) is positive, it confirms that the person is infected with HIV and is capable of transmitting the virus to others. HIV antibody is detectable in at least 95% of people within 3 months after infection (CDC, 2002).

Treatment

The goals of HIV drug therapy are to:

- Decrease the HIV viral load below the level of detection
- Restore the body's ability to fight off pathogens
- Improve the client's quality of life
- Reduce HIV morbidity and mortality (Moreo, 2003)

Often treatment begins with combination HAART therapy at the time of the first infection, when the person's immune system is still intact. The current HAART therapy standard is a triple combination therapy, but some clients may be given a fourth or fifth agent.

There are obvious challenges involved in meeting these goals. The viral load can be reduced much more quickly than the T-cell count can be increased, and this disparity leaves the woman vulnerable to opportunistic infections.

Current therapy to prevent the transmission of HIV to the newborn includes a three-part regimen of having the mother take an oral antiretroviral agent at 14 to 34 weeks of gestation; it is continued throughout pregnancy. During labor, an antiretroviral agent is administered intravenously until delivery. An antiretroviral syrup is administered to the infant within 12 hours after birth.

Dramatic new treatment advances with antiretroviral medications have turned a disease that used to be a death sentence into a chronic, manageable one for individuals who live in countries where antiretroviral therapy is available. Despite these advances in treatment, only a minority of HIV-positive Americans who take antiretroviral medications are receiving the full benefits because they are not adhering to the prescribed regimen. Successful antiretroviral therapy requires nearly perfect adherence to a complex medication regimen; less-than-perfect adherence leads to drug resistance (CDC, 2002).

Adherence is difficult because of the complexity of the regimen and the life-long duration of treatment. A typical antiretroviral regimen may consist of three or more medications taken twice daily. Adherence is made even more difficult because of the unpleasant side effects, such as nausea and diarrhea. Women in early pregnancy already experience these, and the antiretroviral medication only exacerbates them.

Nurses can help to reduce the development of drug resistance and thus treatment failure by identifying the barriers to adherence and can work to help the woman to overcome them. Some of the common barriers include:

- The woman does not understand the link between drug resistance and nonadherence.
- The woman fears revealing her HIV status by being seen taking medication.
- The woman hasn't adjusted emotionally to the HIV diagnosis.
- The woman doesn't understand the dosing regimen or schedule.
- The woman experiences unpleasant side effects frequently.
- The woman feels anxious or depressed (Enriquez & McKinsey, 2004)

Depending on which barriers are causing nonadherence, the nurse can work with the woman by educating her about the dosing regimen, helping her find ways to integrate the prescribed regimen into her lifestyle, and making referrals to social service agencies as appropriate. By addressing barriers on an individual level, the nurse can help the woman to overcome them.

Nursing Management

Consider THIS!

I was thinking of my carefree college days, when the most important thing was having an active sorority life and meeting guys. I had been raised by very strict parents and never allowed to date under their watch. Since I attended an out-of-state college, my parent's outdated advice and rules no longer applied. Abruptly, my past thoughts were interrupted by the HIV counselor asking about my feelings concerning my positive diagnosis. What was there to say at this point? I had a lot of fun but never dreamed it would haunt me for the rest of my life, which was going to be shortened considerably now. I only wish I could turn back the hands of time and listened to my parents' advice, which somehow doesn't seem so outdated now.

Thoughts: All of us have thought back on our lives to better times and wondered how our lives would have changed if we had made better choices or gone down another path. It is a pity that we have only one chance to make good sound decisions at times. What would you have changed in your life if given a second chance? Can you still make a change for the better now?

Nurses can play a major role in caring for the HIV-positive woman by helping her accept the possibility of a shortened life span, cope with others' reactions to a stigmatizing illness, and develop strategies to maintain her physical and emotional health. The nurse can educate the woman about changes she can make in her behavior to prevent spreading HIV to others and can refer her to appropriate community resources such as HIV medical care services, substance abuse, mental health services, and social services. See Nursing Care Plan 5-1: Overview for the Woman With HIV.

Providing Education About Drug Therapy

The goal of antiretroviral therapy is to suppress viral replication so that the viral load becomes undetectable (<400). This is done to preserve immune function and delay disease progression but is a challenge because of the side effects of nausea and vomiting, diarrhea, altered taste, anorexia, flatulence, constipation, headaches, anemia, and fatigue. Although not everyone experiences all of the side effects, the majority do have some of them. Current research hasn't documented the long-term safety of exposure of the fetus to antiretroviral agents during pregnancy, but collection of data is ongoing.

The nurse can educate the woman about the prescribed drug therapy and impress upon her that it is very important to take the regimen as prescribed. Offer suggestions about how to cope with anorexia, nausea, and vomiting by:

Nursing Care Plan 5-1

Overview of the Woman Who Is HIV Positive

Annie, a 28-year-old African-American woman, is HIV positive. She acquired HIV through unprotected sexual contact. She has been inconsistent in taking her antiretroviral medications and presents today stating she is tired and doesn't "feel well."

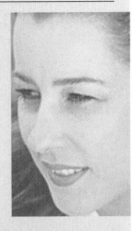

Nursing Diagnosis: Risk for infection related to positive HIV status and inconsistent compliance with antiretroviral therapy

Outcome Identification and *evaluation*

Client will remain free of opportunistic infections as *evidenced by temperature within acceptable parameters and absence of signs and symptoms of opportunistic infections.*

Interventions with *rationales*

Assess CD4 count and viral loads *to determine disease progression* (CD4 counts <500/L and viral loads >10,000 copies/L = increased risk for opportunistic infections).

Assess complete blood count *to identify presence of infection* (>10,000 cells/mm^3 may indicate infection)

Assess oral cavity and mucous membranes for painful white patches in mouth *to evaluate for possible fungal infection.*

Monitor for general signs and symptoms of infections, such as fever, weakness, and fatigue, *to ensure early identification.*

Stress importance of avoiding people with infections when possible *to minimize risk of exposure to infections.*

Teach importance of keeping appointments so her CD4 count and viral load can be monitored *to alert the healthcare provider about her immune system status.*

Instruct her *to reduce her exposure to infections* via:
-Meticulous handwashing
-Thorough cooking of meats, eggs, and vegetables
-Wearing shoes at all times, especially when outdoors

Encourage a balance of rest with activity throughout the day *to prevent overexertion.*

Stress importance of maintaining prescribed antiretroviral drug therapies *to prevent disease progression and resistance.*

If necessary, refer Annie to a nutritionist *to help her understand what constitutes a well-balanced diet with supplements to promote health and ward off infection.*

(continued)

Overview of the Woman Who Is HIV Positive (continued)

Nursing Diagnosis: Knowledge deficit related to HIV infection and possible complications

Outcome Identification and *evaluation*	Interventions with *rationales*
Client will demonstrate increased understanding of HIV infection as *evidenced by verbalizing appropriate health care practices and adhering to measures to comply with therapy and reduce her risk of further exposure and reduce risk of disease progression.*	Assess understanding of HIV and its treatment *to provide a baseline for teaching.* Establish trust and be honest with Annie; encourage her to talk about her fears and impact of the disease *to provide an outlet for her concerns and encourage her to discuss reasons for her noncompliance.* Present a nonjudgmental, accessible, confidential, and culturally sensitive approach *to promote Annie's self-esteem and allow her to feel that she is a priority.* Explain measures, including safer sex practices and birth control options, *to prevent disease transmission;* determine her willingness to practice safer sex to protect others *to determine further teaching needs.* Educate about signs and symptoms of disease progression and potential opportunistic infections *to promote early detection for prompt intervention.* Inform Annie about the availability of community resources and make appropriate referrals as needed *to provide additional education and support.* Encourage Annie to keep scheduled appointments *to ensure follow-up and allow early detection of potential problems.*

- Separating the intake of food and fluids
- Eating dry crackers upon arising
- Eating six small meals daily
- Using high-protein supplements (Boost, Ensure) to provide quick and easy protein and calories
- Eating "comfort foods," which may appeal when other foods don't

Promoting Compliance

Remaining compliant with drug therapy is a huge challenge for many HIV-infected people. Compliance becomes difficult when the same pills that are supposed to thwart the disease are making the person sick. Nausea and diarrhea are just two of the possible side effects. It is often difficult to increase the client's quality of life when so much oral mediation is required. The combination medication therapy is challenging for many people, and staying compliant over a period of years is extremely difficult. The nurse can stress the importance of taking the prescribed antiretroviral drug therapies by explaining that they help prevent replication of the retroviruses and subsequent progression

of the disease, as well as decreasing the risk of perinatal transmission of HIV. In addition, the nurse can provide written materials describing diet, exercise, medications, and signs and symptoms of complications and opportunistic infections. This information should be reinforced at each visit.

Preventing HIV Infection

The lack of information about HIV infection and AIDS causes great anxiety and fear of the unknown. Nurses must take a leadership role in educating the public about risky behaviors in the fight to control this disease.

The core of HIV prevention is to abstain from sex until marriage, to be faithful, and to use condoms. This is all good advice for many women, but some simply do not have the economic and social power or choices or control over their lives to put that advice into practice. Nurses need to recognize that fact and address the factors that will give them more control over their lives by providing anticipatory guidance, giving ample opportunities to practice negotiation techniques and refusal skills in a safe environment, and encouraging the use of female condoms to protect themselves against this deadly virus. Prevention is the key to reversing the current infection trends.

Providing Care During Pregnancy and Childbirth

Voluntary counseling and HIV testing should be offered to all pregnant women as early in the pregnancy as possible to identify HIV-infected women so that treatment can be initiated early. Once identified as being HIV infected, pregnant women should be informed about the risk for perinatal infection. Current evidence indicates that in the absence of antiretroviral medications, 25% of infants born to HIV-infected mothers will become infected with HIV (CDC, 2003). If women do receive a combination of antiretroviral therapies during pregnancy, however, the risk of HIV transmission to the newborn drops below 2% (NIAID, 2004). In addition, HIV can be spread to the infant through breastfeeding, and thus all HIV-infected pregnant women should be counseled to avoid breastfeeding and use formula instead.

In addition, the woman needs instructions in ways to enhance her immune system by following these guidelines during pregnancy:

- Getting adequate sleep each night (7 to 9 hours)
- Avoiding infections (e.g., staying out of crowds, hand washing)
- Decreasing stress in her life
- Consuming adequate protein and vitamins
- Increasing her fluid intake to 2 liters daily to stay hydrated
- Planning rest periods throughout the day to prevent fatigue

Despite the dramatic reduction in perinatal transmission, hundreds of infants will be born infected with HIV. The birth of each infected infant is a missed prevention opportunity. To minimize perinatal HIV transmission, nurses can identify HIV infection in women, preferably before pregnancy; provide information relative to disease prevention; and encourage HIV-infected women to follow the prescribed drug therapy.

Providing Appropriate Referrals

The HIV-infected woman is challenged by coping with the normal activities of daily living with a compromised energy level and decreased physical endurance. She may be overwhelmed by the financial burdens of medical and drug therapies and the emotional responses to a life-threatening condition, as well as concern about her infant's future, if she is pregnant. A case management approach is needed to deal with the complexity of her needs during this time. The nurse can be an empathetic listener but needs to make appropriate referrals for nutritional services, counseling, homemaker services, spiritual care, and local support groups. Many community-based organizations have developed programs to address the numerous issues regarding HIV/AIDS. The national AIDS hotline (1-800-342-AIDS) is a good resource.

Human Papillomavirus

Human papillomavirus (HPV) is the most common viral infection in the United States (CDC, 2005). Genital warts or condylomata (Greek for warts) are caused by HPV. Conservative estimates suggest that in the United States, approximately 20 million people have productive HPV infection, and 5.5 million Americans acquire it annually (CDC, 2005). HPV-mediated oncogenesis is responsible for up to 95% of cervical squamous cell carcinomas and nearly all preinvasive cervical neoplasms (Morris, 2002). More than 40 types of HPV can infect the genital tract.

Clinical Manifestations

Most HPV infections are asymptomatic, unrecognized or subclinical. Visible genital warts usually are caused by HPV types 6 or 11. Other HPV types (16, 18, 31, 33, and 35) have been strongly associated with cervical cancer (CDC, 2005). In addition to the external genitalia, genital warts can occur on the cervix and in the vagina, urethra, anus, and mouth. Depending on the size and location, genital warts can be painful, friable, and pruritic, although most are typically asymptomatic (Fig. 5-8).

Risk factors for HPV include having multiple sex partners, immunosuppression, smoking, age (15 to 25), contraceptive use, pregnancy, concurrent herpes infection, and socioeconomic variables such as poverty, domestic violence, sexual abuse, and inadequate health care (Hatcher et al., 2004).

Diagnosis

Clinically visible warts are diagnosed by inspection. The warts are fleshy papules with a warty, granular surface. Lesions can grow very large during pregnancy, affecting urination, defecation, mobility, and descent of the fetus (Carey & Rayburn, 2002). Large lesions, which may resemble cauliflowers, exist in coalesced clusters and bleed easily.

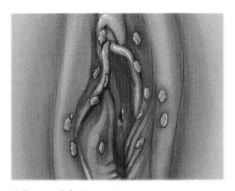

● Figure 5-8 Genital warts.

Diagnostic testing to determine the specific HPV strain may be useful to discriminate between low-risk and high-risk HPV types. A specimen for testing can be obtained with a fluid-phase collection system such as Thin Prep. If the test is positive for the high-risk types, the woman should be referred for colposcopy. Serial Pap smears are done for low-risk women. Regular Pap smears will detect the cellular changes associated with HPV.

Treatment

The primary goal of treatment is to remove the warts and induce wart-free periods for the client. Treatment of genital warts should be guided by the preference of the client and available resources. No single treatment has been found to be ideal for all clients, and most treatment modalities appear to have comparable efficacy. Treatment options for HPV are numerous and may include:

- Topical trichloroacetic acid (TCA) 80% to 90%
- Liquid nitrogen cryotherapy
- Topical imiquimod 5% cream (Aldara)
- Topical podophyllin 10% to 25%
- Laser carbon dioxide vaporization
- Client-applied Podofilox 0.5% solution or gel
- Simple surgical excision
- Loop electrosurgical excisional procedure (LEEP)
- Intralesional interferon therapy (NAIAID, 2004b)

Nursing Management

Education and counseling are important aspects of managing women with genital warts. The woman should know that:

- Even after the warts are removed, the HPV still remains and viral shedding will continue.
- The likelihood of transmission to future partners and the duration of infectivity after treatment is unknown.
- The use of latex condoms has been associated with a lower rate of cervical cancer.
- The recurrence of genital warts within the first few months after treatment is common and usually indicates recurrence rather than reinfection.
- Examination of sex partners is not necessary because there are no data to indicate that reinfection plays a role in recurrences (CDC, 2002).

Because genital warts can proliferate and become friable during pregnancy, they should be removed using a local agent. A cesarean birth is not indicated solely to prevent transmission of HPV infection to the newborn, unless the pelvic outlet is obstructed by warts (CDC, 2002).

Clinical studies have confirmed that HPV is the cause of essentially all cases of cervical cancer, which is the fourth most common cancer in women in the United States following lung, breast, and colorectal cancer

(American Cancer Society, 2003). An HPV infection has many implications for the woman's health, but most women are unaware of HPV and its role in cervical cancer. Recurring warts is a key risk factor for the development of cervical cancer. Nurses can play a significant role in educating women about the link between HPV and cervical cancer prevention. All women should obtain regular Pap smears. The morbidity and mortality associated with cervical cancer can be reduced. Research continues toward the development of HPV immunizations, but at present regular Pap smears and follow-up of any abnormalities is the standard of care (Likes & Itano, 2003).

Vaccine-Preventable STIs
Hepatitis A and B

Hepatitis is an acute, systemic, viral infection that can be transmitted sexually. The viruses associated with hepatitis or inflammation of the liver are hepatitis A, B, C, D, E, and G. *Hepatitis A* (HAV) is spread via the gastrointestinal tract. It can be acquired by drinking polluted water, eating uncooked shellfish from sewage-contaminated waters or food handled by a hepatitis carrier with poor hygiene, and from oral/anal sexual contact. Approximately 33% of the U.S. population has serologic evidence of prior hepatitis A infection; the rate increases directly with age (CDC, 2002).

Hepatitis B (HBV) is transmitted through saliva, blood serum, semen, menstrual blood, and vaginal secretions (Sloane, 2002). In the 1990s, transmission among heterosexual partners accounted for 40% of infections, and transmission among men who have sex with men accounted for 15% of infections. Risk factors for infection include having multiple sex partners, engaging in unprotected receptive anal intercourse, and having a history of other STIs (CDC, 2002). The most effective means to prevent the transmission of hepatitis A or B is preexposure immunization. Vaccines are available for the prevention of HAV and HBV, both of which can be transmitted sexually. Every person seeking treatment for an STI should be considered a candidate for hepatitis B vaccination, and some individuals (e.g., men who have sex with men, and injection-drug users) should be considered for hepatitis A vaccination (CDC, 2002).

Clinical Manifestations and Diagnosis
Hepatitis A produces flulike symptoms with malaise, fatigue, anorexia, nausea, pruritus, fever, and upper right quadrant pain. Symptoms of hepatitis B are similar to those of hepatitis A, but with less fever and skin involvement. The diagnosis of hepatitis A cannot be made on clinical manifestations alone and requires serologic testing. The presence of IgM antibody to HAV is diagnostic of acute HAV infection. Hepatitis B is diagnosed by the presence of hepatitis B surface antibody (HBsAg) (CDC, 2002).

Treatment

Unlike other STIs, HBV and HAV are preventable through immunization. HAV is usually self-limiting and does not result in chronic infection. HBV can result in serious, permanent liver damage. Treatment is generally supportive. No specific treatment for acute HBV infection exists.

Nursing Management

Nurses should encourage all women to be screened for hepatitis when they have their annual Pap smear, or sooner if high-risk behavior is identified. Nurses should also encourage women to undergo HBV screening at their first prenatal visit and repeat screening in the last trimester for women with high-risk behaviors (CDC, 2002). Nurses can also explain that hepatitis B vaccine is given to all infants after birth in most hospitals. The vaccination consists of a series of three injections given within 6 months. The vaccine has been shown to be safe and well tolerated by most recipients (CDC, 2002).

Ectoparasitic Infections

Ectoparasites are a common cause of skin rash and pruritus throughout the world. These infections include infestations of scabies and pubic lice. Since these parasites are easily passed from one person to another during sexual intimacy, clients should be assessed for them when receiving care for other STIs. *Scabies* is an intense pruritic dermatitis caused by a mite. The female mite burrows under the skin and deposits eggs, which hatch, causing intense pruritus. The lesions start as a small papule that reddens, erodes, and sometimes crusts. Diagnosis is based on history and appearance of burrows in the webs of the fingers and the genitalia (Youngkin & Davis, 2004). Aggressive infestation can occur in immunodeficient, debilitated, or malnourished people, but healthy people do not usually suffer sequelae.

Clients with pediculosis pubis (pubic lice) usually seek treatment because of the pruritus, because of a rash brought on by skin irritation from scratching, or because they notice lice or nits in their pubic hair, axillary hair, abdominal and thigh hair, and sometimes in the eyebrows, eyelashes, and beards. Infestation is usually asymptomatic until after a week or so, when bites cause pruritus and secondary infections from scratching (Fig. 5-9). Diagnosis is based on history and the presence of nits (small, shiny, yellow, oval, dewdrop-like eggs) affixed to hair shafts or lice (a yellowish, oval, wingless insect) (Breslin & Lucas, 2003).

Treatment is directed at the infested area, using permethrin cream or lindane shampoo (CDC, 2002). Bedding and clothing should be washed in hot water to decontaminate it. Sexual partners should be treated also, as well as family members who live in close contact with the infected person.

Nursing care of a woman infested with lice or scabies involves a three-tiered approach: eradicating the infesta-

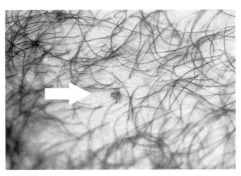

● Figure 5-9 Pubic lice. A small brown living crab louse is seen at the base of hairs (*arrow*). (Source: Goodheart, H. [2003]. *Goodheart's photoguide of common skin disorders*. Philadelphia: Lippincott Williams & Wilkins.)

tion with medication, removing nits, and preventing spread or recurrence by managing the environment. Over-the-counter products containing pyrethrins (RID, Triple X, Pronto, and Kwell) are safe for use and kill the active lice or mites. Nurses should provide education about the products as described in Teaching Guidelines 5-3. The nurse can follow these same guidelines to prevent the healthcare facility from becoming infested.

Prevention of Sexually Transmitted Infections

It is not easy to discuss STI prevention when globally we are failing at it. Knowledge exists on how to prevent every single route of transmission, but the incidence continues to climb. Challenges to prevention of STIs include lack of resources and difficulty in changing the behaviors that contribute to their spread. Regardless of the challenging factors involved, nurses must continue to educate and to meet the needs of all women to promote their sexual health. Successful treatment and prevention of STIs is impossible without education. Successful teaching approaches include giving clear, accurate messages that are age-appropriate and culturally sensitive.

 T E A C H I N G   G U I D E L I N E S   5 - 3

Treating and Minimizing the Spread of Scabies and Pubic Lice

Use the medication according to the manufacturer's instructions.

Remove nits with a fine-toothed nit comb.

Do not share any personal items with others or accept items from others.

Treat objects, clothing, and bedding and wash them in hot water.

Meticulously vacuum carpets to prevent a recurrence of infestation.

Primary prevention strategies include education of all women, especially adolescents, regarding the risk of early sexual activity, the number of sexual partners, and STIs. Sexual abstinence is ideal but often not practiced; therefore, the use of barrier contraception (condoms) should be encouraged.

Secondary prevention involves the need for annual pelvic examinations with Pap smears for all sexually active women, regardless of age. Many women with STIs are asymptomatic, so regular screening examinations are paramount for early detection. Understanding the relationship between poor socioeconomic conditions and poor patterns of sexual and reproductive self-care is significant in disease-prevention and health-promotion strategies.

Every successful form of prevention requires a change in behavior. The nursing role in teaching and rendering quality healthcare is invaluable evidence that the key to reducing the spread of STIs is through behavioral change. Nurses working in these specialty areas have a responsibility to educate themselves, their clients, their families, and the community about STIs and providing compassionate and supportive care to clients. Some strategies nurses can use to prevent the spread of STIs are detailed in Box 5-3.

Behavior Modification

Research validates that changing behaviors does result in a decrease in new STI infections, but it must encompass all

---

BOX 5-3

SELECTED NURSING STRATEGIES TO PREVENT THE SPREAD OF STIs

✓ Provide basic information about STI transmission.
✓ Outline safer sexual behaviors for people at risk for STIs.
✓ Refer to appropriate community resources to reduce risk.
✓ Screen asymptomatic people with STIs.
✓ Identify barriers to STI testing and remove them.
✓ Offer preexposure immunizations for vaccine-preventable STIs.
✓ Respond honestly about testing results and options available.
✓ Counsel and treat sexual partners of persons with STIs.
✓ Educate school administrators, parents, and teens about STIs.
✓ Support youth development activities to reduce sexual risk-taking.
✓ Promote the use of barrier methods (condoms, diaphragms) to prevent the spread of STIs.
✓ Assist clients to gain skills in negotiating safer sex.
✓ Discuss reducing the number of sexual partners to reduce risk.

---

levels—governments, community organizations, schools, churches, parents, and individuals (Miller et al., 2003). Education must address ways to prevent becoming infected, ways to prevent transmitting infection, symptoms of STIs, and treatment. At this point in the STI epidemic, nurses do not have time to debate the relative merits of prevention versus treatment: both are underused and underfunded, and one leads to the other. But being serious about prevention and focusing on the strategies outlined above will bring about a positive change on everyone's part.

Contraception

The spread of STIs could be prevented by access to safe, efficient, appropriate, modern contraception for everyone who wants it. Nurses can play an important role in helping women to identify their risk of STIs and to adopt preventive measures through the dual protection that contraceptives offer. Traditionally, family planning and STI services have been separate entities. Family planning services have addressed a woman's need for contraception without considering her or her partner's risk of STI; meanwhile, STI services have been heavily slanted toward men, ignoring the contraceptive needs of men and their partners.

Many women are at significant risk for unintended pregnancy and STIs, yet with this separation of services, there is limited evaluation of whether they need dual protection—that is, concurrent protection from STIs and unintended pregnancy. This lack of integration of services represents a missed opportunity to identify many at-risk women and to offer them counseling on dual protection (Mantell et al., 2003).

Nurses can expand their scopes in either setting by discussing dual protection by use of a male or female condom alone or by use of a condom along with a nonbarrier contraceptive. Because barrier methods are not the most effective means of fertility control, they have not been typically recommended as a method alone for dual protection. Unfortunately, the most effective pregnancy prevention methods—sterilization, hormonal methods, and IUDs—do not protect against STIs. Dual-method use protects against STIs and pregnancy.

KEY CONCEPTS

● Avoiding risky sexual behaviors may preserve fertility and prevent chronic conditions later in life.
● An estimated 65 million people live with an incurable STI and another 15 million are infected each year.
● The most reliable way to avoid transmission of STIs is to abstain from sexual intercourse (i.e., oral, vaginal, or anal sex) or to be in a long-term mutually monogamous relationship with an uninfected partner.
● Barrier methods of contraception are recommended because they increase protection from contact with

urethral discharge, mucosal secretions, and lesions of the cervix or penis.

- The high rate of asymptomatic transmission of STIs calls for teaching high-risk women the nature of transmission and how to recognize infections.
- The CDC and ACOG recommend that all women be offered group B streptococcal screening by rectovaginal culture at 35 to 37 weeks of gestation, and that colonized women be treated with intravenous antibiotics at the time of labor or ruptured membranes.
- Nurses should practice good handwashing techniques and follow standard precautions to protect themselves and their patients from STIs.
- Nurses are in an important position to promote the sexual health of all women. Nurses should make their clients and the community aware of the perinatal implications and life-long sequelae of STIs.

References

Abbuhl, S., & Reyes, I. (2004). Pelvic inflammatory disease. *EMedicine* [Online]. Available at: http://emedicine.com/emerg/topic410.htm

American Cancer Society (ACS) (2003). *Cancer facts and figures 2003.* Atlanta, GA: Author.

Breslin, E. T., & Lucas, V. A. (2003). *Women's health nursing: toward evidence-based practice.* St. Louis, MO: Saunders.

Brevet, D. B., & Wiggins, M. (2002). Preventing and treating STDs. *Advance for Nurses, 3*(23), 15–18.

Burstein, G. R., Lowry, R., Klein, J. D., & Santelli, J. S. (2003). Missed opportunities for sexually transmitted diseases, human immunodeficiency virus, and pregnancy prevention services during adolescent health supervision visits. *Pediatrics, 111*(5), 996–1001.

Carey, J. C., & Rayburn, W. F. (2002). *Obstetrics and gynecology* (4th ed.). Philadelphia: Lippincott Williams & Wilkins.

Centers for Disease Control and Prevention (CDC) (2002). Sexually transmitted diseases treatment guidelines. *MMWR, 51*(RR-6), 1–77.

Centers for Disease Control and Prevention (CDC) (2002). HIV/AIDS surveillance. General epidemiology. [Online] Available at: http://www.cdc.gov/hiv/graphics/surveill.htm

Centers for Disease Control and Prevention (CDC) (2003). Advancing HIV prevention: new strategies for a changing epidemic—United States. *MMWR, 52*(15), 329.

Centers for Disease Control and Prevention (2004). *Sexually transmitted disease surveillance 2003.* Atlanta, GA: U.S. Department of Health and Human Services.

Centers for Disease Control and Prevention (CDC). (2005). *Genital HPV infection—CDC fact sheet.* [Online] Available at: http://www.cdc.gov/std/HPV/STDFact-HPV.htm

Centers for Disease Control and Prevention (CDC). (2005). *Pelvic inflammatory disease—CDC fact sheet.* [Online] Available at: http://www.cdc.gov/std/PID/STDFact-PID.htm

Enriquez, M., & McKinsey, D. (2004). Readiness for HIV treatment. *American Journal of Nursing, 104*(10), 81–84.

Gibbs, R. S., Sweet, R. L., & Duff, W. P. (2004). Maternal and fetal infectious diseases. In R. K. Creasy, R. Resnik, & J. D. Iams (Eds.), *Maternal-fetal medicine: principles and practice* (5th ed., pp. 741–801). Philadelphia: Saunders.

Gilbert, E. S., & Harmon, J. S. (2003). *Manual of high risk pregnancy & delivery* (3rd ed.). St. Louis, MO: Mosby.

Grella, M. (2005). Chlamydial infections. *eMedicine* [Online]. Available at: http://www.emedicine.com/ped/topic378.htm

Hatcher, R., et al. (2004). *A pocket guide to managing contraception.* Tiger, GA: Bridging the Gap Foundation.

Hemmila, D. (2004). The wait is over. *Nursing Spectrum,* 68–71.

King, J. (2004). *Sexually transmitted infection update.* Lecture presented at The Women's Health Update for Nurse Practitioners & Physicians in Orlando, Florida: Emory University School of Medicine Regional Training Center.

Kirkham, C., Harris, S., & Grzybowski, S. (2005). Evidence-based prenatal care: Part II. Third-trimester care and prevention of infectious diseases. *American Family Physician, 71*(8), 1555–1562.

Likes, W. M., & Itano, J. (2003). Human papillomavirus and cervical cancer: not just a sexually transmitted disease. *Clinical Journal of Oncology Nursing, 7*(3), 271–276.

Lowdermilk, D. L., & Perry, S. E. (2004). *Maternity & women's health care* (8th ed.). St. Louis: Mosby, Inc.

Mantell, J. E., Hoffman, S., Exner, T. M., Stein, Z. A., & Atkins, K. (2003). Family planning providers' perspectives on dual protection. *Perspectives on Sexual and Reproductive Health, 35*(2), 71–78.

Miller, K. E., Ruiz, D. E., & Graves, J. C. (2003). Update on the prevention and treatment of sexually transmitted disease. *American Family Physician, 67*(9), 1915–1922.

Moreo, K. (2003). HIV/AIDS and HIV nephropathy. *Nephrology Nursing Journal, 30*(1), 64–68.

Morris, R. T. (2002). Human papillomavirus and genital neoplasia. In S. B. Ransom, M. P. Dombrowski, M. I. Evans, & K. A. Ginsburg (Eds.), *Contemporary therapy in obstetrics and gynecology.* Philadelphia: W. B. Saunders.

Murray, S. S. & McKinney, E. S. (2006). *Foundations of maternal-newborn nursing* (4th ed.). Philadelphia: W. B. Saunders.

National Institute of Allergy and Infectious Diseases (NIAID) (2004). HIV infection in women. *National Institutes of Health.* [Online] Available at: http://www.niaid.nih.gov/factsheets/womenhiv.htm

National Institute of Allergy and Infectious Diseases (NAIAID). (2004b). Human papillomavirus and genital warts. *National Institutes of Health.* [Online] Available: http://www.niaid.nih.gov/factsheets/stdhpv.htm

Scott, L. D., & Hasik, K. J. (2001). The similarities and differences of endometritis and pelvic inflammatory disease. *JOGNN, 30*(3), 332–341.

Sloane, E. (2002). *Biology of women* (4th ed.). New York: Delmar.

Weglarz, M., & Boland, M. (2005). Family-centered nursing care of the perinatally infected mother and child living with HIV infection. *Journal for Specialists in Pediatric Nursing, 10*(4), 161–170.

White, G., & Mortensen, A. (2003). Counteracting stigma in sexual health care settings. *Journal of Advanced Nursing Practice, 6*(1), 49–59.

Workowski, K., Levine, W., & Wasserheit, J. (2002). U.S. Centers for Disease Control and Prevention guidelines for the treatment of sexually transmitted diseases: an opportunity to unify clinical and public health practice. *Annals of Internal Medicine, 137*(4), 255–262.

Workowski, K. A., & Berman, S. M. (2002). CDC sexually transmitted disease treatment guidelines. *Clinical Infectious Diseases, 35*(Suppl 2): S135–137.

Youngkin, E. Q., & Davis, M. S. (2004). *Women's health: a primary care clinical guide* (3rd ed.). New Jersey: Prentice Hall.

Web Resources

American College of Obstetricians and Gynecologists (ACOG): (202) 863-2518, **http://www.acog.org**

American Psychiatric Association: (202) 682-6000, **http://psych.org**

American Society for Reproductive Medicine: (205) 978-5000, **http://www.asrm.org**

Centers for Disease Control and Prevention: (202) 329-1819, **http://www.cdc.gov**

CDC National AIDS hotline: 1-800-342-2437

Herpes Resource Center: **www.ashastd.org/herpes/hrc**

National Institute of Mental Health: (301) 443-4513, **http://www.nimh.nih.gov**

National Women's Health Resource Center: **http://www.healthywomen.org**

National Women's Information Center (NWHIC): 1-800-994-9662, **http://www.4women.gov**

Resolve, Inc. (Impaired fertility): (617) 623-0744, **http://www.resolve.org**

Chapter WORKSHEET

● MULTIPLE CHOICE QUESTIONS

1. Which of the following contraceptive methods offers protection against sexually transmitted infections (STIs)?

   a. Oral contraceptives

   b. Withdrawal

   c. Latex condom

   d. Intrauterine device

2. In teaching about HIV transmission, the nurse explains that the virus cannot be transmitted by:

   a. Shaking hands

   b. Sharing drug needles

   c. Sexual intercourse

   d. Breastfeeding

3. A woman with HPV is likely to present with which nursing assessment finding?

   a. Profuse, pus-filled vaginal discharge

   b. Clusters of genital warts

   c. Single painless ulcer

   d. Multiple vesicles on genitalia

4. The nurse's discharge teaching plan for the woman with PID should reinforce which of the following potentially life-threatening complications?

   a. Involuntary infertility

   b. Chronic pelvic pain

   c. Depression

   d. Ectopic pregnancy

5. To confirm a finding of primary syphilis, the nurse would observe which of the following on the external genitalia?

   a. A highly variable skin rash

   b. A yellow-green vaginal discharge

   c. A nontender, indurated ulcer

   d. A localized gumma formation

● CRITICAL THINKING EXERCISE

1. Sally, age 17, comes to the Teen Clinic saying that she is in pain and has some "crud" between her legs. The nurse takes her into the examining room and questions her about her symptoms. Sally states she had numerous genital bumps that had been filled with fluid, then ruptured and turned into ulcers with crusts. In addition, she has pain on urination and overall body pain. Sally says she had unprotected sex with several men when she had been drunk at a party a few weeks back, but she thought they were "clean."

   a. What STI would the nurse suspect?

   b. The nurse should give immediate consideration to which of Sally's complaints?

   c. What should be the goal of the nurse in teaching Sally about STIs?

● STUDY ACTIVITIES

1. Select a website at the end of the chapter to explore. Educate yourself about one specific STI thoroughly and share your expertise with your clinical group.

2. Contact your local health department and request current statistics regarding three STIs. Ask them to compare the current number of cases reported to last year's. Are they less or more? What may be some of the reasons for the change in the number of cases reported?

3. Request permission to attend a local STI clinic to shadow a nurse for a few hours. Describe the nurse's counseling role with patients and what specific information is emphasized to patients.

4. Two common STIs that appear together and commonly are treated together regardless of identification of the secondary one are _____ and _____.

5. Genital warts can be treated with which of the following? Select all that apply.

   a. Penicillin

   b. Podophyllin

   c. Imiquimod

   d. Cryotherapy

   e. Antiretroviral therapy

   f. Acyclovir

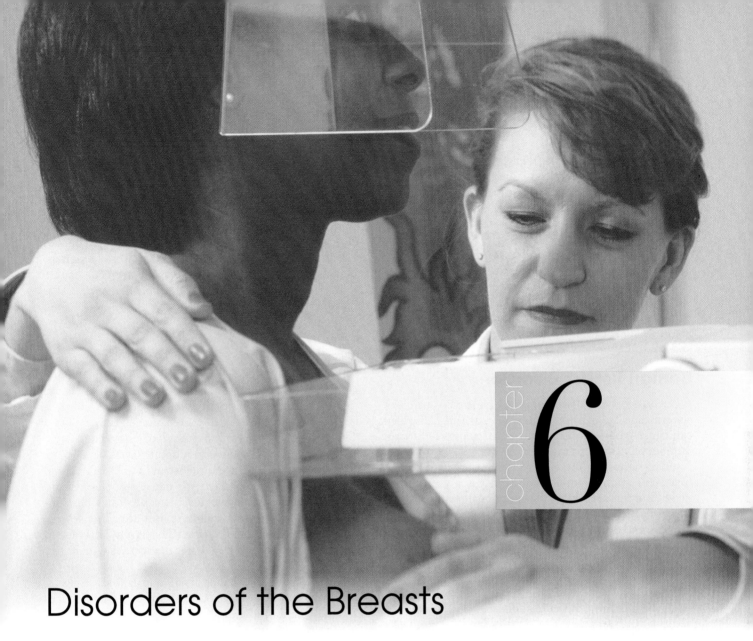

Disorders of the Breasts

chapter 6

KeyTERMS

benign breast disorder
breast cancer
breast-conserving surgery
breast self-examination
carcinoma
chemotherapy
fibroadenomas
fibrocystic breast changes
hormonal therapy
intraductal papilloma
mammary duct ectasia
mammography
mastitis
modified radical
   mastectomy
simple mastectomy

LearningOBJECTIVES

After studying the chapter content, the student should be able to accomplish the following:

1. Define the key terms.
2. Discuss the incidence, risk factors, screening methods, and treatment modalities for benign breast conditions.
3. Outline preventive strategies for breast cancer through lifestyle changes and health screening.
4. Describe the incidence, risk factors, treatment modalities, and nursing considerations related to breast cancer.
5. Develop an educational plan to teach breast self-examination to a group of young women.

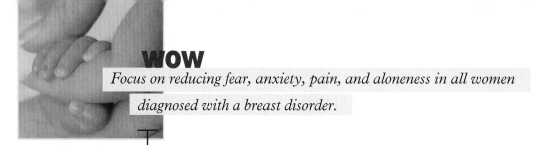

WOW

The female breast is closely linked to womanhood in American culture. Women's breasts act as physical markers for transitions from one stage of life to another, and although the primary function of the breasts is lactation, they are perceived as a symbol of beauty and sexuality.

This chapter will discuss assessments, screening procedures, and management of specific benign and malignant breast disorders. Nurses play a key role in helping women maintain breast health by educating and screening them to improve their health outcomes. A good working knowledge of early detection techniques, diagnosis, and treatment options is essential.

Benign Breast Disorders

A **benign breast disorder** is any noncancerous breast abnormality. Though not life-threatening, benign disorders can cause pain and discomfort and account for a large number of visits to primary care providers.

Depending on the type of benign breast disorder, treatment might or might not be necessary. Although these disorders are benign, the emotional trauma women experience is phenomenal. Fear, anxiety, disbelief, helplessness, and depression are just a few of the reactions that a woman may have when she discovers a lump in her breast. Many women believe that all lumps are cancerous, but actually more than 90% of the lumps discovered are benign and need no treatment (Alexander et al., 2004). Patience, support, and education are essential components of nursing care.

Consider**THIS!**

It was pouring down rain and I was driving alone along dark wet streets to my 8:00 appointment for a breast ultrasound. I recently had my annual mammogram and the radiologist thought he saw something suspicious on my right breast. I was on my way to confirm or refute his suspicions, and I couldn't keep focused on the road ahead. For the past few days I have been a basketcase, fearing the worst. I was playing in my mind what I would do if.... What changes I would make in my life and how I would react when told. I have been through personal turmoil since that doctor announced he wanted "more tests."

Thoughts: This woman is worrying and is emotionally devastated before she even has a conclusive diagnosis. Is this a typical reaction to a breast disorder? Why do women fear the worst? Many women use denial to mask their feelings and hope against hope the doctor made a mistake or misread their mammogram. How would you react if confronted with a breast disorder?

The most commonly encountered benign breast disorders in women include fibrocystic breasts, fibroadenomas, intraductal papilloma, mammary duct ectasia, and mastitis. Although breast disorders are generally benign, fibrocystic breasts and intraductal papillomas carry a cancer risk, with prolific masses and hyperplastic changes within the breasts. Generally speaking, fibroadenomas, mastitis, and mammary duct ectasia carry little cancer risk (DiSaia & Creasman, 2002). Table 6-1 summarizes benign breast conditions.

Fibrocystic Breast Changes

The term **fibrocystic breast changes** does not refer to a disease; rather, it describes a variety of changes in the glandular and structural tissues of the breast. Because this condition affects many women at some point, it is more accurately defined as a "change" rather than a "disease." The cause of fibrocystic changes is related to the way breast tissue responds to monthly levels of estrogen and progesterone. During menstrual cycles, hormonal stimulation of the breast tissue causes the glands and ducts to enlarge and swell. The breasts feel swollen, tender, and lumpy during this time, but after menses the swelling and lumpiness decline. This is why it is best to examine the breasts a week after the menses, when they are not swollen.

Fibrosis, or thickening of the normal breast tissue, occurs in the early stages. Cysts form in the later stages and feel like multiple, smooth, well-delineated tiny pebbles or lumpy oatmeal under the skin (Fig. 6-1). One or both breasts can be involved, and any part of the breast can become tender (Condon, 2004). Fibrocystic changes do not increase the risk of breast cancer for most women. Fibrocystic breast changes are most common in women between the ages of 30 and 50. The condition is rare in postmenopausal women not taking hormone replacement therapy. According to the American Cancer Society (ACS), fibrocystic breast changes affect at least half of all women at some point in their lives (ACS, 2003). It is the most common breast disorder today (Lewis et al., 2004).

Clinical Manifestations

Common manifestations include lumpy, tender breasts, particularly during the week before menses. Changes in breast tissue produce pain by nerve irritation from edema in connective tissue and by fibrosis from nerve pinching. The pain is cyclic and frequently dissipates after the onset of menses. The pain is described as a dull, aching feeling of fullness. Masses or nodularities usually appear in both breasts and are often found in the upper outer quadrants. Some women also experience spontaneous clear to

Table 6-1 Summary of Benign Breast Disorders

Breast Condition	Nipple Discharge	Site	Characteristics/ Age of Client	Tenderness	Dx & Tx
Fibrocystic breast changes	+ or −	Bilateral; upper outer quadrant	Round, smooth Several lesions Cyclic, palpable 30 to 50 years old	+	Aspiration & bx Limit caffeine Ibuprofen Supportive bra
Fibroadenomas	−	Unilateral; nipple area or upper outer quadrant	Round, firm, movable Palpable, rubbery Well delineated Single lesion 15 to 30 years old	−	Mammogram Watch & see Aspiration & bx Surgical excision
Intraductal papilloma	+	Unilateral; near nipple	Small, wartlike Poorly delineated Nonpalpable Can become large 40 to 60 years old	+	Culture discharge Mammogram Ultrasound Surgical excision
Mammary duct ectasia	+	Unilateral; behind nipple	Inflammation Pasty discharge Nonmobile Burning, itching Perimenopausal women	+	Mammogram Ultrasound Culture Surgical excision
Mastitis	−	Unilateral; outer quadrant	Wedge-shaped Warmth, redness Swelling Nipple cracked Breast engorged	+	Antibiotics Warm shower Supportive bra Breastfeeding Increase fluids

Sources: Alexander et al. (2004); Breslin & Lucas (2003); Condon (2004); Lowdermilk & Perry (2004); Mihelic (2003); Olds et al. (2004).

yellow nipple discharge when the breast is squeezed or manipulated.

Diagnosis

On examination of the breasts, a few characteristics might be helpful in differentiating a cyst from a cancerous lesion. Cancerous lesions typically are fixed and painless and may cause skin retraction (pulling). Cysts tend to be mobile and tender and do not cause skin retraction in the surrounding tissue. Mammography can be helpful in distinguishing fibrocystic changes from breast cancer. Ultrasound is a useful adjunct to mammography for breast evaluation because it helps to differentiate a cystic mass from a solid one (Hindle & Gonzalez, 2001). Ultrasound produces images of the breasts by sending sound waves through a gel applied to the breasts. Fine-needle aspiration biopsy can also be done to differentiate a solid tumor, cyst, or malignancy. A fine-needle aspiration biopsy uses a thin needle guided by ultrasound to the mass. In a method called stereotactic needle biopsy, a computer maps the exact location of the mass using mammograms

taken from two angles, and the map is used to guide the needle.

Treatment

Management of the symptoms of fibrocystic breast changes begins with self-care. In severe cases drugs, including bromocriptine, tamoxifen, or danazol, can be used to reduce the influence of estrogen on breast tissue. However, several undesirable side effects, including masculinization, have been documented. Aspiration or surgical removal of breast lumps will reduce pain and swelling by removing the space-occupying mass.

Nursing Management

A nurse caring for a woman with fibrocystic breast changes can teach her about the condition, provide tips for self-care (Teaching Guidelines 6-1), suggest lifestyle changes, and demonstrate how to perform a monthly breast self-examination after her menses to monitor the changes. Nursing Care Plan 6-1 presents a plan of care for a woman with fibrocystic breast changes.

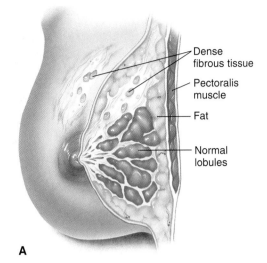

A

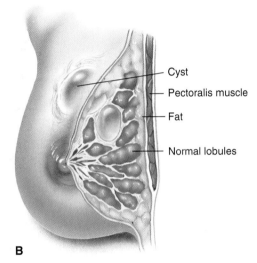

B

● Figure 6-1 (**A**) Fibrocystic breast changes. (**B**) Cysts. (Source: The Anatomical Chart Company. [2002]. *Atlas of pathophysiology*. Springhouse, PA: Springhouse Corporation.)

Fibroadenomas

Fibroadenomas are common benign solid breast tumors that occur in about 10% of all women and account for up to half of all breast biopsies. They are the second most common solid tumors in the breast after carcinoma (Mihelic, 2003). They are considered hyperplastic lesions associated with an aberration of normal development and involution rather than a neoplasm. Fibroadenomas can be stimulated by external estrogen, progesterone, lactation, and pregnancy (Amshel & Sibley, 2001). They are composed of both fibrous and glandular tissue and usually occur in women between 20 and 30 years of age (Alexander et al., 2004). Fibroadenomas are rarely associated with cancer.

Diagnosis

Breast fibroadenomas are usually detected incidentally during clinical or self-examinations and are most often

TEACHING GUIDELINES 6-1

Relieving Symptoms of Fibrocystic Breast Changes

• Wear an extra-supportive bra to prevent undue strain on the ligaments of the breasts to reduce discomfort.
• Avoid caffeine, which is a stimulant. This reduces discomfort for some women.
• Take oral contraceptives, as recommended by a healthcare practitioner, to stabilize the monthly hormonal levels.
• Maintain a low-fat diet rich in fruits, vegetables, and grains to maintain a healthy nutritional lifestyle and ideal weight.
• Apply heat to the breasts to help reduce pain via vasodilation of vessels.
• Take diuretics, as recommended by a healthcare practitioner, to counteract fluid retention and swelling of the breasts.
• Reduce salt intake to reduce fluid retention and swelling in the breasts.
• Take OTC medications, such as aspirin or ibuprofen (Motrin, Advil, Nuprin), to reduce inflammation and discomfort.
• Use thiamine and vitamin E therapy. This has been found helpful for some women, but research has failed to demonstrate a direct benefit from either therapy.
• Take medications as prescribed (e.g., bromocriptine, tamoxifen, or danazol).
• Discuss the possibility of aspiration or surgical removal of breast lumps with a healthcare practitioner.

located in the upper outer quadrants. Several other breast lesions have similar characteristics, so every woman with a breast mass should be evaluated to exclude cancer.

Diagnostic studies include a clinical breast examination by a health care professional; imaging studies (mammography, ultrasound, or both); and some form of biopsy, most often a fine-needle aspiration, core needle biopsy, or stereotactic needle biopsy. The core needle biopsy removes a small cylinder of tissue from the breast mass, more than the fine-needle aspiration biopsy. If additional tissue needs to be evaluated, the advanced breast biopsy instrument (ABBI) is used. This instrument removes a larger cylinder of tissue for examination by using a rotating circular knife. The ABBI procedure removes more tissue than any of the other methods except a surgical biopsy (ACS, 2003).

Clinical Manifestations

Lumps are felt as firm, rubbery, well-circumscribed, freely mobile nodules that might or might not be tender when palpated. Lumps are usually located in the upper outer quadrant of the breast, and more than one may be present (Fig. 6-2). Giant fibroadenomas account for approximately 10% of cases. These masses are frequently larger

Nursing Care Plan 6-1

Overview of the Woman with Fibrocystic Breast Changes

Sheree Rollins is a 37-year-old woman who comes to the clinic for her routine checkup. During the examination, she states, "Sometimes my breasts feel so heavy and they ache a lot. I noticed a couple of lumpy areas in my breast just last week before I got my period. Is this normal? Now they feel like they are almost gone. Should I be worried?" Clinical breast exam reveals two small, pea-sized, mobile, slightly tender nodules in each breast bilaterally. No skin retraction noted. Previous mammogram revealed fibrocystic breast changes.

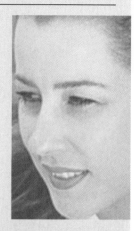

Nursing Diagnosis: Pain related to changes in breast tissue

Outcome identification and *evaluation*	Interventions with *rationales*
Client will demonstrate a decrease in breast pain *as evidenced by a pain rating of 1–2 on a pain rating scale of 0–10 and statements that pain is lessened.*	Ask client to rate her pain using a numeric pain rating scale *to establish a baseline.* Discuss with client any measures used to help relieve pain *to determine effectiveness of the measures.* Encourage use of a supportive bra *to aid in reducing discomfort.* Instruct client in use of over-the-counter analgesics *to promote pain relief.* Advise the client to apply warm compresses or allow warm water from the shower to flow over her breasts *to promote vasodilation and subsequent pain relief.* Tell client to reduce her intake of salt *to reduce risk of fluid retention and swelling leading to increased pain.*

Nursing Diagnosis: Deficient knowledge related to fibrocystic breast changes and appropriate care measures

Client will verbalize understanding of condition *as evidenced by statements about the cause of breast changes and appropriate choices for lifestyle changes, and demonstration of self-care measures.*	Assess client's knowledge of fibrocystic breast changes *to establish a baseline for teaching.* Explain the role of monthly hormonal level changes and describe the signs and symptoms *to promote understanding of this condition.* Teach the client how to perform a breast self-examination after her menstrual period *to monitor for changes.* Encourage client to report any changes promptly *to ensure early detection of problems.*

(continued)

Overview of the Woman with Fibrocystic Breast Changes (continued)

Outcome identification and *evaluation*	Interventions with *rationales*
	Suggest client speak with her primary care provider about the use of oral contraceptives *to help stabilize monthly hormonal levels.*
	Review lifestyle choices, such as avoiding caffeine, eating a low-fat diet rich in fruits, vegetables and grains, and adhering to screening recommendations *to promote health.*
	Discuss measures for pain relief *to minimize discomfort associated with breast changes.*

than 5 cm and occur most often in pregnant or lactating women (Condon, 2004).

Treatment and Nursing Management

Treatment may include a period of "watchful waiting" because many fibroadenomas stop growing or shrink on their own without any treatment. Other growths may need to be surgically removed if they do not regress or if they remain unchanged. Cryoablation, an alternative to surgery, can also be used to remove a tumor. In this procedure, extremely cold gas is piped into the tumor using ultrasound guidance. The tumor freezes and dies. The current trend is toward a more conservative approach to treatment after careful evaluation and continued monitoring. The nurse should urge the client to return for reevaluation in 6 months, perform monthly breast self-examinations, and return annually for a clinical breast examination.

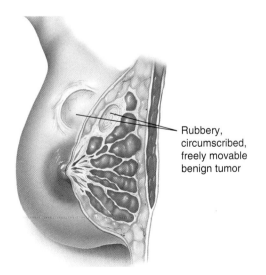

Rubbery, circumscribed, freely movable benign tumor

● Figure 6-2 Fibroadenoma. (Source: The Anatomical Chart Company. [2002]. *Atlas of pathophysiology.* Springhouse, PA: Springhouse Corporation.)

Intraductal Papilloma

An **intraductal papilloma** is a benign, wartlike growth found in the mammary ducts, usually near the nipple. This benign growth is thought to be caused by a proliferation and overgrowth of ductal epithelial tissue. An intraductal papilloma is generally less than 1 cm in diameter and might not be palpable. It produces a spontaneous serous, serosanguineous, or watery nipple discharge (DiSaia & Creasman, 2002). It mostly affects women between the ages of 40 and 60. A single duct or several ducts may be involved.

Diagnosis

The nipple discharge is evaluated for the presence of occult blood using a Hemoccult card; a blue coloration on the card indicates the presence of blood. In addition, a sample of the discharge may be sent for cytologic evaluation to screen for cancer cells. Mammography, ultrasound, or ductography (radiographic dye is instilled into a duct; it outlines the breast ductal system on radiographs) is used to diagnose or differentiate this lesion from a cancerous one. An intraductal papilloma appears as a smooth, lobulated filling defect or a solitary obstructed duct on ductography (Santen & Mansel, 2005).

Clinical Manifestations

A serous, serosanguineous, or watery discharge can be manually expressed from the nipple. If the papilloma is large enough, it can be palpated in the nipple area as a soft, nontender, mobile, poorly delineated mass. The woman might report a feeling of fullness in the breast.

Treatment and Nursing Management

Treatment consists of surgical removal of the papilloma and a part of the duct it is found in, usually through an incision at the edge of the areola. The excised papilloma and duct are sent to the pathology laboratory to rule out cancer (ACS, 2003). The nurse should advise the woman to continue monthly breast self-examinations and yearly clinical breast examinations.

Mammary Duct Ectasia

Mammary duct ectasia is a dilation and inflammation of the ducts behind the nipple. It is most common in perimenopausal women. This benign condition frequently occurs in women who have breastfed their children. The cause is unclear; however, chronic periductal inflammation, fibrosis, and ductal dilatation are associated factors (DiSaia & Creasman, 2002). This condition results in noncyclic breast pain and discharge.

Diagnosis

Mammography, ultrasound, cytology and testing for occult blood on nipple discharge sample, and ductography may be used to assist in the diagnosis of this lesion. In addition, physical examination of the breasts might reveal subareolar redness and swelling, with mild to moderate tenderness on palpation.

Clinical Manifestations

If the ducts have been chronically infected, an erythematous lesion will be present at the edge of the nipple area (ACS, 2003). On breast palpation, tortuous tubular swellings are present beneath the areola, along with nipple retraction and dimpling in some postmenopausal women (Olds et al., 2004). The nipple discharge can be green, brown, straw-colored, reddish, gray, or cream-colored, with the consistency of toothpaste. The woman may report a dull nipple pain, subareolar swelling, or a burning sensation accompanied by pruritus around the nipple (Lowdermilk & Perry, 2004).

Treatment and Nursing Management

This condition frequently improves without any specific treatment, or with warm compresses and antibiotics. If symptoms persist, the abnormal duct is removed through a local incision at the border of the areola. The tissue is sent to the pathology laboratory for evaluation. The nurse should reassure the woman that this condition is benign and should reinforce the importance of monthly self-examinations as well as annual clinical breast examinations by the woman's healthcare provider. This benign breast condition is typically self-limiting; the only intervention needed is reassurance.

Mastitis

Mastitis is an infection of the connective tissue in the breast that occurs primarily in lactating women. The usual causative organisms are *Staphylococcus aureus*, *Haemophilus influenzae*, and *Haemophilus* and *Streptococcus* species (London et al., 2003). Risk factors include poor handwashing, ductal abnormalities, nipple cracks and fissures, lowered maternal defenses due to fatigue, tight clothing,

poor support of pendulous breasts, and failure to empty the breasts properly while breastfeeding or missing feedings.

Clinical Manifestations and Diagnosis

The clinical manifestations may include flulike symptoms, including malaise, fever, and chills. Examination of the breasts reveals increased warmth, redness, tenderness, and swelling. The nipple is usually cracked or abraded and the breast is distended with milk (Fig. 6-3). The diagnosis is made based on history and examination.

Treatment and Nursing Management

Management of mastitis involves the use of oral antibiotics (usually a penicillinase-resistant penicillin or cephalosporin) and acetaminophen (Tylenol) for pain and fever. The nurse should teach the woman about the etiology of mastitis and encourage her to continue to breastfeed, emphasizing that the prescribed medication is safe to take during lactation. Continued emptying of the breast or pumping improves the outcome, decreases the duration of symptoms, and decreases the incidence of breast abscess. Thus, continued breastfeeding is recommended in the presence of mastitis (Youngkin & Davis, 2004). Instructions for the woman with mastitis are detailed in Teaching Guidelines 6-2.

Malignant Breast Disorder

Breast cancer is a neoplastic disease in which normal body cells are transformed into malignant ones (O'Toole, 2003). It is the most common cancer in women and the second leading cause of cancer deaths (lung cancer is

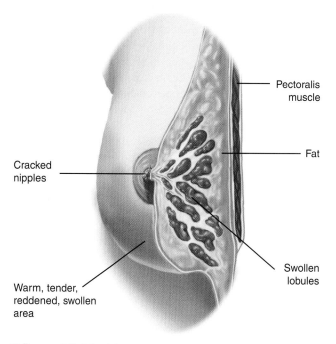

Pectoralis muscle

Fat

Cracked nipples

Swollen lobules

Warm, tender, reddened, swollen area

● Figure 6-3 Mastitis.

TEACHING GUIDELINES 6-2

Caring for Mastitis

- Take medications as prescribed.
- Continue breastfeeding, as tolerated.
- Wear a supportive bra 24 hours a day to support the breasts.
- Increase fluid intake.
- Practice good handwashing techniques.
- Apply warm compresses to the affected breast or take a warm shower before breastfeeding.
- Frequently change positions while nursing.
- Get adequate rest and nutrition to support or improve the immune system.

Modified from Mattson, S., & Smith, J. E. (2004). *Core curriculum for maternal-newborn nursing* (3rd ed.). St. Louis, MO: Elsevier Saunders.

Table 6-2 Estimated Risk of Breast Cancer at Specific Ages

Age 30 to 40	1 out of 262
Age 40 to 50	1 out of 68
Age 50 to 60	1 out of 35
Age 60 to 70	1 out of 27

Modified from National Cancer Institute (NCI). (2004). *Probability of breast cancer in American women.* (Online) Available at: http://cis.nci.nih.gov/fact/5_6.htm

first) among American women. Breast cancer accounts for one of every three cancers diagnosed in the United States (Kessler, 2002). A new case is discovered every 2 minutes (NCI, 2004). It is estimated that one out of every seven women will develop the disease at some time during her life.

In 2004 the ACS estimated that approximately 215,990 women would be diagnosed with breast cancer and 40,110 women would die of it (ACS, 2004). Breast cancer can also affect men, but only 1% of all individuals diagnosed with breast cancer annually are men (ACS, 2004).

Risk Factors

The etiology of breast cancer is unknown, but the disease is thought to develop in response to a number of related factors: aging, delayed childbearing or never bearing children, family history of cancer, late menopause, and hormonal factors (ACS, 2004). Other factors might contribute to breast cancer but have not been scientifically proven.

In 1970, the lifetime risk for developing breast cancer was one in ten; since then, the risk has gradually risen (NCI, 2004). This slight increase in incidence might be explained in a variety of ways—we now have better detection and screening tools, which have identified more cases; women are living to an older age, when their risk increases; and lifestyle changes in American women (having their first pregnancy at an older age, having fewer children, and using hormonal therapy to treat the symptoms of menopause) might have been associated with the higher numbers. Age is a significant risk factor. Because rates of breast cancer increase with age, estimates of risk at specific ages are more meaningful than estimates of lifetime risk. The estimated chance of a woman being diagnosed with breast cancer between the ages of 30 and 70 are detailed in Table 6-2.

Risk factors for breast cancer can be divided into those that cannot be changed (nonmodifiable risk factors) and those that can be changed (modifiable risk factors). Nonmodifiable risk factors (ACS, 2004) are:

- Gender (female)
- Aging (>50 years old)
- Genetic mutations (BRCA-1 and BRCA-2 genes)
- Family history of breast cancer (mother, sister, daughter, grandmother, or aunt)
- Personal history of breast cancer (3- to 4-fold increase in risk for recurrence)
- Race (higher in Caucasian women, but African-American women are more likely to die of it)
- Previous abnormal breast biopsy (atypical hyperplasia)
- Exposure to radiation (radiation damages DNA)
- Previous breast radiation (12 times normal risk)
- Early menarche (<12 years old) or late onset of menopause (>55 years old), which represents increased estrogen exposure over the lifetime

Modifiable risk factors related to lifestyle choices (ACS, 2004) include:

- Not having children at all or not having children until after age 30—this increases the risk of breast cancer by not reducing the number of menstrual cycles
- Postmenopausal use of estrogens and progestins—the recent WHI study (2002) reported increased risks with long-term (>5 years) use of hormone replacement therapy
- Failing to breastfeed for up to a year after pregnancy—increases the risk of breast cancer because it does not reduce the total number of lifetime menstrual cycles
- Alcohol consumption—boosts the level of estrogen in the bloodstream
- Smoking—exposure to carcinogenic agents found in cigarettes
- Obesity and consumption of high-fat diet—fat cells produce and store estrogen, so more fat cells create higher estrogen levels
- Sedentary lifestyle and lack of physical exercise—increases body fat, which houses estrogen

The presence of risk factors, especially several of them, calls for careful ongoing monitoring and evaluation to promote early detection. Even though risk factors are important considerations, 75% of all women with newly diagnosed breast cancer have no known risk factors (DiSaia & Creasman, 2002). While routine mammography and self-examination are prudent for everyone, these precautions may become lifesavers for at-risk individuals.

Clinical Manifestations

Early breast cancer has no symptoms. The earliest sign of breast cancer is often an abnormality seen on a mammogram before the woman or the healthcare professional feels it. As the tumor grows, changes in the breast appearance and contour become apparent (ACS, 2004). These include:

- Continued and persistent changes in the breast
- A lump or thickening in one breast
- Persistent nipple irritation
- Unusual breast swelling or asymmetry
- A lump or swelling in the axilla
- Changes in skin color or texture
- Nipple retraction, tenderness, or discharge

If a lump can be palpated, the cancer has been there for quite some time. Helpful characteristics in evaluating palpable breast masses are described in Box 6-1.

BOX 6-1

CHARACTERISTICS OF BENIGN VS. MALIGNANT BREAST MASSES

- Benign breast masses are described as:
  - Frequently painful
  - Firm, rubbery mass
  - Bilateral masses
  - Induced nipple discharge
  - Regular margins (clearly delineated)
  - No skin dimpling
  - No nipple retraction
  - Mobile, not affixed to the chest wall
  - No bloody discharge
- Malignant breast masses are described as:
  - Hard to palpation
  - Painless
  - Irregularly shaped (poorly delineated)
  - Immobile, fixed to the chest wall
  - Skin dimpling
  - Nipple retraction
  - Unilateral mass
  - Bloody, serosanguineous, or serous nipple discharge
  - Spontaneous nipple discharge

Modified from Makhoul, I., Makhoul, H., Harvey, H., & Souba, W. (2004). Breast Cancer. *EMedicine.* [Online] Available at: http://www. emedicine.com/MED/topic2808.htm; and American Cancer Society (ACS). (2004). Screening guidelines for the early detection of cancer in asymptomatic people. *Cancer prevention & early detection facts & figures 2004,* (p. 31). Atlanta, GA: Author.

Pathophysiology

Cancer is not just one disease, but rather a group of diseases that result from unregulated cell growth. Without regulation, cells divide and grow uncontrollably until they eventually form a tumor. Extensive research has determined that all cancer is the result of changes in DNA or chromosome structure that cause the mutation of specific genes. Most genetic mutations that cause cancer are acquired sporadically, which means they occur by chance and are not necessarily due to inherited mutations (Zawacki & Phillips, 2002). Cancer development is thought to be clonal in nature, which means that each cell is derived from another cell. If one cell develops a mutation, any daughter cell derived from that cell will have that same mutation, and this process continues until a malignant tumor forms.

Breast cancer starts in the epithelial cells that line the mammary ducts within the breast. The growth rate depends on hormonal influences, mainly estrogen and progesterone. The two major categories of breast cancer are noninvasive and invasive. Noninvasive, or in situ, breast cancers are those that have not extended beyond their duct, lobule, or point of origin into the surrounding breast tissue. Conversely, invasive, or infiltrating, breast cancers have extended into the surrounding breast tissue, with the potential to metastasize. Many researchers believe that most invasive cancers probably originate as noninvasive cancers (Weaver, 2002).

By far the most common breast cancer is invasive ductal carcinoma, which represents 70% to 80% of all cases (Makhoul et al., 2004). **Carcinoma** is a malignant tumor that occurs in epithelial tissue; it tends to infiltrate and give rise to metastases. The incidence of this cancer peaks in the sixth decade of life (>60 years old) and spreads rapidly to axillary and other lymph nodes, even while small. Infiltrating ductal carcinoma may take various histologic forms—well differentiated and slow-growing, poorly differentiated and infiltrating, or highly malignant and undifferentiated with numerous metastases. This common type of breast cancer starts in the ducts, breaks through the duct wall, and invades the fatty breast tissue (Penny, 2002).

Invasive lobular carcinomas, which originate in the terminal lobular units of breast ducts, account for 10% to 15% of all cases of breast cancer. The tumor is frequently located in the upper outer quadrant of the breast, and by the time it is discovered the prognosis is usually poor (Youngkin & Davis, 2004). Other invasive types of cancer include tubular carcinoma (2%), which is fairly uncommon and typically occurs in women aged 55 and older. Colloid carcinoma (2% to 4%) occurs in women 60 to 70 years of age and is characterized by the presence of large pools of mucus interspersed with small islands of tumor cells. Medullary carcinoma accounts for 5% to 7% of malignant breast tumors; it occurs frequently in younger women (<50 years of age) and grows into large tumor masses. Inflammatory breast cancer (<4%) often presents with skin edema, redness, and warmth and is associated with a poor prognosis. Paget's disease (2% to 4%) originates in the nipple and typically occurs with invasive ductal carcinoma (Makhoul et al., 2004; Penny, 2002).

Breast cancer is considered to be a highly variable disease. While the process of metastasis is a complex and poorly understood phenomenon, there is evidence to suggest that new vascularization of the tumor plays an important role in the biological aggressiveness of breast cancer (McCready, 2004). Breast cancer metastasizes widely and to almost all organs of the body, but primarily to the bone, lungs, nodes, liver, and brain. The first sites of metastases are usually local or regional, involving the chest wall or axillary supraclavicular lymph nodes or bone (Holmes, 2004).

Breast cancers are classified into three stages based on:

1. Tumor size
2. Extent of lymph node involvement
3. Evidence of metastasis

The purpose of tumor staging is to determine the probability the tumor has metastasized, to decide an appropriate course of therapy, and to assess the client's prognosis. Table 6-3 gives details and characteristics of each stage. The overall 10-year survival rate for a woman with stage I breast cancer is 80% to 90%; for a woman with stage II, it is about 50%. The outlook is not as good for women with stage III or IV disease (Sloane, 2002).

There is no completely accurate way to know whether the cancer has micrometastasized to distant organs, but certain tests can help determine if the cancer has spread. A bone scan can be performed to assess the bones. Magnetic resonance imaging (MRI) can be used to detect metastases to the liver, abdominal cavity, lungs, or brain.

Diagnostic Studies

There are many diagnostic studies performed to make an accurate diagnosis of a malignant breast lump. Diagnostic tests may include:

Table 6-3 Staging of Breast Cancer

Stage	Characteristics
0	In situ, early type of breast cancer
I	Localized tumor <1 inch in diameter
II	Tumor 1–2" in diameter; spread to axillary lymph nodes
III	Tumor 2" or larger and spread to other lymph nodes and tissues
IV	Cancer has metastasized to other body organs

American Cancer Society (ACS). (2004). *Cancer facts and figures 2003*. Atlanta, GA: Author.

- Diagnostic mammography
- Magnetic resonance mammography (MRM)
- Fine-needle aspiration
- Stereotactic needle-guided biopsy
- Sentinel lymph node biopsy
- Hormone receptor status
- DNA ploidy status
- Cell proliferative indices
- HER-2/neu genetic marker (Lewis et al., 2004)

Mammography

Mammography involves taking x-ray pictures of the bare breasts while they are compressed between two plastic plates. This procedure is performed to identify and characterize a breast mass and to detect an early malignancy. A screening mammogram typically consists of four views, two per breast (Fig. 6-4). It can detect lesions as small as 0.5 cm (the average size of a tumor detected by a woman practicing occasional breast self-examination is approximately 2.5 cm) (Willison, 2001). A diagnostic mammogram is performed when the woman has suspicious clinical findings on a breast examination or an abnormality has been found on a screening mammogram. A diagnostic mammogram uses additional views of the affected breast as well as magnification views. Diagnostic mammography provides the radiologist with additional detail to render a more specific diagnosis. A digital mammography, which records images in computer code instead of on x-ray film, can also be used so that images can be transmitted and easily stored.

Most women find the 10-minute mammography procedure uncomfortable but not painful. Teaching Guidelines 6-3 offers tips for a patient to follow before she undergoes this procedure.

Magnetic Resonance Mammography

MRM is a relatively new procedure that might allow for earlier detection because it can detect smaller lesions and provide finer detail. MRM is a highly accurate (>90% sensitivity for invasive carcinoma) but costly tool. Contrast infusion is used to evaluate the rate at which the dye initially enters the breast tissue. The basis of the high sensitivity of MRM is the tumor angiogenesis (vessel growth) that accompanies a majority of breast cancers, even early ones. Malignant lesions tend to exhibit increased enhancement within the first 2 minutes (Wang & Birdwell, 2004). Currently MRM is used only as a complement to mammography and clinical breast examination because it is expensive.

Fine-Needle Aspiration

Fine-needle aspiration (FNA) is done to identify a solid tumor, cyst, or malignancy. It is a simple office procedure that can be performed with or without anesthetic.

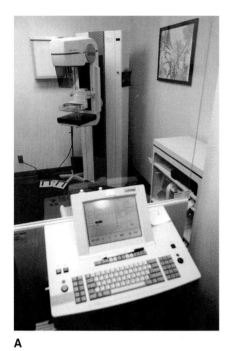

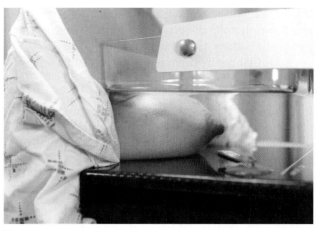

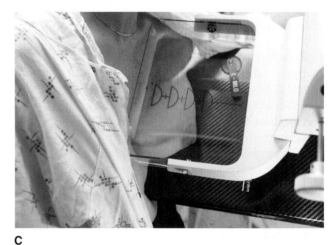

A

B

C

 Figure 6-4 Mammography.
(**A**) Mammography equipment.
(**B**) A top-to-bottom view of the breast.
(**C**) A side view of the breast.

A small (20- to 22-gauge) needle connected to a 10-cc or larger syringe is inserted into the breast mass and suction is applied to withdraw the contents. The aspirate is then sent to the cytology laboratory to be evaluated for abnormal cells.

TEACHING GUIDELINES 6-3

Preparing for a Screening Mammogram

- Schedule the procedure just after menses to reduce breast tenderness.
- Don't use deodorant or powder the day of the procedure, because they can appear on the x-ray film as calcium spots.
- Tylenol or aspirin can relieve any discomfort after the procedure.
- Remove all jewelry from around your neck, because the metal can cause distortions on the film image.
- Select a facility that is accredited by the American College of Radiology (ACR) to ensure appropriate credentialed staff.

Stereotactic Needle-Guided Biopsy

This diagnostic tool is used to target and identify mammographically detected nonpalpable lesions in the breast. This procedure is less expensive than an excisional biopsy. The procedure takes place in a specially equipped room and generally takes about an hour. When proper placement of the breast mass is confirmed by digital mammograms, the breast is locally anesthetized and a spring-loaded biopsy gun is used to obtain two or three core biopsy tissue samples. After the procedure is finished, the biopsy area is cleaned and a sterile dressing is applied.

Sentinel Lymph Node Biopsy

The status of the axillary lymph nodes is an important prognostic indicator in early-stage breast cancer. The presence or absence of malignant cells in lymph nodes is highly significant. The more lymph nodes involved and the more aggressive the cancer, the more powerful chemotherapy will have to be, both in terms of the toxicity of drugs and the duration of treatment (Makhoul et al., 2004). With a sentinel lymph node biopsy, the clinician can determine whether breast cancer has spread to the axillary lymph nodes without having to do a traditional axillary lymph node dissection. Experience has shown that the lymph ducts of the breast typically drain to one lymph node first before draining through the rest of the lymph nodes under the arm. The first lymph node is called the sentinel lymph node.

This procedure can be performed under local anesthesia. A radioactive blue dye is injected 2 hours before the biopsy to identify the afferent sentinel lymph node. The surgeon usually removes one to three nodes and sends them to the pathologist to determine whether cancer cells are present. The sentinel lymph node biopsy is usually performed before a lumpectomy to make sure the cancer has not spread. Removing only the sentinel lymph node can allow women with breast cancer to avoid many of the side effects (lymphedema) associated with a traditional axillary lymph node dissection (McCready, 2004).

Hormone Receptor Status

Normal breast epithelium has hormone receptors and responds specifically to the stimulatory effects of estrogen and progesterone. Most breast cancers retain estrogen receptors, and for those tumors estrogen will retain proliferative control over the malignant cells. It is therefore useful to know the hormone receptor status of the cancer to predict which women will respond to hormone manipulation. Hormone receptor status reveals whether the tumor is stimulated to grow by estrogen and progesterone. Tumors that have estrogen receptors are said to be "ER positive" (ER+) and tumors that do not have estrogen receptors are "ER negative" (ER–). The same terminology applies to progesterone (PR+ or PR–). ER+ and PR+ tumors have a better than 75% response to endocrine therapy in comparison to tumors that are ER+ and PR–, whose response rate is under 35%. Postmenopausal women tend to be ER+; premenopausal women tend to be ER– (Harwood, 2004). Women with these types of tumors generally have a better prognosis. A sample of breast cancer tissue obtained during a biopsy or a tumor removed surgically during a lumpectomy or mastectomy is examined by a cytologist.

DNA Ploidy Status

DNA ploidy status, which correlates with tumor aggressiveness, indicates the amount of DNA in cancer cells. Cancer cells that have the correct amount of DNA (diploid) in contrast with too much or too little DNA (aneuploid) tend not to spread. An aneuploid DNA pattern denotes a greater tendency to metastasize than a diploid one (Penny, 2002). A sample of breast cancer tissue obtained during a biopsy or a tumor removed surgically during a lumpectomy or mastectomy is examined for abnormal amounts of DNA. Using flow cytometry (process of counting and measuring cells), it is possible to measure the DNA content and proliferative activity of a tumor. The number of chromosome sets in the nucleus indicates

the speed of cell replication and tumor growth; a high number predicts a poor outcome.

Cell Proliferative Indices

Research indicates that cell proliferation potential may have prognostic significance. Cell proliferative indices indirectly measure the rate of cell division, which is an indication of how fast the cancer is growing. Flow and image cytometry are used to measure the tumor's cell cycle rate. The percent of tumor cells in S phase (synthesis stage of cell division) of the cell cycle is assessed. S-phase percentages below 10% are considered low, and the tumor has less of a chance of spreading than one with a higher percentage. A tumor with high proliferative activity has a more aggressive metastatic potential (Makhoul et al., 2004).

HER-2/neu Genetic Marker

Molecular and biologic factors are increasingly being used as indicators for prognosis and treatment. Human epidermal growth factor receptor 2 (HER2) whose biological function is associated with cell growth resulting in loss of cell regulation and uncontrolled cell proliferation.

HER-2/neu oncoprotein is a protein that is significant, especially in large tumors. Overexpression of this protein results from an acquired genetic mutation and occurs in approximately 30% of women with metastatic breast cancer. Women whose tumors have high levels of HER-2/neu oncoprotein have a poor prognosis: they have rapid tumor progression, an increased rate of recurrence, a poor response to standard therapies, and a lower survival rate (Schnell et al., 2003). The presence or absence of this oncoprotein helps determine which chemotherapy treatment will be most effective. A breast tissue sample is obtained by a fine-needle or open biopsy and treated with a material that binds to HER-2/neu oncoprotein. A dye is added to the tissue sample and the more uptake of the dye, the higher amount present (Schnell et al., 2003).

Therapeutic Management

Women diagnosed with breast cancer have many treatments available to them. Generally, treatments fall into two categories: local and systemic. Local treatments are surgery and radiation therapy. Effective systemic treatments include chemotherapy, hormonal therapy, and immunotherapy.

Treatment plans are based on multiple factors, primarily on whether the cancer is invasive or noninvasive, the tumor's size and grade, the number of cancerous axillary lymph nodes, the hormone receptor status, and the ability to obtain clear surgical margins (Weaver, 2002). A combination of surgical options and adjunct therapy is often recommended.

Another consideration in making decisions about a treatment plan is genetic testing for BRCA-1 and BRCA-2. This genetic testing became available in 1995 and can pinpoint women who have a significantly increased risk for breast and ovarian cancer: BRCA-1 and BRCA-2 mutations predispose individuals to a 75% lifetime risk of breast cancer and a 30% lifetime risk of ovarian cancer. Most cases of breast and ovarian cancer are sporadic in nature, but approximately 7% of breast cancers and 10% of ovarian cancers are thought to result from genetic inheritance (Zawacki & Phillips, 2002).

Testing positive for a BRCA-1 or BRCA-2 mutation can significantly alter healthcare decisions. In some cases, before genetic testing was available, lumpectomy with radiation or mastectomy was the treatment most often recommended. However, if the woman is found to have a BRCA-1 mutation, she is most likely to be offered the option of contralateral prophylactic mastectomy and possible bilateral oophorectomy (Rebbeck et al., 2004).

Severe psychological distress can occur as a result of genetic testing. Also, many women perceive their breasts as intrinsic to their femininity, self-esteem, and sexuality, and the risk of losing a breast can provoke extreme anxiety (Pasacreta et al., 2002). Nurses need to address the physical, emotional, and spiritual needs of the women they care for, as well as their families, since this mutation is inherited in an autosomal dominant fashion. Based on Mendelian genetics, first-degree relatives of affected women have a 50% risk of having inherited the mutation (Augustine & Bogan, 2004).

Surgical Options

Generally, the first treatment option for the woman diagnosed with breast cancer is surgery. A few women with tumors larger than 5 cm or inflammatory breast cancer may undergo neoadjuvant chemotherapy or radiotherapy to shrink the tumor before surgical removal is attempted (Holmes, 2004). The surgical options depend on the type and extent of cancer. The choices are typically either breast-conserving surgery (lumpectomy with radiation) or mastectomy with or without reconstruction. The overall survival rate with lumpectomy and radiation is about the same as that with modified radical mastectomy (ACS, 2003). Research has shown that the survival rates in women who have had mastectomies versus those who have undergone breast-conserving surgery followed by radiation are the same. However, lumpectomy may not be an option for some women, including those:

- Who have two or more cancer sites that cannot be removed through one incision
- Whose surgery will not result in a clean margin of tissue
- Who have active connective tissue conditions (lupus or scleroderma) that make body tissues especially sensitive to the side effects of radiation
- Who have had previous radiation to the affected breast
- Whose tumors are larger than 5 cm (2 inches) (NCCN, 2004)

These decisions are made jointly between the woman and her surgeon.

Breast-Conserving Surgery

Breast-conserving surgery, the least invasive procedure, is the wide local excision (or lumpectomy) of the tumor along with a 1-cm margin of normal tissue. A lumpectomy is often used for early-stage localized tumors. The goal of breast-conserving surgery is to remove the suspicious mass along with tissue free of malignant cells to prevent recurrence. The results are less drastic and emotionally less scarring to the woman. Women undergoing breast-conserving therapy receive radiation after lumpectomy with the goal of eradicating residual microscopic cancer cells to limit locoregional recurrence. In women who do not require adjuvant chemotherapy, radiation therapy typically begins 3 to 4 weeks after surgery to allow healing of the lumpectomy incision site. Radiation is administered to the entire breast at daily doses over a period of 5 to 6 weeks (Gordils-Perez et al., 2003).

A sentinel lymph node biopsy may also be performed since the lymph nodes draining the breast are located primarily in the axilla. Theoretically, if breast cancer is to metastasize to other parts of the body, it will probably do so via the lymphatic system. If malignant cells are found in the nodes, more aggressive systemic treatment may be needed.

Mastectomy

A **simple mastectomy** is the removal of all breast tissue, the nipple, and the areola. The axillary nodes and pectoral muscles are spared. This procedure would be used for a large or multiple tumors that have not metastasized to adjacent structures or the lymph system.

A **modified radical mastectomy** is another surgical option whose survival rates are comparable to those of radical mastectomy, but it more conducive to breast reconstruction and results in greater mobility and less lymphedema (Alexander et al., 2004). This procedure involves removal of breast tissue, the axillary nodes, and some chest muscles, but not the pectoralis major; thus avoiding a concave anterior chest (DiSaia & Creasman, 2002).

In conjunction with the mastectomy, lymph node surgery (removal of underarm nodes) may need to be done to reduce the risk of distant metastasis and improve a woman's chance of long-term survival. For woman with a positive sentinel node biopsy, the removal of 10 to 20 underarm lymph nodes may be needed. Complications associated with axillary lymph node surgery include nerve damage during surgery, causing temporary numbness down the upper aspect of the arm; seroma formation followed by wound infection; restrictions in arm mobility (some women need physiotherapy); and lymphedema. In many women lymphedema can be avoided by:

- Avoiding using the affected arm for drawing blood, inserting intravenous lines, or measuring blood pressure (can cause trauma and possible infection)
- Seeking medical care immediately if the affected arm swells

- Wearing gloves when engaging in activities such as gardening that might cause injury
- Wearing a well-fitted compression sleeve to promote drainage return

Women having mastectomies must decide whether to have further surgery to "reconstruct" the breast. If the woman decides to have reconstructive surgery, it ideally is performed immediately after the mastectomy. The woman must also determine whether she wants the surgeon to use saline implants or natural tissue from her abdomen (TRAM flap method) or back (LAT flap method).

In the transverse rectus abdominis myocutaneous (TRAM) flap method, the rectus abdominis muscle is transferred from the abdomen via a tunnel under the skin and brought out through a new excision in the breast area. The blood supply is maintained. This tissue is used to reconstruct the breast that has been removed. In the latissimus dorsi (LAT) flap method, tissue from the latissimus dorsi muscle in the upper back is tunneled subcutaneously up to the chest area.

If reconstructive surgery is desired, the ultimate decision regarding the method will be determined by the woman's anatomy (e.g., is there sufficient fat and muscle to permit natural reconstruction?) and her overall health status. Both procedures require a prolonged recovery period.

Some women opt for no reconstruction, and many of them choose to wear breast prostheses. Some prostheses are worn in the bra cup and others fit against the skin or into special pockets made into clothing.

Whether to have reconstructive surgery is an individual and very complex decision. Each woman must be presented with all of the options and then allowed to decide. The nurse can play an important role here by presenting the facts to the woman so that she can make an intelligent decision to meet her unique situation.

Adjunct Therapy

Adjunct therapy is supportive or additional therapy that is recommended after surgery. Adjunct therapies include local therapy such as radiation therapy and systemic therapies using chemotherapy, hormonal therapy, and immunotherapy.

Radiation Therapy

Radiation therapy uses high-energy rays to destroy cancer cells that might have been left behind in the breast, chest wall, or underarm area after the tumor has been removed surgically. Usually serial radiation doses are given 5 days a week to the tumor site for 6 to 8 weeks postoperatively. Each treatment only takes a few minutes, but the dose is cumulative. Women undergoing breast-conserving therapy receive radiation to the entire breast after lumpectomy with the goal of eradicating residual

microscopic cancer cells to reduce the chance of recurrence (Gordils-Perez et al., 2003).

Side effects of traditional radiation therapy include inflammation, local edema, anorexia, swelling, and heaviness in the breast; sunburn-like skin changes in the treated area; and fatigue. Changes to the breast tissue and skin usually resolve in about a year (Lowdermilk & Perry, 2004). This type of therapy can be given several ways: external beam radiation, which delivers a carefully focused dose of radiation from a machine outside the body, or internal radiation, in which tiny pellets that contain radioactive material are placed into the tumor.

Several advances have taken place in the field of radiation oncology for the treatment of women with early-stage breast cancer that assist in reducing the side effects. The treatment position for external radiation has changed from supine to prone, with the arm on the affected side raised above the head, so that the treated breast hangs dependently through the opening of the treatment board. Treatment in the prone position improves dose distribution within the breast and allows for a decrease in the dose delivered to the heart, lung, chest wall, and other breast (NCCN, 2004).

High-dose brachytherapy is another advance that is an alternative to traditional radiation treatment. A balloon catheter is used to insert radioactive seeds into the breast after the tumor is removed surgically. The seeds deliver a concentrated dose directly to the operative site; this is important because most cancer recurrences in the breast (67% to 100%) occur at or near the lumpectomy site. This allows a high dose of radiation to be delivered to a small target volume with a minimal dose to the surrounding normal tissue. This procedure takes 4 to 5 days as opposed to the 4 to 6 weeks traditional radiation therapy takes; it also eliminates the need to delay radiation therapy to allow for wound healing. Brachytherapy is now used as a primary radiation treatment after breast-conserving surgery in selected women as an alternative to whole breast irradiation (Vicini et al., 2002).

Side effects of brachytherapy include redness or discharge around catheters, fever, and infection. Daily cleansing of the catheter insertion site with a mild soap and application of an antibiotic ointment will minimize the risk of infection.

Intensity-modulated radiation therapy (IMRT) offers still another new approach to the delivery of treatment to reduce the dose within the target area while sparing surrounding normal structures. A computed tomography scan is used to create a three-dimensional model of the breast. Based on this model, a series of intensity-modulated beams are produced to the desired dose distribution to reduce radiation exposure to underlying structures. Acute toxicity is thus minimized (Chui et al., 2002). Research is ongoing to evaluate the impact of all of these advances in radiation therapy.

Chemotherapy

Chemotherapy refers to the use of drugs that are toxic to all cells and interfere with a cell's ability to reproduce. They are particularly effective against malignant cells but affect all rapidly dividing cells, especially those of the skin, the hair follicles, the mouth, the gastrointestinal tract, and the bone marrow. Breast cancer is a systemic disease in which small micrometastases are already present in other organs by the time the breast cancer is diagnosed. Chemotherapeutic agents perform a systemic "sweep" of the body to reduce the chances that distant tumors will start growing.

Chemotherapy may be indicated for women with tumors larger than 1 cm, positive lymph nodes, or cancer of an aggressive type. Chemotherapy is prescribed in cycles, with each period of treatment followed by a rest period. Treatment typically lasts 3 to 6 months, depending on the dose used and the woman's health status.

Different classes of drugs affect different aspects of cell division and are used in combinations or "cocktails." The most active and commonly used chemotherapeutic agents for breast cancer include alkylating agents, anthracyclines, antimetabolites, and vinca alkaloids. Fifty or more chemotherapeutic agents can be used to treat breast cancer; however, a combination drug approach versus a single drug treatment appears to be more effective (ACS, 2003).

Side effects of chemotherapy depend on the agents used, the intensity of dosage, the dosage schedule, the type and extent of cancer, and the client's physical and emotional status (Penny, 2002). However, typical side effects include nausea and vomiting, diarrhea or constipation, hair loss, weight loss, stomatitis, fatigue, and immunosuppression. The most serious is bone marrow suppression (myelosuppression). This causes an increased risk of infection, bleeding, and a reduced red-cell count, which can lead to anemia. Treatment of the side effects can generally be addressed through appropriate support medications such as antinausea drugs like granisetron hydrochloride (Kytril) or ondansetron (Zofran). In addition, growth-stimulating factors, such as epoetin alfa (Procrit) and filgrastim (Neupogen), help keep blood counts from dropping too low. Counts that are too low would stop or delay the use of chemotherapy.

An aggressive systemic option, when other treatments have failed or when there is a strong possibility of relapse or metastatic disease, is high-dose chemotherapy with bone marrow and/or stem cell transplant. This therapy involves the withdrawal of bone marrow before the administration of toxic levels of chemotherapeutic agents. The marrow is frozen and then returned to the client after the high-dose chemotherapy is finished. Clinical trials are still researching this experimental therapy (Lowdermilk & Perry, 2004).

Hormonal Therapy

One of estrogen's normal functions is to stimulate the growth and division of healthy cells in the breasts. However, in some women with breast cancer, this normal function contributes to the growth and division of cancer cells.

The objective of hormonal therapy is to block or counter the effect of estrogen. Estrogen plays a central role in the pathogenesis of cancer, and treatment with estrogen deprivation has proven to be effective (Hindle & Gonzalez, 2001). Currently, it is standard for most women with ER+ breast cancer to take a hormone-like medication—known as a selective estrogen receptor modulator (SERM) antiestrogenic agent—daily for 5 years after initial treatment. Certain areas in the female body (breasts, uterus, ovaries, skin, vagina, and brain) contain specialized cells called hormone receptors that allow estrogen to enter the cell and stimulate it to divide. SERMs enter these same receptors and act like keys, turning off the signal for growth inside the cell (Link, 2003). The best-known SERM is tamoxifen (Nolvadex, 20 mg daily for 5 years). Although it works well in preventing further spread of cancer, it is also associated with an increased incidence of endometrial cancer, pulmonary embolus, deep vein thrombosis, hot flashes, vaginal discharge and bleeding, stroke, and cataract formation (Weaver, 2002).

A relatively new SERM is raloxifene (Evista), which has shown promising results. It was originally marketed solely for the prevention and treatment of osteoporosis but is now used as adjunct breast cancer therapy.

Another class of hormonal agents, known as aromatase inhibitors (AIs), stands out as an effective therapy option. AIs work by inhibiting the conversion of androgens to estrogens. AIs includes letozole (Femara, 2.5 mg daily), exemestane (Aromasin, 25 mg daily), and anastrozole (Arimidex, 1 mg daily for 5 years), all of which are taken orally. These are usually given to women with advanced breast cancer or cancers that recur despite the use of tamoxifen (Penny, 2002).

The side effects associated with these endocrine therapies include hot flashes, bone pain, fatigue, nausea, cough, dyspnea, and headache (Harwood, 2004). Women with hormone-sensitive cancers can live for long periods without any intervention other than hormonal manipulation, but quality-of-life issues need to be addressed in the balance between treatment and side effects.

Nurses play an important role in educating women about the use of endocrine therapies, observing women's experiences with treatment, and communicating those observations to their primary care professionals to make dosage adjustments, in addition to contributing to the knowledge base of endocrine therapy in the treatment of breast cancer.

Immunotherapy

Immunotherapy, used as an adjunct to surgery, represents an attempt to stimulate the body's natural defenses to recognize and attack cancer cells. Trastuzumab (Herceptin, 2- to 4-mg/kg intravenous infusion) is the first monoclonal antibody approved for breast cancer (NCCN, 2004). Some tumors produce excessive amounts of HER-2/neu protein, which regulates cancer cell growth. Breast cancers that overexpress the protein HER-2/neu are associated with a more aggressive form of disease and a poorer prognosis. Trastuzumab blocks the effect of this protein to inhibit the growth of cancer cells. It can be used alone or in combination with other chemotherapy to treat clients with metastatic breast disease (Lewis et al., 2004). Adverse effects of trastuzumab include cardiac toxicity, vascular thrombosis, hepatic failure, fever, chills, nausea, vomiting, and pain with first infusion (Spratto & Woods, 2004).

Nursing Management for the Patient With Breast Cancer

When a woman is diagnosed with breast cancer, she faces treatment that may alter her body shape, may make her feel unwell, and may not carry a certainty of cure. Nurses can support women from the time of diagnosis, through the treatments, and through follow-up after the surgical and adjunctive treatments have been completed. Allowing patients time to ask questions and to discuss any necessary preparations for treatment is critical.

Assessment

As our understanding of breast disorders keeps improving, treatments continue to change. Although the goal of treatment remains improved survival, increasing emphasis is focused on prevention (Morrow & Gradishar, 2002). Nurses can have an impact on early detection of breast disorders, treatment, and symptom management (Yarbro, 2003). During assessment, the nurse will take a thorough history of the breast disorder and complete a breast examination to validate the findings. The clinical breast examination involves both inspection and palpation (Nursing Procedure 6-1). Nurses must be cognizant of the impact that breast cancer has on a woman's emotional state, coping ability, and quality of life. Women may experience sadness, anger, fear, and guilt as a result of breast cancer. However, despite potential negative outcomes, many women have a positive outlook for their futures and adapt to treatment modalities with a good quality of life (Kessler, 2002). The nurse should closely monitor clients for their psychosocial adjustment to diagnosis and treatment and should be able to identify those who need further psychological intervention. By giving practical advice, the nurse can help the woman adjust to her altered body image and to accept the changes to her life.

Because family members play a significant role in supporting women through breast cancer diagnosis and treatment, nurses should assess the emotional distress of both partners during the course of treatment and, if needed, make a referral for psychological counseling. By identifying interpersonal strains, negative psychosocial side effects of cancer treatment can be minimized.

A nurse who is involved in the woman's treatment plan from the beginning can effectively offer support throughout the whole experience.

Nursing Diagnosis

Appropriate nursing diagnoses for a woman with a diagnosis of breast cancer might include:

- Disturbed body image related to:
  - Loss of body part (breast)
  - Loss of femininity
  - Loss of hair due to chemotherapy
- Fear related to:
  - Diagnosis of cancer
  - Prognosis of disease
- Educational deficit related to:
  - Cancer treatment options
  - Reconstructive surgery decisions
  - Breast self-examination

Nursing Interventions

Nurses can offer information, support, and perioperative care to women diagnosed with breast cancer who are undergoing treatment. Nurses can also implement health-promotion and disease-prevention strategies to minimize the risk for developing breast cancer and to promote optimal outcomes.

Providing Patient Education

The nurse can help the woman and her partner to prioritize the voluminous amount of information given to them so that they can make informed decisions. All treatment options should be explained in detail so the patient and her family understand them. By preparing an individualized packet of information and reviewing it with the woman and her partner, the nurse can help them understand her specific type of cancer, the diagnostic studies and treatment options she may choose, and the goals of treatment. Providing information is a central role of the nurse. This information can be given via telephone counseling, one-to-one contact, and pamphlets. Telephone counseling with women and their partners may be an effective method to improve symptom management and quality of life (Badger et al., 2004).

Providing Emotional Support

The diagnosis of cancer affects all aspects of life for a woman and her family. The threatening nature of the disease and feelings of uncertainty for the future can lead to anxiety and stress. Nurses must address the woman's needs for:

- Information about diagnosis and treatment
- Physical care while undergoing treatments
- Contact with supportive people
- Education about disease, options, and prevention measures
- Discussion and support by a caring, competent nurse

The nurse should reassure the client and her family that the diagnosis of breast cancer does not necessarily mean imminent death, a decrease in attractiveness, or diminished sexuality. The woman should be encouraged to express her fears and worries. The nurse needs to be available to listen and address the woman's concerns in an open manner to help her toward recovery. All aspects of care must include sensitivity to the patient's personal efforts to cope and heal. Some women will become involved in organizations or charities that support cancer

Nursing Procedure 6-1

Clinical Breast Examination

Purpose: To Assess Breasts for Abnormal Findings

1. Inspect the breast for size, symmetry, and skin texture and color. Inspect the nipples and areola. Ask the client to sit at the edge of the examination table, with her arms resting at her sides (Fig. A).
2. Inspect the breast for masses, retraction, dimpling, or ecchymosis.
   - The client places her hands on her hips (Fig. B).
   - She then raises her arms over her head so the axillae can also be inspected (Fig. C).
   - The client then stands, places her hands on her hips, and leans forward (Fig. D).
3. Palpate the breasts. Assist the client into a supine position with her arms above her head (Fig. E).

Place a pillow or towel under the client's head to help spread the breasts. Three patterns might be used to palpate the breasts:
   - Spiral (Fig. F)
   - Pie-shaped wedges (Fig. G)
   - Vertical strip (Fig. H)
4. Palpate the nipple using the index finger for masses (Fig. I) and discharge (Fig. J)
5. Palpate the axillary area for any tenderness or lymph node enlargement. Have the client sit up and move to the edge of the examination table. While supporting the client's arm, palpate downward from the armpit, palpating toward the ribs just below the breast.

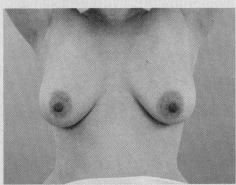

A

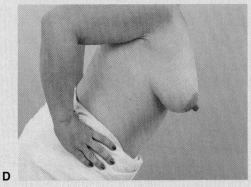

B

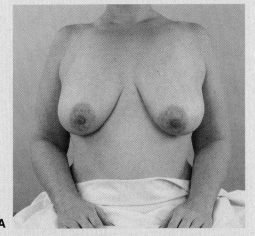

C

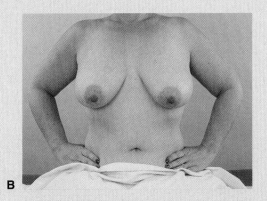

D

(continued)

Nursing Procedure 6-1

Clinical Breast Examination (Continued)

Purpose: To Assess Breasts for Abnormal Findings

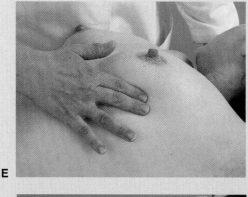

E

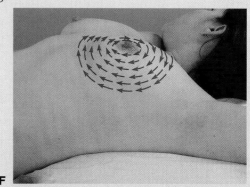

F

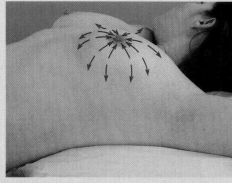

G

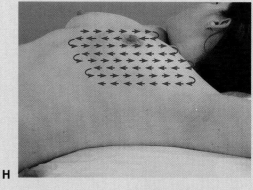

H

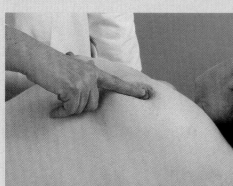

I

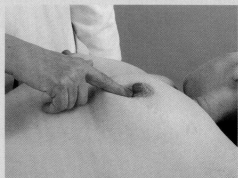

J

Adapted from Rhoads, J. (2006). Advanced health assessment and diagnostic reasoning. Philadelphia: Lippincott Williams & Wilkins.

research; they may participate in breast cancer walks to raise awareness or become a Reach for Recovery volunteer to help others. Each woman copes in her own personal manner, and all of these efforts can be positive motivators for her own healing.

To help women cope with the diagnosis of breast cancer, the American Cancer Society launched Reach to Recovery more than 30 years ago. Specially trained breast cancer survivors give women and their families opportunities to express their feelings, verbalize their fears, and get answers. Most importantly, Reach to Recovery volunteers offer understanding, support, and hope through face-to-face visits or by telephone; they are proof that people can survive breast cancer and live productive lives. National contact information is 1-800-ACS-2345.

Providing Perioperative Care

The following nursing care is needed before surgery and after treatment:

- Pain management (analgesics as needed)
- Affected arm care (the arm should be elevated on a pillow; no treatments to it)

- Wound care (observation and drainage reservoirs emptied as needed)
- Mobility care (active range-of-motion and arm exercises as ordered)
- Respiratory care (turn, cough, and deep breathe every 2 hours)
- Follow-up (information regarding adjunct therapy)
- Emotional care (participate in care and self-empowerment)
- Educational needs (home care and future monitoring strategies)
- Referrals needed (e.g., Reach to Recovery)

Implementing Health-Promotion and Disease-Prevention Strategies

In the past, most women assumed that there was little they could do to reduce their risk of developing breast cancer. However, research has found that the daily choices women make concerning breast cancer screening, diet, exercise, and other health practices have a profound impact on their cancer risk. In the fight against cancer, nurses often assume a variety of roles, such as educator, counselor, advocate, and role model. Nurses need to offer up-to-date information on:

- Prevention
- Early detection
- Resources for screening
- Education for dispelling myths and fears
- Demonstration of self-examination techniques
- Counseling about individual risk status and strategies for risk reduction

Nurses need to be knowledgeable about the most current evidence, familiar with current guidelines based on research, and cognizant of how the media presents this information. Nurses should offer prevention strategies within the context of a woman's life. Factors such as lifestyle choices, economic status, and multiple roles need to be taken into consideration when counseling women. Nurses should advocate for healthy lifestyles and making sound choices to prevent cancer. Nurses, like all health care professionals, should offer guidance from a comprehensive perspective that acknowledges the unique needs of each individual (Morin et al., 2004).

Breast cancer is a frightening experience for women. Like a black cloud hanging over their heads, with little regard for any victim, breast cancer stalks women everywhere they go. Many have a close friend or relative who is battling the disease; many have watched their mothers and sisters die of this dreaded disease. Those with risk factors live with even greater anxiety and fear. No woman wants to hear those chilling words: "The biopsy is positive. You have breast cancer." Nurses can provide women with information about detection and risk factors and should inform them about the new ACS screening guidelines, instruct them on breast self-examination, and outline dietary changes that might reduce their risk of breast cancer.

Awareness is the first step toward a change in habits. Raising the level of awareness about breast cancer is of paramount importance, and nurses are in an ideal position to play an important role in health promotion, disease prevention, and breast education.

Breast Cancer Screening

The three components of early detection are breast self-examination, clinical breast examination, and mammography.

The ACS (2003) has issued breast cancer screening guidelines that, for the first time, offer specific guidance for the women and greater clarification of the role of breast examinations (Table 6-4). ACS screening guidelines are revised about every 5 years to include new scientific findings and developments.

Women are exposed to multiple sources of cancer prevention information, and much of it may not be sound. The benefits, risks, and potential limitations of breast self-examination, clinical breast examination, and mammography should be discussed with each woman and tailored to assessment of her risk factors (Mahon, 2003). Based on the new guidelines, nurses will have to make clinical judgments as to the appropriateness of recommending breast self-examination and should reevaluate the need for teaching the procedure to all women. Perhaps nurses need to focus instead on encouraging regular mammograms, depending of course on the woman's individual risk factors.

Breast self-examination is a technique that enables a woman to detect any changes in her breasts; this could result in early cancer detection. The emphasis is now on awareness of breast changes, not just discovery of cancer.

Table 6-4 American Cancer Society Breast Cancer Screening Guidelines

Woman's Age	Screening Activity
20–39	Breast self-examination (BSE) is optional Clinical breast examination every 3 years
40+	BSE every month is optional Clinical breast examination every year Mammogram every year, continuing for as long as the woman is in good health

Women at increased risk (e.g., family history, genetic tendency, past history of cancer) should discuss with their healthcare professionals the pros and cons of starting mammography screening earlier, undergoing additional diagnostic tests (e.g., ultrasound or MRI), or increasing the frequency of examinations.

American Cancer Society (ACS). (2004). *Cancer facts and figures 2003.* Atlanta, GA: Author.

Research has shown that breast self-examination plays a small role in detecting breast cancer compared with self-awareness. However, doing breast self-examination is one way for women to know how her breasts normally feel so that she can notice any changes that do occur (ACS, 2003).

There are two steps to conducting a breast self-examination: visual inspection and tactile palpation.

The visual part should be done in three separate positions: with the arms up behind the head, with the arms down at the sides, and bending forward. The woman should be instructed to look for:

- Changes in shape, size, contour, or symmetry
- Skin discoloration or dimpling, bumps/lumps
- Sores or scaly skin
- Discharge or puckering of the nipple

In the second part, the tactile examination, the woman feels her breasts in one of three specific patterns: spiral, pie-shaped wedges, or up and down. When using any of the three patterns, the woman should use a circular rubbing motion (in dime-sized circles) without lifting the fingers. She checks not only the breasts but also between the breast and the axilla, the axilla itself, and the area above the breast up to the clavicle and across the shoulder. The pads of the three middle fingers on the right hand are used to assess the left breast; the pads of the three middle fingers on the left hand are used to assess the right breast. The woman should be instructed to use three different degrees of pressure:

- Light (move the skin without moving the tissue underneath)
- Medium (midway into the tissue)
- Hard (down to the ribs)

Once the tactile examination has been completed while standing in front of a mirror, it should be repeated while lying down.

Box 6-2 details breast self-examination.

Nutrition

Nutrition plays a critical role in health promotion and disease prevention (Glanz et al., 2003). Being overweight or obese and consuming a high-fat diet are risk factors for breast cancer in postmenopausal women (Stephenson & Rose, 2003). Healthy People 2010 identified being overweight or obese as one of the 10 leading health indicators and a major health concern (USDHHS, 2000). Almost 62% of women over the age of 20 years are overweight; of these, 33.4% are obese (Flegal et al., 2002). A diet high in fruits, vegetables, and high-fiber carbohydrates and low in fats seems to offer protection against breast cancer as well as weight control. Women who followed these dietary guidelines decreased their risk of breast cancer by 15% (Blackburn et al., 2003).

The American Institute for Cancer Research (AICR), which conducts extensive research, made the following recommendations to reduce a woman's risk for developing breast cancer:

- Engaging in daily moderate exercise and weekly vigorous physical activity
- Consuming at least five servings of fruits and vegetables daily
- Not smoking or using any tobacco products
- Keeping a maximum body mass index (BMI) of 25 and limiting weight gain to no more than 11 pounds since age 18
- Consuming seven or more daily portions of complex carbohydrates, such as whole grains and cereals
- Limiting intake of processed foods and refined sugar
- Restricting red meat intake to approximately 3 ounces daily
- Limiting intake of fatty foods, particularly those of animal origin
- Restricting intake of salted foods and use of salt in cooking (Cerhan et al., 2004).

The medical community is also starting to study the role of phytochemicals in health. The unique geographic variability of breast cancer around the world and the low rate of breast cancer in Asian compared to Western countries prompted this exploration. This area of research appears hopeful for women seeking to prevent breast cancer as well as those recovering from it. Although the mechanism isn't clear, certain foods demonstrate anticancer properties and boost the immune system. Phytochemical-rich foods include:

- Green tea and herbal teas
- Garlic
- Whole grains and legumes
- Onions and leeks
- Soybeans and soy products
- Fruits (citrus, apricots, pumpkin, berries)
- Green leafy vegetables (spinach, collards, romaine)
- Colorful vegetables (carrots, squash, tomatoes)
- Cruciferous vegetables (broccoli, cabbage, cauliflower)
- Flaxseeds (Hu & Knobf, 2004)

Nurses should adopt a holistic approach when addressing the nutritional needs of women with breast cancer. Nutritional assessment should be incorporated into the general overall assessment of all women. Culturally sensitive nutritional assessment tools need to be developed and used to enhance this process. Providing examples of appropriate foods associated with the woman's current dietary habits, relating current health status to nutritional intake, and placing proposed modifications within a realistic personal framework may increase a woman's willingness to incorporate needed changes in her nutritional behavior. Nurses should be able to interpret research results and should stay up to date on nutritional influences so they can transmit this key information to the public.

BOX 6-2

HOW TO PERFORM BREAST SELF-EXAMINATION

Step 1
- Stand before a mirror.
- Check both breasts for anything unusual.
- Look for discharge from the nipple and puckering, dimpling, or scaling of the skin.

The next two steps check for any changes in the contour of your breasts. As you do them, you should be able to feel your muscles tighten.

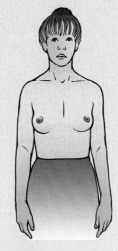

Step 2
- Watch closely in the mirror as you clasp your hands behind your head and press your hands forward.
- Note any change in the contour of your breasts.

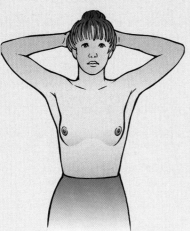

Step 3
- Next, press your hands firmly on your hips and bow slightly toward the mirror as you pull your shoulders and elbows forward.
- Note any change in the contour of your breasts.

Some women perform the next part of the examination in the shower. Your fingers will glide easily over soapy skin, so you can concentrate on feeling for changes inside the breast.

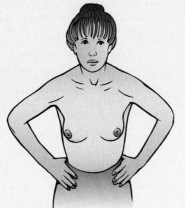

Step 4
- Raise your left arm.
- Use 3 or 4 fingers of your right hand to feel your left breast firmly, carefully, and thoroughly.
- Beginning at the outer edge, press the flat part of your fingers in small circles, moving the circles slowly around the breast.
- Gradually work toward the nipple.
- Be sure to cover the whole breast.
- Pay special attention to the area between the breast and the underarm, including the underarm itself.
- Feel for any unusual lumps or masses under the skin.
- If you have any spontaneous discharge during the month—whether or not it is during your BSE—see your doctor.
- Repeat the examination on your right breast.

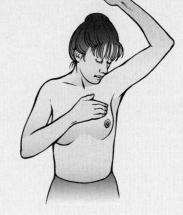

Step 5
- Lie flat on your back with your left arm over your head and a pillow or folded towel under your left shoulder. (This position flattens your breast and makes it easier to check.)
- Repeat the actions of Step 4 in this position for each breast.

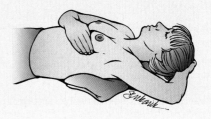

From: Smeltzer, S. C., & Bare, B. (2004). *Brunner and Suddarth's textbook of medical surgical nursing* (10th ed.). Philadelphia: Lippincott Williams & Wilkins. Adapted from U.S. Department of Health and Human Services, Public Health Service, *What you need to know about breast cancer.* Bethesda, MD: National Institutes of Health.

Summary

Teamwork is important in breast screening and caring for women with breast disorders. Treatment is often fragmented between the hospital and community treatment centers, which can be emotionally traumatic for the woman and her family. The advances being made in the diagnosis and treatment of breast disorders mean that guidelines are constantly changing, requiring all health care professionals to keep up to date. Informed nurses can provide support and information and, most importantly, continuity of care for the woman undergoing treatment for a breast problem.

The nurse plays a particularly important role in providing psychological support and self-care teaching to patients with breast cancer. Nurses can influence both physical and emotional recovery, which are both important aspects of care that help in improving the woman's quality of life and the ability to survive. The nurse's role should extend beyond helping clients; spreading the word in the community about screening and prevention is a big part in the ongoing fight against cancer. The community should see nurses as both educators and valued sources of credible information. This role will help improve clinical outcomes while achieving high levels of client satisfaction.

References

Alexander, L. L., LaRosa, J. H., & Bader, H. (2004). *New dimensions in women's health* (3rd ed.). Boston: Jones and Bartlett Publishers.

American Cancer Society (ACS) (2003). Benign breast conditions. [Online] Available at: http://www.cancer.org/docroot/CRI/content/CRI_2_6X_Benign_Breast_Conditions_59.a

American Cancer Society News Center (2003). *Updated breast cancer screening guidelines released* [Online]. Available at: http://www.cancer.org/docroot/MED/content/MED_2_1x_American_Cancer_Society_Is American Cancer Society (ACS) (2004). *Cancer facts and figures 2004.* Atlanta, GA: Author.

American Cancer Society (ACS) (2004). Screening guidelines for the early detection of cancer in asymptomatic people. *Cancer prevention & early detection facts & figures 2004* (p. 31). Atlanta, GA: Author.

American Cancer Society (ACS) (2004). What are the risk factors for breast cancer? *Cancer Reference Information,* [Online] Available at: http://www.cancer.org/docroot/CRI_2_4_2X_What_are_the_risk_factors_fo

American Cancer Society (ACS). (2004). *Cancer facts and figures 2003.* Atlanta, GA: Author.

Amshel, C. E., & Sibley, E. (2001). Multiple unilateral fibroadenomas. *Breast Journal, 7*(3), 189–191.

Augustine, K. M., & Bogan, T. L. (2004). Operating a comprehensive high-risk breast care management program in a community hospital setting. *AWHONN, 8*(5), 434–440.

Badger, T., Segrin, C., Meek, P., Lopez, A. M., & Bonham, E. (2004). A case study of telephone interpersonal counseling for women with breast cancer and their partners. *Oncology Nursing Forum, 31*(5), 997–1003.

Blackburn, G. L., Copeland, T., Khaodhiar, L., & Buckley, R. B. (2003). Diet and breast cancer. *Journal of Women's Health, 12,* 183–192.

Breslin, E. T., & Lucas, V. A. (2003). *Women's health nursing: toward evidence-based practice.* St. Louis, MO: Saunders.

Cerhan, J. R., Potter, J. D., Gilmore, J. M. E., et al. (2004). Adherence to the AICR Cancer Prevention Recommendations and subsequent morbidity and mortality in the Iowa Women's Health Study Cohort. *Cancer Epidemiology, Biomarkers and Prevention, 13,* 1114–1120.

Chui, C. S., Hong, L., Hunt, M., & McCormick, B. (2002). A simplified intensity-modulated radiation therapy technique for the breast. *Medical Physics, 29,* 522–529.

Condon, M. C. (2004) *Women's health: an integrated approach to wellness and illness.* Upper Saddle River, NJ: Prentice Hall.

DiSaia, P. J., & Creasman, W. T. (2002). *Clinical gynecologic oncology* (rev. ed.). St. Louis: Mosby, Inc.

Flegal, K. M., Carroll, M. D., Ogden, C. L., & Johnson, C. L. (2002). Prevalence and trends in obesity among US adults, 1999–2000. *JAMA, 289,* 1723–1727.

Glanz, K., Croyle, R. T., Chollette, V. Y., & Pinn, V. W. (2003). Cancer-related health disparities in women. *American Journal of Public Health, 93,* 292–298.

Gordils-Perez, J., Rawlins-Duell, R., & Kelvin, J. F. (2003). Advances in radiation treatment of patients with breast cancer. *Clinical Journal of Oncology Nursing, 7*(6), 629–636.

Harwood, K. V. (2004). Advances in endocrine therapy for breast cancer: considering efficacy, safety, and quality of life. *Clinical Journal of Oncology Nursing, 8*(6), 629–637.

Hindle, W. H., & Gonzalez, S. (2001). Breast disease: what to do when it's not cancer. *Women's Health in Primary Care, 4*(1), 21–34.

Holmes, S. R. (Aug. 23, 2004). Current protocols for managing breast cancer. *Nursing Spectrum,* 12–13.

Hu, S. A., & Knobf, M. T. (2004). Risks and benefits of soy isoflavones for breast cancer survivors. *Oncology Nursing Forum, 31*(2), 249–263.

Kessler, T. A. (2002). Contextual variables, emotional state, and current and expected quality of life in breast cancer survivors. *Oncology Nursing Forum, 29*(7), 1109–1116.

Lewis, S. M., Heitkemper, M. M., & Dirksen, S. R. (2004). *Medical-surgical nursing: assessment and management of clinical problems* (6th ed.). St. Louis: Mosby, Inc.

Link, J. (2003). *The breast cancer survival manual* (3rd ed.). New York: Henry Holt & Company.

London, M. L., Ladewig, P. W., Ball, J. W., & Bindler, R. C. (2003). *Maternal-newborn & child nursing: family-centered care.* Upper Saddle River, NJ: Prentice Hall.

Lowdermilk, D. L., & Perry, S. E. (2004). *Maternity & women's health care* (8th ed.). St. Louis: Mosby, Inc.

Mahon, S. M. (2003). Evidence-based practice: recommendations for the early detection of breast cancer. *Clinical Journal of Oncology Nursing, 7*(6), 693–696.

Makhoul, I., Makhoul, H., Harvey, H., & Souba, W. (2004). Breast cancer. *EMedicine.* [Online] Available at: http://www.emedicine.com/MED/topic2808.htm

Mattson, S., & Smith, J. E. (2004). *Core curriculum for maternal-newborn nursing* (3rd ed.). St. Louis: Elsevier Saunders.

McCready, T. (2004). Management of patients with breast cancer. *Primary Health Care, 14*(6), 41–49.

McKinney, E. S., James, S. R., Murray, S. S., & Ashwill, J. W. (2005). *Maternal-child nursing* (2nd ed.). Philadelphia: Elsevier Saunders.

Mihelic, E. G. (2003). Diagnosis and management of breast fibroadenomas. *Physician Assistant, 27*(7), 29–32.

Morin, K. H., Stark, M. A., & Searing, K. (2004). Obesity and nutrition in women throughout adulthood. *JOGNN, 33*(6), 823–832.

Morrow, M., & Gradishar, W. (2002). Breast cancer. *British Medical Journal, 324*(7334), 410–415.

National Cancer Institute (NCI) (2004). *Breast cancer: treatment.* [Online] Available at: http://cancer.gov/cancertopics/pdq/treatment/breast/healthprofessional

National Cancer Institute (NCI) (2004). *Probability of breast cancer in American women.* [Online] Available at: http://cis.nci.nih.gov/fact/5_6.htm

National Comprehensive Cancer Network (NCCN) (2004). Breast cancer treatment guidelines. *NCCN patient guidelines.* [Online] Available at: http://www.nccn.org/patients/patient_gls/_english/_breast/5_treatment.asp

Olds, S. B., London, M. L., Ladewig, P. W., & Davidson, M. R. (2004). *Maternal-newborn & women's health care* (7th ed.). Upper Saddle River, NJ: Pearson Prentice Hall.

O'Toole, M. T. (2003) *Miller-Keane encyclopedia and dictionary of medicine, nursing, and allied health* (7th ed.). Philadelphia: Saunders.

Pasacreta, J. V., Jacobs, L., & Cataldo, J. K. (2002). Genetic testing for breast and ovarian cancer risk: the psychosocial issues. *AJN, 102*(12), 40–47.

Penny, J. (2002). Breast cancer overview: the basics. *Nursing Spectrum, 7*(21), 19–24.

Rebbeck, T. R., Friebel, T., Lynch, H. T., et al. (2004). Bilateral prophylactic mastectomy reduces breast cancer risk in BRACA-1 and BRACA-2 mutation carriers: the PROSE Study Group. *Journal of Clinical Oncology, 22*(6), 1055–1062.

Santen, R. J., & Mansel, R. (2005). Benign breast disorders. *New England Journal of Medicine, 353*(3), 275–285.

Schnell, Z. B., Van Leeuwen, A. M., & Kranpitz, T. R. (2003). *Davis's comprehensive handbook of laboratory and diagnostic tests with nursing implications.* Philadelphia: F. A. Davis Company.

Sloane, E. (2002). *Biology of women* (4th ed.). New York: Delmar.

Spratto, G. R., & Woods, A. L. (2004). *2004 edition, PDR nurse's drug handbook.* Clifton Park, NY: Thomson Delmar Learning.

Stephenson, G. D., & Rose, D. P. (2003) Breast cancer and obesity: an update. *Nutrition and Cancer, 45,* 1–16.

U.S. Department of Health and Human Services (USDHHS) (2000). *Healthy people 2010.* Rockville, MD: Author.

Vicini, F., Baglan, K., Kestin, L., et al. (2002). The emerging role of brachytherapy in the management of patients with breast cancer. *Seminars in Radiation Oncology, 12,* 31–39.

Wang, S., & Birdwell, R. (2004). Magnetic resonance mammography. *EMedicine.* [Online] Available at: http://emedicine.com/radio/topic792.htm

Weaver, C. (2002). Breast cancer breakthroughs. *Nursing Management, 33*(11), 28–34.

Willison, K. M. (2001). Mammographic positioning. In V. F. Andolina (Ed.), *Mammographic imaging* (rev. ed.). Baltimore: Lippincott Williams & Wilkins.

Writing Group for Women's Health Initiative Investigators. (2002). Risks and benefits of estrogen plus progestin in healthy menopausal women: principal results for the Women's Health Initiative randomized controlled trial. *JAMA, 288*(3), 321–333.

Yarbro, C. H. (2003). International nursing and breast cancer. *Breast Journal, 9*(3), S98–S100.

Youngkin, E. Q., & Davis, M. S. (2004). *Women's health: a primary care clinical guide* (3rd ed.). Upper Saddle River, NJ: Prentice Hall.

Zawacki, K. L., & Phillips, M. (2002). Cancer genetics and women's health. *JOGNN, 31*(2), 208–216.

Web Resources

American Cancer Society (ACS): 1-800-ACS-2345, **http://www.cancer.org**

Facing Our Risk of Cancer Empowered: **www.facingourrisk.org**

International Society of Nurses in Genetics: **http://nursing.creighton.edu/isong**

Living Beyond Breast Cancer: 1-888-753-5222, **http://www.lbbc.org**

National Alliance of Breast Cancer Organizations: 1-888-80-NABCO, **http://www.nabco.org**

National Cancer Institute (NCI): 1-800-422-6327, **http://www.nci.nih.gov**

Oncology Nursing Society (ONS): 1-866-257-4ONS, **http://www.ons.org**

Susan G. Komen Breast Cancer Foundation: 1-800-462-9273, **http://www.komen.org**

Y-me National Breast Cancer Organization: 1-800-221-2141, **http://www.Y-me.org**

Chapter WORKSHEET

● MULTIPLE CHOICE QUESTIONS

1. Breast self-examinations involve both touching of breast tissue and:

   a. Palpation of cervical lymph nodes

   b. Firm squeezing of both breast nipples

   c. Visualizing both breasts for any change

   d. A mammogram to evaluate breast tissue

2. Which of the following is the strongest risk factor for breast cancer?

   a. Advancing age and being female

   b. High number of children

   c. Genetic mutations in BRCA-1 and BRCA-2

   d. Family history of colon cancer

3. A biopsy procedure that traces radioisotopes and blue dye from the tumor site through the lymphatic system into the axillary nodes is:

   a. Stereotactic biopsy

   b. Sentinel node biopsy

   c. Axillary dissection biopsy

   d. Advanced breast biopsy

4. The most serious potential adverse reaction from chemotherapy is:

   a. Thrombocytopenia

   b. Deep vein thrombosis

   c. Alopecia

   d. Myelosuppression

5. What suggestion would be helpful for the client experiencing painful fibrocystic breast changes?

   a. Increase her caffeine intake.

   b. Take a mild analgesic when needed.

   c. Reduce her intake of leafy vegetables.

   d. Wear a bra bigger than she needs.

6. A postoperative mastectomy client should be referred to which of the following organizations for assistance?

   a. National Women's Association (NOW)

   b. Food and Drug Administration (FDA)

   c. March of Dimes Foundation (MDF)

   d. Reach to Recovery volunteers

● CRITICAL THINKING EXERCISE

1. Mrs. Gordon, 48, presents to the Women's Health Community clinic where you work as a nurse. She is very upset and crying. She tells you that she found lumps in her breast and she knows that "it's cancer and I will die." When you ask her further about her problem, she says she does not routinely check her breasts monthly and hasn't had a mammogram for years because "they're too expensive." She also describes the intermittent pain she experiences.

   a. What specific questions would you ask this client to get a clearer picture?

   b. What education is needed for this client regarding breast health?

   c. What community referrals are needed to meet this client's future needs?

● STUDY ACTIVITIES

1. Discuss with a group of women what their breasts symbolize to them and to society. Do they symbolize something different to each one?

2. When a woman experiences a breast disorder, what feelings might she be experiencing and how can a nurse help her sort them out?

3. Interview a woman who has fibrocystic breast changes and find out how she manages this condition.

4. An infection of the breast connective tissue that frequently occurs in the lactating woman is

   _____.

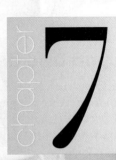

chapter 7

Benign Disorders of the Female Reproductive Tract

KeyTERMS

cystocele
enterocele
Kegel exercises
ovarian cyst
pelvic organ prolapse
pessary
polyps
rectocele
urinary incontinence
uterine fibroids
uterine prolapse

LearningOBJECTIVES

After studying the chapter content, the student should be able to accomplish the following:

1. Define the key terms.
2. Describe the major pelvic relaxation disorders in terms of etiology, management, and nursing interventions.
3. Outline the nursing management needed for the most common benign reproductive disorders in women.

Several benign pelvic disorders increase in incidence as women age. For instance, women may experience pelvic support disorders related to pelvic relaxation or urinary incontinence. These disorders generally develop after years of wear and tear on the muscles and tissues that support the pelvic floor—such as that which occurs with childbearing, chronic coughing, straining, surgery, or simply aging. In addition to pelvic support disorders, woman may also experience various benign neoplasms of the reproductive tract, such as cervical polyps, uterine leiomyomas (fibroids), and ovarian cysts.

This chapter provides an overview of various pelvic support disorders and benign neoplasms, along with assessment, treatment, and potential prevention strategies for each.

Pelvic Support Disorders

Pelvic support disorders such as pelvic organ prolapse and urinary and fecal incontinence are prevalent conditions in aging women. They cause significant physical and psychological morbidity, with obvious detriment to women's social interactions, emotional well-being, and overall quality of life. Because pelvic support disorders increase with age, the problem will grow worse as our population ages. These disorders occur as a result of weakness of the connective tissue and muscular support of pelvic organs due to a number of factors: vaginal childbirth, obesity, lifting, chronic cough, straining at defecation, and estrogen deficiency (McIntosh, 2005). The bony pelvis has an exaggerated lumbar spine curve and downward tilt to it. The bladder rests on the symphysis and the posterior organs rest on the sacrum and coccyx. The pelvis holds the organs, but a woman's erect posture causes a funneling effect and constant downward pressure.

Pelvic Organ Prolapse

Pelvic organ prolapse (from the Latin *prolapsus*, a slipping forth) refers to the abnormal descent or herniation of the pelvic organs from their original attachment sites or their normal position in the pelvis. Pelvic organ prolapse occurs when structures of the pelvis shift and protrude into or outside of the vaginal canal. The Egyptians were the first to describe prolapse of the genital organs. Hippocrates made reference to placing a half of a pomegranate into the vagina for the treatment of organ prolapse (Shaw, 2003). Even today, the treatment and diagnosis of pelvic organ prolapse continues to be problematic.

The four most common types of genital prolapse are cystocele, rectocele, enterocele, and uterine prolapse (Fig. 7-1):

- **Cystocele** occurs when the posterior bladder wall protrudes downward through the anterior vaginal wall.
- **Rectocele** occurs when the rectum sags and pushes against or into the posterior vaginal wall.
- **Enterocele** occurs when the small intestine bulges through the posterior vaginal wall (especially common when straining).
- **Uterine prolapse** occurs when the uterus descends through the pelvic floor and into the vaginal canal. Multiparous women are at particular risk for uterine prolapse.

The extent of uterine prolapse is described in terms of degree:

- First degree: prolapse of the organ into the vaginal canal
- Second degree: cervix descends to the vaginal introitus
- Third degree: cervix is below the vaginal introitus (Youngkin & Davis, 2004)

Incidence and Etiology

It is difficult to determine the incidence of women with pelvic organ prolapse, as the disorder is often asymptomatic and many women do not seek treatment. It has been estimated, however, that at least half of all women who have given birth experience pelvic organ prolapse (Thakar & Stanton, 2002).

Causes of pelvic organ prolapse might include:

- Constant downward gravity because of erect human posture
- Atrophy of supporting tissues with aging and decline of estrogen levels
- Weakening of pelvic support related to childbirth trauma
- Reproductive surgery
- Pelvic radiation
- Increased abdominal pressure secondary to:
  - Lifting of children or heavy objects
  - Straining due to chronic constipation
  - Respiratory problems or chronic coughing
  - Obesity (Lowdermilk & Perry, 2004)

Clinical Manifestations

Pelvic organ prolapse is often asymptomatic, but when symptoms do occur, they are often related to the site and type of prolapse. Symptoms common to all types of prolapses are a feeling of dragging, a lump in the vagina, or something "coming down." Symptoms associated with pelvic organ prolapse are summarized in Box 7-1.

Women present with varying degrees of descent. Uterine prolapse is the most troubling type of pelvic

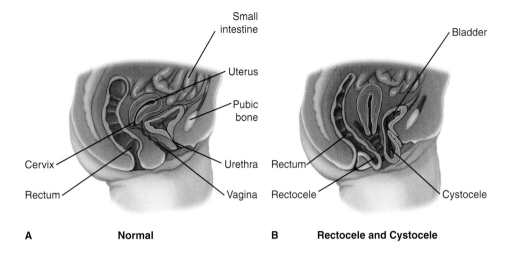

A   **Normal**   B   **Rectocele and Cystocele**

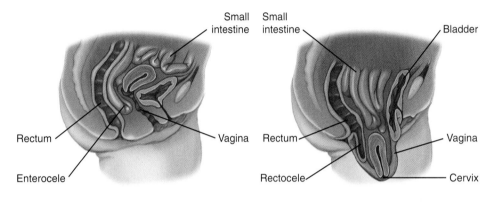

● Figure 7-1 Types of pelvic prolapses. (**A**) Normal. (**B**) Rectocele and cystocele. (**C**) Enterocele. (**D**) Uterine prolapse.

C   **Enterocele**   D   **Uterine Prolapse**

relaxation because it is often associated with concomitant defects of the vagina in the anterior, posterior, and lateral compartments (Lazarou & Scotti, 2004).

Treatment and Nursing Management

Treatment options for pelvic organ prolapse depend on the nature of the symptoms and their effect on the client's quality of life. Important considerations when deciding on nonsurgical or surgical options include the severity of symptoms, the woman's preferences, the woman's health status, age, and suitability for surgery, and the presence of other pelvic conditions (urinary or fecal incontinence). When surgery is being considered, the nature of the procedure and the likely outcome must be fully explained and discussed with the woman and her partner.

Nurses should help clients understand the nature of the condition, the treatment options, and the likely outcomes. Nursing considerations might include the following:

• Describe normal anatomy and causes for pelvic prolapse.
• Assess how this condition has affected the client's life.

• Outline the options available, with the advantages and disadvantages of each.
• Allow the client to make the decision that is right for her.
• Provide education.
• Schedule preoperative activities needed for surgery.
• Reassure the client that there is a solution for her symptoms.
• Provide community education concerning genital prolapse.

Nursing Care Plan 7-1 provides an overview of care for a woman with pelvic organ prolapse.

Nonsurgical Interventions

Nonsurgical interventions for pelvic organ prolapse include Kegel exercises, estrogen replacement therapy, dietary and lifestyle modifications, and use of pessaries.

Kegel Exercises

Kegel exercises strengthen the pelvic-floor muscles to support the inner organs and prevent further prolapse. An American gynecologist, Arnold Kegel, was the first to describe pelvic-floor exercises in the treatment of urinary

SYMPTOMS ASSOCIATED WITH PELVIC ORGAN PROLAPSE

- Urinary symptoms
  - Stress incontinence
  - Frequency (diurnal and nocturnal)
  - Urgency and urge incontinence
  - Hesitancy
  - Poor or prolonged stream
  - Feeling of incomplete emptying
- Bowel symptoms
  - Difficulty in defecation
  - Incontinence of flatus, liquid or solid stool
  - Urgency of defecation
  - Feeling of incomplete evacuation
  - Rectal protrusion or prolapse after defecation
- Sexual symptoms
  - Inability to have frequent intercourse
  - Dyspareunia
  - Lack of satisfaction or orgasm
  - Incontinence during sexual activity
- Other local symptoms
  - Pressure or heaviness in the vagina
  - Pain in the vagina or perineum
  - Low back pain, after long standing
  - Abdominal pressure or pain (Lazarou & Scotti, 2004)

incontinence in women. The purpose of pelvic-floor exercises is to increase the muscle volume, which will result in a stronger muscular contraction. Kegel exercises might limit the progression of mild prolapse and alleviate mild prolapse symptoms, including low back pain and pelvic pressure. They will not, however, help severe uterine prolapse. Nurses should encourage clients to perform Kegel exercises daily (Teaching Guidelines 7-1).

Estrogen Replacement Therapy

Estrogen replacement therapy (orally, transdermally, or vaginally) may help to improve the tone and vascularity of the supporting tissue in perimenopausal and menopausal women by increasing blood perfusion and elasticity to the vaginal wall. Before this therapy is started, each woman must be evaluated based on a thorough medical history to validate her risk for complications (e.g., endometrial cancer, myocardial infarction, stroke, breast cancer, pulmonary emboli, and deep vein thrombosis). Because of these risks, estrogens, with or without progestins, should be taken at the lowest effective doses and for the shortest duration consistent with the treatment goals and risks for the individual woman (Spratto & Woods, 2005).

Controversy still exists regarding the benefits versus the risks of taking estrogen, so the woman must weigh this option carefully (Hendrix et al., 2005). The nurse can discuss current research findings and educate the woman about hormone therapy, allowing the woman to make her own decision on whether to use hormones.

Dietary and Lifestyle Modifications

Dietary and lifestyle modifications may help prevent pelvic relaxation and chronic problems later in life. Dietary habits can exacerbate the prolapse by causing constipation and consequently chronic straining. The stools of a constipated woman are hard and dry, and typically she must strain while bearing down to defecate. This straining to pass a hard stool increases intra-abdominal pressure, which over time causes the pelvic organs to prolapse.

Dietary modifications can help to establish regular bowel movements without discomfort and eliminate flatus and bloating. Nurses should instruct clients to increase dietary fiber and fluids to prevent constipation. A high-fiber diet with an increase in fluid intake alleviates constipation by increasing stool bulk and stimulating peristalsis. It is accomplished by replacing refined, low-fiber foods with high-fiber foods. The recommended daily intake of fiber for women is 25 grams daily (Dudek, 2006). In addition to increasing the amount of fiber in her diet, the nurse should also encourage the woman to drink eight 8-oz glasses of fluid daily and to engage in regular aerobic exercise, which promotes muscle tone and stimulates peristalsis.

Other lifestyle changes that will assist with prolapse include:

- Achieve ideal weight to reduce higher intra-abdominal pressures and strain on pelvic organs, including pressure on the bladder.
- Wear a girdle or abdominal support to help support the muscles surrounding the pelvic organs.
- Avoid lifting heavy objects to reduce the risk of increasing intra-abdominal pressure, which can push the pelvic organs downward.
- Avoid high-impact aerobics, jogging, or jumping repeatedly to minimize the risk of increasing intra-abdominal pressure, which places downward pressure on the organs.
- Give up smoking to minimize the risk for a chronic "smoker's cough," which increases intra-abdominal pressure and forces the pelvic organs downward.

Pessaries

A **pessary** is a hard rubber or plastic device that is placed into the vagina to support the uterus, bladder, and rectum (Fig. 7-2). While there are many types and shapes, the most commonly used pessary is a firm ring that presses against the wall of the vagina and urethra to help decrease

Nursing Care Plan 7-1

Overview of a Woman With Pelvic Organ Prolapse (POP)

Katherine, a 62-year-old multiparous woman, came to her gynecologist with complaints of a chronic dragging or heavy painful feeling in her pelvis, lower backache, constipation, and urine leaking. Her symptoms increase when standing for long periods. She hasn't had menstrual cycles for at least a decade. She states, "I'm not taking any of those menopausal hormones."

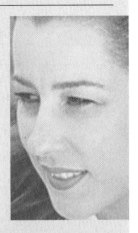

Nursing Diagnosis: Pain related to relaxation of pelvic support and elimination difficulties

Outcome identification and *evaluation*	Interventions with *rationales*
Client will report an acceptable level of discomfort within 1 to 2 hours of intervention as *evidenced by verbalizing a rating of <4 on a 0-to-10 pain scale.*	Obtain a thorough pain history, including ongoing pain experiences, previously used methods of pain control, what worked, what didn't, any allergies to pain medications, and the effect of pain on her activities of daily living *to provide a baseline and enable a systematic approach to pain management.*
	Assess the location, frequency, severity, duration, precipitating factors, and aggravating/alleviating factors *to identify defining characteristics of the client's subjective pain experience to better plan appropriate interventions.*
	Educate client about any medications prescribed as to correct dosage, route, side effects, and potential precautions *to increase understanding of and help promote compliance with therapy.*
	Assess problematic elimination patterns *to aid in identifying underlying factors from which to plan appropriate prevention strategies.*
	Encourage client to increase fluids and fiber in diet and increase physical activity daily *to promote peristalsis.*
	Assist client with establishing regular toileting patterns by setting aside time daily for bowel elimination *to promote regular bowel function and evacuation.*
	Urge client to avoid the routine use of laxatives *to reduce risk of compounding constipation.*

(continued)

Overview of a Woman With Pelvic Organ Prolapse (POP) (continued)

Nursing Diagnosis: Knowledge deficit related to causes of structural disorders and treatment options

Outcome identification and *evaluation*	Interventions with *rationales*
Client will demonstrate understanding of current condition and possible treatments *as evidenced by identifying possible treatment options, making health-promoting lifestyle choices, verbalizing appropriate healthcare practices, and adhering to measures to comply with treatment plan.*	Assess client's understanding of pelvic organ prolapse and its treatment options *to provide a baseline for teaching.* Review information provided about possible surgical procedures and recommendations for healthy lifestyle, obtaining feedback frequently *to validate adequate understanding of instructions.* Discuss association between uterine, bladder, and rectal prolapse and symptoms *to assist client in understanding the etiology of her symptoms and pain.* Have client verbalize and discuss information related to diagnosis, surgical procedure, preoperative routine, and postoperative regimen *to ensure adequate understanding and provide time for correcting or clarifying any misinformation or misconceptions.* Provide written material with pictures *to promote learning and help client visualize what has occurred to her body secondary to aging, weight gain, childbirth, and gravity.* Discuss pros and cons of hormone replacement therapy, osteoporosis prevention, and cardiovascular events common in postmenopausal women *to promote informed decision making by the client about available menopausal therapies.* Inform client about the availability of community resources and make appropriate referrals as needed *to provide additional education and support.* Document details of teaching and learning *to allow for continuity of care and further education, if needed.*

 T E A C H I N G   G U I D E L I N E S   7 - 1

Performing Kegel Exercises

- Squeeze the muscles in your rectum as if you are trying to prevent passing flatus.
- Stop and start urinary flow to help identify the pubococcygeus muscle.
- Tighten the pubococcygeus muscle for a count of three, then relax it.
- Contract and relax the pubococcygeus muscle rapidly 10 times.
- Try to bring up the entire pelvic floor and bear down 10 times.
- Repeat Kegel exercises at least five times daily.

leakage and support a prolapsed vagina or uterus. Pessaries are of two main types:

- Support pessaries, which rest under the symphysis and sacrum and elevate the vagina (e.g., Ring, Gehrung, and Hodge pessaries)
- Space-occupying pessaries, which are designed to manage severe prolapse by supporting the uterus even with a lack of vaginal tone (e.g., cube, donut, and inflatable Gellhorn pessaries)

Indications for pessary use include uterine prolapse or cystocele, especially among elderly clients for whom surgery is contraindicated; younger women with prolapse who plan to have additional children; and women with

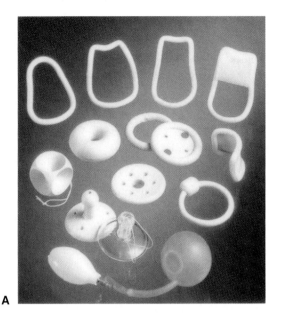

A

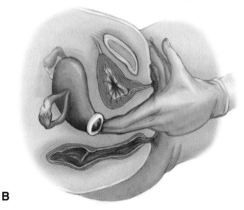

B

● Figure 7-2 Examples of pessaries. (**A**) Various shapes and sizes of pessaries available. (**B**) Insertion of one type of pessary.

marked prolapse who prefer to use a pessary rather than undergo surgery (Brolmann, 2004).

Pessaries are fitted by trial and error. Proper fitting of the pessary often requires the woman to try several sizes or styles. The largest pessary that the woman can wear comfortably is generally the most effective. The woman should be instructed to report any discomfort or difficulty with urination or defecation while wearing the pessary.

Although the pessary is a safe device, it is still a foreign body in the vagina. Because of this, the most common side effects of the pessary are increased vaginal discharge, urinary tract infections, vaginitis, and odor. This can be reduced by douching with dilute vinegar or hydrogen peroxide. Postmenopausal women with thin vaginal mucosa are susceptible to vaginal ulceration with the use of a pessary. Using estrogen cream can make the vaginal mucosa more resistant to erosion and strengthen the vaginal walls. Nurses should discuss these complications as part of their instruction.

Women must be capable of managing use of the pessary, either alone or with the help of a caretaker. The most common recommendations for pessary care include removing the pessary twice weekly and cleaning it with soap and water; using a lubricant for insertion; and having regular follow-up examinations every 6 to 12 months after an initial period of adjustment. Nurses should educate women in the care of their pessaries so that they feel comfortable with all aspects of care before leaving the healthcare facility.

Surgical Interventions

Surgical interventions for genital organ prolapse are designed to correct specific defects, with the goals being restoration of normal anatomy and preservation of function (Lewis et al., 2004). Surgery is not an option for all women. Women who are at high risk of suffering recurrent prolapse after a surgical repair or who have morbid obesity, chronic obstructive pulmonary disease, or medical conditions that would place them at risk for general anesthesia are not good candidates for surgical repair (Kimmons, 2003), and noninvasive treatment strategies should be discussed with them.

Surgical interventions might include anterior or posterior colporrhaphy (to repair a cystocele or rectocele) and vaginal hysterectomy (for uterine prolapse).

An anterior and posterior colporrhaphy may be effective for a first-degree prolapse. This surgical procedure tightens the anterior and posterior vaginal wall, thus repairing a cystocele or rectocele. The pubocervical fascia (supportive tissue between the vagina and bladder) is folded and sutured to bring the bladder and urethra in proper position (Cronje et al., 2004).

A vaginal hysterectomy is the treatment of choice for uterine prolapse because it removes the prolapsed organ that is bringing down the bladder and rectum with it. It can be combined with an anterior and posterior repair if a cystocele or rectocele is present.

Nurses can prepare the woman for surgery by reinforcing the risks and benefits of surgery and describing the postoperative course. The nurse can explain that a Foley catheter will be in place for 1 to 2 days after surgery, and the woman might be unable to urinate due to the swelling after the catheter has been removed. During the recovery period, the nurse should instruct the client to avoid for several weeks activities that cause an increase in abdominal pressure, such as straining, sneezing, and coughing. In addition, she should avoid lifting anything heavy or straining to push anything. Stool softeners and gentle laxatives might be prescribed to prevent constipation and straining with bowel movements. Pelvic rest will be prescribed until the operative area is healed in 6 weeks.

Urinary Incontinence

Urinary incontinence is the involuntary loss of urine sufficient enough to be a social or hygiene problem (Wilson,

2003). This disorder affects approximately 18 million people in the United States, about 11 million of them women (Getliffe & Dolman, 2002). It has been estimated that one in four women experience urinary incontinence at some time in their life, varying from mild to severe leakage (Sloane, 2002). It is more prevalent than diabetes and Alzheimer's disease, both of which receive a great deal of press attention. About half the women with incontinence have never discussed the problem with their healthcare provider because they are too embarrassed to talk about it (Weiss, 2005).

Incontinence can have far-reaching affects on the lives of women who experience it. Some women experience anxiety, depression, social isolation, and disruption in self-esteem and personal dignity. It can cause women to stop working, traveling, socializing, and enjoying sexual relationships. In addition, incontinence can create a tremendous burden for caretakers and is a common reason for admission to a long-term care facility (Weiss, 2005).

Pathophysiology

Urinary continence depends on several factors, including effective functioning of the bladder, adequate pelvic-floor muscles, neural control from the brain, and the integrity of neural connections that facilitate voluntary control. The bladder neck and proximal urethra function as a sphincter. During urination the sphincter relaxes and the bladder empties. The ability to control urination depends on the integrated function of numerous components of the lower urinary tract, which must be structurally sound and function normally. Incontinence can develop if the bladder muscles become overactive due to weakened sphincter muscles, if the bladder muscles become too weak to contract properly, or if signals from the nervous system to the urinary structures are interrupted. A major factor in women that contributes to urinary continence is the estrogen level, because this hormone helps maintain bladder sphincter tone. In perimenopausal or menopausal women, incontinence can be a problem as estrogen levels begin to decline and genitourinary changes occur.

Types of Urinary Incontinence

The three most common types of incontinence are urge incontinence (overactive bladder caused by detrusor muscle contractions), stress incontinence (inadequate urinary sphincter function), and mixed incontinence (involves both stress and urge incontinence) (Guerrero & Sinert, 2004).

Urge incontinence is precipitous loss of urine, preceded by a strong urge to void, with increased bladder pressure and detrusor contraction. Causes might be neurologic, idiopathic, or infectious. Clinical manifestations include urgency, frequency, nocturia, and a large amount of urine loss.

Consider THIS!

It seems that life can be complicated and embarrassing at times when we least expect it. I met a man in church who seemed interested in me, and he asked me out for coffee after Sunday services. I have been alone for 10 years and this prospect seemed exciting to me. We talked for hours over coffee and seemed to have a great deal in common, especially since both of us had lost our spouses to cancer. He asked me to go square dancing with him since that was an activity we both had enjoyed in the past with our spouses. I hadn't been out or physically active for ages and didn't realize how our body changes with age.

It was during the first dance that I noticed a wet sensation between my legs, which I was unable to control. I managed to continue on and pretend that all was fine, but then realized what many of my friends were talking about—stress incontinence. Not being able to control one's urine is very embarrassing and it complicates your life, but I made up my mind that it wasn't going to control me!

Thoughts: Gravity and childbirth take a toll on women's reproductive organs by bringing them downward. It would appear that stress incontinence isn't going to curtail her outside activity, which demonstrates a good attitude. What can be done about her embarrassing accidents? Were there any preventive strategies she could have used at an earlier age?

Stress incontinence is the accidental leakage of urine that occurs with increased pressure on the bladder from coughing, sneezing, laughing, or physical exertion. It develops commonly in women in their 40s and 50s and is usually the result of weakened muscles and ligaments in the pelvis following childbirth. Clinical manifestations include the involuntary loss of a small amount of urine in response to physical activity that raises intra-abdominal pressure.

Treatment

Treatment options depend on the type of urinary incontinence that the woman experiences. Overall, the least invasive procedure with the fewest risks is the first choice for treatment. Surgery is used only if other methods have failed. There is a widespread belief that urinary incontinence is an inevitable problem of getting older and that little or nothing can be done to relieve symptoms or reverse it. Nothing is further from the truth, and attitudes must change so that women feel comfortable seeking help for this embarrassing condition.

For many women with urge incontinence, simple reassurance and lifestyle interventions might help. However, if more than simple lifestyle measures are needed, effective treatments might include:

- Bladder training to establish normal voiding intervals (every 3 to 5 hours)

- Kegel exercises to strengthen the pelvic floor
- Pharmacotherapy to reduce the urge to void. Anticholinergic agents such as oxybutynin (Ditropan) or tolterodine (Detrol) (Balmforth & Cardozo, 2005) might be prescribed.

For women with stress incontinence, treatment is not always a cure, but it can certainly minimize the impact of this condition on the woman's quality of life. Some treatment options for stress incontinence might include:

- Weight loss if needed
- Avoidance of constipation
- Smoking cessation
- Kegel exercises to strengthen the pelvic floor
- Pessaries
- Weighted vaginal cones to improve the tone of pelvic-floor muscles
- Periurethral injection (injecting a bulking agent [collagen] to form a bulge that brings the urethral walls closer together to achieve a better closure)
- Medications such as duloxetine (Yentreve) to increase urethral sphincter contractions during the storage phase of urination cycle
- Estrogen replacement therapy to improve bladder sphincter tone
- Surgery to correct genital prolapse and improve urethral and bladder tone

Nursing Management

Incontinence can be devastating and can cause psychosocial concerns and isolation. Nurses can encourage women with troublesome symptoms to seek help. Nurses should discuss the treatment options with the client, including benefits and potential outcomes, and encourage her to select the continence treatment best for her lifestyle. Nurses can provide education about good bladder habits and strategies to reduce the incidence or severity of incontinence (Teaching Guidelines 7-2). Patients need the nurse's support and encouragement to ensure compliance. Nurses need to remember that aging can increase the risk of incontinence, but incontinence is not an inevitable part of aging. Reviewing the anatomy and physiology of the urinary system and offering simple explanations can help women cope with urinary alterations.

Benign Growths

The most common benign growths of the reproductive tract include cervical, endocervical, and endometrial polyps; uterine fibroids (leiomyomas); and ovarian cysts.

Polyps

Polyps are small benign growths. The etiology underlying polyp growth is not well understood, but they are frequently the result of infection. Polyps might be associated with chronic inflammation, an abnormal local response to

 TEACHING GUIDELINES 7-2

Managing Urinary Incontinence

- Avoid taking in too much fluid (i.e., 1.5 L total daily limit). However, do not decrease intake of fluids and become dehydrated.
- Reduce intake of fluids and foods that are bladder irritants and precipitate urgency: chocolate; caffeine; sodas; alcohol; artificial sweetener; hot, spicy foods; orange juice; tomatoes; and watermelon (Thompson & Smith, 2002).
- Increase fiber and fluids in diet to reduce constipation.
- Control blood glucose levels to prevent polyuria.
- Treat chronic cough.
- Remove any barriers that delay reaching the toilet.
- Practice good perineal hygiene by using mild soap and water. Wipe from front to back to prevent urinary tract infections.
- Increase awareness of adverse drug effects.
- Take medications as prescribed.
- Continue pelvic-floor (Kegel) exercises.

increased levels of estrogen, or local congestion of the cervical vasculature (Chen, 2004). Single or multiple polyps might occur. They are most common among multiparous women. Polyps can appear anywhere but are most common on the cervix and in the uterus (Fig. 7-3).

Cervical polyps often appear after the onset of menstruation. Endocervical polyps are commonly found in multiparous women age 40 to 60. Endocervical polyps are

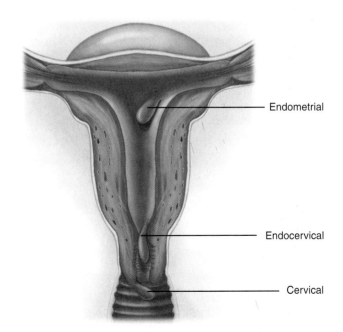

Endometrial

Endocervical

Cervical

● Figure 7-3 Cervical, endocervical, and endometrial polyps.

more common than cervical polyps, with a stalk of varied width and length. Endometrial polyps are benign tumors or localized overgrowths of the endometrium. Most endometrial polyps are solitary, and they rarely occur in women younger than 20 years of age. The incidence of these polyps rises steadily with increasing age, peaks in the fifth decade of life, and gradually declines after menopause. They are present in about 10% to 24% of women being seen for abnormal bleeding (Condon, 2004).

Clinical Manifestations and Diagnosis

Most endocervical polyps are cherry red, while most cervical polyps are grayish-white (Scott, 2004). Typically, cervical polyps are diagnosed when the cervix is visualized through a speculum during the woman's annual gynecologic examination (Youngkin & Davis, 2004). Cervical and endocervical polyps are often asymptomatic, but they can produce mild symptoms such as abnormal vaginal bleeding (after intercourse, douching, between menses) or discharge.

The most frequent clinical manifestation of women with endometrial polyps is *metrorrhagia* (irregular, acyclic uterine bleeding). They are not detected on physical examination, but rather with ultrasound or hysteroscopy (introduction of a small camera through the cervix to visualize the uterine cavity).

Treatment

Treatment of polyps usually consists of simple removal with small forceps done on an outpatient basis, removal during hysteroscopy, or dilatation and curettage (D&C). Removal of the polyp base can be done by laser vaporization. Because many polyps are infected, an antibiotic may be ordered after removal as a preventive measure (prophylactically) or due to early signs of infection.

Although polyps are rarely cancerous, a specimen should be sent after surgery to a pathology laboratory to exclude malignancy. A cervical biopsy typically reveals mildly atypical cells and signs of infection. Polyps rarely return after they are removed. Regularly scheduled Pap smears are suggested for women with cervical polyps to detect any future abnormal growths that may be malignant.

Nursing Management

Nursing management of polyps involves explaining the condition and the rationale for removal and giving follow-up care instructions. The nurse also assists the healthcare provider with any procedure for removal.

Uterine Fibroids

Uterine fibroids, or leiomyomas, are benign tumors composed of muscular and fibrous tissue in the uterus. Fibroids can occur in the submucous layer, the intramural layer, or the subserous layer of the uterus (Fig. 7-4). They are estrogen-dependent and thus grow rapidly during the

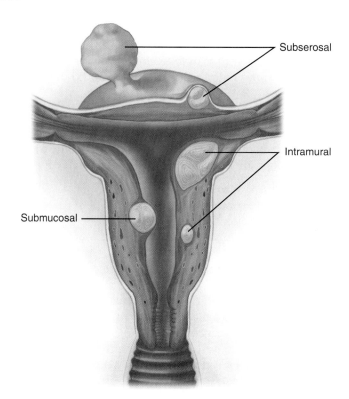

● Figure 7-4 Submucosal, intramural, and subserosal fibroids.

childbearing years, when estrogen is plentiful, but they shrink during menopause, when estrogen levels decline. It is believed that these benign tumors develop in about 25% of all women older than age 30 (Flake et al., 2003). Fibroids are the most common indication for hysterectomy in the United States. The peak incidence occurs around the age of 45, with approximately 8 cases per 1,000 women annually in the United States (Speroff & Fritz, 2005).

Although the cause of fibroids is unknown, several predisposing factors have been identified, including:

• Age (late reproductive years)
• Genetic predisposition
• African-American ethnicity
• Nulliparity
• Obesity (Alexander et al., 2004).

Clinical Manifestations and Diagnosis

Fibroids are usually detected during pelvic examinations because the uterus is enlarged and irregularly shaped. Common symptoms of fibroids depend on the size and location of the tumors and may include:

• Chronic pelvic pain
• Low back pain
• Iron deficiency anemia secondary to bleeding
• Bloating
• Infertility (with large tumors)
• Dysmenorrhea
• Dyspareunia

- Irregular vaginal bleeding (menorrhagia)
- Feeling of heaviness in the pelvic region

Treatment

Treatment depends on the size of the fibroids and the symptoms experienced and may include several options, from watchful waiting to surgery.

Medical Management

The goals of medical therapy are to reduce symptoms and to reduce the tumor size. This can be accomplished with gonadotropin-releasing hormone (GnRH) agonists, which induce reversible menopause, or low-dose mifepristone, a progestin antagonist. Both have produced regression and reduced the size of the tumors without surgery, but long-term therapy is expensive and not tolerated by most women. The side effects of GnRH medications include hot flashes, headaches, mood changes, vaginal dryness, musculoskeletal malaise, bone loss, and depression (Speroff & Fritz, 2005). Long-term mifepristone therapy can result in endometrial hyperplasia, which increases the risk of endometrial malignancy. Once either therapy is stopped, the fibroids typically reoccur.

Uterine artery embolization (UAE) is an option in which polyvinyl alcohol pellets are injected into selected blood vessels via a catheter to block circulation to the fibroid, causing shrinkage of the fibroid and resolution of the symptoms. After treatment, most fibroids are reduced by 50% within 3 months, but they might recur (Todd, 2002). The failure rate is approximately 10% to 15%, and this therapy should not be performed on women desiring to retain their fertility.

Surgical Management

For women with large fibroids or severe menorrhagia, surgery is preferred over medical treatment. Surgical management might involve myomectomy, laser surgery, or hysterectomy.

Myomectomy involves removing the fibroid alone. A myomectomy is performed through a laparoscopic or abdominal incision approach or through a vaginal approach. The advantage is that only the fibroid is removed, and fertility is not jeopardized because this procedure leaves the uterine muscle walls intact. Myomectomy relieves symptoms but does not affect the underlying process; thus, fibroids do grow back, and further treatment is needed in the future.

Laser surgery (or electrocauterization) involves destroying small fibroids with lasers. Laser therapy can be done using a vaginal approach or laparoscopically. The laser treatment preserves the uterus, but the process may cause scarring and adhesions, and fertility may be disturbed (Lowdermilk & Perry, 2004). Fibroids can return after this procedure. Controversy remains as to whether laser treatment weakens the uterine wall and thus may contribute to uterine rupture in the future.

A *hysterectomy* is the surgical removal of the uterus. After cesarean section, it is the second most frequently performed surgical procedure for women in the United States. Approximately 600,000 hysterectomies are performed annually in the United States (CDC, 2005). The top three conditions associated with hysterectomies are fibroids, endometriosis, and uterine prolapse (CDC, 2005). A hysterectomy to remove fibroids eliminates both the symptoms and the risk of recurrence, but it also terminates the woman's ability to bear children. Three types of hysterectomy surgeries are available: vaginal hysterectomy, laparoscopically assisted vaginal hysterectomy, and abdominal hysterectomy.

In a vaginal hysterectomy, the uterus is removed through an incision in the posterior vagina. Advantages include a shorter hospital stay and recovery time and no abdominal scars. Disadvantages include a limited operating space and poor visualization of other pelvic organs.

In a laparoscopically assisted vaginal hysterectomy, the uterus is removed through a laparoscope, through which structures within the abdomen and pelvis are visualized. Small incisions are made in the abdominal wall to permit the laparoscope to enter the surgical site. Advantages include a better surgical field, less pain, less cost, and a shorter recovery time. Disadvantages include potential injury to the bladder and the inability to remove enlarged uteruses and scar tissue.

In abdominal hysterectomy, the uterus and other pelvic organs are removed through an incision in the abdomen. This procedure allows the surgeon to visualize all pelvic organs and is typically used when a malignancy is suspected or a very large uterus is present. Disadvantages include the need for general anesthesia, a longer hospital stay and recovery period, more pain, higher cost, and a visible scar on the abdomen.

Nursing Management

Women considering surgery need information so they can make an informed decision. Nurses can offer a thorough explanation of the procedure and aftercare (Box 7-2). A woman undergoing a hysterectomy for the treatment of fibroids often needs special care.

Ovarian Cysts

An **ovarian cyst** is a fluid-filled sac that forms on the ovary (Fig. 7-5). These very common growths are benign 90% of the time and are asymptomatic in many women (Breslin & Lucas, 2003). Ovarian cysts occur in 30% of women with regular menses, 50% with irregular menses, and 6% of postmenopausal women (Kazzi & Roberts, 2004). When cysts grow large and exert pressure on surrounding structures, women often seek medical help.

The most common benign ovarian cysts include follicular cysts, corpus luteum (lutein) cysts, theca-lutein cysts, and polycystic ovarian syndrome (PCOS).

BOX 7-2
NURSING INTERVENTIONS FOR A WOMAN UNDERGOING A HYSTERECTOMY

Preoperative Care
• Instruct the patient and her family regarding the procedure and aftercare.
• Teach turning, deep breathing, and coughing prior to the surgery to prevent atelectasis and respiratory complications such as pneumonia.
• Encourage discussion of feelings and emotions. Some women equate their femaleness with their reproductive capability, and loss could evoke grieving.
• Complete all preop orders in a timely manner to allow for rest.

Postoperative Care
• Provide comfort measures.
• Administer analgesics promptly or use PCA pump.
• Administer antiemetics to control nausea and vomiting per order.
• Change linens and gown frequently to promote hygiene.
• Change position frequently and use pillows for support to promote comfort and pain management.
• Assess incision, dressing, and vaginal bleeding and report if excessive (soaking perineal pad within an hour).
• Monitor elimination and provide increased fluids and fiber to prevent constipation and potential straining.
• Encourage ambulation and active range of motion when in bed to prevent thrombophlebitis and venous stasis.

• Monitor vital signs to detect early complications for treatment.
• Be open to listening and discussing sexual concerns with client.

Discharge Planning
• Advise client to reduce activity level to avoid fatigue, which might inhibit healing.
• Advise client to rest when tired and increase activity level slowly.
• Educate client on need for pelvic rest (nothing in the vagina) for 6 weeks.
• Instruct client to avoid heavy lifting or straining for about 6 weeks to prevent an increase in intra-abdominal pressure, which may weaken sutures.
• Teach client signs and symptoms of infection.
• Advise showers instead of tub baths to reduce risk for infection.
• Encourage a healthy diet with increased intake of fluids to prevent dehydration and potential fluid and electrolyte imbalance.
• Instruct client to change peri-pad frequently to prevent infection.
• Explain and schedule follow-up care appointments as needed.
• Provide community resources for support/help.

Follicular Cysts

Follicular cysts are caused by the failure of the ovarian follicle to rupture at the time of ovulation. Follicular cysts seldom grow larger than 5 cm in diameter; most regress and require no treatment. They can occur at any age but are more common in reproductive-aged women and are rare after menopause. They are detected by vaginal ultrasound.

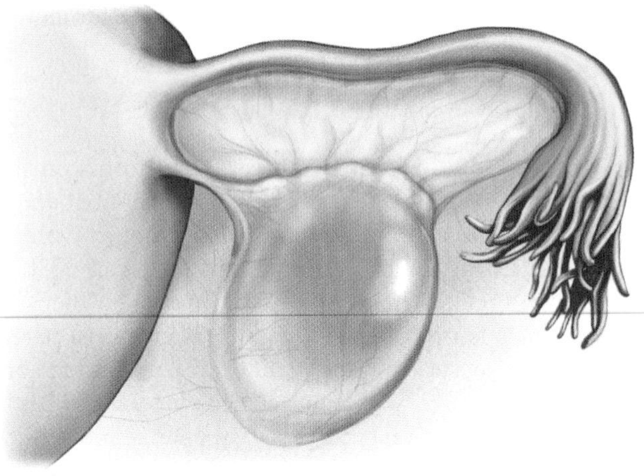

● Figure 7-5 Ovarian cyst.

Corpus Luteum (Lutein) Cyst

A corpus luteum cyst forms when the corpus luteum becomes cystic or hemorrhagic and fails to degenerate after 14 days. These cysts might cause pain and delay the next menses. A pelvic ultrasound helps to make this diagnosis. Typically these cysts appear after ovulation and resolve without intervention.

Theca-Lutein Cysts

Prolonged abnormally high levels of human chorionic gonadotropin (hCG) stimulate the development of theca-lutein cysts. Although rare, these cysts are associated with hydatiform mole, choriocarcinoma, PCOS, and Clomid therapy.

Polycystic Ovarian Syndrome

PCOS involves the presence of multiple inactive follicle cysts within the ovary that interfere with ovarian function. Hyperandrogenism, insulin resistance, and chronic anovulation characterize PCOS. Careful attention should be given to this condition because women with it are at increased risk for long-term health problems such as cardiovascular disease, hypertension, dyslipidemia, type 2 diabetes, and cancer (endometrial, breast, and ovarian) (Speroff & Fritz, 2005). Because this syndrome is complex and of unknown etiology, it can be difficult to manage (Jackson, 2005).

Clinical Manifestations

Common symptoms of large ovarian cysts include:

- Abdominal distention
- Interference with normal voiding patterns
- Altered bowel habits
- Abnormal uterine bleeding
- Dyspareunia
- Pelvic pain (Lowdermilk & Perry, 2004)

The typical clinical picture of a woman with PCOS includes infertility, hyperinsulinemia, obesity, menstrual irregularities (amenorrhea or oligomenorrhea, or menorrhagia), and androgen excess (hirsutism on upper lip, chin, cheeks, and between the breasts, and acne). Making the diagnosis of PCOS is difficult; the diagnosis is primarily one of exclusion because of the diffuse nature of the symptoms and the lack of standard criteria.

Treatment

Treatment of ovarian cysts focuses on differentiating a benign cyst from a solid ovarian malignancy. Transvaginal ultrasound is useful in distinguishing fluid-filled cysts from solid masses. Laparoscopy may be needed to remove the cyst, if it is large and pressing on surrounding structures. For smaller cysts, monitoring with repeat ultrasounds every 3 to 6 months might be in order (Helm, 2004). Oral contraceptives are often prescribed to suppress gonadotropin levels, which may help resolve the cysts. Pain medication is also prescribed if needed.

Management of PCOS includes both drug and non-drug therapy, along with lifestyle modifications. Goals of therapy focus on suppressing hyperandrogenism to decrease hirsutism and acne, restoring reproductive function in women desiring children, and reducing the long-term risk of developing diabetes and cardiovascular disease (Hill, 2003). Treatment modalities for PCOS are highlighted in Box 7-3.

Nursing Management

Nursing care should include education about the condition, treatment options, diagnostic test arrangements, and referral for surgery if needed. Providing support and reassurance during the diagnostic period is vital to allay anxiety in the client and her family. Many women need reassurance that the majority of ovarian cysts are benign, but follow-up care should be stressed regardless. Listening to the woman's concerns about her appearance, infertility, and facial hair growth is important. Offering suggestions on ways to bring about improvement can go a long way in making the woman feel better about herself and her future health.

Nurses can have a positive impact on women with PCOS through counseling and education. They can

---

> **BOX 7-3**
>
> **TREATMENT MODALITIES FOR PCOS**
>
> - Oral contraceptives to treat menstrual irregularities and acne
> - Mechanical hair removal (shaving, waxing, plucking, or electrolysis) to treat hirsutism
> - Glucophage (metformin), which improves insulin uptake by fat and muscle cells, to treat hyper-insulinemia
> - Ovulation induction agents (Clomid) to treat infertility
> - Lifestyle changes (e.g., weight loss; exercise; balanced, low-fat diet)
> - Referral to support groups to help improve emotional state and build self-esteem (ACOG, 2002)

---

provide support for women dealing with negative self-image secondary to the physical manifestations of PCOS. Through education, nurses can help women to understand the syndrome and its associated risk factors to prevent long-term health problems. Nurses should encourage women to make positive lifestyle changes. Making community referrals to local support groups may help the woman build her coping skills.

Summary

Nurses can play a key role in helping women deal with various benign disorders of the reproductive tract by providing pictures or diagrams to explain the disorder and discussing the treatment options available. Much of the time, reassurance might be all that is needed to reduce their fears and anxieties. Offering physical presence and empathetic therapeutic communication will help them through their difficult times. Including the family in the instructional sessions will help strengthen the woman's support system. Nurses must keep up to date on the latest research about treatments so that they can present the most current information to allow the woman to make informed decisions about her healthcare.

References

Alexander, L. L., LaRosa, J. H., Bader, H., & Garfield, S. (2004). *New dimensions in women's health* (3rd ed.). Sudbury, MA: Jones and Bartlett Publishers.

American College of Obstetrics and Gynecology (ACOG) (2002). Polycystic ovary syndrome. Practice bulletin number 41: Clinical management guidelines for obstetrician-gynecologists. *Obstetrics & Gynecology, 100*(6), 1389–1401.

Balmforth, J., & Cardozo, L. (Feb. 5, 2005). Urinary incontinence: what the GP can do. *Clinical Pulse,* 41–46.

Breslin, E. T., & Lucas, V. A. (2003). *Women's health nursing: toward evidence-based practice.* St. Louis, MO: Saunders.

Brolmann, H. (2004). Pelvic floor disorders: diagnosis, management and new developments. *Gynecology Forum.* [Online] Available at: http://www.medforum.nl/gynfo/leading_article10.htm

Centers for Disease Control and Prevention (CDC) (2005). Women's reproductive health: hysterectomy. *CDC Reproductive Health.* [Online] Available at: http://www.cdc.gov/reproductivehealth/WomensRH/Hysterectomy.htm

Chen, P. (2004). Cervical polyps. *Medline Plus.* [Online] Available at: http://www.nlm.nih.gov/medlineplus/ency/article/001494.htm

Condon, M. C. (2004) *Women's health: an integrated approach to wellness and illness.* Upper Saddle River, NJ: Prentice Hall.

Cronje, H. S., De Beer, J. A., & Bam, R. H. (2004). The pathophysiology of an enterocele and its management. *Journal of Obstetrics and Gynecology, 24*(4), 408–413.

Dudek, S. G. (2006). *Nutritional essentials for nursing practice* (5th ed.). Philadelphia: Lippincott Williams & Wilkins.

Eisinger, S. H., Meldrum, S., Fiscella, K., et al. (2003). Low-dose mifepristone for uterine leiomyomata. *Obstetrics & Gynecology, 101*(2), 243–251.

Flake, G. P., Andersen, J., & Dixon, D. (2003). Etiology and pathogenesis of uterine leiomyomas: a review. *Environmental Health Perspectives, 111* (8), 1037–1055.

Getliffe, K., & Dolman, M. (2002). *Promoting continence: a clinical and research source* (2nd ed.). London: Bailliere Tindall.

Guerrero, P., & Sinert, R. (2004). Urinary incontinence. *eMedicine.* [Online] Available at: http://emedicine.com/emerg/topic791.htm

Helm, C. W. (2004). Ovarian cysts. *eMedicine.* [Online] Available at: http://emedicine.com/med/topic1699.htm

Hendrix, S. L., Cochrane, B. C., Nygaard, I. E., et al. (2005). Effects of estrogen with and without progestin on urinary incontinence. *JAMA, 293,* 935–948.

Hill, K. M. (2003). Update: the pathogenesis and treatment of PCOS. *Nurse Practitioner, 28*(7), 8–25.

Jackson, M. L. (2005). Polycystic ovarian syndrome: what nurses need to know about this misunderstood disorder. *AWHONN Lifelines, 8*(6), 512–518.

Kazzi, A. A., & Roberts, R. (2004). Ovarian cysts. *eMedicine.* [Online] Available at: http://www.emedicine.com/EMERG/topic352.htm

Kimmons, B. J. (2003). Female urinary incontinence: diagnosis and noninvasive treatment strategies. *Physician Assistant Journal, 27*(4), 26–36.

Lazarou, G., & Scotti, R. J. (2004). Uterine prolapse. *eMedicine.* [Online] Available at: http://emedicine.com/med/topic3291.htm

Lewis, S. M., Heitkemper, M. M., & Dirksen, S. R. (2004). *Medical-surgical nursing: assessment and management of clinical problems* (6th ed.). St. Louis: Mosby.

Lowdermilk, D. L., & Perry, S. E. (2004). *Maternity & women's health care* (8th ed.). St. Louis: Mosby.

Lumb, J. (2004). Stress urinary incontinence. *Practice Nurse, 28*(9), 38–41.

McIntosh, L. (2005). The role of the nurse in the use of vaginal pessaries to treat pelvic organ prolapse and/or urinary incontinence: a literature review. *Urologic Nursing, 25*(1), 41–49.

Scott, P. J. (2004). Cervix and common cervical abnormalities. *PatientPlus.* [Online] Available at: http://www.patient.co.uk/showdoc/40024690/

Shaw, H. A. (2003). Rectocele. *eMedicine.* [Online] Available at: http://www.emedicine.com/med/topic3325.htm

Sloane, E. (2002). *Biology of women* (4th ed.). New York: Delmar.

Speroff, L., & Fritz, M. A. (2005). *Clinical gynecologic endocrinology and infertility* (7th ed.). Philadelphia: Lippincott Williams & Wilkins.

Spratto, G. R., & Woods, A. L. (2005). *PDR nurse's drug handbook.* Clifton Park, NY: Thomson Delmar Learning.

Thakar, R., & Stanton, S. (2002). Management of genital prolapse. *British Medical Journal, 324*(7348), 1258–1263.

Thompson, D. L., & Smith, D. A. (2002). Continence nursing: a whole person approach. *Holistic Nursing Practice, 16*(2), 14–31.

Todd, A. (2002). An alternative to hysterectomy. *RN, 65*(3), 30–35.

Weiss, B. D. (2005). Selecting medications for the treatment of urinary incontinence. *American Family Physician, 71*(2), 315–322.

Wilson, L. (2003). Continence and older people: the importance of functional assessment. *Nursing Older People, 15*(4), 22–28.

Youngkin, E. Q., & Davis, M. S. (2004). *Women's health: a primary care clinical guide* (3rd ed.). New Jersey: Prentice Hall.

Web Resources

American Cancer Society: (800)-ACS-2345, **www.cancer.org**

American College of Obstetricians and Gynecologists: (202) 863-2518, **www.acog.org**

American Urological Association: (410) 727-1100, **www.auanet.org**

Fibroid Treatment Collective: (310) 794-6645, **www.fibroid.org**

Hysterectomy Educational Resource and Services (HERS): (215) 667-7757, **www.ccon.com/hers**

National Association for Continence: (800) 252-3337, **www.nafc.org**

National Women's Health Information Center: (800) 994-9662, **www.4women.gov**

Polycystic Ovarian Syndrome Association: **www.pcossupport.org**

Sexuality Information and Education Council of the United States: (212) 819-9770, **www.siecus.org**

Chapter WORKSHEET

● MULTIPLE CHOICE QUESTIONS

1. As the nurse interviewing a patient with uterine fibroids, what subjective data would you expect from her history?

   a. Cyclic migraine headaches

   b. Urinary urgency

   c. Chronic pelvic pain

   d. Chronic constipation

2. Treatment options available for women experiencing pelvic organ prolapse are:

   a. Pessaries and Kegel exercises

   b. External pelvic fixation devices

   c. Weight gain and yoga programs

   d. Firm panty and girdle garments

3. Which of the following dietary and lifestyle modifications might the nurse recommend to help prevent pelvic relaxation as women age?

   a. Consume a high-fiber diet to avoid constipation and straining.

   b. Avoid sitting for long periods; get up and walk around frequently.

   c. Limit the amount of exercise to prevent over-developing muscles.

   d. Space children a year apart to reduce wear and tear on uterus.

4. Women experiencing polycystic ovarian syndrome (PCOS) are at increased risk for developing which of the following long-term health problems?

   a. Osteoporosis

   b. Lupus

   c. Type 2 diabetes

   d. Migraine headaches

5. Side effects experienced by women taking gonadotropin-releasing hormone (GnRH) agonists for the treatment of fibroids closely resemble those of:

   a. Osteoporosis

   b. Osteoarthritis

   c. Depression

   d. Menopause

● CRITICAL THINKING EXERCISE

1. Faith, a 42-year-old multiparous woman, presents to the women's health clinic complaining of pelvic pain, menorrhagia, and vaginal discharge. She says she has been experiencing these problems for several months. On examination, her uterus is enlarged and irregular in shape. Her blood studies reveal anemia.

   a. What condition might Faith have, based on her symptoms?

   b. What treatment options are available to address this condition?

   c. What educational interventions should the nurse discuss with Faith?

● STUDY ACTIVITIES

1. Prepare an educational session to teach women how to do Kegel exercises to prevent stress incontinence and pelvic-floor relaxation.

2. In a small group, discuss the personal, social, and sexual issues that might affect a woman with pelvic organ prolapse. How might these issues affect her socialization? How might a support group help?

3. List the symptoms that a woman with uterine fibroids might experience. Discuss how these symptoms might mimic a more frightening condition and why the woman might delay seeking treatment.

4. A bladder that herniates into the vagina is a

   _____.

5. A rectum that herniates into the vagina is a

   _____.

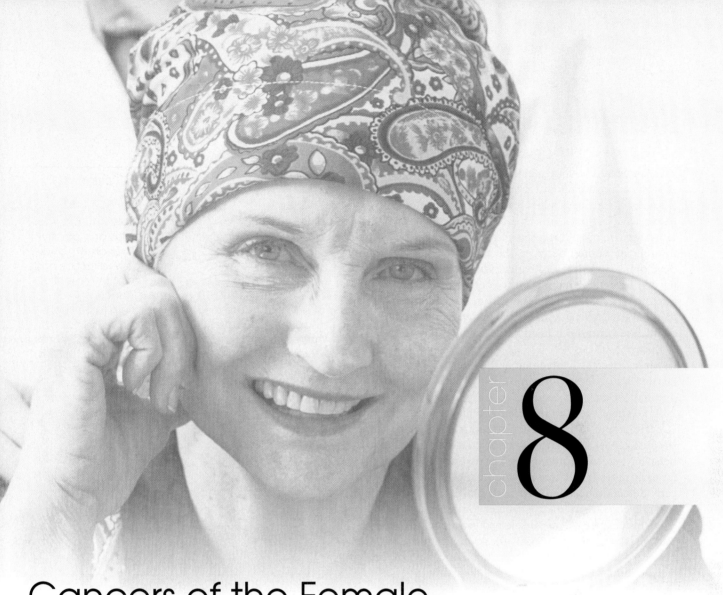

chapter 8

Cancers of the Female Reproductive Tract

KeyTERMS

cervical cancer
cervical dysplasia
colposcopy
cone biopsy
cryotherapy
endometrial cancer
human papillomavirus
ovarian cancer
Papanicolaou (Pap) test
vaginal cancer
vulvar cancer

LearningOBJECTIVES

After studying the chapter content, the student should be able to accomplish the following:

1. Define the key terms.
2. Identify the major modifiable risk factors for reproductive tract cancers.
3. Discuss the risk factors, screening methods, and treatment modalities for cancers of the reproductive tract.
4. Outline the nursing management needed for the most common malignant reproductive disorders in women.
5. Describe lifestyle changes and health screenings needed to reduce risk or prevent reproductive tract cancers.
6. List community resources available for the women undergoing surgery for a malignant reproductive condition.

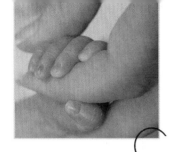

ancer is the second leading cause of death for women in the United States, surpassed only by cardiovascular disease (Youngkin & Davis, 2004). Obviously, cardiovascular disease is and must continue to be a major focus of our efforts in women's health. However, we must not lose sight of the fact that a large number of women between the ages of 35 and 74 are developing and dying of cancer (NCI, 2004). Women have a one in three lifetime risk of developing cancer, and one out of every four deaths is from cancer (Alexander et al., 2004). African-American women have the highest death rates from both heart disease and cancer (Breslin & Lucas, 2003).

It has been estimated that in the United States half of all premature deaths, one third of acute disabilities, and one half of chronic disabilities are preventable (NCI, 2004). Nurses need to put their energies into screening, education, and early detection to reduce these statistics. Because cancer risk is strongly associated with lifestyle and behavior, screening programs are of particular importance for early detection. There is evidence that prevention and early detection have reduced both cancer mortality rates and prevented reproductive cancers (Smith et al., 2004).

This chapter will cover selected cancers of the reproductive system and will identify the appropriate screenings needed. The reproductive cancers to be discussed are cervical, endometrial, ovarian, vaginal, and vulvar.

Cervical Cancer

Cervical cancer is cancer of the uterine cervix. The American Cancer Society (ACS) estimates that over 10,000 cases of invasive cervical cancer will be diagnosed in the United States in 2005. Of that number, approximately 4,000 women will die. Some researchers estimate that noninvasive cervical cancer (carcinoma in situ) is about four times more common than invasive cervical cancer. The 5-year survival rate for all stages of cervical cancer is 73% (ACS, 2005). The median age at diagnosis for cervical cancer is 47 years, and nearly half of all cases are diagnosed before the age of 35 (Waggoner, 2003).

Cervical cancer incidence and mortality rates have decreased noticeably in the past several decades, with most of the reduction attributed to the **Papanicolaou (Pap) test,** which detects cervical cancer and precancerous lesions. Cervical cancer is one of the most treatable cancers when detected at an early stage (ACS, 2005). *Healthy People 2010* (USDHHS, 2000) identifies two goals that address cervical cancer (Healthy People 2010).

National Health Goals Related to Cervical Cancer

Objective	Significance
Goal 3-4—Reduce the death rate from cancer of the uterine cervix from 3 per 100,000 females (1998) to 2 per 100,000 females in 2010.	This will help improve mortality rates and quality of life for women, and reduce healthcare costs related to treatment of malignancies.
Goal 3-11—Increase the proportion of women who received a Pap smear within the preceding 3 years from 79% to 90% by 2010.	This will help to promote screening and early detection. The National Institutes of Health (NIH) reported that half of women diagnosed with invasive cervical cancer have never had a Pap smear and 10% have not had Pap smears during the past 5 years (NIH, 2005).

Pathophysiology

Cervical cancer starts with abnormal changes in the cellular lining or surface of the cervix. Typically these changes occur in the squamous–columnar junction of the cervix. Here, cylindrically shaped secretory epithelial cells (columnar) meet the protective flat epithelial cells (squamous) from the outer cervix and vagina in what is termed the transformation zone. The continuous replacement of columnar epithelial cells by squamous epithelial cells in this area makes these cells vulnerable to take up foreign or abnormal genetic material (Adams, 2002). Figure 8-1 shows the pathophysiology of cervical cancer.

Etiology and Risk Factors

The primary factor in the development of cervical cancer is **human papillomavirus** (HPV), which is acquired through sexual activity (Roye et al., 2003). More than 90% of squamous cervical cancers contain HPV DNA, and the virus is now accepted as a major causative factor in the development of cervical cancer and its precursor, **cervical dysplasia** (disordered growth of abnormal cells).

Risk factors associated with cervical cancer include:

- Early age at first intercourse (within 1 year of menarche)
- Lower socioeconomic status
- Promiscuous male partners
- Unprotected sexual intercourse

Carcinoma in situ   **Squamous cell carcinoma**

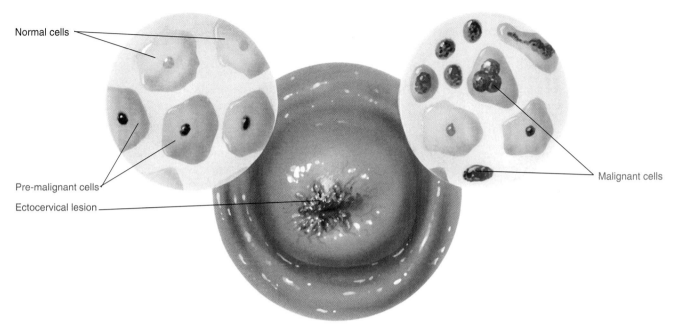

Normal cells

Pre-malignant cells

Ectocervical lesion

Malignant cells

● Figure 8-1 Cervical cancer. (The Anatomical Chart Company. [2002]. *Atlas of pathophysiology.* Springhouse, PA: Springhouse.)

- Family history of cervical cancer (mother or sisters)
- Sexual intercourse with uncircumcised men
- Female offspring of mothers who took diethylstilbestrol (DES)
- Infections with genital herpes or chronic chlamydia
- History of multiple sex partners
- Cigarette smoking
- Immunocompromised state
- HIV infection
- Oral contraceptive use
- Moderate dysplasia on Pap smear within past 5 years
- HPV infection (Grund, 2005)

Clinical Manifestations

Clinically, the first symptom is abnormal vaginal bleeding, usually after sexual intercourse. Vaginal discomfort, malodorous discharge, and dysuria are common manifestations also. Some women with cervical cancer have no symptoms. Frequently it is detected at an annual gynecologic examination and Pap test. Advanced symptoms of cervical cancer may include pelvic, back, or leg pain, weight loss, anorexia, weakness and fatigue, and bone fractures.

Diagnosis

Screening for cervical cancer is very effective because the presence of a precursor lesion, cervical intraepithelial neoplasia (CIN), helps determine whether further tests are needed. Lesions start as dysplasia and progress in a predictable fashion over a long period, allowing ample oppor-

tunity for intervention at a precancerous stage. Progression from low-grade to high-grade dysplasia takes an average of 9 years, and progression from high-grade dysplasia to invasive cancer takes up to 2 years (Jemal et al., 2005).

Widespread use of the Pap test (also known as a Pap smear), a procedure used to obtain cells from the cervix for cytology screening, is credited with saving tens of thousands of women's lives and decreasing deaths from cervical cancer by more than 70% (ACS, 2005) (Nursing Procedure 8-1: Assisting with Collection of a Pap Smear). Despite its outstanding record of success as a screening tool for cervical cancer (it detects approximately 90% of early cancer changes), the conventional Pap smear has a 20% false-negative rate. High-grade abnormalities missed by human screening are frequently detected by computerized instruments (Garcia & Bi, 2004). Thus, many new technologies are being studied and introduced clinically, including:

- *Automated slide thin-layer preparation (Thin-Prep):* In this liquid-based cervical cytology technique, the cervical specimen is placed into a vial of fixative solution rather than on the glass slide.
- *Computer-assisted automated Pap test rescreening (Autopap):* An algorithm-based decision-making technology that identifies slides that should be rescreened by cytopathologists by selecting samples that exceed a certain threshold for the likelihood of abnormal cells
- *HPV-DNA typing (Hybrid Capture):* This system uses the association between certain types of HPV (16, 18, 31, 33,

Nursing Procedure 8-1

Assisting With Collection of a Pap Smear

Purpose: To Obtain Cells From the Cervix for Cervical Cytology Screening

1. Explain procedure to the client (Fig. A).
2. Instruct client to empty her bladder.
3. Wash hands thoroughly.
4. Assemble equipment, maintaining sterility of equipment (Fig. B)
5. Position client on stirrups or foot pedals so that her knees fall outward.
6. Drape client with a sheet for privacy, covering the abdomen but leaving the perineal area exposed.
7. Open packages as needed.
8. Encourage client to relax.
9. Provide support to client as the practitioner obtains a sample by spreading the labia; inserting the speculum; inserting the cytobrush and swabbing the endocervix; and inserting the plastic spatula and swabbing the cervix (Fig. C–H).
10. Transfer specimen to container (Fig. I) or slide. If a slide is used, spray the fixative on the slide.
11. Place sterile lubricant on the practitioner's fingertip when indicated for the bimanual examination.
12. Wash hands thoroughly.
13. Label specimen according to facility policy.
14. Rinse reusable instruments and dispose of waste appropriately (Fig. J).
15. Wash hands thoroughly.

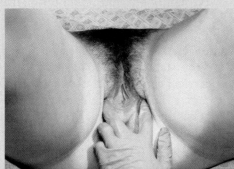

A

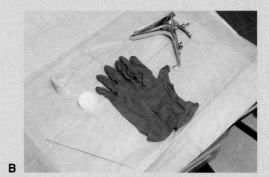

B

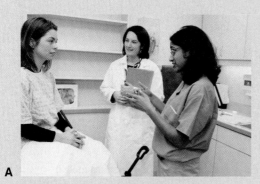

C

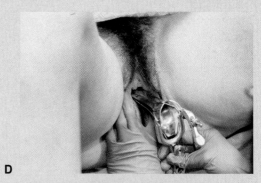

D

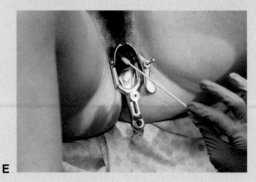

E

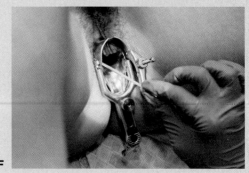

F

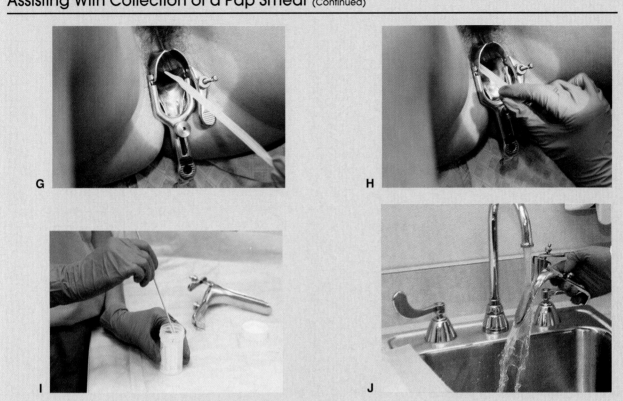

Used with permission from Klossner, N. J. (2006). *Introductory maternity nursing.* Philadelphia: Lippincott Williams & Wilkins.

35, 45, 51, 52, and 56) and the development of cervical cancer. This system can identify high-risk HPV types and improves detection and management.
• *Computer-assisted technology (Cytyc CDS-1000, AutoCyte, AcCell):* These computerized instruments can detect abnormal cells that are sometimes missed by technologists (Anderson & Runowicz, 2002).

Other factors contributing to the high rate of false-negative results include errors in sampling the cervix, in preparing the slide, and in patient preparation. To optimize conditions for Pap smear collection, nurses can offer the instructions provided in Teaching Guidelines 8-1.

Although many professional medical organizations disagree as to the frequency of screening for cervical cancer, the ACS 2003 guidelines suggest that women should begin annual screening for cervical cancer via a Pap test after they initiate sexual activity or at 21 years of age, whichever comes first. If three consecutive Pap smears are negative, a trained healthcare provider may suggest that screening can be performed less frequently. Women ages 65 to 70 with no abnormal tests in the previous 10 years may choose to stop screenings (ACS, 2003).

 TEACHING GUIDELINES 8-1

Strategies to Optimize Pap Smear Results

• Schedule your Pap smear appointment about 2 weeks (10 to 18 days) after the first day of your last menses to increase the chance of getting the best sample of cervical cells without menses.
• Refrain from intercourse for 48 hours before the test because additional matter such as sperm can obscure the specimen.
• Do not douche within 48 hours before the test to prevent washing away cervical cells that might be abnormal.
• Do not use tampons, birth control foams, jellies, vaginal creams, or vaginal medications for 72 hours before the test, as they could cover up or obscure the cervical cell sample.
• Cancel your Pap appointment if vaginal bleeding occurs, because the presence of blood cells interferes with visual evaluation of the sample (Ross, 2003).

For high-risk women, annual Pap smears should continue annually throughout their life (Table 8-1).

Pap smear results are classified using the Bethesda System (Box 8-1), which provides a uniform diagnostic terminology that allows clear communication between the laboratory and the healthcare provider. The healthcare provider receives the laboratory information divided into three categories: specimen adequacy, general categorization of cytologic findings, and interpretation/result (ACS, 2005).

Treatment

Using the 2001 Bethesda system, the following management guidelines were developed by the National Cancer Institute (NCI) to provide direction to healthcare providers and their patients to deal with abnormal Pap smear results:

- ASC-US: Repeat the Pap smear in 4 to 6 months or refer for colposcopy.
- ASC-H: Refer for colposcopy without HPV testing.
- Atypical glandular cells (AGC) and adenocarcinoma in situ (AIS): Immediate colposcopy; follow-up is based on the results of findings.

Colposcopy is a microscopic examination of the lower genital tract using a magnifying instrument called a colposcope. Specific patterns of cells that correlate well with certain histologic findings can be visualized. With the woman in lithotomy position, the cervix is cleansed with acetic acid solution. Acetic acid makes abnormal cells appear white, which is referred to as acetowhite. These white areas are then biopsied and sent to the pathologist for tissue assessment. The examination is not painful, it has no side effects, and it can be performed safely in the healthcare provider's office.

Treatment options available for abnormal Pap smears depend on the severity of the results and the health history of the woman. Therapeutic choices all involve destruction of as many affected cells as possible. Box 8-2 describes treatment options.

Table 8-1 Pap Smear Guidelines

First Pap	Age 21 or within 3 years of first sexual intercourse
Until age 30	Yearly—using glass slide method Every 2 years—using liquid-based method
Age 30–70	Every 2–3 years if last 3 Paps were normal
After age 70	May discontinue if: - Past 3 Paps were normal and - No Paps in the past 10 years were abnormal

American Cancer Society (ACS). (2005). *How Pap test results are reported.* American Cancer Society, Inc. (Online) Available at: http://www.cancer.org/docroot/PED/content/PED_2_3X_Pap_Test.asp.

BOX 8-1

THE 2001 BETHESDA SYSTEM FOR CLASSIFYING PAP SMEARS

Specimen Type: Conventional Pap smear vs. liquid-based
Specimen Adequacy: Satisfactory or unsatisfactory for evaluation
General Categorization: (optional)
- Negative for intraepithelial lesion or malignancy
- Epithelial cell abnormality. See interpretation/result

Automated Review: If case was examined by automated device or not
Ancillary Testing: Provides a brief description of the test methods and report results so healthcare provider understands
Interpretation/Result:
- Negative for intraepithelial lesion or malignancy
- Organisms: *Trichomonas vaginalis;* fungus; bacterial vaginosis; herpes simplex
- Other non-neoplastic findings: Reactive cellular changes associated with inflammation, radiation, IUDs, atrophy
- Other: Endometrial cells in a woman >40 years of age
- Epithelial cell abnormalities:
- *Squamous cell*
  - Atypical squamous cells
    - Of undetermined significance (ASC-US)
    - Cannot exclude HSIL (ASC-H)
  - Low-grade squamous intraepithelial lesion (LSIL)
    - Encompassing HPV/mild dysplasia/CIN-1
  - High-grade squamous intraepithelial lesion (HSIL)
    - Encompassing moderate and severe dysplasia CIS/CIN-2 and CIN-3
    - With features suspicious for invasion
  - Squamous cell carcinoma
- *Glandular Cell:* Atypical
  - Endocervical, endometrial, or glandular cells
  - Endocervical cells—favor neoplastic
  - Glandular cells—favor neoplastic
  - Endocervical adenocarcinoma in situ
  - Adenocarcinoma
    - Endocervical, endometrial, extrauterine
- Other malignant neoplasms (specify)

Educational Notes and Suggestions: (optional)

Sources: NIH, 2002; Apgar & Wright, 2003; ACS, 2005

Nursing Management

The nurse's role involves primary prevention through education of women regarding risk factors and preventive techniques to avoid cervical dysplasia. Secondary prevention focuses on reducing or limiting the area of cervical

TREATMENT OPTIONS FOR CERVICAL CANCER

- *Cryotherapy*—destroys abnormal cervical tissue by freezing with liquid nitrogen, Freon, or nitrous oxide. Studies show a 90% cure rate (Youngkin & Davis, 2004). Healing takes up to 6 weeks, and the client may experience a profuse, watery vaginal discharge for 3 to 4 weeks.
- *Cone Biopsy* or *conization*—removes a cone-shaped section of cervical tissue. The base of the cone is formed by the ectocervix (outer part of the cervix) and the point or apex of the cone is from the endocervical canal. The transformation zone is contained within the cone sample. The cone biopsy is also a treatment and can be used to completely remove any precancers and very early cancers. There are two methods commonly used for cone biopsies:
  - LEEP (loop electrosurgical excision procedure) or LLETZ (large loop excision of the transformation zone)—the abnormal cervical tissue is removed with a wire that is heated by an electrical current. For this procedure, a local anesthetic is used. It is performed in the healthcare provider's office in approximately 10 minutes. Mild cramping and bleeding may persist for several weeks after the procedure.
  - Cold knife cone biopsy—a surgical scalpel or a laser is used instead of a heated wire to remove tissue. This procedure requires general anesthesia and is done in a hospital setting. After the procedure, cramping and bleeding may persist for a few weeks.
- *Laser therapy*—destroys diseased cervical tissue by using a focused beam of high-energy light to vaporize it (burn it off). After the procedure, the woman may experience a watery brown discharge for a few weeks. Very effective in destroying precancers and preventing them from developing into cancers.
- *Hysterectomy*—removes the uterus and cervix surgically
- *Radiation therapy*—delivered by internal radium applications to the cervix or external radiation therapy that includes lymphatics of the pelvis
- *Chemoradiation*—weekly cisplatin therapy concurrent with radiation. Investigation of this therapy is ongoing (ACS, 2005).

---

dysplasia. Tertiary prevention focuses on minimizing disability or spread of cervical cancer. Specific areas of education include:

- Encourage prevention of STIs to reduce risk factors (see Chapter 5: Sexually Transmitted Infections).
- Counsel teenagers to avoid early sexual activity.
- Encourage pelvic rest for a month after any cervical treatment.
- Screen for cervical cancer by annual Pap smears.
- Identify high-risk behavior and how to reduce it.

- Make sure the Pap smear is sent to an accredited laboratory for interpretation.
- Encourage the faithful use of barrier methods of contraception.
- Encourage cessation of smoking and drinking.
- Reinforce guidelines for Pap smears and sample preparation.
- Remind all women about follow-up procedures and times.
- Explain in detail all procedures that might be needed.
- Outline proper preparation before having a Pap smear.
- Provide emotional support throughout the decision-making process.
- Inform all women of community resources available to them.

Nursing Care Plan 8-1: Overview of a Woman With Cervical Cancer highlights specific nursing interventions.

Endometrial Cancer

Endometrial cancer (also known as uterine cancer) is malignant neoplastic growth of the uterine lining. It is the most common gynecologic malignancy and accounts for 6% of all cancers in women in the United States. The NCI estimates that there will be over 40,000 new cases in 2005, of which approximately 7,000 women will die (NCI, 2005). It is uncommon before the age of 40, but as women age their risk of endometrial cancer increases. Approximately 95% of these malignancies are carcinomas of the endometrium. The most common symptom in up to 90% of women is postmenopausal bleeding. Most women recognize the need for prompt evaluation, so the majority of women are diagnosed in an early stage of the disease (Winter & Gosewehr, 2004).

Pathophysiology

Endometrial cancer may originate in a polyp or in a diffuse multifocal pattern. The pattern of spread partially depends on the degree of cellular differentiation. Well-differentiated tumors tend to limit their spread to the surface of the endometrium. Metastatic spread occurs in a characteristic pattern and most commonly involves the lungs, inguinal and supraclavicular nodes, liver, bones, brain, and vagina (NCI, 2005). Early tumor growth is characterized by friable and spontaneous bleeding. Later tumor growth is characterized by myometrial invasion and growth toward the cervix (Fig. 8-2). Adenocarcinoma of the endometrium is typically preceded by hyperplasia. Carcinoma in situ is found only on the endometrial surface. In stage I, it has spread to the muscle wall of the uterus. In stage II, it has spread to the cervix. In stage III, it has spread to the bowel or vagina, with metastases to pelvic lymph nodes. In stage IV, it has invaded the bladder mucosa, with distant metastases to the lungs, liver, and bone (Brose, 2004).

Nursing Care Plan 8-1

Overview of a Woman With Cervical Cancer

Molly, a 28-year-old, thin Native American woman, comes to the free health clinic complaining of a thin, watery vaginal discharge and spotting after sex. She reports being homeless and living "on the streets" for years. Molly admits to having multiple sex partners to pay for her food and cigarettes. She had an abnormal Pap smear a while back but didn't return to the clinic for any follow-up. She hopes nothing "bad" is wrong with her because she just found a job to get off the streets. Cervical cancer is suspected.

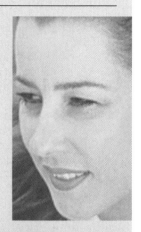

Nursing Diagnosis: Anxiety related to diagnosis and uncertainty of outcome

Outcome Identification and *evaluation*	Interventions with *rationales*
Client will demonstrate measures to cope with anxiety *as evidenced by statements acknowledging anxiety, use of positive coping strategies, and verbalization that anxiety level has decreased.*	Encourage client to express her feelings and concerns *to reduce her anxiety and to determine appropriate interventions.*
	Assess the meaning of the diagnosis to the client, clarify misconceptions, and provide reliable, realistic information *to enhance her understanding of her condition, subsequently reducing her anxiety level.*
	Assess client's psychological status *to determine degree of emotional distress related to diagnosis and treatment options.*
	Identify and address verbalized concerns, providing information about what to expect *to decrease level of uncertainty about the unknown.*
	Assess the client's use of coping mechanisms in the past and their effectiveness *to foster use of positive strategies.*
	Teach client about early signs of anxiety and help her recognize them (for example, fast heartbeat, sweating, or feeling flushed) *to minimize escalation of anxiety.*
	Provide positive reinforcement that the client's condition can be managed *to relieve her anxiety.*

Nursing Diagnosis: Deficient knowledge related to diagnosis, prevention strategies, and treatment

Client will demonstrate understanding of diagnosis, *as evidenced by making health-promoting lifestyle choices, verbalizing appropriate health-care practices, and adhering to measures to comply with therapy.*	Assess client's current knowledge about her diagnosis and proposed therapeutic regimen *to establish a baseline from which to develop a teaching plan.*

Overview of a Woman With Cervical Cancer (continued)

Outcome Identification and *evaluation*	Interventions with *rationales*
	Review contributing factors associated with development of cervical cancer, including possible associated lifestyle behaviors, *to foster an understanding of the the etiology of cervical cancer.*
	Review information provided about possible treatments and procedures and recommendations for healthy lifestyle, obtaining feedback frequently *to validate adequate understanding of instructions.*
	Discuss strategies, including using condoms and limiting the number of sexual partners, *to reduce the risk of transmission of STIs, specifically human papillomavirus (HPV), which is associated with causing cervical cancer.*
	Encourage client to obtain prompt treatment of any vaginal or cervical infections *to minimize the risk for cervical cancer.*
	Urge the client to have an annual Pap smear *to provide for screening and early detection.*
	Provide written material with pictures *to allow for client review and help her visualize what is occurring in her body.*
	Inform client about available community resources and make appropriate referrals as needed *to provide additional education and support.*
	Document details of teaching and learning *to allow for continuity of care and further education, if needed.*

Etiology and Risk Factors

Unopposed endogenous and exogenous estrogens are the major etiologic risk factors associated with the development of this cancer. Other risk factors for endometrial cancer include:

- Nulliparity
- Obesity (>50 pounds overweight)
- Liver disease
- Infertility
- Diabetes mellitus
- Hypertension
- History of pelvic radiation
- Polycystic ovarian syndrome
- Infertility
- Early menarche (<12 years old)
- High-fat diet
- Use of prolonged exogenous unopposed estrogen with an intact uterus
- Endometrial hyperplasia
- Family history of endometrial cancer
- Personal history of hereditary nonpolyposis colon cancer
- Personal history of breast or ovarian cancer
- Late onset of menopause
- Tamoxifen use
- Anovulation (Smith et al., 2004)

Clinical Manifestations and Diagnosis

The major initial symptom of endometrial cancer is abnormal and painless vaginal bleeding. Any episode of bright-red bleeding that occurs after menopause should be investigated. Abnormal uterine bleeding is rarely the result of uterine malignancy in a young woman. In the postmenopausal woman, however, it should be regarded with suspicion. Additional clinical manifestations of advanced disease may include dyspareunia, low back pain, purulent genital discharge, dysuria, pelvic pain, weight loss, and a change in bladder and bowel habits.

Screening for endometrial cancer is not routinely done because it is not practical or cost-effective. The ACS recommends that women should be informed about the risks and symptoms of endometrial cancer at the onset of menopause and strongly encouraged to report any un-

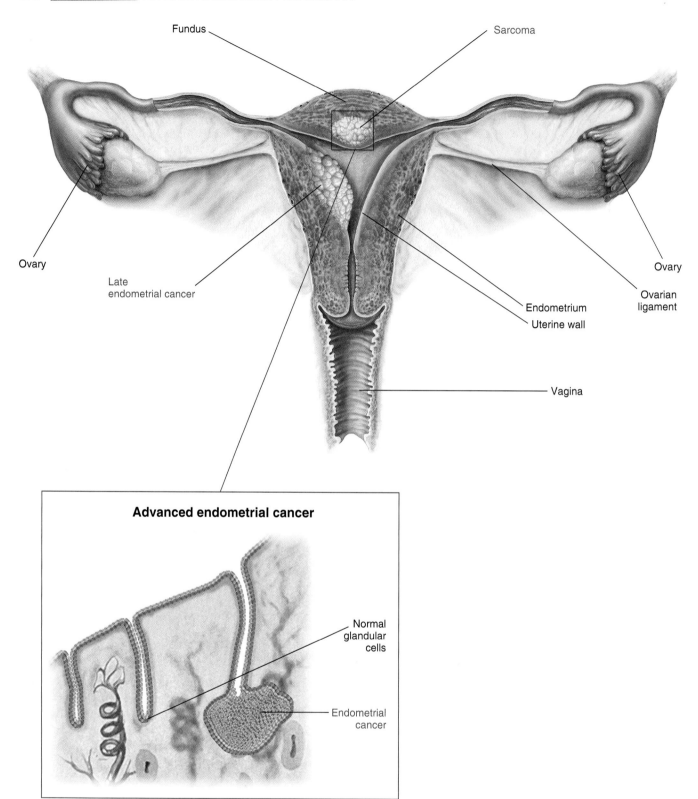

● Figure 8-2 Progression of endometrial cancer. (The Anatomical Chart Company. [2002].
Atlas of pathophysiology. Springhouse, PA: Springhouse.)

expected bleeding or spotting to their healthcare provider (ACS, 2005). A pelvic examination is frequently normal in the early stages of the disease. Changes in the size, shape, or consistency of the uterus or its surrounding supporting structures may exist when the disease is more advanced.

An endometrial biopsy is the procedure of choice to make the diagnosis. It can be done in the healthcare provider's office without anesthesia. A slender suction catheter is used to obtain a small sample of tissue for pathology. It can detect up to 90% of cases of endometrial cancer in the woman with postmenopausal bleeding, depending on the technique and experience of the healthcare provider (Burke, 2005). The woman may experience mild cramping and bleeding after the procedure for about 24 hours, but typically mild pain medication will reduce this discomfort.

Transvaginal ultrasound can be used to evaluate the endometrial cavity and measure the thickness of the endometrial lining. It can be used to detect endometrial hyperplasia. If the endometrium measures less than 4 mm, then the client is at low risk for malignancy (Burke, 2005).

Because endometrial cancer is usually diagnosed in the early stages, it has a better prognosis than cervical or ovarian caner (Brose, 2004).

Treatment

Treatment of endometrial cancer depends on the stage of the disease and usually involves surgery with adjunct therapy based on pathologic findings. Surgery most often involves removal of the uterus (hysterectomy) and the fallopian tubes and ovaries (salpingo-oophorectomy). Removal of the tubes and ovaries is recommended because tumor cells spread early to the ovaries, and any dormant cancer cells could be stimulated to grow by ovarian estrogen. In more advanced cancers, radiation and chemotherapy are used as adjunct therapies to surgery. Routine surveillance intervals for follow-up care are typically every 3 to 4 months for the first 2 years, since 85% of recurrences occur in the first 2 years after diagnosis (Winter & Gosewehr, 2004).

Nursing Management

The nurse should make sure the woman understands all the options available for treatment; listen to any sexual concerns the woman expresses; ensure that follow-up care appointments are scheduled appropriately; refer the patient to a support group; and offer the family explanations and emotional support throughout. The nurse's role is also to educate the patient about preventive measures or follow-up care if she has been treated for cancer (Teaching Guidelines 8-2).

Ovarian Cancer

Ovarian cancer is malignant neoplastic growth of the ovary (Fig. 8-3). It is the seventh most common cancer among women and the fourth most common cause of can-

 TEACHING GUIDELINES 8-2

Preventive and Follow-Up Measures for Endometrial Cancer

- Schedule regular pelvic examinations after the age of 21.
- Visit healthcare practitioner for early evaluation of any abnormal bleeding after menopause.
- Maintain a low-fat diet throughout life.
- Exercise daily.
- Manage weight to discourage hyperestrogenic states, which predispose to endometrial hyperplasia.
- Pregnancy serves as a protective factor by reducing estrogen.
- Ask your doctor about the use of combination estrogen and progestin pills.
- When combination oral contraceptives are taken to facilitate the regular shedding of the uterine lining, take risk-reduction measures.
- Be aware of risk factors for endometrial cancer and make modifications as needed.
- Report any of the following symptoms immediately:
  - Bleeding or spotting after sexual intercourse
  - Bleeding that lasts longer than a week
  - Reappearance of bleeding after 6 months or more of no menses
- After cancer therapy, schedule follow-up appointments for the next few years.
- After cancer therapy, frequently communicate with your healthcare provider concerning your status.
- After surgery, maintain a healthy weight.

cer deaths for women in the United States, accounting for more deaths than any other cancer of the reproductive system (ACS, 2005). The ACS estimates that about 23,000 new cases of ovarian cancer will be diagnosed in the United States during 2005 and 16,000 deaths will occur. A woman's risk of getting ovarian cancer during her lifetime is 1.7%, or about 1 in 58. About 77% of women with ovarian cancer survive 1 year after diagnosis (ACS, 2005). Older women are at highest risk. Ovarian cancer occurs most frequently in women between 55 and 75 years of age, and approximately 25% of ovarian cancer deaths occur in women between 35 and 54 years old (Brose, 2004).

Etiology and Risk Factors

The cause of ovarian cancer is not known. Ovarian cancer can originate from different cell types, although most originate in the ovarian epithelium. They usually present as solid masses that have spread beyond the ovary and seeded into the peritoneum prior to diagnosis. An inherited genetic mutation is the causative factor in 5% to 10% of cases of epithelial ovarian cancer. Two genes, BRCA-1 and BRCA-2, are linked with hereditary breast and ovar-

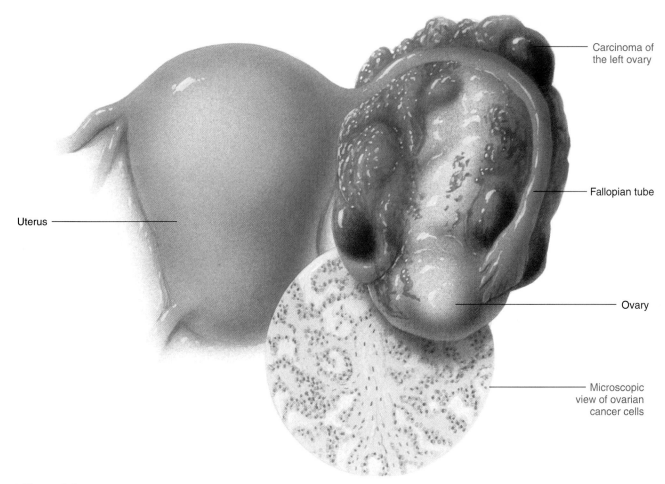

● Figure 8-3 Ovarian cancer. (The Anatomical Chart Company. [2002]. *Atlas of pathophysiology.* Springhouse, PA: Springhouse.)

ian cancers. Blood tests can be performed to assess DNA in white blood cells to detect mutations in the BRCA genes. These genetic markers do not predict whether the person will develop cancer; rather, they provide information regarding the risk of developing cancer. If a woman is BRCA positive, then her lifetime risk of developing ovarian cancer increases to between 16% and 60% versus the general population's risk of 1.7% (O'Rourke & Mahon, 2003). Nurses must know the risk factors associated with ovarian cancer so they can tailor patient care and teaching.

Risk factors for ovarian cancer include:

• Nulliparity
• Early menarche (<12 years old)
• Late menopause (>55 years old)
• Increasing age (>50 years of age)
• High-fat diet
• Obesity
• Persistent ovulation over time
• First-degree relative with ovarian cancer
• Use of perineal talcum powder or hygiene sprays
• Older than 30 years at first pregnancy
• Positive BRCA-1 and BRCA-2 mutations
• Personal history of breast or colon cancer

• Hormone replacement therapy for more than 10 years
• Infertility (Claus et al., 2005)

Clinical Manifestations and Diagnosis

Consider THIS!

I felt I was a lucky woman because I had been in remission from breast cancer for 12 years, and I had been given the gift of life to share with my beloved family. Recently I became ill with stomach problems: pain, indigestion, bloating, and nausea. My doctor treated me for GERD (acid reflux disease), but the symptoms persisted. I then was referred to a gastroenterologist, an urologist, and then a gynecologist, who did an ultrasound, which was negative. I received reassurance from all three that there was nothing wrong with me. As time went by, I experienced more pain, more symptoms, and increased frustration. Six months after seeing all three specialists, a repeat ultrasound revealed I had ovarian cancer, and I needed surgery as soon as possible. I underwent a complete hysterectomy and my surgeon found I was in stage 3. Since then, I have undergone chemotherapy and participated in a clinical cancer study that wasn't successful for me, and now I am facing the fact that I am going to die soon.

Thoughts: This woman has tried everything to save her life, but, alas, time has run out for her with advanced ovarian cancer. Women diagnosed with breast cancer are at a significant risk for developing ovarian cancer later in life. Of the string of doctors she saw, one has to ponder why none ordered a CA-125 blood test with her history of breast cancer. We are haunted with the question: If they had and it was elevated, would she be in stage 3 now? I guess we will never know.

Ovarian cancers are considered the worst of all the gynecologic malignancies, primarily because they sometimes develop slowly and remain silent and without symptoms until the cancer is far advanced. It has been described as "the overlooked disease" or "the silent killer" because women and health care practitioners often ignore or rationalize early symptoms. For example, women may attribute gastrointestinal problems to personal stress and midlife changes. However, vague complaints may precede more obvious symptoms by months. The most common symptoms include unusual bloating, back pain, abdominal fullness, fatigue, urinary frequency, constipation, and abdominal pressure. The less common symptoms include anorexia, dyspepsia, ascites, palpable abdominal mass, weight loss or gain, pelvic pain, and vaginal bleeding (Goff et al., 2004).

Seventy-five percent of ovarian cancers are not diagnosed until the cancer has advanced to stage III or IV, primarily because there is still no adequate screening test. There is no practical and certain way of detecting early cancer of the ovary. Currently available tests are not reliable, sensitive, or affordable enough to be useful in mass screening of all women. Pap smears are generally ineffective, and the cancer is usually found by chance in advanced stages.

Clinical guidelines for the diagnostic screening of ovarian cancer have not been developed, which markedly hinders the diagnosis of ovarian cancer until it is in later stages. The U.S. Preventive Services Task Force (USPSTF) recommends against routine screening for ovarian cancer with serum CA-125 or transvaginal ultrasound because earlier detection would have a small effect, at best, on mortality. The USPSTF concluded that the potential harm from the invasive nature of the diagnostic tests would outweigh the potential benefits (USPSTF, 2004). CA-125 is a biologic tumor marker associated with ovarian cancer. Although levels are elevated in many women with ovarian cancer, it is not specific for this cancer and may be elevated with other malignancies (pancreatic, liver, colon, breast, and lung cancers). Currently, it is not sensitive enough to serve as a screening tool (Speroff & Fritz, 2005).

Women need to have yearly bimanual pelvic examinations and a transvaginal ultrasound to identify ovarian masses in their early stages. After menopause, a mass on an ovary is not a cyst. Physiologic cysts can arise only from a follicle that has not ruptured or from the cystic degeneration of the corpus luteum. There is no such thing as a physiologic cyst in a postmenopausal woman, therefore, because there are no follicles or luteal cysts in the postmenopausal ovary. A small ovarian "cyst" found on ultrasound in an asymptomatic postmenopausal woman should arouse suspicion. Any mass or ovary palpated in a postmenopausal woman should be considered cancerous until proven otherwise (DeGaetano, 2004).

Treatment

Treatment options for ovarian cancer vary depending on the stage and severity of the disease. Usually a laparoscopy (abdominal exploration with an endoscope) is performed for diagnosis and staging, as well as evaluation for further therapy. In stage I the ovarian cancer is limited to the ovaries. In stage II the growth involves one or both ovaries, with pelvic extension. Stage III cancer spreads to the lymph nodes and other organs or structures inside the abdominal cavity. In stage IV, the cancer has metastasized to distant sites (Alexander et al., 2004). Figure 8-4 shows the likely metastatic sites for ovarian cancer.

Surgical intervention remains the mainstay of treatment in the management of ovarian cancer. Surgery generally includes a total abdominal hysterectomy, bilateral salpingo-oophorectomy, peritoneal biopsies, omentectomy, and pelvic para-aortic lymph node sampling to evaluation cancer extension (Garcia, 2004). Because most women are diagnosed with advanced-stage ovarian cancer, aggressive management involving debulking or cytoreductive surgery is the primary treatment. This surgery involves resecting all visible tumors from the peritoneum, taking peritoneal biopsies, sampling lymph nodes, and removing all reproductive organs and the omentum. This aggressive surgery has been shown to improve long-term survival rates.

The most important variable influencing the prognosis is the extent of the disease. Survival depends on the stage of the tumor, grade of differentiation, gross findings on surgery, amount of residual tumor after surgery, and effectiveness of any adjunct treatment postoperatively. Many women with ovarian cancer will experience recurrence despite the best efforts of eradicating the cancer through surgery, radiation, or chemotherapy to eliminate residual tumor cells. The likelihood of long-term survival in the event of recurrence is dismal (Garcia, 2004). The 5-year survival rates (the percentage of women who live at least 5 years after their diagnosis) are shown in Table 8-2 according to stage.

Nursing Management

Although ovarian cancer is a scary disease, a nurse with a positive attitude can be reassuring to the client. The complexities of ovarian cancer make a multidisciplinary ap-

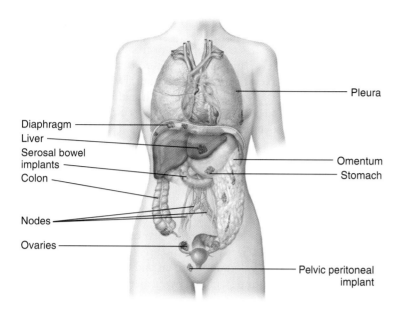

Pleura

Diaphragm

Liver

Serosal bowel implants

Colon

Nodes

Ovaries

Omentum

Stomach

Pelvic peritoneal implant

● Figure 8-4 Common metastatic sites for ovarian cancer. (The Anatomical Chart Company. [2002]. *Atlas of pathophysiology.* Springhouse, PA: Springhouse.)

proach necessary for optimal management. With the insidious nature and high risk of recurrence and mortality of this condition, most women find it an emotionally exhausting and devastating experience. The nurse should focus on activities related to early detection of the disease, information about ovarian cancer, and emotional support for women and their families. The nurse can also carry out the following interventions during all interactions with clients:

- Educate women about the risk factors and common early symptoms.
- Avoid dismissing innocuous symptoms as "just a part of aging."
- Encourage women to describe their nonspecific complaints.
- Advise women about screening options. Emphasize the lack of good screening methods for ovarian cancer.
- Direct women with high personal risk to the appropriate screening strategies.
- Assess the woman's family and personal history for risk factors.

Table 8-2 Five-Year Survival Rates for Ovarian Cancer

Stage	Five-Year Relative Survival Rates
I	80% to 90%
II	65% to 70%
III	30% to 60%
IV	20%

American Cancer Society (ACS). (2005). *What are the key statistics about ovarian cancer?* American Cancer Society, Inc. (Online) Available at: http://www.cancer.org/docroot/ CRI/content/CRI_2_4_1X_What_are_the_key_statistics_for_ ovarian_cancer_33.asp?sitearea=&level=.

- Encourage genetic testing for women with affected family members.
- Outline screening guidelines for women with hereditary cancer syndrome.
- Advise women about risk reduction.
- Explain that pregnancy and use of oral contraceptives reduce the risk of ovarian cancer.
- Stress the importance of maintaining a healthy weight to reduce risk.
- Encourage women to eat a low-fat diet.
- Raise community awareness about risk-reducing behaviors.
- Encourage breastfeeding as a risk-reducing strategy
- Instruct women to avoid the use of talc and hygiene sprays to genitals.
- Try to restore hope to women with ovarian cancer, and stress treatment compliance.
- Teach coping strategies to allow for the best quality of life.
- Outline information about treatment options and the implications of choices.
- Provide one-to-one support for women facing treatment for ovarian cancer.
- Describe in simple terms the tests, treatment modalities, and follow-up needed.
- Discuss the hereditary factors BRCA-1 and BRCA-2 and lifetime risks.
- Listen to and support women contemplating prophylactic oophorectomy.
- Encourage participation in clinical trials to offer hope for all women.
- Encourage open discussion of sexuality and the impact of cancer.
- Offer support for family members coping with grief and sadness.
- Refer the woman and family members to appropriate community resources and support groups.

Vaginal Cancer

Vaginal cancer is malignant tissue growth arising in the vagina. It is rare, representing less than 3% of all genital cancers. The ACS estimates that in 2005, over 2,000 new cases of vaginal cancer will be diagnosed in the United States, and approximately 800 will die of this cancer (ACS, 2005). Vaginal cancer can be effectively treated, and when found early it is often curable. There are several types of vaginal cancer. About 85% are squamous cell carcinomas that begin in the epithelial lining of the vagina. They develop slowly over a period of years, commonly in the upper third of the vagina. They tend to spread early by directly invading the bladder and rectal walls. They also metastasize through blood and lymphatics. About 15% are adenocarcinomas, which differ from squamous cell carcinoma by an increase in pulmonary metastases and supraclavicular and pelvic node involvement (ACS, 2005).

Etiology and Risk Factors

The etiology of vaginal cancer has not been identified. It usually occurs in women over age 50 and is usually of the squamous cell variety. The peak incidence of vaginal cancer occurs at 60 to 65 years of age. Malignant diseases of the vagina are either primary vaginal cancers or metastatic forms from adjacent or distant organs. About 80% of vaginal cancers are metastatic, primarily from the cervix and endometrium. These cancers invade the vagina directly. Cancers from distant sites that metastasize to the vagina through the blood or lymphatic system are typically from the colon, kidneys, skin (melanoma), or breast (Bardawil & Manetta, 2004). Tumors in the vagina commonly occur on the posterior wall and spread to the cervix or vulva.

Direct risk factors for the initial development of vaginal cancer have not been identified. Associated risk factors include advancing age (>60 years old), previous pelvic radiation, exposure to diethylstilbestrol (DES) in utero, vaginal trauma, history of genital warts (HPV infection), HIV infection, cervical cancer, chronic vaginal discharge, smoking, and low socioeconomic level (Lewis et al., 2004).

Clinical Manifestations and Diagnosis

Most women with vaginal cancer are asymptomatic. Those who do present with symptoms have painless vaginal bleeding (often after sexual intercourse), abnormal vaginal discharge, dyspareunia, dysuria, constipation, and pelvic pain (Bardawil & Manetta, 2004). Colposcopy with biopsy of suspicious lesions confirms the diagnosis.

Treatment and Nursing Management

Treatment of vaginal cancer depends on the type of cells involved and the stage of the disease. If the cancer is localized, radiation, laser surgery, or both may be used. If the cancer has spread, radical surgery might be needed, such as a hysterectomy, or removal of the upper vagina with dissection of the pelvic nodes in addition to radiation therapy.

Women undergoing radical surgery need intensive counseling about the nature of the surgery, risks, potential complications, changes in physical appearance and physiologic function, and sexuality alterations. Nursing management for this cancer is similar to that for other reproductive cancers with emphasis on sexuality counseling and referral to local support groups.

The prognosis of vaginal cancer depends largely on the stage of disease and the type of tumor. The overall 5-year survival rate for squamous cell carcinoma is about 42%; that for adenocarcinoma is about 78% (Brose, 2004).

Vulvar Cancer

Vulvar cancer is an abnormal neoplastic growth on the external female genitalia (Fig. 8-5). It is responsible for 1% of all malignancies in women and 4% of all female genital cancers. It is the fourth most common gynecologic cancer, after endometrial, ovarian, and cervical cancers (Youngkin & Davis, 2004). The ACS estimates that in 2005, about 4,000 cancers of the vulva will be diagnosed in the United States and about 870 women will die of this cancer (ACS, 2005). When detected early, it is highly curable. The overall 5-year survival rate when lymph nodes are not involved is 90%, but it drops to 50% to 70% when the lymph nodes have been invaded (ACS, 2005).

Etiology and Risk Factors

Vulvar cancer is found most commonly in older women in their mid-60s to 70s, but the incidence in women younger than 35 years old has increased over the past few decades. The disease has been linked to the presence of genital warts caused by HPV (types 16, 18, 31, 33, 35, and 51), but the exact relationship is unknown (Lowdermilk & Perry, 2004).

Approximately 90% of vulvar tumors are squamous cell carcinomas. This type of cancer forms slowly over several years and is usually preceded by precancerous changes. These precancerous changes are termed vulvar intraepithelial neoplasia (VIN). The two major types of VIN are classic (undifferentiated) and simplex (differentiated). Classic VIN, the more common one, is associated with HPV infection and smoking. It typically occurs in women between 30 and 40 years old. In contrast to classic VIN, simplex VIN usually occurs in postmenopausal women and is not associated with HPV (Edwards et al., 2005).

The following risk factors have been linked to the development of vulvar cancer:

- Exposure to HPV type 16
- Age above 50
- HIV infection
- VIN

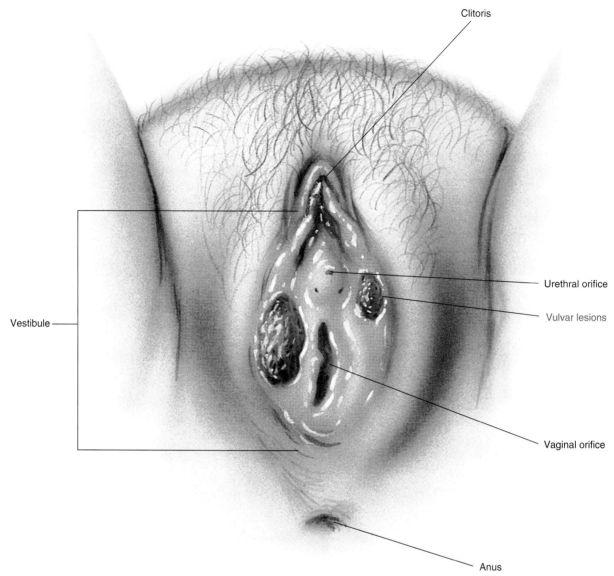

● Figure 8-5 Vulvar cancer. (The Anatomical Chart Company. [2002]. *Atlas of pathophysiology.* Springhouse, PA: Springhouse.)

- Lichen sclerosus
- Melanoma or atypical moles
- Exposure to HSV II
- Multiple sex partners
- Smoking
- History of breast cancer
- Immune suppression
- Hypertension
- Diabetes mellitus
- Obesity (ACS, 2005)

Clinical Manifestations and Diagnosis

The diagnosis of vulvar cancer is often delayed significantly because there is no single specific clinical symptom that heralds it. The most common presentation is persistent vulvar itching that does not improve with the use of creams or ointments. Less common presenting symptoms include vulvar bleeding, discharge, dysuria, and pain. The most common presenting sign of vulvar cancer is a vulvar lump or mass. The vulvar lesion is usually raised and may be fleshy, ulcerated, leukoplakic, or warty (Naumann & Higgins, 2004). The diagnosis of vulvar cancer is made by a biopsy of the suspicious lesion, usually found on the labia majora.

Treatment

Treatment varies depending on the extent of the disease. Laser surgery, cryosurgery, or electrosurgical incision may be used. Larger lesions may need more extensive surgery and skin grafting. The traditional treatment for vulvar cancer has been radical vulvectomy, but more conservative techniques are being used to improve psychosexual outcomes.

Nursing Management

Women with vulvar cancer must clearly understand their disease, treatment options, and prognosis. To accomplish this, nurses must provide information and establish effective communication with the patient and her family. The nurse's role is one of an educator and advocate. Important teaching points are as follows:

- Encourage smoking cessation.
- Teach clients self-examination of genitals.
- Advise clients to avoid tight undergarments.
- Advise clients to avoid using perfumes and dyes in the vulvar region.
- Instruct clients to seek care for any suspicious lesions.
- Educate women to use barrier methods of birth control (e.g., condoms) to reduce the risk of contracting HIV, HSV, and HPV.
- Discuss changes in sexuality if radical surgery is performed.
- Encourage open communication between the client and her partner.
- Refer to appropriate community resources and support groups.
- Instruct clients to complete vulvar examinations monthly between menstrual periods, looking for any changes in appearance (e.g., whitened or reddened patches of skin); changes in feel (e.g., areas of the vulva becoming itchy or painful); or the development of lumps, moles (e.g., changes in size, shape, or color), freckles, cuts, or sores on the vulva. These changes should be reported to the healthcare provider (ACS, 2005).

Nursing Management for Women With Cancer of the Reproductive Tract

Neoplastic conditions often cause extreme emotional distress to women and their families. Nurses, therefore, can play a vital role in the healing process for many patients. Nurses can have a positive impact by providing answers to clients to help guide them through the "medical maze" of diagnostic tests and decision-making.

Assessment

Nurses may assess for cancers of the reproductive tract by considering risk factors, prompting discussion of symptoms, and recording thorough medical and gynecologic histories. Physical assessment centers on the collection of data to rule out or confirm cancer of the reproductive tract. A nurse might recommend further diagnostic procedures or follow-up appointments.

Nursing Diagnosis

Applicable nursing diagnosis might include:

Disturbed body image related to:
- Loss of body part
- Loss of good health
- Altered sexuality patterns

Anxiety related to:
- Threat of malignancy
- Potential diagnosis
- Anticipated pain/discomfort
- Effect of condition or treatment on future

Deficient knowledge related to:
- Disease process and prognosis
- Specific treatment options
- Diagnostic procedures needed

Nursing Interventions

Nurses can arm patients with the facts, which helps to prevent disease and enhance quality of life. Nurses should educate women about the importance of consistent and timely screenings to identify a neoplasm early to improve their overall outcome. Nurses can be instrumental in assisting women to identify lifestyle behaviors that need to be altered to reduce their risk of developing various reproductive tract cancers. Nursing interventions are not limited to preventive education; they also include informing women about the consequences of "doing nothing" about their conditions and what the long-range possibilities might be without treatment. Other nursing interventions for cancers of the reproductive tract may include:

- Promote cancer awareness, prevention, and control.
- Work to improve the availability of cancer-screening services.
- Provide public education about risk factors for pelvic cancers.
- Stress the importance of annual pelvic examinations by a healthcare professional.
- Stress the importance of visiting a healthcare professional if certain symptoms appear:
  ○ Blood in a bowel movement
  ○ Unusual vaginal discharge or chronic vulvar itching
  ○ Persistent abdominal bloating or constipation
  ○ Irregular vaginal bleeding
  ○ Persistent low backache not related to standing
  ○ Elevated or discolored vulvar lesions
  ○ Bleeding after menopause
  ○ Pain or bleeding after sexual intercourse
- Validate the patient's feelings and provide realistic hope.
- Use basic communication skills in a sincere way during all interactions.

- Provide useful, nonjudgmental advice to all women.
- Individualize care to address the client's cultural traditions.
- Carry out postoperative care and instructions as prescribed.
- Discuss postoperative issues, including incision care, pain, and activity level.
- Instruct client on health maintenance activities after treatment.
- Inform the client and family about available support resources.

Nurses have traditionally served as advocates in the health care arena. They must continue to be on the forefront of health education and diagnosis and leaders in the fight against malignancies. Over a half million women in the United States will be diagnosed with cancer this year alone, and more than half will die of it. It is important to get the word out that not only are these deaths preventable, but also many of the cancers themselves are preventable. Nurses need to work to improve the availability and quality of cancer-screening services, as well as make them accessible to underserved and socioeconomically disadvantaged patients. Through consistency, continuity, and collaboration, nurses can offer quality care to all women who experience a malignancy.

A reduction in malignant pelvic disorders can be achieved through a unified effort between health care professionals, health policy experts, government agencies, health insurance companies, the media, educational institutions, and women themselves. Nurses can have a tremendous impact on the lives of many women and their families by stepping forward and meeting the challenges ahead.

KEY CONCEPTS

- Women have a one in three lifetime risk of developing cancer, and one out of every four deaths is from cancer; thus, nurses must focus on screening and educating all women regardless of risk factors.
- Cervical cancer incidence and mortality rates have decreased noticeably in the past several decades, with most of the reduction attributed to the Pap test, which detects cervical cancer and precancerous lesions.
- The nurse's role involves primary prevention of cervical cancer through education of women regarding risk factors and preventive techniques to avoid cervical dysplasia.
- Unopposed endogenous and exogenous estrogens are the major etiologic risk factors associated with the development of endometrial cancer.
- The American Cancer Society (ACS) recommends that women should be informed about risks and symptoms of endometrial cancer at the onset of menopause and strongly encouraged to report any unexpected bleeding or spotting to their health care providers.
- Ovarian cancer is the seventh most common cancer among women and the fourth most common cause of cancer deaths for women in the United States, accounting for more deaths than any other cancer of the reproductive system.
- Ovarian cancer has been described as "the overlooked disease" or "silent killer," because women and/or health care practitioners often ignore or rationalize early symptoms. It is typically diagnosed in advanced stages.
- Vaginal cancer tumors can be effectively treated and, when found early, are often curable.
- Malignant diseases of the vagina are either primary vaginal cancers or metastatic forms from adjacent or distant organs.
- Diagnosis of vulvar cancer is often delayed significantly because there is no single specific clinical symptom that heralds it. The most common presentation is persistent vulvar itching that does not improve with the application of creams or ointments.
- Nurses should educate women about the importance of consistent and timely screenings to identify a neoplasm early to improve their overall outcome.
- Nurses can be very instrumental in assisting women to identify lifestyle behaviors that need to be altered to reduce their risk of developing various reproductive tract cancers.

References

Adams, K. L. (2002). Confronting cervical cancer: screening is the key to stopping this killer. *AWHONN Lifelines, 6*(3), 216–222.

Alexander, L. L., LaRosa, J. H., Bader, H., & Garfield, S. (2004). *New dimensions in women's health* (3rd ed.). Sudbury, MA: Jones and Bartlett Publishers

American Cancer Society (ACS) (2005). *What are the key statistics about cervical cancer?* American Cancer Society, Inc. [Online] Available at: http://www.cancer.org/docroot/CRI/content/CRI_2_4_1X_What_are_the_key_statistics_for_cervical_cancer_8.asp?sitearea=

American Cancer Society (ACS) (2005). *How Pap test results are reported.* American Cancer Society, Inc. [Online] Available at: http://www.cancer.org/docroot/PED/content/PED_2_3X_Pap_Test.asp

American Cancer Society (ACS) (2005). *What are the key statistics about ovarian cancer?* American Cancer Society, Inc. [Online] Available at: http://www.cancer.org/docroot/CRI/content/CRI_2_4_1X_What_are_the_key_statistics_for_ovarian_cancer_33.asp?sitearea=&level=

American Cancer Society (ACS) (2005). *What are the key statistics about vaginal cancer?* American Cancer Society, Inc. [Online] Available at: http://www.cancer.org/docroot/CRI/content/CRI_2_4_1X_What_are_the_key_statistics_for_vaginal_cancer_55.asp?sitearea=

American Cancer Society (ACS) (2005). *What are the key statistics about vulvar cancer?* American Cancer Society, Inc. [Online] Available at: http://www.cancer.org/docroot/cri/content/cri_2_4_1x_what_are_the_key_statistics_for_vulvar_cancer_45.asp?sitearea=&level=

American Cancer Society (ACS) (2005). *Cancer prevention & early detection cancer facts and figures 2005.* Atlanta: ACS.

Anderson, P. S., & Runowicz, C. D. (2002). Beyond the Pap test: new techniques for cervical cancer screening. *Women's Health, 2,* 37–43.

Apgar, B. S., & Wright, T. C. (2003). The 2001 Bethesda System terminology. *American Family Physician, 68*(10), 1992–1998.

Bardawil, T., & Manetta, A. (2004). Surgical treatment for vaginal cancer. *eMedicine.* [Online] Available at: htto://www.emedicine.com/med/topic3330.htm

Breslin, E. T., & Lucas, V. A. (2003). *Women's health nursing: toward evidence-based practice.* St. Louis, MO: Saunders.

Brose, M. S. (2004). Endometrial cancer. *Medline Plus.* [Online] Available at: http://www.nlm.nih.gov/medlineplus/print/ency/article/000910.htm

Brose, M. S. (2004). Ovarian cancer. *Medline Plus.* [Online] Available at: http://www.nlm.nih.gov/medlineplus/print/ency/article/000889.htm

Brose, M. S. (2004). Vaginal tumors. *Medline Plus.* [Online] Available at: http://www.nlm.nih.gov/medlineplus/ency/article/001510.htm

Burke, C. (2005). Endometrial cancer and tamoxifen. *Clinical Journal of Oncology Nursing, 9*(2), 247–249.

Claus, E. B., Petruzella, S., Matloff, E., & Carter, D. (2005). Prevalence of BRCA1 and BRCA2 mutations in women diagnosed with ductal carcinoma in situ. *JAMA, 293*(8), 964–969.

DeGaetano, C. (2004). Ovarian cancer: It whispers . . . so listen. [Online]. Available at: http://nsweb.nursingspectrum.com/ce/ce237.htm

Edwards, Q. T., Saunders-Goldson, S., Morgan, P. D., et al. (2005). Vulvar intraepithelial neoplasia. *Advance for Nurse Practitioners, 13*(3), 49–51.

Garcia, A. A., & Bi, J. (2004). Cervical cancer. *eMedicine.* [Online] Available at: http://www.emedicine.com/med/topic324.htm

Garcia, A. A. (2004). Ovarian cancer. *eMedicine* [Online] Available at: http://www.emedicine.com/med/topic1698.htm

Goff, B., Mandel, L. S., Melancon, C. H., & Muntz, H. G. (2004). Frequency of symptoms of ovarian cancer in women presenting to primary care clinics. *JAMA, 291*(22), 2705–2712.

Grund, S. (2005). Cervical cancer. *Medline Plus.* [Online] Available at: http://www.nlm.nih.gov/medlineplus/ency/article/000893.htm

Jemal, A., Murray, T., Ward, E., et al. (2005). Cancer statistics, 2005. *CA: A Cancer Journal for Clinicians, 55*(1), 10–31.

Lewis, S. M., Heitkemper, M. M., & Dirksen, S. R. (2004). *Medical-surgical nursing: assessment and management of clinical problems* (6th ed.). St. Louis: Mosby.

Lowdermilk, D. L., & Perry, S. E. (2004). *Maternity & women's health care* (8th ed.). St. Louis: Mosby.

National Cancer Institute (NCI) (2004). *Annual report on the status of cancer.* U.S. National Institutes of Health. [Online] Available at: http://www.nci.nih.gov/newscenter/pressreleases/ReportNation2004Release

National Cancer Institute (NCI) (2005). *Endometrial cancer: treatment.* U.S. National Institutes of Health. [Online] Available at: http://www.nci.hih.gov/cancertopics/pdq/treatment/endometrial/HealthProfessional/page1/ . . .

National Institutes of Health (NIH) (2005). *Cervical cancer: prevention.* National Cancer Institute. [Online] Available at: http://www.nci.nih.gov/cancertopics/pdq/prevention/cervical/HealthProfessional/page2

National Institutes of Health News Release. (2002). *Bethesda 2001: a revised system for reporting Pap test results aims to improve cervical cancer screening.* [Online] Available at: http://www.nih.gov/news/pr/apr2002/nci-23.htm

Naumann, R. W., & Higgins, R. V. (2004). Surgical treatment of vulvar cancer. *eMedicine.* [Online] Available at: http://www.emedicine.com/med/topic3328.htm

O'Rourke, J., & Mahon, S. M. (2003). A comprehensive look at the early detection of ovarian cancer. *Clinical Journal of Oncology Nursing, 7*(1), 1–7.

Richart, R. M. (2002). A sea change in diagnosing and managing HPV and cervical disease—part 1. *Contemporary OB/GYN, 5,* 42–56.

Ross, S. H. (2003). *Cervical cancer prevention.* [Online]. Available at: http://nsweb.nursingspectrum.com/ce/ce170.htm

Roye, C. F., Nelson, J., & Stanis, P. (2003). Evidence of the need for cervical cancer screening in adolescents. *Pediatric Nursing, 29*(3), 224–232.

Smith, R. A., Cokkinides, V., & Eyre, H. J. (2004). American Cancer Society guidelines for early detection of cancer, 2004. *CA: A Cancer Journal for Clinicians, 54,* 41–52.

Solomon, D., Davey, D., Kurman, R., et al. (2002). The 2001 Bethesda System: terminology for reporting results of cervical cytology. *JAMA, 287*(16), 2114–2119.

Speroff, L., & Fritz, M. A. (2005). *Clinical gynecologic endocrinology and infertility* (7th ed.). Philadelphia: Lippincott Williams & Wilkins.

U.S. Department of Health and Human Services (USDHHS), Public Health Service. (2000). *Healthy People 2010* (conference edition, in two volumes). U.S. Department of Health and Human Services. Washington, D.C.: U.S. Government Printing Office.

U.S. Preventive Services Task Force (USPSTF). (2004). *Screening for ovarian cancer.* U.S. Preventive Services Task Force Summary of Recommendations. [Online] Available at: http://www.ahrq.gov/clinic/uspstf/uspsovar.htm

Waggoner, S. E. (2003). Cervical cancer. *Lancet, 361*(9376), 2217–2226.

Winter, W. E., & Gosewehr, J. A. (2004). Uterine cancer. *eMedicine.* [Online] Available at: http://www.emedicine.com/med/topic2832.htm

Youngkin, E. Q., & Davis, M. S. (2004). *Women's health: a primary care clinical guide* (3rd ed.). New Jersey: Prentice Hall.

Web Resources

American Cancer Society: 1-800-ACS-2345, **www.cancer.org**

American Urological Association: (410) 727-1100, **www.auanet.org**

Cancer Care, Inc.: (212) 712-8080, **www.cancercare.org**

Gilda Radner Familial Ovarian Cancer Registry: (800) OVARIAN, **www.ovariancancer.com**

Gynecologic Cancer Foundation: (800) 444-4441, **www.wcn.org**

Hysterectomy Educational Resource and Services (HERS): (215) 667-7757, **www.ccon.com/hers**

National Ovarian Cancer Coalition: (888) 682-7426. **www.ovarian.org**

National Women's Health Information Center: (800) 994-9662, **www.4women.gov**

Oncology Nursing Society (ONS): (866) 257-4ONS, **www.ons.org**

Ovarian Cancer Research Fund, Inc.: (800) 873-9569, **www.ocrf.org**

Sexuality Information and Education Counsel of the United States: (212) 819-9770, **www.siecus.org**

SHARE: Self-Help for Women with Breast or Ovarian Cancer: (866) 891-3431, **www.sharecancersupport.org**

Vulvar Health: **www.vulvarhealth.org**

Women's Cancer Network: (312) 644-6610, **www.wcn.org**

Chapter WORKSHEET

● MULTIPLE CHOICE QUESTIONS

1. Ovarian cancer is often not diagnosed early because:

    a. The disease progresses very slowly

    b. The early stages produce very vague symptoms

    c. The disease usually is diagnosed only at autopsy

    d. Clients don't follow up on acute pelvic pain

2. A postmenopausal woman reports that she has started spotting again. The nurse should advise the client to:

    a. Keep a menstrual calendar for the next few months

    b. Not to worry, since this a common but not serious event

    c. Start warm-water douches to promote healing

    d. Visit her doctor for an endometrial biopsy

3. One of the key psychosocial needs of women diagnosed with cancer is:

    a. Providing clear information

    b. Hand-holding

    c. Being cheerful

    d. Offering hope

4. The most effective screening tool for the early detection of cervical cancer is:

    a. Fecal occult blood test

    b. CA-125 blood test

    c. Pap smear

    d. Sigmoidoscopy

5. The deadliest cancer of the female reproductive system is:

    a. Vulvar

    b. Ovarian

    c. Endometrial

    d. Cervical

● CRITICAL THINKING EXERCISES

1. Tammy Scott, a 27-year-old sexually active Caucasian woman, visits the Health Department family planning clinic and requests information about the various methods available. In taking her history, the nurse learns that she started having sex at age 15 and has had multiple sex partners since then. She smokes two packs of cigarettes daily. Because she has been unemployed for a few months, her health insurance policy has lapsed. She has never previously obtained any gynecologic care.

    a. Based on her history, which risk factors for cervical cancer are present?

    b. What recommendations would you make for her and why?

    c. What are this patient's educational needs concerning health maintenance?

2. Jennifer Nappo, a 60-year-old nulliparous woman, presents to the gynecologic oncology clinic after her health care provider palpated an adnexal mass on her right ovary. In taking her history, the nurse learns that Mrs. Nappo has experienced mild abdominal bloating and weight loss for the past several months but felt fine otherwise. She was diagnosed with breast cancer 15 years ago and was treated with a lumpectomy and radiation. She has occasionally used talcum powder in her perineal area over the past 20 years. A transvaginal ultrasound revealed a complex mass in the right adnexa. She underwent a total abdominal hysterectomy and bilateral salpingo-oophorectomy and lymph node biopsy. Pathology confirmed a diagnosis of stage III ovarian cancer with abdominal metastasis and positive lymph nodes.

    a. Is Mrs. Nappo typical for a woman with this diagnosis?

    b. What in her history might increase her risk for ovarian cancer?

    c. What can the nurse do to increase awareness of this cancer for all women?

● STUDY ACTIVITIES

1. During your surgical clinical rotation, interview a female patient undergoing surgery for cancer of her reproductive organs. Ask her to recall the symptoms that brought her to the healthcare provider. Ask her what thoughts, feelings, and emotions went through her mind before and after her diagnosis. Finally, ask her how this experience will change her life in the future.

2. Visit an oncology and radiology treatment center to find out about the various treatment modalities available for cancer. Contrast the various treatment methods and report your findings to your class.

3. Visit one of the websites listed at the end of the chapter to explore a topic of interest concerning reproductive cancers. Critique the web site for correctness, currency, and level of content. Share your assessment with your classmates.

4. Taking oral contraceptives provides protection against _____ cancer.

5. Two genes, BRCA-1 and BRCA-2, are linked with hereditary _____ and _____ cancers.

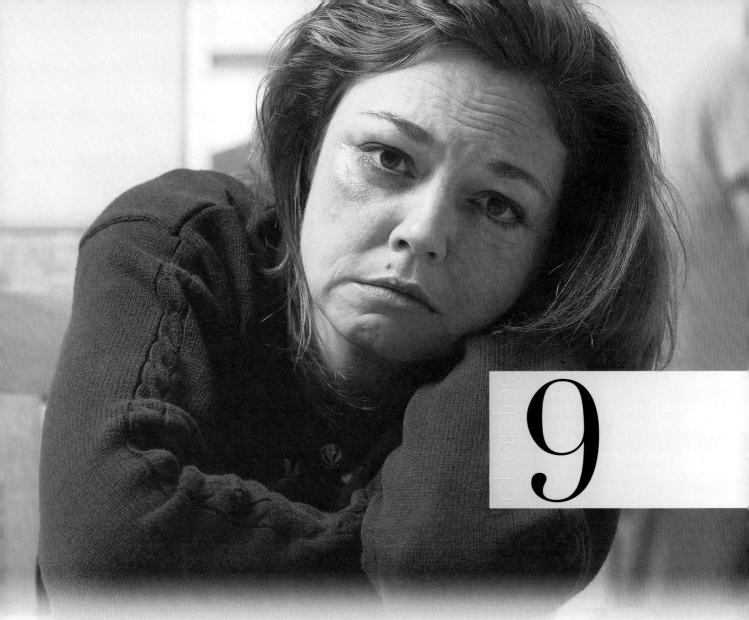

chapter 9

Violence and Abuse

KeyTERMS

acquaintance rape
battered women
  syndrome
cycle of violence
date rape
female genital mutation
human trafficking
incest
intimate partner violence
posttraumatic stress
  disorder
rape
sexual abuse
statutory rape

LearningOBJECTIVES

After studying the chapter content, the student should be able to accomplish the following:

1. Define the key terms.
2. Discuss the incidence of violence in women.
3. Outline the cycle of violence and appropriate interventions.
4. Describe the myths and facts about violence.
5. Identify the dynamics of rape and sexual abuse.
6. List the resources available to women experiencing abuse.
7. Delineate the role of the nurse who cares for abused women.

WOW

If women want to heal, they have to start being honest with themselves and others. They have to admit they were raped or abused to allow other women to come forth.

Violence against women is a significant health and social problem affecting virtually all societies, but often it goes unrecognized and unreported. For all the strides American women have made in the past 100 years, obliterating violence against themselves isn't one of them. Violence against women is a growing problem. In many countries it is still accepted as part of normal behavior. According to the National Violence Against Women Survey, 1 out of 4 U.S. women has been physically assaulted or sexually assaulted by an intimate partner (Tjaden & Thoennes, 2000). Forty percent to 60% of murders of women in North America are committed by intimate partners (Crandall et al., 2004). Federal funding for the problem is trickling down to local programs, but it isn't reaching victims fast enough. In the United States, there are three times more shelters for animals than for battered women (Hessmiller & Ledray, 2004). In many cases, a victim escapes her abuser only to be turned away from a local shelter because it is full. The number of abused women is staggering: one woman is being battered every 12 seconds in the United States (Penny, 2004).

This chapter will address two types of violence against women: intimate partner violence and sexual abuse. Nurses will come in contact with both types in whatever healthcare setting in which they work. Acts of violence against women have devastating and costly consequences for all of society, making the issue ripe for the involvement of nurses. Nurses must be ready to ask the right questions and to act on the answers, because such action could be life-saving.

Intimate Partner Violence

Intimate partner violence is actual or threatened physical or sexual violence or psychological/emotional abuse. It includes threats of physical or sexual violence when the threat is used to control a person's actions (CDC, 2004). Some of the common terms used to describe intimate partner violence are domestic abuse, spouse abuse, domestic violence, battering, and rape. Intimate partner violence affects a distressingly high percentage of the population and has physical, psychological, social, and economic consequences (Fig. 9-1).

A nurse may be the first healthcare professional to discover the signs of intimate partner violence and can have a profound impact on a woman's decision to seek help. It is important for nurses to be able to identify abuse and aid the victim. Domestic violence can leave significant psychological scars, and a well-trained nurse may be able to have a positive impact on the victim's mental and emotional health.

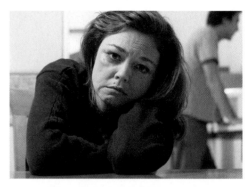

● Figure 9-1 Intimate partner violence has significant physical, psychological, social, and economic consequences. An important role of the health care provider is to identify abusive or potentially abusive situations as soon as possible and provide support for the victim.

Incidence

Although estimates vary, as many as 6 million women are abused annually—one every 12 seconds (CDC, 2004). Even more shocking, 75% of the abused women initially identified in a medical setting go on to suffer repeated abuse, including homicide (CDC, 2004). This may include physical violence, emotional abuse, sexual assault, rape, incest, or elder abuse.

Women are at risk for violence at nearly every stage of their lives. Old, young, beautiful, unattractive, married, single—no woman is completely safe from the risk of intimate partner violence. Current or former husbands or lovers kill over half of the murdered women in the United States. Intimate partner violence against women causes more serious injuries and deaths than automobile accidents, rapes, and muggings combined. The medical cost of intimate partner violence approaches $3 to $5 billion each year (Aggeles, 2004).

Abuse occurs in both heterosexual and homosexual relationships. Violence within gay and lesbian relationships may go unreported for fear of harassment or ridicule. In addition, since gay and lesbian partnerships are not seen as legal in many states, there are few statistics gathered on incident rates.

Background

Until the mid-1970s, our society tended to legitimize a man's power and control over a woman. The U.S. legal and judicial systems considered intervention into family disputes wrong and against the family's right to privacy. Intimate partner violence was often tolerated and even socially acceptable. Fortunately, attitudes and laws have changed to protect women and punish abusers. In *Healthy*

HEALTHY PEOPLE *2010*

Violence Against People

Objectives	Significance
1. Reduce the rate of physical assault by current or former intimate partners.	Will increase women's quality and years of healthy life
	Eliminate health disparities for survivors of violence
2. Reduce the annual rate of rape or attempted rape.	Goal is to have 90% compliance in screening for intimate partner violence by health professionals.
	Meeting these objectives will reflect the importance of early detection, intervention, and evaluation.

Available online: www.healthypeople.gov/ (2000)

People 2010, two key objectives speak to violence against women (Healthy People 2010: Violence Against People).

Characteristics of Abuse

Generation-to-Generation Continuum of Violence

Violence is a learned behavior that, without intervention, is self-perpetuating. It is a cyclical health problem. The long-term effects of violence on victims and children can be profound. Children who witness one parent abuse another are more likely to become delinquents or batterers themselves. They see abuse as an integral part of a close relationship. Thus, an abusive relationship between father and mother can perpetuate future abusive relationships (Thompson, 2005).

Childhood maltreatment is a major health problem that is associated with a wide range of physical conditions and leads to high rates of psychiatric morbidity and social problems in adulthood. Women who were physically or sexually abused as children have an increased risk of victimization and experience adverse mental health conditions such as depression, anxiety, and low self-esteem in adulthood (Nelson et al., 2004).

In 50% to 75% of the cases when a parent is abused, the children are abused as well (Holtrop et al., 2004). Exposure to violence has a negative impact on children's physical, emotional, and cognitive well-being. The cycle insinuates itself into another generation through learned responses and violent acting out. While there are always exceptions, most children deprived of their basic physical, psychological, and spiritual needs do not develop healthy personalities. They grow up with feelings of fear, inadequacy, anxiety, anger, hostility, guilt, and rage. They often lack coping skills, blame others, demonstrate poor

impulse control, and generally struggle with authority. Unless this cycle is broken, more than half become abusers themselves (Holtrop et al., 2004).

The Cycle of Violence

In an abusive relationship, the **cycle of violence** includes three distinct phases: the tension-building phase, the acute battering phase, and the reconciliation or honeymoon phase (Watts, 2004). The cyclic behavior begins with a time of tension-building arguments, progresses to violence, and settles into a making-up or calm period. With time, this cycle of violence increases in frequency and severity as it is repeated over and over again. The cycle can cover a long or short period of time.

Phase 1: Tension-Building

During the first—and usually the longest—phase of the overall cycle, tension escalates between the couple. Excessive drinking, jealousy, or other factors might lead to name-calling, hostility, and friction. The woman might sense that her partner is reacting to her more negatively, that he is on edge and reacts heatedly to any trivial frustration. A woman often will accept her partner's building anger as legitimately directed toward her. She internalizes what she perceives as her responsibility to keep the situation from exploding. In her mind, if she does her job well, he remains calm. If she fails, the resulting violence is her fault.

Phase 2: Acute Battering

The second phase of the cycle is the explosion of violence. The batterer loses control both physically and emotionally. This is when the victim may be assaulted or killed. After a battering episode, most victims consider themselves lucky that the abuse was not worse, no matter how severe their injuries. They often deny the seriousness of their injuries and refuse to seek medical treatment.

Phase 3: Reconciliation

The third phase of the cycle is a period of calm, loving, contrite behavior on the part of the batterer. The batterer may be genuinely sorry for the pain he caused his partner. He attempts to make up for his brutal behavior and believes he can control himself and never hurt the woman he loves. The victim wants to believe that her partner really can change. She feels responsible, at least in part, for causing the incident, and she feels responsible for her partner's well being (Box 9-1).

Types of Abuse

Abusers may use whatever it takes to control a situation—from emotional abuse and humiliation to physical assault. Victims often tolerate mental, physical, and sexual abuse. Many remain in abusive relationships because they believe they deserve the abuse.

Mental Abuse

Mental abuse includes:

- Promising, swearing, or threatening to hit the victim
- Forcing the victim to perform degrading or humiliating acts
- Threatening to harm children or close friends
- Attacking or destroying pets or valued possessions
- Making demeaning remarks about the victim
- Controlling the victim's every move

Physical Abuse

Physical abuse includes:

- Hitting or grabbing the victim so hard that it leaves marks
- Throwing things at the victim
- Pushing, choking, or shoving the victim
- Kicking or punching the victim, or slamming her against things
- Attacking the victim with a knife, gun, rope, or electrical cord

Sexual Abuse

Sexual abuse includes:

- Forcing the woman to have vaginal, oral, or anal intercourse against her will
- Biting the victim's breasts or genitals
- Shoving objects into the victim's vagina
- Forcing the victim to perform sexual acts on other people or animals

Myths and Facts About Intimate Partner Violence

Many myths surround intimate partner violence and shape attitudes and policies regarding it. As healthcare providers it is important to dispel these myths, which lead to misunderstanding and disbelief. Table 9-1 outlines common myths and facts about violence.

Table 9-1 Common Myths and Facts About Violence

Myths	Facts
Battering of women occurs only in lower socioeconomic classes.	Violence occurs in all socioeconomic classes.
Substance abuse causes the violence.	Violence is a learned behavior and can be changed. The presence of drug and alcohol can make a bad problem worse.
Violence occurs to only a small percentage of women.	One in four women will be victims of violence.
Women can easily choose to leave the abusive relationship.	Women stay in the relationship because they feel they have no options.
Only men with mental health problems commit violence against women.	Abusers often seem normal and don't appear to suffer from personality disorders or other forms of mental illness.
Pregnant women are protected from abuse by their partners.	One in five women is physically abused during pregnancy. Effect on infant outcomes: preterm delivery, fetal distress, low birthweight, and child abuse.
Women provoke their partners to abuse them.	Women may be willing to blame themselves for someone else's bad behavior, but nobody deserves to be beaten.
Violent tendencies have gone on for generations and are accepted.	The police, justice system, and society are beginning to make domestic violence socially unacceptable.

Modified from McKinney et al., 2005; Watts, 2004; Thompson, 2005; Tjaden & Thoennes, 2000.

Abuse Profiles

Victims

Ironically, victims rarely describe themselves as abused. **Battered woman syndrome** describes a woman who has experienced deliberate and repeated physical or sexual assault at the hands of an intimate partner. The woman responds with terror, entrapment, and helplessness. She feels alone and reacts to any expression of anger or threat by avoidance and withdrawal behavior.

Some women attribute the cause of their abuse to a personality flaw or inadequacy (e.g., inability to keep the man happy within the relationship). These feelings of failure are reinforced and exploited by their partners. After being told repeatedly that they are "bad," some women begin to believe it. Many victims were abused as children and may have poor self-esteem, depression, insomnia, or a history of suicide attempts, injury, or drug and alcohol abuse (Aggeles, 2004).

Abusers

Abusers come from all walks of life and often have feelings of insecurity, powerlessness, and helplessness that are not in line with the male image they would like to project. The abuser's violence typically occurs within the confines of the home and is usually directed toward his intimate partner or the children who reside there. The abuser expresses his feelings of inadequacy through violence or aggression toward others (Tilley & Brackley, 2004).

Abusers refuse to share power with a partner or family member and choose violence to control their victims. They often exhibit childlike aggression or antisocial behaviors. They may fail to accept responsibility or blame others for their own problems. They might also have substance abuse problems, mental illness, prior arrests, troubled relationships, obsessive jealousy, controlling behaviors, erratic employment history, and financial problems.

Violence During Pregnancy

Women are at a higher risk for violence during pregnancy. Pregnancy is often the start or escalation of violence. The strongest predictor of abuse during pregnancy is prior abuse (Watts, 2004). For many women, the beating and violence during pregnancy is "business as usual" for them. Pregnant women are vulnerable during this time and abusers can take advantage of it.

Various factors may lead to battering during pregnancy, including:

- Inability of the couple to cope with the stressors of pregnancy
- Resentment toward the interference of the growing fetus and change in the woman's shape
- Doubt about his partner's fidelity during pregnancy
- Perception of the baby as a competitor once born

- Outside attention the pregnancy brings to the woman
- The woman's new interest in herself and her unborn baby
- Insecurity and jealousy of the pregnancy and the responsibilities it brings
- Financial burden related to expense of pregnancy and loss of income
- Stress of role transition from adult man to becoming the father of a child
- Physical and emotional changes of pregnancy that make the woman vulnerable
- Previous isolation from family and friends that limit the couple's support system

Physical abuse during pregnancy puts the unborn child at risk as well. Women assaulted during pregnancy are more likely to suffer chronic anxiety, miscarriage, stillbirth (death of the baby before it is born), poor nutrition, insomnia, smoking and substance abuse, late entry into prenatal care, preterm labor, chorioamnionitis, vaginitis, sexually transmitted infections, and urinary tract infections and give birth to premature, low-birthweight infants (Schoening et al., 2004). Frequently the fear of harm to her unborn child will motivate a woman to escape an abusive relationship.

The main health effect specific to abuse during pregnancy is the threat to the health of the mother, fetus, or both from trauma. Physical violence to the pregnant woman brings injuries to the head, face, neck, thorax, breasts, and abdomen (Dunn & Oths, 2004). The mental health consequences of violence are significant. Several studies now confirm the relationship between abuse and poor mental health, especially depression (Salmon et al., 2004). For the pregnant woman, this most often manifests itself as postpartum depression.

Sexual Violence

Sexual violence is both a public health problem and a human rights violation. More than once every 3 minutes, 78 times an hour, 1,871 times a day, girls and women in America are raped (Medicine Net, 2005). Rape has been reported against females from age 6 months to 93 years, but it still remains one of the most underreported violent crimes in the United States. Estimates suggest that, somewhere in the United States, a woman is sexually assaulted every 2.5 minutes (RAINN, 2005). The National Center for Prevention and Control of Sexual Assault estimates that one out of three women will be sexually assaulted sometime in her life, and two thirds of these assaults will not be reported (CDC, 2005). Over the course of their lives, women may experience more than one type of violence.

Many rape survivors seek treatment in the hospital emergency rooms, where they often wait for hours in public waiting rooms. To make matters worse, many emergency room doctors and nurses have little training in how to treat rape survivors or in collecting evidence from rape survivors. Because of the long delays in stressful emergency waiting rooms, some sexual assault survivors leave the hospital altogether, never to receive treatment or supply the evidence needed to arrest and convict their assailants.

Sexual violence can have a variety of devastating short- and long-term effects. Women can experience psychological, physical, and cognitive symptoms that affect them daily. They can include chronic pelvic pain, headaches, backache, sexually transmitted infections, pregnancy, anxiety, denial, fear, withdrawal, sleep disturbances, guilt, nervousness, phobias, substance abuse, depression, sexual dysfunction, and posttraumatic stress disorder (CDC, 2005). Sexual violence has been called a "tragedy of youth" because more than half of all rapes (54%) of women occur before age 18 (Medicine Net, 2005).

Characteristics and Types of Sexual Violence

Assailants, like their victims, come from all walks of life and all ethnic backgrounds; there is no "typical profile." More than half are under 25, and the majority are married and leading "normal" sex lives. Why do men rape? No theory provides a satisfactory explanation. So few assailants are caught and convicted that a clear profile is not possible. What is known is that many assailants have trouble dealing with the stresses of daily life. Such men become angry and experience feelings of powerlessness. They commit a sexual assault as an expression of power and control (Maurer & Smith, 2005).

Sexual violence is a broad term that can be used to describe sexual abuse, incest, rape, female genital mutilation, and human trafficking.

Sexual Abuse

Sexual abuse occurs when a woman is forced to have sexual contact of any kind (vaginal, oral, or anal) without her consent. Childhood sexual abuse is any type of sexual exploitation that involves a child younger than 18 years old, which might include disrobing, nudity, masturbation, fondling, digital penetration, and intercourse (Lowdermilk & Perry, 2004).

Childhood sexual abuse has a lifelong impact on its survivors. Women who were sexually abused during childhood are at a heightened risk for repeat abuse. This is because the early abuse lowers their self-esteem and their ability to protect themselves and set firm boundaries. Childhood sexual abuse is a trauma that influences the way victims live their lives: form relationships, deal with adversity, cope with daily problems, relate to their children and peers, protect their health, and live joyfully. Studies have shown that the more victimization a woman experiences, the more likely it is she will be re-victimized (Hobbins, 2004).

Incest

Incest is any type of sexual exploitation between blood relatives or surrogate relatives before the victim reaches 18 years of age. Survivors of incest involving an adult are often tricked, coerced, or manipulated. All adults appear to be powerful to children. Perpetrators might threaten victims so that they are afraid to disclose the abuse or might tell them the abuse is their fault. Often these threats serve to silence victims.

Consider THIS!

At 53 years old, I stood and looked at myself in the mirror. The image staring back at me was one of a frightened, middle-aged, cowardly woman hiding her past. I had been sexually abused by my father for many years as a child and never told anyone. My mother knew of the abuse but felt helpless to make it stop. I married right out of high school to escape and felt I lived a 'happy normal life' with my husband and three children. My children have left home and live away, and my husband recently died of a sudden heart attack. I am now experiencing dreams and thoughts about my past abuse and feeling afraid again.

Thoughts: This woman suppressed her abusive past for most of her life and now her painful experience has surfaced. What can be done to reach out to her at this point? Did her healthcare providers miss the "red flags" that are common to women with a history of childhood sexual abuse all those years?

Rape

Rape is an act of violence rather than a sexual act. Rape is a legal rather than a medical term. It denotes penile penetration (vagina, mouth, or rectum) of the female or male without consent. It might or might not include the use of a weapon. **Statutory rape** is sexual activity between an adult and a person under the age of 18 and is considered to have occurred despite the willingness of the underage person (Shah & Imhoff, 2005). Rape is not an act of lust or an overzealous release of passion: rape is a violent, aggressive assault on the victim's body and integrity. Nine out of every 10 rape victims are female (Alexander et al., 2004).

Many people believe that rape usually occurs on a dark night when a stranger assaults a provocatively dressed, promiscuous woman. They believe that rapists are sex-starved people seeking sexual gratification. Such myths and the facts are presented in Table 9-2.

Acquaintance rape involves someone being forced to have sex by a person he or she knows. Rape by a co-worker, professor, teacher, a husband's friend, or boss is considered acquaintance rape. **Date rape,** an assault that occurs within a dating relationship or marriage without consent of one of the participants, is a form of acquaintance rape. Acquaintance and date rapes are commonly found on college campuses. They are physically and emotionally devastating for the victims.

Table 9-2 Common Myths and Facts About Sexual Violence

Myths	Facts
Women who are raped get over it quickly.	It can take several years to recover emotionally and physically from rape.
Most sexual violence victims tell someone about it.	The majority of women never tell anyone about it. In fact, almost two thirds of victims never report it to the police.
Once the rape is over, a survivor can again feel safe in her life.	The victim feels vulnerable, betrayed, and insecure afterwards.
If a woman does not want to be raped, it cannot happen.	A woman can be forced and overpowered by most men.
Women who feel guilty after having sex then say they were raped.	Few women falsely cry "rape." It is very traumatizing to be a victim.
Victims should report the violence to the police and judicial system.	Only 1% of rapists are arrested and convicted.
Women blame themselves for the rape, believing they did something to provoke the rape.	Women should never blame themselves for being the victim of someone else's violence.
Women who wear tight, short clothes are "asking for it."	No victim invites sexual assault, and what she wears is irrelevant.
Women have rape fantasies and want to be raped.	Reality and fantasy are different. Dreams have nothing to do with the brutal violation of rape.
Medication could help women forget about this.	Initially medication can help, but counseling is needed.

Sources: Rogers, 2002; CDC, 2005; MedicineNet, 2005.

Although acquaintance and date rape do not always involve drugs, a rapist might use alcohol or other drugs to sedate his victim. In 1996 the federal government passed a law making it a felony to give an unsuspecting person a "date rape drug" with the intent of raping him or her. Even with penalties of large fines and up to 20 years in prison, the use of date rape drugs is growing (U.S. DHHS, 2004).

Date rape drugs are also known as "club drugs" because of their use at dance clubs, fraternity parties, and all-night raves. The most common is Rohypnol, also known as roofies, forget pills, and the drop drug. It comes in the form of a liquid or pill that quickly dissolves in liquid with no odor, taste, or color. This drug is 10 times as strong as diazepam (Valium) and produces memory loss for up to 8 hours. Gamma hydroxybutyrate (GHB) is called "liquid ecstasy" or "easy lay" because it produces euphoria, an out-of-body high, sleepiness, increased sex drive, and memory loss. It comes in a white powder or liquid and may cause unconsciousness, depression, and coma. The third date rape drug is ketamine, known as Special K, vitamin K, or super acid. It acts on the central nervous system to separate perception and sensation. Combining ketamine with other drugs can be fatal.

Date rape drugs can be very dangerous, and there are a variety of ways to guard against the risk of receiving them (Teaching Guidelines 9-1).

Female Genital Mutilation

Female genital mutilation, also known as female circumcision, is a cultural practice carried out predominantly in countries of southern Africa and in some areas of the Middle East and Asia. The World Health Organization (WHO) defines female genital mutilation as all procedures involving the partial or total removal or other injury to the female genital organs, whether for cultural or other non-therapeutic purposes (Taylor, 2003). More than 140 million girls are estimated to have undergone female genital mutilation and another 2 million are at risk annually, approximately 6,000 daily (Dare et al., 2004). Many immigrants moving to Europe, Canada, New Zealand, Australia, and the United States have gone through this

 TEACHING GUIDELINES 9-1

Protecting Yourself Against Date Rape Drugs

• Avoid parties where alcohol is being served.
• Never leave a drink of any kind unattended.
• Don't accept a drink from someone else.
• Don't drink from a punch bowl or a keg.
• If you think someone drugged you, call 911.

procedure. Nurses need to know about this cultural practice and its impact on women's reproductive health.

Reasons for performing the ritual reflect the ideology and cultural values of each community that practices it. Some consider it a rite of passage into womanhood; others use it as a means of preserving virginity until marriage. In cultures where it is practiced, it is an important part of culturally defined gender identity. In any case, all the reasons are cultural and traditional and are not rooted in any religious texts (RAINBO, 2004). Female genital mutilation causes absolute injury to women and does not benefit them.

Female genital mutilation is usually performed when the girl is between 4 and 10 years old, an age when she cannot give informed consent for a procedure with lifetime health consequences (Little, 2003). In its mildest form, the clitoris is partially or totally removed. In the most extreme form, called infibulation, the clitoris, labia minora, labia majora, and the urethral and vaginal openings are cut away. The vagina is then stitched or held together, leaving a small opening for menstruation and urination. Cutting and restitching may be necessary to permit the woman to have sexual intercourse and bear children. Box 9-2 lists types of female genital mutilation procedures.

Untrained village practitioners, using no form of anesthesia, generally perform the operation. Cutting instruments may include broken glass, knives, tin lids, scissors, unspecialized razors, or other crude instruments. In addition to causing intense pain, the procedure carries with it a number of health risks, including:

- Pelvic infections
- Hemorrhage

BOX 9-2

FOUR MAJOR TYPES OF FEMALE GENITAL MUTILATION PROCEDURES

Type I	Excision of the prepuce with or without excision of part or all of the clitoris
Type II	Excision of the clitoris and part or all of the labia minora
Type III	(Infibulation) Excision of all or part of the external genitalia and stitching/narrowing of the vaginal opening
Type IV	Pricking, piercing, or incision of the clitoris or labia
	Stretching of the clitoris and/or labia
	Cauterizing by burning the clitoris and surrounding tissues
	Scraping or cutting the vaginal orifice
	Introduction of corrosive substance into the vagina
	Placing herbs into the vagina to narrow it (WHO, 2002)

- HIV infection (Wellard, 2003)
- Damage to the urethra, vagina, and anus
- Recurrent vaginitis
- Urinary tract infections
- Incontinence
- Posttraumatic stress disorder
- Panic attacks
- Keloid formation
- Dermoid cysts
- Vulvar abscesses
- Dysmenorrhea
- Dyspareunia
- Increased morbidity and mortality during childbirth (Condon, 2004)

Helping women who have had one of these procedures requires good communication skills and often an interpreter, since many may not speak English. Nurses have the opportunity to educate patients by providing accurate information and positive healthcare experiences. Make sure that you are comfortable with your own feelings about this practice before dealing with patients. Some guidelines are as follows:

- Speak clearly and slowly, using simple, accurate terms.
- Never use the term "female genital mutilation." Rather, use the term "female circumcision."
- Use pictures and diagrams to assist the woman's understanding.
- Be patient in allowing the client to answer questions.
- Let the client know you are concerned and interested and want to help.
- Repeat back your understanding of her statements.
- Always look and talk directly to the client, not the interpreter.
- Place no judgment on the cultural practice.
- Encourage the client to express herself freely.
- Maintain strict confidentiality.
- Provide culturally competent care to all women.

From a Western perspective, female genital mutilation is hard to comprehend. Because it is not talked about openly in communities that practice it, women who have undergone it accept it without question and assume it is done to all girls (Wellard, 2003).

This issue has drawn increasing global attention over the past several years. Nongovernmental organizations such as Amnesty International are conducting research and campaign work on the practice. The U.S. government has taken steps to criminalize the practice in America and now considers asylum applications in light of mutilation practices in the country of origin (Wilkinson, 2003). The WHO, the United Nations Population Fund, and the United Nations Children's Fund have issued a joint plea for the eradication of the practice, saying it would be a major step forward in the promotion of human rights worldwide (Wilkinson, 2003).

Human Trafficking

A girl who was just 14 years old was held captive in a tiny trailer room, where she was forced to have sex with as many as 30 men a day. On her night stand was a teddy bear that reminded her of her childhood in Mexico.

The girl's scenario describes **human trafficking,** the enslavement of immigrants for profit in America. Human trafficking is a modern form of slavery that affects nearly 1 million people worldwide and approximately 20,000 persons in the United States annually (U.S. Department of State, 2003). Women and children are the primary victims of human trafficking, many in the sex trade as described above and others through forced-labor domestic servitude.

The United States is a profitable destination country for traffickers, and these profits contribute to the development of organized criminal enterprises worldwide. According to findings from the Victims of Trafficking and Violence Protection Act of 2000:

- Victims are primarily women and children who lack education, employment, and economic opportunities in their own countries.
- Traffickers promise victims employment as nannies, maids, dancers, factory workers, sales clerks, or models in the United States.
- Traffickers transport the victims from their counties to unfamiliar destinations away from their support systems.
- Once they are here, traffickers coerce them, using rape, torture, starvation, imprisonment, threats, or physical force, into prostitution, pornography, sex trade, forced labor, or involuntary servitude.

These victims are exposed to serious and numerous health risks, such as rape, torture, HIV/AIDS, sexually transmitted infections, violence, hazardous work environments, poor nutrition, and drug and alcohol addiction (U.S. Department of State, 2003). Healthcare is one of the most pressing needs of these victims, and there isn't any comprehensive care available for undocumented immigrants. As a nurse it is important to be alert for trafficking victims in any setting and to recognize cues that would increase your suspicion (Box 9-3).

If you suspect a trafficking situation, obtain the victim's consent to proceed with any intervention before following through by notifying local law enforcement and a regional social service organization that has experience in dealing with trafficking victims. It is imperative to reach out to these victims and stop the cycle of abuse by following through on your suspicions.

Impact of Sexual Violence

Sexual violence can have a variety of devastating short- and long-term effects. Women may experience many psychological, physical, and cognitive symptoms that affect them daily. A traumatic experience not only damages a woman's sense of safety in the world, but it can also reduce her self-

---

BOX 9-3

IDENTIFYING VICTIMS OF HUMAN TRAFFICKING

Cues

Look beneath the surface and ask yourself: Is this person . . . .

- Female or a child in poor health?
- Foreign-born and doesn't speak English?
- Lacking immigration documents?
- Giving an inconsistent explanation of injury?
- Reluctant to give any information about self, injury, home, or work?
- Fearful of authority figure or "sponsor" if present? ("Sponsor" might not leave victim alone with healthcare provider.)
- Living with the employer (Spear, 2004)?

Sample questions to ask the potential victim of human trafficking:

- Can you leave your job or situation if you wish?
- Can you come and go as you please?
- Have you been threatened if you try to leave?
- Has anyone threatened your family with harm if you leave?
- What are your working and living conditions?
- Do you have to ask permission to go to the bathroom, eat, or sleep?
- Is there a lock on your door so you cannot get out?
- What brought you to the United States? Are your plans the same now?
- Are you free to leave your current work or home situation?
- Who has your immigration papers? Why don't you have them?
- Are you paid for the work you do?
- Are there times you feel afraid?
- How can your situation be changed?

Modified from http://www.rainn.org/statistics.html.

---

esteem and her ability to continue her education, to earn money and be productive, to have children and, if she has children, to nurture and protect them (Maurer & Smith, 2005).

A significant proportion of women who are sexually assaulted or raped experience symptoms of **post-traumatic stress disorder** (PTSD). PTSD develops when an event outside the range of normal human experience occurs that produces marked distress in the person. Symptoms of PTSD are grouped into three clusters:

- *Intrusion* (re-experiencing the trauma, including nightmares, flashbacks, recurrent thoughts)
- *Avoidance* (avoiding trauma-related stimuli, social withdrawal, emotional numbing)
- *Hyperarousal* (increased emotional arousal, exaggerated startle response, irritability)

Rape survivors take a long time to heal from their traumatic experience. Rape is viewed as a situational crisis that the survivor is unprepared to handle because it is an unforeseen event. Survivors usually go through four phases of recovery following rape (Table 9-3).

Nursing Management

Violence against women has become a major public health problem in the United States. Nurses play a major role in assisting women who have suffered some type of violence. Often, after a woman is victimized, she will complain about physical ailments that will give her the opportunity to visit a health care setting. A visit to a health care agency is an ideal time for women to be assessed for violence. Because nurses are viewed as trustworthy and sensitive about very personal subjects, women often feel comfortable in confiding or discussing these issues with them.

Nurses encounter thousands of these victims each year in their practice settings, but many victims continue to slip through the cracks. There are many things that nurses can do to help victims of this tragedy. Action is essential: early recognition and interventions can significantly reduce the morbidity and mortality associated with intimate partner violence. If abuse is identified, nurses can undertake interventions that can increase the woman's safety and improve her health. Remember, abuse is a risk factor for many health-related problems, but the causes and extent of such risk are only beginning to be understood. The accompanying Nursing Care Plan highlights a sample plan of care for a victim of rape.

Assessment

Nurses need to recognize the factors that increase the risk of violence toward women and know the cues that could signal abuse. Some basic assessment guidelines follow.

Screen for Abuse During Every Health Care Visit

Although screening for violence takes only a few minutes, it can have an enormously positive effect on the outcome for the abused woman. Any woman could be a victim. No single sign marks patients as abuse victims, but the following clues may be helpful:

- Injuries: bruises, scars from blunt trauma, or weapon wounds on the face, head, and neck
- Injury sequelae: headaches, hearing loss, joint pain, sinus infections, teeth marks, clumps of hair missing, dental trauma, pelvic pain, breast or genital injuries
- The reported history of the injury doesn't seem to add up to the actual presenting problem.
- Mental health problems: depression, anxiety, substance abuse, eating disorders, suicidal ideation or suicide attempts
- Frequent health care visits for chronic, stress-related disorders such as chest pain, headaches, back or pelvic pain, insomnia, and gastrointestinal disturbances
- Partner's behavior at the health care visit: appears overly solicitous or overprotective, unwilling to leave her alone with the healthcare provider, answers questions for her, and attempts to control the situation in the health care setting (Aggeles, 2004).

Isolate Patient Immediately From Family

If abuse is detected, immediately isolate her to provide privacy and prevent potential retaliation from the abuser. Asking about abuse in front of a possible abuser may trigger an abusive episode. Even if there isn't an incident at the time of the interview, the abuser might punish the woman when she returns home. Ways to ensure her safety and achieve isolation would be to take the victim to an area away from the abuser to ask questions. The assessment can take place anywhere (x-ray area, ultrasound room, elevator, ladies' room, laboratory) that is private and physically away from the possible abuser.

If abuse is detected, the nurse can do the following to enhance the nurse–client relationship:

- Educate the patient about the connection between the violence and her symptoms.

Table 9-3 Four Phases of Rape Recovery

Phase	Survivor's Response
Acute phase (disorganization)	Shock, fear, disbelief, anger, shame, guilt, feelings of uncleanliness. Also insomnia, nightmares, and sobbing.
Outward adjustment phase (denial)	Appears outwardly composed and returns to work or school; refuses to discuss the assault and denies need for counseling
Reorganization	Denial and suppression don't work, and the survivor attempts to make life adjustments by moving or changing jobs and uses emotional distancing to cope.
Integration and recovery	Survivor begins to feel safe and starts to trust others. May become an advocate for other rape victims.

Nursing Care Plan 9-1

Overview of the Woman Who Is a Victim of Rape

Lucia, a 20-year-old college junior, was admitted to the emergency room after police found her when a passerby called 911 to report an assault. She stated, "I think I was raped a few hours ago while I was walking home through the park." Assessment reveals the following:

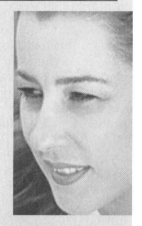

- Numerous cuts and bruises of varying sizes on her face, arms, and legs; lip swollen and cut; right eye swollen and bruised
- Jacket and shirt ripped and bloodied
- Hair matted with grass and debris
- Vital signs within acceptable parameters
- Client tearful, clutching her clothing, and trembling
- Perineal bruising and tearing noted

Nursing Diagnosis: Rape-trauma syndrome related to report of recent sexual assault

Outcome identification and *evaluation*	Interventions with *rationales*
Client will demonstrate adequate coping skills related to effects of rape as evidenced by *her ability to discuss the event, verbalize her feelings and fears, and exhibit appropriate actions to return to her pre-crisis level of functioning.*	Stay with the client *to promote feelings of safety.* Explain the procedures to be completed based on facility's policy *to help alleviate client's fear of the unknown.* Assist with physical examination for specimen collection *to obtain evidence for legal proceedings.* Administer prophylactic medication as ordered *to prevent pregnancy and sexually transmitted infections.* Provide care to wounds as ordered *to prevent infection.* Assist client with hygiene measures as necessary *to help promote self-esteem.* Allow client to describe the events as much as possible *to encourage ventilation of feelings about the incident;* engage in active listening and offer nonjudgmental support *to facilitate coping and demonstrate understanding of the client's situation and feelings.* Help the client identify positive coping skills and personal strengths used in the past *to aid in effective decision making.* Assist client in developing additional coping strategies and teach client relaxation techniques *to help deal with the current crisis and anxiety.* Contact the rape counselor in the facility *to help the client deal with the crisis.* Arrange for follow-up visit with rape counselor *for continued support and to promote continuity of care.* Encourage the client to contact a close friend, partner, or family member *to accompany her home for support.* Provide the client with the telephone number of a counseling service or community support groups *to assist with coping and obtaining ongoing support.* Provide written instructions related to follow-up appointments, care, and testing *to ensure adequate understanding.*

• Assist her in acknowledging what has happened to her and begin to deal with the situation.
• Offer her referrals so she can get the help that will allow her to begin to heal.

Research underscores the profound and complex trauma experienced by rape survivors. They should be provided with a safe and comfortable environment for a forensic examination that includes a change of clothes, access to a shower and toiletries, and a private waiting area for family and friends. The survivor should be brought to an isolated area away from family and friends so she can be open and honest when asked about the assault. Once initial treatment and evidence collection are completed, follow-up care should include counseling, medical treatment, and crisis intervention. There is mounting evidence that early intervention and immediate counseling speed a rape survivor's recovery.

Ask Direct or Indirect Questions About Abuse

Questions to screen for abuse should be routine and handled just like any other question regarding the patient's care. Many nurses feel uncomfortable asking questions of this nature, but broaching the subject is important even if the answer comes later. Just knowing that someone else knows about the abuse offers a victim some relief. Communicating support through a nonjudgmental attitude, or telling her that no one deserves to be abused, is the first step in establishing trust and rapport.

Choose the type of question that makes you most comfortable. Direct and indirect questions produce the same results. "Does your partner hit you?" or "Have you ever been or are you now in an abusive relationship?" are direct questions. If that approach feels uncomfortable, try indirect questions: "We see many women with injuries or complaints like yours and often they are being abused. Is that what is happening to you?" or "Many women in our community experience abuse from their partners. Is anything like that happening in your life?" With either approach, nurses need to maintain a nonjudgmental acceptance of whatever answer the woman offers.

SAVE is a model screening protocol for nurses to use when assessing women for violence (Box 9-4).

Assess Survivors of Rape for PTSD

Nurses can begin to assess the extent to which a survivor is suffering from PTSD by asking the following questions:

• To assess the presence of intrusive thoughts:
  • Do upsetting thoughts and nightmares of the trauma bother you?
  • Do you feel as though you are actually reliving the trauma?
  • Does it upset you to be exposed to anything that reminds you of that event?
• To assess the presence of avoidance reactions:
  • Do you find yourself trying to avoid thinking about the trauma?

BOX 9-4

SAVE MODEL

SCREEN all of your patients for violence by asking:
• Do you feel safe in your home?
• Do you feel you are in control of your life?
• Have you ever been sexually or physically abused?
• Can you talk about your abuse with me now?

ASK direct questions in a nonjudgmental way:
• Begin by normalizing the topic to the woman.
• Make continuous eye contact with the woman.
• Stay calm; avoid emotional reactions to what she tells you.
• Never blame the woman, even if she blames herself.
• Don't dismiss or minimize what she tells you, even if she does.
• Wait for each answer patiently. Don't rush to the next question.
• Do not use formal, technical, or medical language.
• Use a nonthreatening, accepting approach.

VALIDATE the patient by telling her:
• You believe her story.
• You do not blame her for what happened.
• It is brave of her to tell you this.
• Help is available for her.
• Talking with you is a hopeful sign and a first big step.

EVALUATE, educate, and refer this patient by asking her:
• What type of violence was it?
• Is she now in any danger?
• How is she feeling now?
• Does she know that there are consequences to violence?
• Is she aware of community resources available to help her?

Source: Rogers, 2002.

• Do you stay away from situations that remind you of the event?
• Do you have trouble recalling exactly what happened?
• Do you feel numb emotionally?
• To assess the presence of physical symptoms:
  • Are you having trouble sleeping?
  • Have you felt irritable or experienced outbursts of anger?
  • Do you have heart palpitations and sweating?
  • Do you have muscle aches and pains all over? (Clark, 2005)

Document and Report Your Findings

If the interview reveals a history of abuse, accurate documentation is critical because this evidence may support the woman's case in court. Documentation must include details as to the frequency and severity of abuse; the location, extent, and outcome of injuries; and a description of any treatments or interventions. When documenting, use direct quotes and be very specific: "He choked me." Describe any visible injuries, and use a body map (outline of a woman's body) to show where the injuries are. Obtain photos (with informed consent) or document her refusal if the woman declines photos. Pictures or diagrams can be worth a thousand words. Figure 9-2 shows a sample documentation form for intimate partner violence.

Laws in many states require health care providers to alert the police to any injuries that involve knives, firearms, or other deadly weapons or that present life-threatening emergencies. If assessment reveals suspicion or actual indication of abuse, you can explain to the woman that you are required by law to report it.

Assess Immediate Safety

The Danger Assessment Tool helps women and health care providers assess the potential for homicidal behavior within an ongoing abusive relationship. It is based on research that showed several risk factors for abuse-related murders:

- Increased frequency or severity of abuse
- Presence of firearms
- Sexual abuse
- Substance abuse
- Generally violent behavior outside of the home
- Control issues (e.g., daily chores, friends, job, money)
- Physical abuse during pregnancy
- Suicide threats or attempts (victim or abuser)
- Child abuse (Dienemann et al., 2003)

Nursing Diagnosis

When violence is suspected or validated, the nurse needs to formulate nursing diagnoses based on the completed assessment. Examples of potential nursing diagnoses related to violence against women might include the following:

- Deficient knowledge related to understanding the cycle of violence and availability of resources
- Fear related to possibility of severe injury to self or children during cycle of violence
- Low self-esteem related to feelings of worthlessness
- Hopelessness related to prolonged exposure to violence
- Compromised individual and family coping related to persistence of victim–abuser relationship

Interventions

The goal of intervention is to enable the victim to gain control of her life. Provide sensitive, predictable care in an accepting setting. Offer step-by-step explanations of procedures. Provide educational materials about violence. Allow the victim to actively participate in her care and have control over all healthcare decisions. Pace your nursing interventions and allow the woman to take the lead. Communicate support through a nonjudgmental attitude.

Carefully document assessment findings and nursing interventions.

Depending on when the nurse encounters the abused woman in the cycle of violence, interventional goals may fall into three groups:

- Primary prevention: aimed at breaking the abuse cycle through community educational initiatives by nurses, physicians, law enforcement, teachers, and clergy
- Secondary prevention: focuses on dealing with victims and abusers in early stages, with the goal of preventing progression of abuse
- Tertiary prevention: activities are geared toward helping severely abused women and children recover and become productive members of society and rehabilitating abusers to stop the cycle of violence. These activities are typically long-term and expensive.

An essential element in the care of rape survivors involves offering them the treatment they need to prevent pregnancy. After unprotected intercourse, including rape, pregnancy can be prevented by using emergency contraceptive pills, sometimes called postcoital contraception. Emergency contraceptive pills are high doses of the same oral contraceptives that millions of women take every day. The emergency regimen consists of two doses: the first dose is taken within 72 hours of the unprotected intercourse and the second dose is taken 12 hours after the first dose or sooner. Emergency contraception works by preventing ovulation, fertilization, or implantation. It does not disrupt an established pregnancy and should not be confused with mifepristone (RU-486), a drug approved by the Food and Drug Administration for abortion in the first 49 days of gestation. Emergency contraception is most effective if the first dose is taken within 12 hours of the rape; it becomes less effective with every 12 hours of delay thereafter.

Establishing a therapeutic and trusting relationship will help women disclose and describe their abuse. A tool developed by Holtz and Furniss (1993) provides a framework for sensitive nursing interventions—the ABCDES of caring for the abused women (Box 9-5).

Specific nursing interventions for the abused woman include educating her about community services, providing emotional support, and offering a safety plan.

Educate the Woman About Community Services

A wide range of support services is available to meet the needs of victims of violence. Nurses should be prepared to help the woman take advantage of these opportunities. Services will vary by community but might include psychological counseling, legal advice, social services, crisis services, support groups, hotline services, housing, vocational training, and other community-based referrals.

Refer the woman to community shelters or services available, even if she initially rejects it. Give the woman the National Domestic Violence hotline number:

INTIMATE PARTNER VIOLENCE DOCUMENTATION FORM

Explain to Client: The majority of what you tell me is confidential and cannot be shared with anyone without your written permission. However, I am required by law to report information pertaining to child or adult abuse and gunshot wounds or life-threatening injuries.

STEP 1–Establish total privacy to ask screening questions. Safety is the first priority. Client must be alone, or if the client has a child with her, the child must not be of verbal age. ONLY complete this form if YOU CAN assure the client's safety, privacy, and confidentiality.

STEP 2–Ask the client screening questions.

"Because abuse is so common, we are now asking all of our female clients:

Are you in a relationship in which you are being hurt or threatened, emotionally or physically?
___Yes ___ No

Do you feel unsafe at home?"
___Yes ___ No

If both screening questions are NO in STEP 2, and you are not concerned that the client may be a victim, sign and date the form in the signature block directly below. Provide information and resources as appropriate.

Signature _____ Title _____ Date _____

If both screening answers are NO and you are concerned that the client may be a victim, go to STEP 5. If the client answers YES to either question, proceed to STEP 3 below. Sign and date the signature block on the back of the form after completing STEP 6.

STEP 3–Assess the abuse and safety of the client and any children

Say to client: "From the answers you have just given me, I am worried for you."

    "Has the relationship gotten worse, or is it getting scarier?"   ___Yes ___ No

    "Does your partner ever watch you closely, follow you, or stalk you?" ___Yes ___ No

Ask the following question in clinic settings only. Do not ask in home settings:

"If your partner is here with you today, are you afraid to leave with him/her?"   ___Yes ___ No

"Is there anything else you want to tell me?" _____
_____
_____
_____

            Name: _____

            ID No: _____

            Date of Birth: _____

DH 3202, 2/03
Stock Number: 5744-000-3202-2

● Figure 9-2 Intimate partner violence documentation form. (Florida Department of Health.)

"Are there children in the home?" ___Yes ___ No

If the answer to the question above is "yes," say to client: "I'm concerned for your safety and the safety of your children. You and your children deserve to be at home without feeling afraid."

"Have there been threats of abuse or direct abuse of the children?" ___Yes ___ No

STEP 4—Assess client's physical injuries and health conditions, past and present

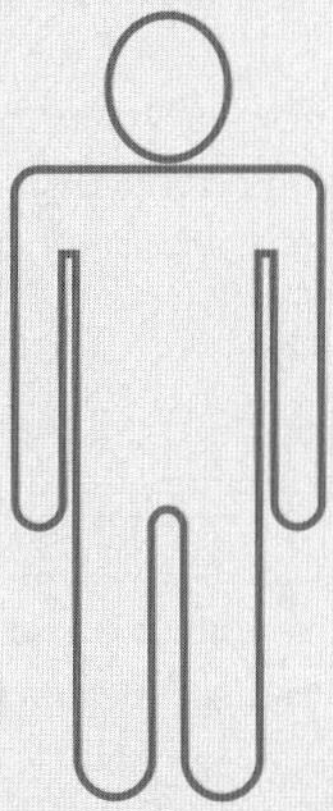

Observations/Comments/Interventions:

_____

_____

_____

_____

_____

_____

_____

_____

_____

_____

_____

STEP 5—If both screening answers are NO, and you ARE CONCERNED that the client may be a victim:

a. Say to the client: "All of us know of someone at some time in our lives who is abused. So, I am providing you with information in the event you or a friend may need it in the future."

b. Document under comments in Step 6.

STEP 6—Information, referrals or reports made

Yes No

___ ___ 1. Client given domestic violence information including safety planning
___ ___ 2. Reviewed domestic violence information including safety planning
___ ___ 3. State Abuse Hotline (1-800-96-ABUSE) and State Domestic Violence
              Hotline number (1-800-500-1119) given to the client
___ ___ 4. Client called hotline during visit
___ ___ 5. Client seen by advocate during visit
___ ___ 6. Report made. If yes, to whom: _____

Comments

_____

_____

_____

_____

_____

_____

Signature _____ Title _____ Date _____

● Figure 9-2 (continued)

THE ABCDES OF CARING FOR ABUSED WOMEN

- **A** is reassuring the woman that she is not *alone*. The isolation by her abuser keeps her from knowing that others are in the same situation and that healthcare providers can help her.
- **B** is expressing the *belief* that violence against women is not acceptable in any situation and that it is not her fault.
- **C** is *confidentiality*, since the woman might believe that if the abuse is reported, the abuser will retaliate.
- **D** is *documentation*, which includes the following:
  1. A clear quoted statement about the abuse
  2. Accurate descriptions of injuries and the history of them
  3. Photos of the injuries (with the woman's consent)
- **E** is *education* about the cycle of violence and that it will *escalate*.
- **S** is *safety*, the most important aspect of the intervention, to ensure that the woman has resources and a plan of action to carry out when she decides to leave.

(800) 799-7233. Since 1992, guidelines from the Joint Commission on Accreditation of Healthcare Organizations (JCAHO) have required emergency departments to maintain lists of community referral agencies that deal with the victims of intimate partner violence (JCAHO, 2002).

Provide Emotional Support

Providing reassurance and support to a victim of abuse is key if the violence is to end. Nurses in all clinical settings can assist victims to feel a sense of personal power and provide them with a safe and supportive environment. Appropriate action can help victims to express their thoughts and feelings in constructive ways, manage stress, and move on with their lives. Interventions appropriate to promote this are:

- Strengthen the woman's sense of control over her life by:
  - Teaching coping strategies to manage her stress
  - Assisting with activities of daily living to improve her lifestyle
  - Allowing her to make as many decisions as she can
  - Educating her about the symptoms of PTSD and their basis
- Encourage the woman to establish realistic goals for herself by:
  - Teaching problem-solving skills
  - Encouraging social activities to connect with other people
- Provide support and allow the woman to grieve for her losses by:
  - Listening to and clarifying her reactions to the traumatic event

- Discussing shock, disbelief, anger, depression, and acceptance
- Explain to the woman that:
  - Abuse is never OK. She didn't ask for it and she doesn't deserve it.
  - She is not alone and help is available.
  - Abuse is a crime and she is a victim.
  - Alcohol, drugs, money problems, depression, or jealousy does not cause violence. However, these things can give the abuser an excuse for losing control and abusing her.
  - The actions of the abuser are not her fault.
  - Her history of abuse is believed.
  - Making a decision to leave an abusive relationship can be very hard and takes time.

Offer a Safety Plan

The choice to leave must rest with the victim. Nurses cannot choose a life for the victim; they can only offer choices. Leaving is a process, not an event. Victims may try to leave their abusers as many as seven or eight times before succeeding.

Women planning to leave an abusive relationship should have a safety plan, if possible (Teaching Guidelines 9-2).

Summary

The causes of violence against women are complex. Many women will experience some type of violence in their lives, and it can have a debilitating affect on their health and future relationships. Violence frequently leaves a "legacy of pain" to future generations. Nurses can empower women and encourage them to move forward and take

 TEACHING GUIDELINES 9-2

Safety Plan for Leaving an Abusive Relationship

- When leaving an abusive relationship, take the following items:
  - Driver's license or photo ID
  - Social security number or green card/work permit
  - Birth certificates for you and your children
  - Phone numbers for social services or women's shelter
  - The deed or lease to your home or apartment
  - Any court papers or orders
  - A change of clothing for you and your children
  - Pay stubs, checkbook, credit cards, and cash
  - Insurance cards (Domestic Violence, 2000)
- If you need to leave a domestic violence situation immediately, turn to authorities for assistance in gathering this material.
  - Develop a "game plan" for leaving and rehearse it.
  - Don't use phone cards—they leave a trail to follow.

control of their lives. When women live in peace and security and free from violence, they have an enormous potential to contribute to their own communities and to the national and global society. Violence against women is not normal, legal, or acceptable and it should never be tolerated or justified. It can and must be stopped by the entire world community.

KEY CONCEPTS

● Violence against women is a major public health and social problem because it violates a woman's very being and causes numerous mental and physical health sequelae.

● Every woman has the potential to become a victim of violence.

● Several *Healthy People 2010* objectives focus on reducing the rate of physical assaults and the number of rapes and attempted rapes.

● Abuse may be mental, physical, or sexual in nature or a combination.

● The cycle of violence includes three phases: tension-building, acute battering, and reconciliation.

● Many women experience posttraumatic stress disorder (PTSD) after being sexually assaulted. PTSD can inhibit a survivor from moving on with her life.

● Pregnancy can cause violence toward the woman to start or escalate.

● The nurse's role in dealing with survivors of violence is to open up lines of communication and assess all women they encounter in practice.

References

Aggeles, T. B. (2004). *Domestic violence advocacy, Florida, update* [On-line]. Available at: http://nsweb.NursingSpectrum.com/ce/ce294b.html

Alexander, L. L., LaRosa, J. H., Bader, H., & Garfield, S. (2004). *New dimensions in women's health* (3rd ed.). Sudbury, MA: Jones and Bartlett Publishers

Centers for Disease Control and Prevention (CDC) (2004). *Intimate partner violence: fact sheet.* National Center for Injury Prevention and Control. [Online] Available at: http://www.cdc.gov/ncipc/factsheets/ipvfacts.htm

Centers for Disease Control and Prevention (CDC) (2005). *Sexual violence: fact Sheet.* National Center for Injury Prevention and Control. [Online] Available at: http://www.cdc.gov/ncipc/factsheets/svfacts.htm

CDC/National Center for Injury Prevention and Control (2004). *Tips for handling domestic violence.* [On-line]. Available at: http://www.cdc.gov/communication/tips/domviol.htm

Clark, C. C. (2005). Posttraumatic stress disorder, part I: an overview. *Nursing Spectrum,* [Online]. Available at: http://nsweb.nursingspectrum.com/ce/ce117d.htm.

Domestic Violence. (2000) The CareNotes System. Englewood, CO: MICROMEDEX, Inc.

Condon, M. C. (2004). *Women's health: an integrated approach to wellness and illness.* Upper Saddle River, NJ: Prentice Hall.

Crandall, M., Nathens, A. B., Kernic, M. A., et al. (2004). Predicting future injury among women in abusive relationships. *Journal of Trauma-Injury Infection & Critical Care, 56*(4), 906–912.

Dare, F. O., Oboro, V. O., Fadiora, S. O., et al. (2004). Female genital mutilation: an analysis of 522 cases in South-Western Nigeria. *Journal of Obstetrics and Gynecology, 24*(3), 281–283.

Dienemann, J., Campbell, J., Wiederhorn, N., et al. (2003) A critical pathway for intimate partner violence across the continuum of care. *JOGNN, 32*(5), 594–602.

Dunn, L. L., & Oths, K. S. (2004). Prenatal predictors of intimate partner abuse. *JOGNN, 33*(1), 54–63.

Healthy People 2010 (2000) [On-line]. Available at: http://www.healthypeople.gov/document/HTML/Volume2/15Injury.htm#_Toc490549392

Hessmiller, J. M., & Ledray, L. E. (2004). Violence. In M. C. Condon, *Women's health: an integrated approach to wellness and illness* (pp. 516–536). Upper Saddle River, NJ: Prentice Hall.

Hobbins, D. (2004). Survivors of childhood sexual abuse: implications for perinatal nursing care. *JOGNN, 33*(4), 485–496.

Holtrop, T. G., Fischer, H., Gray, S. M., et al. (2004). Screening for domestic violence in a general pediatric clinic: be prepared! *Pediatrics, 114*(5), 1253–1257.

Holtz, H., & Furniss, K. K. (1993). The health care provider's role in domestic violence. *Trends in Health Care Law and Ethics, 15,* 519–522.

Joint Commission on Accreditation of Healthcare Organizations. (2002). *The Joint Commission accreditation manual for hospitals.* Chicago, IL: JCAHO.

Little, C. (2003). Female genital circumcision: medical and cultural considerations. *Journal of Cultural Diversity, 10*(1), 30–34.

Lowdermilk, D. L., & Perry, S. E. (2004). *Maternity & women's health Care* (8th ed.). St. Louis: Mosby, Inc.

Maurer, F. A., & Smith, C. M. (2005). *Community public health nursing practice: health for families and populations.* St. Louis, MO: Elsevier Saunders.

McKinney, E. S., James, S. R., Murray, S. S., & Ashwill, J. W. (2005). *Maternal-child nursing* (2nd ed.). Philadelphia: W. B. Saunders Co.

Medicine Net (2005). *Sexual assault.* [Online] Available at: http://www.medicinenet.com/script/main/art.asp?articlekey=46498&pf=3

Nelson, H. D., Nygren, P., McInerney, Y., & Klein, J. (2004). Screening women and elderly adults for family and intimate partner violence: a review of the evidence for the U.S. Preventive Services Task Force. *Annuals of Internal Medicine, 104*(5), 387–396.

Penny, J. (2004). Domestic violence: 2004 update. *Vital Signs, 14*(8), 13–16.

Research Action and Information Network for the Bodily Integrity of Women (RAINBO) (2004). *Caring for women with circumcision: fact sheet for physicians* [Online] Available at: http://www.rainbo.org/factsheet.html

Rape, Abuse, and Incest National Network (RAINN) (2005). *RAINN statistics.* [On-line]. Available at: http://www.rainn.org/statistics.html

Rogers, D. (2002). *Screening your patients for sexual assault.* Florida Council Against Sexual Violence, Tallahassee, Florida.

Salmon, D., Baird, K., Price, S., & Murphy, S. (2004). *An evaluation of the Bristol Pregnancy and Domestic Violence Program to promote the introduction of routine antenatal enquiry for domestic violence at North Bristol NHS Trust.* Research Center for Public Health & Primary Care Development, University of the West of England.

Schoening, A. M., Greenwood, J. L., McNichols, J. A., et al. (2004). Effect of an intimate partner violence educational program on attitudes of nurses. *JOGNN, 33*(5), 572–579.

Shah, S., & Imhoff, V. (2005). Statutory rape: reporting myths and facts. The Cochran Firm. [Online] Available at: http://www.criminalattorney.com/pages/firm_articles_rape_myths.htm

Spear, D. L. (2004). Human trafficking: a health care prospective. *AWHONN Lifelines, 8*(4), 314–321.

Taylor, V. (2003). Female genital mutilation: cultural practice or child abuse? *Pediatric Nursing, 15*(1), 31–34.

Thompson, R. (2005). Intimate partner violence: a culturally sensitive approach. *Advance for Nurse Practitioners, 13*(5), 57–59.

Tilley, D. S., & Brackley, M. (2004). Violent lives of women: critical points for intervention—phase I focus groups. *Perspectives in Psychiatric Care, 40*(4), 157–176.

Tjaden, P., & Thoennes, N. (2000). *Full report of the prevalence, incidence, and consequences of intimate partner violence against women: findings from the National Violence Against Women Survey.* Report for grant 93-IJ-CX-0012, funded by the National Institute of Justice and the Centers for Disease Control and Prevention. Washington, D.C.

U.S. Department of Health and Human Services (U.S. DHHS) (2004). *Frequently asked questions about date rape drugs.* The National Women's Health Information Center. [Online] Available at: http://www.4woman.gov/faq/rohypnol.pdf

U.S. Department of State. (2003). *Trafficking in persons report.* U.S. Department of State Publication No. 11057, p. 7. Washington, D.C: Author.

Victims of Trafficking and Violence Protection Act of 2000, Pub. Law No. 106-386 [H.R. 3244] (2000). [Online] Available at: http://ojp. gov/vawo/laws/vawo2000/stitle_a.htm

Watts, N. (2004). Screening for domestic violence: a team approach for maternal/newborn nurses. *AWHONN Lifelines, 8*(3), 210–219.

Wellard, S. (2003). Culture and cruelty. *Community Care, 1455,* 32–34.

Wilkinson, R. (2003). Female genital mutilation. *Human rights: The essential reference.* [Online] Available at: http://www. humanrightsreference.com/chap8b.html

Web Resources

Boat People S.O.S., Inc.: **www.bpsos.org**

Center for the Prevention of Sexual and Domestic Violence: (206) 634-1903, **www.cpsdv.org**

Coalition to Abolish Slavery and Trafficking: **www.trafficked-women.org**

Domestic Violence Handbook: **www.domesticviolence.org**

Immigrant & Refugee Community Organization: **www.irco.org/irco**

National Coalition Against Sexual Assault (NCADV): (303) 839-1852, **www.ncadv.org**

National Domestic Violence Hotline: (800) 799-SAFE (7233), **www.ndvh.org**

Protection Project: **www.protectionproject.org**

Rape, Abuse, and Incest National Network (RAINN): (800) 656-HOPE, **www.rainn.org**

SAGE Project: **www.sageinc.org**

Trafficking Information and Referral Hotline: (888) 373-7888, **www.acf.hhs.gov/trafficking**

U.S. Department of Health Human Services: **aaqui@acf.hhs.gov**

U.S. Department of Labor, Women's Bureau: **www.dol.gov.dol/wb**

Violence Against Women Office, U.S. Department of Justice: (202) 616-8894, **www.raw.umn.edu**

Chapter WORKSHEET

● MULTIPLE CHOICE QUESTIONS

1. The primary goal of intervention in working with abused women is to:

   a. Set up an appointment with a mental health counselor for the victim

   b. Convince them to set up a safety plan to use when they leave

   c. Help them to develop courage and financial support to leave the abuser

   d. Empower them and improve their self-esteem to regain control of their lives

2. The first phase of the abuse cycle is characterized by:

   a. The woman provokes the abuser to bring about battering

   b. Tension-building and verbal or minor battery

   c. A honeymoon period that lulls the victim into forgetting

   d. An acute episode of physical battering

3. Women recovering from abusive relationships need to learn ways to improve their:

   a. Cooking skills and provide more nutritious meals for their children

   b. Creativity so as to improve their decorating skills within the home

   c. Communication and negotiation skills to increase their assertiveness

   d. Personal appearance by losing weight and exercising more

4. Which of the following statements might empower abuse victims to take action?

   a. "You deserve better than this."

   b. "Your children deserve to grow up in a two-parent family."

   c. "Try to figure out what you do to trigger his abuse and stop it."

   d. "Give your partner more time to come to his senses about this."

● CRITICAL THINKING EXERCISE

1. Mrs. Boggs has three children under the age of 5 and is 6 months pregnant with her fourth child. She has made repeated unscheduled visits to your clinic with vague somatic complaints regarding the children as well as herself, but has missed several scheduled prenatal appointments. On occasion she has worn sunglasses to cover bruises around her eyes. As a nurse you sense there is something else bothering her, but she doesn't seem to want to discuss it with you. She appears sad and the children cling to her when they are with her.

   a. Outline your conversation when you broach the subject of abuse with Mrs. Boggs.

   b. What is your role as a nurse in caring for this family in which you suspect abuse?

   c. What ethical/legal considerations are important in planning care for this family?

● STUDY ACTIVITIES

1. Visit the BellaOnline website for victims of violence (www.bellaonline.com). Discuss what you discovered on this site and your reactions to it.

2. Research the statistics about violence against women in your state. Are law enforcement and community interventions reducing the incidence of sexual assault and intimate partner violence?

3. Attend a dorm orientation at a local college to hear about measures in place to protect women's safety on campus. Find out the number of sexual assaults reported and what strategies the college uses to reduce this number.

4. Volunteer to spend a weekend evening at the local sheriff's department 911 hotline desk to observe the number and nature of calls received reporting domestic violence. Interview the dispatch operator about the frequency and trends of these calls.

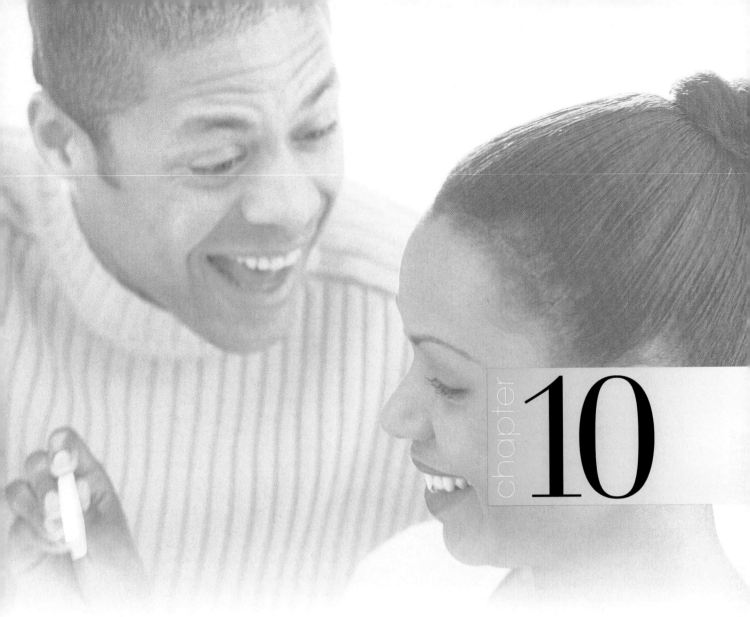

chapter 10

Fetal Development and Genetics

LearningOBJECTIVES

After studying the chapter content, the student should be able to accomplish the following:

1. Define the key terms.
2. Describe the process of fertilization, implantation, and cell differentiation.
3. Explain the functions of the placenta, umbilical cord, and amniotic fluid.
4. Outline normal fetal development from conception through birth.
5. Discuss the education/counseling needs of patients undergoing genetic testing.
6. Delineate the role of the nurse involved in genetic-related activities.

Human reproduction is one of the most intimate spheres of an individual's life. For conception to occur, a healthy ovum from the woman has to be released from the ovary; pass into a normal, open fallopian tube; and start being transported downward. Sperm from the male must be deposited into the vagina and be able to swim approximately seven inches to meet the ovum and penetrate its hard cover to begin the wondrous human life. All this activity takes place within a 5-hour time span, during which the sperm reaches the outer portion of the fallopian tube, where **fertilization** takes place (Gilbert & Harmon, 2003).

Nurses caring for the childbearing family need to have a basic understanding of conception and prenatal development to be able to identify problems/variations and to initiate appropriate interventions should any problems occur. This chapter presents an overview of fetal development, beginning with conception. It also discusses hereditary influences on fetal development and the nurse's role in **genetic counseling.**

Fetal Development

Fetal development during pregnancy is measured in number of weeks after fertilization. The duration of pregnancy is about 40 weeks from the time of fertilization. This equates to 9 calendar months or approximately 266 to 280 calendar days. The three different stages of fetal development during pregnancy are

1. **Preembryonic stage:** fertilization through the second week
2. **Embryonic stage:** end of the second week through the eighth week
3. **Fetal stage:** end of the eighth week until birth

Fetal circulation is a significant aspect of fetal development that spans all three stages.

Preembryonic Stage

The preembryonic stage begins with fertilization, also called *conception.* Fertilization is defined as the union of ovum and sperm, which starts the onset of pregnancy. Fertilization typically occurs around 2 weeks after the last normal menstrual period in a 28-day cycle (Dillon, 2003). Fertilization requires a timely interaction between the release of the mature ovum at ovulation and the ejaculation of enough healthy, mobile sperm to survive the hostile vaginal environment through which they must travel to meet the ovum. All things considered, the act of conception is difficult at best. To say merely that it occurs when the sperm unites with the ovum is deceptively simple. Getting them both together at the right time involves an intricate interplay of hormonal preparation and an overwhelming number of natural barriers. A human being is truly an amazing outcome of this elaborate process.

Prior to fertilization, the ovum and the spermatozoon undergo the process of meiosis. The primary oocyte completes its first meiotic division before ovulation. The secondary oocyte begins its second meiotic division just before ovulation. Primary and secondary spermatocytes undergo meiotic division while still in the testes (Fig. 10-1).

Although more than 200 million sperm/mL are contained in the ejaculated semen, only one is able to enter the female ovum to fertilize it. All others are blocked by the clear protein layer called the **zona pellucida.** The zona pellucida disappears in about 5 days. Once the sperm gets to the plasma membrane, the ovum resumes meiosis and forms a nucleus with half the number of **chromosomes** (23). When the nucleus from the ovum and the nucleus of the sperm make contact, they lose their respective nuclear membranes and combine their maternal and paternal chromosomes. Because each nucleus contains a haploid number of chromosomes (23), this union restores the diploid number (46). The resulting **zygote** begins the process of a new life. This genetic information from both ovum and sperm establishes the unique physical characteristics of the individual. Sex determination is also determined at fertilization and depends on whether the ovum is fertilized by a Y-bearing sperm or an X-bearing sperm. An XX zygote will become a female and an XY zygote will become a male (Fig. 10-2).

Fertilization takes place in the outer third of the ampulla of the fallopian tube. When the ovum is fertilized by the sperm (now called a *zygote*), a great deal of activity immediately takes place. Mitosis, or *cleavage*, takes place as the zygote is slowly transported into the uterine cavity as a result of tubal muscular movements (Fig. 10-3). After there are four cleavages, the 16 cells appear as a solid ball of cells or **morula,** meaning "little mulberry." The morula reaches the uterine cavity about 72 hours after fertilization (Sloane, 2002).

With additional cell division, the morula divides into specialized cells that will later form fetal structures. Within the morula, an off-center, fluid-filled space appears, transforming it into a hollow ball of cells called **blastocysts** (Fig. 10-4). The inner surface of the blastocysts will form the embryo and amnion. The outer layers of cells surrounding the blastocyst cavity are called **trophoblasts.** Eventually, the trophoblast develops into one of the embryonic membranes, the chorion, and helps to form the **placenta.**

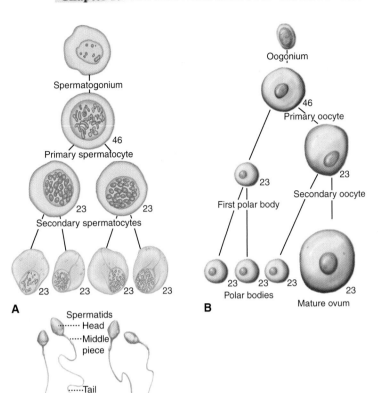

A

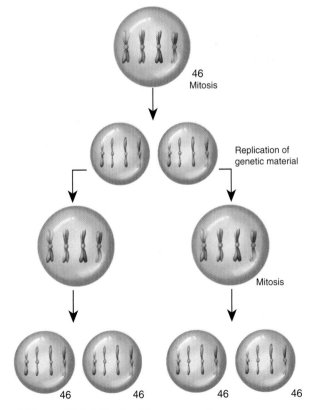

B

● Figure 10-1 The formation of gametes by the process of meiosis is known as gametogenesis. (**A**) Spermatogenesis. One spermatogonium gives rise to four spermatozoa. (**B**) Oogenesis. From each oogonium, one mature ovum and three abortive cells are produced. The chromosomes are reduced to one-half the number characteristic for the general body cells of the species. In humans, the number in the body cells is 46, and that in the mature spermatozoon and secondary oocyte is 23.

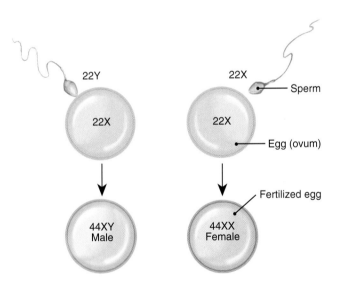

● Figure 10-2 Inheritance of gender. Each ovum contains 22 autosomes and an X chromosome. Each spermatozoon (sperm) contains 22 autosomes and either an X chromosome or a Y chromosome. The gender of the zygote is determined at the time of fertilization by the combination of the sex chromosomes of the sperm (either X or Y) and the ovum (X).

● Figure 10-3 Mitosis of the stoma cells.

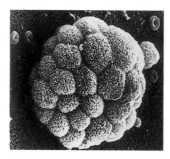

● Figure 10-4 Blastocyst.

By now the developing blastocyst needs to receive more food and oxygen to keep growing. The trophoblast attaches itself to the surface of the endometrium for further nourishment. Normal implantation occurs in the upper uterus (fundus). This location is best because it has a rich supply of blood and strong muscular fibers, which clamp down on blood vessels after the placenta separates from the inner wall of the uterus. Also, the lining is thickest here so the placenta cannot attach so strongly that it remains attached after birth (McKinney, James, Murray, & Ashwill, 2005). Figure 10-5 describes the process of fertilization and implantation.

Concurrent with the development of the trophoblast and implantation there is further differentiation of the inner cell mass. Some of the cells become the embryo itself, and others give rise to the membranes that surround and protect it. Three embryonic layers of cells are formed as follows:

1. Ectoderm—forms the central nervous system, special senses, skin, and glands
2. Mesoderm—forms skeletal, urinary, circulatory, and reproductive organs
3. Endoderm—forms respiratory system, liver, pancreas, and digestive system

These three layers are formed at the same time as the embryonic membranes, and all tissues, organs, and organ systems develop from these three primary germ cell layers (London, Ladewig, Ball, & Bindler, 2003).

Despite all the dramatic activities that go on internally to create a human life, many women are not aware right away that a potential pregnancy has been initiated. Several weeks will pass before even one of the presumptive signs of pregnancy—missing the first menstrual period—will take place. Box 10-1 provides a summary of preembryonic development.

Embryonic Stage

The embryonic stage of development begins at day 15 after conception and continues through week 8. Basic structures

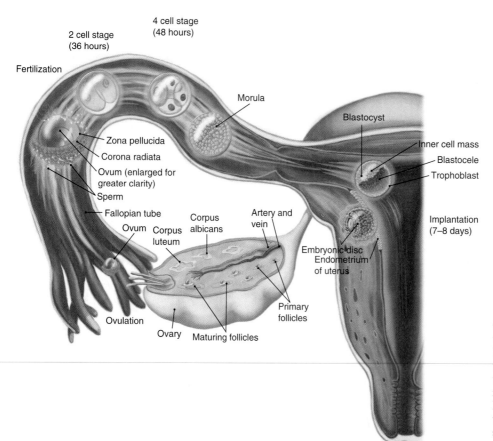

● Figure 10-5 Fertilization and tubal transport of the zygote. From fertilization to implantation, the zygote travels through the fallopian tube, experiencing rapid mitotic division (cleavage). During the journey toward the uterus the zygote evolves through several stages, including morula and blastocyst.

of all major body organs and the main external features are completed during this time period. See Table 10-1 and Figure 10-6 for a summary of embryonic development.

The embryonic membranes (Fig. 10-7) begin to form around the same time of implantation. The chorion consists of trophoblast cells and a mesodermal lining. It has finger-like projections called *chorionic villi* on its surface. The amnion originates from the ectoderm germ layer during the early stages of embryonic development. It is a thin protective membrane that contains amniotic fluid. As the embryo grows, the amnion expands until it touches the chorion. These two fetal membranes form the fluid-filled amniotic sac, or bag of waters, that protects the floating embryo (Littleton & Engebretson, 2005).

Amniotic fluid surrounds the embryo and increases in volume as the pregnancy progresses, reaching approximately a liter in volume by term. Amniotic fluid is derived from two sources: fluid transported from the maternal blood across the amnion and fetal urine. It is constantly changing in volume as the fetus swallows and voids into it. Sufficient amounts of amniotic fluid help maintain a constant body temperature for the fetus, permit symmetric growth and development, cushion the fetus from trauma, allow the **umbilical cord** to be relatively free of compression, and promote fetal movement to enhance musculoskeletal development. It is made up of 98% water and 2% organic matter. It is slightly alkaline and contains albumin, urea, uric acid, creatinine, bilirubin, lecithin, sphingomyelin, epithelial cells, vernix, and fine hair called *lanugo* (Lowdermilk & Perry, 2004).

The volume of amniotic fluid is important in determining fetal well-being. It gradually fluctuates throughout the course of the pregnancy. Alterations in normal amniotic fluid volume can relate to potential problems in the fetus. Having a deficiency in the amount of amniotic fluid (<500 mL at term) is called *oligohydramnios* and is associated with utero placental insufficiency and fetal renal abnormalities. Having an excessive amount of amniotic fluid (>2000 mL at term) is termed *hydram-*

nios and is associated with maternal disease such as diabetes, neural tube defects, chromosomal deviations, and malformations of the central nervous system and/or gastrointestinal tract that prevent normal swallowing of amniotic fluid by the fetus (Olds, London, Ladewig, & Davidson, 2004).

At the same time the placenta is developing (end of the second week), the umbilical cord is also formed from the amnion. It is the lifeline from the mother to the growing embryo. It contains one large vein and two small arteries. Wharton's jelly (a specialized connective tissue) surrounds these three blood vessels in the umbilical cord to prevent compression, which would choke off the blood supply and nutrients to the growing life inside. At term, the average umbilical cord is 22 inches long and about an inch in width (Olds et al., 2004).

The precursor cells of the placenta—the trophoblasts—first appear 4 days after fertilization as the outer layer of cells of the blastocyst. These early blastocyst trophoblasts differentiate into all the cells that form the placenta. When fully developed, the placenta serves as the interface between the mother and the developing fetus. As early as 3 days after conception, the trophoblasts make human chorionic gonadotropin (hCG), a hormone, which ensures that the endometrium will be receptive to the implanting embryo. During the next few weeks the placenta begins to make hormones that control the basic physiology of the mother in such a way that the fetus is supplied with the necessary nutrients and oxygen needed for successful growth. The placenta also protects the fetus from immune attack by the mother, removes waste products from the fetus, induces the mother to bring more food to the placenta, and, near the time of delivery, produces hormones that mature fetal organs in preparation for life outside the uterus (Kilman, 2003).

At no time during pregnancy is there any direct contact between the blood of the fetus and the blood of the mother, so there is no mixing of blood. There are always layers of fetal tissue that separate the maternal blood and the fetal blood. These fetal tissues are called the *placental barrier.* Materials can be interchanged only through diffusion. The maternal uterine arteries deliver the nutrients and the mother's uterine veins carry oxygen and the fetal waste products away. The structure of the placenta is usually completed by week 12.

The placenta is not only a transfer organ but a factory as well. It produces several hormones necessary for normal pregnancy:

- *Human chorionic gonadotropin* (or hCG)—preserves the corpus luteum and its progesterone production so that the endometrial lining of the uterus is maintained; is the basis for pregnancy tests
- *Human placental lactogen* (hPL)—modulates fetal and maternal metabolism, participates in the development of

(text continues on page 218)

Table 10-1 Embryonic and Fetal Development

Week 3
Beginning development of brain, spinal cord, and heart
Beginning development of the gastrointestinal tract
Neural tube forms, which later becomes the spinal cord
Leg and arm buds appear and grow out from body

Week 4
Brain differentiates
Limb buds grow and develop more

4 weeks

Week 5
Heart now beats at a regular rhythm
Beginning structures of eyes and ears
Some cranial nerves are visible
Muscles innervated

Week 6
Beginning formation of lungs
Fetal circulation established
Liver produces RBCs
Further development of the brain
Primitive skeleton forms
Central nervous system forms
Brain waves detectable

Week 7
Straightening of trunk
Nipples and hair follicles form
Elbows and toes visible
Arms and legs move
Diaphragm formed
Mouth with lips and early tooth buds

Week 8
Rotation of intestines
Facial features continue to develop
Heart development complete
Resembles a human being
  (Ratner, 2002)

8 weeks

Weeks 9–12
Sexual differentiation continues
Buds for all 20 temporary teeth laid down
Digestive system shows activity

Head comprises nearly half the fetus size
Face and neck are well formed
Urogenital tract completes development
Red blood cells are produced in the liver
Urine begins to be produced and excreted
Fetal gender can be determined by week 12
Limbs are long and thin; digits are well formed

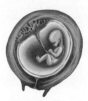

12 weeks

Weeks 13–16
A fine hair develops on the head called *lanugo*
Fetal skin is almost transparent
Bones become harder
Fetus makes active movement
Sucking motions are made with the mouth
Amniotic fluid is swallowed
Fingernails and toenails present
Weight quadruples
Fetal movement (also know as *quickening*) detected
  by mother

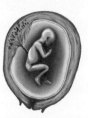

16 weeks

Weeks 17–20
Rapid brain growth occurs
Fetal heart tones can be heard with stethoscope
Kidneys continue to secret urine into amniotic fluid
Vernix caseosa, a white greasy film, covers the fetus
Eyebrows and head hair appear
Brown fat deposited to help maintain temperature
Nails are present on both fingers and toes
Muscles are well developed

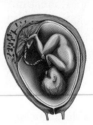

20 weeks

(continued)

Table 10-1 Embryonic and Fetal Development (continued)

Weeks 21–24
Eyebrows and eyelashes are well formed
Fetus has a hand grasp and startle reflex
Alveoli forming in lungs
Skin is translucent and red
Lungs begin to produce *surfactant*

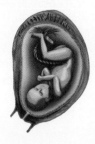

25 weeks

Weeks 25–28
Fetus reaches a length of 15 inches
Rapid brain development
Eyelids open and close
Nervous system controls some functions
Fingerprints are set
Blood formation shifts from spleen to bone marrow
Fetus usually assumes head-down position

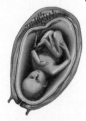

28 weeks

Weeks 29–32
Rapid increase in the amount of body fat
Increased central nervous system control over body
     functions
Rhythmic breathing movements occur
Lungs are not fully mature
Fetus stores iron, calcium, and phosphorus

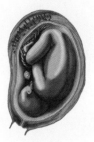

32 weeks

Weeks 33–38
Testes are in scrotum of male fetus
Lanugo begins to disappear
Increase in body fat
Fingernails reach the end of fingertips
Small breast buds are present on both sexes
Mother supplies fetus with antibodies against disease
Fetus is considered full term at 38 weeks
Fetus fills uterus (Bailey, 2003)

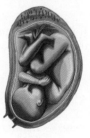

37 weeks

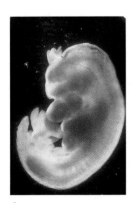
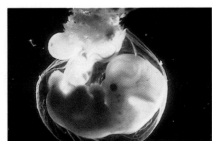
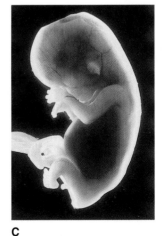

A   B   C

● Figure 10-6 Embryonic development. (**A**) 4-week embryo; (**B**) 5-week embryo;
(**C**) 6-week embryo.

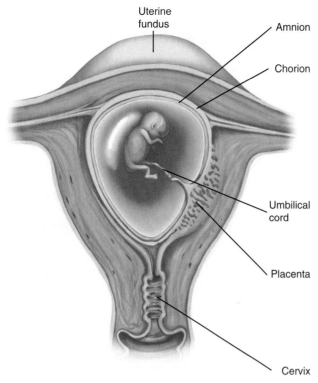

Uterine fundus

Amnion

Chorion

Umbilical cord

Placenta

Cervix

● Figure 10-7 The embryo is floating in amniotic fluid surrounded by the protective fetal membranes (amnion and chorion).

maternal breasts for lactation, and decreases maternal insulin sensitivity to increase its availability for fetal nutrition

- *Estrogen* (estriol)—causes enlargement of a woman's breasts, uterus, and external genitalia; stimulates myometrial contractility
- *Progesterone* (progestin)—maintains the endometrium, decreases the contractility of the uterus, stimulates maternal metabolism and breast development, provides nourishment for the early conceptus
- *Relaxin*—acts synergistically with progesterone to maintain pregnancy, causes relaxation of the pelvic ligaments, softens the cervix in preparation for birth (Condon, 2004)

The placenta should not be thought of as a barrier between mother and conceptus, but rather as a pass-through in which almost everything the mother ingests (food, alcohol, drugs) "passes through" to the developing conceptus. This is why it is so important to advise pregnant women not to take unauthorized substances (drugs, alcohol, tobacco), because they can be harmful to the conceptus.

During the embryonic stage, rapid growth of the conceptus takes place as all organs and structures are forming. It is during this critical period of differentiation when the growing embryo is most susceptible to damage from external sources, including teratogens (substances that cause birth defects such as alcohol and drugs), infections (such as rubella or cytomegalovirus), radiation, and nutritional deficiencies.

Fetal Stage

The average pregnancy lasts 280 days from the first day of the last menstrual period. The fetal stage is from the end of the eighth week until birth. It is the longest period of prenatal development. It is during this period that the conceptus is sufficiently developed to be called a fetus. Although all major systems are present in their basic form, dramatic growth and refinement of all organ systems take place during the fetal period (Table 10-1). Figure 10-8 depicts a 12- to 15-week fetus.

Fetal Circulation

The circulation through the fetus during uterine life is different than ours. Fetal circulation encompasses the circulation of blood from the placenta to and through the fetus, and back to the placenta. Fetal circulation is one of the first organ systems needed to be able to function properly to sustain the fetus. Before it develops, nutrients and oxygen diffuse through the extraembryonic coelom and the yolk sac from the placenta. As the embryo increases in size, its nutrient needs increase and the amount of tissue easily reached by diffusion increases. Thus, the circulation must develop quickly and accurately (Everett & Hammill, 2002).

The circulatory system of the fetus functions much differently from that of a newborn. The most significant difference is that oxygen is received from the placenta during fetal life and via the lungs after birth. In addition, the fetal liver does not have the metabolic functions that it will have after birth because the mother's body performs these functions. Three shunts are present in fetal life:

1. *Ductus venosus*—connects the umbilical vein to the inferior vena cava
2. *Ductus arteriosus*—connects the main pulmonary artery to the aorta
3. *Foramen ovale*—anatomic opening between the right and left atrium

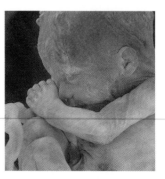

● Figure 10-8 Fetal development: 12- to 15-week fetus.

The whole function of fetal circulation is to carry highly oxygenated blood to vital areas (e.g., heart, brain) while first shunting it away from less vital ones (e.g., lungs, liver). The placenta essentially takes over the functions of the lungs and liver during fetal life, and therefore large volumes of oxygenated blood are not needed. Fetal circulation can be traced as follows: The oxygenated blood is carried from the placenta to the fetus via the umbilical vein. About half of this blood passes through the hepatic capillaries and the rest flows through the *ductus venosus* into the inferior vena cava. Blood from the vena cava is mostly deflected through the *foramen ovale* into the left atrium, then to the left ventricle, into the ascending aorta, and on to the head and upper body. This allows the fetal coronary circulation and brain to receive the blood with the highest level of oxygenation.

Deoxygenated blood from the superior vena cava flows into the right atrium, right ventricle, and then into the pulmonary artery. Because of high pulmonary vascular resistance, only a small percentage (5–10%) of the blood in the pulmonary artery flows to the lungs, the majority of it being shunted through the patent *ductus arteriosus* and then down the descending aorta (O'Toole, 2003). The fetal lungs are essentially nonfunctional and filled with fluid. The presence of this fluid makes the lungs resistant to the flow of blood into them and they receive only enough blood as required for proper nourishment. Finally, two umbilical arteries carry the unoxygenated blood from the descending aorta back to the placenta.

At birth, a dramatic change in the fetal circulatory pattern occurs. The foramen ovale, ductus arteriosus, ductus venosus, and the umbilical vessels are no longer needed. When the newborn takes a first breath at birth, the lungs inflate, which tends to draw blood into them from the right ventricle. The increase in blood flow into and out of the lungs increases pressure in the left atrium. This causes a one-way flap on the left side of the foramen ovale, called the *septum primum,* to press against the opening, effectively separating the two atria. This also increases blood flow to the lungs, because blood entering the right atrium can no longer bypass the right ventricle, which pumps it into the pulmonary artery and on to the lungs. The ductus venosus closes with the clamping of the umbilical cord and inhibition of blood flow through the umbilical vein. The ductus arteriosus constricts partly in response to higher arterial oxygen levels that occur after the first few breaths. This closure prevents blood from the aorta from entering the pulmonary artery (Sabella, 2003). Thus, the newborn is left with the adult pattern of circulation, in which deoxygenated blood enters the right atrium and is pumped through the right atrium to the pulmonary arteries. In the lungs it is oxygenated to be returned to the left atrium of the heart via the pulmonary veins. Oxygenated blood can then be pumped to all parts of the body by the left ventricle. See Figure 10-9 for a summary of the fetal circulation pattern.

Genetics

Genetics is the study of the patterns of inheritance of specific traits (O'Toole, 2003). Traditionally, genetics has been associated with childbearing decision making and caring for children with genetic disorders. Recent genetic and technologic advances are helping to expand our understanding of how genetic changes affect human diseases such as diabetes, cancer, Alzheimer disease, and other multifactorial diseases that are prevalent in adults (Greco & Mahon, 2002). Genetic science has the potential to revolutionize health care with regard to national screening programs, predisposition testing, detecting genetic disorders, and pharmacogenetics. Today, nurses are required to have basic skills and knowledge in genetics so they can take on new roles and help patients understand the personal and societal effects of genetic information (Burton, 2003).

Advances in Genetic Science

Recent advances in genetic knowledge and technology have affected all areas of health. These advances have increased the number of health interventions that can be undertaken with regard to genetic disorders. For example, genetic diagnosis is now possible before conception and earlier in pregnancy. Genetic testing can now identify presymptomatic conditions in children and adults. Gene therapy can be used to replace or repair defective or missing **genes** with normal ones. Gene therapy has been used for a variety of disorders, including cystic fibrosis, melanoma, HIV, and hepatitis (Lewis, Heitkemper, & Dirksen, 2004). It may also treat many chronic illnesses. The potential exists for creation of increased intelligence and size through genetic intervention. Genetic agents may replace drugs, general surgery may be replaced by gene surgery, and genetic intervention may replace radiation (Terzioglu & Dinc, 2004).

The information gained from the Human Genome Project, an international 13-year effort begun in 1990 by the Department of Energy and National Institutes of Health, has brought new advances in genetic testing (Lea & Williams, 2002). These advances will have a profound effect on the diagnosis, treatment, and prevention of diseases. The goal of this project was to map the human genome (complete set of genetic instructions in the nucleus of each human cell) by 2005. A substantially complete version of this project was announced in 2002. Two key findings from the project were found: (1) All human beings are 99.9% identical at the DNA level and (2) approximately 30,000 genes make up the human genome (International Human Genome Sequencing Consortium, 2004). An individual's genome represents their genetic blueprint, which determines genotype (the gene pairs inherited from parents) and phenotype (physical characteristics and manifestations) (Edgar, 2004).

Research from the Human Genome Project has provided a better understanding of the genetic contribution to disease. It is now recognized that most common human

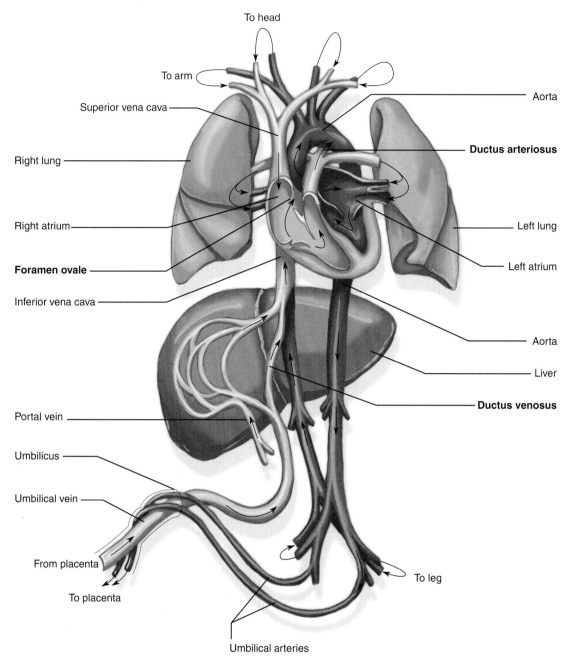

To head

To arm

Superior vena cava

Right lung

Right atrium

Foramen ovale

Inferior vena cava

Portal vein

Umbilicus

Umbilical vein

From placenta

To placenta

Umbilical arteries

Aorta

Ductus arteriosus

Left lung

Left atrium

Aorta

Liver

Ductus venosus

To leg

● Figure 10-9 Fetal circulation. Arrows indicate the path of blood. The umbilical vein carries oxygen-rich blood from the placenta to the liver and through the ductus venosus. From there it is carried to the inferior vena cava to the right atrium of the heart. Some of the blood is shunted through the foramen ovale to the left side of the heart where it is routed to the brain and upper extremities. The rest of the blood travels down to the right ventricle and through the pulmonary artery. A small portion of the blood travels to the non-functioning lungs, while the remaining blood is shunted through the ductus arteriosus into the aorta to supply the rest of the body.

diseases such as myocardial infarction, cancer, mental illness, diabetes, and Alzheimer disease are a result of complex interactions between a number of factors, including the influence of one or more genes and a variety of environmental exposures (Greco & Mahon, 2002).

The potential benefits of these discoveries are vast, but so is the potential for misuse. These benefits challenge all healthcare professionals to consider the many

ethical, legal, and social ramifications of genetics knowledge in human lives. In the near future, individual risk profiling based on an individual's unique genetic makeup will be used to tailor prevention, treatment, and ongoing management of health conditions. This profiling will raise issues associated with patient privacy and confidentially related to workplace discrimination and access to health insurance. Issues of autonomy are equally problematic as society considers how to address injustices that will inevitably surface when disease risk can be determined years in advance of its occurrence. Nurses will certainly play an important role in developing new policies and charting a course in this bold new world of genetics. Nurses, however, must know the basics of genetics to do this.

Basics of Genetics

The nucleus within the cell is the controlling factor in all cellular activities because it contains chromosomes, which are made up of genes—the "how-to" units of instruction for building. Each person has a unique genetic constitution, or genotype, made up of 30,000 to 40,000 genes. An individual *gene* is a unit of heredity. Each gene has a segment of DNA with a specific set of instructions for making proteins needed by body cells for proper functioning. Genes control the types of proteins made and the rate at which they are produced (Sloane, 2002) (Fig. 10-10). Any change in gene structure or location leads to a **mutation,**

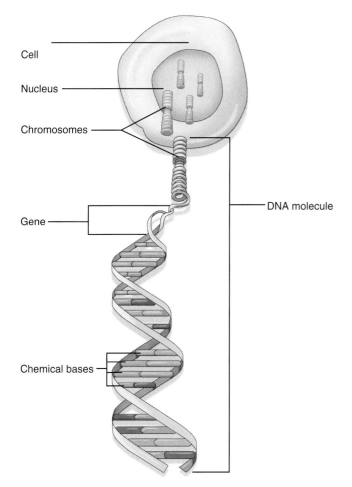

● Figure 10-10 DNA is made up of four chemical bases. Tightly coiled strands of DNA are packaged in units called chromosomes, housed in the cell's nucleus. Working subunits of DNA are known as genes. (From the National Institute of Health and National Cancer Institute. [1995]. *Understanding gene testing* [NIH Pub. No. 96-3905]. Washington, DC: U.S. Department of Human Services.)

which may alter the type and amount of protein produced (Fig. 10-11). Genes never act in isolation; they always interact with other genes and the environment. They are arranged in a specific linear formation along a chromosome. Genes carry instructions for either dominant or recessive traits, which determine the color of eyes and hair, body build, and the growth and development of every physical and biochemical system (Lea, 2003).

A chromosome is a filament-like nuclear structure consisting of chromatin that stores genetic information as base sequences in DNA, and with a number that is constant in each species. Each chromosome is composed of varying numbers of genes. A total of 22 chromosome pairs are autosomes, and the 23rd pair comprises the sex chromosomes. Humans have 46 paired chromosomes that are found in all cells of the body—except the ovum and sperm cells, which have just 23 chromosomes. In males and females, 22 of the chromosome pairs are the same (autosomes). The last pair is the sex chromosomes—two X chromosomes in females, and an X chromosome and a Y chromosome in males. Offspring receive one chromosome of each of the 23 pairs from each parent.

DNA stores genetic information and encodes the instructions for synthesizing specific proteins needed to maintain life. The structure of DNA is double stranded and is identified as a double helix. The side pieces of the double helix are made up of a sugar, deoxyribose, and a phosphate, occurring in alternating groups. The cross-connections or rungs of the ladder are attached to the sides and are made up of four nitrogenous bases: adenine, cytosine, thymine, and guanine. The sequence of the base pairs as they form each rung of the ladder is referred to as the *genetic code* (Sloane, 2002).

Regulation and expression of the thousands of human genes is very complex and is the result of many intricate interactions within each cell. Alterations in gene structure, function, transcription, translation, and protein synthesis can influence an individual's health (Lea, 2002). Gene mutations are a permanent change in the sequence of DNA. Some mutations have no significant affect, whereas others can have a tremendous impact on the health status of the individual. Several genetic disorders can result from these mutations, such as cystic fibrosis, sickle-cell disease, phenylketonuria, or hemophilia.

The pictorial analysis of the number, form, and size of an individual's chromosomes is termed *karyotype.* White blood cells and fetal cells in amniotic fluid are commonly analyzed. The chromosomes are numbered from the largest to the smallest, 1 to 22, and the sex chromosomes are designated by the letter X or Y. A female karyotype is designated as 46,XX and a male karyotype is designated as 46,XY. See Figure 10-12 for an example of a karyotyping pattern.

Just as there are maternal and paternal copies of each chromosome, there are also maternal and paternal copies of each gene. The sequence of the maternal and paternal gene pair may be *homozygous* (identical) or *heterozygous*

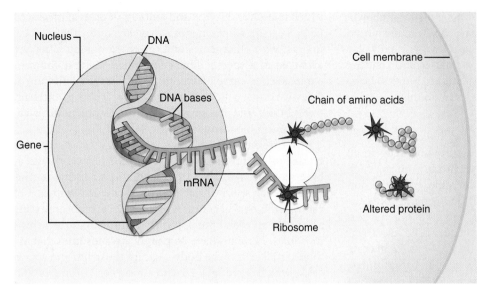

● Figure 10-11 When a gene contains a mutation, the protein encoded by that gene will be abnormal. Some protein changes are insignificant, others are disabling. (From the National Institutes of Health and National Cancer Institute. [1995]. *Understanding gene testing* [NIH Pub. No. 96-3905]. Washington, DC: U.S. Department of Human Services.)

(different). Homozygous means both alleles (a different form of the same gene copy) for a trait are the same. For example, WW stands for homozygous dominant; ww stands for homozygous recessive. Heterozygous indicates members of the allelic pair are different, such as Ww. For example, an offspring inherits blood type AB. The type A allele (gene copy) came from one parent and the type B allele from the other parent. This would therefore be considered heterozygous for the gene pair. If the offspring inherited blood type O, this would be considered a homozygous gene pairing because both parents gave the same gene pair (B) (Black & Hawks, 2005).

Chromosomal Abnormalities

The mechanisms underlying cell division are so complex that an occasional error is not unexpected. Errors resulting in chromosomal abnormalities can occur during mitosis

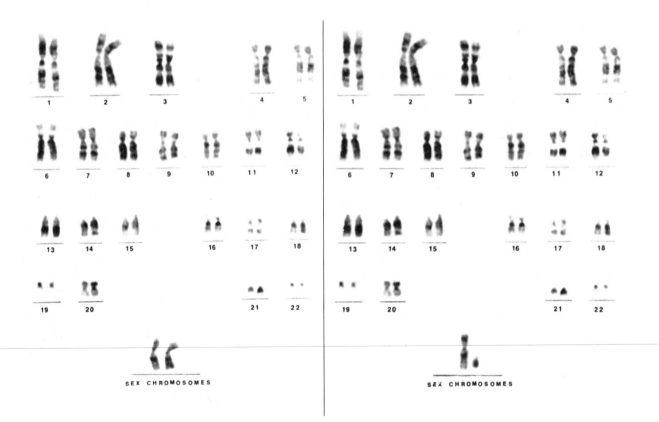

● Figure 10-12 Karyotype pattern. (**A**) Normal female karyotype. (**B**) Normal male karyotype.

or meiosis. These errors can occur in either the autosomes or sex chromosomes. About 1 in 160 live-born infants is born with a chromosomal abnormality (March of Dimes, 2005). These often cause major defects because they involve added or missing genes. There are two major kinds of autosomal errors: changes in the number of chromosomes or changes in the structure of the chromosomes.

Numeric Abnormalities

- Entire single added chromosome (trisomy)
- Entire single chromosome missing (monosomy)
- One or more added sets of chromosomes (polyploidy)

Structural Abnormalities

- Part of a chromosome missing or added
- Rearrangements of material within the chromosomes
- Two chromosomes that adhere to each other
- Fragility of a specific site on the X chromosome (Murray & McKinney, 2006)

Numeric Abnormalities

Numeric abnormalities of chromosomes are most commonly seen as **trisomies, monosomies,** and **polyploidy.** All involve added or missing single chromosomes, or multiple sets of chromosomes.

Trisomies

Trisomies are the product of the union of a normal ovum or sperm with a gamete that contains an extra chromosome. This means there will be 47 chromosomes instead of the normal 46. Down syndrome is an example of a trisomy. Individuals with Down syndrome have three copies of chromosome 21. Down syndrome affects 1 in 800 to 1000 live-born babies. The risk of this and other trisomies increases with maternal age. The risk of having a baby with Down syndrome is about 1 in 1250 for a woman at age 25, 1 in 1000 at 30, 1 in 400 at 35, and 1 in 100 at age 40 (March of Dimes, 2004). Individuals with Down syndrome have characteristic features that are usually identified at birth (Fig. 10-13). These common characteristics include

- Small, low-set ears
- Hyperflexibility
- Muscle hypotonia
- Deep crease across palm (termed *simian crease*)
- Flat facial profile
- Small white, crescent-shaped spots on irises
- Open mouth with protruding tongue
- Broad, short fingers (Littleton & Engebretson, 2005)

The outlook for children with Down syndrome is much brighter now than it was years ago. Most children with Down syndrome have mental retardation in the mild to moderate range. With early intervention and special education, many learn to read and write, and participate in diverse childhood activities (March of Dimes, 2004). Despite modern medical technology, the individual with Down syndrome has a shortened life expectancy, with 22% dying in the first decade and 50% dying by the age of 60, mostly from cardiac and malignant conditions (Littleton & Engebretson, 2005).

Another chromosomal disorder involving an extra chromosome is Klinefelter syndrome, which occurs only in males. About 1 in 400 males born have Klinefelter syndrome. There is an extra X chromosome (XXY) present. The extra genetic material causes abnormal development

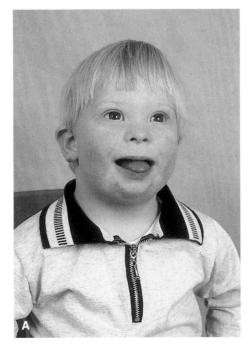
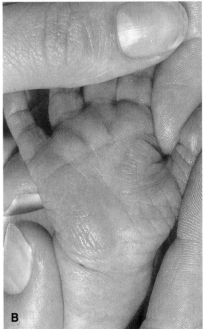

● Figure 10-13 **(A)** Typical facial features of the child with Down syndrome. **(B)** A simian line, a horizontal crease seen in children with Down syndrome.

of the testicles, resulting in decreased production of sperm and male sex hormones. Clinical manifestations may include

• Mild mental retardation
• Small testicles
• Infertility
• Long arms and legs
• Enlarged breast tissue (gynecomastia)
• Scant facial and body hair
• Decreased sex drive (libido) (Mayo Clinic, 2002)

No treatment can correct this genetic abnormality, but testosterone replacement therapy can improve symptoms resulting from a deficiency. Most males with Klinefelter syndrome (XXY) are diagnosed after their 14th year of life after experiencing a late onset of puberty. Infertility is common and life expectancy is normal (Verklan & Walden, 2004).

Two other common trisomies are trisomy 18 and trisomy 13. Trisomy 18 and trisomy 13 are, respectively, the second and third most commonly diagnosed autosomal trisomies in live-born infants. Although these conditions are associated with a high degree of infant mortality, 5 to 10% of children with these conditions survive beyond the first year of life (Rasmussen, Wong, Yang, May, & Friedman, 2003). Trisomy 18 or Edward syndrome occurs in 1 of every 5000 newborns, with advanced maternal age as a causative factor. Prenatally, there are several findings apparent on ultrasound, which includes intrauterine growth restriction (IUGR), hydramnios or oligohydramnios, cardiac malformations, single umbilical artery, and decrease in fetal movement. Additionally, trisomy 18 has been associated with an decrease in maternal serum levels of maternal serum alpha-fetoprotein (MSAFP) and hCG. Most affected newborns are female, with a 4:1 ratio to males. Affected newborns have 47 chromosomes (three at chromosome 18) and are characterized by severe mental retardation, growth deficiency of cranium (microcephaly), low-set ears, small for gestational age, seizures, drooping eyelids, webbing of fingers, congenital heart defects, rocker-bottom feet, and severe hypotonia (Sterk, 2004). Infants with trisomy 18 have multiple anomalies that are severe, and life expectancy is greatly reduced beyond a few months.

Trisomy 13 or Patau syndrome affects 1 of 12,000 newborns with 47 chromosomes (three of chromosome 13) present. Maternal age is also thought to be a causative factor in this genetic disorder (Lea, 2003). The common abnormalities associated with trisomy 13 are microcephaly, cardiac defects, central nervous system anomalies, polydactyly (Fig. 10-14), severe mental retardation, severe hypotonia, and seizures (Lowdermilk & Perry, 2004). Life expectancy is only a few months for most infants with trisomy 13. Care is supportive in nature for these infants.

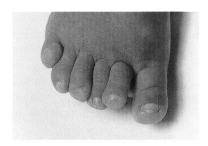

● Figure 10-14 An infant with trisomy 13 has supernumerary digits (polydactyly).

Monosomies

Monosomies exist when each body cell has a missing chromosome, with a total number of 45. The only monosomy compatible with life is Turner syndrome, or monosomy X. It affects about 1 in 2000 newborn girls (March of Dimes, 2005). Clinical manifestations include low posterior hair line and webbing of the neck, short stature, broad skeletal abnormalities, shield-like chest with widely spaced nipples, puffy feet, no toenails, underdeveloped secondary sex characteristics, and infertility (Postellon, 2005). Only about a third are diagnosed as newborns with this syndrome, with the remaining two thirds being diagnosed in early adolescence when they experience primary amenorrhea. Most females with Turner syndrome are of normal intelligence and usually live essentially normal lives (Sterk, 2004).

Polyploidy

Polyploidy causes an increase in the number of haploid sets (23) of chromosomes in a cell. Triploidy refers to three whole sets of chromosomes in a single cell (in humans, a total of 69 chromosomes per cell); tetraploidy refers to four whole sets of chromosomes in a single cell (in humans, a total of 92 chromosomes per cell). Polyploidy usually results in an early spontaneous abortion and is incompatible with life.

Structural Abnormalities

Structural abnormalities involve only part of the chromosome and generally occur as deletions or translocations. Part of the chromosome may be missing or added, or DNA within the chromosome may be rearranged. They include the **cri du chat syndrome, fragile X syndrome,** and many others.

Cri du Chat Syndrome

Cri du chat syndrome, *or cry of the cat,* is caused by a missing piece of chromosome 5. It was named cri du chat based on the distinctive cry in newborns associated with a laryngeal defect, which sounds like a mewing cat. Incidence of the disorder is thought to be approximately 1 in 50,000 live births (Chen, 2005). It is characterized by a cat-like, high-pitched cry in infancy; severe mental retardation; microcephaly; low birth weight and slow growth; hypotonia; failure to thrive; wide-set eyes; small jaw; low-set ears; and various organ malformations. No specific treatment is available for this syndrome. With contemporary interventions, the chance of survival to adulthood is possible. Currently, death occurs in 6 to 8% of the overall population affected with the syndrome. Pneumonia, aspiration pneumonia, and congenital heart defects are the common causes of death (Chen, 2005). Parents should be referred for genetic counseling (Brooks, 2003).

Fragile X Syndrome

Fragile X syndrome, also termed *Martin–Bell syndrome,* is an X-linked chromosomal abnormality. The X chromosome demonstrates breaks and gaps. The syndrome is usually diagnosed by molecular DNA studies. Conservative estimates report that fragile X syndrome affects approximately 1 in 4000 males and 1 in 8000 females. The rate of the female carrier state has been estimated to be as high as 1 in 250 (Jewell, 2004). Typically, a female becomes the carrier and will be mildly affected. The male who receives the X chromosome that has a fragile site will exhibit the full effects of the syndrome. Transmission occurs through carrier mothers and not through unaffected carrier fathers (McKinney et al., 2005). It is characterized by mental retardation, hyperactivity, short attention span, hand flapping, strabismus, hypotonia, speech delay, inflexible behavior, autistic-like behavior, poor eye contact, tactile defensiveness, double jointedness, and perseverative speech (continued repetition of words or phrases). Fragile X syndrome is the most common form of male retardation (Jewell, 2005). Aside from the morbidity associated with mental retardation and cognitive/behavioral/neuropsychological problems, the life span of an individual with fragile X syndrome is unaffected by the disorder. There is no cure for this disorder. Referrals to speech, occupational, and physical therapy are needed, as well as special education and counseling (Hockenberry, 2005).

Inheritance Patterns

Genetic disorders can be categorized into autosomal dominant, autosomal recessive, X linked, or multifactorial. If the mutation occurs on the autosome, the genetic disorder is termed *autosomal.* If the defect is on the X chromosome, the genetic disorder is called *X linked.* Inherited characteristics are passed from parent to child by the genes in each chromosome. These traits are classified as dominant (strong) or recessive (weak).

Autosomal Dominant Inherited Disorders

Autosomal dominant inherited disorders occur when an abnormal gene pair (heterozygous) from one parent is capable of causing disease even though the match-

ing gene from the other parent is normal. The abnormal gene dominates the outcome of the gene pair (Fig. 10-15). The following are characteristics of autosomal dominant inheritance:

- Individuals are affected in succeeding generations.
- Affected individuals will have an affective parent.
- Children will have a 50% chance of being affected.
- Male and female family members are equally affected.
- Severity of the inherited disorder varies among family members.
- Having the gene mutation does not mean an individual will have the disease (Lewis et al., 2004).

Examples of autosomal dominant inherited disorders are familial hypercholesterolemia, neurofibromatosis, breast and ovarian cancer related to BRCA genes, Huntington disease, and hereditary nonpolyposis colorectal cancer (Lea, 2002).

Autosomal Recessive Inherited Disorders

Autosomal recessive inherited disorders are caused by mutations of two gene pairs (homozygous) on a chromosome. Recessive inheritance occurs when both genes of a pair are abnormal, which then produce disease. If only one gene in the pair is abnormal, the disease is not manifested or is only mildly manifested. However, a person with a single defective gene is called a *carrier* (meaning the disease can be passed on to the children; Fig. 10-16). Autosomal recessive inherited disorders are generally seen among particular ethnic groups (e.g., Tay–Sachs disease, which is highest among Jewish people of central and eastern European descent) and tend to occur more often in children whose parents are related by blood (e.g., first cousins). These types of conditions have a horizontal, rather than vertical, inheritance pattern, with relatives in a

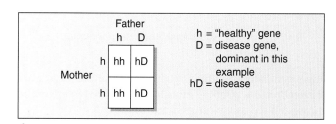

● Figure 10-15 Autosomal dominant inheritance.

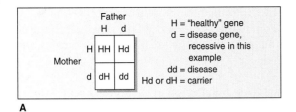

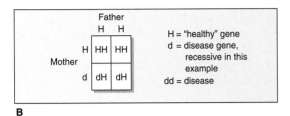

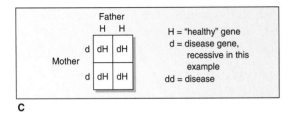

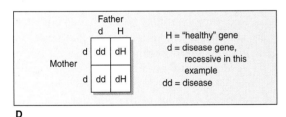

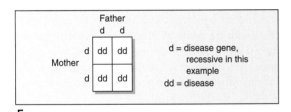

● Figure 10-16 Autosomal recessive inheritance.

X-Linked Inherited Disorders

X-linked inherited disorders can follow dominant or recessive patterns; however, in each case, the gene mutation is on the X chromosome. Usually only men are affected by these disorders because women who carry the mutated gene on one X chromosome have another X chromosome to compensate for the mutation. However, women who carry the mutated gene can transmit the mutated gene to their offspring (Fig. 10-17) (Lewis et al., 2004). The following are characteristics of X-linked inheritance:

- Affected individuals are usually males.
- Females are affected by the condition if it is a dominant X-linked disorder.
- Most affected individuals will have unaffected parents.
- Daughters of an affected male are usually carriers.
- Female carriers have a 50% chance of transmitting the disorder to their sons.
- Sons of an affected male are usually unaffected (Spahis, 2002).

Examples of X-linked disorders are hemophilia, Duchenne dystrophy (childhood muscular dystrophy), and color blindness (red–green).

Multifactorial Inherited Disorders

Multifactorial inherited disorders, or polygenic disorders, are caused by a combination of polygenic (several genes) and environmental factors. Not all conditions are transmitted via a single gene. In multifactorial conditions,

single generation tending to have the condition (Littleton & Engebretson, 2005). The following are characteristics of autosomal recessive inheritance:

- Usually there is a negative family history of the disorder.
- Males and females are equally affected.
- Affected offspring have unaffected parents who are heterozygous.
- Each pregnancy carries a 25% risk of transmitting the condition.
- Offspring have a 50% chance of becoming a trait carrier (Lea, 2002).

Examples of autosomal recessive disorders include sickle-cell disease, thalassemia, phenylketonuria, Tay–Sachs disease, and cystic fibrosis.

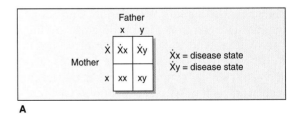

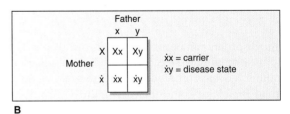

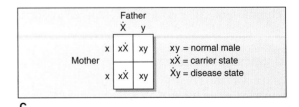

● Figure 10-17 X-linked inheritance.

more than one gene is involved and environmental factors are also involved. Environmental factors might include health status, age of the parents, and/or exposure to pollution. These disorders tend to run in families, but do not show the same inherited characteristics as the single-gene mutation conditions. The cause of many birth defects and common adult-onset health conditions, such as arthritis, diabetes, and cancer, is multifactorial and complex. The following are characteristics of multifactorial inheritance:

- There is an additive effect by having more family members affected.
- Fewer genes are involved if environmental influences are great.
- There is a tendency for gender bias in occurrence rates for some disorders such as pyloric stenosis in males and congenital hip dysplasia in females.
- It is difficult to determine or predict the risk factors of disorders to offspring.
- The disorders vary from mild to severe (Spahis, 2002).

Examples of multifactorial inherited disorders are cleft lip, soft palate, congenital heart disease, neural tube defects, pyloric stenosis, hypertension, diabetes, some heart diseases, cancer, and mental illness (Lowdermilk & Perry, 2004).

Nursing Management

The nurse is likely to interact with the patient and her family in a variety of ways related to genetics—taking a family history, scheduling genetic testing, explaining the purposes of all screening and diagnostic tests, answering questions, and addressing concerns raised by family members.

Nursing Assessment

Nurses in any practice setting can obtain a patient's genetic history during the initial encounter. The purpose is to gather patient and family information that may provide clues regarding whether the patient has a genetic trait, inherited condition, or inherited predisposition (Lea, 2002). At a basic level, all nurses should be able to take a family medical history to assist in identifying those at risk for hereditary conditions, and make a referral to a genetic specialist when appropriate.

At least three generations should be spanned when taking a family history during the initial patient encounter. Box 10-2 presents focused assessment questions to be asked of each family member. Based on the information gathered from the genetic history, the nurse must decide whether a referral is necessary to a genetic specialist or whether further evaluation is needed. Prenatal testing to assess for genetic risks and defects might be used to identify genetic disorders. These tools are described in Table 10-2.

Genetic Counseling

Genetic counseling provides detailed information on the occurrence or risk of recurrence of a genetic disease in

---

BOX 10-2

FOCUSED HEALTH ASSESSMENT: GENETIC HISTORY

What was the cause and age of death for deceased family members?

Does any consanguinity exist between relatives?

Do any serious illnesses or chronic conditions exist? If so, what was the age of onset?

Do any female family members have a history of miscarriages, stillbirths, or diabetes?

Do any female members have a history of alcohol or drug use during pregnancy?

What were the ages of female members during childbearing, especially if older than 35?

Do any family members have mental retardation or developmental delays?

Do any family members have a known or suspected metabolic disorder such as PKU?

Do any family members have an affective disorder such as bipolar disorder?

Have any close relatives been diagnosed with any type of cancer?

What is your ethnic background (explore as related to certain disorders)?

Do any family members have a known or suspected chromosomal disorder?

Do any family members have a progressive neurologic disorder?

Source: Lea, 2003.

---

that family (Greco & Mahon, 2002). Genetic counselors help families make informed decisions about their future based on the assessment of their current risk profile.

When all the previous information has been processed and analyzed, the genetic counselor discusses with the family all the implications of the findings, presents options, and outlines possible outcomes. Genetic counseling is a nondirective process in that family members are given the facts to make their own decisions. Paramount in this whole process is the fact that family members are the ones who have to live with their decisions, and therefore healthcare professionals must respect and support them throughout this period.

Nursing responsibilities related to genetic counseling include

- Interviewing and active listening skills to identify genetic concern
- Knowing basic genetic terminology and inheritance patterns
- Explaining basic concepts of probability and disorder susceptibility
- Safeguarding privacy and confidentiality of patients' genetic information
- Providing complete informed consent to facilitate decisions about genetic testing

Table 10-2 Prenatal Tests to Assess Risk for Genetic Disorders?

Test	Description	Indication	Timing
Family pedigree	A visual representation of a family history	To identify an inheritance pattern that needs further evaluation	Ideally prior to conception; however, may be mapped anytime during pregnancy
Alpha-fetoprotein	A sample of the woman's blood is drawn to evaluate plasma protein that is produced by the fetal liver, yolk sac, and GI tract, and crosses from the amniotic fluid into the maternal blood.	Increased levels might indicate a neural tube defect, Turner syndrome, tetralogy of Fallot, multiple gestation, omphalocele gastroschisis, or hydrocephaly. Decreased levels might indicate Down syndrome or trisomy 18.	Typically performed between 15 and 18 weeks' gestation
Amniocentesis	Amniotic fluid aspirated from the amniotic sac; safety concerns include infection, pregnancy loss, and fetal needle injuries	To perform chromosome analysis, alpha-fetoprotein, DNA markers, viral studies, karyotyping; and identify inborn errors of metabolism	Usually performed between 15 and 20 weeks' gestation to allow for adequate amniotic fluid volume to accumulate; results take 2 to 4 weeks
Chorionic villus sampling	Removal of small tissue specimen from the fetal portion of the placenta, which reflects the fetal genetic makeup; main complications include severe transverse limb defects and spontaneous pregnancy loss	To detect fetal karyotype, sickle-cell anemia, phenylketonuria, Down syndrome, Duchenne muscular dystrophy, and numerous other genetic disorders	Typically performed between 10 and 12 weeks' gestation, with results available in less than a week
Percutaneous umbilical blood sampling	Insertion of a needle directly into a fetal umbilical vessel under ultrasound guidance; two potential complications: fetal hemorrhage and risk of infection	Used for prenatal diagnosis of inherited blood disorders such as hemophilia A, karyotyping, detection of fetal infection, determination of acid–base status, and assessment and treatment of isoimmunization	Generally performed after 16 weeks' gestation

(continued)

Table 10-2 Prenatal Tests to Assess Risk for Genetic Disorders? (continued)

Test	Description	Indication	Timing
Fetal nuchal translucency (FNT)	An intravaginal ultrasound that measures fluid collection in the subcutaneous space between the skin and the cervical spine of the fetus	To identify fetal anomalies; abnormal fluid collection can be associated with genetic disorders (trisomies 13, 18, and 21), Turner syndrome, cardiac deformities, and/or physical anomalies. When the FNT is greater than 2.5 mm, the measurement is considered abnormal.	Performed between 10 and 14 weeks' gestation
Level II ultrasound/fetal scan	Use of high-frequency sound waves to visualize the fetus	Enables evaluation of structural changes to be identified early	Typically performed after 18 weeks' gestation
Triple marker test	Serum screening test using the levels of three maternal serum markers—MSAFP, unconjugated estriol, and hCG—in combination with maternal age to calculate risk	To identify risk for Down syndrome, neural tube defects, and other chromosomal disorders. Elevated hCG combined with lower than normal estriol and MSAFP levels indicate increased risk for Down syndrome or other trisomy condition.	Performed between 16 and 18 weeks' gestation

Sources: Agarwal, 2003; Lowdermilk & Perry, 2004; Littleton & Engebretson, 2005; Mattson & Smith, 2004. Terzioglu & Dinc, 2004; Wald, Rodeck, Hackshaw, Walters, Chitty, & Mackinson, 2003; Youngkin & Davis, 2004.

- Discussing costs of genetic services, benefits, and risks of using health insurance for payment of genetic services; and potential risks of discrimination
- Recognizing and defining ethical, legal, and social issues
- Providing accurate information about risks and benefits of genetic testing
- Providing culturally appropriate media to convey genetic information
- Monitoring patients' emotional reactions after receiving genetic analysis
- Providing information on appropriate local support groups
- Knowing your own limitations and making appropriate referrals (Cook, 2003)

ConsiderTHIS!

As I waited for the genetic counselor to come into the room, my mind was filled with numerous fears and questions. What does an inconclusive amniocentesis really mean? What if this pregnancy produced an abnormal baby? How would I cope with a special child in my life? If only I had gone to the midwife sooner when I thought I was pregnant, but still in denial. Why did I wait so long to admit this pregnancy and get prenatal care? If only I had started to take my folic acid pills when prescribed. Why didn't I research my family's history to know of any hidden genetic conditions? What about my sister with a Down syndrome child? What must I have been thinking? I guess I could play the "what-if" game forever and never come up with answers. It was too late to do anything about this pregnancy because I was in my last trimester. I started to pray silently when the counselor opened the door. . . .

Thoughts: This woman is reviewing the last several months, looking for answers to her greatest fears. Inconclusive screenings can introduce emotional torment for many women as they wait for validating results. Are these common thoughts and fears for many women facing potential genetic disorders? What supportive interventions might the nurse offer?

One of the most important aspects of genetic counseling in which the nurse is involved is follow-up counseling after the couple has been to the specialist. The nurse is in an ideal position to help families review what has been discussed during the genetic counseling sessions and to answer any additional questions they might have. The nurse can provide helpful information, support families in their decisions, and make appropriate referrals within their community.

Summary

Nurses have entered a new era in which the reality of genetic advances and knowledge affects the practice of every nurse. Understanding the contribution of genetic factors to the development of disease is fundamental to the practice of every nurse. The future of genetic technology is here with genetic testing, gene therapy, pharmacogenetics, genetic selection, and other challenges to nursing practice. Nurses need to be ready by educating themselves about conception, fetal development, and genetics to assist their patients in their decision-making process for their future health and welfare.

Genetic advances pose new and unique ethical dilemmas to the issues of privacy, confidentially, access to and justice in health care, and informed health decisions. For nurses, this means ensuring the privacy and confidentiality of genetic information derived from assessments, genetic tests, and other interventions. Nurses will be instrumental in providing patients and their families with the information to make knowledgeable decisions about their reproductive health and their personal lives. Nurses will need additional education in genetics so they can assume their potential roles in the ever-growing field of genetics.

KEY CONCEPTS

- Fertilization takes place in the outer third of the ampulla of the fallopian tube.
- Three embryonic layers of cells are formed as follows:
  - Ectoderm—forms central nervous system, special senses, skin, and glands
  - Mesoderm—forms skeletal, urinary, circulatory, and reproductive systems
  - Endoderm—forms respiratory system, liver, pancreas, and digestive system
- Amniotic fluid surrounds the embryo and increases in volume as the pregnancy progresses, reaching approximately a liter in volume by term.
- At no time during pregnancy is there any direct connection between the blood of the fetus and the blood of the mother, so there is no mixing of blood.
- A specialized connective tissue known as Wharton's jelly surrounds the three blood vessels in the umbilical cord to prevent compression, thus choking off the blood supply and nutrients to the growing life inside.

- The placenta protects the fetus from immune attack by the mother, removes waste products from the fetus, induces the mother to bring more food to the placenta, and, near the time of delivery, produces hormones that mature fetal organs in preparation for life outside the uterus.
- The purpose of fetal circulation is to carry highly oxygenated blood to vital areas (heart and brain) while first shunting it away from less vital ones (lungs and liver).
- Humans have 46 paired chromosomes that are found in all cells of the body, except the ovum and sperm cells, which have just 23 chromosomes.
- Genetic science has the potential to revolutionize health care with regard to national screening programs, predisposition testing, detecting genetic disorders, and pharmacogenetics.
- Research from the Human Genome Project has provided a better understanding of the genetic contribution to disease.
- Each person has a unique genetic constitution, or genotype, made up of approximately 30,000 to 40,000 genes.
- Humans have 46 paired chromosomes that are found in all cells of the body, except the ovum and sperm cells, which have just 23 chromosomes.
- Genetic disorders can be categorized as autosomal dominant, autosomal recessive, X-linked recessive, or multifactorial.
- Genetic counselors help families make informed decisions about their future based on the assessment of their current risk profile.

References

Agarwal, R. (2003). Prenatal diagnosis of chromosomal anomalies: Pictorial essay. *Indian Journal of Radiology and Imaging, 13*, 173–187.

Bailey, V. L. (2003). Fetal development: the story of a baby. *American Collegians Life.* [Online]. Available at www.aclife.org/education/development.html.

Black, J. M., & Hawks, J. H. (2005). *Medical–surgical nursing: Clinical management for positive outcomes* (7th ed.). St. Louis: Elsevier Saunders.

Brooks, D. G. (2003). *Cri du chat syndrome. Medical encyclopedia.* [Online] Available at www.nlm.nih.gov/medlineplus/ency/article/001593.htm.

Burton, H. (2003). Genetics education for primary healthcare nurses. *Primary Healthcare, 13*, 35–38.

Chen, H. (2005). Cri-du-chat syndrome. *eMedicine.* [Online] Available at www.emedicine.com/ped/topic504.htm.

Condon, M. C. (2004). *Women's health: an integrated approach to wellness and illness.* Upper Saddle River, NJ: Pearson Prentice Hall.

Cook, S. S. (2003). Decoding DNA: Understanding genetic implications in nursing care. *AWHONN Lifelines, 7*, 140–144.

Dillon, P. M. (2003). *Nursing health assessment: A critical thinking, case studies approach.* Philadelphia: FA Davis.

Edgar, D. A. (2004). Advances in genetics: Implications for children, families and nurses. *Paediatric Nursing, 16*, 26–29.

Everett, A. D., & Hammill, W. (2002). *Fetal circulation.* Cove Point Foundation. [Online]. Available at www.pted.org/htms/fetal1.htm.

Gilbert, E. S., & Harmon, J. S. (2003). *Manual of high-risk pregnancy & delivery* (3rd ed.). St. Louis: Mosby.

Greco, K. E., & Mahon, S. M. (2002). Genetics: nursing practice enters a new era with credentialing. *Journal of Advanced Nursing Practice, 5*, 99.

Hockenberry, M. J. (2005). *Wong's essentials of pediatric nursing* (7th ed.). St. Louis: Elsevier Mosby.

International Human Genome Sequencing Consortium. (2004). Finishing the euchromatic sequence of the human genome. *Nature, 431*, 931–945.

Jewell, J. (2005). Fragile X syndrome. *eMedicine.* [Online] Available at www.emedicine.com/PED/topic800.htm.

Kilman, H. J. (2003). *From trophoblast to human placenta: encyclopedia of reproduction.* New Haven, CT: Yale University School of Medicine.

Lea, D. H. (2002). What nurses need to know about genetics. *Dimensions of Critical Care Nursing, 21*, 50–62.

Lea, D. H. (2003). How genetics changes daily practice. *Nursing Management, 34*, 19–25.

Lea, D. H., & Williams, J. K. (2002). Genetic testing and screening. *American Journal of Nursing, 102*, 36–49.

Lewis, S. M., Heitkemper, M. M., & Dirksen, S. R. (2004). *Medical–surgical nursing* (6th ed.). St. Louis: Mosby.

Littleton, L. Y., & Engebretson, J. C. (2005). *Maternity nursing care.* Clifton Park, NY: Thomson Delmar Learning.

London, M. L., Ladewig, P. W., Ball, J. W., & Bindler, R. C. (2003). *Maternal–newborn & child nursing: family-centered care.* Upper Saddle River, NJ: Prentice Hall.

Lowdermilk, D. L., & Perry, S. E. (2004). *Maternity & women's healthcare* (8th ed.). St. Louis: Mosby.

March of Dimes. (2005). *Chromosomal abnormalities: Fact sheet.* [Online] Available at http://modimes.org/professionals/ 681_1209.asp.

Mattson, S., & Smith, J. E. (2004). *Core curriculum for maternal–newborn nursing* (3rd ed.). St. Louis: Elsevier Saunders.

Mayo Clinic. (2002). *Klinefelter's syndrome.* [Online] Available at www.mayoclinic.com/invoke.cfm?id=HQ00976.

McKinney, E. S., James, S. R., Murray, S. S., & Ashwill, J. W. (2005). *Maternal–child nursing* (2nd ed.). Philadelphia: Elsevier Saunders.

Murray, S. S., & McKinney, E. S. (2006). *Foundations of maternal–newborn nursing* (4th ed.). Philadelphia: W. B. Saunders.

Olds, S. B., London, M. L., Ladewig, P. A., & Davidson, M. R. (2004). *Maternal–newborn nursing & women's health care* (7th ed.). Upper Saddle River, NJ: Pearson Prentice Hall.

O'Toole, M. T. (2003). *Encyclopedia & medical dictionary of medicine, nursing & allied health* (7th ed.). Philadelphia: W. B. Saunders.

Postellon, D. (2005). Turner syndrome. *eMedicine.* [Online] Available at http://www.emedicine.com/ped/topic2330.htm.

Rasmussen, S. A., Wong, L. C., Yang, Q., May, K. M., & Friedman, J. M. (2003). Population-based analysis of mortality in trisomy 13 and trisomy 18. *Pediatrics, 111*, 777–784.

Ratner, A. (2002). *Fetal development.* Medline plus. [Online] Available at www.nlm.nih.gov/medlineplus/ency/article/002398.htm.

Sabella, J. (2003). Fetal circulation: a review. *Tulane Pulmonary Center.* [Online] Available at www.mcl.tulane.edu/departments/ peds_respcare/Fetcir.htm.

Sloane, E. (2002). *Biology of women* (4th ed.). New York: Delmar.

Spahis, J. (2002). Human genetics: Constructing a family pedigree. *American Journal of Nursing, 102*, 44–49.

Sterk, L. (2004). Congenital anomalies. In M. T. Verklan & M. Walden (Eds.), *Core curriculum for neonatal intensive care nursing* (3rd ed., pp. 858–892). St. Louis: Elsevier Saunders.

Terzioglu, F., & Dinc, L. (2004). Nurses views on their role in genetics. *Journal of Obstetric, Gynecologic, and Neonatal Nursing, 33*, 756–764.

Verklan, M. T., & Walden, M. (2004). *Core curriculum for neonatal intensive care nursing* (3rd ed.). St. Louis: Elsevier Saunders.

Wald, N. J., Rodeck, C., Hackshaw, A. K., Walters, J., Chitty, L., & Mackinson, A. M. (2003). First and second trimester antenatal screening for Down's syndrome: The results of the serum, urine, and ultrasound screening study (SURUSS). *Journal of Medical Screening, 10*, 56–104.

Youngkin, E. Q., & Davis, M. S. (2004). *Women's health: A primary care clinical guide.* Upper Saddle River, NJ: Prentice Hall.

Web Resources

American Society of Human Genetics, **www.faseb.org/genetics/ashg/ashgmenu.htm**
CDC: Office of Genetics, **www.cdc.gov/genetics/activities/ogdp.htm**
5p–Society (Cat Cry Syndrome), **www.fivepminus.org/**
Gene Clinics, **www.geneclinics.org**
Gene Tests, **www.genetests.org**
Genetic Alliance, **www.geneticalliance.org**
Human Genome Project of the US Department of Energy, **www.ornl.gov/hgmis**
International Society of Nurses in Genetics, **www.nursing.creighton.edu/isong**
Klinefelter Syndrome and Associates, **http://genetic.org/ks/**
National Coalition for Health Professional Education in Genetics, **www.nchpeg.org**
National Down Syndrome Society, **www.ndss.org/**
National Human Genome Research Institute, **www.nhgri.gov**
Turner Syndrome Society of the United States, **www.turner-syndrome-us.org**
Virtual Library on Genetics, **www.ornl.gov/TechResources/Human_Genome/genetics.html**
Visible Embryo, **www.visembryo.ucsf.edu**

ChapterWORKSHEET

● MULTIPLE CHOICE QUESTIONS

1. Fertilization usually occurs in the

   a. Fundus of the uterus

   b. Endometrium of the uterus

   c. Upper portion of fallopian tube

   d. Follicular tissue of the ovary

2. Pregnancy tests detect the presence of which hormone in the maternal blood or urine?

   a. hPL

   b. hCG

   c. FSH

   d. TSH

3. Which of the following prenatal tests is used to detect neural tube defects such as spina bifida or anencephaly?

   a. Alpha-fetoprotein

   b. Fetoscopy

   c. CT scan

   d. Coombs test

4. Most health conditions are believed to result from which of the following?

   a. Unrelated to human genetics

   b. Have no underlying cause of disease

   c. Caused by poor lifestyle choices

   d. Have both genetic and environmental factors

5. The first step in establishing the genetic risk for a condition is to

   a. Observe the patient and family over time

   b. Conduct extensive psychological testing

   c. Obtain a thorough family health history

   d. Complete an extensive exclusionary list

6. Increased risk of having offspring with chromosomal abnormalities is greater in women who are

   a. Expecting twins or triples

   b. Emotionally distressed over the pregnancy

   c. Experiencing their first pregnancy

   d. 35 years or older

7. Which of the following is characteristic of Down syndrome?

   a. The infant has 46 paired chromosomes

   b. The male infant has only 23 chromosomes

   c. The female has two extra YY chromosomes

   d. The infant has an extra chromosome number 21

● CRITICAL THINKING EXERCISE

1. Mr. and Mrs. Martin wish to start a family, but they can't agree on something important. Mr. Martin wants his wife to be tested for cystic fibrosis (CF) to see if she is a carrier. Mr. Martin had a brother with CF and watched his parents struggle with the hardship and the expense of caring for him for years, and he doesn't want to experience it in his own life. Mr. Martin has found out he is a CF carrier. Mrs. Martin doesn't want to have the test because she figures that once a baby is in their arms, they will be glad, no matter what.

   a. What information/education is needed for this couple to consider before deciding whether to have the test?

   b. How can you assist this couple in their decision-making process?

   c. What is your role in this situation if you don't agree with their decision?

● STUDY ACTIVITIES

1. Obtain/rent the video entitled *Miracle of Life* and view it for the spectacular photography showing conception and fetal development. What are your impressions? Is the title of this video realistic?

2. Arrange a visit to a local hospital obstetric ultrasound department. Request permission to observe several obstetric ultrasounds and discuss with the technician what the findings may indicate (after the patient has left).

3. Select one of the Helpful Informational Resource Web sites to explore the topic of genetics. Critique the information presented. Was it understandable to a lay person? What specifically did you learn?

Share your findings with your classmates during a discussion group.

4. Draw your own family pedigree representing your family history that identifies their inheritance patterns. Share it with your family to validate its accuracy. What did you discover about your family's past health?

5. Select one of the various prenatal screening tests (alpha-fetoprotein, amniocentesis, chorionic villus sampling, or fetal nuchal translucency) and research it in depth. Role-play with another nursing student how you would explain its purpose, procedure, and potential findings to an expectant couple at risk for a potential fetal abnormality.

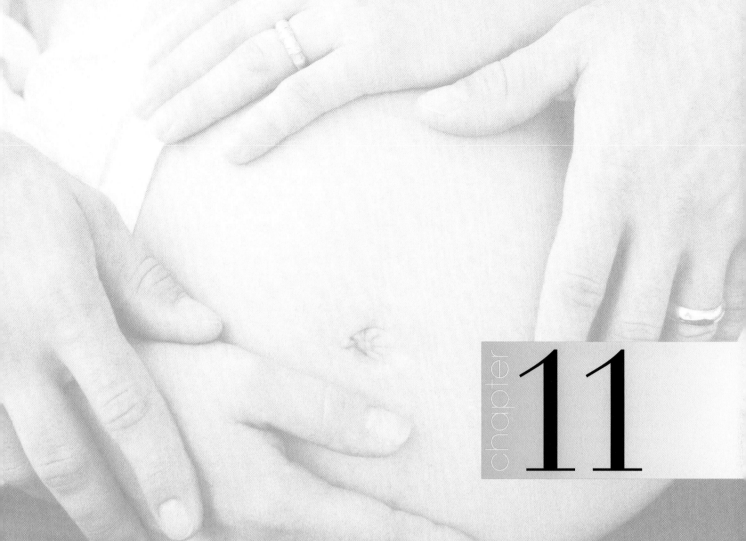

Maternal Adaptation During Pregnancy

ballottement
Braxton Hicks contractions
Chadwick's sign
Goodell's sign
Hegar's sign
linea nigra
physiologic anemia of
    pregnancy
quickening
trimester

LearningOBJECTIVES

After studying the chapter content, the student should be able to accomplish the following:

1. Define the key terms.
2. Discuss maternal physiologic changes that occur during pregnancy.
3. Differentiate between subjective (presumptive), objective (probable), and diagnostic (positive) signs of pregnancy.
4. Explain the emotional and psychological changes that occur during pregnancy.

Pregnancy is a normal life event that involves considerable physical and psychological adjustments for the mother. A pregnancy is described within specific time frames. A **trimester** is a division of pregnancy into three equal parts of 13 weeks each (Lowdermilk & Perry, 2004). Within each time frame or trimester, numerous adaptations take place that facilitate the growth of the fetus. The most obvious are physical changes to accommodate the growing fetus. However, pregnant women also undergo psychological changes as they prepare for parenthood.

Signs and Symptoms of Pregnancy

Traditionally, signs and symptoms of pregnancy have been grouped into the following categories: presumptive, probable, and positive (Table 11-1). The only signs that can determine a positive pregnancy with 100% accuracy, however, are positive signs.

Subjective (Presumptive) Signs

Presumptive signs are those signs experienced by the woman herself. The most obvious presumptive sign of pregnancy is the absence of menstruation. However, just being late or even skipping a period is not a reliable sign

of pregnancy. But if it is accompanied by consistent nausea, fatigue, breast tenderness, and urinary frequency, pregnancy would seem very likely. Presumptive changes are the least reliable indicators of pregnancy because any one of them can be caused by conditions other than pregnancy (Murray et al., 2006).

For example, amenorrhea can be caused by early menopause, endocrine dysfunction, malnutrition, anemia, diabetes mellitus, long-distance running, cancer, or stress. Nausea and vomiting can also have alternative causes such as gastrointestinal disorders, food poisoning, acute infections, or eating disorders. Fatigue could be caused by anemia, stress, or viral infections. Breast tenderness may result from chronic cystic mastitis, premenstrual changes, or the use of oral contraceptives. Lastly, urinary frequency could have a variety of causes outside of pregnancy, such as infection, cystocele, structural disorders, pelvic tumors, or emotional tension (Olds et al., 2004).

Objective (Probable) Signs

Probable signs of pregnancy are those that are apparent on physical examination by a healthcare professional. Common probable signs of pregnancy include softening of the lower uterine segment or isthmus (**Hegar's sign**), softening of the cervix (**Goodell's sign**), and a bluish-purple coloration of the vaginal mucosa and cervix

Table 11-1 Signs and Symptoms of Pregnancy

Presumptive (Time of Occurrence)	Probable (Time of Occurrence)	Positive (Time of Occurrence)
Fatigue (12 wk)	Braxton Hicks contractions (16–28 wk)	Ultrasound verification of embryo or fetus (4–6 wk)
Breast tenderness (3–4 wk)	Positive pregnancy test (4–12 wk)	Fetal movement felt by experienced clinician (20 wk)
Nausea and vomiting (4–14 wk)	Abdominal enlargement (14 wk)	Auscultation of fetal heart tones via Doppler (10–12 wk)
Amenorrhea (4 wk)	**Ballottement** (16–28 wk)	
Urinary frequency (6–12 wk)	Goodell's sign (5 wk)	
Hyperpigmentation of the skin (16 wk)	Chadwick's sign (6–8 wk)	
Fetal movements (quickening; 16–20 wk)	Hegar's sign (6–12 wk)	
Uterine enlargement (7–12 wk)		
Breast enlargement (6 wk)		

Sources: Pillitteri (2003), Matteson (2001), Murray et al. (2006), Wong et al. (2002), and Youngkin & Davis (2004).

(**Chadwick's sign**). Other probable signs include changes in the shape and size of the uterus, abdominal enlargement, and **Braxton Hicks contractions.**

Along with these physical signs, pregnancy tests are also considered a probable sign of pregnancy. Several pregnancy tests are available (Table 11-2). The tests vary in sensitivity, specificity, and accuracy, influenced by the length of gestation, specimen concentration, presence of blood, and some drugs (Youngkin & Davis, 2004).

Human chorionic gonadotropin (hCG) is the earliest biochemical marker for pregnancy, and many pregnancy tests are based on the recognition of hCG or a beta subunit of hCG (Lowdermilk & Perry, 2004). hCG levels in normal pregnancy usually double every 48 to 72 hours until they reach a peak at approximately 60 to 70 days after fertilization, then decrease to a plateau at 100 to 130 days of pregnancy (Youngkin & Davis, 2004). This elevation of hCG corresponds to the morning sickness period of approximately 6 to 12 weeks during early pregnancy.

Home pregnancy tests are available over the counter and have become quite popular since their introduction in 1975. These tests are very sensitive, cost-effective, and faster than traditional laboratory pregnancy tests. Enzyme-linked immunosorbent assay (ELISA) technology is the basis for most home pregnancy tests. More than 20 brands have become available. Many manufacturers claim that the tests are accurate more than 99% of the time, but recent research has not validated their claims (Cole et al., 2004). Therefore, clients are advised to have their pregnancy test repeated and confirmed by their health care provider.

Although probable signs suggest pregnancy and are more reliable than presumptive signs, they still are not 100% reliable in confirming a pregnancy. For example, uterine tumors, polyps, infection, and pelvic congestion can cause changes to uterine shape, size, and consistency. And, although pregnancy tests are used to establish the diagnosis of pregnancy when the physical signs are still inconclusive, they are not completely reliable, because conditions other than pregnancy (e.g., ovarian cancer, choriocarcinoma, hydatidiform mole) can also elevate hCG levels.

Consider THIS!

Jim and I decided to start our family so I stopped taking the pill 3 months ago. One morning when I got out of bed to take the dog out, I felt queasy and light-headed. I sure hoped I wasn't coming down with the flu. By the end of the week, I was feeling really tired and started taking naps in the afternoon. In addition, I seemed to be going to the bathroom frequently, despite not drinking much fluid. When my breasts started to tingle and ache, I decided to make an appointment with my doctor to see what "illness" I had contracted.

After listening to my list of physical complaints, the office nurse asked me if there would be a chance that I might be pregnant. My eyes opened wide and I somehow thought I had missed the link between my symptoms with pregnancy. I started to think about when my last period was and it had been 2 months ago. The office ran a pregnancy test and much to my surprise—it was positive!

Table 11-2 Selected Pregnancy Tests

Type	Specimen	Example	Remarks
Agglutination inhibition tests	Urine	Pregnosticon, Gravindex	If hCG is present in urine, agglutination does not occur, which is positive for pregnancy; reliable 14–21 days after conception; 95% accuracy in diagnosing pregnancy
Radioimmunoassay	Blood serum or urine	Hospital laboratories	Uses radioisotopes to detect beta subunit of hCG; reliable 1 week after conception; 99% accuracy in diagnosing pregnancy
Radioreceptor assay	Blood serum	Biocept-G	Measures ability of blood sample to inhibit the binding of radiolabeled hCG to receptors; reliable 6–8 days after conception; 99% accuracy in diagnosing pregnancy
Enzyme-linked immunosorbent assay	Blood serum or urine	Over-the-counter home/office pregnancy tests; Precise	Uses an enzyme to bond with hCG in the urine if present; reliable 4 days after implantation; 99% accuracy if hCG specific

Sources: Hatcher et al. (2004), Cunningham et al. (2005), Pagana & Pagana (2003), and Schnell et al. (2003).

Thoughts: Many women stop contraceptives in an attempt to achieve pregnancy, but miss the early signs. This woman was experiencing several signs of early pregnancy—urinary frequency, fatigue, morning nausea, and breast tenderness. What advice can the nurse give this woman to ease these symptoms? What additional education related to her pregnancy would be appropriate at this time?

Positive Signs

Usually within 2 weeks after a missed period, enough subjective symptoms are present so that a woman can be reasonably sure she is pregnant. However, an experienced healthcare professional can confirm her suspicions by identifying positive signs of pregnancy. The positive signs of pregnancy confirm that a fetus is growing in the uterus. Visualizing the fetus by ultrasound, palpating for fetal movements, and hearing a fetal heartbeat are all signs that make the diagnosis of pregnancy a certainty.

Once pregnancy is confirmed, the healthcare professional will set up a schedule of prenatal visits to assess the woman and her fetus throughout the entire pregnancy. Beginning with the initial visit, the process of assessment and education then continues throughout the pregnancy (see Chapter 13).

Physiologic Adaptations During Pregnancy

Every system of a woman's body changes during pregnancy, with startling rapidity to accommodate the needs of the growing fetus. The physical aspects of pregnancy occur within a variable time frame and are sometimes uncomfortable. In addition, every woman reacts uniquely to the myriad changes that occur.

Reproductive System Adaptations

Uterus

During the first few months of pregnancy, estrogen stimulates uterine growth, with the uterus undergoing a tremendous increase in size throughout pregnancy. At full term, the uterus weighs 2 lb, is about five to six times larger than the nonpregnant uterus, and has increased its capacity by 2000 times to accommodate the developing fetus (Sloan, 2002). To put this growth into perspective, please note the following:

- Size has increased 20 times that of nonpregnant size
- Walls thin to 1.5 cm or less from a solid globe to a hollow vessel
- Weight increases from 2 oz to approximately 2 lb at term
- Volume capacity increases from 2 tsp to 1 gal (Mattson & Smith, 2004)

Uterine growth occurs as a result of both hyperplasia and hypertrophy of the myometrial cells, which do not increase much in number but do increase in size. Blood vessels elongate, enlarge, dilate, and sprout new branches to support and nourish the growing muscle tissue, and the increase in uterine weight is accompanied by a large increase in uterine blood flow necessary to perfuse the uterine muscle and accommodate the growing fetus (Matteson, 2001).

Uterine contractility is evidently enhanced as well. Spontaneous, irregular, and painless contractions, called Braxton Hicks contractions, begin during the first trimester. These contractions continue throughout pregnancy, becoming especially noticeable during the last month, when they function in thinning out or effacing the cervix before birth (see Chapter 13 for more information).

Changes in the uterus occurring during the first 6 to 8 weeks of gestation produce some of the typical findings, including a positive Hegar's sign. This softening and compressibility of the lower uterine segment results in exaggerated uterine anteflexion during the early months of pregnancy, which adds to urinary frequency (Lowdermilk & Perry, 2004).

The uterus remains in the pelvic cavity for the first 3 months of pregnancy, after which it progressively ascends into the abdomen (Fig. 11-1). As the uterus grows, it

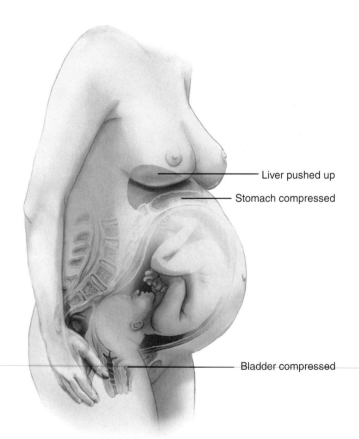

Liver pushed up

Stomach compressed

Bladder compressed

● Figure 11-1 The growing uterus in the abdomen.

presses on the urinary bladder and causes the increased frequency of urination experienced during early pregnancy.

Uterine enlargement occurs in a linear fashion (1 cm/week), and the uterus remains globular and ovoid in shape (Youngkin & Davis, 2004). By 20 weeks' gestation, the fundus, or top of the uterus, is at the level of the umbilicus and measures 20 cm. A monthly measurement of the height of the top of the uterus in centimeters, which corresponds to the number of gestational weeks, is commonly used to date the pregnancy. After 36 weeks' gestation, this measurement is no longer reliable because of the beginning of fetal descent.

The fundus reaches its highest level at the xiphoid process at approximately 36 weeks. Between 38 to 40 weeks, fundal height drops as the fetus begins to descend and engage into the pelvis. Because it pushes against the diaphragm, many women experience shortness of breath. By 40 weeks, the fetal head begins to descend and engage in the pelvis, which is termed *lightening*. For the woman who is pregnant for the first time, lightening usually occurs at approximately 2 weeks before the onset of labor; for the woman who is experiencing her second or subsequent pregnancy, this usually occurs at the onset of labor. Although breathing becomes easier because of this descent, the pressure on the urinary bladder now increases, and women experience urinary frequency again.

Cervix

Between weeks 6 and 8 of pregnancy, the cervix begins to soften (Goodell's sign) due to vasocongestion. Along with the softening, the endocervical glands increase in size and number, and produce more cervical mucus. Under the influence of progesterone, a thick mucous plug is formed that blocks the cervical os and protects the opening from bacterial invasion. At about the same time, increased vascularization of the cervix causes Chadwick's sign.

Vagina

During pregnancy, there is increased vascularity because of estrogen influences, resulting in pelvic congestion and hypertrophy of the vagina in preparation for the distention needed for birth. The vaginal mucosa thickens, the connective tissue begins to loosen, the smooth muscle begins to hypertrophy, and the vaginal vault begins to lengthen (Lowdermilk & Perry, 2004).

Vaginal secretions become more acidic, white, and thick. Most women experience an increase in a whitish vaginal discharge, called *leukorrhea*, during pregnancy. This is normal except when it is accompanied by itching and irritation, possibly suggesting *Candida albicans,* a monilial vaginitis, which is a very common occurrence in this glycogen-rich environment (Murray et al., 2006). Monilial vaginitis is a benign fungal condition that is uncomfortable for women, but it can be transmitted from an infected mother to her newborn at birth. Neonates develop an oral infection known as thrush, which presents as white patches on the mucus membranes of their mouths. It is self-limiting and is treated with local antifungal agents.

Ovaries

The increased blood supply to the ovaries causes them to enlarge until approximately the 12th to 14th week of gestation. The ovaries are not palpable after that time because the uterus fills the pelvic cavity. Ovulation ceases during pregnancy because of the elevated levels of estrogen and progesterone, which block secretion of FSH and luteinizing hormone (LH) from the anterior pituitary. The ovaries are very active in hormone production to support the pregnancy until about weeks 6 to 7, when the corpus luteum regresses and the placenta takes over the major production of progesterone.

Breasts

The breasts increase in fullness, become tender, and grow larger throughout pregnancy under the influence of estrogen and progesterone. The breasts become highly vascular, and veins become visible under the skin. The nipples will become larger and more erect. Both the nipples and surrounding areola become deeply pigmented, and sebaceous glands become prominent. These sebaceous glands keep the nipples lubricated for breast-feeding.

Changes that occur in the connective tissue of the breasts, along with the tremendous growth, can lead to striae (stretch marks) in approximately half of all pregnant women (Littleton & Engebretson, 2005). Initially they appear as pink-to-purple lines on the skin and eventually fade to a sliver color. Although they become less conspicuous in time, they never completely disappear.

Creamy, yellowish breast fluid called *colostrum* can be expressed by the third trimester. This fluid provides nourishment for the breast-feeding newborn during the first few days of life (see Chapters 15 and 16 for more information).

General Body System Adaptations

In addition to changes in the reproductive system, the pregnant woman also experiences changes in virtually every other body system in response to the growing fetus.

Gastrointestinal System

The gastrointestinal (GI) system begins in the oral cavity and ends at the rectum. During pregnancy, the gums become hyperemic, swollen, and friable with a tendency to bleed easily. This change is influenced by estrogen and increased proliferation of blood vessels and circulation to the mouth. In addition, the saliva produced in the mouth becomes more acidic. Some women complain about excessive salivation, termed *ptyalism*, which may be caused by the decrease in unconscious swallowing by the woman when nauseated (Cunningham et al., 2005).

Smooth muscle relaxation and decreased peristalsis occur related to the progesterone influence. Elevated progesterone levels cause smooth muscle relaxation, which results in delayed gastric emptying and decreased peristalsis. Transition time of food throughout the GI tract may be so much slower that more water than normal is reabsorbed, leading to bloating and constipation. Constipation can also result from low-fiber food choices, reduced fluid intake, use of iron supplements, decreased activity level, and intestinal displacement secondary to a growing uterus. Constipation, increased venous pressure, and the pressure of the gravid uterus contribute to the formation of hemorrhoids.

The slowed gastric emptying combined with relaxation of the cardiac sphincter allows reflux, which causes heartburn. Acid indigestion or heartburn (*pyrosis*) seems to be a universal problem for most pregnant women. It is caused by regurgitation of the stomach contents into the upper esophagus and may be associated with the generalized relaxation of the entire digestive system. Over-the-counter antacids will usually relieve the symptoms. They should be taken with the healthcare provider's awareness and only as directed.

The emptying time of the gallbladder is prolonged secondary to the smooth muscle relaxation from progesterone. Hypercholesterolemia can follow, increasing the risk of gallstone formation (Olds et al., 2004).

Nausea and vomiting, better known as *morning sickness,* plagues about 50 to 80% of pregnant women (Sloan, 2002). Although it occurs most often in the morning, the nauseated feeling can last all day in some women. The highest incidence of morning sickness is between 6 to 12 weeks. The physiologic basis for morning sickness is still debatable. It has been linked to the high levels of hCG, high levels of circulating estrogens, reduced stomach acidity, and the lowered tone and motility of the digestive tract (Condon, 2004).

Cardiovascular System

Cardiovascular changes occur early during pregnancy to meet the demands of the enlarging uterus and the placenta for more blood and more oxygen. Perhaps the most striking cardiac alteration occurring during pregnancy is the increase in blood volume.

Blood Volume

Blood volume increases by approximately 1500 mL, or 40 to 50% above nonpregnant levels (Cunningham et al., 2005). The increase is made up of 1000 mL plasma plus 450 mL red blood cells (RBCs). It begins at weeks 10 to 12, peaks at weeks 32 to 34, and decreases slightly at week 40.

The increase in blood volume is needed to provide adequate hydration of fetal and maternal tissues, to supply blood flow to perfuse the enlarging uterus, and to provide a reserve to compensate for blood loss at birth and during postpartum (Hockenberry, 2005). Additionally, this increase is necessary to meet the increased metabolic needs of the mother and to meet the need for increased perfusion of other organs, especially the woman's kidneys, because she is excreting waste products for herself and the fetus.

Cardiac Output and Heart Rate

Cardiac output is the product of stroke volume and heart rate. It increases from 30 to 50% over the nonpregnant rate by the 32nd week of pregnancy and declines to about a 20% increase at 40 weeks' gestation (Lowdermilk & Perry, 2004). Heart rate increases by 10 to 15 bpm between 14 and 20 weeks of gestation and persists to term. There is slight hypertrophy or enlargement of the heart during pregnancy. This is probably to accommodate the increase in blood volume and cardiac output. The heart works harder and pumps more blood to supply the oxygen needs of the fetus as well as those of the mother. A woman with preexisting heart disease may become symptomatic and begin to decompensate during the time the blood volume peaks. She warrants close monitoring during 28 to 35 weeks' gestation.

Blood Pressure

Blood pressure declines slightly during pregnancy as a result of peripheral vasodilation caused by progesterone, reaching a low point at 22 weeks' gestation, and thereafter increasing to prepregnant levels until term (Sloan, 2002). During the first trimester, blood pressure typically remains at the prepregnancy level. During the second trimester, the blood pressure decreases 5 to 10 mmHg and thereafter returns to first trimester levels (Hockenberry, 2005).

When the pregnant woman assumes a supine position, most commonly during the third trimester, the expanding uterus exerts pressure on the inferior vena cava, causing a reduction in blood flow to the heart. Called *supine hypotension syndrome,* the woman experiences dizziness, clamminess, and a marked decrease in blood pressure. Placing the woman in the left lateral recumbent position will correct this syndrome and optimize cardiac output and uterine perfusion.

Blood Components

The number of RBCs also increases about 30%, depending on the amount of iron available. This increase is necessary to transport the additional oxygen required during pregnancy. Although there is an increase in RBCs, there is a greater increase in the plasma volume as a result of hormonal factors and sodium and water retention. Because the plasma increase exceeds the increase of RBC production, normal hemoglobin and hematocrit values decrease. This state of hemodilution is referred to as **physiologic anemia of pregnancy** (Lowdermilk & Perry, 2004).

Iron requirements during pregnancy increase because of the demands of the growing fetus and increase in maternal blood volume. The fetal tissues take predominance over the mother's tissues with respect to use of iron stores. With the accelerated production of RBCs, iron is necessary for hemoglobin formation, the oxygen-carrying component of RBCs. Many women enter pregnancy in a depleted iron state and thus need supplementation to meet the extra demands of their growth state.

Both fibrin and plasma fibrinogen levels increase, along with various blood-clotting factors. These factors make pregnancy a hypercoagulable state. These changes, coupled with venous stasis secondary to venous pooling, which occurs during late pregnancy after long periods of standing in the upright position with the pressure exerted by the uterus on the large pelvic veins, contribute to slowed venous return, pooling, and dependent edema. These factors also increase the woman's risk for venous thrombosis (Ladewig, London, & Davidson, 2006).

Respiratory System

The growing uterus and the increased production of the hormone progesterone cause the lungs to function differently during pregnancy. During the course of the pregnancy, the length of space available to house the lungs decreases as the uterus puts pressure on the diaphragm and causes it to shift upward. The growing uterus does change the size and shape of the thoracic cavity, but diaphragmatic excursion increases, chest circumference increases by 2 to 3 in, and the transverse diameter increases by an inch, allowing a larger tidal volume, as evidence by deeper breathing (Littleton & Engebretson, 2005). Tidal volume or the volume of air inhaled increases gradually by 30 to 40% as the pregnancy progresses. As a result of these changes, the women's breathing becomes more diaphragmatic than abdominal (Matteson, 2001).

A pregnant woman breathes faster and more deeply because more oxygen is needed for herself and the fetus. Changes in the structures of the respiratory system take place to prepare the body for the enlarging uterus and increased lung volume (Mattson & Smith, 2004). All these structural alterations are temporary and revert back to their prepregnant state at the conclusion of the pregnancy.

Increased vascularity of the respiratory tract is influenced by increased estrogen levels, leading to congestion. This congestion gives rise to nasal and sinus stuffiness, epistaxis (nosebleed), and changes in the tone and quality of the woman's voice (Youngkin & Davis, 2004).

Renal/Urinary System

Changes in renal structure occur from hormonal influences of estrogen and progesterone, pressure from an enlarging uterus, and an increase in maternal blood volume. Like the heart, the kidneys work harder throughout the pregnancy. Changes in kidney function occur to accommodate a heavier workload while maintaining a stable electrolyte balance and blood pressure. As more blood flows to the kidneys, the glomerular filtration rate (GFR) increases, leading to an increase in urine flow and volume, substances delivered to the kidneys, and filtration and excretion of water and solutes (Littleton & Engebretson, 2005).

Anatomically, the kidneys enlarge during pregnancy. Each kidney increases in length and weight as a result of

hormonal effects that cause increased tone and decreased motility of the smooth muscle. The renal pelvis becomes dilated. The ureters (especially the right ureter) elongate, widen, and become more curved above the pelvic rim as early as the 10th gestational week (Ladewig, London, & Davidson, 2006). Progesterone is thought to cause both these changes because of its relaxing influence on smooth muscle.

Blood flow to the kidneys increases by 35 to 60% as a result of the increase in cardiac output. This in turn leads to an increase in the GFR by as much as 50% starting during the second trimester. This elevation continues until birth (Littleton & Engebretson, 2005).

The activity of the kidneys normally increases when a person lies down and decreases on standing. This difference is amplified during pregnancy, which is one reason a pregnant woman feels the need to urinate frequently while trying to sleep. Late in the pregnancy, the increase in kidney activity is even greater when a pregnant woman lies on her side rather than her back. Lying on the side relieves the pressure that the enlarged uterus puts on the vena cava carrying blood from the legs. Subsequently, venous return to the heart increases, leading to increased cardiac output. Increased cardiac output results in increased renal perfusion and glomerular filtration (Mattson & Smith, 2004).

Musculoskeletal System

Changes in the musculoskeletal system are progressive, resulting from the influence of hormones, fetal growth, and maternal weight gain. By the 10th to 12th week of pregnancy, the ligaments that hold the sacroiliac joints and the pubis symphysis in place begin to soften and stretch, and the articulations between the joints widen and become more movable (Sloan, 2002). The relaxation of the joints maximizes by the beginning of the third trimester. The purpose of these changes is to increase the size of the pelvic cavity and to make delivery easier.

The postural changes of pregnancy—an increased swayback and an upper spine extension to compensate for the enlarging abdomen—coupled with the loosening of the sacroiliac joints may result in lower back pain. The woman's center of gravity shifts forward, requiring a realignment of the spinal curvatures. An increase in the normal lumbosacral curve (lordosis) occurs and a compensatory curvature in the cervicodorsal area develops to assist her in maintaining her balance (Fig. 11-2). In addition, relaxation and increased mobility of joints occur because of the hormones progesterone and relaxin, which lead to the characteristic "waddle gait" that pregnant women demonstrate toward term. Increased weight gain can add to this discomfort by further accentuating the lumbar and dorsal curves (Lowdermilk & Perry, 2004).

Integumentary System

The skin of pregnant women undergoes hyperpigmentation primarily as a result of estrogen, progesterone, and

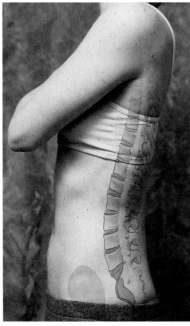

A. Early pregnancy

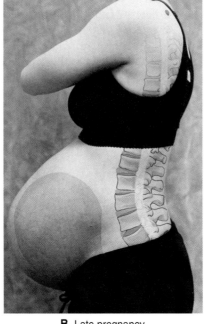

B. Late pregnancy

● Figure 11-2 Postural changes during (**A**) the first trimester and (**B**) the third trimester.

melanocyte-stimulating hormone levels. These changes are mainly seen on the nipples, areolae, umbilicus, perineum, and axillae. Although many integumentary changes disappear after giving birth, some only fade. Many pregnant women express concern about stretch marks, skin color changes, and their hair falling out. Unfortunately, little is known about how to avoid these changes.

Complexion changes are not unusual. The increased pigmentation that occurs on the breasts and genitalia also develops on the face to form the "mask of pregnancy," or facial melasma. This is a blotchy, brownish pigment that covers the forehead and cheeks in dark-haired women. Fortunately most fade as the hormones subside at the end of the pregnancy, but some may linger beyond the pregnancy. The skin in the middle of the abdomen may develop a pigmented line called **linea nigra,** which extends from the umbilicus to the pubic area (Fig. 11-3).

Striae gravidarum, or stretch marks, are irregular reddish streaks that may appear on the abdomen, breasts, and buttocks in about half of pregnant women after month 5 of gestation. They result from reduced connective tissue strength resulting from the elevated adrenal steroid levels and stretching of the structures secondary to growth (Ladewig, London, & Davidson, 2006).

Another skin manifestation, believed to be secondary to high estrogen levels, is the appearance of small, spiderlike blood vessels called *vascular spiders.* They may appear in the skin, usually above the waist and on the neck, thorax, face, and arms. They are especially obvious in white women and typically disappear after childbirth (Sloan, 2002). Palmar erythema is a well-delineated pinkish area on the palmar surface of the hands. This integu-

mentary change is also related to elevated estrogen levels (Lowdermilk & Perry, 2004).

Some women also notice a decline in hair growth during pregnancy. The hair follicles normally undergo a growing and resting phase. The resting phase is followed by a loss of hairs, which is then replaced by new ones. During pregnancy, fewer hair follicles go into the resting phase. After delivery, the body catches up with subsequent hair loss for several months (Ladewig, London, & Davidson, 2006).

Endocrine System

The endocrine system undergoes many changes during pregnancy, because hormonal changes are essential in meeting the needs of the growing fetus. Hormonal changes play a major role in controlling the supplies of maternal glucose, amino acids, and lipids to the fetus. Although estro-

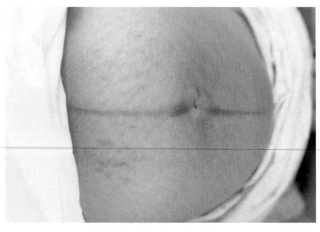

● Figure 11-3 Linea nigra.

gen and progesterone are the main hormones involved in pregnancy changes, other endocrine glands and hormones change during pregnancy.

Thyroid Gland

The thyroid gland enlarges slightly and becomes more active during pregnancy as a result of increased vascularity and hyperplasia. Increased gland activity results in an increase in thyroid hormone secretion starting during the first trimester and tapering off within a few weeks after birth to return to normal limits (Ladewig, London, & Davidson, 2006). With an increase in the secretion of thyroid hormones, the basal metabolic rate (BMR; the amount of oxygen consumed by the body over a unit of time in milliliters per minute) progressively increases by 25% along with heart rate and cardiac output (Littleton & Engebretson, 2005).

Pituitary Gland

The pituitary gland, also known as the *hypophysis*, is a small, oval gland about the size of a pea that is connected to the hypothalamus by a stalk called the *infundibulum*. During pregnancy, the pituitary gland enlarges and returns to normal size after birth.

The anterior lobe of the pituitary is glandular tissue and produces multiple hormones. The release of these hormones is regulated by releasing and inhibiting hormones produced by the hypothalamus.

Some of these anterior pituitary hormones induce other glands to secrete their hormones. The increase in blood levels of the hormones produced by the final target glands (e.g., the ovary or thyroid) inhibits the release of anterior pituitary hormones as follows:

- FSH and LH secretion are inhibited during pregnancy, probably as a result of hCG produced by the placenta and corpus luteum, and the increased secretion of prolactin by the anterior pituitary gland. They remain decreased until after delivery.
- Thyroid-stimulating hormone (TSH) is reduced during the first trimester but usually returns to normal for the remainder of the pregnancy. Decreased TSH is thought to be one of the factors, along with elevated hCG levels, associated with morning sickness, nausea, and vomiting during the first trimester.
- Growth hormone (GH) is an anabolic hormone that promotes protein synthesis. It stimulates most body cells to grow in size and divide, facilitating the use of fats for fuel and conserving glucose. During pregnancy, there is a decrease in the number of GH-producing cells and a corresponding decrease in GH blood levels. The action of human placental lactogen (hPL) is thought to decrease the need for and use of GH.
- During pregnancy, an increase in the number of prolactin-secreting cells (lactotrophs) and a significant increase in the blood level of this hormone occur. Prolactin stimulates the glandular production of colostrum.

During pregnancy, the ability of prolactin to produce milk is opposed by progesterone. As soon as the placenta is delivered, the opposition is removed, and lactation can begin. Levels of prolactin decrease after delivery, even in the lactating mother. Prolactin is produced in spurts, in response to the infant's sucking (Cunningham et al., 2005).

- Melanocyte-stimulating hormone (MSH), another anterior pituitary hormone, increases during pregnancy. For many years, its increase was thought to be responsible for many of the skin changes of pregnancy, particularly changes in skin pigmentation (e.g., darkening of the areola, melasma, and linea nigra). However, current belief attributes the skin changes to estrogen (and possibly progesterone) as well as the increase in MSH.

The two hormones oxytocin and antidiuretic hormone (ADH) released by the posterior pituitary are actually synthesized in the hypothalamus. They migrate along nerve fibers to the posterior pituitary and are stored until stimulated to be released into the general circulation.

Oxytocin is released by the posterior pituitary gland, and its production gradually increases as the fetus matures (Mattson & Smith, 2004). Oxytocin is responsible for uterine contractions, both before and after delivery. The muscle layers of the uterus (myometrium) become more sensitive to oxytocin near term. Toward the end of a term pregnancy, levels of progesterone decline and contractions that were previously suppressed by progesterone begin to occur more frequently and with stronger intensity. This change in the hormonal levels is believed to be one of the initiators of labor.

Oxytocin is responsible for stimulating uterine contractions that bring about delivery. Contractions lead to cervical thinning and dilation. They also exert pressure, helping the fetus to descend in the pelvis for eventual delivery. After delivery, oxytocin secretion continues, causing the myometrium to contract and helping to constrict the uterine blood vessels, decreasing the amount of vaginal bleeding after delivery.

Oxytocin is also responsible for milk ejection during breast-feeding. Stimulation of the breasts through sucking or touching stimulates the secretion of oxytocin from the posterior pituitary gland. Oxytocin causes contraction of the myoepithelial cells in the lactating mammary gland. With breast-feeding, uterine cramping often occurs, which signals that oxytocin is being released.

Vasopressin (ADH) functions to inhibit or prevent the formation of urine via vasoconstriction, which results in increased blood pressure. Vasopressin also exhibits an antidiuretic effect and plays an important role in the regulation of water balance (Olds et al., 2004).

Pancreas

The pancreas is an exocrine organ, supplying digestive enzymes and buffers, and an endocrine organ. The endocrine pancreas consists of islets of Langerhans, which are groups of cells scattered throughout, each containing four cells types. One of the cell types is the beta cell, which produces insulin. Insulin lowers blood glucose by increasing the rate of glucose uptake and utilization by most body cells. The growing fetus has large needs for glucose, amino acids, and lipids. Even during early pregnancy the fetus makes demands on the maternal glucose stores. Ideally, hormonal changes of pregnancy help meet fetal needs without putting the mother's metabolism out of balance.

Women's insulin secretion works on a "supply-versus-demand" mode. As the demand to meet the needs of pregnancy increase, more insulin is secreted. Maternal insulin does not cross the placenta, so the fetus must produce his or her own supply to maintain glucose control (see Box 11-1 for information about pregnancy, glucose, and insulin).

During the first half of pregnancy, much of the maternal glucose is diverted to the growing fetus and thus the mother's glucose levels are low. hPL and other hormonal antagonists increase during the second half of pregnancy.

BOX 11-1

PREGNANCY, INSULIN, AND GLUCOSE

- During early pregnancy, there is a decrease in maternal glucose levels because of the heavy fetal demand for glucose. The fetus is also drawing amino acids and lipids from the mother, decreasing the mother's ability to synthesize glucose. Maternal glucose is diverted across the placenta to assist the growing embryo/fetus during early pregnancy, and thus levels decline in the mother. As a result, maternal glucose concentrations decline to a level that would be considered "hypoglycemic" in a nonpregnant woman. During early pregnancy there is also a decrease in maternal insulin production and insulin levels.
- The pancreas is responsible for the production of insulin, which facilitates entry of glucose into cells. Although glucose and other nutrients easily cross the placenta to the fetus, *insulin does not*. Therefore, the fetus must produce its own insulin to facilitate the entry of glucose into its own cells.
- After the first trimester, hPL from the placenta and steroids (cortisol) from the adrenal cortex act against insulin. hPL acts as an antagonist against maternal insulin, and thus more insulin must be secreted to counteract the increasing levels of hPL and cortisol during the last half of pregnancy.
- Prolactin, estrogen, and progesterone are also thought to oppose insulin As a result, glucose is less likely to enter the mother's cells and is more likely to cross over the placenta to the fetus (Cunningham et al., 2005).

Therefore, the mother must produce more insulin to overcome the resistance by these hormones.

If the mother has normal beta cells of the islets of Langerhans, there is usually no problem meeting the demands for extra insulin. However, if a woman has inadequate numbers of beta cells, she may be unable to produce enough insulin and will develop glucose intolerance during pregnancy. If the woman has glucose intolerance, she is not able to meet the increasing demands and her blood glucose level increases.

Adrenal Glands

Pregnancy does not cause much change in the size of the adrenal glands themselves, but there are changes in some secretions and activity. One of the key changes is the marked increase in cortisol secretion, which regulates carbohydrate and protein metabolism and is helpful in times of stress. Although pregnancy is considered a normal condition, it is a time of stress for a woman's body. Cortisol increases in response to increased estrogen levels throughout pregnancy and returns to normal levels within 6 weeks postpartum (Ladewig, London, & Davidson, 2006).

During the stress of pregnancy, cortisol

- Helps keep up the level of glucose in the plasma by breaking down noncarbohydrate sources, such as amino and fatty acids, to make glycogen. Glycogen, stored in the liver, is easily broken down to glucose when needed so that glucose is available in times of stress.
- Breaks down proteins to repair tissues and manufacture enzymes
- Has anti-insulin, anti-inflammatory, and antiallergic actions
- Is needed to make the precursors of adrenaline, which the adrenal medulla produces and secretes (Cunningham et al., 2005)

Aldosterone, also secreted by the adrenal glands, is increased during pregnancy. It normally regulates absorption of sodium from the distal tubules of the kidney. During pregnancy, progesterone allows salt to be "wasted" (or lost) in the urine. Aldosterone is produced in increased amounts by the adrenal glands as early as 15 weeks of pregnancy (Dickey, 2003).

Prostaglandin Secretion During Pregnancy

Prostaglandins are not protein or steroid hormones; they are chemical mediators, or "local" hormones. Although hormones circulate in the blood to influence distant tissues, prostaglandins act locally on adjacent cells. The fetal membranes of the amniotic sac—the amnion and chorion—are both believed to be involved in the production of prostaglandins. Various maternal and fetal tissues, as well as the amniotic fluid itself, are considered to be sources of prostaglandins, but details about their composition and sources are limited. It is widely believed that prostaglandins play a part in softening the cervix, initiating and/or maintaining labor, but the exact mechanism is unclear.

Placental Secretion

The placenta is a unique kind of endocrine gland; it has a feature possessed by no other endocrine organ— the ability to form protein and steroid hormones. Very early during pregnancy, the placenta begins to produce hormones:

- hCG
- hPL
- Relaxin
- Progesterone
- Estrogen

Table 11-3 summarizes the role of these hormones.

Immune System

During pregnancy, the immune system also undergoes changes. These changes include

- Decreased resistance to infection resulting from the depressed leukocyte function
- Improvement in certain autoimmune conditions resulting from the depressed leukocyte function
- Decreased maternal immunoglobulin G (IgG) levels secondary to cross-placental transfer to the fetus starting at about 16 weeks' gestation
- Stable maternal IgA and IgM levels (Mattson & Smith, 2004)

Table 11-3 Placental Hormones

Hormone	Description
hCG	• Responsible for maintaining the maternal corpus luteum, which secretes progesterone and estrogens, with synthesis occurring before implantation • Production by fetal trophoblast cells until the placenta is developed sufficiently to take over that function • Basis for early pregnancy tests because it appears in the maternal bloodstream soon after implantation • Production peaking at 8 weeks and then gradually declining
hPL (also known as human chorionic somatomammotropin (hCS))	• Preparation of mammary glands for lactation and involvement in the process of making glucose available for fetal growth by altering maternal carbohydrate, fat, and protein metabolism • Antagonist of insulin because it decreases tissue sensitivity or alters the ability to use insulin • Increase in the amount of circulating free fatty acids for maternal metabolic needs and decrease in maternal metabolism of glucose to facilitate fetal growth
Relaxin	• Secretion by the placenta as well as the corpus luteum during pregnancy • Thought to act synergistically with progesterone to maintain pregnancy • Increase in flexibility of the pubic symphysis, permitting the pelvis to expand during delivery • Dilation of the cervix, making it easier for the fetus to enter the vaginal canal; thought that it suppresses the release of oxytocin by the hypothalamus, thus delaying the onset of labor contractions (Ladewig, London, & Davidson, 2006)
Progesterone	• Often called *the hormone of pregnancy* because of the critical role it plays in supporting the endometrium of the uterus • Support of the endometrium to provide an environment conducive to fetal survival • Production by the corpus luteum during the first few weeks of pregnancy and then by the placenta until term • Initially, thickening of the uterine lining in anticipation of implantation of the fertilized ovum. From then on, it maintains the endometrium, inhibits uterine contractility, and assists in the development of the breasts for lactation (Matteson, 2001).
Estrogen	• Promotion of the enlargement of the genitals, uterus, and breasts, and increased vascularity, causing vasodilatation. • Relaxation of pelvic ligaments and joints (Lowdermilk & Perry, 2004) • Association with hyperpigmentation, vascular changes in the skin, increased activity of the salivary glands, and hyperemia of the gums and nasal mucous membranes (Murray et al., 2006) • Aid in developing the ductal system of the breasts in preparation for lactation (Ladewig, London, & Davidson, 2006)

Psychosocial Adaptations During Pregnancy

Pregnancy is a unique time in a woman's life. It is a time of dramatic alterations in her body and her appearance, as well as a time of change in her social status. All these changes occur simultaneously. Concurrent with her physiologic changes within her body systems are psychosocial changes within the mother and family members as they face significant role and lifestyle changes.

Maternal Emotional Responses

Motherhood, perhaps more than any role in society, has acquired a special significance for women: Women should find fulfillment and satisfaction in the role of the "ever-bountiful, ever-giving, self-sacrificing mother" (Kruger, 2003). With such high expectations, many pregnant women experience various emotions throughout their pregnancy. The woman's approach to these emotions is influenced by her emotional makeup, her sociologic and cultural background, her acceptance or rejection of the pregnancy, and her support network (Olds et al., 2004).

Despite the wide-ranging emotions associated with the pregnancy, many women experience similar responses. These responses commonly include ambivalence, introversion, acceptance, mood swings, and changes in body image.

Ambivalence

The realization of a pregnancy can lead to fluctuating responses, possibly at the opposite ends of the spectrum. For example, regardless of whether the pregnancy was planned, the woman may feel proud and excited at her achievement while at the same time fearful and anxious of the implications. The reactions are influenced by several factors, including the way the woman was raised by her family, her current family situation, the quality of the relationship with the expectant father, and her hopes for the future. Some women express concern over the timing of the pregnancy, wishing that goals and life objectives had been met before becoming pregnant. Other women may question how a newborn or infant will affect their career or their relationships with friends and family. These feelings can cause conflict and confusion about the impending pregnancy.

Ambivalence, or having conflicting feelings at the same time, is a universal feeling and is considered normal when preparing for a lifestyle change and new role. Pregnant women commonly experience ambivalence during the first trimester. Usually ambivalence evolves into acceptance by the second trimester, when fetal movement is felt. The woman's personality, her ability to adapt to changing circumstances, and the reactions of her partner will affect her adjustment to being pregnant and her acceptance of impending motherhood.

Introversion

Introversion, or focusing on oneself, is common during the early part of pregnancy. The woman may withdraw and become increasingly preoccupied with herself and her fetus. As a result, her participation with the outside world may be less, and she will appear passive to her family and friends.

This introspective behavior is a normal psychological adaptation to motherhood for most women. Introversion seems to heighten during the first and third trimesters when the woman's focus is on behaviors that will ensure a safe and health pregnancy outcome. Couples need to be aware of this behavior and be informed about measures to maintain and support the focus on the family.

Acceptance

During the second trimester, as the pregnancy progresses, the physical changes of the growing fetus with an enlarging abdomen and fetal movement bring reality and validity to the pregnancy. There are many tangible signs that someone separate from herself is present. The pregnant woman feels fetal movement and may hear the heartbeat. She may see the fetal image on an ultrasound screen and feel distinct parts, recognizing independent sleep and awake patterns. She becomes able to identify the fetus as a separate individual and accepts this.

Many women will verbalize positive feelings of the pregnancy and will conceptualize the fetus. The woman may accept her new body image and talk about the new life within. Generating a discussion about the woman's feelings and offering support and validation at prenatal visits are important.

Mood Swings

Emotional liability is characteristic throughout most pregnancies. One moment a woman can feel great joy, and within a short time span feel shock and disbelief. Frequently, pregnant women will start to cry without any apparent cause. To some, they feel as though they are riding an "emotional roller-coaster." These extremes in emotion can make it difficult for partners and family members to communicate with the pregnant woman without placing blame on themselves for their mood changes. Clear explanations about mood swings as common during pregnancy are key.

Change in Body Image

The way in which pregnancy affects a woman's body image varies greatly from person to person. Some women feel as if they have never been more beautiful, whereas others spend their pregnancy feeling overweight and uncomfortable. For some women pregnancy is a relief from worrying about weight, whereas for others it only exacerbates their fears of weight gain. Changes in body image are normal but can be very stressful for the pregnant woman. Offering a thorough explanation and initiating discussion of the expected bodily changes may be helpful in assisting the family to cope with them.

Maternal Role Tasks

Reva Rubin (1984) identified maternal tasks that a woman must accomplish to incorporate the maternal role successfully into her personality. Accomplishment of these tasks helps the expectant mother develop her self-concept as a mother. They form a mutually gratifying relationship with her infant. These tasks include

- Ensuring safe passage throughout pregnancy and birth
  - Primary focus of the woman's attention
  - First trimester: woman focusing on herself, not on the fetus
  - Second trimester: woman developing attachment of great value to her fetus
  - Third trimester: woman having concern for herself and her fetus as a unit
  - Participation in positive self-care activities related to diet, exercise, and overall well-being
- Seeking acceptance of infant by others
  - First trimester: acceptance of pregnancy by herself and others
  - Second trimester: family needing to relate to the fetus as member
  - Third trimester: unconditional acceptance without rejection
- Seeking acceptance of self in maternal role to infant ("binding in")
  - First trimester: mother accepting idea of pregnancy, but not of infant
  - Second trimester: with sensation of fetal movement (**quickening**), mother acknowledging fetus as a separate entity within her
  - Third trimester: mother longing to hold infant and becoming tired of being pregnant
- Learning to give of oneself
  - First trimester: identification of what must be given up to assume new role
  - Second trimester: identification with infant, learning how to delay own desires
  - Third trimester: questioning her ability to become a good mother to infant (Rubin, 1984)

Pregnancy and Sexuality

The way a pregnant woman feels and experiences her body during pregnancy can affect her sexuality. The woman's changing shape, emotional status, fetal activity, changes in breast size, pressure on the bladder, and other discomforts of pregnancy result in increased physical and emotional demands. These can produce stress on the sexual relationship between the pregnant woman and her partner. As the changes of pregnancy ensue, many partners become confused, anxious, and fearful of how the relationship may be affected.

Sexual desire of pregnant women may change throughout the pregnancy. During the first trimester, the woman may be less interested in sex because of fatigue, nausea, and fear of disturbing the early embryonic development. During the second trimester, her interest may increase because of the stability of the pregnancy. During the third trimester, her enlarging size may produce discomfort during sexual activity (Littleton & Engebretson, 2005).

A woman's sexual health is intimately linked to her own self-image. Sexual positions to increase comfort as the pregnancy progresses as well as alternative noncoital modes of sexual expression, such as cuddling, caressing, and holding, should be discussed. Giving permission to talk about and then normalizing sexuality can help enhance the sexual experience during pregnancy and, ultimately, the couple's relationship. If avenues of communication are open regarding sexuality during pregnancy, any fears and myths the couple may have can be dispelled.

Pregnancy and the Partner

Reactions to pregnancy and to the psychological and physical changes by the woman's partner varies vary greatly. Some enjoy the role of being the nurturer, whereas others experience alienation and may seek comfort or companionship elsewhere. Some expectant fathers may view pregnancy as proof of their masculinity and assume the dominant role, whereas others see their role as minimal, leaving the pregnancy up to the woman entirely. Each expectant partner reacts uniquely.

Emotionally and psychologically, expectant partners may undergo less visible changes than women, but most remain unexpressed and unappreciated (Buist et al., 2003). Expectant partners too experience a multitude of adjustments and concerns. Physically, they may gain weight around the middle and experience nausea and other GI disturbances, indicative of what is termed *couvade syndrome*—a sympathetic response to their partner's pregnancy. They also experience ambivalence during early pregnancy, with extremes of emotions (e.g., pride and joy versus an overwhelming sense of impending responsibility).

During the second trimester of pregnancy, partners go through acceptance of their role of breadwinner, caretaker, and support person. They come to accept the reality of the fetus when movement is felt and they experience confusion when dealing with the woman's mood swings and introspection.

During the third trimester, the expectant partner prepares for the reality of this new role and negotiates what the role will be during the labor and birthing process. Many may express their concern about being the primary support person during labor and birth, and how they will react when faced with their loved one in pain. Expectant partners share many of the same anxieties as their pregnant partners. However, revealing these anxieties to the pregnant partner or health care professionals is uncommon.

Pregnancy and Siblings

A sibling's reaction to pregnancy is age dependent. Some children might express excitement and anticipation, whereas others might verbalize negative reactions. The introduction of a new infant into the family is often the beginning of sibling rivalry, which results from the child's fear of change in the security of their relationships with their parents (Olds et al., 2004).

Preparation of the siblings for the anticipated birth is imperative and must be designed according to the age and life experiences of the sibling at home. Constant reinforcement of love and caring will help to reduce their fear of change and possible replacement by the new family member.

If possible, parents are urged to include siblings at home in this event and make them feel part of preparing for the new infant (Fig. 11-4). Sibling preparation is important, but parents' focus must also continue on the older sibling after the birth to reduce regressive or aggressive behavior that might manifest toward the newborn.

KEY CONCEPTS

- Pregnancy is a normal life event that involves considerable physical, psychosocial, emotional, and relationship adjustments.
- The sign and symptoms of pregnancy have been grouped into those that are subjective (*presumptive*) and experienced by the woman herself, those that are objective (*probable*) and observed by the health-care professional, and those that are the *positive*, beyond-the-shadow-of-a-doubt signs.
- Physiologically, almost every system of a woman's body changes during pregnancy with startling rapidity to accommodate the needs of the growing fetus. A majority of the changes are influenced by hormonal changes.

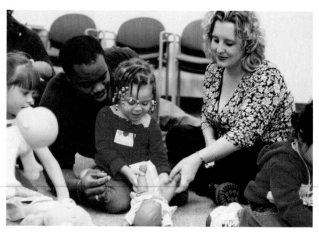

● Figure 11-4 Parents preparing sibling for the birth of a new baby.

- The placenta is a unique kind of endocrine gland; it has a feature possessed by no other endocrine organ—the ability to form protein and steroid hormones.
- Occurring in conjunction with the physiologic changes in the woman's body systems are psychosocial changes occurring within the mother and family members as they face significant role and lifestyle changes.
- Commonly experienced emotional responses to pregnancy in the woman include ambivalence, introversion, acceptance, mood swings, and changes in body image.
- Reactions of expectant partners to pregnancy and to the physical and psychological changes in the woman vary greatly.
- A sibling's reaction to pregnancy is age dependent. The introduction of a new infant to the family is often the beginning of sibling rivalry, which results from the established child's fear of change in security of their relationships with their parents. Therefore, preparation of the siblings for the anticipated birth is imperative.

References

Buist, A., Morse, C. A., & Durkin, S. (2003). Men's adjustment to fatherhood: implications for obstetric health care. *JOGNN, 32,* 172–180.

Cole, L. A., et al. (2004). Accuracy of home pregnancy tests at the time of missed menses. *American Journal of Obstetrics and Gynecology, 190,* 100–105.

Condon, M. C. (2004). *Women's health: an integrated approach to wellness and illness.* Upper Saddle River, NJ: Prentice Hall.

Cunningham, F., et al. (2005). *William's obstetrics* (22nd ed.). New York: McGraw-Hill.

Dickey, N. W. (2003). *Hormones during pregnancy.* Loyola University Health System. [Online] Available at www.luhs.org/health/topics/pregnant/hormone.htm.

Hatcher, R., et al. (2004). *A pocket guide to managing contraception.* Tiger, GA: Bridging the Gap Foundation.

Hockenberry, M. J. (2005). *Wong's essentials of pediatric nursing* (7th ed.). St. Louis: Mosby, Inc.

Kruger, L. M. (2003). *Narrating motherhood: The transformative potential of.*

Ladewig, P. A., London, M. L., & Davidson, M. R. (2006). *Contemporary maternal–newborn nursing care* (6th ed.). Upper Saddle River, NJ: Pearson Prentice Hall.

Littleton, L. Y., & Engebretson, J. C. (2005). *Maternity nursing care.* Clifton Park, NY: Thomson Delmar Learning.

Lowdermilk, D. L., & Perry, S. E. (2004). *Maternity & women's health care* (8th ed.). St. Louis: Mosby.

Matteson, P. S. (2001). *Women's health during the childbearing years: a community-based approach.* St. Louis: Mosby.

Mattson, S., & Smith, J. E. (2004). *Core curriculum for maternal–newborn nursing* (3rd ed.). St. Louis: Elsevier Saunders.

Murray, S. S., & McKinney, E. S. (2006). *Foundations of maternal–newborn nursing* (4th ed.). Philadelphia: WB Saunders.

Olds, S. B., London, M. L., Ladewig, P. A., & Davidson, M. R. (2004). *Maternal–newborn nursing & women's health care* (7th ed.). Upper Saddle River, NJ: Pearson Prentice Hall.

Pagana, K., & Pagana, T. (2003). *Mosby's diagnostic and laboratory test reference* (6th ed.). St. Louis: Mosby.

Pillitteri, A. (2003). *Maternal & child health nursing: care of the childbearing and childrearing family* (4th ed.). Philadelphia: Lippincott Williams & Wilkins.

Rubin, R. (1984). *Maternal identity and the maternal experience.* New York: Springer.

Schnell, Z. B., Van Leeuwen, A. M., & Kranpitz, T. R. (2003). *Davis' comprehensive handbook of laboratory and diagnostic tests with nursing implications.* Philadelphia: FA Davis.

Sloan, E. (2002). *Biology of women* (4th ed.). New York: Delmar.

Youngkin, E. Q., & Davis, M. S. (2004). *Women's health: a primary care clinical guide* (3rd ed.). Upper Saddle River, NJ: Prentice Hall.

Web Resources

American College of Nurse Midwives, 202-347-5445, **www.acnm.org**
American College of Obstetricians and Gynecologists, **www.acog.com**
Association of Women's Health, Obstetrics & Neonatal Nurses, **www.awhonn.org**
International Childbirth Education Association, **www.icea.org**
March of Dimes, **www.modimes.org**
Mayo Clinic Pregnancy Center, **www.mayoclinic.org**
National Center for Education in Maternal and Child Health, **www.ncemch.org**

ChapterWORKSHEET

● MULTIPLE CHOICE QUESTIONS

1. When teaching a client about hormones, which would the nurse identify as responsible for calming the uterus and preventing contractions during early pregnancy?

   a. Estrogen

   b. Progesterone

   c. Oxytocin

   d. Prolactin

2. When assessing a client, which of the following would the nurse identify as a presumptive sign or symptom of pregnancy?

   a. Restlessness

   b. Elevated mood

   c. Urinary frequency

   d. Low backache

3. When obtaining a blood test for pregnancy, which hormone would the nurse expect the test to measure?

   a. hCG

   b. hPL

   c. FSH

   d. LH

4. A universal feeling expressed by most women upon learning they are pregnant is

   a. Acceptance

   b. Depression

   c. Jealousy

   d. Ambivalence

5. Reva Rubin identified four major tasks that the pregnant woman undertakes to form the basis for a mutually gratifying relationship with her infant. Which one describes binding in?

   a. Ensuring safe passage through pregnancy, labor, and birth

   b. Seeking of acceptance of this infant by others

   c. Seeking acceptance of self as mother to the infant

   d. Learning to give of oneself on behalf of one's infant

● CRITICAL THINKING EXERCISES

1. When interviewing a woman at her first prenatal visit, the nurse asks about her feelings. The woman replies, "I am frightened and confused. I don't know whether I want to be pregnant or not. Being pregnant means changing our whole life, and now having somebody to care for all the time. I'm not sure I would be a good mother. Plus I'm a bit afraid of all the changes that would happen to my body. Is this normal? Am I okay?"

   a. How should the nurse answer her question?

   b. What specific information is needed to support the client during this pregnancy?

2. Sally, age 23, is 9 weeks pregnant. At her clinic visit she says, "I'm so tired that I can barely make it home from work. Then once I'm home, I don't have the energy to make dinner." Sally's current lab work is within normal limits.

   a. What explanation can the nurse offer Sally regarding her fatigue?

   b. What interventions can the nurse offer to Sally?

3. Bringing a new infant into the family affects the siblings.

   a. What strategies can a nurse discuss with a concerned mother when she asks how to deal with this?

● STUDY ACTIVITIES

1. Go to your local health department's maternity clinic and interview several women regarding their feelings and bodily changes that have taken place since their acknowledgment of pregnancy. Based on your findings, place them into appropriate trimesters of their pregnancy.

2. Complete a Web search for information regarding psychological changes occurring during pregnancy and share your Web sites with your clinical group.

3. During pregnancy, the plasma volume increases by 50% and the RBC volume only increases by 18 to 30%. This disproportion is manifested as

   _____.

4. When a pregnant woman in her third trimester lies on her back and experiences dizziness and light-headedness, the underlying cause of this is

   _____.

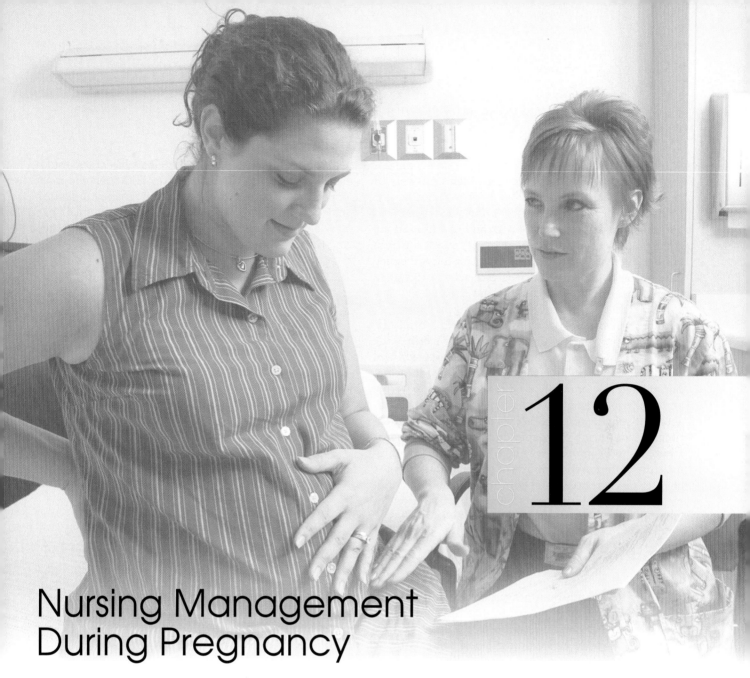

Nursing Management During Pregnancy

KeyTERMS

alpha fetoprotein
amniocentesis
biophysical profile
chorionic villus sampling
   (CVS)
dietary reference intakes
   (DRIs)
doula
gravida
high-risk pregnancy
natural childbirth
para
perinatal education
pica
preconception care

LearningOBJECTIVES

After studying the chapter content, the student should be able to accomplish the following:

1. Define the key terms.
2. Identify the information typically collected at the initial prenatal visit.
3. Describe the assessments completed at follow-up prenatal visits.
4. List the tests used to assess maternal and fetal well-being, including nursing management for each.
5. Summarize the nutritional needs of the pregnant woman and her fetus.
6. Outline appropriate nursing management to promote maternal self-care and minimize the common discomforts of pregnancy.
7. Discuss the key components of perinatal education.

The secret of human touch is simple, showing a sincere liking and interest in people. Nurses need to use touch often.

Pregnancy is a time of many physiologic and psychological changes that can positively or negatively affect the woman, her fetus, and her family. Misconceptions, inadequate information, and unanswered questions about pregnancy, birth, and parenthood are common. The ultimate goal of any pregnancy is the birth of a healthy newborn. Nurses play a major role in helping the pregnant woman and her partner achieve this goal. Ongoing assessment and education are essential.

This chapter describes the nursing management required during pregnancy. It begins with a brief discussion of preconception care and then describes the assessment of the woman at the first prenatal visit and on follow-up visits. The chapter presents key information related to commonly used tests to assess maternal and fetal well-being, including specific nursing management related to each test. It also addresses nutritional needs during pregnancy and identifies important strategies to promote the woman's self-care and minimize the common discomforts of pregnancy. Lastly the chapter discusses perinatal education, including childbirth education, birthing options, and preparation for labor and birth.

Preconception Care

Ideally, couples thinking about having a child should schedule a visit with their healthcare provider for preconception counseling to ensure that the couple is in the best possible state of health before pregnancy. **Preconception care** is the promotion of the health and well-being of a woman and her partner before pregnancy. The goal of preconception care is to identify any areas such as health problems, lifestyle habits, or social concerns that might unfavorably affect pregnancy (Frey, 2002).

The period of greatest environmental sensitivity and consequent risk for the developing embryo is between days 17 and 56 after conception. Traditionally, the first prenatal visit, which is usually a month or later after a missed menstrual period, may occur too late to affect reproductive outcomes associated with abnormal organogenesis secondary to poor lifestyle choices. In some cases, such as with unplanned pregnancies, women may delay seeking health care, denying that they are pregnant. However, as the pregnancy progresses and the woman's abdomen visibly increases in size, denial no longer is effective.

In addition, commonly used prevention practices may begin too late to avert the morbidity and mortality associated with congenital anomalies and low birthweight (Moos, 2003a, 2003b). To address these issues and foster the overall well-being of pregnant women and their

fetuses, specific National Health Goals have been established (see Healthy People 2010). Although the most opportune window for improving pregnancy outcomes may be missed, appropriate nursing management can have a positive impact on the health of pregnant women and their unborn children.

Nursing Management

Preconception care involves obtaining a complete health history and physical examination of the woman and her partner. Key areas addressed include:

HEALTHY PEOPLE *2010*

National Health Goals Related to Prenatal Care

Objective	Significance
1. Increase the proportion of pregnant women who receive early and adequate prenatal care: Increase the number of women receiving maternal prenatal care beginning in the first trimester of pregnancy from a baseline of 83% to 90% of live births. Increase the number of women receiving early and adequate prenatal care from a baseline of 74% to 90% of live births.	Will help to contribute to reduced rates of perinatal illness, disability, and death by helping to identify possible risk factors and implementing measures to lessen these factors that contribute to poor outcomes
2. Increase the proportion of pregnant women who attend a series of prepared childbirth classes.	Will help contribute to a more pleasant birthing experience because women will be prepared for what they will face; also help in reducing pain and anxiety
3. Increase abstinence from alcohol, cigarettes, and illicit drugs among pregnant women.	Will help to reduce the wide-ranging effects, such as spontaneous abortion, low birthweight, and preterm birth associated with prenatal substance use

(DHHS, 2000)

- Immunization status
- Underlying medical conditions, such as cardiovascular or respiratory problems or genetic disorders
- Reproductive health data such as pelvic examinations, use of contraceptives, and sexually transmitted infections (STIs)
- Sexuality and sexual practices, such as safer-sex practices and body image issues
- Nutrition
- Lifestyle practices, including occupation and recreational activities
- Psychosocial issues such as levels of stress, exposure to abuse and violence
- Medication and drug use, including use of tobacco, alcohol, over-the-counter and prescription medications, and illicit drugs
- Support system including family, friends, and community (see Fig. 12-1 for a sample screening tool)

This information provides a foundation from which nurses can plan health-promotion activities and education. For example, to have a positive impact on the pregnancy, the nurse should:

- Stress the importance of taking folic acid to prevent neural tube defects.
- Urge the woman to achieve optimal weight before a pregnancy.
- Ensure that the woman's immunizations are up to date.
- Address substance use issues, including smoking and drugs.
- Identify victims of violence and assist them to get help.
- Manage chronic conditions such as diabetes and asthma.
- Educate the woman about environmental hazards, including metals and herbs.
- Offer genetic counseling to identify carriers.
- Suggest the availability of support systems, if needed (Cullum, 2003).

Nurses can act as advocates and educators, creating healthy, supportive communities for women and their partners in the childbearing phases of their lives. Nurses can enter into a collaborative partnership with a woman and her partner, enabling them to examine their own health and its influence on the health of their future baby. The information provided by the nurse will allow the woman and her partner to make an informed decision about having a baby, although the decision solely rests with the couple. "Preconception care should be integrated into the women's health care continuum to achieve high levels of lifetime wellness for all women" (Moos, 2003b, p. 552).

The First Prenatal Visit

Once a pregnancy is suspected and, in some cases, tentatively confirmed by a home pregnancy test, the woman should seek prenatal care to promote a healthy outcome.

The assessment process begins at this initial prenatal visit and continues throughout the pregnancy. The initial visit is an ideal time to screen for factors that might place the woman and her fetus at risk for problems such as preterm delivery or other poor outcomes. The initial visit also is an optimal time to begin educating the client about changes that will affect her life.

Counseling and education of the pregnant woman and her partner are critical to healthy outcomes for mother and her infant. Pregnant women and their partners frequently have questions, misinformation, or misconceptions about what to eat, weight gain, physical discomforts, drug and alcohol use, sexuality, and the birthing process. The nurse needs to allow time to answer questions and provide anticipatory guidance during the pregnancy and to make appropriate community referrals to meet the needs of this client.

Comprehensive Health History

During the initial visit, a comprehensive health history is obtained. Often, using a prenatal history form (Fig. 12-2) is the best way to document the data collected (Wong et al., 2002).

The initial health history typically includes questions about three major areas: the reason for seeking care; the client's past medical, surgical, and personal history, including that of the family and her partner; and the client's reproductive history. During the history-taking process, the nurse and client establish the foundation of a trusting relationship and jointly develop a plan of care for the pregnancy. This plan is tailored to the client's lifestyle as much as possible and focuses primarily on education for overall wellness during the pregnancy. The ultimate goal is early detection and prevention of any problems that occur during the pregnancy (Youngkin & Davis, 2004).

Reason for Seeking Care

The woman commonly comes for prenatal care based on the suspicion that she is pregnant: she may report that she has missed her menstrual period or has had a positive result on a home pregnancy test. Ask the woman for the date of her last menstrual period (LMP). Also ask about any presumptive or probable signs of pregnancy that she might be experiencing. Typically a urine or blood test to check for evidence of human chorionic gonadotropin (hCG) is done to provide initial confirmation of the pregnancy.

Past History

Ask about the woman's past medical and surgical history. This information is important because conditions that the woman experienced in the past (e.g., urinary tract infections) may recur or be exacerbated during the pregnancy. Also, chronic illnesses, such as diabetes or heart disease, can increase the risk for complications during

(text continues on page 259)

PRECONCEPTION SCREENING AND COUNSELING CHECKLIST

NAME	BIRTHPLACE	AGE

DATE: / /   ARE YOU PLANNING TO GET PREGNANT IN THE NEXT SIX MONTHS? ___ Y ___N

IF YOUR ANSWER TO A QUESTION IS YES, PUT A CHECK MARK ON THE LINE IN FRONT OF THE QUESTION. FILL IN OTHER INFORMATION THAT APPLIES TO YOU.

DIET AND EXERCISE

What do you consider a healthy weight for you?_____
___Do you eat three meals a day?
___Do you follow a special diet (vegetarian, diabetic, other)?
___Which do you drink (__ coffee __ tea __ cola __ milk __ water __ soda/pop
    other_____)?
___Do you eat raw or undercooked food (meat, other)?
___Do you take folic acid?
___Do you take other vitamins daily (__ multivitamin __ vitamin A __ other)?
___Do you take dietary supplements (__ black cohosh __ pennyroyal __ other)?
___Do you have current/past problems withh eating disorders?
___Do you exercise? Type/frequency:_____
Notes:

LIFESTYLE

___Do you smoke cigarettes or use other tobacco products?
    How many cigarettes/packs a day?_____
___Are you exposed to second-hand smoke?
___Do you drink alcohol?
    What kind?_____How often?_____How much?_____
___Do you use recreational drugs (cocaine, heroin, ecstasy, meth/ice, other?
    List:_____
___Do you see a dentist regularly?
    What kind of work do you do?_____
___Do you work or live near possible hazards (chemicals, x-ray or other radiation,
    lead)? List:_____
___Do you use saunas or hot tubs?
Notes:

MEDICATION /DRUGS

___Are you taking prescribed drugs (Accutane, valproic acid, blood thinners)? List
    them_____
___Are you taking non-prescribed drugs?
    List them:_____
___Are you using birth control pills?
___Do you get injectable contraceptives or shots for birth control?
___Do you use any herbal remedies or alternative medicine?
    List:_____
NOTES:

MEDICAL/FAMILY HISTORY

Do you have or have you ever had:
___Epilepsy?
___Diabetes?
___Asthma?
___High blood pressure?
___Heart disease?
___Anemia?
___Kidney or bladder disorders?
___Thyroid disease?
___Chickenpox?
___Hepatitis C?
___Digestive problems?
___Depression or other mental health problem?
___Surgeries?
___Lupus?
___Scleroderma?
___Other conditions?
Have you ever been vaccinated for:
___Measles, mumps, rubella?
___Hepatitis B?
___Chickenpox?
NOTES:

WOMEN'S HEALTH

___Do you have any problems with your menstrual cycle?
___How many times have you been pregnant?
    What was/ were the outcomes(s)?_____
___Did you have difficulty getting pregnant last time?
___Have you been treated for infertility?
    Have you had surgery on your uterus, cervix, ovaries, or tubes?
___Did you mother take the hormone DES during pregnancy?
    Have you ever had HPV, genital warts or chlamydia?
___Have you ever been treated for a sexually transmitted infection (genital herpes,
    gonorrhea, syphilis, HIV/AIDS, other)? List:_____
NOTES:

GENETICS

Does your family have a history of   Or   Your partner's family
___Hemophilia?   ___
___Other bleeding disorders?   ___
___Tay-Sachs disease?   ___
___Blood diseases (sickle cell, thalassemia, other)?   ___
___Muscular dystrophy?   ___
___Down syndrome/mental retardation?   ___
___Cystic fibrosis?   ___
___Birth defects (spine/heart/kidney)?   ___
Your ethnic background is:_____
Your partner's ethnic background is: _____
NOTES:

HOME ENVIRONMENT

___Do you feel emotionally supported at home?
___Do you have help from relatives or friends if needed?
___Do you feel you have serious money/financial worries?
___Are you in a stable relationship?
___Do you feel safe at home?
___Does anyone threaten or physically hurt you?
___Do you have pets (cats, rodents, exotic animals)? List:_____
___Do have any contact with soil, cat litter, or sandboxes?

Baby preparation (if planning pregnancy):
___Do you have a place for a baby to sleep?
___Do you need any baby items?
NOTES:

OTHER

IS THERE ANYTHING ELSE YOU'D LIKE ME TO KNOW?

ARE THERE ANY QUESTIONS YOU'D LIKE TO ASK ME?

● Figure 12-1 Sample preconception screening tool. (Used with permission. Copyright
March of Dimes.)

Health History Summary
Maternal/Newborn Record System

Page 1 of 2

Patient's name _____

ID. No. _____

_____

_____

Demographic data

Date of birth _____ Age _____ Language ☐ _____ Interpreter ☐ _____
☐ English ☐ None
☐ N/A

Religion ☐ _____ Race/ethnicity _____

Marital status S M SEP D W   Name of baby's father _____

Education	Occupation	Full	Part	Self	Unemp	Work Tel No	Home Tel No
Patient		☐	☐	☐	☐		
Father of baby		☐	☐	☐	☐		

Allergy/sensitivity

☐ None ☐ Latex

☐ Other _____

_____

Primary/referring physician

Menstrual history	**Menarche** yrs	**Interval** days	**Length** days	**Abnormalities** ☐ None		**EDD**		
							By dates ___/___/___	
	Certain ☐ Yes ☐ No		Positive	☐ Blood			By ultrasound ___/___/___	
LMP ___/___/___	Normal ☐ Yes ☐ No		pregnancy test ___/___/___	☐ Urine			Date of ultrasound ___/___/___	

Pregnancy history	Gravida	Full term	Premature	Spontaneous Ab	Induced Ab	Ectopic	Multiple births	Live

No	Month/ year	Infant sex	Weight at birth	Wks gest	Hours in labor	Type of delivery	Anesthesia	Comments/complications
1								
2								
3								
4								
5								
6								
7								

Medical history

Obstetric Patient

1. Anemia _____ ☐
2. Fetal/neonatal death or anomaly _____ ☐
3. Gestational diabetes _____ ☐
4. Hemorrhage _____ ☐
5. Hyperemesis _____ ☐
6. Incompetent cervix _____ ☐
7. Intrauterine growth retardation _____ ☐
8. Isoimmunization _____ ☐
9. Polyhydramnios _____ ☐
10. Postpartum depression _____ ☐
11. Pregnancy-induced hypertension _____ ☐
12. Preterm labor or birth _____ ☐
13. PROM-chorioamnionitis _____ ☐
14. Rhogam given _____ ☐
15. RH neg _____ ☐

Gynecologic

16. Contraceptive use _____ ☐
17. Abnormal PAP _____ ☐
18. Fibroids _____ ☐
19. Gyn· surgery _____ ☐

Check and detail positive findings below. Use reference numbers.

Gynecologic (cont'd.) Patient

20. Infertility _____ ☐
21. In utero exposure to DES ____ ☐
22. Uterine/cervical anomaly _____ ☐

Sexually transmitted diseases

23. Chlamydia _____ ☐
24. Gonorrhea _____ ☐
25. Herpes (HSV) _____ ☐
26. Syphilis _____ ☐

Vaginal/genital infections

27. Trichomonas _____ ☐
28. Condylomata _____ ☐
29. Candidiasis _____ ☐

Other infections

30. Toxoplasmosis _____ ☐
31. Group B streptococcus _____ ☐
32. Rubella or immunization _____ ☐
33. Varicella or immunization ____ ☐
34. Cytomegalovirus (CMV) _____ ☐
35. AIDS (HIV) _____ ☐
36. Hepatitis (type ___) _____ ☐ or immunization (type _____)

● Figure 12-2 Sample prenatal history form. (Used with permission. Copyright Briggs Corporation, 2001.) *(continued)*

Health History Summary
Maternal/newborn record system

Page 2 of 2

Patient's name _____

ID. No. _____

_____

_____

Check and detail positive findings below. Use reference numbers.

Cardiovascular
	Patient	Family
37. Myocardial infarction	☐	☐
38. Heart disease	☐	☐
39. Rheumatic fever	☐	
40. Valve disease	☐	
41. Chronic hypertension	☐	☐
42. Disease of the aorta	☐	☐
43. Varicosities Thrombophlebitis	☐	☐
44. Previous pulmonary embolism	☐	
45. Blood disorders	☐	☐
46. Anemia/ hemoglobinopathy	☐	☐
47. Blood transfusions	☐	
48. Other	☐	

Pulmonary
	Patient	Family
49. Asthma	☐	
50. Tuberculosis	☐	☐
51. Chronic obstructive pulmonary disease	☐	☐

Endocrine
	Patient	Family
52. Diabetes	☐	☐
53. Thyroid dysfunction	☐	☐
54. Maternal PKU	☐	
55. Endocrinopathy	☐	☐
56. Gastrointestinal	☐	
57. Liver disease	☐	

Renal disease
	Patient	Family
58. Cystitis	☐	
59. Pyelonephritis	☐	
60. Asymptomatic bacteriuria	☐	
61. Chronic renal disease	☐	☐
62. Autoimmune disease	☐	☐
63. Cancer	☐	☐

Neurologic disease
	Patient	Family
64. Cerebrovascular accident	☐	☐
65. Seizure disorder	☐	☐
66. Migraine headaches	☐	☐
67. Degenerative disease	☐	☐
68. Other	☐	

Psychological/surgical
	Patient	Family
69. Psychiatric disease Mental lillness	☐	☐
70. Physical abuse or neglect	☐	☐
71. Emotional abuse or neglect	☐	☐
72. Addiction (drug, alcohol, nicotine)	☐	☐
73. Major accidents	☐	
74. Surgery	☐	
75. Anesthetic complications	☐	
76. Non-surgical hospitalization	☐	
77. Other	☐	
78. **No known disease/problems**	☐	

Genetic history
	Patient	Father of baby	Family
79. Age 35 or older (female) 50 or older (male)	☐	☐	☐
80. Cerebral palsy	☐	☐	☐
81. Cleft lip/palate	☐	☐	☐
82. Congenital anomalies	☐	☐	☐
83. Congenital heart disease	☐	☐	☐
84. Consanguinity	☐	☐	☐
85. Cystic fibrosis	☐	☐	☐
86. Down's syndrome	☐	☐	☐
87. Hemophilia	☐	☐	☐
88. Huntington's chorea	☐	☐	☐
89. Mental retardation	☐	☐	☐
90. Muscular dystrophy	☐	☐	☐
91. Neural tube defect	☐	☐	☐
92. Sickle cell disease or trait	☐	☐	☐
93. Tay-sachs disease	☐	☐	☐
94. Test for fragile X	☐	☐	☐
95. Thalassemia A or B	☐	☐	☐
96. Other	☐	☐	☐
97. Other	☐	☐	☐
98. Other	☐	☐	☐

Historical risk status   ☐ No risk factors noted
☐ **At risk (identify)**

Signature

● Figure 12-2 *(continued)*

pregnancy for the woman and her fetus. Ask about any history of allergies to medications, foods, or environmental substances. Gather similar information about the woman's family and her partner.

The woman's personal history also is important. Ask about her occupation, possible exposure to teratogens, exercise and activity level, recreational patterns (including the use of substances such as alcohol, tobacco, and drugs), use of alternative and complementary therapies, sleep patterns, nutritional habits, and general lifestyle. Each of these may have an impact on the outcome of the pregnancy. For example, if the woman smokes during pregnancy, nicotine in the cigarettes causes vasoconstriction in the mother, leading to reduced placental perfusion. As a result, the newborn may be small for gestational age. The newborn will also go through nicotine withdrawal soon after birth. No safe level of alcohol ingestion in pregnancy has been determined. Many fetuses exposed to heavy alcohol levels during pregnancy develop fetal alcohol syndrome, a collection of deformities and disabilities in the newborn.

Reproductive History

The woman's reproductive history includes a menstrual, obstetric, and gynecologic history. Typically, this history begins with a description of the woman's menstrual cycle, including her age at menarche, number of days in her cycle, typical flow characteristics, and any discomfort

experienced. The use of contraception also is important, including when the woman last used any contraception.

Ask the woman the date of her LMP to determine the estimated or expected date of birth (EDB) or delivery (EDD). Several methods may be used to estimate the date of birth. Nagele's rule can be used to establish the EDD or EDB. Using this rule, subtract 3 months and then add 7 days to the first day of the LMP. Then correct the year by adding 1 to it. This date has a margin of error of plus or minus 2 weeks. For instance, if a woman reports that her LMP was Oct. 14, 2005, you would subtract 3 months (July) and add 7 days (21), then add 1 year (2006). The woman's EDD or EDB is July 21, 2006.

Because of the normal variations in women's menstrual cycles, differences in the normal length of gestation between ethnic groups, and errors in dating methods, there is no such thing as an exact due date. In general, a birth 2 weeks before or 2 weeks after the EDD or EDB is considered normal. Nagele's rule is less accurate if the woman's menstrual cycles are irregular, if the woman conceives while breastfeeding or before her regular menstrual cycle is established, if she is ovulating although she is amenorrheic, or after she discontinues oral contraceptives (Condon, 2004).

A gestational or birth calculator or wheel can also be used to calculate the due date instead of using Nagele's rule (Fig. 12-3). Still other practitioners use ultrasound

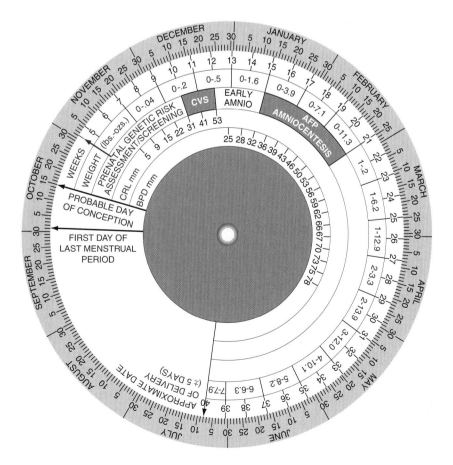

● Figure 12-3 EDB using a birth wheel. The first day of the woman's LNMP was October 1. Using the birth wheel, her EDB would be approximately July 8 of the following year. (Used with permission. Copyright March of Dimes, 2003.)

to more accurately determine the gestational age and date the pregnancy.

Typically, an obstetric history provides information about the woman's past pregnancies, including any problems encountered during the pregnancy, labor, delivery, and afterward. Such information can provide clues to problems that might develop in the current pregnancy. Some common terms used to describe and document an obstetric history include:

- Gravid: the state of being pregnant
- **Gravida:** a pregnant woman; gravida I (primigravida) during the first pregnancy, gravida II (secundigravida) during the second pregnancy, and so on
- **Para:** a woman who has produced one or more viable offspring carrying a pregnancy 20 weeks or more; thus, a primipara is a woman who has given birth once after a pregnancy of at least 20 weeks, commonly referred to as a "primip" in clinical practice. A multipara is a woman who has had two or more pregnancies resulting in viable offspring, commonly referred to as a "multip." Nullipara (para 0) is a woman who has not produced a viable offspring.

Other systems may be used to document a woman's obstetric history. These systems often break down the category of para more specifically (Box 12-1).

Information about the woman's gynecologic history is important. Ask about any reproductive tract surgeries the woman has undergone. For example, surgery on the uterus may affect its ability to contract effectively during labor. A history of tubal pregnancy increases the woman's risk for another tubal pregnancy. Also ask about safer-sex practices and any history of STIs.

Physical Examination

The next step in the assessment process is the physical examination, which detects any physical problems that may affect the pregnancy outcome. The initial physical examination provides the baseline for evaluating changes during future visits.

Preparation

Instruct the client to undress and put on a gown. Also ask her to empty her bladder and in doing so to collect a urine specimen. Typically this specimen is a clean-catch urine specimen that is sent to the laboratory for a urinalysis to detect a possible urinary tract infection.

Begin the physical examination by obtaining vital signs, including blood pressure, respiratory rate, temperature, and pulse (Fig. 12-4). Also measure the client's height and weight. Abnormalities such as an elevated blood pressure (140/90 or higher) may suggest pregestational hypertension, requiring further evaluation. Abnormalities in pulse rate and respiration require further investigation for possible cardiac or respiratory disease and possible treatment. If the woman weighs less than 100 pounds or greater than 200 pounds or there has been a sudden weight gain, report these findings to the primary care provider. Medical treatment or nutritional counseling may be necessary.

Head-to-Toe Assessment

A complete head-to-toe assessment is usually performed by the healthcare professional. Every body system is assessed. Some of the major areas are discussed here (Fig. 12-5). Throughout the assessment, be sure to drape the client appropriately to ensure privacy and prevent chilling.

BOX 12-1

OBSTETRIC HISTORY TERMS

GTPAL or TPAL
G = gravida, T = term births, P = preterm births, A = abortions, L = living children

  G—the current pregnancy
  T—the number of pregnancies ending >37 weeks' gestation, at term
  P—the number of preterm pregnancies ending >20 weeks or viability but before completion of 37 weeks
  A—the number of pregnancies ending before 20 weeks or viability
  L—the number of children currently living

Consider this example:
Mary Johnson is pregnant for the fourth time. She had one abortion at 8 weeks' gestation. She has a daughter who was born at 40 weeks' gestation and a son born at 34 weeks. Mary's obstetric history would be documented as follows:

Using the gravida/para method: Gravida 4, para 2
Using the TPAL method: 1112 (T = 1 [daughter born at 40 weeks]; P = 1 [son born at 34 weeks], A = 1 [abortion at 8 weeks]; L = 2 [two living children])

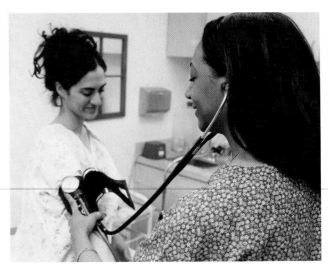

● Figure 12-4 Obtaining vital signs on the first prenatal visit.

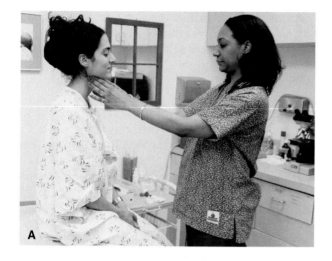

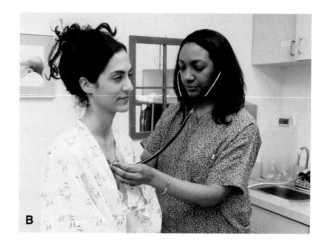

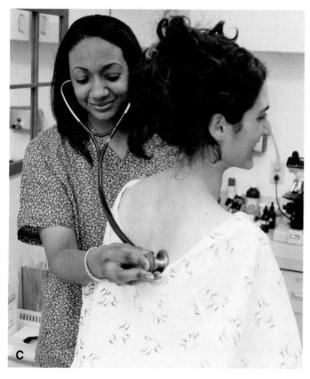

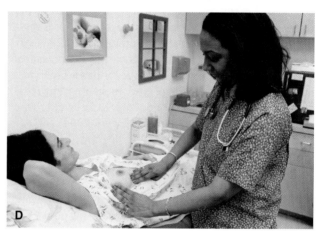

● Figure 12-5 Performing the physical examination. (**A**) Head and neck assessment. (**B**) Heart auscultation. (**C**) Lung auscultation. (**D**) Breast examination.

Head and Neck

Assess the head and neck area for any previous injuries and sequelae. Evaluate for any limitations in range of motion. Palpate for any enlarged lymph nodes or swelling. Note any edema of the nasal mucosa or hypertrophy of gingival tissue in the mouth; these are typical responses to increased estrogen levels in pregnancy. Palpate the thyroid gland for enlargement. Slight enlargement is normal, but marked enlargement may indicate hyperthyroidism, requiring further investigation and possible treatment.

Chest

Auscultate heart sounds, noting any abnormalities. A soft systolic murmur caused by the increase in blood volume may be noted. Anticipate an increase in heart rate by 10 to

15 beats per minute secondary to increases in cardiac output and blood volume. The body adapts to the increase in blood volume with peripheral dilatation to maintain blood pressure. Progesterone causes peripheral dilatation.

Auscultate the chest for breath sounds, which should be clear. Also note symmetry of chest movement and thoracic breathing patterns. Estrogen promotes relaxation of the ligaments and joints of the ribs, with a resulting increase in the anteroposterior chest diameter. Expect a slight increase in respiratory rate to accommodate the increase in tidal volume and oxygen consumption.

Inspect and palpate the breasts. Increases in estrogen and progesterone and blood supply make the breasts feel full and more nodular, with increased sensitivity to touch. Blood vessels become more visible and there is an increase in breast size. Striae gravidarum (stretch marks) may be visible in women with large breasts. Darker pigmentation of the nipple and areola is present, along with enlargement of Montgomery's glands. Use this opportunity to reinforce and teach breast self-examination.

Abdomen

The appearance of the abdomen depends on the number of weeks of gestation. The abdomen enlarges progressively as the fetus grows. Palpate the abdomen, which should be rounded and nontender. A decrease in muscle tone may be noted due to the influence of progesterone. Inspection also may reveal striae gravidarum (stretch marks) and linea nigra, depending on the duration of the pregnancy.

Typically, the height of the fundus is measured when the uterus arises out of the pelvis to evaluate fetal growth. At 12 weeks' gestation the fundus can be palpated at the symphysis pubis. At 16 weeks' gestation the fundus is midway between the symphysis and the umbilicus. At 20 weeks the fundus can be palpated at the umbilicus and measures approximately 20 cm. By 36 weeks the fundus is noted just below the ensiform cartilage and measures approximately 36 cm. The uterus maintains a globular/ovoid shape throughout pregnancy (Youngkin & Davis, 2004).

Extremities

Inspect and palpate both legs for dependent edema, pulses, and varicose veins. If edema is present in early pregnancy, further evaluation may be needed to rule out pregnancy-induced hypertension. Assess for calf pain (positive Homans' sign) when dorsiflexing the foot to identify deep vein thrombophlebitis (DVT). High levels of estrogen during pregnancy place women at higher risk for DVT.

Pelvic Examination

The pelvic examination provides information on the health of the internal and external reproductive organs. In addition, it aids in assessing some of the presumptive and probable signs of pregnancy and allows for determination of pelvic adequacy. During the pelvic examination, remain in the examining room to assist the healthcare provider with any specimen collection, fixation, and labeling. Also provide comfort and emotional support for the woman, who might be anxious. Throughout the examination, explain what is happening and why, and answer any questions as necessary.

External Genitalia

After the client is placed in the lithotomy position and draped appropriately, the external genitalia are visually inspected. They should be free from lesions, discharge, hematomas, varicosities, and inflammation upon inspection. A culture for STIs may be collected at this time.

Internal Genitalia

Next, the internal genitalia are examined via a speculum. The cervix should be smooth, long, thick, and closed.

Because of increased pelvic congestion, the cervix will softened (Goodell's sign), the uterine isthmus will be softened (Hegar's sign), and there will be a bluish coloration of the cervix and vaginal mucosa (Chadwick's sign).

The uterus typically is pear-shaped and mobile, with a smooth surface. It will undergo cell hypertrophy and hyperplasia to enlarge throughout the pregnancy to accommodate the growing fetus.

During the pelvic examination, a Papanicolaou (Pap) smear may be obtained. Additional cultures, such as for gonorrhea and chlamydia screening and group B streptococcus screening, also may be obtained. Ensure that all specimens obtained are labeled correctly and sent to the laboratory for evaluation.

A rectal examination is done last to assess for lesions, masses, prolapse, or hemorrhoids.

Once the examination of the internal genitalia is completed and the speculum is removed, a bimanual examination is performed to estimate the size of the uterus to confirm dates and to palpate the ovaries to assess for any masses. The ovaries should be small and nontender, without masses. At the conclusion of the bimanual examination, the healthcare professional reinserts the index finger into the vagina and the middle finger into the rectum to assess the strength and regularity of the posterior vaginal wall.

Pelvic Shape

The size and shape of the women's pelvis can affect her ability to deliver vaginally. Pelvic shape is typically classified as one of four types: gynecoid, android, anthropoid, and platypelloid (Fig. 12-6).

The *gynecoid* pelvis is considered the normal-shaped female pelvis. It offers the optimal diameters in all three planes of the pelvis and is considered the best pelvic type for a vaginal birth (Sloan, 2002). This type of pelvis allows early and complete fetal internal rotation during labor. A gynecoid pelvis occurs in approximately 50% of all women.

The *android* pelvis is considered the male-shaped pelvis and is characterized by a funnel shape. It occurs in approximately 20% of women. (Olds et al., 2004). The pelvic inlet is heart-shaped and the posterior segments are reduced in all pelvic planes. Transverse arrest of labor and fetal head rotation failure are common with this pelvic shape. The prognosis for labor is poor, subsequently leading to caesarean birth.

The *anthropoid* ("ape-like") pelvis is wider front to back (anterior to posterior) than it is side to side (transverse). Approximately 25% of women have this type of pelvic shape. The pelvis inlet is oval, with a short transverse diameter. Vaginal birth is more favorable with this pelvic shape compared to the android or platypelloid shape (Mattson & Smith, 2004).

The *platypelloid* or flat female pelvis is the least common pelvic shape, occurring in approximately 5% of

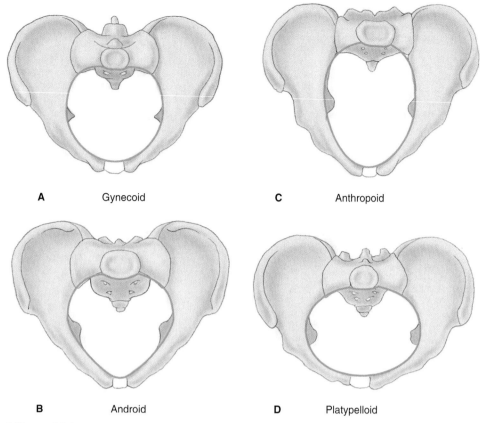

● Figure 12-6 Pelvic shapes. (**A**) Gynecoid. (**B**) Android. (**C**) Anthropoid. (**D**) Platypelloid.

women. Arrest of labor at the pelvic inlet is common. The prognosis for vaginal birth is poor and cesarean birth often is necessary (Mattson & Smith, 2004).

Pelvic Measurements

Taking internal pelvic measurements determines the actual diameters of the inlet and outlet through which the fetus will pass. This is extremely important if the woman has never given birth vaginally. Taking pelvic measurements is unnecessary for the woman who has given birth vaginally before (unless she has experienced some type of trauma to the area) because vaginal delivery demonstrates that the pelvis is adequate for the passage of the fetus.

Three measurements are assessed: diagonal conjugate, true conjugate, and ischial tuberosity (Fig. 12-7). The *diagonal conjugate* is the distance between the anterior surface of the sacral prominence and the anterior surface of the inferior margin of the symphysis pubis (Engstrom, 2004). This measurement, usually 12.5 cm or greater, indicates the anteroposterior diameter of the pelvic inlet. The diagonal conjugate is the most useful measurement for estimating pelvic size because a misfit with the fetal head occurs if it is too small.

The *true conjugate*, also called the obstetric conjugate, is the measurement from the anterior surface of the sacral prominence to the posterior surface of the inferior margin

of the symphysis pubis. This diameter cannot be measured directly; rather, it is estimated by subtracting 1 to 2 cm from the diagonal conjugate measurement. The average true conjugate diameter is at least 11.5 cm (Wong et al., 2002). This measurement is important because it is the smallest front-to-back diameter through which the fetal head must pass when moving through the pelvic inlet.

The *ischial tuberosity* diameter is the transverse diameter of the pelvic outlet. This measurement is made outside the pelvis at the lowest aspect of the ischial tuberosities. A diameter of 10.5 cm or more is considered adequate for passage of the fetal head (Youngkin & Davis, 2004).

Laboratory Tests

A series of tests are generally ordered during the initial visit so that baseline data can be obtained, allowing for early detection and prompt intervention if any problems occur. Tests that are generally conducted for all pregnant women include urinalysis and blood studies. The urine is analyzed for albumin, glucose, ketones, and bacteria casts. Blood studies usually include a complete blood count (hemoglobin, hematocrit, red and white blood cell counts, and platelets), blood typing and Rh factor, a rubella titer, hepatitis B surface antibody antigen, HIV, VDRL and RPR tests, and cervical smears to detect STIs (Table 12-1).

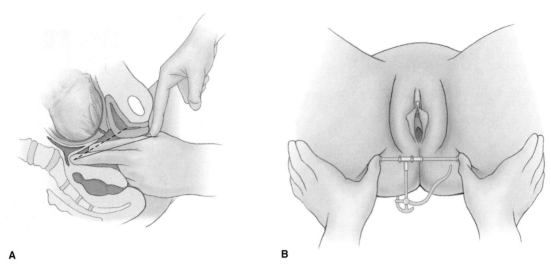

A **B**

● Figure 12-7 Pelvic measurements. (**A**) Diagonal conjugate (*solid line*) and true conjugate (*dotted line*). (**B**) Ischial tuberosity diameter.

Table 12-1 Common Tests for the Initial Prenatal Visit

Test	Comments
Complete blood cell count (CBC)	Evaluates hemoglobin (12–14 g) and hematocrit (42% (±5%)) levels and red blood cell count (4.2–5.4 million/mm³) to detect presence of anemia; identifies WBC (5,000–10,000/mm³), which if elevated may indicate an infection; determines platelet count (150,000–450,000 cubic mL) to assess clotting ability
Blood typing	Determines woman's blood type and Rh status to rule out any blood incompatibility issues early; Rh-negative mother would likely receive RhoGAM (at 28 weeks) if she is Rh sensitive via indirect Coombs test
Rubella titer	Detects antibodies for the virus that causes German measles; if titer is 1:8 or less, the woman is not immune, requires immunization after birth, and is advised to avoid people with undiagnosed rashes
Hepatitis B	Determines if mother has hepatitis B by detecting presence of hepatic antibody surface antigen (HbsAg) in her blood
HIV testing	Detects HIV antibodies and if positive requires more specific test, counseling, and treatment during pregnancy with antiretroviral medications to prevent transmission to fetus
Syphilis screening Venereal Disease Research Laboratory (VDRL) or rapid plasma reagin (RPR) serologic tests	Detects syphilis so that treatment can be initiated early to prevent transmission to fetus
Cervical smears	Detects abnormalities such as cervical cancer (Pap test) or infections such as gonorrhea, chlamydia, group B streptococcus so that treatment can be initiated if positive

Sources: Engstrom, 2004; Matteson, 2001; Murray et al., 2006

In addition, most offices and clinic facilities have ultrasound facilities so that women can be evaluated to validate an intrauterine pregnancy and assess early fetal growth.

The need for additional laboratory studies is determined by a woman's history, physical examination findings, current health status, and risk factors identified in the initial interview. Additional tests can be offered and encouraged, but ultimately the woman and her partner make the decision about undergoing additional studies. The nurse educates the client and her partner about the tests, including the rationale. In addition, the nurse supports the client and her partner in their decision-making process, regardless of whether the nurse agrees with the couple's decision. The couple's decisions about their healthcare are based on the ethical principle of autonomy, which allows an individual the right to make decisions about his or her own body.

Follow-Up Visits

Continuous prenatal care is important for a successful outcome. The recommended schedule for a healthy pregnant woman is as follows:

- Every 4 weeks up to 28 weeks (7 months)
- Every 2 weeks from 29 to 36 weeks
- Every week from 37 weeks to birth

At each subsequent prenatal visit the following assessments are completed:

- Weight and blood pressure, which are compared to baseline values
- Urine testing for protein, glucose, ketones, and nitrites
- Fundal height measurement to assess fetal growth
- Assessment for quickening/fetal movement to determine well-being
- Assessment of fetal heart rate (should be 120 to 160 bpm)

With each follow-up visit, the nurse answers questions, provides anticipatory guidance and education, reviews nutritional guidelines, and evaluates the client for compliance with prenatal vitamin therapy. Throughout the pregnancy, the nurse also encourages the woman's partner to participate if possible.

Fundal Height Measurement

Fundal height is the distance (in cm) measured with a tape measure from the top of the pubic bone to the top of the uterus (fundus) with the client lying on her back with her knees slightly flexed (Fig. 12-8). Measurement in this way is termed the McDonald's method. Fundal height typically increases as the pregnancy progresses; it reflects the progress of fetal growth and provides a gross estimate of the duration of the pregnancy.

At about 12 to 14 weeks' gestation, the fundus can be palpated above the symphysis pubis. The fundus reaches

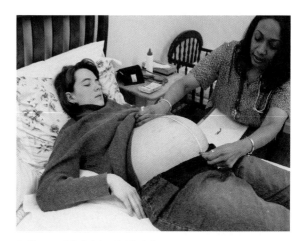

● Figure 12-8 Fundal height measurement.

the level of the umbilicus at approximately 20 weeks and measures 20 cm. Fundal measurement should approximately equal the number of weeks of gestation until week 36. For example, a fundal height of 24 cm suggests a fetus at 24 weeks' gestation. After 36 weeks, the fundal height then drops due to lightening and may no longer correspond with the week of gestation.

Measurement of fundal height is used as an indicator of fetal growth. In addition, it provides a gross estimate of the duration of the pregnancy. It is expected that the fundal height will increase progressively throughout the pregnancy, reflecting fetal growth, but if the growth curve flattens or stays stable, it may indicate the presence of intrauterine growth restriction (IUGR). If the fundal height measurement is greater than 4 cm from the estimated gestational age, further evaluation is warranted if a multifetal gestation has not been diagnosed or the presence of hydramnios has not been ruled out (Dillon, 2003).

Fetal Movement Determination

Fetal movement is usually perceived by the client at 16 to 20 weeks' gestation (Youngkin & Davis, 2004). Perceived fetal movement is most often related to trunk and limb motion and rollovers, or flips (Walsh, 2001). Fetal movement is a gross indicator of fetal well-being. Decreased fetal movement may indicate asphyxia and IUGR. If compromised, the fetus decreases its oxygen requirements by decreasing activity (Littleton & Engebretson, 2005). A decrease in fetal movement may be related to other factors as well, such as maternal use of central nervous system depressants, fetal sleep cycles, hydrocephalus, bilateral renal agenesis, and bilateral hip dislocation (Druzin et al., 2002).

Two suggested techniques for determining fetal movement, also called fetal movement counts, are the Cardiff technique and the Sadovsky technique (Box 12-2). Fetal movement is a noninvasive method of screening and can be easily taught to all pregnant women. Both techniques require client participation.

BOX 12-2

TECHNIQUES FOR FETAL MOVEMENT COUNTS

Maternal perception of fetal movements or counting fetal movements is an inexpensive, noninvasive method of assessing fetal well-being. Several different techniques, two of which are described below, can be used. Scientific evidence has not shown that one technique is better than another. However, the amount of time required for the client to complete the count varies. Additionally, because counts are highly subjective on the mother's part, consistency is essential when performing fetal movement counts. Fetal movement counts should be done at approximately the same time each day, and further testing should be initiated within 12 hours of a client's perception of decreased activity (Littleton & Engebretson, 2005).

With the *Cardiff* technique, the woman lies or sits and concentrates on fetal movements until she records 10 movements. She must record the length of time during which the 10 movements occurred. She is instructed to notify her healthcare provider if she doesn't feel at least 10 movements within 1 hour. Further follow-up testing is indicated.

With the *Sadovsky* technique, the woman lies down on her left side for 1 hour after meals and concentrates on fetal movement. Four movements should be felt within 1 hour. If four movements have not been felt within 1 hour, then the woman should monitor movement for a second hour. If after 2 hours, four movements haven't been felt, the client should contact her healthcare provider.

Instruct the client about how to count fetal movements, the reasons for doing so, and the significance of decreased fetal movements. Urge the client to perform the counts in a relaxed environment and a comfortable position, such as semi-Fowler's or side-lying. Provide the client with detailed information concerning fetal movement count and stress the need for consistency in monitoring (at approximately the same time each day) and the importance of informing the health care provider promptly of any reduced movements. Providing clients with "fetal kick count" charts to record movement is helpful in promoting compliance. There is no established number of fetal movements that indicates fetal well-being, but instruct the woman to report a count of less than three fetal movements within an hour. Further investigation with a nonstress test or biophysical profile is usually warranted (Littleton & Engebretson, 2005).

Fetal Heart Rate Measurement

Fetal heart rate measurement is integral to fetal surveillance throughout the pregnancy. Auscultating the fetal heart rate with a handheld Doppler at each prenatal visit helps confirm that the intrauterine environment is still supportive to the growing fetus. The purpose of assessing fetal heart rate is to determine rate and rhythm. Nursing Procedure 12-1 lists the steps involved in measuring fetal heart rate.

Follow-Up Visit Intervals and Assessments

Up to 28 weeks' gestation, follow-up visits involve assessment of the client's blood pressure and weight. The urine

---

Nursing Procedure 12-1

Measuring Fetal Heart Rate

Purpose: To Assess Fetal Well-Being

1. Assist the woman onto the examining table and have her lie down.
2. Cover her with a sheet to ensure privacy, and then expose her abdomen.
3. Palpate the abdomen to determine the fetal lie, position, and presentation.
4. Locate the back of the fetus (the ideal position to hear the heart rate).
5. Apply lubricant gel to abdomen in the area where the back has been located.
6. Turn on the handheld Doppler device and place it on the spot over the fetal back.
7. Listen for the sound of the amplified heart rate, moving the device slightly from side to side as

necessary to obtain the loudest sound. Assess the woman's pulse rate and compare it to the amplified sound. If the rates appear the same, reposition the Doppler device.

8. Once the fetal heart rate has been identified, count the number of beats in one minute and record the results.
9. Remove the Doppler device and wipe off any remaining gel from the woman's abdomen and the device.
10. Record the heart rate on the woman's medical record.
11. Provide information to the woman regarding fetal well-being based on findings.

is tested for protein and glucose. Fundal height and fetal heart rate are assessed at every office visit. Between weeks 24 to 28, a blood glucose level is obtained using a 50-g glucose load followed by a 1-hour plasma glucose determination. If the result is more than 140 mg/dL, further testing, such as with a 3-hour 100-g glucose tolerance test, is warranted to determine whether gestational diabetes is present.

During this time, review the common discomforts of pregnancy, evaluate any client complaints, and answer questions from the couple. Reinforce appropriate nutrition and use of prenatal vitamins, along with daily exercise.

Between 29 and 36 weeks' gestation, all the assessments of previous visits are completed, along with assessment for edema. Special attention is focused on the presence and location of edema during the last trimester. Pregnant women commonly experience dependent edema of the lower extremities from constriction of blood vessels secondary to the heavy gravid uterus. Periorbital edema around the eyes, edema of the hands, and pretibial edema are abnormal and could be signs of pregnancy-induced hypertension. Inspecting and palpating both extremities, listening for complaints of tight rings on fingers, and observing for swelling around the eyes are important assessments. Abnormal findings in any of these areas need to be reported.

If the mother is Rh negative, her antibody titer is reevaluated. RhoGAM is given if indicated. The client also is evaluated for risk of preterm labor. At each visit ask if she is experiencing any common signs or symptoms of preterm labor (e.g., uterine contractions, dull backache, feeling of pressure in the pelvic area or thighs, increased vaginal discharge, menstrual-like cramps, vaginal bleeding). A pelvic examination is performed to assess the cervix for position, consistency, length, and dilation. If the woman has had a previous preterm birth, she is at risk for another and warrants close monitoring.

Counsel the woman about choosing a healthcare provider for the newborn, if she has not selected one yet. Along with completion of a breast assessment, discuss the choice of breastfeeding versus bottle-feeding. Reinforce the importance of daily fetal movement monitoring as an indicator of fetal well-being. Reevaluate hemoglobin and hematocrit levels to assess for anemia.

Between 37 and 40 weeks' gestation, the same assessments are done as for the previous weeks. In addition, screening for group B streptococcus, gonorrhea, and chlamydia is done. Fetal presentation and position (via Leopold's maneuvers) are assessed. Review the signs and symptoms of labor and forward a copy of the prenatal record to the hospital labor department for future reference. Review the client's desire for family planning after birth as well as her decision to breastfeed or bottle-feed. Remind the client that an infant car seat is required by law.

Assessment of Fetal Well-Being

During the antepartum period, several tests are performed to monitor fetal well-being as well as to detect possible problems. When a **high-risk pregnancy** (one in which the life or health of the mother or infant is jeopardized by a disorder coincidental with or unique to pregnancy; Wong et al., 2002) is identified, additional antepartum testing can be initiated to promote positive maternal, fetal, and neonatal outcomes. High-risk pregnancies include those that are complicated by maternal or fetal conditions that jeopardize the health status of the mother and put the fetus at risk for uteroplacental insufficiency, hypoxia, and death. However, antepartum fetal testing should take place only when the results obtained will guide future care, whether it is reassurance, more frequent testing, admission to the hospital, or the immediate need to deliver (Davies, 2000).

Ultrasonography

Since its introduction in the late 1950s, ultrasonography has become a very useful diagnostic tool in obstetrics. Real-time scanners can produce a continuous picture of the fetus on a monitor screen. A transducer that emits high-frequency sound waves is placed on the mother's abdomen and moved to visualize the fetus (Fig. 12-9). The fetal heartbeat and any malformations in the fetus can be assessed and measurements can be made accurately from the picture on the monitor screen.

Ultrasound, which is noninvasive, is considered a safe, accurate, and cost-effective tool. It provides important information about fetal activity, growth, and gestational age, assesses fetal well-being, and acts as a guide for the need for invasive intrauterine tests (Brown, 2004).

There are no hard-and-fast rules as to the number of ultrasounds a woman should have during her pregnancy. An ultrasound usually is performed in the first trimester to confirm pregnancy, exclude ectopic or molar pregnancies, and confirm cardiac pulsation. A second scan may be performed at about 18 to 20 weeks to look for congenital malformations, exclude multifetal pregnancies, and verify dates and growth. A third scan may be done at around 34 weeks to evaluate fetal size, assess fetal growth, and verify placental position (Woo, 2004). An ultrasound is used to confirm placental location during amniocentesis and provide visualization during chorionic villus sampling. An ultrasound is also ordered whenever an abnormality is suspected based on clinical grounds.

Nursing Management

Nursing management focuses on educating the woman about the ultrasound test and reassuring her that she will not experience any sensation from the sound waves during the test. No special client preparation is needed prior to performing the ultrasound, although in early preg-

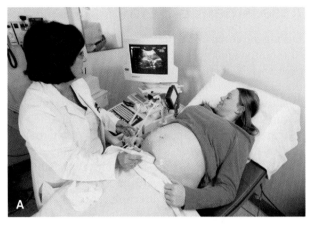 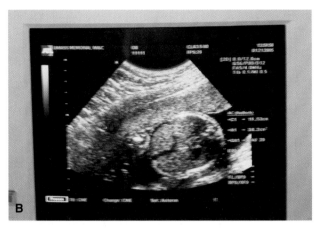

● Figure 12-9 Ultrasound. (**A**) Ultrasound device being applied to client's abdomen.
(**B**) View of monitor.

nancy the woman may need to have a full bladder. Inform
her that she may experience some discomfort from the
pressure on the full bladder during the scan, but it will
last only a short time. Tell the client that a conducting gel
is used on the abdomen during the scan and that it may
feel cold initially.

Doppler Flow Studies

Doppler flow studies can be used to measure the velocity
of blood flow via ultrasound. The color images produced
help to identify abnormalities in diastolic flow within the
umbilical vessels. The velocity of the fetal red blood cells
can be determined by measuring the change in the frequency of the sound wave reflected off the cells. Thus,
Doppler flow studies can detect the movement of red
blood cells in vessels (Littleton & Engebretson, 2002). In
pregnancies complicated by hypertension or IUGR, diastolic blood flow may be absent or even reversed (Opipari
& Johnson, 2000). Doppler flow studies also can be
used to evaluate the blood flow through other fetal blood
vessels, such as the aorta and those in the brain.

Doppler flow studies can detect fetal compromise in
high-risk pregnancies. The test is noninvasive and has no
contraindications. Research continues to determine the
indications for Doppler flow studies to improve pregnancy outcomes.

Nursing Management
Nursing management of the woman undergoing Doppler
flow studies is similar to that described for an ultrasound.

Alpha-Fetoprotein Analysis

Alpha-fetoprotein (AFP) is a substance produced by
the fetal liver between weeks 13 and 20 of gestation.
AFP analysis is a blood test that measures AFP levels
(Alexander et al., 2004). About 30 years ago, elevated levels of maternal serum AFP or amniotic fluid AFP were
first linked to the occurrence of fetal neural tube defects.
This biomarker screening test is now recommended for all
pregnant women (ACOG, 2003).

AFP is present in amniotic fluid in low concentrations between 10 and 14 weeks of gestation and can be
detected in maternal serum beginning approximately at
12 to 14 weeks of gestation (Gilbert & Harmon, 2003).
If a developmental defect, such as failure of the neural
tube to close, exists, more AFP escapes into amniotic
fluid from the fetus. AFP then enters the maternal circulation by crossing the placenta, and the level in maternal
serum can be measured. The optimal time for AFP
screening is 16 to 18 weeks of gestation (ACOG, 2001).
Correct information about gestational dating, maternal
weight, race, number of fetuses, and insulin dependency
is necessary to ensure the accuracy of this screening test.

A variety of situations can lead to elevation of maternal
serum AFP, including open neural tube defect, under-
estimation of gestational age, the presence of multiple
fetuses, gastrointestinal defects, low birthweight, oligohydramnios, and decreased maternal weight (Miller & Isabel,
2002). Lower-than-expected maternal serum AFP levels are seen when fetal gestational age is overestimated or
in cases of fetal death, hydatidiform mole, increased
maternal weight, maternal type I diabetes, and fetal trisomy 21 (Down syndrome) or trisomy 18 (Edward's
syndrome) (Graves et al., 2002).

Measurement of maternal serum AFP is minimally
invasive, requiring a venipuncture for a blood sample.
It detects approximately 80% of all open neural tube
defects and open abdominal wall defects in early pregnancy (Lowdermilk & Perry, 2004). AFP has now been
combined with other biomarker screening tests to determine risks of neural tube defects or Down syndrome. If
incorrect maternal information is submitted or the blood
specimen is not drawn during the appropriate timeframe,
false-positive results may occur, increasing the woman's
anxiety. Subsequently, further testing might be ordered

based on an inaccurate interpretation, resulting in additional financial and emotional costs to the woman.

Nursing Management

Prepare the woman for this screening test by gathering accurate information about the date of her LMP, weight, race, and gestational dating. Accurately determining the window of 16 to 18 weeks' gestation will help to ensure that the test results are correct. Also explain that the test involves a blood specimen.

Marker Screening Tests

Two other screening tests may be used to determine risk: the triple-marker screen and the addition of a fourth marker, inhibin A, which is used to enhance the accuracy of screening for Down syndrome in women younger than 35 years of age. Low inhibin A levels indicate the possibility of Down syndrome (ACOG, 2001). These tests combine three or four procedures to enhance the ability to determine a diagnosis. These biomarkers are merely screening tests and identify women who need further definitive procedures to make a diagnosis of neural tube defects (anencephaly, spina bifida, and encephalocele) or Down syndrome in this fetus. Most screening tests are performed between 15 to 22 weeks of gestation (16 to 18 weeks is ideal) (ACOG, 2001).

The triple-marker screening or triple screening test is performed at 16 to 18 weeks of gestation. It uses the levels of three maternal serum markers (AFP, unconjugated estriol, and hCG), in combination with maternal age, to calculate risk (Lowdermilk & Perry, 2004). With this screening, low maternal serum AFP and unconjugated estriol levels and a high hCG level suggests the possibility of Down syndrome.

The screening test using four maternal markers is also used to screen for Down syndrome. It uses maternal age at term and the concentration of four biomarkers in maternal serum: AFP, unconjugated estriol, hCG, and inhibin A. This test is done at 14 to 22 weeks of pregnancy and is reported to detect 85% of trisomy 21 cases; the triple screen was reported to detect only 69% (Wald et al., 2003). Like other screening tests, abnormal values do not diagnose a defect, but they may help in identifying potential high-risk conditions that require additional tests such as an amniocentesis and genetic counseling.

Nursing Management

Prenatal screening has become standard in prenatal care. However, for many couples it remains confusing, emotionally charged, and filled with uncertain risks. Offer a thorough explanation of the test, reinforcing the information given by the healthcare professional. Provide couples with a description of the risks and benefits of performing these screens, emphasizing that these tests are for screening purposes only. Remind the couple that a definitive

diagnosis is not made without further tests such as an amniocentesis. Answer any questions about these prenatal screening tests and respect the couple's decision if they choose not to have them done. Many couples may wish not to know because they would not consider an abortion regardless of the test results.

Amniocentesis

Amniocentesis involves a transabdominal perforation of the amniotic sac to obtain a sample of amniotic fluid for analysis. The fluid contains fetal cells that are examined to detect chromosomal abnormalities and several hereditary metabolic defects in the fetus before birth. In addition, amniocentesis is used to confirm a fetal abnormality when other screening tests detect a possible problem.

Amniocentesis is performed in the second trimester of pregnancy, usually between weeks 16 and 18. It can be done as early as week 14 or as late as week 20 (Engstrom, 2004). Over 40 different chromosomal abnormalities, inborn errors of metabolism, and neural tube defects can be diagnosed with amniocentesis. It can replace a genetic probability with a diagnostic certainty and provide the option of therapeutic abortion.

Amniocentesis can be performed in any of the three trimesters of pregnancy. An early amniocentesis (performed between weeks 11 and 14) is done to detect genetic anomalies, but early amniocentesis has been associated with a greater risk of spontaneous miscarriage and postprocedural amniotic fluid leakage compared with transabdominal chorionic villus screening (Alfirevic, 2001). ACOG (2004) has issued a position statement on first-trimester screening methods, recommending chorionic villus sampling and nuchal translucency to detect Down syndrome rather than amniocentesis because of the increased risks associated with the early procedure. However, early screening and diagnosis can provide the couple with time to make decisions about the pregnancy outcome.

In the second trimester the procedure is performed between 15 and 20 weeks (ACOG, 2001) to detect chromosomal abnormalities, evaluate the fetal condition when the woman is sensitized to the Rh-positive blood, diagnose intrauterine infections, and investigate amniotic fluid AFP when the maternal serum AFP level is elevated (Murray et al., 2006).

In the third trimester amniocentesis is most commonly indicated to determine fetal lung maturity after the 35th week of gestation via analysis of lecithin-to-sphingomyelin ratios and to evaluate the fetal condition with Rh isoimmunization.

Table 12-2 lists amniotic fluid analysis findings and their implications.

The second trimester is the most common time to have an amniocentesis for any prenatal diagnosis since it carries such high risk if done earlier. By week 14 to 16 of gestation, there is sufficient amniotic fluid for sampling yet enough time for a safe abortion, if desired. Amniocentesis is offered to women who are 35 years of age or older, women who have a child with a neural tube defect, and women with elevated maternal serum AFP levels. It also may be used to detect chromosomal aberrations when a parent has a chromosomal abnormality or is a carrier for a metabolic disease (O'Toole, 2003).

Amniocentesis is performed after an ultrasound examination identifies an adequate pocket of amniotic fluid free of fetal parts, umbilical cord, or the placenta (Fig. 12-10). The health care provider inserts a long pudendal or spinal needle, a 22-gauge, 5-inch needle, into the amniotic cavity and aspirates amniotic fluid, which is placed in an amber or foil-covered test tube to protect it from light. When the desired amount of fluid has been withdrawn, the needle is removed and slight pressure is applied to the site. If there is no evidence of bleeding, a sterile bandage is applied to the needle site. The specimens are then sent to the laboratory immediately for the cytologist to evaluate.

Examining a sample of fetal cells directly produces a definitive diagnosis rather than a "best guess" diagnosis based on indirect screening tests. It is an invaluable diagnostic tool, but the risks include spontaneous abortion (1 in 200), maternal or fetal infection, fetal-maternal hemorrhage, leakage of amniotic fluid, and maternal discomfort after the procedure. The test results may take up to 3 weeks.

Nursing Management

When preparing the woman for an amniocentesis, explain the procedure and encourage her to empty her bladder just before the procedure to avoid the risk of bladder puncture. Inform her that a 20-minute electronic fetal monitoring strip usually is obtained to evaluate fetal well-being

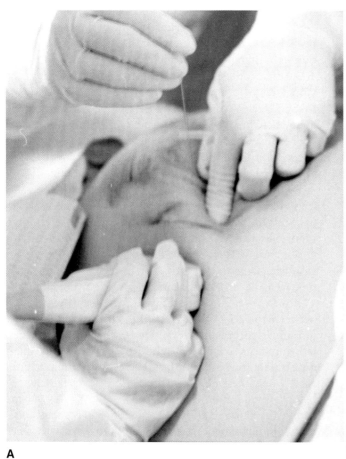

A

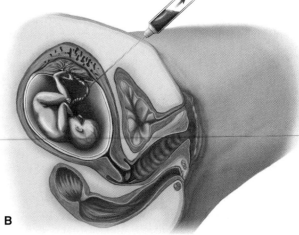

B

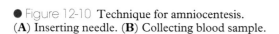

● Figure 12-10 Technique for amniocentesis.
(**A**) Inserting needle. (**B**) Collecting blood sample.

Table 12-2 Amniotic Fluid Analysis and Implications

Test Component	Normal Findings	Fetal Implications of Abnormal Findings
Color	Clear with white flecks of vernix caseosa in a mature fetus	Blood of maternal origin is usually harmless. "Port wine" fluid may indicate abruptio placentae. Fetal blood may indicate damage to the fetal, placental, or umbilical cord vessels.
Bilirubin	Absent at term	High levels indicate hemolytic disease of the neonate in isoimmunized pregnancy.
Meconium	Absent (except in breech presentation)	Presence indicates fetal hypotension or distress.
Creatinine	More than 2 mg/dL in a mature fetus	Decrease may indicate immature fetus (less than 37 weeks).
Lecithin–sphingomyelin ratio	More than 2 generally indicates fetal pulmonary maturity	A ratio of less than 2 indicates pulmonary immaturity and subsequent respiratory distress syndrome.
Phosphatidylglycerol	Present	Absence indicates pulmonary immaturity.
Glucose	Less than 45 mg/dL	Excessive increases at term or near term indicate hypertrophied fetal pancreas and subsequent neonatal hypoglycemia.
Alpha-fetoprotein	Variable, depending on gestation age and laboratory technique, highest concentration (about 18.5 μg/mL) occurs at 13 to 14 weeks	Inappropriate increases indicate neural tube defects, such as spina bifida or anencephaly, impending fetal death, congenital nephrosis, or contamination of fetal blood.
Bacteria	Absent	Presence indicates chorioamnionitis
Chromosome	Normal karyotype	Abnormal karyotype may indicate fetal sex and chromosome disorders.
Acetylcholinesterase	Absent	Presence may indicate neural tube defects, exomphalos, or other serious malformations.

From Engstrom, J. (2004). *Maternal-neonatal nursing.* Philadelphia: Lippincott Williams & Wilkins, p. 179.

and obtain a baseline to compare after the procedure is completed. Obtain and record maternal vital signs.

After the procedure, assist the woman to a position of comfort and administer RhoGAM intramuscularly if the woman is Rh negative to prevent potential sensitization to fetal blood. Assess maternal vital signs and fetal heart rate every 15 minutes for an hour after the procedure. Observe the puncture site for bleeding or drainage. Instruct the client to rest after returning home and remind her to report fever, leaking amniotic fluid, vaginal bleeding, or uterine contractions or any changes in fetal activity (increased or decreased) to the healthcare provider.

When the test results return, be available to offer support, especially if a fetal abnormality is found. Also prepare the woman and her partner for the necessity of genetic counseling. Trained genetic counselors can provide accurate medical information and help couples to interpret the results of the amniocentesis so they can make the decisions that are right for them as a family.

Chorionic Villus Sampling

Chorionic villus sampling (CVS) is a procedure for obtaining a sample of the chorionic villi for prenatal evaluation of chromosomal disorders, enzyme deficiencies, and fetal gender determination and to identify sex-linked disorders such as hemophilia, sickle cell anemia, and Tay-Sachs disease (O'Toole, 2003). Chorionic villi are finger-like projections that cover the embryo and anchor it to the uterine lining before the placenta is developed. Because they are of embryonic origin, sampling provides information about the developing fetus. CVS can be used to detect numerous genetic disorders, with the exception of neural tube defects (Cavanaugh, 2003).

There has been an impetus to develop earlier prenatal diagnostic procedures so that couples can expand their options if the pregnancy outcome is not optimal. Early prenatal diagnosis by CVS was proposed as an alternative to routine amniocentesis, which carries fewer risks if done later in the pregnancy.

CVS is performed between 8 and 12 weeks. First, an ultrasound is done to confirm gestational age and viability. Then, with continuous ultrasound guidance, CVS is performed using either a transcervical or transabdominal approach. With the transcervical approach, the woman is placed in the lithotomy position and a sterile catheter is introduced through the cervix and inserted in the placenta, where a sample of chorionic villi is aspirated. This approach requires the client to have a full bladder to push the uterus and placenta into a position that is more accessible to the catheter. A full bladder also helps in better visualization of the structures. With the transabdominal approach, an 18-gauge spinal needle is inserted through the abdominal wall into the placental tissue and a sample of chorionic villi is aspirated. Regardless of the approach used, the sample is sent to the cytogenetics laboratory for analysis.

CVS can be performed as early as the eighth week of pregnancy, thus permitting the couple to make an early decision to terminate the pregnancy if an anomaly is confirmed. Results are available sooner than amniocentesis results, usually within 48 hours. Potential complications of CVS include mild vaginal bleeding and cramping, miscarriage, rupture of membranes, chorioamnionitis, and fetal-maternal hemorrhage (Harris et al., 2004). In addition, women who are Rh negative should receive immune globulin (RhoGAM) to avoid isoimmunization (Gilbert & Harmon, 2003).

Nursing Management

Explain to the woman that the procedure will last about 15 minutes. An ultrasound will be done first to localize the embryo, and a baseline set of vital signs will be taken prior to starting. Make sure she is informed of the risks related to the procedure, including their incidence.

If a transabdominal CVS procedure is planned, advise her to fill her bladder by drinking increased amounts of water. Inform her that a needle will be inserted through her abdominal wall and samples will be collected. Once the samples are collected, the needle will be withdrawn and the samples will be sent to the genetics laboratory for evaluation.

For transcervical CVS, instruct the woman to void immediately prior to the procedure. Inform her that a speculum will be placed into the vagina under ultrasound guidance. Then the vagina is cleaned and a small catheter is inserted through the cervix. The samples obtained through the catheter are then sent to the laboratory.

After either procedure, assist the woman to a position of comfort and clean any excess lubricant or secretions from the area. Instruct her about signs to watch for and report, such as fever, cramping, and vaginal bleeding. Urge her not to engage in any strenuous activity for the next 48 hours. Assess fetal heart rate for changes and administer RhoGAM to an unsensitized Rh-negative woman after the procedure.

Percutaneous Umbilical Blood Sampling

Percutaneous umbilical blood sampling (PUBS) permits the collection of a blood specimen directly from the fetal circulation. Under continuous ultrasound guidance, a fine needle is inserted through the mother's abdomen and uterine wall into an umbilical cord vessel. Specimens can be evaluated for coagulation studies, blood group typing, complete blood count, karyotyping, and blood gas analysis (Ghezzi et al., 2001). Fetal infection, Rh incompatibility, and fetal acid–base status can be determined. The blood sample is usually drawn late in the second trimester to assist in medical management, but PUBS can be done anytime after 16 weeks of gestation. This test allows for rapid chromosomal analysis to achieve a timely diagnosis. It is done specifically for women at risk for genetic anomalies and those with potential blood disorders, such as blood incompatibility or hemoglobinopathies.

Although the information gained from this procedure is valuable and can be life-saving for many fetuses, PUBS is not without risks. Potential complications include leaking of blood from the puncture site, cord laceration, cord hematomas, transient fetal bradycardia, infection, thromboembolism in the umbilical cord, preterm labor, infection, and premature rupture of membranes (Simpson, 2002).

Nursing Management

Explain the procedure thoroughly to the woman. Position her properly on the examination table and help clean the area for needle insertion. Monitoring vital signs and fetal heart rate throughout the procedure. At the conclusion of the procedure, closely monitor the mother and fetus for changes. Assess fetal heart rate continuously and perform external fetal monitoring for up to 2 hours before the woman is discharged from the outpatient area. A repeat ultrasound is usually done within an hour after the procedure to rule out bleeding or hematoma formation.

Prior to discharge, instruct the woman to report signs of infection, an increase in contractions, or a change in fetal activity level from normal. Reinforce the need to count fetal movements, and review the technique, so she can assess them when she is discharged home.

Nonstress Test

The nonstress test (NST) is an indirect measurement of uteroplacental function. Unlike the fetal movement counting done by the mother alone, this procedure requires specialized equipment and trained personnel. The basis for the nonstress test is that the normal fetus produces characteristic fetal heart rate patterns in response to fetal movements. In the healthy fetus there is an acceleration of the fetal heart rate with fetal movement. Currently, a NST is recommended twice weekly (after 28 weeks of gestation) for clients with diabetes and other high-risk conditions, such as IUGR, preeclampsia, postterm pregnancy, renal disease, and multifetal pregnancies (Wong et al., 2002). Before the procedure the client eats a meal. Then she is placed in the left lateral recumbent position to avoid supine hypotension syndrome. An external electronic fetal monitoring device is applied to her abdomen. The device consists of two belts, each with a sensor. One of the sensors records uterine activity; the second sensor records fetal heart rate. The client is handed an "event marker" with a button that she pushes every time she perceives fetal movement. When the button is pushed, the fetal monitor strip is marked to identify that fetal movement has occurred. The procedure usually lasts 20 to 30 minutes.

NST is a noninvasive test that requires no initiation of contractions. It is quick to perform and there are no known side effects. However, it is not as sensitive to fetal oxygen reserves as the contraction stress test, and there is a high false-positive rate (Gilbert & Harmon, 2003).

Nursing Management

Prior to the NST, explain the testing procedure and have the woman empty her bladder. Position her in a semi-Fowler's position and apply the two external monitor belts. Document the date and time the test is started, patient information, the reason for the test, and the maternal vital signs. Obtain a baseline fetal monitor strip over 15 to 30 minutes.

During the test, observe for signs of fetal activity with a concurrent acceleration of the fetal heart rate. Interpret the NST as reactive or nonreactive. A "reactive" NST includes at least two fetal heart rate accelerations from the baseline of at least 15 bpm for at least 15 seconds within the 20-minute recording period. If the test does not meet these criteria after 40 minutes, it is considered nonreactive. A "nonreactive" NST is characterized by the absence of two fetal heart rate accelerations using the 15-by-15 criterion in a 20-minute timeframe. A nonreactive test has been correlated with a higher incidence of fetal distress during labor, fetal mortality, and IUGR (Sloan, 2002). Additional testing, such as a contraction stress test or biophysical profile, should be considered (Davies, 2000).

After the NST procedure, assist the woman off the table, provide her with fluids, and allow her to use the restroom. Typically the results are discussed with the woman at this time by the health care provider. Provide teaching about signs and symptoms to report. If serial NSTs are being done, schedule her next testing session.

Contraction Stress Test

Because blood flow to the uterus and placenta is slowed during uterine contractions, the contraction stress test (CST), also called the oxytocin-challenge test (OCT), is a diagnostic procedure performed to determine the fetal heart rate response under stress, such as during contractions. The goal of the test is to achieve three uterine contractions in a 10-minute period. This can occur spontaneously with the aid of nipple stimulation, which causes the release of endogenous oxytocin, or through the use of an oxytocin infusion (Harrison, 2002).

A CST is indicated in pregnancies in which placental insufficiency is suspected—preeclampsia, IUGR, diabetes mellitus, postterm pregnancy, a previous stillbirth— or when an irregularity of the fetal heart rate has been observed (Davies, 2000).

The client is positioned in a semi-Fowler's position and an external electronic fetal monitoring device is attached. A 20-minute NST is performed to establish a baseline. Then uterine contractions are induced via nipple stimulation or with an intravenous oxytocin infusion. With nipple stimulation, the client is instructed to stroke her nipple for 2 minutes, followed by a 5-minute rest period. The cycle is repeated until adequate contractions are observed. If oxytocin is used, the infusion is initiated at 0.5 to 1.0 mU/min and doubled in strength every 15 to 20 minutes until the desired contraction pattern is achieved (Youngkin & Davis, 2004). Once adequate contractions are achieved, the infusion is discontinued.

The CST is more cumbersome to perform and presents more risks to the woman and fetus compared with the NST. However, it may identify fetuses who are only marginally compromised by assessing their reserve when subjected to the stress of uterine contractions. The CST determines fetal ability to endure labor. If the fetus cannot tolerate the stress of contractions in a short controlled testing environment, then it is unlikely the fetus could tolerate the stress of labor over several hours. Therefore, this screening helps to avoid fetal distress in a true labor situation. Caution is needed when using the CST before 37 weeks' gestation in clients at risk for preterm labor because of the potential to cause hyperstimulation and uncontrolled contractions (Engstrom, 2004).

Nursing Management

Explaining the testing procedure thoroughly and instruct the woman to empty her bladder. Position her in a semi-Fowler's position. A wedge may be placed under her right hip to prevent supine hypotension syndrome, if applicable. After applying the external monitor belts and documenting the time, vital signs, client data, and the reason for the test, obtain a 20-minute baseline fetal monitoring strip to gain information about uterine contraction status and fetal heart rate characteristics. Then instruct the client on nipple stimulation or begin the intravenous oxytocin infusion.

During the CST, observe for uterine hyperstimulation and monitor the woman's blood pressure every 15 minutes and when the test is over. Discontinue the intravenous infusion of oxytocin when three or more contractions lasting more than 40 seconds within a 10-minute period are achieved.

Interpreting a CST requires three contractions, lasting at least 40 seconds each, within a 10-minute period. The test is considered negative if no late decelerations (a decrease in fetal heart rate that occurs after the peak of a contraction and returns to baseline after the contraction has subsided) are observed with contractions. It is considered positive if late decelerations are detected in more than 50 percent of the contractions (two out of three). The test should raise suspicion if an occasional late deceleration is seen.

At the conclusion of the CST testing period, promptly give the healthcare provider the fetal monitoring strip for interpretation. Then assist the woman into a position of comfort and provide her with fluids and a snack. Remain with the woman and continue to monitor the uterine and fetal heart rate until they have returned to the pre-CST state. Additional testing should be scheduled if needed.

Biophysical Profile

A **biophysical profile** uses a real-time ultrasound to allow assessment of various parameters of fetal well-being: fetal tone, breathing, and motion and amniotic fluid volume. These four parameters, together with the NST, constitute the biophysical profile. Each parameter is controlled by a different structure in the fetal brain: fetal tone by the cortex; fetal movements by the cortex and motor nuclei; fetal breathing movements by the centers close to the fourth ventricle; and the NST by the posterior hypothalamus and medulla. The amniotic fluid is the result of fetal urine volume. Not all facilities perform an NST unless other parameters of the profile are abnormal (Gilbert & Harmon, 2003). The biophysical profile is based on the concept that a fetus that experiences hypoxia loses certain behavioral parameters in the reverse order in which they were acquired during fetal development (normal order of development: tone at 8 weeks; movement at 9 weeks; breathing at 20 weeks; and fetal heart rate reactivity at 24 weeks).

The biophysical profile is a scored test with five components, each worth 2 points if present. A total score of 10 is possible if the NST is used. Thirty minutes are allotted for testing, although fewer than 10 minutes are usually needed. The following criteria must be met to obtain a score of 2; anything less is scored as 0 (Gilbert & Harmon 2003):

- Body movements: three or more discrete limb or truck movements
- Fetal tone: one or more instances of full extension and flexion of a limb or trunk
- Fetal breathing: one or more fetal breathing movements more than 30 seconds
- Amniotic fluid volume: one or more pockets of fluid measuring 2 cm
- NST: normal NST = 2 points; abnormal NST = 0 points

Interpretation of the biophysical profile score can be complicated, depending on several fetal and maternal variables. Because it is indicated as a result of a nonreassuring finding from previous fetal surveillance tests, this test can be used to quantify the interpretation, and intervention can be initiated if appropriate. One of the important factors is the amniotic fluid volume, taken in conjunction with the results of the NST. Amniotic fluid is largely composed of fetal urine. As placental function decreases, perfusion of fetal organs, such as kidneys, decreases, and this can lead to a reduction of amniotic fluid. If oligohydramnios or decreased amniotic fluid is present, the potential exists for antepartum or intrapartum fetal compromise (Mattson & Smith, 2004).

Overall, a score of 8 to 10 is considered normal if the amniotic fluid volume is adequate. A score of 6 or below is suspicious, possibly indicating a compromised fetus; further investigation is needed.

Because the biophysical profile is an ultrasonographic assessment of fetal behavior, it requires more extensive equipment and more highly trained personnel than other testing modalities. The cost is much greater than with less sophisticated tests. It permits conservative therapy and prevents premature or unnecessary intervention. There are fewer false-positive results than with the NST or CST (ACOG, 2002).

Nursing Management

Nursing management focuses primarily on offering the client support and answering her questions. Expect to complete the NST before scheduling the biophysical profile, and explain why further testing might be needed. Tell the woman that the ultrasound will be done in the diagnostic imaging department.

Nursing Management to Promote Self-Care

Pregnancy is considered a time of health, not illness. Health promotion and maintenance activities are key to promoting an optimal outcome for the woman and her fetus.

Pregnant women commonly have many questions about the changes occurring during pregnancy, how these changes affect their usual routine, such as working, traveling, exercising, or engaging in sexual activity, how the changes influence their typical self-care activities, such as bathing, perineal care, or dental care, and whether these changes are signs of a problem. Women may have heard stories about or been told by others what to do and what not to do during this time, leading to many misconceptions and much misinformation.

Nurses can play a major role in providing anticipatory guidance and teaching to foster the woman's responsibility for self-care, helping to clarify misconceptions and correct any misinformation. Educating the client to identify threats to safety posed by her lifestyle or environment and proposing ways to modify them to avoid a negative outcome are important. Counseling should also include healthy ways to prepare food and advice to avoid medications unless they are prescribed for her and identify teratogens within her environment or at work and make changes to reduce her risk from exposure. The pregnant client can better care for herself and the fetus if her concerns are anticipated and identified by the nurse and are incorporated into teaching sessions at each prenatal visit.

Personal Hygiene

Hygiene is a necessity for the maintenance of good health. Cleansing the skin removes dirt, bacteria, sweat, dead skin cells, and body secretions. Counsel women to wash their hands frequently throughout the day to lower the bacterial count on their hands and under their fingernails. During pregnancy a woman's sebaceous (sweat) glands become more active under the influence of hormones, and sweating is more profuse. This increase may make it necessary to use a stronger deodorant and shower more frequently. The cervical and vaginal glands also produce more secretions during pregnancy. Taking showers twice daily helps to keep the area dry and promotes better hygiene. Encourage the use of cotton underwear to allow greater air circulation. Taking a tub bath in early pregnancy is permitted, but closer to term, when the woman's center of gravity shifts, it is safer to shower to prevent the risk of slipping.

Hot Tubs and Saunas

Pregnant women should avoid using hot tubs, saunas, whirlpools, and tanning beds during pregnancy. The heat may cause fetal tachycardia as well as raise the maternal temperature. Exposure to bacteria in hot tubs that have not been cleaned sufficiently is another reason to avoid them during pregnancy.

Perineal Care

The glands in the cervical and vaginal areas become more active during pregnancy secondary to hormonal influences. This increase in activity will produce more vaginal secretions, especially in the last trimester. Advise pregnant women to shower frequently and wear all-cotton underwear to minimize the effects of these secretions. Pregnant women should not douche, because douching can increase the risk of infection. Pregnant women should not wear panty liners, which block air circulation and promote moisture. They should also avoid perfumed soaps, lotions, perineal sprays, and harsh laundry detergents to help prevent irritation and potential infection.

Dental Care

Research has established that the elevated levels of estrogen and progesterone during pregnancy cause women to be more sensitive to the effects of bacterial dental plaque, which can cause gingivitis, an oral infection characterized by swollen and bleeding gums (Wener & Lavigne, 2004). Brushing and flossing teeth daily will help reduce bacteria in the mouth. Advise the woman to visit her dentist early in the pregnancy to address any dental caries and have a thorough cleaning to prevent possible infection later in the pregnancy. Advise her to avoid exposure to x-rays by informing the hygienist of the pregnancy. If x-rays are necessary, the abdomen should be shielded with a lead apron.

Researchers are exploring a link between prematurity and periodontitis, an oral infection that spreads beyond the gum tissues to invade the supporting structures of the teeth. Periodontitis is characterized by bleeding gums, loss of tooth attachment, loss of supporting bone, and bad breath due to pus formation. Unfortunately, because this infection is chronic and often painless, women frequently don't realize they have it. According to the March of Dimes Foundation (2004), preterm births have increased by almost 30% since 1981 and are the number-one obstetric problem in the United States.

Additional guidelines that the nurse should stress regarding maintaining dental health include:

- Seek professional dental care during the first trimester for assessment and care.
- Obtain treatment for dental pain and infection promptly during pregnancy.
- Brush twice daily for 2 minutes, especially before bed, with fluoridated toothpaste and rinse well. Use a soft-bristled toothbrush and be sure to brush at the gumline to remove food debris and plaque to keep gums healthy.
- Eat healthy foods, especially those high in vitamins A, C, and D and calcium.
- Avoid sugary snacks.
- Chew sugar-free gum for 10 minutes after a meal if brushing isn't possible.
- After vomiting, rinse your mouth immediately with baking soda (1/4 teaspoon) and warm water (1 cup) to neutralize the acid (Wilkins, 2004).

Breast Care

Since the breasts enlarge significantly and become heavier throughout pregnancy, stress the need to wear a firm, supportive bra with wide straps to balance the weight of the breasts. Instruct the woman to anticipate buying a larger-sized bra about halfway through her pregnancy because of the increasing size of the breasts. Advise her to avoid using soap on the nipple area because it can be very drying. Encourage her to rinse the nipple area with plain water while bathing to keep it clean. The Montgomery glands secrete a lubricating substance that keeps the nipples moist and discourages growth of bacteria. There is no need to use alcohol or other antiseptics on the nipples.

If the mother has chosen to breastfeed, nipple preparation is unnecessary unless her nipples are inverted and do not become erect when stimulated. Breast shells can be worn during the last 2 months to address this issue (Youngkin & Davis, 2004).

Around week 16 of pregnancy, colostrum secretion begins, which the woman may notice as moisture in her bra. Advise the woman to place breast pads or a cotton cloth in her bra and change them frequently to prevent build-up, which may lead to excoriation.

Clothing

Many contemporary clothes are loose-fitting and layered, so the woman may not need to buy an entirely new wardrobe to accommodate her pregnancy. Some pregnant women may continue to wear tight clothes. Point out that loose clothing will be more comfortable for the client and her expanding waistline.

Pregnant women should avoid wearing constricting clothes and girdles that compress the growing abdomen. Urge the woman to avoid knee-high hose, which might impede lower-extremity circulation and increase the risk of developing deep vein thrombosis. Low-heeled shoes will minimize pelvic tilt and possible backache. Wearing layered clothing may be more comfortable, especially toward term, when the woman may feel overheated.

Exercise

Exercise is well tolerated by a healthy woman during pregnancy. It promotes a feeling of well-being, improves circulation, promotes relaxation and rest, and relieves the lower back discomfort that often arises as the pregnancy progresses (Wong et al., 2002). However, the duration and difficulty of exercise should be modified throughout pregnancy because of a decrease in performance efficiency with gestational age. Some women continue to push themselves to maintain their prior level of exercise, but most find that as their shape changes and their abdominal area enlarges, they must modify their exercise routines. Modification also helps to reduce the risk of injury caused by laxity of the joints and connective tissue due to the hormonal effects (Leonard, 2002).

Exercise during pregnancy is contraindicated in women with preterm labor, poor weight gain, anemia, facial and hand edema, pain, hypertension, threatened abortion, dizziness, shortness of breath, incompetent cervix, multiple gestation, decreased fetal activity, cardiac disease, and palpitations (Nolan, 2003).

The American College of Obstetrics and Gynecology (ACOG) has stated that healthy pregnant women can perform the same activity recommended for the general population: 30 minutes or more of moderate exercise every day (ACOG, 2002; Fig. 12-11). It is believed that pregnancy is a unique time for behavior modification, and that healthy behaviors maintained or adopted during pregnancy may improve the woman's health for the rest of her life. The excess weight gained in pregnancy, which some women never lose, is a major public health problem (Schnirring, 2002).

Exercise during pregnancy helps return a woman's body to good health after the baby is born. The long-term benefits of exercise that begin in early pregnancy include improved posture, weight control, and improved muscle tone; exercise also aids in the prevention of osteoporosis after menopause (Leiferman & Evenson, 2003). Teaching Guidelines 12-1 highlights recommendations for exercise during pregnancy.

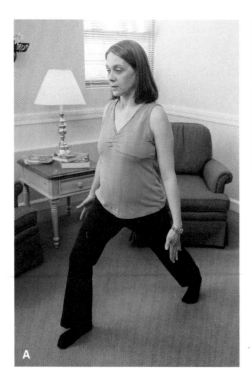

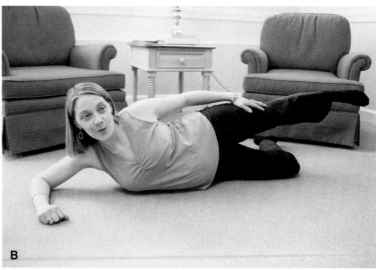

● Figure 12-11 Exercising during pregnancy.

TEACHING GUIDELINES 12-1

Teaching to Promote Exercise During Pregnancy

During pregnancy, follow these general exercise guidelines:

- Consume liquids before, during, and after exercising.
- Exercise 3 or 4 times each week, not sporadically.
- Engage in brisk walking, swimming, biking, low-impact aerobics; these are considered ideal activities.
- Avoid getting overheated during exercise periods.
- Reduce the intensity of workouts in late pregnancy.
- Avoid jerky, bouncy, or high-impact movements.
- Avoid lying flat after fourth month because of hypotensive effect.
- Use pelvic tilt and pelvic rocking to help relieve backache.
- Start with 5 to 10 minutes of stretching exercises.
- Rise slowly following an exercise session to avoid dizziness.
- Avoid activities such as skiing, surfing, scuba diving, and ice hockey.
- Never exercise to the point of exhaustion (ACOG, 2002).

Sleep and Rest

Getting enough sleep helps a person feel better and promotes optimal performance levels during the day. The body releases its greatest concentration of growth hormone during sleep, helping the body repair damaged tissue and grow. Also, with the increased metabolic demands during pregnancy, fatigue is a constant challenge to many pregnant women, especially during the first and third trimesters.

The following tips can help promote adequate sleep:

- Stay on a regular schedule by going to bed and waking up at the same times.
- Eat regular meals at regular times to keep external body cues consistent.
- Take time to unwind and relax before bedtime.
- Establish a bedtime routine or pattern and follow it.
- Create a proper sleep environment by reducing the light and lowering the room temperature.
- Go to bed when you feel tired; if sleep doesn't occur, read a book until you are sleepy.
- Reduce caffeine intake close to bedtime.
- Limit fluid intake after dinner to minimize trips to the bathroom.
- Exercise daily to improve circulation and well-being.
- Use a modified Sims position to improve circulation in the lower extremities.
- Avoid lying on your back, which may compromise circulation to the uterus.
- Avoid sharply bending your knees, which promotes venous stasis below the knees.
- Keep anxieties and worries out of the bedroom. Set aside a specific area in the home or time of day for them.

Sexual Activity and Sexuality

Pregnancy is characterized by intense biological, psychological, and social changes. These changes have direct and indirect, conscious and unconscious effects on a woman's sexuality. The woman experiences dramatic alterations in her physiology, her appearance, and her body, as well as her relationships. A woman's sexual responses during pregnancy vary widely. Common symptoms such as fatigue, nausea, vomiting, breast soreness, and urinary frequency may reduce her desire for sexual intimacy. However, many women report enhanced sexual desire due to increasing levels of estrogen. Fluctuations in sexual desire are normal and a highly individualized response throughout pregnancy.

The physical and emotional adjustments of pregnancy can cause changes in body image, fatigue, mood swings, and sexual activity. The woman's changing shape, emotional status, fetal activity, changes in breast size, pressure on the bladder, and other common discomforts of pregnancy result in increased physical and emotional demands. These can produce stress on the sexual relationship of the pregnant woman and her partner. However, most women adjust well to the alterations and experience a satisfying sexual relationship (Mattson & Smith, 2004).

Often pregnant women ask whether sexual intercourse is allowed during pregnancy or whether there are specific times when they should refrain from having sex. This is a good opportunity to educate clients about sexual behavior during pregnancy and also to ask about their expectations and individual experience related to sexuality and possible changes. It is also a good time for nurses to address the impact of the changes associated with pregnancy on sexual desire and behavior. For example, some women experience increased sexual desire while others experience less. Couples may enjoy sexual activity more because there is no fear of pregnancy and no need to disrupt spontaneity by using birth control. An increase in pelvis congestion and lubrication secondary to estrogen influence may heighten orgasm for many women. Some women have a decrease in desire because of a negative body image, fear of harming the fetus by engaging in intercourse, and fatigue, nausea, and vomiting (Mattson & Smith, 2004). A couple may need assistance to adjust to the various changes brought about by pregnancy.

Reassure the women and her partner that sexual activity is permissible during pregnancy unless there is a history of any of the following:

- Vaginal bleeding
- Placenta previa
- Risk of preterm labor
- Multiple gestation
- Incompetent cervix
- Premature rupture of membranes
- Presence of infection (Trupin, 2004)

Inform the couple that the fetus will not be injured by intercourse. Suggest alternative positions that may be more comfortable (e.g., woman on top, side-lying), especially during the later stages of pregnancy, when the woman's abdomen increases in size.

Many women feel a particular need for closeness during pregnancy, and she should communicate this need to her partner (Wong et al., 2002). Emphasize to the couple that closeness and cuddling need not culminate in intercourse, and that other forms of sexual expression, such as mutual masturbation, foot massage, holding hands, kissing, and hugging, can be very satisfying (DeJudicibus & McCabe, 2002).

Women will experience a myriad of symptoms, feelings, and physical sensations during their pregnancy. Having a satisfying sexual relationship during pregnancy is certainly possible, but it requires honest communication between partners to determine what works best for them, and a good relationship with their health care provider to ensure safety (March of Dimes, 2004).

Employment

For the most part, women can continue working until delivery if they have no complications during their pregnancy and the workplace does not present any special hazards (ACOG, 2000). Hazardous occupations include health care workers, day care providers, laboratory technicians, chemists, painters, hairstylists, veterinary workers, and carpenters (ACOG, 2000). Jobs requiring strenuous work such as heavy lifting, climbing, carrying heavy objects, and standing for prolonged periods place a pregnant woman at risk if modifications are not instituted.

Assess for environmental and occupational factors that place a pregnant women and her fetus at risk for injury. Interview the woman about her employment environment. Ask about possible exposure to teratogens (substances with the potential to alter the fetus permanently in form or function) and the physical demands of employment: Is she exposed to temperature extremes? Does she need to stand for prolonged periods in a fixed position? A description of the work environment is important in providing anticipatory guidance to the woman. Stress the importance of taking rest periods throughout the day because constant physically intensive workloads increase the likelihood of low birthweight and preterm labor and birth (Cunningham et al., 2005).

Due to the numerous physiologic and psychosocial changes that women experience during their pregnancies, the employer may need to make special accommodations to reduce the pregnant woman's risk of hazardous exposures and heavy workloads. The employer may need to provide adequate coverage so that the woman can take rest breaks; remove the woman from any areas where she might be exposed to toxic substances; and avoid work assignments that require heavy lifting, hard physical labor, continuous standing, or constant moving. Some recom-

mendations for working while pregnant are highlighted in Teaching Guidelines 12-2.

Travel

Pregnancy does not curtail a woman's ability to travel in a car or in a plane. However, women should follow a few safety guidelines to minimize risk to themselves and their fetuses. According to ACOG, pregnant women can travel safely throughout their pregnancy, although the second trimester is perhaps the best time to travel because there is the least chance of complications (ACOG, 2001). Pregnant women considering international travel should evaluate the potential problems that could occur during the journey as well as the quality of medical care available at the destination. In general, pregnant women with serious underlying illnesses should not travel to developing countries (CDC, 2003). Pregnant women should be aware of the potential for injuries and trauma related to traveling and should be educated on ways to prevent them.

Teaching Guidelines 12-3 offers tips for safe travel on planes and to foreign areas.

When traveling by car, the major risk is a car accident. The impact and momentum can lead to traumatic separation of the placenta from the wall of the uterus. Shock and massive hemorrhage might result (Walling, 2004). Tips that nurses can offer to promote safety during ground travel include:

- Always wear a three-point seat belt, no matter how short the trip, to prevent ejection or serious injury from collision.

 TEACHING GUIDELINES 12-2

Teaching for the Pregnant Working Woman

Use the following guidelines for working during your pregnancy:
- Plan to take two 10- to 15-minute breaks within an 8-hour work day.
- Be sure that there is a place available for you to rest, preferably in the side-lying position, with a restroom readily available.
- Avoid jobs that require strenuous workloads; if this is not possible, then request a modification of work duties (lighter tasks) to reduce your workload.
- Change your position from standing to sitting or vice versa at least every 2 hours.
- Ensure that you are allowed time off without penalty, if necessary, to ensure a healthy outcome for you and your fetus.
- Make sure the work environment is free of toxic substances.
- Ensure the work environment is smoke-free so passive smoking isn't a concern.
- Minimize heavy lifting if associated with bending.

TEACHING GUIDELINES 12-3

Teaching to Promote Safe Travel on Planes
and in Foreign Countries

When traveling by plane or to foreign countries during pregnancy, follow these general tips:

• Bring along a copy of the prenatal record if your travel plans are prolonged in case there is a medical emergency away from home.
• When traveling abroad, carry a foreign dictionary that includes words or phrases for the most common pregnancy emergencies.
• Travel with at least one companion at all times for personal safety.
• Check with your healthcare provider before receiving any immunizations necessary for foreign travel; some may be harmful to the fetus.
• When in a foreign country, be careful to avoid fresh fruit, vegetables, and local water.
• Avoid any milk that is not pasteurized.
• Eat only meat that is well cooked to avoid exposure to toxoplasmosis.
• Request an aisle seat and walk about the airplane every 2 hours.
• While sitting on long flights, practice calf-tensing exercises to improve circulation to the lower extremities.
• Be aware of typical problems encountered by pregnant travelers, such as fatigue, heartburn, indigestion, constipation, vaginal discharge, leg cramps, urinary frequency, and hemorrhoids.
• Always wear support hose while flying to prevent the development of blood clots.
• Drink plenty of water to keep well hydrated throughout the flight (ACOG, 2001).

• Apply a nonpadded shoulder strap properly; it should cross between the breasts and over the upper abdomen, above the uterus (Fig. 12-12).
• If no seat belts are available (buses or vans), ride in the back seat of the vehicle.
• Use a lap belt that crosses over the pelvis below the uterus.
• Deactivate the airbag if possible. If you can't, move the seat as far back from the dashboard as possible to minimize impact on the abdomen.
• Avoid using a cellular phone while driving to prevent distraction.
• Avoid driving when very fatigued in the first and third trimesters.
• Avoid late-night driving, when visibility might be compromised.

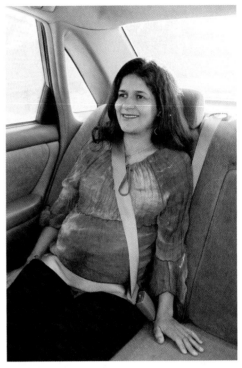

● Figure 12-12 Proper application of a seat belt during pregnancy.

• Direct a tilting steering wheel away from the abdomen (Smith, 2002).

Immunizations and Medications

Ideally clients should receive all childhood immunizations before conception to protect the fetus from any risk of congenital anomalies. If the client comes for a preconception visit, immunizations such as measles, mumps, and rubella (MMR), hepatitis B, and diphtheria/tetanus (every 10 years) should be discussed and given at this time if needed.

The risk to a developing fetus from vaccination of the mother during pregnancy is primarily theoretical. Routine immunizations are not usually indicated during pregnancy. However, no evidence exists of risk from vaccinating pregnant women with inactivated virus or bacterial vaccines or toxoids. A number of other vaccines have not been adequately studied, and thus theoretical risks of vaccination must be weighed against the risks of the disease to mother and fetus (Sur et al., 2003). Pregnant women should be advised to avoid live virus vaccines (MMR and varicella) and should also avoid becoming pregnant within 1 month of having received one of these vaccines because of the theoretical risk of transmission to the fetus (CDC, 2004). CDC guidelines for vaccine administration are highlighted in Box 12-3.

CDC GUIDELINES FOR VACCINE ADMINISTRATION DURING PREGNANCY

Vaccines that should be considered if otherwise indicated:
- Hepatitis B
- Influenza (inactivated)
- Tetanus/diphtheria
- Meningococcal
- Rabies

Vaccines contraindicated during pregnancy:
- Influenza (live, attenuated vaccine)
- Measles
- Mumps
- Rubella
- Varicella (CDC, 2004)

FDA PREGNANCY RISK CLASSIFICATION OF DRUGS

The FDA has classified drugs into five categories based on their risk

Category A: These drugs have been tested and found safe during pregnancy
- Folic acid, vitamin B6, and thyroid medicine

Category B: These drugs have been used frequently during pregnancy and do not appear to cause major birth defects or other fetal problems
- Antibiotics, acetaminophen (Tylenol), aspartame (artificial sweetener)
- Famotidine (Pepcid), prednisone (cortisone), insulin, and ibuprofen

Category C: These drugs are more likely to cause problems and safety studies have not been completed.
- Prochlorperazine (Compazine), fluconazole (Diflucan), ciprofloxacin (Cipro), and some antidepressants

Category D: These drugs have clear health risks for the fetus
- Alcohol, lithium (treats bipolar disorders), phenytoin (Dilantin)
- All chemotherapeutic agents used to treat cancer

Category X: These drugs have been shown to cause birth defects and should never be taken during pregnancy
- Accutane (treats cystic acne), androgens (treat endometriosis), Coumadin (prevents blood clots), antithyroid medications for overactive thyroid
- Radiation therapy (cancer treatment), Tegison or Soriatane (treats psoriasis), streptomycin (treats tuberculosis)
- Thalidomide (treats insomnia), diethylstilbestrol (DES) (treats menstrual disorders), and organic mercury from contaminated food (Trupin, 2004)

It is best to advise pregnant women not to take any medications. At the very least, encourage them to discuss with the healthcare provider their current medications and any herbal remedies they take so that they can learn about any potential risks should they continue to take them during pregnancy. Generally, if the woman is taking medicine for seizures, high blood pressure, asthma, or depression, the benefits of continuing the medicine during pregnancy outweigh the risks to the fetus. The safety profile of some medications may change according to the gestational age of the fetus (Black & Hill, 2003).

The Food and Drug Administration has developed a system of ranking drugs that appears on the labels and in the package inserts. These risk categories are summarized in Box 12-4. Always advise women to check with the healthcare provider for guidance.

A common concern of many pregnant women involves the use of over-the-counter (OTC) medications and herbal agents. Many women consider OTC medications benign simply because they are available without prescription (Tillett et al., 2003). While herbal medications are commonly thought of as "natural" alternatives to other medicines, they can be just as potent as some prescription medications. A major concern about herbal medicine is the lack of consistent potency in the active ingredients in any given batch of product, making it difficult to know the exact strength by reading the label. Also, many herbs may contain chemicals that cross the placenta and cause harm to the fetus.

Nurses are often asked about the safety of OTC medicines and herbal agents. Unfortunately, many drugs have not been evaluated in controlled studies, and it is difficult to make general recommendations for OTC and herbal medications. Therefore, encourage pregnant women to check with their health care provider before taking any-

thing. Questions about the use of OTC and herbal products are part of the initial prenatal interview.

Nursing Management for the Common Discomforts of Pregnancy

Most women experience common discomforts during pregnancy and ask a nurse's advice about ways to minimize them. However, other women will not bring up their concerns unless asked. Therefore, the nurse needs to address the common discomforts that occur in each trimester at each prenatal visit and provide realistic measures to help the client deal with them (Teaching Guidelines 12-4). Nursing Care Plan 12-1 applies the nursing process to the care of a woman experiencing some discomforts of pregnancy.

Consider THIS!

One has to wonder sometimes why women go through what they do. During my first pregnancy I was sick for the first 2 months. I would experience waves of nausea from the moment I got out of bed until midmorning. Needless to say, I wasn't the happiest camper around. After the third month, my life seemed to settle down and I was beginning to think that being pregnant wasn't too bad after all. I was fooled momentarily, though. During my last 2 months, another wave of discomfort struck—heartburn and constipation—a double whammy! I now feared eating anything that might trigger acid indigestion and also remain in my body too long. I literally had to become the "fiber queen" to combat these two challenges. Needless to say, my "suffering" was well worth our bright-eyed baby girl in the end.

Thoughts: Despite the various discomforts associated with pregnancy, most women wouldn't change their end result. Do most women experience these discomforts? What suggestions could be made to reduce them?

 TEACHING GUIDELINES 12-4

Teaching to Manage the Discomforts of Pregnancy

While you are pregnant, use these suggestions to help deal with some of the more common discomforts of pregnancy.

Urinary frequency or incontinence

- Try Kegel exercises to increase control over leakage.
- Empty your bladder when you first feel a full sensation.
- Avoid caffeine drinks, which stimulate voiding patterns.
- Reduce your fluid intake after dinner to reduce nighttime urination.

Fatigue

- Attempt to get a full night's sleep, without interruptions.
- Eat a healthy balanced diet.
- Schedule a nap in the early afternoon daily.
- When you are feeling tired, rest.

Nausea and vomiting

- Avoid an empty stomach at all times.
- Munch on dry crackers/toast in bed before arising.
- Eat several small meals throughout the day.
- Drink fluids between meals rather than with meals.
- Avoid greasy, fried foods or ones with a strong odor, such as cabbage or Brussels sprouts.

Backache

- Avoid standing or sitting in one position for long periods.
- Apply heating pad (low setting) to small of your back.
- Support your lower back with pillows when sitting.
- Stand with your shoulders back to maintain correct posture.

Leg cramps

- Elevate legs above the heart level frequently throughout the day.
- If you get a cramp, straighten both legs and flex your feet toward your body.
- Ask your health care provider about taking additional calcium supplementation, which may be helpful to reduce leg spasms.

Varicosities

- Walk daily to improve circulation to extremities.
- Elevate both legs above heart level while resting.
- Avoid standing in one position for long periods of time.
- Don't wear constrictive stockings and socks.
- Don't cross the legs when sitting for long periods.
- Wear support stockings to promote better circulation.

Hemorrhoids

- Establish a regular time for daily bowel elimination.
- Prevent straining by drinking plenty of fluids and eating fiber-rich foods and exercising daily.
- Use warm sitz baths and cool witch hazel compresses for comfort.

Constipation

- Increase your intake of foods high in fiber and drink at least eight 8-ounce glasses of fluid daily.
- Exercise each day (brisk walking) to promote movement through the intestine.
- Reduce the amount of cheese consumed.

Heartburn/indigestion

- Avoid spicy or greasy foods and eat small frequent meals.
- Sleep on several pillows so that your head is elevated.
- Stop smoking and caffeine drinks to reduce stimulation.
- Avoid lying down for at least two hours after meals.
- Try drinking sips of water to reduce burning sensation.
- Take antacids *sparingly* if burning sensation is severe.

Braxton Hicks contractions

- Keep in mind that these contractions are a normal sensation.
- Try changing your position or engaging in mild exercise to help reduce the sensation.
- Drink more fluids if possible.

Nursing Care Plan 12-1

Overview of the Woman Experiencing Common Discomforts of Pregnancy

Alicia, a 32-year-old, G1 P0, at 10 weeks' gestation, comes to the clinic for a visit. During the interview, the client states, "I'm running to the bathroom to urinate it seems like all the time, and I'm so nauseous that I'm having trouble eating." Client denies any complaints of burning or pain on urination. Vital signs within acceptable limits.

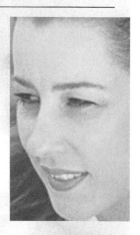

Nursing Diagnosis: Impaired urinary elimination related to frequency secondary to physiologic changes of pregnancy

Outcome identification and *evaluation*	Interventions with *rationales*
Client will report a decrease in urinary complaints, *as evidenced by a decrease in the number of times she uses the bathroom to void, reports that she feels her bladder is empty after voiding, and use of Kegel exercises.*	Assess client's usual bladder elimination patterns *to establish a baseline for comparison.* Obtain a urine specimen for analysis *to rule out infection or glucosuria.* Review with client the physiologic basis for the increased frequency during pregnancy; inform client that frequency should abate during the second trimester and that it most likely will return during her third trimester *to promote understanding of the problem.* Encourage the client to empty her bladder when first feeling a sensation of fullness *to minimize risk of urinary retention.* Suggest client avoid caffeinated drinks, *which can stimulate the need to void.* Have client reduce her fluid intake for 2 to 3 hours before bedtime *to reduce nighttime urination.* Urge client to keep perineal area clean and dry *to prevent irritation and excoriation from any leakage.* Instruct client in Kegel exercises *to increase perineal muscle tone and control over leakage.* Teach client about the signs and symptoms of urinary tract infection and to report them should they occur *to ensure early detection and prompt intervention.*

Overview of the Woman Experiencing Common Discomforts of Pregnancy (continued)

Nursing Diagnosis: Imbalanced nutrition, less than body requirements related to nausea and vomiting

Outcome identification and *evaluation*	Interventions with *rationales*
Client will ingest adequate amounts of nutrients for maternal and fetal well-being as evidenced by *acceptable weight gain pattern and statements indicating an increase in food intake with a decrease in the number of episodes of nausea and vomiting.*	Obtain weight and compare to baseline *to determine effects of nausea and vomiting on nutritional intake.* Review client's typical dietary intake over 24 hours *to determine nutritional intake and patterns for individualizing suggestions.* Encourage client to eat 5 or 6 small frequent meals throughout the day *to prevent her stomach from becoming empty.* Suggest that she munch on dry crackers, toast, cereal, or cheese or drink a small amount of lemonade before arising *to help minimize nausea.* Encourage client to arise slowly from bed in the morning and avoid sudden movements *to reduce stimulation of the vomiting center.* Advise client to drink fluids between meals rather than with meals *to avoid overdistention of the abdomen and subsequent increase in abdominal pressure.* Encourage her to increase her intake of foods high in vitamin B6 such as meat, poultry, bananas, fish, green leafy vegetables, peanuts, raisins, walnuts, and whole grains, as tolerated, *to ensure adequate nutrient intake.* Advise the client to avoid greasy, fried, or highly spiced foods and to avoid strong odors, including foods such as cabbage, *to minimize gastrointestinal upset.* Encourage the client to avoid tight or restricting clothes *to minimize pressure on the expanding abdomen.* Arrange for consultation with nutritionist as necessary *to assist with diet planning.*

First-Trimester Discomforts

During the first 3 months of pregnancy, the woman's body is undergoing numerous changes. Some women experience many discomforts and others have few. These discomforts are caused by the changes taking place within the body and pass as the pregnancy progresses.

Urinary Frequency or Incontinence

Urinary frequency or incontinence is common in the first trimester because the growing uterus compresses the bladder. For this same reason, it also is a common com-

plaint during the third trimester, especially when the fetal head settles into the pelvis. However, the discomfort tends to improve in the second trimester when the uterus becomes an abdominal organ and moves away from the bladder region.

After infection and gestational diabetes have been ruled out as causative factors, suggest that the woman decrease her fluid intake 2 to 3 hours before bedtime and limit her intake of caffeinated beverages. Without any pain or burning, increased voiding is normal, but encourage the client to report any pain or burning. Also explain that the symptom may subside as she enters her second trimester, only to recur in the third trimester. Teach the client to perform Kegel exercises throughout the day to help strengthen perineal muscle tone, thereby enhancing urinary control and decreasing the possibility of incontinence.

Fatigue

Fatigue plagues all pregnant women, primarily in the first and third trimesters (the highest energy levels typically occur during the second trimester), even if they get their normal amount of sleep at night. First-trimester fatigue most often is related to the vast physical changes (e.g., increased oxygen consumption, increased levels of progesterone and relaxin, increased metabolic demands) and psychosocial changes (e.g., mood swings, multiple role demands). Third-trimester fatigue can be caused by sleep disturbances from increased weight (many women may be unable to find a comfortable sleeping position due to the enlarging abdomen), physical discomforts, such as heartburn, and insomnia due to mood swings, multiple role anxiety, and a decrease in exercise (Youngkin & Davis, 2004).

Once anemia, infection, and blood dyscrasias have been ruled out as contributing to the client's fatigue, advise her to arrange work, childcare, and other demands in her life to permit additional rest periods. Work with the client to devise a realistic schedule for rest. Encourage her to use good posture and to wear low-heeled shoes to prevent backache. Using pillows for support in the side-lying position relieves pressure on major blood vessels that supply oxygen and nutrients to the fetus when resting (Fig. 12-13). Also recommend the use of relaxation techniques, providing instruction as necessary, and suggest she increase her daily exercise level.

Nausea and Vomiting

Nausea and vomiting are common discomforts during the first trimester: at least 50% of women experience nausea during pregnancy (Engstrom, 2004). The physiologic

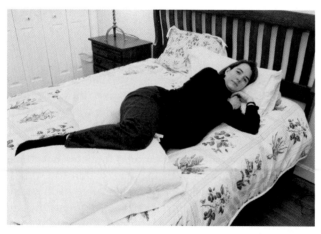

● Figure 12-13 Using pillows for support in the side-lying position.

changes that cause nausea and vomiting are unknown, but research suggests that unusually high levels of estrogen, progesterone, and hCG and a vitamin B6 deficiency may be contributing factors. Symptoms generally last until the second trimester and are generally associated with a positive pregnancy outcome (Cunningham et al., 2005).

To help the client alleviate her nausea and vomiting, advise her to eat small, frequent meals (five or six a day) to prevent her stomach from becoming completely empty. Other helpful suggestions include eating dry crackers, Cheerios, lemonade, or cheese before getting out of bed in the morning and increasing her intake of foods high in vitamin B6 such as meat, poultry, bananas, fish, green leafy vegetables, peanuts, raisins, walnuts, and whole grains, or making sure she is receiving enough vitamin B6 by taking her prescribed prenatal vitamins. Other helpful tips to deal with nausea and vomiting include:

- Get out of bed in the morning very slowly.
- Avoid sudden movements.
- Open a window to remove odors of food being cooked.
- Limit intake of fluids or soups during meals (drink them between meals).
- Avoid fried foods and foods cooked with grease, oils, or fatty meats, for they tend to upset the stomach.
- Avoid highly seasoned foods such as those cooked with garlic, onion, pepper, and chili.
- Drink a small amount of caffeine-free carbonated beverage (ginger ale) if nauseated.
- Avoid strong smells.
- Avoid wearing tight or restricting clothes, which might place increased pressure on the expanding abdomen.
- Avoid stress (Leonard, 2002).

Breast Tenderness

Due to increased estrogen and progesterone levels, which cause the fat layer of breasts to thicken and the number of milk ducts and glands to increase during the first trimester, many women experience breast tenderness. Offering a thorough explanation to the woman about the reasons for the breast discomfort is important. Wearing a larger bra with good support can help alleviate this discomfort. Advise her to wear a supportive bra, even while sleeping. As her breasts increase in size, advise her to change her bra size to ensure adequate support.

Constipation

With increasing levels of progesterone leading to decreased contractility of the gastrointestinal tract, movement of substances through the colon slows, allowing an increase in water absorption that leads to constipation. Lack of exercise or too little fiber or fluids in the diet can also promote constipation. In addition, the large bowel is mechanically compressed by the enlarging uterus, adding to this discomfort. The iron and calcium in prenatal vitamins can also contribute to constipation during the first and third trimesters.

Explain how pregnancy exacerbates the symptoms of constipation and offer the following suggestions:

• Eat fresh or dried fruit daily.
• Eat more raw fruits and vegetables, including their skins.
• Eat whole-grain cereals and breads such as raisin bran or bran flakes.
• Participate in physical activity on a daily basis.
• Eat meals at regular intervals.
• Establish a time of day to defecate, and elevate your feet on a stool to avoid straining.
• Drink six to eight glasses of water daily.
• Decrease your intake of refined carbohydrates.
• Drink warm fluids on arising to stimulate bowel motility.
• Decrease your consumption of sugary sodas.
• Avoid eating large amounts of cheese.

If the suggestions above are ineffective, the woman may use a bulk-forming laxative such as Metamucil.

Nasal Stuffiness, Bleeding Gums, Epistaxis

Increased levels of estrogen cause edema of the mucous membranes of the nasal and oral cavities. Advise the woman to drink extra water for hydration of the mucous membranes or to use a cool mist humidifier in her bedroom at night. If she needs to blow her nose to relieve nasal stuffiness, advise her to blow gently, one nostril at a time. Advise her to avoid the use of nasal decongestants and sprays.

If a nosebleed occurs, advise the woman to loosen the clothing around her neck, sit with her head tilted forward, pinch her nostrils with her thumb and forefinger for 10 to 15 minutes, and apply an ice pack to the bridge of her nose.

If the woman has bleeding gums, encourage her to practice good oral hygiene by using a soft toothbrush and flossing daily. Warm saline mouthwashes can relieve discomfort. If the gum problem persists, instruct her to see her dentist.

Cravings

Desires for certain foods and beverages are likely to begin during the first trimester but do not appear to reflect any physiologic need. Foods with a high sodium or sugar content often are the ones craved. At times, some women crave non-food substances such as clay, cornstarch, laundry detergent, baking soda, soap, paint chips, dirt, ice, or wax. This craving for non-food substances, termed *pica,* may indicate a severe dietary deficiency of minerals or vitamins, or it may have cultural roots (Monti, 2004). Pica is discussed further later in this chapter.

Leukorrhea

Increased vaginal discharge begins during the first trimester and continues throughout pregnancy. The physiologic changes behind leukorrhea arise from the high levels of estrogen, which cause increased vascularity and hypertrophy of cervical glands as well as vaginal cells (Cunningham et al., 2005). The result is progressive vaginal secretions throughout pregnancy.

Advise the woman to keep the perineal area clean and dry, washing the area with mild soap and water during her daily shower. Also recommend that she avoid wearing pantyhose and other tight-fitting nylon clothes that prevent air from circulating to the genital area. Encourage the use of cotton underwear and suggest wearing a nightgown rather than pajamas to allow for increased air flow. Also instruct the woman to avoid douching and tampon use.

Second-Trimester Discomforts

A sense of well-being typically characterizes the second trimester for most women. By this time, the fatigue, nausea and vomiting, and fatigue have subsided and the uncomfortable changes of the third trimester are a few months away. Not every woman experiences the same discomforts during this time, so nursing assessments and interventions must be individualized.

Backache

Backache, experienced by many women during the second trimester, is due to a shift in the center of gravity caused by the enlarging uterus. Muscle strain results. In addition, a high level of circulating progesterone softens cartilage and loosens joints, thus increasing discomfort. Upper back pain also can be caused by increased breast size (ACOG, 2000).

After exploring other reasons that might cause backache, such as uterine contractions, urinary tract infection, ulcers, or musculoskeletal back disorders, the following instructions may be helpful:

• Maintain correct posture, with head up and shoulders back.
• Use good body mechanics when lifting objects.
• When sitting, use foot supports and pillows behind the back.
• Try pelvic tilt or rocking exercises to strengthen the back (Murray et al., 2006).

The pelvic tilt or pelvic rock is used to alleviate pressure on the lower back during pregnancy by stretching the lower back muscles. It can be done sitting, standing, or on all fours. To do it on all fours, the hands are positioned directly under the shoulders and the knees under the hips. The back should be in a neutral position with the head and neck aligned with the straight back. The woman then presses up with the lower back and holds this position for a few seconds, then relaxes to a neutral position. This action of pressing upward is repeated frequently throughout the day to prevent a sore back (VanderLaan, 2004).

Leg Cramps

Leg cramps occur primarily in the second and third trimesters and could be related to the pressure of the gravid uterus on pelvic nerves and blood vessels (Curtis & Schuler, 2000). Diet can also be a contributing factor if the woman is not consuming enough of certain minerals, such as calcium and magnesium. The sudden stretching of leg muscles may also play a role in causing leg cramps (Condon, 2004).

Encourage the woman to gently stretch the muscle by dorsiflexing the foot up toward the body. Wrapping a warm, moist towel around the leg muscle can also help the muscle to relax. Advise the client to avoid stretching her legs, pointing her toes, and walking excessively. Stress the importance of wearing low-heeled shoes and support hose and arising slowly from a sitting position. If the leg cramps are due to deficiencies in minerals, the condition can be remedied by eating more foods rich in these nutrients. Also instruct the woman on calf-stretching exercises: have her stand 3 feet from the wall and lean toward it, resting her lower arms against it, while keeping her heels on the floor. This may help reduce cramping if it is done before going to bed.

Elevating the legs throughout the day will help relieve pressure and minimize strain. Wearing support hose and avoiding curling the toes may be helpful to relieve leg discomfort. Also instruct the client to avoid standing in one spot for a prolonged period or crossing her legs. If she must stand for prolonged periods, suggest that she change her position at least every 2 hours by walking or sitting to reduce the risk of leg cramps. Encourage her to drink an adequate amount of fluids (eight 8-ounce glasses of fluid daily) throughout the day to ensure adequate hydration.

Varicosities of the Vulva and Legs

Varicosities of the vulva and legs are associated with the increased venous stasis caused by the pressure of the gravid uterus on pelvic vessels and the vasodilation resulting from increased progesterone levels. Progesterone relaxes the vein walls, making it difficult for blood to return to the heart from the extremities; thus, pooling can result. Genetic predisposition, inactivity, obesity, and poor muscle tone are contributing factors. Encourage the client to wear support hose and teach her how to apply them properly. Advise her to elevate her legs above her heart while lying on her back for 10 minutes before she gets out of bed in the morning, thus promoting venous return before she applies the hose. Instruct the client to avoid crossing her legs and avoid wearing knee-high stockings. They cause constriction of leg vessels and muscles and contribute to venous stasis. Also encourage the client to elevate both legs above the level of the heart for 5 to 10 minutes at least twice a day (Fig. 12-14); to wear low-heeled shoes; and to avoid long periods of standing or sitting, frequently changing her position.

If the client has vulvar varicosities, suggest she apply ice packs to the area when she is lying down.

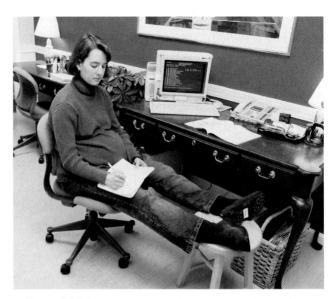

● Figure 12-14 Woman elevating her legs while working.

Hemorrhoids

Hemorrhoids are varicosities of the rectum and may be external (outside the anal sphincter) or internal (above the sphincter) (Murray et al., 2002). They occur as a result of progesterone-induced vasodilation and from pressure of the enlarged uterus on the lower intestine and rectum. Hemorrhoids are more common in women with constipation, poor fluid intake or poor dietary habits, smokers, or those with a previous history of hemorrhoids (Tiran, 2003).

Instruct the client in measures to prevent constipation, including increasing fiber intake and drinking at least 2 liters of fluid per day. Recommend the use of topical anesthetics (e.g., Preparation H, Anusol, witch hazel compresses) to reduce pain, itching, and swelling, if permitted by the healthcare provider. Teach the client about local comfort measures such as warm sitz baths, witch hazel compresses, or cold compresses. To minimize her risk of straining while defecating, suggest that she elevate her feet on a stool. Also encourage her to avoid prolonged sitting or standing (ACOG, 2000).

Flatulence With Bloating

The physiologic changes that result in constipation (reduced gastrointestinal motility and dilation secondary to progesterone's influence) may result in increased flatulence. As the enlarging uterus compresses the bowel, it delays the passage of food through the intestines, thus allowing more time for gas to be formed by bacteria in the colon. The woman usually reports increased passage of rectal gas, abdominal bloating, or belching. Instructing the woman to avoid gas-forming foods, such as beans, cabbage, and onions, as well as foods that have a high content of white sugar, will help to decrease flatus. Adding more fiber to the diet, increasing fluid intake, and increasing physical exercise are also helpful. In addition, reducing the swallowing of air when chewing gum or smoking will reduce gas build-up. Reducing the intake of carbonated beverages and cheese and using mints can also be helpful in reducing flatulence during pregnancy (Florida Department of Health, 2003).

Third-Trimester Discomforts

As women enter into their third trimester, their appearance is changing. What many find is a return of the first-trimester discomforts: fatigue, urinary frequency, and leukorrhea. These discomforts are secondary to the ever-enlarging uterus compressing adjacent structures, increasing hormone levels, and the metabolic demands of the fetus. In addition to these discomforts, many women experience shortness of breath, constipation, heartburn and indigestion, swelling, and Braxton Hicks contractions.

Shortness of Breath and Dyspnea

The increasing growth of the uterus prevents complete lung expansion late in pregnancy. As the uterus enlarges upward, the expansion of the diaphragm is limited. Dyspnea can occur when the woman lies on her back and the pressure of the gravid uterus against the vena cava reduces venous return to the heart (ACOG, 2000).

Explain to the woman that her dyspnea is normal and will improve when the fetus drops into the pelvis (lightening). Instruct her to adjust her body position to allow for maximum expansion of the chest and to avoid large meals, which increase abdominal pressure. Raising the head of the bed on blocks or placing pillows behind her back is helpful too. Stress that lying on her side will displace the uterus off the vena cava and improve her breathing. Advise the woman to avoid exercise that precipitates dyspnea, to rest after exercise, and to avoid overheating in warm climates. If she still smokes, encourage her to stop.

Constipation

During pregnancy, constipation is usually attributed to the relaxing effects of progesterone on the gastrointestinal tract, leading to reduced peristalsis, and to compression of the bowel by the enlarging uterus. In addition, prenatal vitamins containing iron or calcium typically prescribed during pregnancy can contribute to constipation.

Stress the need for lifestyle changes such as increasing her exercise level and setting a regular time for bowel movements by ensuring privacy and barring interruptions. Advise the client to eat foods high in fiber (e.g., fresh fruits and vegetables, whole-grain breads and cereals) and to decrease her intake of refined carbohydrates, such as white bread, pasta, white rice, and cornflakes. Also encourage fluid intake (at least eight 8-ounce glasses of fluid per day). Suggest drinking warm fluids on arising to stimulate peristalsis (Youngkin & Davis, 2004).

Heartburn and Indigestion

Heartburn and indigestion result when high progesterone levels cause relaxation of the cardiac sphincter, allowing food and digestive juices to flow backward from the stomach into the esophagus. Irritation of the esophageal lining occurs, causing the burning sensation known as heartburn (Engstrom, 2004). The pain may radiate to the neck and throat. It worsens when the woman lies down, bends over after eating, or wears tight clothes. Indigestion, vague abdominal discomfort after meals, results from eating too much or too fast; from eating when tense, tired, or emotionally upset; from food that is too fatty or spicy; and from heavy food or food that has been badly cooked or processed (O'Toole, 2003). In addition, the stomach is displaced upward and compressed by the large uterus in the third trimester, thus limiting the stomach's capacity to empty quickly. Food sits, causing heartburn and indigestion.

Review the client's usual dietary intake and offer suggestions to limit or avoid gas-producing or fatty foods and large meals. Encourage the client to maintain proper posture and remain in the sitting position after eating to prevent reflux of gastric acids into the esophagus by gravity. Urge the client to eat slowly, chewing her food thoroughly to prevent excessive swallowing of air, which can lead to increased gastric pressure. Instruct the client to avoid highly spiced foods, chocolate, coffee, alcohol, sodas, and spearmint or peppermint. These items stimulate the release of gastric digestive acids, which may cause reflux into the esophagus.

Dependent Edema

Swelling is the result of increased capillary permeability caused by elevated hormone levels and by the increased in blood volume. Sodium and water are retained and thirst increases. Edema occurs most often in dependent areas such as the legs and feet throughout the day due to gravity; it improves after a night's sleep. Warm weather or prolonged standing or sitting may increase edema. Generalized edema, appearing in the face, hands and feet, can signal preeclampsia if accompanied by dizziness, blurred vision, headaches, upper quadrant pain, or nausea (Condon, 2004). This edema should be reported to the healthcare provider.

Appropriate suggestions to help minimize dependent edema include:

- Elevate your feet and legs above the level of the heart.
- Wear support hose when standing or sitting for long periods.
- Change position frequently throughout the day.
- Walk at a sensible pace to help contract leg muscles to promote venous return.
- When taking a long car ride, stop to walk around every 2 hours.
- When standing, rock from the ball of the foot to the toes to stimulate circulation.

- Lie on your left side to keep the gravid uterus off the vena cava to return blood to the heart.
- Avoid foods high in sodium, such as lunch meats, potato chips, and bacon.
- Avoid wearing knee-high stockings.
- Drink six to eight glasses of water daily to replace fluids lost through perspiration.
- Avoid high intake of sugar and fats, because they cause water retention.

Braxton Hicks Contractions

Braxton Hicks contractions are irregular, painless contractions that occur without cervical dilation. Typically they intensify in the third trimester in preparation for labor. In reality, they have been present since early in the pregnancy but have gone unnoticed. They are thought to increase the tone of uterine muscles for labor purposes (ACOG, 2000).

Reassure the client that these contractions are normal. Instruct the client in how to differentiate between Braxton Hicks and labor contractions. Tell her that true labor contractions usually grow longer, stronger, and closer together and occur at regular intervals. Walking usually strengthens true labor contractions, whereas Braxton Hicks contractions tend to decrease in intensity and taper off. Advise the client to keep herself well hydrated and to rest in a side-lying position to help relieve the discomfort. Suggest that she use breathing techniques such as Lamaze techniques to ease the discomfort.

Nursing Management to Meet Nutritional Needs

Healthy eating during pregnancy enables optimal gestational weight gain and reduces complications, both of which are associated with positive birth outcomes. During pregnancy, maternal nutritional needs change to meet the demands of the pregnancy. Healthy eating can help ensure that adequate nutrients are available for both mother and fetus.

Since the requirements for so many nutrients increase during pregnancy, pregnant women should take a vitamin and mineral supplement daily. Prenatal vitamins are routinely prescribed as a safeguard against a less-than-optimal diet.

In particular, iron and folic acid need to be supplemented because their increased requirements during pregnancy are usually too great to be met through diet alone (Florida Department of Health, 2003). Iron and folic acid are needed to form new blood cells for the expanded maternal blood volume and prevent anemia. Folic acid is necessary before and after pregnancy to prevent neural tube defects in the fetus. For most pregnant women, supplements of 30 mg of ferrous iron and 600 mcg of folic acid per day are recommended by the **dietary reference intakes** (DRIs) (Institute of Medicine [IOM], 2002).

Women with a previous history of a fetus with a neural tube defect are often prescribed a higher dose.

Nutritional intake during pregnancy has a direct effect on fetal well-being and birth outcome. Inadequate nutritional intake, for example, is associated with preterm birth, low birthweight, and congenital anomalies. Excessive nutritional intake is connected with fetal macrosomia (>4,000 g), leading to a difficult birth, neonatal hypoglycemia, and continued obesity in the mother (Fowles, 2002).

There is an abundance of conflicting advice about nutrition and what is good or bad to eat. What constitutes a healthy diet for the pregnant woman? Overall, the following guidelines can be helpful:

- Increase your consumption of fruits and vegetables.
- Replace saturated fats with unsaturated ones.
- Avoid hydrogenated or partially hydrogenated fats.
- Use reduced-fat spreads and dairy products instead of full-fat ones.
- Eat at least two servings of fish weekly, with one of them being an oily fish.
- Consume at least 2 quarts of water daily (Engstrom, 2004).

The current DRIs developed by the IOM suggest an increase in the pregnant woman's intake of protein from 60 to 80 g per day, iron from 18 to 27 g per day, and folate from 400 to 600 mcg per day, along with an increase of 300 calories per day (IOM, 1997, 1998, 2000, 2001, 2002) over the recommended intake of 1,800 to 2,200 calories for nonpregnant women.

It is important for a woman to understand that a healthy diet should begin before pregnancy so she will start the pregnancy in optimal health. While most women recognize the importance of healthy eating, some find it challenging to achieve. Many women say they have little time and energy to devote to meal planning and preparation. Another barrier to healthy eating is conflicting messages from various sources, resulting in a lack of clear, reliable, and relevant information. Moreover, many women are eating less in an effort to control their weight, putting them at greater risk of inadequate nutrient intake.

In the months before conception, food choices are key. The foods and vitamins consumed can ensure that the woman and her fetus will have the nutrients that are essential for the very start of pregnancy.

Nutritional Requirements

Pregnancy is one of the most nutritionally demanding periods of a woman's life. Gestation involves rapid cell division and organ development, and an adequate supply of nutrients is essential to support this tremendous fetal growth.

Most women are usually motivated to eat properly during pregnancy for the sake of the fetus. The Food and

Nutrition Board of the National Research Council has made recommendations for nutrient intakes for people living in the United States. The DRIs are more comprehensive than previous nutrient guidelines issued by the board. They have replaced previous recommendations because they are not limited to preventing deficiency diseases; rather, the DRIs incorporate current concepts about the role of nutrients and food components in reducing the risk of chronic disease, developmental disorders, and other related problems. The DRIs can be used to plan and assess diets for healthy people (Dudek, 2006).

These dietary recommendations also include information for women who are pregnant or lactating, because growing fetal and maternal tissues require increased quantities of essential dietary components (Table 12-3). For a pregnant woman to meet recommended DRIs, it is important for her to eat according to the USDA's Food Guide Pyramid (Fig. 12-15).

An eating plan that follows the pyramid should provide sufficient nutrients for a healthy pregnancy. Except for iron, folic acid, and calcium, most of the nutrients a woman needs during pregnancy can be obtained by making healthy food choices. However, a vitamin and mineral supplement may be prescribed. If so, it should be taken only as directed.

Fish and shellfish are an important part of a healthy diet because they contain high-quality protein, are low in saturated fat, and contain omega-3 fatty acids. However, nearly all fish and shellfish contain traces of mercury and some contain higher levels of mercury that may harm a developing fetus if ingested by pregnant women in large amounts. With this in mind, the FDA and the Environmental Protection Agency (EPA) are advising women who may become pregnant, pregnant women, and nursing mothers to do the following:

- Avoid eating shark, swordfish, king mackerel, and tilefish.
- Eat up to 12 ounces (two average meals) weekly of these fish:
  - Shrimp, canned light tuna, salmon
  - Pollock and catfish
- Check local advisories about the safety of fish caught by family and friends in local lakes, rivers, and coastal areas (FDA, EPA, 2004).

Maternal Weight Gain

The amount of weight gain during pregnancy is not as important as what the mother eats. A woman can lose extra weight after a pregnancy, but she can never replace a poor nutritional status during the pregnancy. Currently,

Table 12-3 Dietary Recommendations for the Pregnant and Lactating Woman

Nutrient	Nonpregnant Woman	Pregnant Woman	Lactating Woman
Calories	2,200	2,500	2,700
Protein	60 g	80 g	80 g
Water/fluids	6–8 glasses daily	8 glasses daily	8 glasses daily
Vitamin A	700 mcg	770 mcg	1,300 mcg
Vitamin C	75 mg	85 mg	120 mg
Vitamin D	5 mcg	5 mcg	5 mcg
Vitamin E	15 mcg	15 mcg	19 mcg
B1 (thiamine)	1.1 mg	1.5 mg	1.5 mg
B2 (riboflavin)	1.1 mg	1.4 mg	1.6 mg
B3 (niacin)	14 mg	18 mg	17 mg
B6 (pyridoxine)	1.3 mg	1.9 mg	2 mg
B12 (cobalamin)	2.4 mcg	2.6 mcg	2.8 mcg
Folate	400 mcg	600 mcg	500 mcg
Calcium	1,000 mg	1,000 mg	1,000 mg
Phosphorus	700 mg	700 mg	700 mg
Iodine	150 mcg	220 mcg	290 mcg
Iron	18 mg	27 mg	9 mg
Magnesium	310 mg	350 mg	310 mg
Zinc	8 mg	11 mg	12 mg

Sources: Institute of Medicine, 1997, 1998, 2000, 2001, 2002.

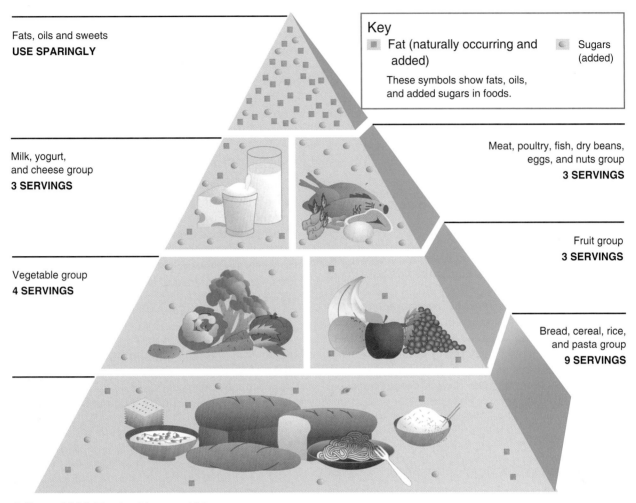

● Figure 12-15 Food guide pyramid for pregnancy.

the ACOG recommends a 25- to 35-pound weight gain during pregnancy. Table 12-4 summarizes the distribution of weight gain during pregnancy.

The best way to measure whether a pregnant woman is consuming enough calories is to follow her pattern of weight gain. If she is gaining in a steady, gradual manner, then she is taking in enough calories. However, consuming an adequate amount of calories doesn't guarantee that her nutrients are sufficient. It is critical to evaluate both the quantity and the quality of the foods eaten.

The IOM has issued recommendations for weight gain during pregnancy based on prepregnancy body mass index (BMI; Box 12-5). A woman who is underweight before pregnancy or who has a low maternal weight gain pattern should be monitored carefully, for she is at risk of giving birth to a low-birthweight infant (<2,500 g or 5.5 pounds). Frequently these women simply need advice on what to eat to add weight. Encourage the woman to eat snack foods that are high in calories such as nuts, peanut butter, milkshakes, cheese, fruit yogurt, and ice cream. Any woman who has a prepregnancy BMI of less than 19.8 is considered to be high risk and should be

Table 12-4 Normal Distribution of Weight Gain During Pregnancy

Component	Weight
Fetus	7.5–8.5 pounds
Blood	4 pounds
Uterus	2 pounds
Breasts	1 pound
Placenta and umbilical cord	1.5 pounds
Fat and protein stores	7.5 pounds
Tissue fluids	2.7 pounds
Amniotic fluid	1.8 pounds
Approximate total weight gain	29 pounds

Mahan & Escott-Stump, 2004; McKinney et al., 2005; Lowdermilk & Perry, 2004.

Body Mass Index (BMI) provides an accurate estimate of total body fat and is considered a good method to assess overweight and obesity in people. BMI is a weight-to-height ratio calculation that can be determined by dividing a woman's weight in kilograms by her height in meters squared. BMI can also be calculated by weight in pounds divided by the height in inches squared, multiplied by 704.5.

The Centers for Disease Control and Prevention (CDC) categorizes BMI as follows:
• Underweight: less than 18.5
• Healthy weight: 18.5 to 24.9
• Overweight: 25 to 29.9
• Obese: 30 or higher (CDC, 2003)

Use this example to calculate BMI:
Mary is 5′ 5″ tall and weighs 150 pounds.
1. Convert weight into kilograms 150 ÷ 2.2 lb/kg = 68.18 kg.
2. Convert height into meters
   a. 5′ 5″ = 65″ × 2.54 cm/in = 165.1 cm
   b. 165.1 cm ÷ 100 cm = 1.65 m
3. Then square the height in meters 1.65 × 1.65 = 2.72
4. Calculate BMI 68.18 ÷ 2.72 = **25**

referred to a nutritionist. These women are encouraged to gain 28 to 40 pounds during the pregnancy (IOM, 2002).

Conversely, women who start a pregnancy being overweight (BMI >25 to 29) run the risk of a high-birth-weight infant with resulting cephalopelvic disproportion and a surgical birth. Dieting during pregnancy is never recommended, even for women who are obese. Severe restriction of caloric intake is associated with a decrease in birthweight. Because of the expansion of maternal blood volume and development of fetal and placental tissues, some weight gain is essential for a healthy pregnancy. Women who gain more than the recommended weight during pregnancy and who fail to lose this weight 6 months after giving birth are at much higher risk of being obese nearly a decade later (ACOG, 2002). Mothers who are overweight when beginning a pregnancy should gain no more than 15 to 25 pounds during the pregnancy, depending on their nutritional status and degree of obesity (Cesario, 2003).

All pregnant women should aim for a steady rate of weight gain throughout pregnancy. During the first trimester, for women whose prepregnant weight is within the normal weight range, weight gain should be about 3.5 to 5 pounds. For underweight women, weight gain should be at least 5 pounds. For overweight women, weight gain should be about 2 pounds. Much of the weight gained

during the first trimester is caused by growth of the uterus and expansion of the blood volume.

During the second and third trimesters, the following pattern is recommended. For women whose prepregnant weight is within the normal weight range, weight gain should be about 1 pound per week. For underweight women, weight gain should be slightly more than 1 pound per week. For overweight women, weight gain should be about two thirds of a pound per week (Florida Department of Health, 2003).

Nutrition Promotion

Through education, nurses can play an important role in ensuring adequate nutrition for pregnant women. During the initial prenatal visit, healthcare providers conduct a thorough assessment of a woman's typical dietary practices and address any conditions that may affect intake of adequate nutrition, such as nausea and vomiting or lack of access to adequate food. Assess and reinforce dietary information at every prenatal visit to promote good nutrition. A normal pregnancy and a well-balanced diet generally provide most of the recommended nutrients except iron and folate, both of which must be supplemented.

The Food Guide Pyramid, developed in 1992 by the U.S. Department of Agriculture, is the typical tool used for nutritional education and is recognized by the general population as the gold standard for healthy eating patterns (Fowles, 2004). Use this well-known tool as a basis for dietary instruction and tailor it to meet each woman's individual needs (Teaching Guidelines 12-5).

 TEACHING GUIDELINES 12-5

Teaching to Promote Optimal Nutrition
During Pregnancy

Use the following guidelines to ensure the best nutrition possible during your pregnancy:
• Follow the Food Guide Pyramid and select a variety of foods from each group.
• Gain weight in a gradual and steady manner as follows:
   a. Normal-weight woman—25 to 35 pounds
   b. Underweight woman—28 to 40 pounds
   c. Overweight woman—15 to 25 pounds
   d. Obese woman—15 pounds
• Take your prenatal vitamin/mineral supplementation daily.
• Avoid weight-reduction diets during pregnancy.
• Do not skip meals; eat three meals with one or two snacks daily.
• Limit the intake of sodas and caffeine-rich drinks.
• Avoid the use of diuretics during pregnancy.
• Do not restrict the use of salt unless instructed to do so by your healthcare provider.
• Engage in reasonable physical activity daily.

Special Nutritional Considerations

Many factors play an important role in shaping a person's food habits, and these factors must be taken into account if nutritional counseling is to be realistic and appropriate. Nurses need to be aware of these factors to ensure individualized teaching and care.

Cultural Variations and Restrictions

Food is important to every cultural group. It is often part of celebrations and rituals. When working with women from various cultures, the nurse needs to adapt American nutritional guidelines to meet their nutritional needs within their cultural framework. Food pyramid choices and variations for different cultures might include the following:

- Bread, cereal, rice, and pasta group
  - African-American: biscuits, cornbread, grits
  - Asian: barley, dumplings, rice, hau jaun (Chinese)
  - Hispanic: bolello, tortilla (Mexican), taco shell, rice
  - Native American: blue corn, flour tortillas, fry bread
- Vegetable group
  - African-American: greens, okra, sweet potatoes
  - Asian: bamboo shoots, bok choy, water chestnuts
  - Hispanic: cabbage, jicama, carrots, agave, onions, squash
  - Native American: wild celery and onion, squash, zucchini
- Protein group
  - African-American: legumes, fish, chicken, beef
  - Asian: bean paste, eggs, shellfish, duck, beef, chicken
  - Hispanic: beef, legumes, lamb, pork, tripe, eggs, fish
  - Native American: blood sausage, deer, processed meats
- Fruit group
  - African-American: apples, bananas, watermelon
  - Asian: Chinese beans, guava, kumquats, papaya
  - Hispanic: apples, guava, mango, plantain, zapate, pineapple
  - Native American: catabopy, casabas, yucca fruit, watermelon
- Milk and dairy products group
  - African-American: buttermilk, cheese, ice cream, pudding
  - Asian: buffalo's milk, soybean milk, yogurt, cow's milk
  - Hispanic: custard, cheese, ice cream
  - Native American: cheese, goat or cow milk (Moore & Moos, 2003)

Lactose Intolerance

The best source of calcium is milk and dairy products, but for women with lactose intolerance, adaptations are necessary. Women with lactose intolerance lack an enzyme (lactase) needed for the breakdown of lactose into its component simple sugars, glucose and galactose. Without adequate lactase, lactose passes through the small intestine undigested and causes abdominal discomfort, gas, and diarrhea. Lactose intolerance is especially common among women of African, Asian, and Middle Eastern descent (Marchiano & Ural, 2004).

Additional or substitute sources of calcium may be necessary. These may include peanuts, almonds, sunflower seeds, broccoli, salmon, kale, and molasses (Mahan & Escott-Stump, 2000). In addition, encourage the woman to drink lactose-free dairy products or calcium-enriched orange juice or soy milk.

Vegetarians

Vegetarian diets are becoming increasing prevalent in the United States. People choose a vegetarian diet for various reasons, including environmental, animal rights, philosophical, religious, and health (Monti & Kehler, 2001). Vegetarians choose not to eat meat, chicken, and fish. Their diets consist mostly of plant-based foods, such as legumes, vegetables, whole grains, nuts, and seeds. Vegetarians fall into groups defined by the types of foods they eat. Lacto-ovo-vegetarians omit red meat, fish, and poultry but eat eggs, milk, and dairy products, in addition to plant-based foods. Lacto-vegetarians consume milk and dairy products along with plant-based foods; they omit eggs, meat, fish, and poultry. Vegans eliminate all foods from animals, including milk, eggs, and cheese, and eat only plant-based foods (Dudek, 2006).

The concern with any form of vegetarianism, especially during pregnancy, is that the diet may be inadequate in nutrients. Other risks of vegetarian eating patterns during pregnancy may include low gestational weight gain, iron-deficiency anemia, compromised protein utilization, and decreased mineral absorption (Florida Department of Health, 2003). A diet can become so restrictive that a woman is not gaining weight or is consistently not eating enough from one or more of the food groups. Generally, the more restrictive the diet, the greater the chance of nutrient deficiencies.

Well-balanced vegetarian diets that include dairy products provide adequate caloric and nutrient intake and do not require special supplementation; however, vegan diets do not include any meat, eggs, or dairy products. Pregnant vegetarians must pay special attention to their intake of protein, iron, calcium, and vitamin B_{12}. Suggestions include:

- For protein: substitute soy foods, beans, lentils, nuts, grains, and seeds.
- For iron: eat a variety of meat alternatives, along with vitamin C-rich foods.
- For calcium: substitute soy, calcium-fortified orange juice, and tofu.
- For vitamin B_{12}: eat fortified soy foods and a B_{12} supplement.

The woman may also take a multivitamin prenatal supplement (Monti & Kehler, 2001).

Pica

Many women experience unusual food cravings during their pregnancy. Having cravings during pregnancy is perfectly normal. Sometimes, however, women crave substances that have no nutritional value and can even be dangerous to themselves and their developing fetus. **Pica** is the compulsive ingestion of nonfood substances. Pica is derived from the Latin term for magpie, a bird that is known to consume a variety of non-food substances. Unlike the bird, pregnant women who develop a pica habit typically have one or two specific cravings.

The exact cause of pica is not known. Many theories have been advanced to explain it, but none has been scientifically proven. The incidence of pica is difficult to determine, since it is underreported. It is more common in the United States among African-American women than other ethnicities, but the practice of pica is not limited to any one geographic area, race, creed, or culture (Corbett et al., 2003). In the United States, pica is also common in women from rural areas and women with a family history of it (Lowdermilk & Perry, 2004).

The three main substances consumed by women with pica are soil or clay (geophagia), ice (pagophagia), and laundry starch (amylophagia). Nutritional implications include:

- Soil: replaces nutritive sources and causes iron-deficiency anemia
- Clay: produces constipation; can contain toxic substances and cause parasitic infection
- Ice: can cause iron-deficiency anemia, tooth fractures, freezer burn injuries
- Laundry starch: replaces iron-rich foods and leads to iron deficiencies and replaces protein metabolism, thus depriving the fetus of amino acids needed for proper development (Ellis & Schnoes, 2005).

Clinical manifestations of anemia often precede the identification of pica because it is rarely addressed by the health care provider and the woman does not usually volunteer such information (Littleton & Engebretson, 2005). Secrecy surrounding this habit makes research and diagnosis difficult because some women fail to view their behavior as anything unusual, harmful, or worth reporting. Compulsive ingestion of non-food substances is not rare or bound by culture, race, or socioeconomic status; instead, it is vastly underreported and underdiagnosed (Ellis & Schnoes, 2005). Because of the clinical implications, pica should be discussed with all pregnant women as a preventive measure. The topic can be part of a general discussion of cravings, and the nurse should stress the harmful effects outlined above.

Suspect the possibility of pica when the woman exhibits anemia although her dietary intake is appropriate. Ask about her usual dietary intake, and include questions about the ingestion of non-food substances. Consider the potential negative outcomes for the pregnant woman and her fetus, and take appropriate action.

Perinatal Education

Childbirth today is a very different experience from childbirth in previous generations. In the past, women were literally "put to sleep" with anesthetics, and they woke up with a baby. Most never remembered the details. The woman had a passive role in childbirth, as the physician delivered her newborn. In the 1950s, consumers began to insist on taking a more active role in their health care, and couples desired to be together during the extraordinary event of childbirth. Beginning in the 1970s, the father or significant other support person remained with the mother throughout labor and birth (McKinney et al., 2005).

Childbirth education began because women demanded to become more involved in their birthing experience rather than simply turning control over to a health care provider. Nurses played a pivotal role in bringing about this change by providing information and supporting clients and their families, fostering a more active role in and preparation for the upcoming birth.

Perinatal education includes breastfeeding, infant care, transition to parenthood, relationship skills, family health promotion, and sexuality (Littleton & Engebretson, 2005). Traditionally, childbirth education classes focused on developing and practicing techniques for use in managing pain and facilitating the progress of labor. Recently, the focus has broadened to include preparation for pregnancy and family adaptation to the new parenting roles. Subjects commonly addressed in perinatal education include:

- Anatomy and physiology of reproduction
- Fetal growth and development
- Prenatal maternal exercise
- Physiologic and emotional changes during pregnancy
- Sex during pregnancy
- Infant growth and development
- Nutrition and healthy eating habits during pregnancy
- Teratogens and impact on the fetus
- Signs and symptoms of labor
- Preparation for labor and birth (for parents, siblings, and other family members)
- Options for birth
- Infant nutrition, including preparation for breastfeeding
- Infant care, including safety, CPR, and first aid
- Family planning (March of Dimes, 2005)

Childbirth Education Classes

Childbirth education classes teach pregnant women and their support person about pregnancy, birth, and parenting in a series of instructional classes offered in their local communities or online. The classes are usually taught by certified childbirth educators.

Most childbirth classes support the concept of **natural childbirth** (a birth without pain-relieving medications) so that the woman can be in control throughout the experience as much as possible. The classes differ in their approach to specific comfort techniques and breathing patterns. The three most common childbirth methods are the Lamaze (psychoprophylactic) method, the Bradley (partner-coached childbirth) method, and the Dick-Read (natural childbirth) method.

Lamaze Method

Lamaze is a psychoprophylactic ("mind prevention") method of preparing for labor and birth that promotes the use of specific breathing and relaxation techniques. Dr. Fernand Lamaze, a French obstetrician, popularized this method of childbirth preparation in the 1960s. Lamaze believed that conquering fear through knowledge and support was important. He also believed women needed to alter the perception of suffering during childbirth. This perception change would come about by learning conditioned reflexes that, instead of signaling pain, would signal the work of producing a child, and thus would carry the woman through labor awake, aware, and in control of her own body (Leonard, 2002). Lamaze felt strongly that all women have the right to deliver their babies with minimal or no medication while maintaining their dignity, minimizing their pain, maximizing their self-esteem, and enjoying the miracle of birth.

Lamaze classes include information on toning exercises, relaxation exercises and techniques, and breathing methods for labor. The breathing techniques are used in labor to enhance relaxation and to reduce the woman's perception of pain. The goal is for women to become aware of their own comfortable rate of breathing in order to maintain relaxation and adequate oxygenation of her fetus. Breathing techniques are an effective attention-focusing strategy to reduce pain.

Paced breathing describes breathing techniques used to decrease stress responses and therefore decrease pain. This type of breathing implies self-regulation by the woman. The woman starts off by taking a cleansing breath at the onset and end of each contraction. This cleansing breath symbolizes freeing her mind from worries and concerns. This breath enhances oxygenation and puts the woman in a relaxed state.

Slow-paced breathing is associated with relaxation and should be half the normal breathing rate (6 to 9 breaths per minute). This type of breathing is the most relaxed pattern and is recommended throughout labor. Abdominal or chest breathing may be used. It is generally best to breathe in through the nose and breathe out either through the nose or mouth, whichever is more comfortable for the woman.

Modified-paced breathing can be used for increased work or stress during labor to increase alertness or focus attention or when slow-paced breathing is no longer effective in keeping the woman relaxed. The woman's respiratory rate increases, but it does not exceed twice her normal rate. Modified-paced breathing is a quiet upper chest breath that is increased or decreased according to the intensity of the contraction. The inhalation and the exhalation are equal. This breathing technique should be practiced during pregnancy for optimal use during labor.

Patterned-paced breathing is similar to modified-paced breathing but with a rhythmic pattern. It uses a variety of patterns, with an emphasis on the exhalation breath at regular intervals. Different patterns can be used, such as 4/1, 6/1, 4/1. A 4/1 rhythm is four upper chest breaths followed by an exhalation (a sighing out of air, like blowing out a candle). Random patterns can be chosen for use as long as the basic principles of rate and relaxation are met.

Couples practice these breathing patterns typically during the last few months of the pregnancy until they feel comfortable using them. Focal points (visual fixation on a designated object), effleurage (light abdominal message), massage, and imagery (journey of the mind to a relaxing place) are also added to aid in relaxation. From the nurse's perspective, the woman is encouraged to breathe at a level of comfort that allows her to cope. Always remain quiet during the woman's periods of imagery and focal point visualization to avoid breaking her concentration.

Bradley Method (Partner-Coached)

The Bradley method uses various exercises and slow, controlled abdominal breathing to accomplish relaxation. Dr. Robert Bradley, a Denver-based obstetrician, advocated a completely unmedicated labor and birth experience. The Bradley method emphasizes the pleasurable sensations of childbirth, teaching women to concentrate on these sensations while "turning on" to their own bodies (Leonard, 2002). In 1965, he wrote *Husband-Coached Childbirth,* which advocated the active participation of the husband as labor coach.

A woman is conditioned to work in harmony with her body using breath control and deep abdominopelvic breathing to promote general body relaxation during labor. This method stresses that childbirth is a joyful, natural process and emphasizes the partner's involvement during pregnancy, labor, birth, and the early newborn period. Thus, the training techniques are directed toward the coach, not the mother. The coach is educated in massage/comfort techniques to use on the mother throughout the labor and birth process.

Dick-Read Method

In 1944 Grantly Dick-Read, a British obstetrician, wrote *Childbirth Without Fear.* He believed that the attitude of a woman toward her birthing process had a considerable influence on the ease of her labor, and he believed that fear is the primary pain-producing agent in an otherwise normal labor. He felt that fear builds a state of tension, creating an antagonistic effect on the laboring muscles of the uterus, which results in pain. Pain causes more fear, which further increases the tension, and the vicious cycle of "fear–tension–pain" is established (Leonard, 2002). Dick-Read sought to interrupt the circular pattern of fear, tension, and pain during the labor and birthing process. He promoted the belief that the degree of fear could be diminished with increased understanding of the normal physiologic response to labor (Murray et al., 2006).

Dick-Read believed that prenatal instruction was essential for pain relief and that emotional factors during labor interfered with the normal labor progression. The woman achieves relaxation and reduces pain by arming herself with the knowledge of normal childbirth and using abdominal breathing during contractions.

Nursing Management and Childbirth Education

Childbirth education is less about methods than about mastery. The overall aim of any of the methods is to promote an internal locus of control that will enable each woman to yield her body to the process of birth. As the woman gains success and tangible benefits from the exercises she is taught, she begins to reframe her beliefs and gains practical knowledge, and the impetus will be there for her to engage in the conscious use of the techniques (Fig. 12-16). Nurses play a key role in supporting and encouraging each couple's use of the techniques taught in childbirth education classes.

Every woman's labor is unique, and it is important for nurses not to generalize or stereotype women. The most effective support a nurse can offer couples using prepared childbirth methods is encouragement and presence. These nursing measures must be adapted to each individual throughout the labor process. Offering encouraging phrases such as "great job" or "you can do it" helps to reinforce their efforts and at the same time empowers them to continue. Using eye-to-eye contact to engage the woman's total attention is important if she appears overwhelmed or appears to lose control during the transition phase of labor.

Nurses play a significant role in enhancing the couple's relationship by respecting the involvement of the partner and demonstrating concern for his needs throughout labor. Offering to stay with the woman to give him a break periodically allows him to meet his needs while at the same time still actively participating. Nurses can offer anticipatory guidance to the couple and assist during critical times in labor. The nurse can demonstrate many of the coping techniques to the partner and praise their successful use, which increases self-esteem. Focus on their strengths and the positive elements of the labor experience. Congratulating the couple for a job well done is paramount.

Throughout the labor experience, demonstrate personal warmth and project a friendly attitude. Frequently, a nurse's touch may help to prevent a crisis by reassuring the mother that she is doing fine.

Options for Birth

From the moment a woman discovers she is pregnant, numerous decisions await her—where the infant will be born, what birth setting is best, and who will assist with the birth. The great majority of women are well and healthy and can consider the full range of birth settings—hospital, birth center, or home setting—based on knowledge about each to ensure the most informed decision.

Hospitals are the most common site for birth in the United States. If the woman has a serious medical condition or is at high risk for developing one, she will probably need to plan to give birth in a hospital setting under the care of an obstetrician. Giving birth in a hospital is advantageous for several reasons. Hospitals are best equipped to diagnose and treat women and newborns with complications; trained personnel are available if necessary; and no transportation is needed if a complication should arise during labor or birth. Disadvantages include the high-tech atmosphere, strict policies and restrictions that might limit who can be with the woman, and the medical model of care.

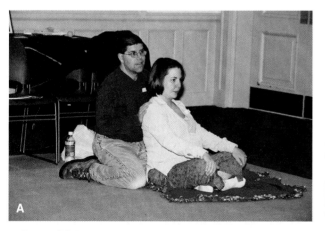
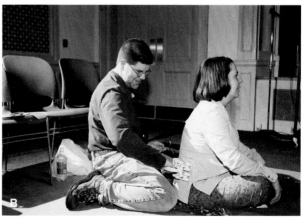

● Figure 12-16 A couple practicing the techniques taught in a childbirth education class.

Within the hospital setting, however, choices do exist regarding birth environments. The *conventional delivery room* resembles an operating room, where the healthcare professional delivers the newborn from the women, who is positioned in stirrups. The woman is then transferred to the recovery area on a stretcher and then again to the postpartum unit. The *birthing suite* is the other option within the hospital setting; the woman and her partner remain in one place for labor, birth, and recovery. The birthing suite is a private room decorated to look as homelike as possible: the bed converts to allow for various birthing positions, and there may be a rocking chair or an easy chair for the woman's partner. Despite the homey atmosphere, the room is still equipped with emergency resuscitative obstetric equipment and electronic fetal monitors in case they are needed quickly (Fig. 12-17). Such settings provide a more personal childbirth experience in a less formal and intimidating atmosphere compared to the traditional delivery room.

A *freestanding birth center* (Fig. 12-18) can be a good choice for a woman who wants more personalized care than in a hospital but does not feel comfortable with a home birth. In contrast to the institutional environment in hospitals, most freestanding birth centers have a homelike atmosphere, and many are in fact located in converted homes. Some are located on hospital property and are affiliated with them. Birth centers are designed to provide maternity care to women judged to be at low risk for obstetric complications. Women are allowed to give birth in the position most comfortable for them. Care in birth centers is often provided by midwives and is more relaxed, with no routine intravenous lines, fetal monitoring, and restrictive protocols. A disadvantage of the birth center is the need to transport the woman to a hospital quickly if an emergency arises; emergency equipment is not readily available. In a research study comparing home-like to conventional institutional settings, the author concluded that there appeared to be some benefits from home-like

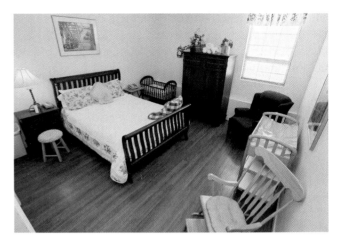

● Figure 12-18 Birthing center.

settings for childbirth, although increased support from caregivers may be more important (Hodnett, 2004).

Most women who choose a *home birth* believe that birth is a natural process that requires little medical intervention (Kennedy & Shannon, 2004). Home births can be safe if there are qualified, experienced attendants and an emergency transfer system in place in case of serious complications. Many women choose the home setting out of a strong desire to control the kind of childbirth and to give birth surrounded by family members. Most home birth caregivers are midwives who have provided continuous care to the woman throughout the pregnancy. Disadvantages include the need to transport the woman to the hospital during or after labor if a problem arises, and the limited pain management available in the home setting.

Care Providers

While most women in the United States still receive pregnancy care from an obstetrician, an increasing number are opting for a midwife for their care. The difference is a matter of degrees. Obstetricians must finish a 4-year residency in obstetrics and gynecology in addition to medical school. Certified nurse-midwives complete 1 to 2 years of graduate work in midwifery following nursing school. Obstetricians can handle high-risk pregnancies and delivery emergencies, can administer or order pain-relief drugs, and are assisted by a support staff in the hospital setting. Midwives work in hospitals, birthing centers, and home settings to deliver care. They believe in the normalcy of birth and tolerate wide variations of what is considered normal during labor, which leads to fewer interventions applied during the childbirth process (Kennedy & Shannon, 2004). They are not able to handle high-risk births and some birth emergencies.

In addition to the woman's primary health care professional, some women hire a **doula** to be with them during labor. *Doula* is a Greek word that means "woman's

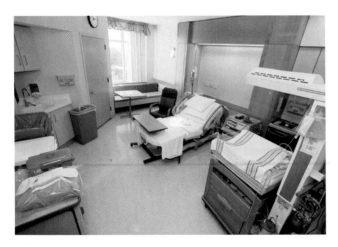

● Figure 12-17 Birthing suite.

servant." A doula is a laywoman trained to provide women and their families with encouragement, emotional and physical support, and information through late pregnancy, labor, and birth. Doulas provide the woman with continuous support throughout labor but do not perform any clinical procedures.

Preparation for Bottle or Breastfeeding

One could say that lactation and breastfeeding are so natural that they should just happen on their own accord, but this is not the case. Pregnant women are faced with a decision about which method of feeding to choose. The nurse needs to educate the pregnant client about the advantages and disadvantages of each method, allowing the woman and her partner to make an informed decision about the best method for their situation. Providing the client and her partner with this information will increase the likelihood of a successful experience.

Substantial scientific evidence exists documenting the health benefits of breastfeeding for newborns. Human milk provides an ideal balance of nutrients for newborns (Landers, 2003). Breastfeeding is advantageous for the following reasons:

- Human milk is digestible, economical, and requires no preparation.
- Bonding between mother and child is promoted.
- Cost is less than purchasing formula.
- Ovulation is suppressed (however, this is not a reliable birth control method).
- The risk of ovarian cancer and the incidence of premenopausal breast cancer are reduced.
- Extra calories are used, which promotes weight loss gradually without dieting.
- Oxytocin is released to promote more rapid uterine involution with less bleeding.
- Sucking helps to develop the muscles in the infant's jaw.
- Absorption of lactose and minerals in the newborn is improved.
- The immunologic properties of breast milk help prevent infections in the baby.
- The composition of breast milk adapts to meet the infant's changing needs.
- Constipation in the baby is not a problem with adequate intake.
- Food allergies are less likely to develop in the breastfed baby.
- The incidence of otitis media and upper respiratory infections in the infant is reduced.
- Breastfed babies are less likely to be overfed, thus reducing the risk of adult obesity.
- Breastfed newborns are less prone to vomiting (McKinney et al., 2005).

Encouraging a woman to attend a La Leche League class, providing her with sources of information about infant feeding, and suggesting that she read a good reference book about lactation will also help in her decision-making process.

Breastfeeding also has disadvantages. These include breast discomfort, sore nipples, mastitis, engorgement, vaginal dryness, and decreased libido (Youngkin & Davis, 2004). Nipple preparation is not necessary during the prenatal period unless the nipples are inverted and do not become erect when stimulated. Assess for this by placing the forefinger and thumb above and below the areola and compressing behind the nipple. If it flattens or inverts, advise the client to wear breast shields during the last 2 months of pregnancy. Breast shields exert a continuous pressure around the areola, pushing the nipple through a central opening in the inner shield (Curtis & Schuler, 2000). The shields are worn inside the bra. Initially the shields are worn for 1 hour, and then the woman progressively increases the wearing time up to 8 hours daily. The client maintain this schedule until after delivery, and then she wears the shield 24 hours a day until the infant latches on easily (Youngkin & Davis, 2004). In addition, suggest that the woman wear a supportive nursing bra 24 hours a day.

Bottle-feeding an infant isn't just a matter of "open, pour and feed." Parents need information on types of formulas, preparation and storage of formula, equipment, and feeding positions. It is recommended that normal full-term infants receive conventional cow's milk-based formula, and this choice should be directed by the physician. If the infant has a reaction (diarrhea, vomiting, abdominal pain, excessive gas) to the first formula, another formula should be tried. Frequently a soy-based formula is substituted. In terms of preparation of formula and its use, the following information applies:

- Equipment must be obtained and maintained.
- Supplies are needed: six 4-ounce bottles, eight 8-ounce bottles, and nipples.
- Consistency is important. Stay with a nipple that is comfortable to the infant.
- Frequently assess nipples for any loose pieces of rubber at the opening.
- The average speed of flow from the bottle is one drop per second.
- Formula preparation is critical to the health and development of the infant.
- Formula is available in three forms: ready-to-feed, concentrate, and powder.
- Reading the formula label thoroughly is important before mixing.
- Correct formula dilution is important:
  - Ready-to-use: use as is without dilution
  - Concentrated formulas: dilute with equal parts of water
  - Powdered formulas: mix one scoop of powder with 2 ounces of water

- If the water supply is safe, sterilization is not necessary.
- Bottles and nipples should be washed in hot, sudsy water using a bottle brush.
- Formula should be served at room temperature.
- If the water supply is questionable, water should be boiled for 5 minutes before use.
- Formula should not be heated in a microwave oven, because it is heated unevenly.
- Formula can be prepared for 24 hours ahead of time and stored in the refrigerator.

The formula-fed infant should be fed in a semi-upright position using the cradle hold in the arms. This position allows for face-to-face contact between the infant and caretaker. Advise the parents to hold the bottle so that the nipple is kept full of formula to prevent excessive air swallowing. Instruct the parents to feed the infant every 3 to 4 hours and adapt the feeding times to the infant's needs. Frequent burping of the infant (every ounce) helps prevent gas build-up in the stomach. Caution parents not to prop the bottle, to prevent choking (McKinney et al., 2005).

Feeding an infant from a bottle should mirror breastfeeding as closely as possible. While nutrition is important, so are the emotional and interactive components of feeding. Encourage the parents to cuddle the infant closely and position the infant so that his or her head is in a comfortable position. Also encourage the parents to communicate with the infant during feedings. Warn parents about the danger of putting the infant to bed with a bottle; this can lead to "baby bottle tooth decay" because sugars in the formula stay in contact with the infant's developing teeth for prolonged periods.

Preparation for Labor and Birth

The nurse has played a supportive/education role for the couple throughout the pregnancy and now needs to assist in preparing them for their "big event" by making sure they have made informed decisions and completed the following checklist:

- Attended childbirth preparation classes and practiced breathing techniques
- Purchased an infant safety seat to bring their newborn home in
- Selected a feeding method (bottle or breast) they feel comfortable with
- Made a decision regarding circumcision if they have a boy
- Selected a birth setting and made arrangements there
- Toured the birthing facility
- Selected a family planning method to use after the birth
- Communicated their needs and desires concerning pain management
- Have been instructed on signs and symptoms of labor and what to do

- Made arrangements to have other siblings taken care of during labor
- Discussed the possibility of a cesarean birth if complications occur
- Packed a suitcase to take to the birthing facility when labor starts
- Discussed possible names for the newborn
- Know what to expect during labor and birth
- Know what to do if membranes rupture prior to going into labor
- Know how to reach their healthcare professional when labor starts
- Decided on a pediatrician
- Have items needed to prepare for the newborn's homecoming:
  - Infant clothes in several sizes
  - Nursing bras
  - Infant crib with spaces between the slats that are 2–3/8 inches or less
  - Diapers (cloth or disposable)
  - Feeding supplies (bottles and nipples if formula feeding)
  - Infant thermometer

At each prenatal visit the nurse has had the opportunity to discuss and reinforce the importance of being prepared for the birth of the child with the parents. It is now up to the parents to use the nurse's guidance and put it into action to be ready for their upcoming "main event."

Danger Signs of Pregnancy

In promoting safety for the client, it is also important to educate her about danger signs related to pregnancy that need further evaluation. If she experiences any of the following signs or symptoms, she should contact her healthcare provider:

- *During the first trimester:* spotting or bleeding (miscarriage), painful urination (infection), severe persistent vomiting (hyperemesis gravidarum), fever higher than 100°F (infection), and lower abdominal pain with dizziness and accompanied by shoulder pain (ruptured ectopic pregnancy)
- *During the second trimester:* regular uterine contractions (preterm labor); pain in calf, often increased with foot flexion (blood clot in deep vein); sudden gush or leakage of fluid from vagina (premature rupture of membranes); and absence of fetal movement for more than 24 hours (possible fetal distress or demise)
- *During the third trimester:* sudden weight gain; periorbital or facial edema, severe upper abdominal pain, or headache with visual changes (pregnancy-induced hypertension); and a decrease in fetal daily movement for more than 24 hours (possible demise). Any of the previous warning signs and symptoms can also be present in this last trimester (Youngkin & Davis, 2004).

One of the warning signs that should be emphasized is early contractions, which can lead to preterm birth. All pregnant women need to be able to recognize early signs of contractions to prevent preterm labor, which is a major public health problem in the United States. Approximately 12% of all live births—or one out of eight babies—is born too soon (Katz, 2003). These preterm infants (born <37 weeks' gestation) can suffer life-long health consequences, such as mental retardation, chronic lung disease, cerebral palsy, seizure disorders, and blindness, among other problems (Katz, 2003). Preterm labor can happen to any pregnant women at any time. In many cases it can be stopped with medications if it is recognized early, before significant cervical dilation has taken place. If the woman experiences menstrual-like cramps occurring every 10 minutes accompanied by a low, dull backache, she should stop what she is doing and lie down on her left side for 1 hour and drink two or three glasses of water. If the symptoms worsen or don't subside after 1 hour, she should contact her healthcare provider for further instructions.

KEY CONCEPTS

- Preconception care is the promotion of the health and well-being of a woman and her partner before pregnancy. The goal of preconception care is to identify any areas such as health problems, lifestyle habits, or social concerns that might unfavorably affect pregnancy.

- A thorough history and physical examination is performed on the initial prenatal visit.

- A primary aspect of nursing management during the antepartum period is counseling and educating the pregnant women and her partner to promote healthy outcomes for all involved.

- Nagele's rule can be used to establish the estimated date of birth. Using this rule, subtract 3 months, then add 7 days to the first day of the last normal menstrual period. Then correct the year by adding 1 to it. This date is within plus or minus 2 weeks (margin of error).

- Pelvic shape is typically classified as one of four types: gynecoid, android, anthropoid, and platypelloid. The gynecoid type is the typical female pelvis and offers the best shape for a vaginal delivery.

- Continuous prenatal care is important for a successful outcome. The recommended schedule is every 4 weeks up to 28 weeks (7 months); every 2 weeks from 29 to 36 weeks; and every week from 37 weeks to birth.

- The height of the fundus is measured when the uterus arises out of the pelvis to evaluate fetal growth. The fundus reaches the level of the umbilicus at approximately 20 weeks and measures 20 cm. Fundal measurement should approximately equal the number of weeks of gestation until week 36.

- At each visit the woman is asked whether she is having any common signs or symptoms of preterm labor, which might include uterine contractions, dull backache, pressure in the pelvic area or thighs, increased vaginal discharge, menstrual-like cramps, and vaginal bleeding.

- Prenatal screening has become standard in prenatal care to detect neural tube defects and genetic abnormalities.

- The nurse should address common discomforts that occur in each trimester matter-of-factly at all prenatal visits and should provide realistic measures to help the client deal with them effectively.

- The pregnant client can better care for herself and the fetus if her concerns are anticipated by the nurse and incorporated into guidance sessions at each prenatal visit.

- Iron and folic acid need to be supplemented because their increased requirements during pregnancy are usually too great to be met through diet alone.

- The American College of Obstetricians and Gynecologists recommends a 25- to 35-pound weight gain during pregnancy.

- For a pregnant woman to meet recommended dietary reference intakes (DRIs), it is important for her to eat according to the USDA's Food Guide Pyramid.

- Throughout pregnancy, a well-balanced diet is critical for a healthy baby.

- Perinatal education has broadened its focus to include preparation for pregnancy and family adaptation to the new parenting roles. Childbirth education began because of increasing pressure from consumers who wanted to become more involved in their birthing experience.

- Three common childbirth education methods are Lamaze (psychoprophylactic), Bradley (partner-couched childbirth), and Dick-Read (natural childbirth).

- The great majority of women in the United States are well and healthy and can consider the full range of birth settings: hospital, birth center, or home setting.

- All pregnant women need to be able to recognize early signs of contractions to prevent preterm labor.

References

Alexander, L. L., LaRosa, J. H., Bader, H., & Garfield, S. (2004). *New dimensions in women's health* (3rd ed.). Sudbury, MA: Jones and Bartlett Publishers.

Alfirevic, Z. (2001). Early amniocentesis verses transabdominal chorion villus sampling for prenatal diagnosis (Cochrane Review). In *The Cochrane Library*, Issue 3.

American College of Obstetricians and Gynecologists (2000). *Planning for your pregnancy and birth* (3rd ed.). Washington, D.C.: Author.

American College of Obstetricians and Gynecologists (2001). *Prenatal diagnosis of fetal chromosomal abnormalities*, Practice Bulletin, No. 27. Washington, D.C.: ACOG.

American College of Obstetricians and Gynecologists (2001). *Air travel during pregnancy* (ACOG Committee Opinion No. 264). Washington, D.C: Author.

American College of Obstetricians and Gynecologists (2002). *Guidelines for perinatal care* (5th ed.). Elk Grove Village, IL and Washington, D.C: Author.

American College of Obstetricians and Gynecologists (2002). Excess weight gain during pregnancy = obesity years later. *ACOG News Release.* [Online] Available at: http://www.acog.org/from_home/ publications/press_releases/nr07-31-02-1.cfm

American College of Obstetricians and Gynecologists (ACOG). (2003). Neural tube defects. (ACOG practice bulletin no. 44). [Online] Available at http://www.guideline.gov/summary/ summary.aspx?ss=15&doc_id=3994&nbr=3131

American College of Obstetricians and Gynecologists (2004). ACOG issues position on first-trimester screening methods. *ACOG News Release.* [Online] Available at: http://acog.org/from_home/ publications/press_releases/nr06-30-04.cfm

American College of Obstetricians and Gynecologists Committee on Obstetric Practice (2002). Exercise during pregnancy and the postpartum period. *International Journal of Gynecology & Obstetrics, 77*(1), 79–81.

Anderson, M. (2001). Pica: is it being overlooked? *Physician Assistant, 25*(9), 19–24.

Black, R. A., & Hill, D. A. (2003). Over-the-counter medications in pregnancy. *American Family Physician, 67*(12), 2517–2525.

Brown, J. J. (2004). pregnancy ultrasound. *Medline Plus.* [Online] Available at: http://www.nlm.nih.gov/medlineplus/ency/ article/003778.htm.

Cavanaugh, B. M. (2003). *Nurse's manual of laboratory and diagnostic tests* (4th ed.). Philadelphia: F. A. Davis Company.

Centers for Disease Control and Prevention (CDC) (2003). *BMI for adults: Body mass index calculator.* [Online] Available at: http://www.cdc.gov/nccdphp/dnpa/bmi/calc-bmi.htm

Centers for Disease Control and Prevention (CDC) (2003). Pregnancy, breast-feeding and travel: factors affecting the decision to travel. *Traveler's Health,* [Online] Available at: http://www.cdc. gov/travel/pregnant.htm

Centers for Disease Control and Prevention (CDC) (May 7, 2004). Spina bifida and anencephaly before and after folic acid mandate—United States, 1995–1996 and 1999–2000. *MMWR, 53*(17), 362–365.

Centers for Disease Control and Prevention (CDC) (2004). Guidelines for vaccinating pregnant women. Recommendations of the Advisory Committee on Immunization Practices (ACIP). Atlanta, GA: CDC.

Cesario, S. K. (2003). Obesity in pregnancy: what every nurse should know. *AWHONN Lifelines, 7,* 119–125.

Condon, M. C. (2004). *Women's health: an integrated approach to wellness and illness.* Upper Saddle River, NJ: Prentice Hall.

Corbett, R. W., Ryan, C., & Weinrich, S. P. (2003). Pica in pregnancy: does it affect pregnancy outcome? *American Journal of Maternal Child Nursing, 28*(3), 183–189.

Cullum, A. S. (2003) Changing provider practices to enhance preconception wellness. *JOGNN, 32*(4), 543–549.

Cunningham, F., et al. (2005). *William's obstetrics* (22nd ed.). New York: McGraw-Hill.

Curtis, G. B., & Schuler, J. (2000). *Your pregnancy week by week* (4th ed.). Tucson, AZ: Fisher Books.

Davies, G. A. L. (2000). Antenatal fetal assessment. *Journal of Society of Obstetrics and Gynecology of Canada, 22*(6), 456–462.

DeJudicibus, M. A., & McCabe, M. P. (2002). Psychological factors and the sexuality of pregnant and postpartum women. *Journal of Sex Research, 39*(2), 94–104.

Dillon, P. M. (2003). *Nursing health assessment: a critical thinking, case studies approach.* Philadelphia: F. A. Davis Company.

Druzin, M., Gabbe, S., & Reed, K. (2002). Antepartal fetal evaluation. In S. Gabbe, J. Niebyl, & J. L. Simpson (Eds.), *Obstetrics: normal and problem pregnancies* (pp. 313–352). New York: Churchill Livingstone.

Dudek, S. G. (2006). *Nutrition essentials for nursing practice* (5th ed.). Philadelphia: Lippincott Williams & Wilkins.

Engstrom, J. (2004). *Maternal-neonatal nursing made incredibly easy.* Philadelphia: Lippincott Williams & Wilkins.

Florida Department of Health (2003). *Prenatal & postpartum nutrition module,* Bureau of WIC and Nutritional Services. Tallahassee, FL: Florida Department of Health.

Food and Drug Administration (FDA) and Environmental Protection Agency (EPA) (2004). What you need to know about mercury in fish and shellfish. [Online] Available at: www.cfsan.fda.gov/ seafood1.html and www.epa.gov/ost/fish

Fowles, E. (2002). Comparing pregnant women's nutritional knowledge to their actual diet intake. *MCN, 27*(3), 171–177.

Fowles, E. R. (2004). Prenatal nutrition and birth options. *JOGNN, 33*(6), 809–822.

Frey, K. A. (2002). Preconception care by the nonobstetricial provider. *Mayo Clinic Proceedings, 77,* 469–473.

Ghezzi, F., Romero, R., Maymon, E., et al. (2001). Fetal blood sampling. In A. Fleisher, F. Manning, P. Jeanty, & R. Romero (Eds.), *Sonography in obstetrics and gynecology* (pp. 775–804). New York: McGraw-Hill.

Gilbert, E. S., & Harmon, J. S. (2003). *Manual of high-risk pregnancy and delivery* (3rd ed.). St. Louis: Mosby.

Graves, J. C., Miller, K. E., & Sellers, A. D. (2002). Maternal serum triple analyte screening in pregnancy. *American Family Physician, 65*(5), 915–922.

Harris, R. A., Washington, A. E., Nease, R. F., & Kuppermann, M. (2004). Cost utility of prenatal diagnosis and the risk-based threshold. *Lancet, 363,* 276–282.

Harrison, J. (2002). Monitoring uteroplacental insufficiency. *British Journal of Midwifery, 10*(11), 680–686.

Hodnett, E. D. (2004). Home-like versus conventional institutional settings for birth (Cochrane Review). In: *The Cochrane Library,* Issue 4, Chichester, UK: John Wiley & Sons, Ltd.

Institute of Medicine (1992). *Nutrition during pregnancy. Part I: weight gain. Part II: nutrient supplements.* National Academy of Sciences. Washington, D.C.: National Academy Press.

Institute of Medicine (1997). *Dietary reference intakes for calcium, phosphorus, magnesium, vitamin D and fluoride.* Washington, D.C.: National Academy Press.

Institute of Medicine (1998). *Dietary reference intakes for thiamine, riboflavin, niacin, vitamin B6, vitamin B 12, pantothenic acid, biotin, and choline.* Washington, D.C: National Academy Press.

Institute of Medicine (2000). *Dietary reference intakes for vitamin C, vitamin E, selenium, and carotenoids.* Washington, D.C.: National Academy Press.

Institute of Medicine (2001). *Dietary reference intakes for vitamin A, vitamin K, arsenic, boron, chromium, copper, iodine, manganese, molybdenum, nickel, silicon, vanadium, and zinc.* Washington, D.C.: National Academy Press.

Institute of Medicine (2002). *Dietary reference intakes for energy, carbohydrates, fiber, protein and amino acids.* Washington, D.C.: National Academy Press.

Kaiser, L. L., & Allen, L. (2002). Position of the American Dietetic Association: nutrition and lifestyle for a healthy pregnancy outcome. *Journal of the American Dietetic Association, 102*(10), 1479–1490.

Katz, A. (2003). Preventing premature birth. *AWHONN Lifelines, 7*(4), 361.

Kennedy, H. P., & Shannon, M. T. (2004). Keeping birth normal: research findings on midwifery care during childbirth. *JOGNN, 33*(5), 554–560.

Kim, S. Y., Khandelwal, M., Gaughan, J. P., et al. (2003). Is the intrapartum biophysical profile useful? *Obstetrics & Gynecology, 102*(3), 471–476.

Landers, S. (2003). Maximizing the benefits of human milk feeding. *Pediatric Annals, 32*(5), 298–305.

Leiferman, J. A., & Evenson, K. R. (2003). The effect of regular leisure physical activity on birth outcomes. *Maternal & Child Health Journal, 7*(1), 59–65.

Leonard, P. (2002). Childbirth education: a handbook for nurses. *Nursing Spectrum.* [Online] Available at: http://nsweb. nursingspectrum.com/ce/m350a.htm

Littleton, L. Y., & Engebretson, J. C. (2002). *Maternal, neonatal, and women's health nursing.* New York: Delmar.

Littleton, L. Y., & Engebretson, J. C. (2005). *Maternity nursing care.* Clifton Park, NY: Thompson Delmar Learning.

London, M. L., Ladewig, P. W., Ball, J. W., & Bindler, R. C. (2003). *Maternal-newborn & child nursing: family-centered care.* New Jersey: Prentice Hall.

Lowdermilk, D. L., & Perry, S. E. (2004). *Maternity & women's health care* (8th ed.). St. Louis: Mosby, Inc.

Mahan, L. K., & Escott-Stump, S. (2004). *Krause's food, nutrition, & diet therapy* (11th ed.). Philadelphia: W. B. Saunders.

March of Dimes (2004). The joy of sex during pregnancy. [Online] Available at: http://www.marchofdimes.com/printableArticles/159_516.asp?printable=true

March of Dimes. (2005). Childbirth educational classes. [Online] Available at: http://www.marchofdimes.com/pnhec/159_12929.asp

March of Dimes Foundation (2004). *Prematurity: the answers can't come soon enough.* [Online] Available at: http://www.marchofdimes.com/prematurity

Marchiano, D., & Ural, S. R. (2004). Prenatal nutrition. *eMedicine* [Online] Available at: http://www.emedicine.com/med/topic3234.htm

Matteson, P. S. (2001). *Women's health during the childbearing years: a community-based approach.* St. Louis: Mosby.

Mattson, S., & Smith, J. E. (2004). *Core curriculum for maternal-newborn nursing* (3rd ed.). St. Louis: Elsevier Saunders.

McKinney, E. S., James, S. R., Murray, S. S., & Ashwill, J. W. (2005). *Maternal-child nursing* (2nd ed.). St. Louis: Elsevier Saunders.

Miller, S. M., & Isabel, J. M. (2002). *Prenatal screening tests facilitate risk assessment* [Online] Available at: www.mlo-online.com

Monti, D. (2004). Nutrition news: "I'm craving dirt . . . I must be going crazy!" *International Journal of Childbirth Education, 19*(1), 8–9.

Monti, D., & Kehler, L. (2001). The vegetarian alternative. *International Journal of Childbirth Education, 16*(3), 8–9.

Moore, M. L., & Moos, M. K. (2003). *Cultural competence in the care of childbearing families.* March of Dimes Nursing Module. White Plains, NY: Education Services, March of Dimes.

Moos, M. K. (2003a). Preconception care. *JOGNN, 32*(4), 514–515.

Moos, M. K. (2003b). Preconception wellness as a routine objective for women's health care: an integrative strategy. *JOGNN, 32*(4), 550–556.

Murray, S. S., & McKinney, E. S. (2006). *Foundations of maternal-newborn nursing* (3rd ed.). Philadelphia: W. B. Saunders.

National Academy of Sciences (2002). *Dietary reference intakes for energy, carbohydrates, fiber, fat, protein and amino acids (macronutrients).* Washington, D.C.: National Academies Press, pp. 5–64.

Nolan, M. (2003). Effects of antenatal exercise on psychological well-being, pregnancy and birth outcome. *Journal of Advanced Nursing, 41*(6), 623.

Olds, S. B., London, M. L., Ladewig, P. A. W., & Davidson, M. R. (2004). *Maternal-newborn nursing & women's health care* (7th ed.). Upper Saddle River, NJ: Pearson Prentice Hall.

Opipari, A. W., & Johnson, T. R. B. (2000). Fetal assessment. In S. B. Ransom, M. P. Dombrowski, S. G. McNeeley, et al. (Eds.), *Practical strategies in obstetrics and gynecology* (pp. 224–233). Philadelphia: W. B. Saunders.

O'Toole, M. T. (2003). *Encyclopedia & dictionary of medicine, nursing & allied health* (7th ed.). Philadelphia: Saunders.

Schnirring, L. (2002). New ACOG recommendations encourage exercise in pregnancy. *Physician & Sportsmedicine, 30*(8), 9–10.

Simpson, J. (2002). Genetic counseling and prenatal diagnosis. In S. Gabbe, J. Niebyl, & J. Simpson (Eds.), *Obstetrics: normal and problem pregnancies* (4th ed.). New York: Churchill Livingstone.

Sloan, E. (2002). *Biology of women* (4th ed.). New York: Delmar.

Smith, L. (2002). The pregnant trauma patient. In K. A. McQuillan, K. T. Von Rueden, R. L. Hartsock, et al. (Eds.), *Trauma nursing: from resuscitation through rehabilitation* (3rd ed., pp. 718–746). Philadelphia: Saunders.

Sur, D. K., Wallis, D. H., & O'Connell, T. X. (2003). Vaccinations in pregnancy. *American Family Physician, 68*(2), 299–309.

Tillett, J., Kostich, L. M., & VandeVusse, L. (2003). Use of over-the-counter medications during pregnancy. *Journal of Perinatal and Neonatal Nursing, 17*(1), 3–18.

Tiran, D. (2003). Self-help for constipation and hemorrhoids in pregnancy. *British Journal of Midwifery, 11*(9), 579–581.

Trupin, S. R. (2004). Common pregnancy complaints and questions. *eMedicine* [Online] Available at: http://emedicine.com/med/topic3238.htm

Tucker, S. (2000). *Pocket guide to fetal monitoring and assessment* (4th ed.). St. Louis: Mosby.

U.S. Department of Health and Human Services (2000). *Healthy people 2010.* Washington, D.C.: US Department of Health and Human Services.

VanderLaan, J. (2004). Pelvic rocking. *Birthing Naturally* [Online] Available at: http://www.birthingnaturally.net/exercise/preg/pelvicrock.html

Wald, N. J., Huttly, W. J., & Hackshaw, A. K. (2003). Antenatal screening for Down's syndrome with the quadruple test. *Lancet, 361*(9360), 835–837.

Walling, A. D. (2004). Effects of automobile crashes occurring during pregnancy. *American Family Physician, 69*(5), 1281–1283.

Walsh, L. (2001). *Midwifery: community-based care during the childbearing year.* Philadelphia: W. B. Saunders.

Wener, M. E., & Lavigne, S. E. (2004). Can periodontal disease lead to premature delivery? *AWHONN Lifelines, 8*(5), 422–432.

Wilkins, E. M. (2004). *Clinical practice of the dental hygienist* (9th ed.). Baltimore: Lippincott Williams & Wilkins.

Wong, D. L., Perry, S. E., & Hockenberry, M. J. (2002). *Maternal child nursing care* (2nd ed.). St. Louis: Mosby.

Woo, J. (2004). Obstetric ultrasound: a comprehensive guide to ultrasounds in pregnancy. [Online] Available at: http://www.ob-ultrasound.net

Youngkin, E. Q., & Davis, M. S. (2004). *Women's health: a primary care clinical guide* (3rd ed.). New Jersey: Prentice Hall.

Web Resources

American Academy of Husband-Coached Childbirth: **www.bradleybirth.com**

American College of Nurse Midwives: (202) 347-5445, **www.acnm.org**

American College of Obstetricians and Gynecologists (ACOG): **www.acog.com**

Association of Women's Health, Obstetrics & Neonatal Nurses: **www.awhonn.org**

Dietary Guidelines for Americans: **http://www.nal.usda.gov/fnic/dga**

Doulas of North America (DONA): (206) 324-5440, **www.dona.com**

International Childbirth Education Association: **www.icea.org**

International Lactation Consultation Association (ILCA): **www.ilca.org**

LaLeche League International: (800) 525-3243, **www.lalacheleague.org**

Lamaze International: (800) 368-4404, **www.lamaze-childbirth.com**

March of Dimes: **www.modimes.org**

Mayo Clinic Pregnancy Center: **www.mayoclinic.org**

National Center for Education in Maternal and Child Health: **www.ncemch.org**

Nutrition during Pregnancy and Breastfeeding: **www.nal.usda.gov/fnic/pubs/topics/pregnancy/precom.html**

Prepared Childbirth Education: **www.childbirtheducation.org**

Special Supplemental Nutrition Program for Women, Infants, and Children (WIC): **www.usda.gov/fns/wic.html**

Vegan Diet during Pregnancy: **www.vrg.org/nutrition/veganpregnancy.htm**

Weight Gain during Pregnancy: **www.marchofdimes.com/pnhec/159_153.asp**

ChapterWORKSHEET

● MULTIPLE CHOICE QUESTIONS

1. When teaching a pregnant woman about nutrition, the nurse would urge her to ingest foods containing which vitamin to prevent the risk of neural tube defects (NTDs)?

   a. Folic acid

   b. Vitamin A

   c. Vitamin C

   d. Vitamin K

2. The nurse teaches the pregnant client how to perform Kegel exercises as a way to accomplish which of the following?

   a. Prevent perineal lacerations

   b. Stimulate postdates labor

   c. Increase pelvic muscle tone

   d. Lose pregnancy weight quickly

3. During a clinic visit, a pregnant client at 30 weeks' gestation states, "I've had some mild contractions, I think. They come and go pretty irregularly. They feel similar to a menstrual cramp. What does this mean?" The nurse responds to the client based on the interpretation that which of the following is occurring?

   a. The contractions that the client is feeling suggest that she is experiencing the beginning of labor in the very early stages.

   b. These contractions are an ominous finding that indicate that the client is about to abort the fetus.

   c. The contractions are related to overhydration in the client.

   d. These are Braxton Hicks contractions. They occur throughout pregnancy but aren't usually felt until the third trimester.

4. The nurse teaches a pregnant woman about exercise and activity, including activities not recommended during pregnancy. The nurse determines that the teaching was effective when the pregnant woman states which of the following activities is not recommended during pregnancy?

   a. Swimming

   b. Walking

   c. Scuba diving

   d. Bike riding

5. A pregnant client's last normal menstrual period was on August 10. Using Nagele's rule, the nurse calculates that her estimated date of birth (EDB) will be which of the following?

   a. June 23

   b. July 10

   c. July 30

   d. May 17

● CRITICAL THINKING EXERCISES

1. Mary Jones comes to the Women's Health Center where you work as a nurse.

   She is in her first trimester of pregnancy and tells you her main complaint is extreme fatigue, to the point that she wants to sleep most of the time. She appears pale and tired. Her mucous membranes are pale. She reports that she gets 8 to 9 hours of sleep each night but still can't seem to stay awake and alert at work. She reports that she doesn't eat like she should because she doesn't have time. Her hemoglobin and hematocrit are abnormally low.

   a. What subjective and objective data do you have to make your assessment?

   b. What is your impression of this woman?

   c. What nursing interventions would be appropriate for this client?

   d. How will you evaluate the effectiveness of your interventions?

2. Monica, a 16-year-old African-American high school student, is here for her first prenatal visit. Her last normal menstrual period was 2 months ago, and she states she has been "sick ever since." She is 5-foot-6 tall and weighs 110 pounds. In completing her dietary assessment, the nurse asks about her intake of milk and dairy products. Monica reports that she doesn't like "that stuff" and doesn't want to put on too much weight because it "might ruin my figure."

   a. In addition to the routine obstetric assessments, which additional ones might be warranted for this teenager?

   b. What dietary instruction should be provided to this teenager based on her history?

   c. What follow-up monitoring should be included in subsequent prenatal visits?

3. Maria, a 27-year-old Hispanic woman in her last trimester of pregnancy (34 weeks), complains to the clinic nurse that she is constipated and feels miserable most of the time. She reports that she has started taking laxatives, but mostly they don't help her. When questioned about her dietary habits, she replies that she eats beans and rice and drinks tea with most meals. She says she has tried to limit her fluid intake so she doesn't have to go to the bathroom so much, because she doesn't want to miss any of her daytime soap operas on television.

a. What additional information would the nurse need to assess her complaint?

b. What interventions would be appropriate for Maria?

c. What adaptations will Maria need to make to alleviate her constipation?

● **STUDY ACTIVITIES**

1. Visit a freestanding birth center and compare it to a traditional hospital setting in terms of restrictions, type of pain management available, and costs.

2. Arrange to shadow a nurse-midwife for a day to see her role in working with the childbearing family.

3. Select two of the websites supplied at the end of this chapter and note their target audience, the validity of information offered, and their appeal to expectant couples. Present your findings.

4. Request permission to attend a childbirth education class in your local area and help a woman without a partner practice the paced breathing exercise. Present the information you learned and how you can apply it while taking care of a woman during labor.

5. A laywoman with a specialized education and experience in assisting women during labor is a

_____.

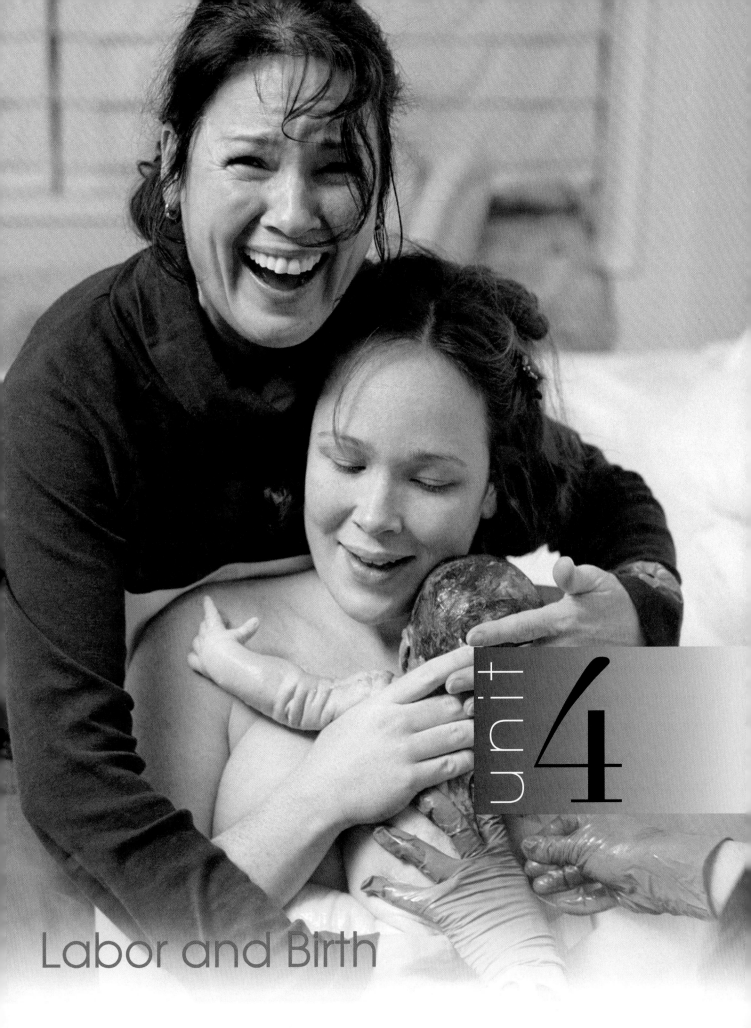

Labor and Birth

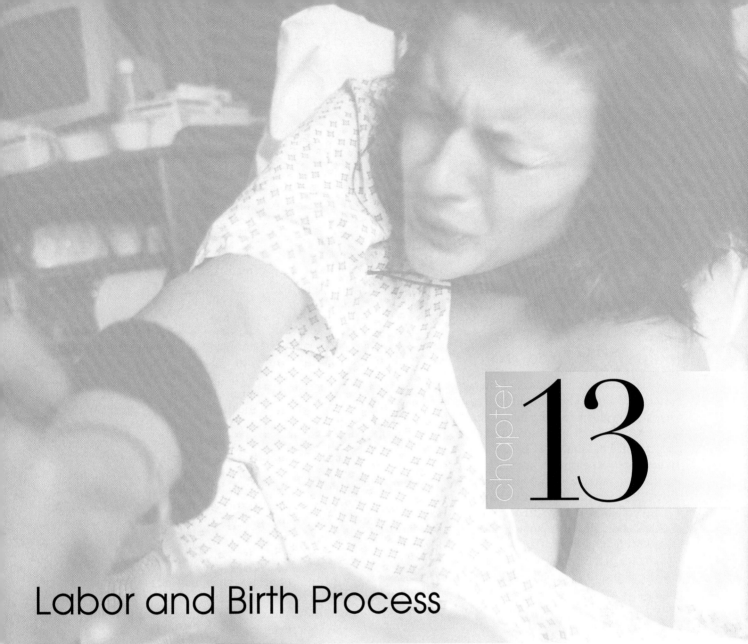

chapter **13**

Labor and Birth Process

KeyTERMS

attitude
dilation
doula
duration
effacement
engagement
frequency
intensity
lie
lightening
molding
position
presentation
station

LearningOBJECTIVES

After studying the chapter content, the student should be able to accomplish the following:

1. Outline premonitory signs of labor.
2. Compare and contrast true versus false labor.
3. Discuss the critical factors affecting labor and birth.
4. List the cardinal movements of labor.
5. Identify the maternal and fetal responses to labor and birth.
6. Describe the stages of labor and the critical events occurring during each stage.
7. Recognize the normal physiologic/psychological changes occurring during all four stages of labor.
8. Describe the concept of pain as it relates to the woman in labor.

The process of labor and birth involves more than the delivery of a newborn. Numerous physiologic and psychological events occur that ultimately result in the birth of a newborn and the creation or expansion of the family.

This chapter describes labor and birth as a process. It addresses the premonitory signs of labor, including true and false labor, critical factors affecting labor and birth, maternal and fetal response to the laboring process, and the four stages of labor. The chapter also identifies specific criteria related to each stage of labor.

Initiation of Labor

Labor is a complex, multifaceted interaction between the mother and fetus. Thus, it is difficult to determine exactly why labor begins and what initiates it. Although several theories have been proposed to explain the onset and maintenance of labor, it is widely believed that labor is influenced by a combination of factors, including uterine stretch, progesterone withdrawal, increased oxytocin sensitivity, and increased release of prostaglandins.

Several theories have been advanced to explain what initiates labor. However, none of these have been proved scientifically. One theory suggests that labor is initiated by a change in the estrogen-to-progesterone ratio. During the last trimester of pregnancy, estrogen levels increase and progesterone levels decrease. This change leads to an increase in the number of myometrium gap junctions. Gap junctions are proteins that connect cell membranes and facilitate coordination of uterine contractions and myometrial stretching (Gilbert & Harmon, 2003).

Prostaglandin levels increase late during pregnancy secondary to elevated estrogen levels. Prostaglandins stimulate smooth muscle contraction of the uterus. An increase in prostaglandins leads to myometrial contractions and to a reduction in cervical resistance. Subsequently, the cervix softens, thins out, and dilates during labor.

Although physiologic evidence for the role of oxytocin in the initiation of labor is inconclusive, the number of oxytocin receptors in the uterus increases at the end of pregnancy. This creates an increased sensitivity to oxytocin. Estrogen, the levels of which are also rising, increases myometrial sensitivity to oxytocin. With the increasing levels of oxytocin in the maternal blood in conjunction with fetal production, initiation of uterine contractions can occur. Oxytocin also aids in stimulating prostaglandin synthesis through receptors in the decidua. Prostaglandins lead to additional contractions, cervical softening, gap junction induction, and myometrial sensitization, thereby leading to a progressive cervical dilation (Blackburn & Loper, 2003).

Premonitory Signs of Labor

Before the onset of labor, a pregnant woman's body undergoes several changes in preparation for the birth of the newborn. The changes that occur often lead to characteristic signs and symptoms that suggest that labor is near. These premonitory signs and symptoms can vary, and not every woman experiences every one of these signs and symptoms.

Cervical Changes

Before labor begins, cervical softening and possible cervical **dilation** with descent of the presenting part into the pelvis occurs. This stage can begin 1 month to 1 hour before actual labor begins.

As the time for labor approaches, the cervix changes from an elongated structure to a shortened, thinned segment. Cervical collagen fibers undergo enzymatic rearrangement into smaller, more flexible fibers that facilitate water absorption, leading to a softer, more stretchable cervix. These changes occur secondary to the effects of prostaglandins and pressure from Braxton Hicks contractions (Burst et al., 2004).

Lightening

Lightening occurs when the fetal presenting part begins to descend into the maternal pelvis. The uterus lowers and moves into a more anterior position. The shape of the abdomen changes as a result of the change in the uterus. With this descent, the woman usually notes that her breathing is much easier. However, she may complain of increased pelvic pressure, cramping, and low back pain. She also may note edema of the lower extremities as a result of the increased stasis of blood pooling, an increase in vaginal discharge, and more frequent urination. In primiparas, lightening can occur 2 weeks or more before labor begins, and among multiparas it may be as late as during labor (Youngkin & Davis, 2004).

Increased Energy Level

Some women report a sudden increase in energy before labor. This is sometimes referred to as *nesting*, because many women will focus this energy toward childbirth preparation by cleaning, cooking, preparing the nursery, and spending extra time with other children in the household. The increased energy level usually occurs 24 to 48 hours before the onset of labor. It is thought to be the result of an increase in epinephrine release caused by a decrease in progesterone (Mattson & Smith, 2004).

Bloody Show

At the onset of labor, the mucous plug that fills the cervical canal during pregnancy is expelled as a result of cervical softening and increased pressure of the presenting part. The exposed cervical capillaries release a small amount of blood that mixes with mucus, resulting in pink-tinged secretions known as *bloody show*.

Braxton Hicks Contractions

Braxton Hicks contractions, which the woman may have been experiencing throughout the pregnancy, may become stronger and increase in **frequency.** These contractions aid in moving the cervix from a posterior position to an anterior position. They also help in ripening and softening the cervix. However, the contractions are irregular and diminish by walking, voiding, eating, increasing fluid intake, or changing position.

Braxton Hicks contractions are typically felt as a tightening or pulling sensation of the top of the uterus. They occur primarily in the abdomen and groin areas and gradually spread downward before relaxing. In contrast, true labor contractions are more commonly felt in the lower back.

Braxton Hicks contractions will usually last about 30 seconds but can persist for as long as 2 minutes. As birth draws near and the uterus becomes more sensitive to oxytocin, the frequency and **intensity** of these contractions increase. However, if the contractions last more than 30 seconds and occur more than four to six times an hour, the woman should contact her healthcare provider so that she can be evaluated for possible preterm labor, especially if she is less than 35 weeks pregnant.

Spontaneous Rupture of Membranes

One in four women will experience spontaneous rupture of the membranes before the onset of labor (Engstrom, 2004). The rupture of membranes can result in either a sudden gush or a steady leakage of amniotic fluid. Although much of the amniotic fluid is lost when the rupture occurs, a continuous supply is produced to ensure protection of the fetus until birth.

After the amniotic sac has ruptured, the barrier to infection is gone and an ascending infection is possible. In addition, there is danger of cord prolapse if **engagement** has not occurred with the sudden release of fluid and pressure with rupture. With these potential complications, women are advised to notify their healthcare provider and go in for an evaluation.

True Versus False Labor

False labor is a condition occurring during the latter weeks of some pregnancies in which irregular uterine contractions are felt, but the cervix is not affected. In contrast, true labor is characterized by contractions occurring at regular intervals that increase in frequency, **duration,** and intensity. True labor contractions bring about progressive cervical dilation and **effacement.** Table 13-1 summarizes the differences between true and false labor. False labor, prodromal labor, and Braxton Hicks contractions are all names for contractions that do not contribute in a measurable way toward the delivery goal.

Many women fear being sent home from the hospital with "false labor." All women feel anxious when they feel contractions, but should be informed that labor could be a long process, especially if it is their first pregnancy. With

Table 13-1 Differences between True and False Labor

Parameters	True Labor	False Labor
Contraction timing	Regular, becoming closer together, usually 4–6 minutes apart, lasting 30–60 seconds	Irregular, not occurring close together
Contraction strength	Become stronger with time, vaginal pressure is usually felt	Frequently weak, not getting stronger with time or alternating (a strong one followed by weaker ones)
Contraction discomfort	Starts in the back and radiates around toward the front of the abdomen	Usually felt in the front of the abdomen
Position changes	Contractions continue no matter what positional change is made	Contractions may stop or slow down with walking or making a position change
Stay or go?	Staying home until contractions are 5 minutes apart, lasting 45–60 seconds, and strong enough so that a conversation during one is not possible—go to hospital	Drinking fluids and walking to assess if there is any change; if diminish—stay home

Sources: Leonard (2002), Mattson & Smith (2004), Condon (2004); Breslin & Lucas (2003).

first pregnancies, the cervix can take up to 20 hours to dilate completely (Lowdermilk & Perry, 2004).

Factors Affecting the Labor Process

In many references, the critical factors that affect the process of labor and birth are outlined as the five Ps:

1. Passageway (birth canal)
2. Passenger (fetus and placenta)
3. Powers (contractions)
4. Position (maternal)
5. Psychological response

These critical factors are commonly accepted and discussed by health care professionals. However, there may be five additional factors that affect the labor process as well:

1. Philosophy (low tech, high touch)
2. Partners (support caregivers)
3. Patience (natural timing)
4. Patient preparation (childbirth knowledge base)
5. Pain control (comfort measures)

These five additional "Ps" are helpful in planning care for the laboring family. These patient-focused factors are an attempt to foster labor that can be managed through the use of high touch, patience, support, knowledge, and pain management.

Passageway

The birth passageway is the route through which the fetus must travel to be delivered vaginally. The passageway consists of the maternal pelvis and soft tissues. Of the two, however, the maternal bony pelvis is more important because it is relatively unyielding (except for the coccyx).

Typically the pelvis is assessed during the first trimester, often at the first visit to the healthcare provider, to identify any abnormalities or barriers that might hinder a successful vaginal delivery. As the pregnancy progresses, the hormones relaxin and estrogen cause the connective tissues to become more relaxed and elastic, and cause the joints to become more flexible to prepare the mother's pelvis for birth. Additionally, the soft tissues usually yield to the forces of labor.

Bony Pelvis

The maternal bony pelvis can be divided into the *true* and *false* portions. The false (or greater) pelvis is composed of the upper flared parts of the two iliac bones with their concavities and the wings of the base of the sacrum. The false pelvis is divided from the true pelvis by an imaginary line drawn from the sacral prominence at the back to the superior aspect of the symphysis pubis at the front of the pelvis. This imaginary line is called the *linea terminalis*. The false pelvis lies above this imaginary line; the true pelvis lies below it (Fig. 13-1).

The true pelvis is the bony passageway through which the fetus must travel. It is made up of three planes: the inlet, the mid pelvis (cavity), and the outlet.

Pelvic Inlet

The pelvic inlet allows entrance to the true pelvis. It is bounded by the sacral prominence in the back, the ileum on the sides, and the superior aspect of the symphysis pubis in the front (Pillitteri, 2003). The pelvis inlet is heart shaped and is wider in the transverse aspect (sideways) than it is from front to back.

Mid Pelvis

The mid pelvis (cavity) occupies the space between the inlet and outlet. It is through this snug, curved-shaped space that the fetus must navigate to reach the outside.

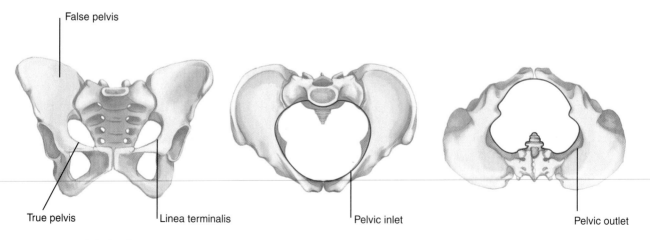

False pelvis

True pelvis   Linea terminalis   Pelvic inlet   Pelvic outlet

Anterior view   Superior view   Inferior view

● Figure 13-1 The bony pelvis.

As the fetus passes through this small area, its chest is compressed, causing lung fluid and mucus to be expelled. This expulsion removes the space-occupying fluid so that air can enter the lungs with the newborn's first breath.

Pelvic Outlet

The pelvic outlet is bound by the ischial tuberosities, the lower rim of the symphysis pubis, and the tip of the coccyx. In comparison with the pelvic inlet, the outlet is wider from front to back. For the fetus to pass through the pelvis, the outlet must be of adequate size.

To ensure the adequacy of the pelvic outlet for vaginal delivery, the following pelvic measurements are assessed:

- Diagonal conjugate of the inlet (distance between the anterior surface of the sacral prominence and the anterior surface of the inferior margin of the symphysis pubis)
- Transverse or ischial tuberosity diameter of the outlet (distance at the medial and lowermost aspect of the ischial tuberosities, at the level of the anus; a known hand span or clenched-fist measurement is generally used to obtain this measurement)
- True or obstetric conjugate (distance estimated from the measurement of the diagonal conjugate; 1.5 cm is subtracted from the diagonal conjugate measurement. For more information about pelvic measurements, see Chapter 12.)

If the diagonal conjugate measures at least 11.5 cm, and the true or obstetric conjugate measures 10 cm or more (1.5 cm less than the diagonal conjugate, or about 10 cm), then the pelvis is adequate for a vaginal birth of what would be considered a normal-size newborn.

Pelvic Shape

In addition to size, the shape of a woman's pelvis is a determining factor for a vaginal delivery. The pelvis is divided into four main shapes: anthropoid, android, gynecoid, and the platypelloid (refer back to Fig. 12-6).

The anthropoid pelvis is common in men and occurs in 20 to 30% of women (Sloane, 2002). The pelvic inlet is oval and the sacrum is long, producing a deep pelvis. This pelvic shape is usually favorable for a vaginal delivery.

The android pelvis is also common in men and occurs in approximately 20% of women. It has a heart-shaped inlet with narrow side walls. This pelvic type is also called a *funnel pelvis*, and it produces difficulty in vaginal delivery. Descent of the fetal head into the pelvis is slow, and failure of the fetus to rotate is common. Labor prognosis is poor.

The gynecoid pelvis is less common in men and is considered the true female pelvis, although only about half of all women have this type (Sloane, 2002). Vaginal birth is most favorable with this type of pelvis because the inlet is round and the outlet is roomy. This shape offers the optimal diameters in all three planes of the pelvis.

The platypelloid or flat pelvis is the least common type of pelvic structure among men and women, with an approximate incidence of 5% (Mattson & Smith, 2004). The pelvic cavity is shallow, but widens at the pelvic outlet, making it difficult for the fetus to descend through the mid pelvis. It is not favorable for a vaginal birth unless the fetal head can pass through the inlet. Women with this type of pelvis usually require cesarean delivery.

Many women have a combination of these four basic pelvis types with no two pelves being exactly the same. An important principle is that most pelves are not purely defined, but occur in nature as mixed types. Regardless of the shape, the newborn will be born if size and positioning remain compatible. The narrowest part of the fetus attempts to align itself with the narrowest pelvic dimension (e.g., biparietal to interspinous diameters, which means the fetus generally tends to rotate to the most ample portion of the pelvis).

Soft Tissues

The soft tissues of the passageway consist of the cervix, the pelvic floor muscles, and the vagina. The cervix effaces (thins) and dilates (opens) to allow the presenting fetal part to descend into the vagina, similar to pulling a turtleneck sweater over your head. The pelvic floor muscles help the fetus to rotate anteriorly as it passes through the birth canal. The soft tissues of the vagina expand to accommodate the fetus during birth.

Passenger

The fetus (with placenta) is the passenger. The fetal skull (size and presence of **molding**), fetal **attitude** (degree of body flexion), fetal **lie** (relationship of body parts), fetal **presentation** (first body part), fetal **position** (relationship to maternal pelvis), fetal **station,** and fetal engagement are all important factors that have an affect on the ultimate outcome in the birthing process.

Fetal Skull

The fetal head is the largest and least compressible fetal structure, making it an important factor in relation to labor and birth. Considerable variation in the size and diameter of the fetal skull is often seen. Some diameters shorten whereas others lengthen as the head is molded during the labor and birthing process.

Compared with an adult, the fetal head is large in proportion to the rest of the body, usually about one quarter of the body surface area (Hait, 2002). The bones that make up the face and cranial base are fused and essentially fixed. However, the bones that make up the rest of the cranium (two frontal bones, two parietal bones, and the occipital bone) are not fused; rather, they are soft and pliable with gaps between the plates of bone. These gaps, which are membranous spaces between the cranial bones, are called *sutures*, and the intersections of these sutures are called *fontanelles*. Sutures are important because they allow the cranial bones to overlap in order for the head to adjust in shape (elongate) when pressure is exerted on it by uterine contractions or the maternal bony pelvis. (These sutures close as the bones grow and the brain reaches its full growth.)

The changed shape of the fetal skull as a result of overlapping of the cranial bones is known as *molding.* This malleability of the fetal skull may decrease fetal skull dimensions by 0.5 to 1 cm (Mattson & Smith, 2004).

Along with molding, fluid can also collect in the scalp (caput succedaneum) or blood can collect beneath the scalp (cephalohematoma), further distorting the shape and appearance of the fetal head. Parents may become concerned about this distortion. However, reassurance that the oblong shape is only temporary is usually all that is needed to reduce their anxiety.

Sutures also play a role in helping to identify the position of the fetal head during a vaginal exam. See Figure 13-2 for a view of a fetal skull.

The *coronal sutures* are located between the frontal and parietal bones, and extend transversely on both sides of the anterior fontanelles. The *frontal suture* is located between the two frontal bones. The *lambdoidal sutures* are located between the occipital bone and the two parietals, extending transversely on either side of the posterior fontanelles. The *sagittal suture* is located between the parietal bones and divides the skull into the right and left halves. During a pelvic examination, palpation of these sutures by the examiner reveals the position of the fetal head and the degree of rotation that has occurred.

The anterior and posterior fontanelles, also useful in helping to identify the position of the fetal head, allow for molding. In addition, the fontanelles are important when evaluating the newborn. The anterior fontanelle is the famous "soft spot" of the newborn's head. It is diamond shaped and measures about 2 to 3 cm. It remains open for 12 to 18 months after birth to allow for growth of the brain (Ladewig et al., 2006). The posterior fontanelle corresponds to the anterior one but is located at the back of the

fetal head and is triangular in shape. This one closes within 8 to 12 weeks after birth and measures, on average, 0.5 to 1 cm at its widest diameter (Mattson & Smith, 2004).

The diameter of the fetal skull is an important consideration during the labor and birth process. Fetal skull diameters are measured between the various landmarks of the skull. Diameters include occipitofrontal, occipitomental, suboccipitobregmatic, and biparietal (Fig. 13-3). The two most important diameters that can affect the birth process are the suboccipitobregmatic (approximately 9.5 cm at term) and the biparietal (approximately 9.25 cm at term) diameters. The suboccipitobregmatic diameter, measured from the base of the occiput to the center of the anterior fontanelle, identifies the smallest anteroposterior diameter of the fetal skull. The biparietal diameter measures the largest transverse diameter of the fetal skull: the distance between the two parietal bones. In a cephalic (head-first) presentation, which occurs in 95% of all term births, if the fetus presents in a flexed position in which the chin is resting on the chest, the optimal or smallest fetal skull dimensions for a vaginal birth are demonstrated. If the fetal head is not fully flexed at birth, the anteroposterior diameter increases. This increase in dimension might prevent the fetal skull from entering the maternal pelvis.

Fetal Attitude

Fetal attitude is another important consideration related to the passenger. Fetal attitude refers to the posturing (flexion or extension) of the joints and the relationship of fetal parts to one another. The most common fetal attitude when labor begins is with all joints flexed—the fetal back is rounded, the chin is on the chest, the thighs are flexed on the abdomen, and the legs are flexed at the knees (Fig. 13-4). This normal fetal position is most favorable for vaginal birth, presenting the smallest fetal skull diameters to the pelvis.

When the fetus presents to the pelvis with abnormal attitudes (no flexion or extension), the diameter can increase the diameter of the presenting part as it

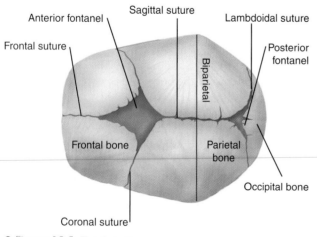

● Figure 13-2 Fetal skull.

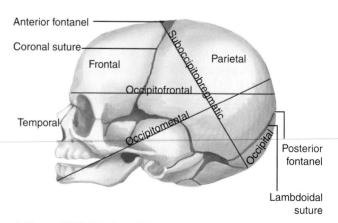

● Figure 13-3 Fetal skull diameters.

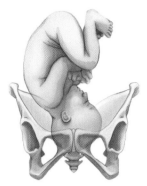

● Figure 13-4 Fetal attitude: Full flexion. Note that the smallest diameter presents to the pelvis.

passes through the pelvis, increasing the difficulty of birth. Extension tends to present larger fetal skull diameters, which may make birth difficult.

Fetal Lie

Fetal lie refers to the relationship of the long axis (spine) of the fetus to the long axis (spine) of the mother. There are two primary lies: longitudinal (which is the most common) and transverse (Fig. 13-5).

A longitudinal lie occurs when the long axis of the fetus is parallel to that of the mother (fetal spine to maternal spine side-by-side). A transverse lie occurs when the long axis of the fetus is perpendicular to the long axis of

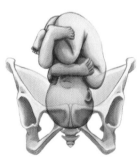

A. Longitudinal lie

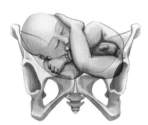

B. Transverse lie

● Figure 13-5 Fetal lie.
(**A**) Longitudinal lie.
(**B**) Transverse lie.

the mother (fetus spine lies across the maternal abdomen and crosses her spine). A fetus in a transverse lie position cannot be delivered vaginally (Wong et al., 2002).

Fetal Presentation

Fetal presentation refers to the body part of the fetus that enters the pelvic inlet first (the "presenting part"). This is the fetal part that lies over the inlet of the pelvis or the cervical os. Knowing which fetal part is coming first with birth is critical for planning and initiating appropriate interventions.

The three main fetal presentations are cephalic (head first), breech (pelvis first), and shoulder (scapula first). The majority of term newborns (95%) enter into this world in a cephalic presentation; breech presentation accounts for 3% of term births, whereas shoulder presentations account for approximately 2% of term births (Mattson & Smith, 2004).

In a *cephalic presentation,* the presenting part is usually the occiput portion of the fetal head. This would be the portion of the head that is covered by wearing a beanie cap (Fig. 13-6). This presentation is also referred to as a *vertex presentation.* Variations in a vertex presentation include the military, brow, and face presentations.

The *breech presentation* occurs when the fetal buttocks or feet enter the maternal pelvis first and the fetal skull enters last. This abnormal presentation poses several challenges at birth. Primarily, the largest part of the fetus (skull) is born last and may become "hung up" in the pelvis. In addition, the umbilical cord can become compressed between the fetal skull and the maternal pelvis after the fetal chest is born because the head is the last to exit. Moreover, unlike the hard fetal skull, the buttocks are soft and are not as effective as a cervical dilator when compared with a cephalic presentation. Also, there is the possibility of trauma to the after-coming head as a result of the lack of opportunity for molding.

The types of breech presentations are determined by the positioning of the fetal legs (Fig. 13-7). In a frank breech (50–70%), the buttocks present first with both legs extended up toward the face, similar to a pike position. In a full or complete breech (5–10%), the fetus sits crossed-legged above the cervix similar to a cannonball position. In a footling or incomplete breech (10–30%), one or both legs are presenting. Breech presentations are associated with prematurity, placenta previa, multiparity, uterine abnormalities (fibroids), and some congenital anomalies such as hydrocephaly (Fischer, 2004).

A shoulder presentation occurs when the fetal shoulders present first, with the head tucked inside. Odds of a shoulder presentation are one in 1,000 (Cunningham et al., 2005). The fetus is in a transverse lie with the shoulder as the presenting part (denominator is scapula). Conditions associated with shoulder presentation including placenta previa, multiple gestation, or fetal anomalies. A cesarean birth is typically necessary (McKinney et al., 2005).

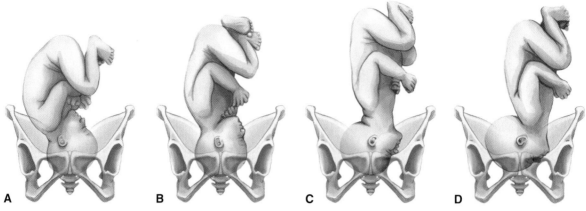

● Figure 13-6 Fetal presentation: cephalic presentations (**A**) Vertex. (**B**) Military. (**C**) Brow. (**D**) Face.

Fetal Position

Fetal position describes the relationship of a given point on the presenting part of the fetus to a designated point of the maternal pelvis (O'Toole, 2003). The landmark fetal presenting parts include the occipital bone (O), which designates a vertex presentation; the chin (mentum [M]), which designates a face presentation; the buttocks (sacrum [S]), which designate a breech presentation; and the scapula (acromion process [A]), which designates a shoulder presentation.

In addition, the maternal pelvis is divided into four quadrants: right anterior, left anterior, right posterior, and left posterior. These quadrants designate whether the presenting part is directed toward the front, back, left, or right of the pelvis. Fetal position is determined first by identifying the presenting part and then the maternal quadrant the presenting part is facing. Position is indicated by a three-letter abbreviation as follows:

- The first letter defines whether the presenting part is tilted toward the left (L) or the right (R) side of the maternal pelvis.
- The second letter represents the particular presenting part of the fetus: O for occiput, S for sacrum (buttocks), M for mentum (chin), A for acromion process, and D for dorsal (refers to the fetal back) when denoting the fetal position in shoulder presentations (Olds et al., 2004).
- The third letter defines the location of the presenting part in relation to the anterior (A) portion of the maternal pelvis or the posterior (P) portion of the maternal pelvis. If the presenting part is directed to the side of the maternal pelvis, the fetal presentation is designated as transverse (T).

For example, if the occiput is facing the left anterior quadrant of the pelvis, then the position is termed left occipitoanterior and is recorded as LOA. LOA is the most common fetal position for birthing today, followed by

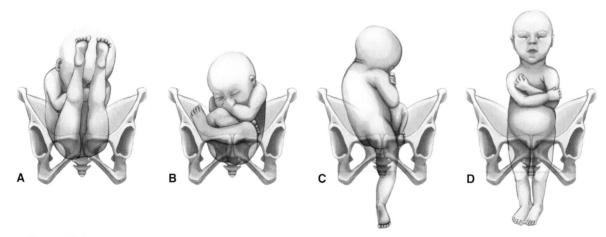

● Figure 13-7 Breech presentations. (**A**) Frank breech. (**B**) Complete breech. (**C**) Single footling breech. (**D**) Double footling breech.

right occipitoanterior (ROA). See Box 13-1 for a list of the various fetal positions.

Fetal Station

Station refers to the relationship of the presenting part to the level of the maternal pelvic ischial spines. Fetal station is measured in centimeters and is referred to as a minus or plus, depending on its location above or below the ischial spines. Typically, the ischial spines are the most narrow part of the pelvis and are the natural measuring point for the delivery progress.

Zero (0) station is designated when the presenting part is at the level of the maternal ischial spines. When the presenting part is above the ischial spines, the distance is recorded as minus stations. When the presenting part is below the ischial spines, the distance is recorded as plus stations. For instance, if the presenting part is above the ischial spines by 1 cm, it is documented as being a −1 station; if the presenting part is below the ischial spines by 1 cm, it is documented as being a +1 station. An easy way to understand this concept is to think in terms of meeting the goal, which is the birth. If the

fetus is descending downward (past the ischial spines) and moving toward meeting the goal of birth, then the station is positive and the centimeter numbers grow bigger from +1 to +5. If the fetus is not descending past the ischial spines, then the station is negative and the centimeter numbers grow bigger from −1 to −5. The farther away the presenting part from the outside, the larger the negative number (−5 cm). The closer the presenting part to the outside, the larger the positive number (+5 cm). See Figure 13-8 for stations of presenting part.

Fetal Engagement

Along with station, which measures the degree of fetal presenting part descent, engagement occurs also. Engagement is determined by pelvic examination and it signifies the entrance of the largest diameter of the fetal presenting part (usually the fetal head) into the smallest diameter of the maternal pelvis (O'Toole, 2003). The fetus is said to be "engaged" in the pelvis when the presenting part reaches 0 station. Engagement is determined by vaginal examination.

The largest diameter of the fetal head is the biparietal diameter. It extends from one parietal prominence to the other. It is an important factor in the navigation through the maternal pelvis. Engagement typically occurs in primigravidas 2 weeks before term, whereas multiparas may experience engagement several weeks before the onset of labor or not until labor begins. The term *floating* is used when engagement has not occurred, because the presenting part is freely movable above the pelvic inlet.

Cardinal Movements of Labor

The fetus goes through many positional changes as it navigates through the passageway. These positional changes are known as *cardinal movements of labor.* They are deliberate, specific, and very precise movements that allow the smallest diameter of the fetal head to pass through a corresponding diameter of the mother's pelvic structure. Although cardinal movements are conceptualized

---

BOX 13-1

SELECTED FETAL POSITIONS

Vertex Presentation (Occiput)
• Left occipitoanterior (LOA)
• Left occipitotransverse (LOT)
• Left occipitoposterior (LOP)
• Right occipitoanterior (ROA)
• Right occipitotransverse (ROT)
• Right occipitoposterior (ROP)

Face Presentation (Mentum)
• Left mentoanterior (LMA)
• Left mentotransverse (LMT)
• Left mentoposterior (LMP)
• Right mentoanterior (RMA)
• Right mentotransverse (RMT)
• Right mentoposterior (RMP)

Breech Presentation (Sacrum)
• Complete breech—all-body flexion
• Left sacroanterior (LSA)
• Left sacrotransverse (LST)
• Left sacroposterior (LSP)
• Right sacroanterior (RSA)
• Right sacroposterior (RSP)

Shoulder Presentation (Acromion)
• Left acromion dorsal anterior (LADA)
• Left acromion dorsal posterior (LADP)
• Right acromion dorsal anterior (RADA)
• Right acromion dorsal posterior (RADP;
  Olds et al., 2003)

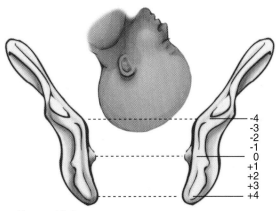

● Figure 13-8 Fetal stations.

as separate and sequential, the movements are typically concurrent (Figs. 13-9 and 13-10).

Engagement

Engagement occurs when the greatest transverse diameter of the head in vertex (biparietal diameter) passes through the pelvic inlet (usually 0 station). The head usually enters the pelvis with the sagittal suture aligned in the transverse diameter.

Descent

Descent is the downward movement of the fetal head until it is within the pelvic inlet. Descent occurs intermittently with contractions and is brought about by one or more forces: pressure of the amniotic fluid, direct pressure of the fundus on the fetus' buttocks or head (depending on which part is located in the top of the uterus), contractions of the abdominal muscles (second stage), and extension and straightening of the fetal body. It occurs throughout labor, ending with birth. During this time, the mother experiences discomfort, but she is unable to isolate this particular fetal movement from her overall discomfort.

Flexion

Flexion occurs as the vertex meets resistance from the cervix, walls of the pelvis, or the pelvic floor. As a result,

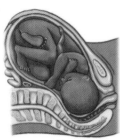
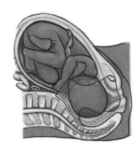

Engagement, Descent, Flexion

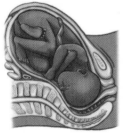
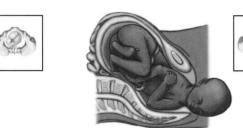

Internal Rotation

External Rotation (restitution)

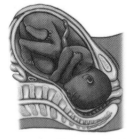
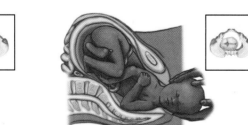

Extension Beginning (rotation complete)

External Rotation (shoulder rotation)

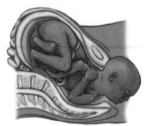
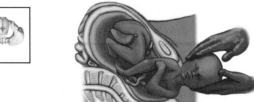

Extension Complete

Expulsion

● Figure 13-9 Cardinal movements of labor.

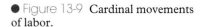

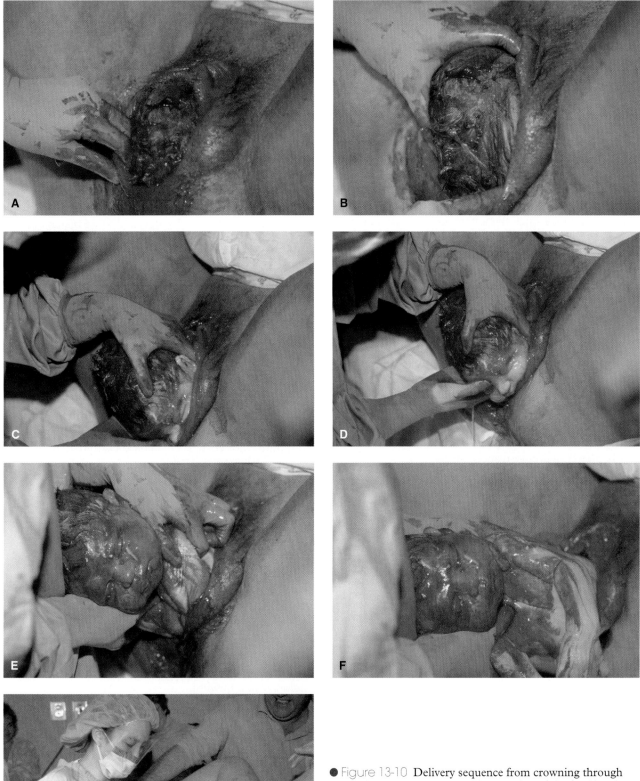

● Figure 13-10 Delivery sequence from crowning through birth of the newborn. (**A**) Early crowning of the fetal head. Notice the bulging of the perineum. (**B**) Late crowning. Notice that the fetal head is appearing face down. This is the normal OA position. (**C**) As the head extends, you can see that the occiput is to the mother's right side—ROA position. (**D**) The cardinal movement of extension. (**E**) The shoulders are born. Notice how the head has turned to line up with the shoulders—the cardinal movement of external rotation. (**F**) The body easily follows the shoulders. (**G**) The newborn is held for the first time! (© B. Proud.)

the chin is brought into contact with the fetal thorax and the presenting diameter is changed from occipitofrontal to suboccipitobregmatic (9.5 cm), which achieves the smallest fetal skull diameter presenting to the maternal pelvic dimensions.

Internal Rotation

After engagement, as the head descends, the lowermost portion of the head (usually the occiput) meets resistance from one side of the pelvic floor. As a result, the head rotates about 45° anteriorly to the midline under the symphysis. This movement is known as *internal rotation.* Internal rotation brings the anteroposterior diameter of the head in line with the anteroposterior diameter of the pelvic outlet. It aligns the long axis of the fetal head with the long axis of the maternal pelvis. The widest portion of the maternal pelvis is the anteroposterior diameter, and thus the fetus must rotate to accommodate the pelvis.

Extension

With further descent and full flexion of the head, the nucha (the base of the occiput) becomes impinged under the symphysis. Resistance from the pelvic floor causes the fetal head to extend so that it can pass under the pubic arch. Extension occurs after internal rotation is complete. The head emerges through extension under the symphysis pubis along with the shoulders. The bregma, brow, nose, mouth, and chin are born successively.

External Rotation (Restitution)

After the head is born and is free of resistance, it untwists, causing the occiput to move about 45° back to its original left or right position (restitution). The sagittal suture has now resumed its normal right-angle relationship to the transverse (bisacromial) diameter of the shoulders (i.e., the head realigns with the position of the back in the birth canal). External rotation of the fetal head allows the shoulders to rotate internally to fit the maternal pelvis.

Expulsion

Expulsion of the rest of the body occurs more smoothly after the delivery of the head, and the anterior and posterior shoulders (Littleton & Engebretson, 2005).

Powers

The primary stimulus powering labor is uterine contractions. Contractions cause complete dilation and effacement of the cervix during the first stage of labor. The secondary powers in labor involve the use of intraabdominal pressure (voluntary muscle contractions) exerted by the woman as she pushes and bears down during the second stage of labor.

Uterine Contractions

Uterine contractions are involuntary and therefore cannot be controlled by the woman experiencing them, regardless of whether the contractions are spontaneous or induced. Uterine contractions are rhythmic and intermittent, with a period of relaxation between contractions. This pause allows the woman and the uterine muscles to rest. In addition, this pause restores blood flow to the uterus and placenta, which is temporarily reduced during each uterine contraction.

Uterine contractions are responsible for thinning and dilating the cervix, and they thrust the presenting part toward the lower uterine segment. With each uterine contraction, the upper segment of the uterus becomes shorter and thicker, whereas the lower passive segment and the cervix become longer, thinner, and more distended. The division between the contractile upper portion (fundus) of the uterus and the lower portion is described as the *physiologic retraction ring.* Longitudinal traction on the cervix by the fundus as it contracts and retracts leads to cervical effacement and dilation. Uterine contractions cause the upper uterine segment to shorten, making the cervix paper thin when it becomes fully effaced.

The cervical canal reduces in length from 2 cm to a paper-thin entity and is described in terms of percentages from 0 to 100%. This thinning out process is termed *effacement.* In primigravidas, effacement typically starts before the onset of labor and usually begins before dilation; whereas, in multiparas, neither effacement nor dilation may start until labor ensues. On clinical examination the

- Cervical canal equal to 2 cm in length would be described as 0% effaced
- Cervical canal equal to 1 cm in length would be described as 50% effaced
- Cervical canal equal 0 cm in length would be described as 100% effaced

The opening or enlargement of the external cervical os is termed *dilation.* Its opening is dependent on the pressure of the presenting part and the contraction and retraction of the uterus. The diameter of the cervical os increases from less than 1 cm to approximately 10 cm to allow for birth. When the cervix is fully dilated, it is no longer palpable on vaginal examination. Descriptions may include the following:

- External cervical os closed: 0 cm dilated
- External cervical os half open: 5 cm dilated
- External cervical os fully open: 10 cm dilated

During early labor, uterine contractions are described as mild, they last about 30 seconds, and they occur about every 5 to 7 minutes. As labor progresses, contractions last longer (60 seconds), occur more frequently (2–3 minutes apart), and are described as being moderate to high in intensity.

Each contraction has three phases: *increment* (buildup of the contraction), *acme* (peak or highest intensity), and *decrement* (descent or relaxation of the uterine muscle fibers; Fig. 13-11).

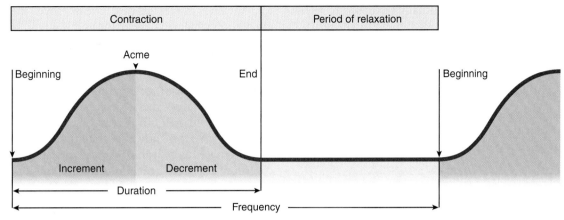

● Figure 13-11 The three phases of a uterine contraction.

Uterine contractions are monitored and assessed according to three parameters: frequency, duration, and intensity:

1. Frequency refers to how often the contractions occur and is measured from the increment of one contraction to the increment of the next contraction.
2. Duration refers to how long a contraction lasts and is measured from the beginning of the increment to the end of the decrement for the same contraction.
3. Intensity refers to the strength of the contraction determined by manual palpation or measured by an internal intrauterine catheter.

Accurate assessment of contraction intensity can only be measured internally by means of an intrauterine pressure catheter (IUPC), which is positioned in the uterine cavity through the cervix after the membranes have ruptured. The IUPC reports intensity by measuring the pressure of the amniotic fluid inside the uterus in millimeters of mercury (Littleton & Engebretson, 2005).

Intra-Abdominal Pressure

Increased intraabdominal pressure (voluntary muscle contractions) compresses the uterus and adds to the power of the expulsion forces of the uterine contractions (Lowdermilk & Perry, 2004). Coordination of these forces in unison promotes delivery of the fetus, fetal membranes, and placenta from the uterus. Interference with these forces (such as when a woman is highly sedated or extremely anxious) can affect the effectiveness of these powers.

Psychological Response

Childbearing can be one of the most life-altering experiences for a woman. The experience of childbirth goes beyond the physiologic aspects. This experience influences a woman's self-confidence, self-esteem, and her view of life, her relationships, and her children. Her state of mind (psyche) throughout the entire process is critical to evoke a positive outcome for her and her family. Factors influencing a positive birth experience include

- Clear information on procedures
- Positive support, not being alone
- Sense of mastery, self-confidence
- Trust in staff caring for her
- Positive reaction to the pregnancy
- Personal control over breathing
- Preparation for the childbirth experience

Having a strong sense of self and meaningful support from others can often help women manage labor well. Feelings of safety and security typically promote feelings of control and ability to withstand the challenges of the childbearing experience. Anxiety and fear, however, decrease a woman's ability to cope with the discomfort of labor. Maternal catecholamines are secreted in response to anxiety and fear and can inhibit uterine blood flow and placental perfusion. In contrast, relaxation can augment the natural process of labor (Murray et al., 2006). Preparing mentally for childbirth is important for women to enable them to work with, rather than against, the natural forces of labor.

Position (Maternal)

Maternal positioning during labor historically has been a topic of interest, but has only recently been the subject of well-controlled research that validates that nonmoving, back-lying positions during labor are not healthy (Simkin, 2002). Despite the scientific evidence to the contrary, most women lie flat on their backs. Why is this so? Some of the reasons may include the following:

- Laboring women need to conserve their energy and not tire themselves.
- Nurses cannot keep track of the whereabouts of ambulating women.
- The supine position facilitates vaginal examinations and external belt adjustment.

- A bed is simply where one is usually supposed to be in a hospital setting.
- Blind routine practice is convenient for the delivering health professional.
- Laboring women are "connected to things" that impede movement (Declercq et al., 2002).

Although many labor and birthing facilities claim that all women are allowed to adopt any position of comfort during their laboring experience, the great majority of women spend their time on their backs during labor and birth. If the only furniture provided is a bed, this is what the woman will use. Furnishing rooms with comfortable chairs, bean bags, and other props fosters a woman's ability to choose a variety of positions and be free to move during labor. Using the research available can bring better outcomes, heightened professionalism, and evidence-based practice to childbearing practices (Livingston & Dennedy, 2002).

Changing positions and moving around during labor and birth do offer several benefits. Maternal position can influence pelvic size and contours. Changing position and walking affect the pelvis joints, and they facilitate fetal descent and rotation. Squatting enlarges the pelvic outlet by approximately 25%, whereas a kneeling position removes pressure on the maternal vena cava and assists to rotate the fetus in the posterior position (Breslin & Lucas, 2003). The use of any upright or lateral position, compared with supine or lithotomy positions, may

- Reduce the duration of the second stage of labor
- Reduce the number of assisted deliveries (vacuum and forceps)
- Reduce episiotomies and perineal tears
- Contribute to fewer abnormal fetal heart rate patterns
- Increase comfort/reduce requests for pain medication
- Enhance a sense of control reported by mothers
- Alter the shape and size of the pelvis, which assists descent
- Assist gravity to move the fetus downward
- Reduce the length of labor (Gupta & Hofmeyr, 2003)

Philosophy

Birth in the 21st century for many women has become "intervention intensive"—designed to start, continue, and end labor through medical management rather than allowing the normal, natural process of birth to unfold. Not everyone views childbirth the same way. A philosophical continuum exists that extends from viewing labor as a natural process to viewing labor as a disease process. One philosophy assumes that women are capable, reasoning individuals who can actively participate in their birth experience. The other philosophy assumes that women are unable to manage the birth experience adequately, and therefore need constant expert monitoring and management.

Advances in medical care have improved the safety for women with high-risk pregnancies. However, the routine use of IV therapy, electronic fetal monitoring, augmentation, and epidural anesthesia has not necessarily improved birth outcomes for all women (Lothian et al., 2003). Perhaps a middle-of-the-road philosophy for intervening when circumstances dictate, along with weighing the risks and benefits before doing so, may be appropriate.

The current health care system view in the United States appears to be leaning toward the latter philosophy, commonly applying technologic interventions to most mothers who enter the hospital system. During the 1970s, FCMC was developed in response to the consumer reaction to the depersonalization of birth. The hope was to shift the philosophy from "technologization" to personalization to humanize childbirth. The term *family-centered birthing* is more appropriate today to denote the low-tech, high-touch approach requested by many childbearing women. Thus, childbirth is viewed as a natural process.

No matter what the philosophy, it is critical that everyone—from the health care provider to the birthing mother—share the same philosophy toward the birth process.

Partners

Throughout the world, few women are left to labor totally alone or in isolation. Women support other women in childbirth worldwide. Emotional, physical, or spiritual support during labor would appear to be the norm for most cultures (Hodnett et al., 2003). The use of massage, light touch, acupressure, hand-holding, stroking, relaxation, helping women communicate their wishes to caregivers, warm water or lotions, and providing a continuous presence by caring partners can all help bring some degree of comfort to the laboring woman (Hodnett et al., 2003). Although a father's presence at the birth provides special emotional support to the birthing experience, a partner can be anyone who is present to support the woman throughout the experience.

One important type of support that often may be used is a **doula.** This is a female support person who is an experienced labor companion. The doula provides the woman and her partner with emotional, informational, and physical support throughout the entire labor and birth experience.

The Cochrane Review (2003) of women supporting women reported that the continuous presence of a female trained support person (doula) reduced the incidence of medication for pain relief, use of vacuum or forceps, and cesarean births. Continuous support was also associated with a slight reduction in the length of labor (Hodnett et al., 2003). A similar study in the United States found that nursing care has been shown to decrease the likelihood of negative evaluations of the childbirth experience, feelings of tenseness during labor, and finding labor worse than expected. Also reported were less perineal trauma, reduced difficulty in mothering, and reduced likelihood of early cessation of breast-feeding (Trainor, 2002).

Women in labor desire support and to be cared for by a caregiver. Caregivers can convey emotional support through their continued presence and words of encouragement. Most women want to be included in the decision-making process during childbirth.

Given the many benefits associated with intrapartum support, laboring women should always have the option to receive partner support, whether from nurses, doulas, significant others, or family. This support partner should provide a continuous presence and hands-on comfort and encouragement.

Patience

The delivery process takes time. If more time were allowed for women to labor naturally without intervention, the cesarean birth rate would most likely be reduced (Larimore & Cline, 2000). The literature suggests that interventional delay can be helpful in affording a woman enough time to progress in labor and reduce the need for surgical intervention (American College of Obstetricians and Gynecologists [ACOG], 2000a). The cesarean birth rate in the United States (26%) is now the highest reported rate since these data first became available from birth certificates in 1989 (Hamilton et al., 2003). Cesarean birth is associated with increased morbidity and mortality for both mother and infant, as well as increased inpatient length of stay and healthcare costs (Rayburn & Zhang, 2002).

It is difficult to predict how a labor will progress and, therefore, equally difficult to determine how long a woman's labor will last before delivery. There is no way to estimate the likely strength and frequency of uterine contractions, the extent to which the cervix will soften and dilate, and how much the fetal head will mold to fit the birth canal. Equally, we cannot know beforehand whether the complex fetal rotation needed for an efficient labor will take place properly. All these factors are unknowns when a woman starts labor. There is a trend in health care, however, to limit the length of labor through medical means such as artificial rupture of membranes and augmentation of labor with oxytocin (Bricker & Luckas, 2003).

As a testament to this, the labor induction rate has increased dramatically in the United States since the 1980s (Rayburn & Zhang, 2002). In fact, since 1989 it has doubled and then increased steadily since that same year (Munson & Sutton, 2005).

Approximately one in five women are induced or have their labors augmented with uterine-stimulating drugs or artificial rupture of membranes to accelerate their progress (Munson & Sutton, 2005). An amniotomy (artificial rupture of the fetal membranes) may be performed to augment or induce labor when the membranes have not ruptured spontaneously. Doing so allows the fetal

head to have more direct contact with the cervix to dilate it. This procedure is performed with the fetal head at −2 station or lower, with the cervix dilated to at least 3 cm. Synthetic oxytocin (Pitocin) is also used to induce or augment labor by stimulating uterine contractions. It is administered piggybacked into the primary IV line with an infusion pump titrated to uterine activity.

There is compelling evidence that elective induction of labor significantly increases the risk of cesarean birth, especially for nulliparous women (Simpson & Atterbury, 2003). The belief is that a large number of cesarean births could be avoided if women were allowed to labor longer and permit time for the natural labor process to complete the job. The longer wait (using the intervention of patience) usually results in less intervention.

The ACOG attributes the dramatic increase in inductions in part to pressure from women, convenience for physicians, and liability concerns. They recommend a "cautious approach" regarding elective induction until clinical trials can validate a more liberal use of labor inductions (ACOG, 2002). There are medical indications for inducing labor, such as spontaneous rupture of membranes and when labor does not start, a pregnancy more than 42 weeks' gestation, maternal hypertension, diabetes or lung disease, and a uterine infection (ACOG, 2000b).

Patient Preparation

Basic prenatal education can help women manage their labor process and feel in control of their birthing experience. The literature indicates that if a woman is prepared before the labor and birth experience, the labor is more likely to remain normal or natural (without the need for medical intervention) (Larimore & Cline, 2000). An increasing body of evidence in the literature also indicates that the well-prepared woman, with good labor support, is less likely to need analgesia or anesthesia and is unlikely to require cesarean birth (Hodnett, 2002).

Prenatal education helps teach women about the childbirth experience and increases a woman's sense of control, who then works as an active participant during the labor experience (Maestas, 2003). The research also suggests that prenatal preparation may affect intrapartum and postpartum psychosocial outcomes. For example, prenatal education covering parenting communication classes had a significant affect on postpartum anxiety and postpartum adjustment (Buckley, 2001).

Having the knowledge to understand labor and birth allows women and couples to express their needs and preferences, enhance their confidence, and improve communication between themselves and the staff.

Pain Control

Labor and birth, although a normal physiologic process, can produce significant pain. Pain during labor is a nearly universal experience for childbearing women. Controlling the pain of labor without harm to the fetus or labor process is the major focus of pain management during the childbearing experience.

Pain is a subjective experience involving a complex interaction of physiologic, spiritual, psychosocial, cultural, and environmental influences (Leeman et al., 2003a). Cultural values and learned behaviors influence perception and response to pain, as do anxiety and fear, both of which tend to heighten the sense of pain (Poole & White, 2003). The challenge for care providers is to find the right combination of pain management methods to keep the pain manageable while minimizing the negative affect on the fetus, the normal physiology of labor, maternal–infant bonding, breast-feeding, and a woman's perception of the labor itself (Primeau et al., 2003).

Physiologic Responses to Labor

Labor is the physiologic process by which the uterus expels the fetus and placenta from the body. During pregnancy, progesterone secreted from the placenta suppresses the spontaneous contractions of a typical uterus, keeping the fetus within the uterus. In addition, the cervix remains firm and noncompliant. At term, however, changes occur in the cervix that make it softer, and uterine contractions that become more frequent and regular, signaling the onset of labor.

The labor process comprises a series of rhythmic, involuntary, usually quite uncomfortable uterine muscle contractions that bring about a shortening that causes effacement and dilation of the cervix, and a bursting of the fetal membranes. Then, accompanied by both reflex and voluntary contractions of the abdominal muscles (pushing), the uterine contractions result in the birth of the baby (Sloane, 2002). During the laboring process, the mother and fetus make several physiologic adaptations.

Maternal Responses

As the woman experiences and progresses through childbirth, numerous physiologic responses occur that assist her to adapt to the laboring process. The labor process stresses several of the woman's body systems and they react through numerous compensatory mechanisms. Maternal physiologic responses include

- Increased heart rate by 10 to 18 bpm (Chin, 2001)
- Increased cardiac output by 10 to 15% during the first stage of labor and increased by 30 to 50% during the second stage of labor (Blackburn & Loper, 2003)
- Increased blood pressure by 10 to 30 mm Hg during uterine contractions in all labor stages
- Increase in white blood cell count to 25,000 to 30,000 cells/mm^3 perhaps as a result of tissue trauma
- Increased respiratory rate along with greater oxygen consumption related to the increase in metabolism

- Decreased gastric motility and food absorption, which may increase the risk of nausea and vomiting during the transition stage of labor
- Decreased gastric emptying and gastric pH, which increases the risk of vomiting with aspiration
- Slight elevation in temperature possibly as a result of an increase in muscle activity
- Muscular aches/cramps as a result of a stressed musculoskeletal system involved in the labor process
- Increased BMR and decreased blood glucose levels because of the stress of labor (Pagana & Pagana, 2002)

A woman's ability to adapt to the stress of labor is influenced by her psychologic state. Many factors affect her coping ability. Some influencing factors may include her previous birth experiences and their outcomes, current pregnancy experience (planned versus unplanned, discomforts experienced, age, high-risk status of pregnancy), cultural considerations (values and beliefs about health status), involvement of support system (presence and support of a valued partner during labor), childbirth preparation (attended childbirth classes and has practiced paced breathing techniques), her expectations of this birthing experience, anxiety level, fear of labor experience, loss of control, and fatigue and weariness (Turley, 2004).

Fetal Responses

Although the focus during labor may be on assessing the mother's adaptations, several physiologic adaptations occur in the fetus as well. The fetus is experiencing labor along with the mother. If the fetus is healthy, the stress of labor usually has no adverse effects. The nurse needs to be alert to any abnormalities in the fetus' adaptation to labor. Fetal responses to labor include

- Periodic fetal heart rate accelerations and slight decelerations related to fetal movement, fundal pressure, and uterine contractions
- Decrease in circulation and perfusion to the fetus secondary to uterine contractions (A healthy fetus is able to compensate for this drop.)
- Increase in arterial carbon dioxide pressure (PCO_2)
- Decrease in fetal breathing movements throughout labor
- Decrease in fetal oxygen pressure with a decrease in the partial pressure of oxygen (PO_2) (Lowdermilk & Perry, 2004)

All the respiratory changes help prepare the fetus for extrauterine respiration immediately after birth.

Stages of Labor

Labor is typically divided into four stages that are unequal in length. The four stages of labor are the dilation stage, the expulsive stage, the placental stage, and the restorative stage.

The first stage is the longest of all the stages and it begins with the first true contraction and ends with full dilation (opening) of the cervix. Because this stage lasts so long, it is divided into three distinct phases of the first stage of labor: latent phase, active phase, and the transitional phase. Each phase corresponds to the progressive dilation of the cervix.

Stage two of labor, or the expulsive stage, begins when the cervix is completely dilated and ends with the birth of the newborn. The expulsive stage can last from minutes to hours until the birth takes place.

The third stage, or placental stage, starts after the newborn is born and ends with the separation and delivery of the placenta. Continued uterine contractions cause the placenta to be expelled within 5 to 30 minutes typically.

The fourth stage, or restorative stage, lasts from 1 to 4 hours after birth. This period is when the mother's body begins to stabilize after the hard work of labor and the loss of the products of conception. The fourth stage is often not recognized as a true stage of labor, but it is a critical period for maternal physiologic transition as well as new family attachment (Condon, 2004). Box 13-2 summarizes the major events of each stage.

First Stage

During the first stage of labor, the fundamental change underlying the process is progressive dilation of the cervix. Cervical dilation is gauged subjectively by vaginal examination and is expressed in centimeters. The first stage ends when the cervix is dilated to 10 cm in diameter and is large enough to permit the passage of a fetal head of average size. The fetal membranes, or bag of waters, usually rupture during the first stage, but they may have burst earlier or may even remain intact until birth. For the woman having her first birth, the average duration of the first stage of labor is about 12 hours. However, this time can vary widely. For the multiparous woman, the duration of the first stage is usually about half the time of that for a nullipara.

During the first stage of labor, women usually perceive the visceral pain of diffuse abdominal cramping and uterine contractions. Pain during the first stage of labor is primarily a result of the dilation of the cervix and lower uterine segment, and the distention, stretching, and tearing of these structures during contractions. The first stage is divided into three phases: latent phase, active phase, and transition phase.

Latent Phase

The latent phase gives rise to the familiar signs and symptoms of labor. This phase begins with the start of regular contractions and ends when rapid cervical dilation begins. Cervical effacement occurs during this phase and the cervix dilates from 0 to 3 cm.

Contractions usually occur every 5 to 10 minutes, last 30 to 45 seconds, and are described as mild by palpation.

BOX 13-2
STAGES AND PHASES OF LABOR

- First stage of labor goes from 0 to 10 cm dilation; consists of three phases
  - Latent phase lasts from 0 to 3 cm dilation; mild contractions
    - Cervical dilation 0 to 3 cm
    - Cervical effacement from 0 to 40%
    - Nullipara lasting up to 9 hours; multipara lasting up to 5 to 6 hours
    - Contraction frequency every 5 to 10 minutes
    - Contraction duration 30 to 45 seconds
    - Contraction intensity mild to palpation
  - Active phase lasts from 4 to 7 cm dilation; moderate contractions
    - Cervical dilation between 4 to 7 cm
    - Cervical effacement between 40 to 80%
    - Nullipara lasting up to 6 hours; multipara lasting up to 4 hours
    - Contraction frequency every 2 to 5 minutes
    - Contraction duration 45 to 60 seconds
    - Contraction intensity moderate to palpation
  - Transition phase is from 8 to 10 cm dilation; strong contractions
    - Cervical dilation from 8 to 10 cm
    - Cervical effacement from 80 to 100%
    - Nullipara lasting up to 1 hour; multipara lasting up to 30 minutes
    - Contraction frequency every 1 to 2 minutes
    - Contraction duration 60 to 90 seconds
    - Contraction intensity hard by palpation
- Second stage is from complete dilation (10 cm) to birth of newborn; lasts up to 1 hour
  - Pelvic phase: period of fetal descent
  - Perineal phase: period of active pushing
  - Nullipara lasts up to 1 hour; multipara lasts up to 30 minutes
  - Contraction frequency every 2 to 3 minutes or less
  - Contraction duration 60 to 90 seconds
  - Contraction intensity strong by palpation
  - Strong urge to push during the later perineal phase
- Third stage (or placental stage) is separation and delivery of placenta
  - Placental separation: detaching from uterine wall
  - Placental expulsion: coming outside the vaginal opening
- Fourth stage is 1 to 4 hours after birth; time of maternal physiologic adjustment

---

Effacement of the cervix is from 0 to 40%. Most women are very talkative during this period, perceiving their contractions similar to menstrual cramps. Women may remain at home during this phase, contacting their health care professional about their onset of labor.

For the nulliparous woman, the latent phase typically lasts about 9 hours, whereas in the multiparous woman, it lasts approximately 6 hours (Littleton & Engebretson, 2005). During this phase, women are apprehensive but excited about the start of their labor after their long gestational period.

Active Phase

Cervical dilation begins to occur more rapidly during the active phase. The cervix usually dilates from 3 to 7 cm with 40% to 80% effacement taking place. This phase can last for as long as 6 hours in for the nulliparous woman and 4.5 hours for the multiparous woman (Smith, 2004). The fetus descends farther in the pelvis. Contractions become more frequent (every 2–5 minutes) and increase in duration (45–60 seconds). The woman's discomfort intensifies (moderate to strong by palpation). She becomes more intense and inwardly focused, absorbed in the serious work of her labor. She limits interactions with those in the room. If she and her partner have attended childbirth education classes, she will begin to use the relaxation and paced breathing techniques learned to cope with the contractions. The suggested dilation rate for the nulliparous woman is 1.2 cm/hour; for the multiparous woman, 1.5 cm/hour (Cunningham et al., 2005).

Transition Phase

The transition phase is the last phase of the first stage of labor. During this phase, dilation slows, progressing from 8 to 10 cm, with effacement from 80% to 100%. The transition phase is the most difficult and, fortunately, the shortest phase for the woman, lasting approximately 1 hour in the first birth and perhaps 15 to 30 minutes in successive births (Sloane, 2002). During transition, the contractions are stronger (hard by palpation), more painful, more frequent (every 1–2 minutes), and last longer (60–90 seconds). The average rate of fetal descent is 1 cm/hour in nulliparous women and 2 cm/hour in multiparous women. Pressure on the rectum is great, and there is a strong desire to contract the abdominal muscles and push.

Other maternal features that are manifested during this transitional phase include nausea and vomiting, trembling extremities, backache, increased apprehension and irritability, restless movement, increased bloody show from the vagina, inability to relax, diaphoresis, feelings of loss of control, and being overwhelmed (with the woman often stating, "I can't take it any more"). This phase should not last longer than 3 hours for nulliparas and 1 hour for multiparas (Cunningham et al., 2005).

Second Stage

The second stage of labor begins with complete cervical dilation (10 cm) and effacement, and ends with the birth of the newborn. Although the previous stage of labor primarily involved the thinning and opening of the cervix, this stage involves moving the fetus through the birth canal and out of the body. The cardinal movements of labor occur during the early phase of passive descent in the second stage of labor.

Contractions occur every 2 to 3 minutes, last 60 to 90 seconds, and are described as strong by palpation. The average length of the second stage of labor in a nullipara is approximately 1 hour and less than half that time for the multipara woman. During this expulsive stage, the mother usually feels more in control and less irritable and agitated. She is focused on the work of pushing. Traditionally, women have been taught to hold their breath to the count of 10, inhale again, push again, and repeat the process several times during a contraction. This sustained, strenuous style of pushing has been shown to lead to hemodynamic changes in the mother and interfere with oxygen exchange between the mother and the fetus. In addition, it is associated with pelvic floor damage: the longer the push, the more damage to the pelvic floor (Chalk, 2004). The newest protocol from the Association of Women's Health and Newborn Nursing (AWHONN) recommends an open-glottis method in which air is released during pushing to prevent the build up of intrathoracic pressure. Doing so also supports mother's involuntary bearing-down efforts (Smith, 2004).

During the second stage of labor, pushing can either follow the mother's spontaneous urge or be directed by the caregiver. Much debate still exists between spontaneous and directed pushing during the second stage of labor. Although directed pushing is common practice in hospitals, there is evidence to suggest that directed pushing be avoided. Research seems to support spontaneous pushing—when the woman is allowed to follow her own instincts (Chalk, 2004).

The second stage of labor has two phases related to the existence and quality of the maternal urge to push and to obstetric conditions related to fetal descent. The early phase of the second stage is called the *pelvic phase*, because it is during this phase that the fetal head is negotiating the pelvis, rotating and advancing in descent. The later phase is called the *perineal phase*, because at this point the fetal head is lower in the pelvis and is distending the perineum. The occurrence of a strong urge to push characterizes the later phase of the second stage and has also been called *the phase of active pushing* (Roberts, 2003).

The later perineal phase occurs when there is a tremendous urge to push by the mother as the fetal head is lowered and is distending the perineum. The perineum bulges and there is an increase in bloody show. The fetal head becomes apparent at the vaginal opening, but disappears between contractions. When the top of the head no longer regresses between contractions, it is said to have *crowned*. The fetus rotates as it maneuvers out. The second stage commonly lasts up to 3 hours in a first labor and up to an hour in subsequent ones.

During the second stage of labor, the woman experiences a sharper, more continuous somatic pain in the perineum. Pressure or nerve entrapment caused by the fetus' head can cause back or leg pain at this time (Leeman et al., 2003a).

Third Stage

The third stage of labor begins with the birth of the newborn and ends with the separation and delivery of the placenta. It consists of two phases: placental separation and placental expulsion.

Placental Separation

After the infant is born, the uterus continues to contract strongly and can now retract, decreasing markedly in size. These contractions cause the placenta to pull away from the uterine wall. The following signs of separation indicate that the placenta is ready to deliver:

• The uterus rises upward
• The umbilical cord lengthens
• A sudden trickle of blood is released from the vaginal opening
• The uterus changes its shape to globular

Spontaneous delivery of the placenta occurs in one of two ways: the fetal side (shiny gray side) presenting first (called *Schultz's mechanism* or more commonly called *shiny Schultz's*) or the maternal side (red raw side) of the placenta presenting first (termed *Duncan's mechanism* or *dirty Duncan*).

Placental Expulsion

After separation of the placenta from the uterine wall, continued uterine contractions cause the placenta to be expelled within 5 to 30 minutes unless there is gentle external traction to assist. After the placenta is expelled, the uterus is massaged briefly by the attending physician or midwife until it is firm in order to constrict uterine blood vessels and minimize the possibility of hemorrhage. Normal blood volume blood loss is approximately 500 mL per vaginal birth and 1000 mL per cesarean birth (Poole & White, 2003).

If the placenta does not spontaneously deliver, the healthcare professional assists with its removal by manual extraction. On expulsion, the placenta is inspected for its intactness by the healthcare professional and the nurse to make sure all sections are present. If any piece is left still attached to the uterine wall, it places the woman at risk for a postpartum hemorrhage, because it becomes a space-occupying object that interferes with the ability of the uterus to contract fully and effectively.

Fourth Stage

The fourth stage begins with completion of the delivery of the placenta and membranes, and ends with the initial physiologic adjustment and stabilization of the mother (1–4 hours after birth). This stage initiates the postpartum period. The mother usually feels a sense of peace and excitement, is wide awake, and is very talkative initially. The attachment process begins with her inspecting her newborn and desiring to cuddle and breast-feed him or her. The mother's fundus should be firm and well contracted. Typically it is located at the midline between the umbilicus and the symphysis, but then slowly rises to the level of the umbilicus during the first hour after birth (Smith, 2004). If the uterus becomes boggy, it is then massaged to keep it firm. The lochia (vaginal discharge) is red in color, mixed with small clots and of moderate flow. If the woman has experienced an episiotomy during the second stage of labor, it should be intact, with the edges approximated, clean, and no redness or edema present.

The focus of this stage is to monitor the mother closely to prevent hemorrhage, bladder distention, and venous thrombosis. Usually the mother is thirsty and hungry during this time, and may request food and drink. Her bladder is hypotonic and thus the mother has limited sensation to acknowledge a full bladder or to void. The vital signs, amount and consistency of the vaginal discharge (lochia), and palpation of the uterine fundus are usually monitored every 15 minutes for a minimum of an hour. The woman will be experiencing cramp-like discomfort during this time secondary to the uterine contraction status.

KEY CONCEPTS

● Labor is a complex, multifaceted interaction between the mother and fetus. Thus, it is difficult to determine exactly why labor begins and what initiates it.

● Before the onset of labor, a pregnant woman's body undergoes several changes in preparation for the birth of the newborn, often leading to characteristic signs and symptoms that suggest that labor is near. These changes include cervical changes, lightening, increased energy level, bloody show, Braxton Hicks contractions, and spontaneous rupture of membranes.

● False labor is a condition seen during the latter weeks of some pregnancies in which irregular uterine contractions are felt, but the cervix is not affected.

● The critical factors in labor and birth are designated as the 10 Ps: passageway (birth canal), passenger (fetus and placenta), powers (contractions), psychological response, maternal position, philosophy (low tech, high touch), partners (support caregivers), patience (natural timing), patient preparation (childbirth knowledge base), and pain control (comfort measures).

● The size and shape of a woman's pelvis are determining factors for a vaginal delivery. The female pelvis is divided into four main groups: anthropoid, android, gynecoid, and the platypelloid.

● The labor process is comprised of a series of rhythmic, involuntary, usually quite uncomfortable uterine muscle contractions that bring about a shortening (effacement) and opening (dilation) of the cervix, and a bursting of the fetal membranes. Important parameters of uterine contractions are frequency, duration, and intensity.

- The diameters of the fetal skull vary considerably, with some diameters shortening and others lengthening as the head is molded during the labor and birth process.

- Pain during labor is a nearly universal experience for childbearing women. Having a strong sense of self and meaningful support from others can often help women manage labor well and reduce their sensation of pain.

- Preparing mentally for childbirth is important for women to enable them to work with the natural forces of labor and not against them.

- As the woman experiences and progresses through childbirth, numerous physiologic responses occur that assist her adaptation to the laboring process.

- Labor is typically divided into four stages that are unequal in length.

- During the first stage, the fundamental change underlying the process is progressive dilation of the cervix. It is further divided into three phases: latent phase, active phase, and transition.

- The second stage of labor is from complete cervical dilation (10 cm) and effacement through the birth of the infant.

- The third stage is that of separation and delivery of the placenta. It consists of two phases: placental separation and placental expulsion.

- The fourth stage begins after the delivery of the placenta and membranes, and ends with the initial physiologic adjustment and stabilization of the mother (1–4 hours).

References

American College of Obstetricians and Gynecologists (ACOG). (2000a). *Evaluation of cesarean delivery.* Washington, DC: ACOG.

American College of Obstetricians and Gynecologists (ACOG). (2000b). *Planning your pregnancy and birth.* Washington, DC: ACOG.

American College of Obstetricians and Gynecologists (ACOG). (2002). *ACOG news release commentary—nonmedical indications help fuel rise in induction rate.* [Released June 30, 2002.] Washington, DC: ACOG.

Blackburn, S. T., & Loper, D. L. (2003). *Maternal, fetal and neonatal physiology: a clinical perspective* (2nd ed.). Philadelphia: WB Saunders.

Breslin, E. T., & Lucas, V. A. (2003). *Women's health nursing: toward evidence-based practice.* St. Louis: Saunders.

Bricker, L., Luckas, M. (2000). Amniotomy alone for induction of labor. *The Cochrane Database of Systematic Reviews, 4.* Art No.: CD002862. DOI: 1002/14651858.CD002862.

Buckley, S. (2001). A natural approach to the third stage of labor. *Midwife Today, 59,* 33–37.

Burst, H. V., Kriebs, J. M., Gegor, C. L., & Varney, H. (2004). *Varney's midwifery* (4th ed.). Boston, MA: Blackwell Scientific.

Chalk, A. (2004). Spontaneous versus directed pushing. *British Journal of Midwifery, 12,* 626–630.

Chin, H. G. (2001). *On-call obstetrics and gynecology* (2nd ed.). Philadelphia: WB Saunders.

Condon, M. C. (2004). *Women's health: an integrated approach to wellness and illness.* Upper Saddle River, NJ: Prentice Hall.

Cunningham, G., Gant, N. F., Leveno, K. J., Gilstrap, L. C., Hauth, J. C., & Wenstrom, K. D. (2005). *Williams obstetrics* (22nd ed.). New York: McGraw-Hill.

Declercq, E. R., Sakala, C., Corry, M. P., Applebaum, S., & Risher, P. (2002). *Listening to mothers: report of the first national U.S. survey of women's childbearing experiences.* New York: Maternity Center Association.

Engstrom, J. (2004). *Maternal–neonatal nursing made incredibly easy!* Philadelphia: Lippincott Williams & Wilkins.

Fischer, R. (2004). Breech presentation. *EMedicine.* [Online] Available at wwwemedicine.com/med/topic3272.htm.

Gilbert, E. S., & Harmon, J. S. (2003). *Manual of high risk pregnancy & delivery.* St. Louis: Mosby.

Gupta, J. K., & Hofmeyr, G. J. (2003). Position in the second stage of labor for women without epidural anesthesia. *The Cochrane Database of Systematic Reviews, 3.* Art. No. CD002006.pub2. DOI: 10.1002/14651858.CD002006.pub2.

Hait, E. (2002). *Newborn head molding.* [Online] Available at www.nlm.nih.gov/medlineplus/ency/article/002270.htm.

Hamilton, B. E., Martin, J. A., & Sutton, P. D. (2003). Births: preliminary data for 2002. *National Vital Statistics Report, 51,* 1–20.

Hodnett, E. D. (2002). Pain and women's satisfaction with the experience of childbirth: a systematic review. *American Journal of Obstetrics and Gynecology, 186,* 60–172.

Hodnett, E. D., Gates, S., Hofmeyr, G. J., & Sakala, C. (2003). Continuous support for women during childbirth. *The Cochrane Database of Systematic Reviews, 3.* Art. No. CD003766 DOI: 10.1002/14651858.CD003766.

Kennedy, H. P., & Shannon, M. T. (2004). Keeping birth normal: Research findings on midwifery care during childbirth. *JOGNN, 33*(5), 554–560.

Ladewig, P. W. (2003). *Maternal–newborn & child nursing: family-centered care.* Upper Saddle River, NJ: Prentice Hall.

Larimore, W. L., & Cline, M. K. (2000). Keeping normal labor normal. *Primary Care, 27,* 221–236.

Leeman, L., Fontaine, P., King, V., Klein, M. C., & Ratcliffe, S. (2003a). The nature and management of labor pain: part I. Nonpharmacologic pain relief. *American Family Physician, 68,* 1109–1112.

Leeman, L., Fontaine, P., King, V., Klein, M. C., & Ratcliff, S. (2003b). The nature and management of labor pain: part II. Pharmacologic pain relief. *American Family Physician, 68,* 1115–1120.

Leonard, P. (2002). Childbirth education: a handbook for nurses. *Nursing Spectrum.* [Online] Available at http://nsweb.nursingspectrum.com/ce/m350b.htm

Littleton, L. Y., & Engebretson, J. C. (2005). *Maternity nursing care.* Clifton Park, NY: Thomson Delmar Learning.

Livingston, C., & Dennedy, S. (2002). *CAPPA position paper: evidence-based practice in childbirth education.* CAPPA Directors of Childbirth Education. Lawrenceville, GA: CAPPA.

Lowdermilk, D. L., & Perry, S. E. (2004). *Maternity & women's health care* (8th ed.). St. Louis: Mosby.

Maestas, L. M. (2003). The effect of prenatal education on the beliefs and perceptions of childbearing women. *International Journal of Childbirth Education, 18,* 17–22.

Mattson, S., & Smith, J. E. (2004). *Core curriculum for maternal–newborn nursing* (3rd ed.). St. Louis: Elsevier Saunders.

McKinney, E. S., James, S. R., Murray, S. S., & Ashwill, J. W. (2005). *Maternal–child nursing.* St. Louis: Elsevier Saunders.

Munson, M. L., & Sutton, P. D. (2005). Births, marriages, divorces, and deaths: Provisional data for April, 2005. *National Vital Statistics Reports (NVSR), 54*(6).

Murray, S. S. & McKinney, E. S. (2006). *Foundations of maternal–newborn nursing* (4th ed.). Philadelphia: WB Saunders.

Olds, S. B., London, M. L., Ladewig, P. W., & Davidson, M. R. (2004). *Maternal–newborn nursing & women's health care* (7th ed.). Upper Saddle River, NJ: Pearson Prentice Hall.

O'Toole, M. T. (2003). *Miller–Keane encyclopedia & dictionary of medicine, nursing, and allied health* (7th ed.). Philadelphia: Saunders.

Pagana, K., & Pagana, T. (2002). *Mosby's manual of diagnostic and laboratory tests* (2nd ed.). St. Louis: Mosby.

Pillitteri, A. (2003). *Maternal & child health nursing: care of the child-bearing and childrearing family* (4th ed.). Philadelphia: Lippincott Williams & Wilkins.

Poole, J., & White, D. (2003). *March of Dimes nursing modules: obstetrical emergencies for the perinatal nurse.* White Plains, NY: March of Dimes Birth Defects Foundation.

Primeau, M. R., Lucey, K. A., & Crotty, P. M. (2003). Managing the pain of labor. *Advances in Nursing, 4,* 15–19.

Rayburn, W. F., & Zhang, J. (2002). Raising rates of labor induction: present concerns and future strategies. *Obstetrics and Gynecology, 100,* 164–167.

Roberts, J. E. (2003). A new understanding of the second stage of labor: implications for nursing care. *JOGNN, 32,* 794–801.

Simkin, P. (2002). Supportive care during labor: a guide for busy nurses. *JOGNN, 1,* 721–732.

Simkin, P. (2003). Maternal positions and pelves revisited. *Birth, 30,* 130–132.

Simpson, K. R., & Atterbury, J. (2003). Trends and issues in labor induction in the United States: implications for clinical practice. *JOGNN, 32,* 767–779.

Sloane, E. (2002). *Biology of women* (4th ed.). Albany, NY: Delmar.

Smith, K. V. (2004). Normal childbirth. In Mattson, S., & Smith, J. E. (Eds.), *AWHONN: maternal–newborn nursing* (3rd ed., pp. 271–302). Philadelphia: Elsevier Saunders.

Trainor, C. L. (2002). Valuing labor support. *AWHONN Lifelines, 6,* 387–389.

Turley, G. M. (2004). Essential forces and factors in labor. In Mattson, S., & Smith, J. E. (Eds.), *AWHONN: maternal–newborn nursing* (3rd ed., pp. 227–270). Philadelphia: Elsevier Saunders.

Wong, D. L., Perry, S. E., & Hockenberry, M. J. (2002). *Maternal child nursing care* (2nd ed.). St. Louis: Mosby.

Youngkin, E. Q., & Davis, M. S. (2004). *Women's health: a primary care clinical guide* (3rd ed.). Upper Saddle River, NJ: Prentice Hall.

Web Resources

Academy of Breast-feeding Medicine, **www.bfmed.org**
Academy for Guided Imagery, Inc., **www.interactiveimagery.com/**
American College of Obstetricians and Gynecologists, **www.acog.org**
American Public Health Association, **www.apha.org**
Association of Labor Assistants and Childbirth Educators, **www.alace.org**
Association of Women's Health, Obstetric and Neonatal Nurses (AWHONN), **www.awhonn.org**
Birthworks, **www.birthworks.org**
BMJ publication: *Evidence-Based Nursing,* **www.evidencebasednursing.com**
Childbirth Organization, **www.childbirth.org**
Diversity Rx, **www.diversityrx.org**
Doulas of North America (DONA), **www.dona.org**
HypnoBirthing Institute, **www.hypnobirthing.com**
International Childbirth Education Association, **www.icea.org**
Lamaze International, **www.lamaze-childbirth.com**
National Association of Childbearing Centers (NACC), **www.birthcenters.org**

Chapter WORKSHEET

● MULTIPLE CHOICE QUESTIONS

1. When determining the frequency of contractions, the nurse would measure which of the following?

   a. Start of one contraction to the start of the next contraction

   b. Beginning of one contraction to the end of the same contraction

   c. Peak of one contraction to the peak of the next contraction

   d. End of one contraction to the beginning of the next contraction

2. Which fetal lie is most conducive for a spontaneous vaginal birth?

   a. Transverse

   b. Longitudinal

   c. Perpendicular

   d. Oblique

3. Which of the following observations would suggest that placental separation is occurring?

   a. Uterus stops contracting altogether

   b. Umbilical cord pulsations stop

   c. Uterine shape changes from discord to globular

   d. Maternal blood pressure drops

4. While preparing to assist with an amniotomy, the nurse understands that this procedure will

   a. Stimulate contractions

   b. Reduce the risk of infection

   c. Increase fetal heart accelerations

   d. Decrease painful contractions

5. The shortest but most intense phase of labor is the

   a. Latent phase

   b. Active phase

   c. Transition phase

   d. Placental expulsion phase

● CRITICAL THINKING EXERCISES

1. Cindy, a 20-year old primipara, calls the birthing center where you work as a nurse and reports she thinks she is in labor because she feels labor pains. Her due date is this week. The midwives have been giving her prenatal care throughout this pregnancy.

   a. What additional information do you need to respond appropriately?

   b. What suggestions/recommendations would you make to her?

   c. What instructions need to be given to guide her decision making?

2. Based on Cindy, the young woman described in the previous scenario, consider the following:

   a. What other premonitory signs of labor might the nurse ask about?

   b. What manifestations would be found if Cindy is experiencing true labor?

3. You are assigned to lead a community education class for women in their third trimester of pregnancy to prepare them for their upcoming birth. Prepare an outline of topics that should be addressed.

● STUDY ACTIVITIES

1. During clinical post conference, share with the other nursing students how the critical forces of labor influenced the length of labor and the birthing process for a laboring woman assigned to you.

2. The cardinal movements of labor include which of the following? Select all that apply.

   a. Extension and rotation

   b. Descent and engagement

   c. Presentation and position

   d. Attitude and lie

   e. Flexion and expulsion

3. Interview a woman on the mother–baby unit who has given birth within the last few hours. Ask her to describe her experience and examine psychological factors that may have influenced her laboring process.

4. On the following illustration, identify the parameters of uterine contractions by marking an "X" where the nurse would measure the duration of the contraction.

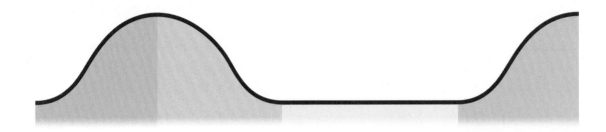

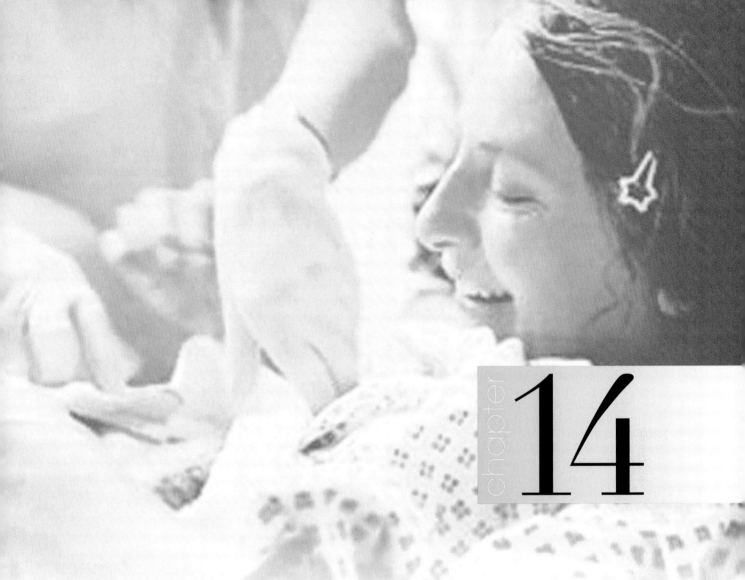

chapter 14

Nursing Management During Labor and Birth

KeyTERMS

accelerations
artifact
baseline fetal heart rate
baseline variability
crowning
deceleration
electronic fetal monitoring
episiotomy
Leopold's maneuvers
neuraxial
    analgesia/anesthesia
periodic baseline changes

LearningOBJECTIVES

After studying the chapter content, the student should be able to accomplish the following:

1. Define the key terms.
2. Describe the assessment data collected on admission to the perinatal unit.
3. Identify the measures used to evaluate maternal status during labor and birth.
4. Compare and contrast the advantages and disadvantages of external and internal fetal monitoring, including the appropriate use for each.
5. Describe appropriate nursing interventions to address nonreassuring fetal heart rate patterns.
6. Outline the nurse's role in fetal assessment.
7. Explain the various comfort-promotion and pain-relief strategies used during labor and birth.
8. Discuss the ongoing assessment involved in each stage of labor and birth.
9. Delineate the nurse's role throughout the labor and birth process.

The laboring and birthing process is a life-changing event for many women. Nurses need to be respectful, available, encouraging, supportive, and professional in dealing with all women. The nursing management for labor and birth should include comfort measures, emotional support, information and instruction, advocacy, and support for the partner (Simkin, 2002).

Consider THIS!

Since I was expecting my first child, I was determined to put my best foot forward and do everything right, for I was an experienced OB nurse and in my mind it was expected behavior. I was already 2 weeks past my "calculated due date" and I was becoming increasingly worried. Today I went to work with a backache but felt no contractions. I managed to finish my shift but felt wiped out. As I walked to my car outside the hospital, my water broke and I felt the warm fluid run down my legs. I went back inside to be admitted for this much-awaited event.

Although I had helped thousands of women go through their childbirth experience, I was now the one in the bed and not standing alongside it. My husband and I had practiced our breathing techniques to cope with the discomfort of labor, but this "discomfort" in my mind was more than I could tolerate. So despite my best intentions of doing everything right, within an hour I begged for a "painkiller" to ease the pain. While the medication took the edge off my pain, I still felt every contraction and truly now appreciate the meaning of the word "labor." Although I wanted to use natural childbirth without any medication, I know that I was a full participant in my son's birthing experience, and that is what "doing everything right" was for me!

Thoughts: Doing what is right varies for each individual, and as nurses we need to support whatever that is. Having a positive outcome from the childbirth experience is the goal, not the means it takes to achieve it. How can nurses support women in making their personal choices to achieve a healthy outcome? Are any women "failures" if they ask for pain medication to tolerate labor? How can nurses help women overcome this stigma of being a "wimp"?

The health of mothers and their infants is of critical importance, both as a reflection of the current health status of a large segment of our population and as a predictor of the health of the next generation. *Healthy People 2010* (DHHS, 2000) addresses maternal health in two objectives for reducing maternal deaths and for reducing maternal illness and complications due to pregnancy. In addition, another objective addresses increasing the proportion of pregnant women who attend a series of prepared childbirth classes. (See Chapters 12 and 22 for more information on these objectives.)

This chapter provides information about nursing management during labor and birth. It describes the necessary data to be obtained with the admission assessment and methods to evaluate labor progress and maternal and fetal status. The chapter also describes the major methods for comfort promotion and pain management. The chapter concludes with a discussion of the nursing management specific to each stage of labor, including key nursing measures that focus on maternal and fetal assessments and pain relief.

Admission Assessments

The nurse usually first comes in contact with the woman either by phone or in person. It is important to ascertain whether the woman is in true or false labor and whether she should be admitted or sent home.

If the initial contact is by phone, the nurse needs to establish a therapeutic relationship with the woman. This is facilitated by speaking in a calm, caring tone. When completing a phone assessment, include questions about the following:

- Estimated date of birth, to determine if term or preterm
- Fetal movement (frequency in the past few days)
- Other premonitory signs of labor experienced
- Parity, gravida, and previous childbirth experiences
- Time from start of labor to birth in previous labors
- Characteristics of contractions, including frequency, duration, and intensity
- Appearance of any vaginal bloody show
- Membrane status (ruptured or intact)
- Presence of supportive adult in household or if she is alone

When speaking with the woman over the telephone, review the signs and symptoms that denote true versus false labor, and suggest various positions she can assume to provide comfort and increase placental perfusion. Also suggest walking, massaging, and taking a warm shower to promote relaxation. Outline what foods and fluids are appropriate for oral intake in early labor. Throughout the phone call, listen to the woman's concerns and answer any questions clearly.

Reducing the risk of liability exposure and avoiding preventable injuries to mothers and fetuses during labor and birth can be accomplished by adhering to two basic tenets of clinical practice: (1) use applicable evidence and/or published standards and guidelines as the foundation of care, and (2) whenever a clinical choice is presented, chose client safety (Simpson & Knox, 2003). With this advice in mind, advise the woman on the phone to contact her healthcare provider for further instructions or to come to the facility to be evaluated, since ruling out true labor and possible maternal-fetal complications cannot be done accurately over the phone.

Additional nursing responsibilities associated with a phone assessment include:

- Consult the woman's prenatal record for parity status, estimated date of birth, and untoward events.
- Call the healthcare provider to inform him or her of the woman's status.
- Prepare for admission to the perinatal unit to ensure adequate staff assignment.
- Notify the admissions office of a pending admission.

If the nurse's first encounter with the woman is in person, an assessment is completed to determine whether she should be admitted to the perinatal unit or sent home until her labor advances. Entering a facility is often an intimidating and stressful event for women since it is an unfamiliar environment. Giving birth for the first time is a pivotal event in the lives of most women. Therefore, demonstrate respect when addressing the client and thoroughly listen and express interest and concern. Nurses must value and respect women and promote their self-worth by allowing them to participate in making decisions and fostering a sense of control (Matthews & Callister, 2004).

An admission assessment includes maternal health history, physical assessment, fetal assessment, laboratory studies, and assessment of psychological status. Usually the facility has a specialized form that can be used throughout labor and birth to document assessment findings (Fig. 14-1).

Maternal Health History

A maternal health history should include typical biographical data such as the woman's name and age and the name of delivering healthcare provider. Other information that is collected includes the prenatal record data, including the estimated date of birth, a history of the current pregnancy, and the results of any laboratory and diagnostic tests, such as blood type and Rh status; past pregnancy and obstetric history; past health history and family history; prenatal education; list of medications; risk factors such as diabetes, hypertension, use of tobacco, alcohol, or illicit drugs; reason for admission, such as labor, cesarean birth, or observation for a complication; history of potential domestic violence; history of previous preterm births; allergies; time of last food ingestion; method chosen for infant feeding; name of birth attendant and pediatrician; and pain management plan.

Ascertaining this information is important to develop an individualized plan of care for the woman. If, for example, the woman's due date is still 2 months away, it is important to establish this information so interventions can be initiated to arrest the labor immediately or notify the intensive perinatal team to be available. In addition, if the woman is a diabetic, it is critical to monitor her glucose levels during labor, to prepare for a surgical birth if dystocia of labor occurs, and to alert the newborn nursery of potential hypoglycemia in the newborn after birth. By collecting important information about each woman they care for, nurses can help improve the outcomes for all concerned.

Be sure to observe the woman's emotions, support system, verbal interaction, body language and posture, perceptual acuity, and energy level. Also note her cultural background and language spoken. This psychosocial information provides cues about the woman's emotional state, culture, and communication systems. For example, if the woman arrives at the labor and birth suite extremely anxious, alone, and unable to communicate in English, how can the nurse meet her needs and plan her care appropriately? It is only by assessing each woman physically and psychosocially that the nurse can make astute decisions regarding proper care. In this case, an interpreter would be needed to assist in the communication process between the healthcare staff and the woman to initiate proper care.

It is important for the nurse to acknowledge and try to understand the cultural differences in women with cultural backgrounds different from that of the nurse. Attitudes toward childbirth are heavily influenced by the culture in which the woman has been raised. As a result, within every society, specific attitudes and values shape the woman's childbearing behaviors. Be aware of what these are. When carrying out a cultural assessment during the admission process, ask questions (Box 14-1) to help plan culturally competent care during labor and birth.

Physical Examination

The physical examination typically includes a generalized assessment of the woman's body systems, including hydration status, vital signs, auscultation of heart and lung sounds, and measurement of height and weight. The physical examination also includes the following assessments:

- Fundal height measurement
- Uterine activity, including contraction frequency, duration, and intensity
- Status of membranes (intact or ruptured)
- Cervical dilatation and degree of effacement
- Fetal status, including heart rate, position, and station
- Pain level

These assessment parameters (described in greater detail later in this chapter), form a baseline against which the nurse can compare all future values throughout labor. The findings should be similar to those of the woman's prepregnancy and pregnancy findings, with the exception

ADMISSION ASSESSMENT OBSTETRICS

▲ PATIENT IDENTIFICATION ▲

ADMISSION DATA

Date	Time	Via
		☐ Ambulatory ☐ Wheelchair ☐ Stretcher

Grav.	Term	Pre-term	Ab.	Living	EDC	LMP	GA

Prev. adm. date _____ Reason _____

Obstetrician _____ Pediatrician _____

Ht. _____ Wt. _____ Wt. gain _____

Allergies (meds/food) ☐ None _____ ☐ Hx latex sensitivity

BP _____ T _____ P _____ R _____

FHR _____ Vag exam _____

Reason for Admission

☐ Labor / SROM ☐ Induction _____

☐ Primary C/S _____ ☐ Repeat C/S

☐ Observation

☐ OB / Medical complication _____

Onset of labor: ☐ Not in labor

Date _____ Time _____

Membranes: ☐ Intact

☐ Ruptured / Date _____ Time _____

☐ Clear ☐ Meconium ☐ Bloody ☐ Foul

Vaginal bleeding: ☐ None

☐ Normal show ☐ _____

Current Pregnancy Labs   ☐ NPC

☐ POL ☐ PPROM ☐ Cerclage

☐ PIH ☐ Chr. HTN ☐ Other _____

☐ Diabetes _____ Diet _____

☐ Insulin _____

☐ Amniocentesis _____ Results _____

Bld type / RH _____ Date Rhogam _____

Antibody screen ☐ Neg ☐ Pos

Rubella ☐ Non-immune ☐ Immune

Diabetic screen ☐ Normal ☐ Abnormal

Recent exposure to chick pox ☐

Current meds: _____

_____

	Pos	Neg	Tested
Hepatitis B	☐	☐	☐ No
HIV	☐	☐	☐ No
Group B strep	☐	☐	☐ No
GC	☐	☐	☐ No
Chlamydia	☐	☐	☐ No
RPR	☐	☐	☐ No

Previous OB History

☐ POL ☐ Multiple gestation

☐ Prev C/S type _____ Reason _____

☐ PIH ☐ Chronic HTN ☐ Diabetes _____

☐ Stillbirth/demise ☐ Neodeath ☐ Anomalies

☐ Precipitous labor (<3 H) ☐ Macrosomia

☐ PP Hemorrhage

☐ Hx Transfusion reaction ☐ Yes ☐ No

☐ Other _____

Latest risk assessment ☐ None

1. _____ 3. _____

2. _____ 4. _____

Date _____

Signature _____ Time _____

NEUROLOGICAL

☐ WNL

Variance: ☐ HA

☐ Scotoma / visual changes

Reflexes ☐ < 2 + ☐ > 2 +

☐ Clonus ____ bts

☐ Numbness ☐ Tingling

☐ Hx Seizures

☐ _____

PESPIRATORY

☐ WNL

Variance: ☐ Hx Asthma ☐ URI

Respirations: ☐ < 12 ☐ > 24

Effort: ☐ SOB

☐ Shallow ☐ Labored

Auscultation:

☐ Diminished ☐ Crackles

☐ Wheezes ☐ Rhonchi

	No	Yes
Cough for greater than 2 weeks?	☐	☐
Is the cough productive?	☐	☐
Blood in the sputum?	☐	☐
Experiencing any fever or night sweats?	☐	☐
Ever had TB in the past?	☐	☐
Recent exposure to TB?	☐	☐
Weight loss in last 3 weeks?	☐	☐

If the patient answers yes to any three of the above questions implement policy and procedure # 5725-0704.

GASTROINTESTINAL

☐ WNL

Variance: ☐ Heartburn

☐ Epigastric pain ☐ Nausea

☐ Vomiting ☐ Diarrhea

☐ Constipation ☐ Pain

☐ Wt. Gain < 2lbs / month**

☐ Recent change in appetite of < 50% of usual intake for > 5 days

☐ _____

INTEGUMENTARY

☐ WNL

Variance: ☐ Rash ☐ Lacerations

☐ Abrasion ☐ Swelling

☐ Uticaria ☐ Bruising

☐ Diaphoretic/hot

☐ Clammy/cold

☐ Scars

☐ _____

FETAL ASSESSMENT

☐ WNL

Variance:

☐ NRFS

FHR ☐ < 110 ☐ > 160

LTV ☐ Absent ☐ Minimal

☐ Increased

STV Absent

Decelerations: _____

☐ Decreased fetal movement

☐ IUGR

☐ _____

CARDIOVASCULAR

☐ WNL

Variance:

☐ MVP

Heart rate: ☐ < 60 ☐ > 100

B/P: Systolic: ☐ < 90 ☐ > 140

Diastolic: ☐ < 50 ☐ > 90

☐ Edema _____

☐ Chest pain / palpitations

☐ _____

MUSCULOSKELETAL

☐ WNL

Variance:

☐ Numbness ☐ Tingling

☐ Paralysis ☐ Deformity

☐ Scoliosis

☐ _____

GENITOURINARY

☐ WNL

Variance: ☐ Albumin _____

Output: ☐ < 30 cc/Hr.

☐ UTI ☐ Rx ☐ Frequency

☐ Dysuria ☐ Hematuria

☐ CVA Tenderness

☐ Hx STD

☐ Vag. discharge _____

☐ Rash ☐ Blisters

☐ Warts ☐ Lesions

☐ _____

EARS, NOSE, THROAT, AND EYES

☐ WNL

Variance:

☐ Sore throat ☐ Eyeglasses

☐ Runny nose ☐ Contact lenses

☐ Nasal congestion

☐ _____

PSYCHOSOCIAL

☐ WNL

Variance: ☐ Hx depression

☐ Yes ☐ No

☐ Emotional behavioral care

Affect: ☐ Flat ☐ Anxious

☐ Uncooperative ☐ Combative

Living will ☐ Yes ☐ No

☐ On chart

Healthcare surrogate ☐ Yes ☐ No

☐ On chart

Are you being hurt, hit, frightened by anyone at home or in your life? ☐ Yes ☐ No

Religious preference _____

Tobacco use	☐ Denies	☐ Yes	Amt _____
Alcohol use	☐ Denies	☐ Yes	Amt _____
Drug use	☐ Denies	☐ Yes	Amt type ___
Primary language	☐ English	☐ Spanish	

PAIN ASSESSMENT

1. Do you have any ongoing pain problems? ☐ No ☐ Yes
2. Do you have any pain now? ☐ No ☐ Yes
3. If any of the above questions are answered yes, the patient has a positive pain screening.
4. Patient to be given pain management education material. Complete pain / symptom assessment on flowsheet.
5. Please proceed to complete pain assessment.

● Figure 14-1 Sample documentation form used for admission to the perinatal unit. (Used with permission. Briggs Corporation, 2001.)

334

of her pulse rate, which might be elevated secondary to her anxious state with beginning labor.

Laboratory Studies

On admission, laboratory studies typically are done to establish a baseline. Although the exact tests may vary among facilities, they usually include a urinalysis via clean-catch urine specimen and complete blood count (CBC). Blood typing and Rh factor analysis may be necessary if the results of these are unknown or unavailable. Other tests that may be done include syphilis screening, hepatitis B (HbsAg) screening, HIV testing (if woman gives consent), and possible drug screening if history is positive.

Evaluation of Labor Progress

Childbirth, a physiologic process that is fundamental to all human existence, is one of the most significant cultural, psychological, spiritual, and behavioral events in a woman's life. Although the act of giving birth is a uni-versal phenomenon, it is a unique experience for each woman. Continuous evaluation and appropriate intervention for women during labor are key to promoting a positive outcome for the family.

The nurse's role in childbirth is to ensure a safe environment for the mother and the birth of her newborn. Nurses begin evaluating the mother and fetus during the admission procedures at the healthcare agency and continue throughout labor. It is critical to provide anticipatory guidance and explain each procedure (fetal monitoring, intravenous therapy, medications given, and expected reactions) and what will happen next. This will prepare the woman for the upcoming physical and emotional challenges, thereby helping to reduce her anxiety. Acknowledging her support systems (family or partner) helps allay their fears and concerns, thereby assisting them in carrying out their supportive role. Knowing how and when to evaluate a woman during the various stages of labor is essential for all labor and birth nurses to ensure a positive maternal experience and a healthy newborn.

Maternal Assessment

During labor and birth, various techniques are used to assess maternal status. These techniques provide an ongoing source of data to determine the woman's response to and her progress in labor. Assess maternal vital signs, including temperature, blood pressure, pulse, respiration, and pain, which are primary components of the physical examination and ongoing assessment (Fig. 14-2). Also review the prenatal record to identify risk factors that may contribute to a decrease in uteroplacental circulation during labor. Monitor vital signs (blood pressure, pulse, and respirations) every 4 hours in the latent phase of labor, hourly in the active phase, and every 15 to 30 minutes during the transition phase of labor. Monitor temperature every 4 hours until the membranes have ruptured, and then every 1 to 2 hours thereafter. Assess uterine activity and fetal heart rate (FHR) every 30 to 60 minutes in the first stage of labor and every 15 to 30 minutes in the active

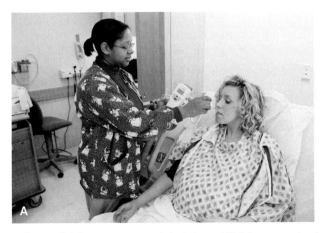
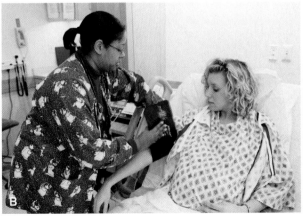

● Figure 14-2 Assessment of vital signs. (**A**) Nurse monitoring temperature. (**B**) Nurse assessing blood pressure.

and transition phases. If there is no vaginal bleeding on admission, a vaginal examination is performed to assess cervical dilation, after which it is monitored periodically as necessary to identify progress. Evaluate maternal pain and the effectiveness of pain-management strategies at regular intervals during labor and birth.

Vaginal Examination

Although not all nurses perform vaginal examinations on laboring women in all practice settings, most nurses working in community hospitals do so because physicians are not routinely present in labor and birth suites. Since most newborns in the United States are born in community hospitals, nurses are performing vaginal examinations (AHA, 2003). Vaginal examinations are also performed by midwives and physicians. It is an assessment skill that takes time and experience to develop; only by doing it frequently in clinical practice can the practitioner's skill level improve.

The purpose of performing a vaginal examination is to assess the amount of cervical dilation, percentage of cervical effacement, and fetal membrane status and gather information on presentation, position, station, degree of fetal head flexion, and presence of fetal skull swelling or molding (Fig. 14-3). Prepare the woman by informing her about the procedure, what information will be obtained from it, how she can assist with the procedure, how it will be performed, and who will be performing it.

The woman is typically on her back during the vaginal examination. The vaginal examination is performed gently, with concern for the woman's comfort. If it is the initial vaginal examination to check for membrane status, water is used as a lubricant. If membranes have already ruptured, an antiseptic solution is used to prevent an ascending infection. After donning sterile gloves, the examiner inserts his or her index and middle fingers into the vaginal introitus. Next, the cervix is palpated to assess dilation, effacement, and position (e.g., posterior or anterior). If the cervix is open to any degree, the presenting fetal part, fetal position, station, and presence of molding can be assessed. In addition, the membranes can be evaluated and described as intact, bulging, or ruptured.

At the conclusion of the vaginal examination, the findings are discussed with the woman and her partner to bring them up to date about labor progress. In addition, the findings are documented either electronically or in writing and reported to the primary healthcare professional in charge of the case.

Cervical Dilation and Effacement

The amount of cervical dilation and the degree of cervical effacement are key areas assessed during the vaginal examination as the cervix is palpated with the gloved index finger. Although this finding is somewhat subjective, experienced examiners typically come up with similar findings. The width of the cervical opening determines dilation, and the length of the cervix assesses effacement. The information yielded by this examination serves as a basis for determining which stage of labor the woman is in and what her ongoing care should be.

Fetal Descent and Presenting Part

In addition to cervical dilation and effacement findings, the vaginal examination can also determine fetal descent (station) and presenting part. During the vaginal examination, the gloved index finger is used to palpate the fetal skull (if vertex presentation) through the opened cervix or the buttocks in the case of a breech presentation. Station is assessed in relation to the maternal ischial spines and the presenting fetal part. These spines are not sharp protrusions but rather blunted prominences at the midpelvis. The ischial spines serve as landmarks and have been designated as zero station. If the presenting part is palpated higher than the maternal ischial spines, a negative number is assigned; if the presenting fetal part is felt below the maternal ischial spines, a plus number is assigned, denoting how many centimeters below zero station.

Progressive fetal descent (−5 to +4) is the expected norm during labor—moving downward from the negative stations to zero station to the positive stations in a timely manner. If progressive fetal descent does not occur, a disproportion between the maternal pelvis and the fetus might exist and needs to be investigated.

Rupture of Membranes

The integrity of the membranes can be determined during the vaginal examination. Typically, if intact, the membranes will be felt as a soft bulge that is more prominent during a contraction. If the membranes have ruptured, the woman may have reported a sudden gush of fluid. Membrane rupture also may occur as a slow trickle of fluid.

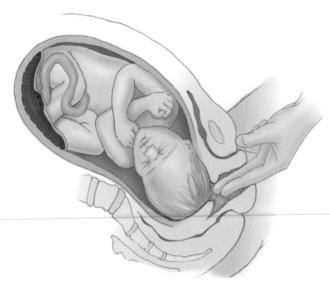

● Figure 14-3 Vaginal examination to determine cervical dilation and effacement.

To confirm that membranes have ruptured, a sample of fluid is taken from the vagina and tested with Nitrazine paper to determine the fluid's pH. Vaginal fluid is acidic, whereas amniotic fluid is alkaline and turns Nitrazine paper blue. Sometimes, however, false-positive results may occur, especially in women experiencing a large amount of bloody show, because blood is alkaline. The membranes are most likely intact if the Nitrazine test tape remains yellow to olive green, with pH between 5 and 6. The membranes are probably ruptured if the Nitrazine test tape turns a blue-green to deep blue, with pH ranging from 6.5 to 7.5 (Olds et al., 2004).

If the Nitrazine test is inconclusive, an additional test, called the fern test, can be used to confirm rupture of membranes. With this test, a sample of fluid is obtained, applied to a microscope slide, and allowed to dry. Using a microscope, the slide is examined for a characteristic fern pattern that indicates the presence of amniotic fluid.

Uterine Contractions

The primary power of labor is uterine contractions, which are involuntary. Uterine contractions increase intrauterine pressure, causing tension on the cervix. This tension leads to cervical dilation and thinning, which in turn eventually forces the fetus through the birth canal. Normal uterine contractions have a contraction (systole) and a relaxation (diastole) phase. The contraction resembles a wave, moving downward to the cervix and upward to the fundus of the uterus. Each contraction starts with a building up (increment), gradually reaching an acme (peak intensity), and then a letting down (decrement). Each contraction is followed by an interval of rest, which ends when the next contraction begins. At the acme (peak) of the contraction, the entire uterus is contracting, with the greatest intensity in the fundal area. The relaxation phase follows and occurs simultaneously throughout the uterus.

Uterine contractions during labor are monitored by palpation and by electronic monitoring. Assessment of the contractions includes frequency, duration, intensity, and uterine resting tone (see Chapter 13 for a more detailed discussion).

Uterine contractions with an intensity of 30 mm Hg or greater initiate cervical dilation. During active labor, the intensity usually reaches 50 to 80 mm Hg. Resting tone is normally between 5 and 10 mm Hg in early labor and between 12 and 18 mm Hg in active labor (Gilbert & Harmon, 2003).

To palpate the fundus for contraction intensity, place the pads of your fingers on the fundus and describe how it feels: like the tip of the nose (mild), like the chin (moderate), or like the forehead (strong). Palpation of intensity is a subjective judgment of the indentability of the uterine wall; a descriptive term is assigned (mild, moderate, or strong (Fig. 14-4). Frequent clinical experience is needed to gain accuracy in assessing the intensity of uterine contractions.

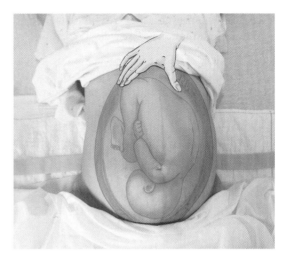

● Figure 14-4 Nurse palpating the woman's fundus during a contraction.

The second method used to assess the intensity of uterine contractions is electronic monitoring, either external or internal. Both methods provide an accurate measurement of the actual intensity of uterine contractions. Although the external fetal monitor is sometimes used to estimate the intensity of uterine contractions, it is not as accurate an assessment tool.

For woman at risk for preterm birth, home uterine activity monitoring can be used to screen for prelabor uterine contractility so that escalating contractility can be identified, allowing earlier intervention to prevent preterm birth. The home uterine activity monitor consists of a pressure sensor attached to a belt that is held against the abdomen and a recording/storage device that is carried on a belt or hung from the shoulder. Uterine activity is typically recorded by the woman for one hour twice daily, while performing routine activities. The stored data are transmitted via telephone to a perinatal nurse, where a receiving device prints out the data. The woman is contacted if there are any problems.

Although in theory identifying early contractions to initiate interventions to arrest the labor sounds reasonable, research shows that uterine activity monitoring in asymptomatic high-risk women is inadequate for predicting preterm birth (Newman, 2003). This practice continues even though numerous randomized trials have found no relationship between monitoring and actual reduction of preterm labor. The value of monitoring uterine contraction frequency as a predictor of preterm delivery remains unclear (Iams et al., 2002).

Leopold's Maneuvers

Leopold's maneuvers are a method for determining the presentation, position, and lie of the fetus through the use of four specific steps. This method involves inspection and palpation of the maternal abdomen as a screening assessment for malpresentation. A longitudinal lie is expected, and the presentation can be cephalic, breech, or shoulder. Each maneuver answers a question:

• What fetal part (head or buttocks) is located in the fundus (top of the uterus)?
• On which maternal side is the fetal back located? (Fetal heart tones are best auscultated through the back of the fetus.)

• What is the presenting part?
• Is the fetal head flexed and engaged in the pelvis? (Nursing Procedure 14-1)

Fetal Assessment

A fetal assessment identifies well-being and signs indicative of compromise. It primarily focuses on determining the

---

Nursing Procedure 14-1

Performing Leopold's Maneuvers

Purpose: To Determine Fetal Presentation, Position, and Lie

1. Place the woman in the supine position and stand beside her.
2. Perform the first maneuver to determine presentation.
   a. Facing the woman's head, place both hands on the abdomen to determine fetal position in the uterine fundus.
   b. Feel for the buttocks, which will feel soft and irregular (indicates vertex presentation); feel for the head, which will feel hard, smooth, and round (indicates a breech presentation).

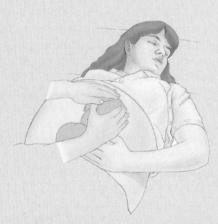

First maneuver

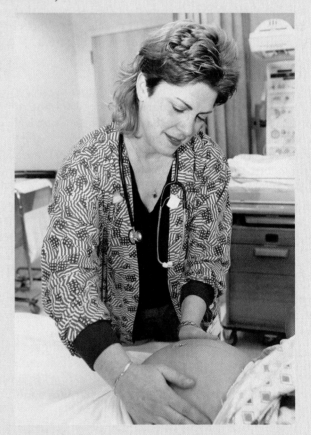

Second maneuver

3. Complete the second maneuver to determine position.
   a. While still facing the woman, move hands down the lateral sides of the abdomen to palpate on which side the back is (feels hard and smooth).
   b. Continue to palpate to determine on which side the limbs are located (irregular nodules with kicking and movement).

4. Perform the third maneuver to confirm presentation.
   a. Move hands down the sides of the abdomen to grasp the lower uterine segment and palpate the area just above the symphysis pubis.
   b. Place thumb and fingers of one hand apart and grasp the presenting part by bringing fingers together.
   c. Feel for the presenting part. If the presenting part is the head, it will be round, firm, and ballottable; if it is the buttocks, it will feel soft and irregular.

Nursing Procedure 14-1

Performing Leopold's Maneuvers (continued)

Purpose: To Determine Fetal Presentation, Position, and Lie

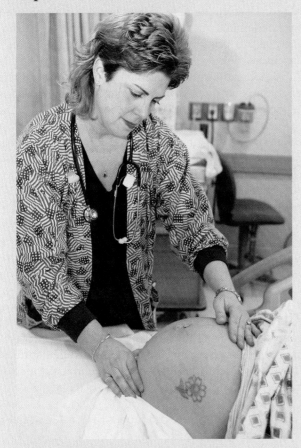

Third maneuver

b. Move fingers toward each other while applying downward pressure in the direction of the symphysis pubis. If you palpate a hard area on the side opposite the fetal back, the fetus is in flexion, because you have palpated the chin. If the hard area is on the same side as the back, the fetus is in extension, because the area palpated is the occiput.

c. Also, note how your hands move. If the hands move together easily, the fetal head is not descended into the woman's pelvic inlet. If the hands do not move together and stop because of resistance, the fetal head is engaged into the woman's pelvic inlet (Dillon, 2003).

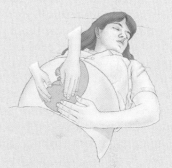

Fourth maneuver

5. Perform the fourth maneuver to determine attitude.
   a. Turn to face the client's feet and use the tips of the first three fingers of each hand to palpate the abdomen.

FHR pattern, but the character of the amniotic fluid is also assessed. Amniotic fluid should be clear when membranes rupture, either spontaneously or artificially through an amniotomy (a disposable plastic hook [Amnihook] is used to perforates the amniotic sac). Cloudy or foul-smelling amniotic fluid indicates infection, whereas green fluid indicates that the fetus has passed meconium secondary to transient hypoxia (McKinney et al., 2005).

Analysis of the FHR is one of the primary evaluation tools used to determine fetal oxygen status indirectly. FHR assessment can be done intermittently using a fetoscope (a modified stethoscope attached to a headpiece) or a Doppler (ultrasound) device or continuously with an electronic fetal monitor applied externally or internally.

Intermittent FHR Monitoring

Intermittent FHR monitoring involves auscultation via a fetoscope or a hand-held Doppler device that uses ultrasound waves that bounce off the fetal heart, producing echoes or clicks that reflect the rate of the fetal heart (Fig. 14-5). Traditionally, a fetoscope was used to assess fetal heart rate, but the Doppler device has been found to have a greater sensitivity than the fetoscope (Engstrom, 2004); thus, at present it is more commonly used.

Doppler devices are relatively low in cost and are not used only in hospitals. Pregnant women can purchase them to aid in reducing anxiety between clinical examinations if they had a previous problem during pregnancy (Mainstone, 2004).

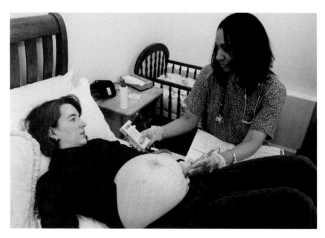

● Figure 14-5 Auscultating fetal heart rate.

Intermittent FHR monitoring affords the advantage of mobility for the woman in the first stage of labor. She is free to move around and change position at will since she is not attached to a stationary electronic fetal monitor. However, intermittent monitoring does not document how the fetus responds to the stress of labor and does not provide a continuous recording of the fetal heart rate. In addition, it does not show the fetal response during the acme of a contraction, because intermittent monitoring is typically done after a contraction, when the uterus is relaxed. The pressure of the device during a contraction is uncomfortable and can distract the woman from using her paced-breathing patterns.

Intermittent FHR auscultation can be used to detect FHR baseline and rhythm and changes from baseline. However, it cannot detect variability and types of decelerations, as electronic fetal monitoring can (Feinstein et al., 2003). During intermittent auscultation to establish a baseline, the FHR is assessed for a full minute after a contraction. From then on, unless there is a problem, listening for 30 seconds and multiplying the value by two is sufficient. If the woman experiences a change in condition during labor, auscultation assessments should be more frequent. Changes in condition include ruptured membranes or the onset of bleeding. In addition, more frequent assessments occur after periods of ambulation, after a vaginal examination, after administration of pain medications, or other clinical important events (SOGC, 2002).

The FHR is heard most clearly at the fetal back. In a cephalic presentation, the FHR is best heard in the lower quadrant of the maternal abdomen. In a breech presentation, it is heard at or above the level of the maternal umbilicus (Fig. 14-6). As labor progresses, the FHR location will change accordingly as the fetus descends lower into the maternal pelvis for the birthing process. To ensure that the maternal heart rate is not confused with the fetal heart rate, palpate the client's radial pulse simultaneously while the FHR is being auscultated through the abdomen.

The procedure for using a fetoscope or Doppler device to assess FHR is similar (see Nursing Procedure 12-1 in Chapter 12). The main difference is that a small amount of water-soluble gel is applied to the woman's abdomen or ultrasound device before auscultation to promote sound wave transmission. This gel is not needed when a fetoscope is used. Usually the FHR is best heard in the woman's lower abdominal quadrants, but if it is not found quickly, it may help to locate the fetal back by performing Leopold's maneuvers.

Although the intermittent method of FHR assessment allows the client to move about during her labor, the information obtained fails to provide a complete picture of the well-being of the fetus moment to moment. This leads to the question of what the fetal status is during the times that are not assessed. For women who are considered at low risk for complications, this period of non-assessment is not a problem. However, for the undiagnosed high-risk woman, it might prove ominous.

National professional organizations have provided general guidelines for the frequency of assessments based on existing evidence. The American College of Obstetricians and Gynecologists (ACOG), the Institute for Clinical Systems Improvement (ICSI), and the Association of Women's Health, Obstetric, and Neonatal Nurses (AWHONN) have published guidelines designed to assist clinicians in caring for laboring clients. Their recommendations are supported by large controlled studies. They recommend the following guidelines for assessing FHR:

- Initial 10- to 20-minute continuous FHR assessment on entry into labor/birth area
- Completion of a prenatal and labor risk assessment on all clients
- Intermittent auscultation every 30 minutes during active labor for a low-risk woman and every 15 minutes for a high-risk woman
- During the second stage of labor, every 15 minutes for the low-risk woman and every 5 minutes for the high-risk woman and during the pushing stage (ACOG, 2005; AWHONN, 2000; ICSI, 2003).

In several randomized controlled studies comparing intermittent auscultation with electronic monitoring in both low- and high-risk clients, no difference in intrapartum fetal death was found. However, in each study a nurse–client ratio of 1:1 was consistently maintained during labor (ICSI, 2003). This suggests that adequate staffing is essential with intermittent FHR monitoring to ensure optimal outcomes for the mother and fetus. Although there is insufficient evidence to indicate specific situations where continuous electronic fetal monitoring might result in better outcomes when compared to intermittent assessment, for pregnancies involving an increased risk of peri-

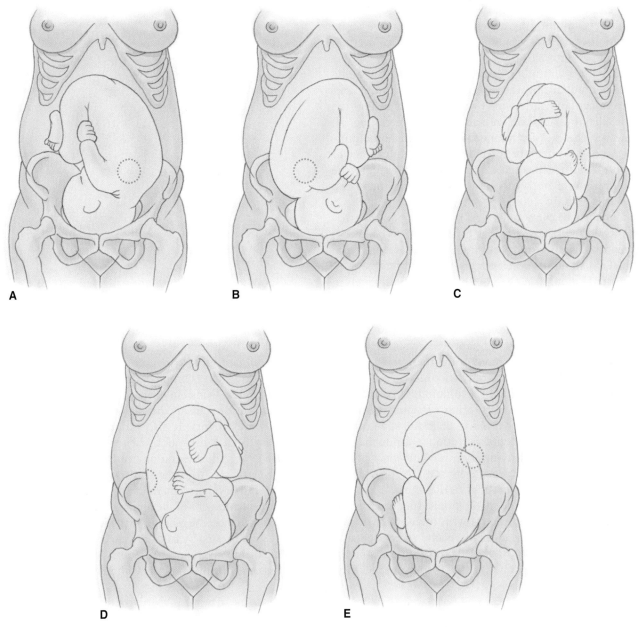

● Figure 14-6 Locations for auscultating fetal heart rate based on fetal position. (**A**) Left occiput anterior (LOA). (**B**) Right occiput anterior (ROA). (**C**) Left occiput posterior (LOP). (**D**) Right occiput posterior (ROP). (**E**) Left sacral anterior (LSA).

natal death, cerebral palsy, or neonatal encephalopathy and use of oxytocin for induction or augmentation, it is recommended that continuous electronic fetal monitoring be used rather than intermittent fetal auscultation (SOGC, 2002, p. 6).

Continuous Electronic Fetal Monitoring

Electronic fetal monitoring uses a machine to produce a continuous tracing of the FHR. When the monitoring device is in place, an audible sound is produced with each heartbeat. In addition, a graphic record of the FHR pattern is produced.

Current methods of continuous electronic fetal monitoring were introduced in the United States during the 1960s, specifically for use in clients considered to be high risk. However, the use of these methods gradually increased and they eventually came to be used for women considered to be high or low risk. This increased use has become controversial, because it was suspected of being associated with unnecessary cesarean birth, rates of which have climbed steadily (Sisk, 2002). The efficacy of electronic fetal monitoring depends on the accurate interpretation of the tracings, not necessarily which method (external vs. internal) is used.

Having a continuous assessment of fetal well-being documented during the stress of labor is important. The concept of hearing and evaluating every beat of the fetus's heart to allow for early intervention seems logical. However, the use of continuous electronic fetal monitoring has had no demonstrated effect on the incidence of newborns born with neurologic damage. Furthermore, the rate of preterm birth and cesarean births has increased markedly (Priddy, 2004).

The use of continuous fetal monitoring for all pregnant clients, whether high risk or low risk, has been criticized by various groups within the medical community. Concerns about the efficiency and safety of routine electronic fetal monitoring in labor have led expert panels in the United States to recommend that such monitoring be limited to high-risk pregnancies. However, its use in low-risk pregnancies continues globally (Thacker & Stroup, 2003). This remains an important research issue.

With electronic fetal monitoring, there is a continuous record of the fetal heart rate, and thus no gaps exist, as they do with intermittent auscultation. On the downside, using continuous monitoring can limit maternal movement and encourages her to lie in the supine position, which reduces placental perfusion. Despite the criticism, electronic fetal monitoring remains an accurate method for determining fetal health status by providing a moment-to-moment printout of FHR status.

Continuous electronic fetal monitoring can be performed externally (indirectly) with attachment to the maternal abdominal wall or internally (directly) with attachment to the fetus. Both methods provide a continuous printout of the FHR, but they differ in their specificity.

External Monitoring

In external or indirect monitoring, two ultrasound transducers, each of which is attached to a belt, are applied around the woman's abdomen. They are similar to the hand-held Doppler device. One transducer, called a tocotransducer, detects changes in uterine pressure and converts the pressure registered into an electronic signal that is recorded on graph paper (Pillitteri, 2003). The tocotransducer is placed over the uterine fundus in the area of greatest contractility to monitor uterine contractions. The other ultrasound transducer records the baseline FHR, long-term variability, accelerations, and decelerations. It is positioned on the maternal abdomen in the midline between the umbilicus and the symphysis pubis. The diaphragm of the ultrasound transducer is moved to either side of the abdomen to obtain a stronger sound and then attached to the second elastic belt. This transducer converts the fetal heart movements into audible beeping sounds and records them on graph paper (Fig. 14-7).

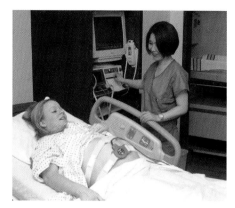

● Figure 14-7 Continuous external EFM device applied to the woman in labor.

Good continuous data are provided on the FHR. External monitoring can be used while the membranes are still intact and the cervix is not yet dilated. It is non-invasive and can detect relative changes in abdominal pressure between uterine resting tone and contractions. External monitoring also measures the approximate duration and frequency of contractions, providing a permanent record of FHR (Feinstein et al., 2003).

However, external monitoring can restrict the mother's movements. It also cannot detect short-term variability. Signal disruptions can occur due to maternal obesity, fetal malpresentation, and fetal movement, as well as by artifact. **Artifact** describes irregular variations or absence of FHR on the fetal monitor record, resulting from mechanical limitations of the monitor or electrical interference. For instance, the monitor may pick up transmissions from CB radios used by truck drivers on nearby roads and translate them into a signal. Additionally, gaps in the monitor strip can occur periodically without explanation.

Continuous Internal Monitoring

Continuous internal monitoring is usually indicated for women or fetuses considered high risk. Possible conditions might include multiple gestation, decreased fetal movement, abnormal FHR on auscultation, intrauterine growth restriction (IUGR), maternal fever, preeclampsia, dysfunctional labor, preterm birth, or medical conditions such as diabetes or hypertension. It involves the placement of a spiral electrode into the fetal presenting part, usually the head, to assess FHR and a pressure transducer internally to record uterine contractions (Fig. 14-8). The fetal spiral electrode is considered the most accurate method of detecting fetal heart characteristics and patterns because it involves directly receiving a signal from the fetus (Feinstein et al., 2003).

Both the FHR and the duration and interval of uterine contractions are recorded on the graph paper. This method permits evaluation of baseline heart rate and changes in rate and pattern.

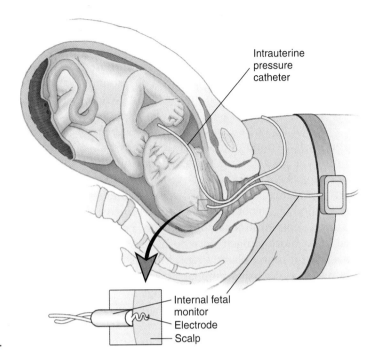

● Figure 14-8 Continuous internal EFM.

Four specific criteria must be met for this type of monitoring to be used:

- Ruptured membranes
- Cervical dilation of at least 2 cm
- Presenting fetal part low enough to allow placement of the scalp electrode
- Skilled practitioner available to insert spiral electrode (Ladewig, London, & Davidson, 2006)

Compared to external monitoring, continuous internal monitoring can accurately detect both short-term (moment-to-moment changes) and long-term variability (fluctuations within the baseline) and FHR dysrhythmias. In addition, it allows for maternal positional changes and movement that doesn't interfere with the quality of the tracing.

FHR Patterns

Assessment parameters of the FHR are classified as baseline rate, baseline variability (long-term and short-term), and periodic changes in the rate (accelerations and decelerations). The nurse must be able to interpret the various FHR parameters to determine if the pattern is reassuring (indicating fetal well-being) or nonreassuring (indicating fetal problems) to care for the woman effectively during labor and birth. Table 14-1 summarizes these patterns.

Baseline FHR

Baseline fetal heart rate refers to the average FHR that occurs during a 10-minute segment that excludes periodic or episodic rate changes, such as tachycardia or

Table 14-1 Interpreting FHR Patterns

FHR Pattern	
Reassuring FHR signs	• Normal baseline (110–160 bpm) • Moderate bradycardia (100–120 bpm); good variability • Good beat-to-beat variability and fetal accelerations
Nonreassuring signs	• Fetal tachycardia (>160 bpm) • Moderate bradycardia (100–110 bpm); lost variability • Absent beat-to-beat variability • Marked bradycardia (90–100 bpm) • Moderate variable decelerations
Ominous signs	• Fetal tachycardia with loss of variability • Prolonged marked bradycardia (<90 bpm) • Severe variable decelerations (<70 bpm) • Persistent late decelerations

Sources: Moses, 2003; Littleton & Engebretson, 2005; Feinstein et al., 2003; Engstrom, 2004; Tucker, 2004.

bradycardia. It is assessed when the woman has no contractions and the fetus is not experiencing episodic FHR changes. The normal baseline FHR ranges between 110 and 160 beats per minute (bpm). The normal baseline FHR can be obtained by auscultation, ultrasound, or Doppler, or by a continuous internal direct fetal electrode.

Fetal bradycardia occurs when the FHR is below 110 bpm and lasts 10 minutes or longer. It can be the initial response of a healthy fetus to asphyxia. Causes of fetal bradycardia might include fetal hypoxia, prolonged maternal hypoglycemia, fetal acidosis, administration of drugs to the mother, hypothermia, maternal hypotension, prolonged umbilical cord compression, and fetal congenital heart block (Engstrom, 2004). Bradycardia may be benign if it is an isolated event, but it is considered an ominous sign when accompanied by a decrease in long-term variability and late decelerations.

Fetal tachycardia is a baseline FHR greater than 160 bpm that lasts for 10 minutes or longer. It can represent an early compensatory response to asphyxia. Other causes of fetal tachycardia include fetal hypoxia, maternal fever, maternal dehydration, amnionitis, drugs (e.g., cocaine, amphetamines, nicotine), maternal hyperthyroidism, maternal anxiety, fetal anemia, prematurity, fetal heart failure, and fetal arrhythmias (Ladewig, London, & Davidson, 2006). Fetal tachycardia is considered an ominous sign if it is accompanied by a decrease in variability and late decelerations (Ladewig, London, & Davidson, 2006).

Baseline Variability

Baseline variability is defined as the fluctuations of the FHR observed along the baseline in the absence of contractions, decelerations, and accelerations (Cypher et al., 2003). It represents the interplay between the parasympathetic and sympathetic nervous systems. The constant interplay (push-and-pull effect) on the FHR from the parasympathetic and sympathetic systems produces a moment-to-moment change in the FHR. Because variability is in essence the combined result of autonomic nervous system branch function, its presence implies that the both branches are working and receiving adequate oxygen (Feinstein et al., 2003). Thus, variability is one of the most important characteristics of the FHR. Two components of baseline variability are described: short-term and long-term.

Short-term variability is the beat-to-beat change in FHR. It represents the variations or fluctuations of the baseline that, when seen on the fetal monitor tracing, produces the irregularity within the baseline. It can be measured by internal monitoring and is classified as either present or absent. The presence of short-term variability typically indicates a well-oxygenated, nonacidemic fetus (Murray, 2004). The most practical way to determine the presence or absence of short-term variability is visually. The fetal heart tracing line is evaluated for roughness or smoothness. If roughness is present in the baseline, short-term variability is present; if smoothness is present, it is absent.

Long-term variability is the waviness or rhythmic fluctuations, which are described as cycles per minute. The frequency of cycles is 3 to 6 per minute. It is classified as absent (<3 bpm), decreased or minimal (3 to 5 bpm), average or moderate (6 to 25 bpm), and marked or salutatory (>25 bpm) (Cypher et al., 2003) (Fig. 14-9).

FHR variability is an important clinical indicator that is predictive of fetal acid–base balance and cerebral tissue perfusion (Baird & Ruth, 2002). As the central nervous system is desensitized by hypoxia and acidosis, FHR decreases until a smooth baseline pattern appears. Loss of variability may be associated with a poor outcome. Some causes of decreased variability include fetal hypoxia/acidosis, drugs that depress the central nervous system, congenital abnormalities, fetal sleep, prematurity, and fetal tachycardia (Pillitteri, 2003).

External electronic fetal monitoring is not able to assess short-term variability. Therefore, if external monitoring shows a baseline that is smoothing out, use of an internal spiral electrode should be considered to gain a more accurate picture of the fetal health status.

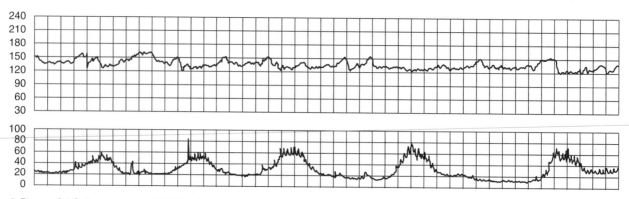

● Figure 14-9 Long-term variability (average or moderate).

Periodic Baseline Changes

Periodic baseline changes are temporary, recurrent changes made in response to a stimulus such as a contraction. The FHR can demonstrate patterns of acceleration or deceleration in response to most stimuli. Fetal **accelerations** are transitory increases in the FHR above the baseline associated with sympathetic nervous stimulation. They are visually apparent, with elevations of FHR of at least 15 bpm above the baseline, and usually last longer than 15 seconds but not for longer than 2 minutes (King & Simpson, 2001). Their appearance provides evidence of fetal well-being and is generally considered reassuring and requires no interventions. Accelerations denote fetal movement and fetal well-being and are the basis for nonstress testing.

A **deceleration** is a transient fall in FHR caused by stimulation of the parasympathetic nervous system. Decelerations are described by their shape and association to a uterine contraction. They are classified as early, late, variable, and prolonged (Fig. 14-10).

Early decelerations are characterized by a gradual decrease in the FHR in which the nadir (lowest point) occurs at the peak of the contraction. They rarely decrease more than 30 to 40 bpm below the baseline. Early decelerations mirror the appearance of the uterine contraction

below it on the fetal tracing. They are most often seen during the active stage of any normal labor, during pushing, crowning, or vacuum extraction. They are thought to be a result of fetal head compression that results in a reflex vagal response with a resultant slowing of the FHR during uterine contractions. Early decelerations are not indicative of fetal distress and do not require intervention.

Late decelerations are transitory decreases in FHR that occur after a contraction begins. The FHR does not return to baseline levels until well after the contraction has ended. Delayed timing of the deceleration occurs, with the nadir of the uterine contraction. Late decelerations are associated with uteroplacental insufficiency, which occurs when blood flow within the intervillous space is decreased to the extent that fetal hypoxia exists (McKinney et al., 2005). Conditions that may decrease uteroplacental perfusion with resultant decelerations include maternal hypotension, gestational hypertension, placental aging secondary to diabetes and postmaturity, hyperstimulation via oxytocin infusion, maternal smoking, anemia, and cardiac disease. They imply some degree of fetal hypoxia. Repetitive late decelerations and late decelerations with decreasing baseline variability are nonreassuring signs. Box 14-2 highlights interventions for decelerations.

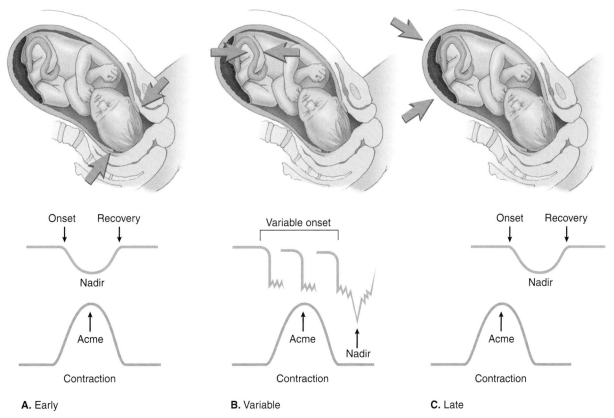

A. Early	**B.** Variable	**C.** Late

● Figure 14-10 Decelerations. (**A**) Early. (**B**) Variable. (**C**) Late.

Variable decelerations have an unpredictable shape on the FHR baseline, possibly demonstrating no consistent relationship to uterine contractions. The shape of variable decelerations may be U, V, or W, or they may not resemble other patterns (Feinstein et al., 2003). Variable decelerations usually occur abruptly with quick deceleration. They are the most common deceleration pattern found in the laboring woman and are usually transient and correctable (Garite, 2002). Variable decelerations are associated with cord compression. However, they become a nonreassuring sign when the FHR decreases to less than 60 bpm, persists at that level for at least 60 seconds, and is repetitive (ICSI, 2003). The pattern of variable deceleration consistently related to the contractions with a slow return to FHR baseline is also nonreassuring.

Prolonged decelerations are abrupt FHR declines of at least 15 bpm that last longer than 2 minutes but less than 10 minutes. The rate usually drops to less than 90 bpm. Many factors are associated with this pattern, including prolonged cord compression, abruptio placentae, cord prolapse, supine maternal position, vaginal examination, fetal blood sampling, maternal seizures, regional anes-

thesia, or uterine rupture (Mattson & Smith, 2004). Prolonged decelerations can be remedied by identifying the underlying cause and correcting it.

Combinations of FHR patterns obtained by electronic fetal monitoring during labor are not infrequent. Nonreassuring patterns are more significant if they are mixed and persist for long periods of time. Other nonreassuring patterns include prolonged late decelerations, absent or minimal variability, bradycardia or tachycardia, and prolonged variable decelerations lower than 60 bpm. The likelihood of fetal compromise is increased if various nonreassuring patterns coexist, particularly those associated with decreased baseline variability or abnormal contraction patterns (ICSI, 2003).

Other Fetal Assessment Methods

In situations suggesting the possibility of fetal compromise, such as inconclusive or nonreassuring FHR patterns, further ancillary testing such as fetal scalp sampling, fetal pulse oximetry, and fetal stimulation may be used to validate the FHR findings and assist in planning interventions.

Fetal Scalp Sampling

Fetal scalp sampling was developed as a means of measuring fetal distress in conjunction with electronic fetal monitoring to make critical decisions about the management of labor and to prevent unnecessary operative interventions resulting from the use of electronic fetal monitoring alone. Nonreassuring FHR patterns may not necessarily indicate fetal hypoxia or acidosis. Therefore, assessing fetal acid–base status through fetal scalp sampling may help to prevent needless surgical intervention.

A sample of fetal scalp blood is obtained to measure the pH. Sampling requires that the woman have ruptured membranes, cervical dilation of at least 3 to 5 cm, and a vertex presentation at −1 station (Torgersen, 2004). Normal fetal blood pH is 7.25 to 7.35. When the fetal scalp pH is below 7.15, the majority of neonates will have an Apgar score of less than 6 (Torgersen, 2004).

During the past decade, the use of fetal scalp sampling has decreased, being replaced by less invasive techniques that yield similar information.

Fetal Oxygen Saturation Monitoring (Fetal Pulse Oximetry)

Fetal pulse oximetry measures fetal oxygen saturation directly and in real time. It is used with electronic fetal monitoring as an adjunct method of assessment when the FHR pattern is nonreassuring or inconclusive. Normal oxygen saturation of a healthy fetus is 30% to 70% (Sisk, 2002). If the fetal oxygen saturation is reassuring (a trend of >30% between contractions), unnecessary cesarean births, invasive procedures such as fetal blood sampling, and operative vaginal births can be minimized (Simpson,

2003). Any reduction in unnecessary interventions during labor and birth has the potential to improve maternal and fetal outcomes and reduce costs.

Adequate maintenance of fetal oxygenation is necessary for fetal well-being. Fetal oxygen saturation monitoring is used for a singleton term fetus in a vertex presentation, at a −2 station or below, and with a nonreassuring FHR pattern. In addition, the fetal membranes must be ruptured and the cervix dilated at least 2 cm (Simpson & Porter, 2001). A soft sensor is introduced through the dilated cervix and placed on the cheek, forehead, or temple of the fetus. It is held in place by the uterine wall. The sensor then is attached to a special adaptor on the fetal monitor that provides a real-time recording that is displayed on the uterine activity panel of the tracing. It is a noninvasive, safe, and accurate method for assessing fetal oxygenation.

The fetal pulse oximetry traces along the contraction portion of the monitoring strip, so it is easy to see how the saturation changes with the contraction. This adjunct test can help support decisions to allow labor to continue or to intervene surgically. Observing the trend of oxygen saturation on the tracing and documenting the values on the labor flow sheet or other medical record forms is crucial. The physician or midwife must be notified if the fetal oxygen saturation becomes nonreassuring (<30% between contractions) in conjunction with a nonreassuring FHR pattern. Ongoing communication is needed between the nurse and the primary care provider to enhance the maternal-fetus status.

Fetal Stimulation

An indirect method used to evaluate fetal oxygenation and acid–base balance to identify fetal hypoxia is fetal scalp stimulation and vibroacoustic stimulation. If the fetus does not have adequate oxygen reserves, carbon dioxide builds up, leading to acidemia and hypoxemia. These metabolic states are reflected in nonreassuring FHR patterns as well as fetal inactivity. Fetal stimulation is performed to promote fetal movement with the hope that FHR accelerations will accompany the movement.

Fetal movement can be stimulated with a vibroacoustic stimulator (artificial larynx) applied to the woman's lower abdomen and turned on for a few seconds to produce sound and vibration or by tactile stimulation via pelvic examination and stimulation of the fetal scalp with the gloved fingers. A well-oxygenated fetus will respond when stimulated (tactile or by noise) by moving in conjunction with an acceleration of 15 bpm above the baseline heart rate that lasts at least 15 seconds. This FHR acceleration reflects a pH of more than 7 and a fetus with an intact central nervous system. Fetal scalp stimulation is not done if the fetus is preterm, or if the woman has an intrauterine infection, a diagnosis of placenta previa (which could lead to hemorrhage), or a fever (which increases the risk of an ascending infection) (McKinney et al., 2005).

Comfort Promotion and Pain Management

Pain during labor is a universal experience, although the intensity of the pain may vary. Although labor and childbirth are viewed as natural processes, both can produce significant pain and discomfort. The physical causes of pain during labor include cervical stretching, hypoxia of the uterine muscle due to a decrease in perfusion during contractions, pressure on the urethra, bladder, and rectum, and distention of the muscles of the pelvic floor (Leonard, 2002). A woman's pain perception can be influenced by her previous experiences with pain, fatigue, pain anticipation, positive or negative support system, labor and birth environment, cultural expectations, and level of emotional stress and anxiety (Hodnett, 2002a).

The techniques used to manage the pain of labor vary according to geography and culture. For example, some Appalachian women believe that placing a hatchet or knife under the bed of a laboring woman may help "cut the pain of childbirth" and a woman from this background may wish to do so in the hospital setting (Stephens, 2003). Cherokee, Hmong, and Japanese women will often remain quiet during labor and birth and not complain of pain because outwardly expressing pain is not appropriate in their cultures. Never interpret their quietness as freedom from pain (Moore & Moos, 2003).

Today, women have many safe nonpharmacologic and pharmacologic choices for the management of pain during labor and birth, which may be used separately or in combination with one another.

Nurses are in an ideal position to provide childbearing women with balanced, clear, concise information regarding effective nonpharmacologic and pharmacologic measures to relieve pain. Pain management standards issued by JCAHO mandate that pain be assessed in all clients admitted to a healthcare facility. Thus, it is important for nurses to be knowledgeable about the most recent scientific research on labor pain-relief modalities, to make sure that accurate and unbiased information about effective pain-relief measures is available to laboring women, to be sure that the woman determines what is an acceptable labor pain level for her, and to allow the woman the choice of pain-relief method.

Nonpharmacologic Measures

Nonpharmacological measures may include continuous labor support, hydrotherapy, ambulation and position changes, acupuncture and acupressure, attention focusing and imagery, therapeutic touch and massage, and breathing techniques and effleurage. Most of these methods are based on the "gate control" theory of pain, which proposes that local physical stimulation can interfere with pain stimuli by closing a hypothetical gate in the spinal cord, thus blocking pain signals from reaching the brain (Engstrom, 2004). It has long been a standard of care for labor nurses to first provide or encourage a variety of non-pharmacologic measures before moving to the pharmacologic interventions.

Nonpharmacologic measures are usually simple, safe, and inexpensive to use. Many of these measures are taught in childbirth classes, and women should be encouraged to try a variety of methods prior to the real labor. Many of the measures need to be practiced for best results and coordinated with the partner/coach. The nurse provides support and encouragement for the woman and her partner using nonpharmacologic methods. Although women can't consciously direct the contractions occurring during labor, they can control how they respond to them, thereby enhancing their feelings of control.

Continuous Labor Support

Continuous labor support involves offering a sustained presence to the laboring woman by providing emotional support, comfort measures, advocacy, information and advice, and support for the partner (Trainor, 2002). This continuous presence can be provided by a woman's family, a midwife, a nurse, a doula, or anyone else close to the woman. A support person can assist the woman to ambulate, reposition herself, and use breathing techniques. A support person can also aid with the use of acupressure, massage, music therapy, or therapeutic touch. During the natural course of childbirth, a laboring woman's functional ability is limited secondary to pain, and she often has trouble making decisions. The support person can help make them based on his or her knowledge of the woman's birth plan and personal wishes.

Research has validated the value of continuous labor support versus intermittent support in terms of lower operative deliveries, cesarean births, and requests for pain medication (Hodnett, 2002b; Hunter, 2002). The human presence is of immeasurable value to make the laboring woman feel secure.

Hydrotherapy

Hydrotherapy is a nonpharmacologic measure in which the woman immerses herself in warm water for relaxation and relief of discomfort. Upon entering the warm water, the warmth and buoyancy help to release muscle tension and can impart a sense of well-being (Primeau et al., 2003). Warm water provides soothing stimulation of nerves in the skin, promoting vasodilatation, reversal of sympathetic nervous response, and a reduction in catecholamines (Leeman et al., 2003a). Contractions are usually less painful in warm water because the warmth and buoyancy of the water have a relaxing effect.

There are a wide range of hydrotherapy options available, from ordinary bathtubs to whirlpool baths and showers, combined with low lighting and music.

Many hospitals provide showers and whirlpool baths for laboring women for pain relief. However, hydrotherapy is more commonly practiced in birthing centers managed by midwives. The recommendation for initiating hydrotherapy is that that women be in active labor (>5 cm dilated) to prevent the slowing of labor contractions secondary to muscular relaxation. The woman's membranes can be intact or ruptured. Women are encouraged to stay in the bath or shower as long as they feel they are comfortable. The water temperature should not exceed body temperature, and the bath time typically is limited to 1 to 2 hours (Simkin & O'Hara, 2002).

Hydrotherapy is an effective pain-management option for many women. Women who are experiencing a healthy pregnancy can be offered this option, but the potential benefits or risks to the woman are still not known (Campbell, 2004).

Ambulation and Position Changes

Ambulation and position changes during labor are another extremely useful comfort measure. Historically, women adopted a variety of positions during labor, rarely using the recumbent position until recently. The medical profession has favored recumbent positions during labor, but without evidence to demonstrate their appropriateness (Chalk, 2004).

Changing position frequently (every 30 minutes or so)—sitting, walking, kneeling, standing, lying down, getting on hands and knees, and using a birthing ball—helps relieve pain (Fig. 14-11). Position changes also may help to speed labor by adding benefits of gravity and changes to the shape of the pelvis. Research reports that position and frequency of position change have a profound effect on uterine activity and efficiency. Allowing the woman to obtain a position of comfort frequently facilitates a favorable fetal rotation by altering the alignment of the presenting part with the pelvis. As the mother continues to change position based on comfort, the optimal presentation is afforded (Gilbert & Harmon, 2003). Supine and sitting positions should be avoided, since they may interfere with labor progress and can cause compression of the vena cava and decrease blood return to the heart.

Swaying from side to side, rocking, or other rhythmic movements may also be comforting. If labor is progressing slowly, ambulating may speed it up again. Upright positions such as walking, kneeling forward, or doing the lunge on the birthing ball give most women a greater sense of control and active movement than just lying down. Table 14-2 highlights some of the more common positions that can be used during labor and birth.

Acupuncture and Acupressure

Acupuncture and acupressure can be used to bring about pain relief during labor. Although controlled research studies of these methods are limited, there is adequate evi-

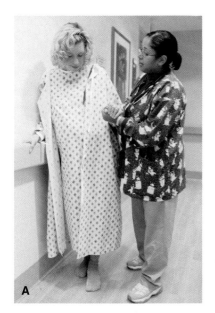
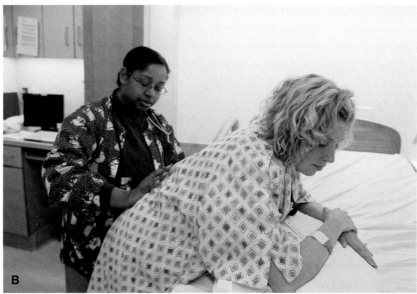
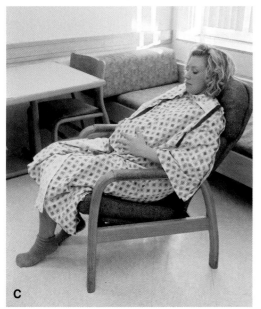
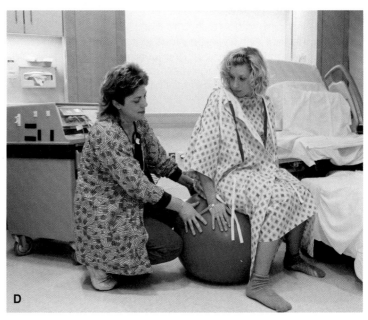

●Figure 14-11 Various positions for use during labor. (**A**) Ambulation. (**B**) Leaning forward. (**C**) Sitting in a chair. (**D**) Using a birthing ball.

dence that both are useful in relieving pain associated with labor and birth. However, both methods require a trained, certified clinician, and such a person is not available in many birth facilities (Skilnand et al., 2002).

Acupuncture involves stimulating key trigger points with needles. This form of Chinese medicine has been practiced for approximately 3,000 years. Classical Chinese teaching holds that throughout the body there are meridians or channels of energy (*qi*) that when in balance regulate body functions. Pain reflects an imbalance or obstruction of the flow of energy. The purpose of acupuncture is to restore *qi,* thus diminishing pain (Eappen & Robbins,

2002). Stimulating the trigger points causes the release of endorphins, reducing the perception of pain.

Acupressure involves the application of a firm finger or massage at the same trigger points to reduce the pain sensation. The amount of pressure is important. The intensity of the pressure is determined by the needs of the woman. Holding and squeezing the hand of a woman in labor may trigger the point most commonly used for both techniques (Engstrom, 2004). Some acupressure points are found along the spine, neck, shoulder, toes, and soles of the feet (Lowdermilk & Perry, 2004).

Table 14-2 Common Positions for Use During Labor and Birth

Standing	• Takes advantage of gravity during and between contractions • Makes contractions feel less painful and be more productive • Helps fetus line up with angle of maternal pelvis • Helps to increase urge to push in second stage of labor
Walking	• Has the same advantages as standing • Causes changes in the pelvic joints, helping the fetus move through the birth canal
Standing and leaning forward on partner, bed, birthing ball	• Has the same advantages as standing • Is a good position for a backrub • May feel more restful than standing • Can be used with electronic fetal monitor
Slow dancing (standing with woman's arms around partner's neck, head resting on his chest or shoulder, with his hands rubbing your lower back; sway to music and breathe in rhythm if it helps)	• Has the same advantages as walking • Back pressure helps relieve back pain • Rhythm and music help you relax and provide comfort
The lunge (standing facing a straight chair with one foot on the seat with knee and foot to the side; bending raised knee and hip, and lunging sideways repeatedly during a contraction, holding each lunge for 5 seconds; partner holds chair and helps with balance)	• Widens one side of the pelvis (the side toward lunge) • Encourages rotation of baby • Can also be done in a kneeling position
Sitting upright	• Helps promote rest • Has more gravity advantage than lying down • Can be used with electronic fetal monitor
Sitting on toilet or commode	• Has the same advantages as sitting upright • May help relax the perineum for effective bearing down
Semi-sitting (setting the head of the bed at a 45-degree angle with pillows used for support)	• Has the same advantages as sitting upright • Is an easy position if on a bed
Rocking in a chair	• Has the same advantages as sitting upright • May help speed labor (rocking movement)
Sitting, leaning forward with support	• Has the same advantages as sitting upright • Is a good position for back rubbing
On all fours, on your hands and knees	• Helps relieve backache • Assists rotation of baby in posterior position • Allows for pelvic rocking and body movement • Relieves pressure on hemorrhoids • Allows for vaginal exams • Is sometimes preferred as a pushing position by women with back labor
Kneeling, leaning forward with support on a chair seat, the raised head of the bed, or on a birthing ball	• Has the same advantages as all-fours position • Puts less strain on wrists and hands
Side-lying	• Is a very good position for resting and convenient for many kinds of medical interventions • Helps lower elevated blood pressure • May promote progress of labor when alternated with walking • Is useful to slow a very rapid second stage • Takes pressure off hemorrhoids • Facilitates relaxation between contractions

Table 14-2 Common Positions for Use During Labor and Birth (continued)

Squatting	• May relieve backache • Takes advantage of gravity • Requires less bearing-down effort • Widens pelvic outlet • May help fetus turn and move down in a difficult birth • Helps if the woman feels no urge to push • Allows freedom to shift weight for comfort • Offers an advantage when pushing, since upper trunk presses on the top of the uterus
Supported squat (leaning back against partner, who supports woman under the arms and takes the entire woman's weight; standing up between contractions)	• Requires great strength in partner • Lengthens trunk, allowing more room for fetus to maneuver into position • Lets gravity help
Dangle (partner sitting high on bed or counter with feet supported on chairs or footrests and thighs spread; woman leaning back between partner's legs, placing flexed arms over partner's thighs; partner gripping sides with his thighs; woman lowering herself and allowing partner to support her full weight; standing up between contractions)	• Has the same advantages of a supported squat • Requires less physical strength from the partner

Sources: Simkin, 2002; Simkin, 2003; Simkin & Ancheta, 2000; McKinney et al., 2005.

Attention Focusing and Imagery

Attention focusing and imagery uses many of the senses and the mind to focus on stimuli. The woman can focus on tactile stimuli such as touch, massage, or stroking. She may focus on auditory stimuli such as music, humming, or verbal encouragement. Visual stimuli might be any object in the room, or the woman can imagine the beach, a mountaintop, a happy memory, or even the contractions of the uterine muscle pulling the cervix open and the fetus pressing downward to open the cervix. Some women focus on a particular mental activity such as a song, a chant, counting backwards, or a Bible verse. Breathing, relaxation, positive thinking, and positive visualization work well for mothers in labor. The use of these techniques keeps the sensory input perceived during the contraction from reaching the pain center in the cortex of the brain (Simkin, 2002).

Therapeutic Touch and Massage

Therapeutic touch and massage use the sense of touch to promote relaxation and pain relief. Massage works as a form of pain relief by increasing the production of endorphins in the body. Endorphins reduce the transmission of signals between nerve cells and thus lower the perception of pain (Duddridge, 2002). In addition, touching and massage offer the woman a distraction from discomfort.

Therapeutic touch is based on the premises that the body contains energy fields that lead to either good or ill health and that the hands can be used to redirect the energy fields that lead to pain (Engstrom, 2004). To be done cor-

rectly, this technique must be learned and practiced. Some women prefer a light touch, while others find a firmer touch more soothing. Massage of the neck, shoulders, back, thighs, feet, and hands can be very comforting. The use of firm counterpressure in the lower back or sacrum is especially helpful for back pain during contractions (Fig. 14-12). Contraindications for massage include skin rashes, varicose veins, bruises, or infections (Leonard, 2002).

Effleurage is a light, stroking, superficial touch of the abdomen, in rhythm with breathing during contractions. It is used as a relaxation and distraction technique from discomfort. The external fetal monitor belts may interfere with her ability to accomplish this.

Breathing Techniques

Breathing techniques are effective in producing relaxation and pain relief through the use of distraction. If the woman is concentrating on slow-paced rhythmic breathing, she isn't likely to fully focus on contraction pain. Breathing techniques are often taught in childbirth education classes (see Chapter 12 for additional information).

Breathing techniques use controlled breathing to reduce the pain experienced through a stimulus-response conditioning. The woman selects a focal point within her environment to stare at during the first sign of a contraction. This focus creates a visual stimulus that goes directly to her brain. The woman takes a deep cleansing breath, which is followed by rhythmic breathing. Verbal commands from her partner supply an ongoing auditory stimulus to her brain. Effleurage can be combined with the

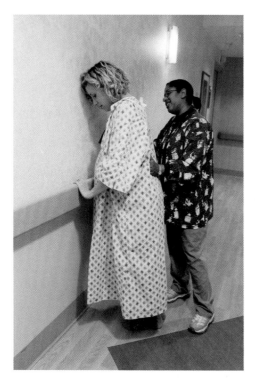

● Figure 14-12 Nurse massaging the client's back during a contraction while she ambulates during labor.

breathing to provide a tactile stimulus, all blocking pain sensations to her brain.

There are five levels of breathing a woman can use depending on the intensity of each contraction:

- First level: slow chest breathing involves 6 to 12 full respirations per minute; used in early labor; starting off and ending with a cleansing breath, which is taking a large volume of air into the lungs and letting it out slowly
- Second level: breathing heavy enough to expand the rib cage but light enough so the diaphragm barely moves; rate can be up to 40 breaths per minute; used during labor when cervical dilation is 4 to 6 cm
- Third level: shallow, sternal breathing, usually at a rate of 50 to 70 breaths per minute; used during transition phase of labor
- Fourth level: pant-blow pattern of breathing involves taking three to four quick breaths in and out and then forcefully exhaling
- Fifth level: continuous chest panting involves taking shallow breaths at a rate of about 60 breaths per minute; used during strong contractions to prevent pushing too early

The last two levels of breathing patterns are used when the previous level is no longer effective. The levels progress with the discomfort of the contractions.

Pharmacologic Measures

With varying degrees of success, generations of women have sought ways to relieve the pain of childbirth. Pharma-cologic pain relief during labor includes systemic analgesia and regional or local anesthesia. Women have seen dramatic changes in pharmacologic pain management options over the years. Methods have evolved from biting down on a stick to a more complex pharmacologic approach such as epidural/intrathecal analgesia. Systemic analgesia and regional analgesia/anesthesia have become less common, while the use of newer neuraxial analgesia/anesthesia techniques involving minimal motor blockade have become more popular. **Neuraxial analgesia/anesthesia** is the administration of analgesic (opioids) or anesthetic (medication capable of producing a loss of sensation in an area of the body) agents, either continuously or intermittently, into the epidural or intrathecal space to relieve pain (Poole, 2003a). Low-dose and ultra-low-dose epidural analgesia, spinal analgesia, and combined spinal-epidural analgesia have replaced the once "traditional" epidural for labor (Poole, 2003).

The shift in pain management allows a woman to be an active participant during labor. Regardless of which approach is used during labor, the woman has the right to choose the methods of pain control that will best suit her and meet her needs.

Systemic Analgesia

Systemic analgesia involves the use of one or more drugs administered orally, intramuscularly, or intravenously that become distributed throughout the body via the circulatory system. Depending on which administration routine is used, the therapeutic effect of pain relief can occur within minutes and last for several hours. The most important complication associated with the use of this class of drugs is respiratory depression. Therefore, women given these drugs require careful monitoring. Opioids given close to the time of birth can cause central nervous system depression in the newborn, necessitating the administration of naloxone (Narcan) to reverse the depressant effects of the opioids.

Several drug categories may be used for systemic analgesia:

- Ataractics: such as hydroxyzine (Vistaril) or promethazine (Phenergan)
- Barbiturates: such as secobarbital (Seconal) or pentobarbital (Nembutal)
- Benzodiazepines: such as diazepam (Valium) or midazolam (Versed)
- Opioids: such as butorphanol (Stadol), nalbuphine (Nubain), meperidine (Demerol), or fentanyl (Sublimaze)

Drug Guide 14-1 highlights some of the major drugs used for systemic analgesia.

Systemic analgesics are typically administered parenterally, usually through an existing intravenous (IV) line. Nearly all medications given during labor cross the placenta and have a depressant effect on the fetus; there-

Drug Guide 14-1 Common Agents Used for Systemic Analgesia

Type	Drug	Comments
Opioids	Morphine 2–5 mg IV	May be given IV, intrathecally, or epidurally Rapidly crosses the placenta Can cause maternal and neonatal CNS depression Decreases uterine contractions
	Meperidine (Demerol) 25–50 mg IV	May be given IV or epidurally with maximal fetal uptake 2–3 hours after administration Can cause CNS depression Decreases fetal variability
	Butorphanol (Stadol) 1 mg IV q 3–4h	Is given IV Is rapidly transferred across the placenta Causes neonatal respiratory depression
	Nalbuphine (Nubain) 10 mg IV	Is given IV Causes less maternal nausea and vomiting Causes decreased FHR variability, fetal bradycardia and respiratory depression
	Fentanyl (Sublimaze) 25–50 mcg IV	Is given IV or epidurally Can cause maternal hypotension, maternal and fetal respiratory depression Rapidly crosses placenta
Ataractics	Hydroxyzine (Vistaril) 50 mg IM	Does not relieve pain but reduces anxiety and potentiates opioid analgesic effects Is used to decrease nausea and vomiting
	Promethazine (Phenergan) 25 mg IV	Is used for antiemetic effect when combined with opioids Causes sedation and reduces apprehension May contribute to maternal hypotension and neonatal depression
Benzodiazepines	Diazepam (Valium) 2–5 mg IV	Is given to enhance pain relief of opioid and cause sedation May be used to stop eclamptic seizures Decreases nausea and vomiting Can cause newborn depression; therefore, lowest possible dose should be used
	Midazolam (Versed) 1–5 mg IV	Is not used for analgesic but amnesia effect Is used as adjunct for anesthesia Is excreted in breast milk
Barbiturates	Secobarbital (Seconal) 100 mg PO/IM Pentobarbital (Nembutal) 100 mg PO/IM	Causes sedation Is used in very early labor to alter a dysfunctional pattern Is not used for pain relief in active labor Crosses placenta and is secreted in breast milk

Sources: Primeau, Lacey, & Crotty, 2003; Poole, 2003b; Florence & Palmer, 2003; Pitter & Preston, 2001; Spratto & Woods, 2004; Mahlmeister, 2003.

fore, it is important for the woman to receive the least amount of systemic medication as possible to relieve her discomfort so that it does not cause any harm to the fetus (Florence & Palmer, 2003). Historically opioids have been administered by nurses, but in the past decade there has been increasing use of client-controlled intravenous analgesia (patient-controlled analgesia [PCA]). With this system, the woman is given a button connected to a computerized pump on the IV line. When the woman desires analgesia, she presses the button and the pump delivers a preset amount of medication. This system provides the woman with a sense of control over her own pain management and active participation in the childbirth process.

Ataractics

The ataractic group of medications is used in combination with an opioid to decrease nausea and vomiting and lessen anxiety. These adjunct drugs help potentiate the effectiveness of the opioid so that a lesser dose can be given. They may also be used to increase sedation. Promethazine

(Phenergan) can be given IV, but hydroxyzine (Vistaril) must be given by mouth or by intramuscular injection into a large muscle mass. Neither drug affects the progress of labor, but either may cause a decrease in FHR variability and possible newborn depression (Poole, 2003b).

Barbiturates

The barbiturate drug group is used only in early labor or in a prolonged latent phase that produces enough discomfort that the woman cannot sleep. Barbiturates are given orally or intramuscularly to produce a light sleep to alter a dysfunctional labor pattern or to calm a very anxious woman in early labor. The goal in giving a barbiturate is to promote therapeutic rest for a few hours to enhance the woman's ability to cope with active labor. These drugs cross the placenta and cause central nervous system depression in the newborn (Poole, 2003a).

Benzodiazepines

Benzodiazepines are used for minor tranquilizing and sedative effects. Diazepam (Valium) also is given IV to stop seizures due to pregnancy-induced hypertension. However, it is not used during labor itself. It can be administered to calm a woman who is out of control, thereby enabling her to relax enough so that she can participate effectively during her labor process rather than fighting against it. Lorazepam (Ativan) can also be used for its tranquilizing effect, but increased sedation is experienced with this medication (Bricker & Lavender, 2002). Midazolam (Versed), also given IV, produces good amnesia but no analgesia. It is most commonly used as an adjunct for anesthesia. Diazepam and midazolam cause central nervous system depression for both the woman and the newborn.

Opioids

Opioids are morphine-like medications that are most effective for the relief of moderate to severe pain. Opioids typically are administered IV. Of all of the synthetic opioids (butorphanol [Stadol], nalbuphine [Nubain], fentanyl [Sublimaze], and meperidine [Demerol]), meperidine is the most commonly used opioid for the management of pain during labor. Opioids are associated with newborn respiratory depression, decreased alertness, inhibited sucking, and a delay in effective feeding (Leeman et al., 2003b).

Opioids decrease the transmission of pain impulses by binding to receptor site pathways that transmit the pain signals to the brain. The effect is increased tolerance to pain and respiratory depression related to a decrease in sensitivity to carbon dioxide (Skidmore-Roth, 2004).

All opioids are considered good analgesics. However, respiratory depression can occur in the mother and fetus depending on the dose given. They may also cause a decrease in FHR variability identified on the fetal monitor strip. This FHR pattern change is usually transient. Other systemic side effects include nausea, vomiting, pruritus,

delayed gastric emptying, drowsiness, hypoventilation, and newborn depression. To reduce the incidence of newborn depression, birth should occur within 1 hour or after 4 hours of administration to prevent the fetus from receiving the peak concentration (Poole, 2003b).

Opioid antagonists such as naloxone (Narcan) are given to reverse the effects of the central nervous system depression, including respiratory depression, caused by opioids. Opioid antagonists also are used to reverse the side effects of neuraxial opioids, such as pruritus, urinary retention, nausea, and vomiting, without significantly decreasing analgesia (Poole, 2003b).

Consult a current drug guide for more specifics on these drug categories.

Regional Analgesia/Anesthesia

Regional analgesia/anesthesia provides pain relief without loss of consciousness. It involves the use of local anesthetic agents, with or without added opioids, to bring about pain relief or numbness through the drug's effects on the spinal cord and nerve roots. Obstetric regional analgesia generally refers to a partial or complete loss of pain sensation below the T8 to T10 level of the spinal cord (ACOG, 2002).

The routes for regional pain relief include epidural block, combined spinal-epidural block, local infiltration, pudendal block, and intrathecal (spinal) analgesia/anesthesia. Local and pudendal routes are used during birth for episiotomies; epidural and intrathecal routes are used for pain relief during active labor and birth. The major advantage of regional pain-management techniques is that the woman can participate in the birthing process and still have good pain control.

Epidural Block

Approximately 60% of laboring women in the United States receive an epidural block for pain relief during labor. In urban areas, many hospitals approach 90% use of epidurals (Eltzschig et al., 2003).

An epidural block involves the injection of a drug into the epidural space, which is located outside the dura mater between the dura and the spinal canal. The epidural space is typically entered through the third and fourth lumbar vertebrae with a needle, and a catheter is threaded into the epidural space. The needle is removed and the catheter is left in place to allow for continuous infusion or intermittent injections of medicine (Fig. 14-13). An epidural block provides analgesia and anesthesia and can be used for both vaginal and cesarean births. It has evolved from a regional block producing total loss of sensation to analgesia with minimal blockade. The effectiveness of epidural analgesia depends on the technique and medications used. It is usually started after labor is well established, typically when cervical dilation is greater than 5 cm.

Theoretically, epidural local anesthetics could block 100 percent of labor pain if used in large volumes and high

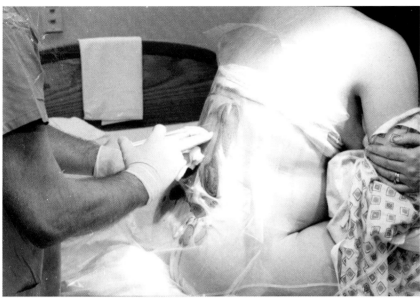

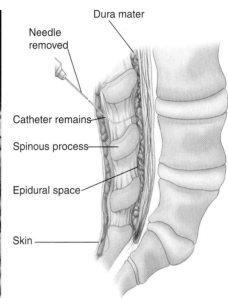

Dura mater

Needle removed

Catheter remains

Spinous process

Epidural space

Skin

A   **B**

● Figure 14-13 Epidural catheter insertion. (**A**) A needle is inserted into the epidural space. (**B**) A Catheter is threaded into the epidural space; the needle is then removed. The catheter allows medication to be administered intermittently or continuously to relieve pain during labor and childbirth.

concentrations. However, pain relief is balanced against other goals such as walking during the first stage of labor, pushing effectively in the second stage, and minimizing maternal and fetal side effects.

An epidural is contraindicated for women with a previous history of spinal surgery or spinal abnormalities, coagulation defects, infections, and hypovolemia. It also is contraindicated for the woman who is receiving anticoagulation therapy.

Complications include nausea and vomiting, hypotension, fever, pruritus, intravascular injection, and respiratory depression. Effects on the fetus during labor include fetal distress secondary to maternal hypotension (Mayberry et al., 2002). Ensuring that the woman avoids a supine position after an epidural catheter has been placed will help to minimize hypotension.

Changes in epidural drugs and techniques have been made to optimize pain control while minimizing side effects. Today most women receive a continuous lumbar epidural infusion of a local anesthetic, typically a drug whose name ends in "caine," and an opioid. To decrease motor blockade, bupivacaine (Sensorcaine) and ropivacaine (Naropin) have replaced lidocaine (Xylocaine), and drug concentrations have been lowered (Caton et al., 2002).

The addition of opioids, such as fentanyl or morphine, to the local anesthetic helps decrease the amount of motor block obtained. Continuous infusion pumps are used to administer the epidural analgesia, allowing the woman to be in control and administer a bolus dose on demand (Mitchell, 2002).

Combined Spinal-Epidural Analgesia

Another epidural technique is combined spinal-epidural (CSE) analgesia. This technique involves inserting the epidural needle into the epidural space and subsequently inserting a small-gauge spinal needle through the epidural needle into the subarachnoid space. An opioid, without a local anesthetic, is injected into this space. The spinal needle is then removed and an epidural catheter is inserted for later use.

CSE is advantageous because of its rapid onset of pain relief (within 3 to 5 minutes) that can last up to 3 hours. It also allows the woman's motor function to remain active. Her ability to bear down during the second stage of labor is preserved because the pushing reflex is not lost, and her motor power remains intact. The CSE technique provides greater flexibility and reliability for labor than either spinal or epidural analgesia alone (Landau, 2002). When compared with traditional epidural or spinal analgesia, which often keeps the woman lying in bed, CSE allows her to ambulate ("walking epidural") (Leeman et al., 2003b). Ambulating during labor provides several benefits: it may help control pain better, shorten the first stage of labor, increase the intensity of the contractions, and decrease the possibility of an operative vaginal or cesarean birth.

Although women can walk with CSE, they often choose not to because of sedation and fatigue. Often healthcare providers don't encourage or assist women to ambulate for fear of injury (Mayberry et al., 2002). Currently, anesthesiologists are performing walking epidurals using continuous infusion techniques as well as CSE and patient-controlled epidural analgesia (PCEA) (Pitter & Preston, 2001).

Complications include maternal hypotension, intravascular injection, accidental intrathecal blockade, postdural puncture headache, inadequate or failed block, and pruritus. Hypotension and associated FHR changes are managed with maternal positioning (semi-Fowler's position), intravenous hydration, and supplemental oxygen (Lieberman & O'Donoghue, 2002).

Patient-Controlled Epidural Analgesia

Patient-controlled epidural analgesia (PCEA) involves the use of an indwelling epidural catheter with an infusion of medication and a programmed pump that allows the woman to control the dosing. This method allows the woman to have a sense of control over her pain and reach her own individually acceptable analgesia level. When compared with the traditional epidural analgesia, PCEA provides equivalent analgesia with lower anesthetic use, lower rates of supplementation, and higher client satisfaction (Paech, 2000).

With PCEA, the woman uses a hand-held device connected to an analgesic agent that is attached to an epidural catheter (Fig. 14-14). When she pushes the button, a bolus dose of agent is administered via the catheter to reduce her pain. This method allows her to manage her pain at will without having to ask a staff member to provide pain relief.

Local Infiltration

Local infiltration involves the injection of a local anesthetic, such as lidocaine, into the superficial perineal nerves to numb the perineal area. This technique is done by the physician or midwife just before performing an **episiotomy** (surgical incision into the perineum to facilitate birth) or suturing a laceration. Local infiltration does not alter the pain of uterine contractions, but it does numb the immediate area of the episiotomy or laceration. Local infiltration does not cause side effects for the woman or her newborn.

Pudendal Nerve Block

A pudendal nerve block refers to the injection of a local anesthetic agent (e.g., bupivacaine, ropivacaine) into the pudendal nerves near each ischial spine. It provides pain relief in the lower vagina, vulva, and perineum (Fig. 14-15).

A pudendal block is used for the second stage of labor, an episiotomy, or an operative vaginal birth with outlet forceps or vacuum extractor. It must be administered about 15 minutes before it would be needed to ensure its full effect. A transvaginal approach is generally used to inject an anesthetic agent at or near the pudendal nerve branch. Neither maternal nor fetal complications are common.

Spinal (Intrathecal) Analgesia/Anesthesia

The spinal (intrathecal) pain-management technique involves injection of an anesthetic "caine" agent, with or without opioids, into the subarachnoid space to provide pain relief during labor or cesarean birth. The contraindications are similar to those for the epidural block. Adverse reactions for the woman include hypotension and spinal headache.

The subarachnoid injection of opioids alone, a technique termed *intrathecal narcotics,* has been gaining popularity since it was introduced in the 1980s. A narcotic is injected into the subarachnoid space, providing rapid pain relief while still maintaining motor function and sensation (Breslin & Lucas, 2003). An intrathecal narcotic is given during the active phase (>5 cm dilation) of labor. Compared with epidural blocks, intrathecal narcotics are easy to administer, provide rapid-onset pain relief, are less likely to cause newborn respiratory depression, and do not cause motor blockade (Fontaine et al., 2002). Although pain relief is rapid with this technique, it is limited by the narcotic's duration of action, which may be only a few hours and not last through the labor. Additional pain measures may be needed to sustain pain management.

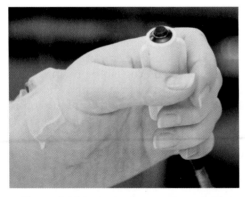

● Figure 14-14 Using a PCEA pump. Here the client holds the button that delivers a dose of medication.

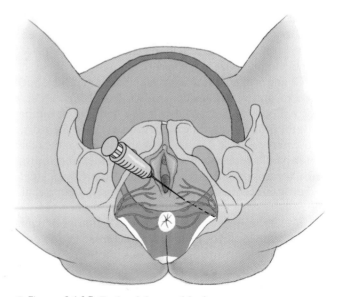

● Figure 14-15 Pudendal nerve block.

General Anesthesia

General anesthesia is typically reserved for emergency cesarean births when there is not enough time to provide spinal or epidural anesthesia or if the woman has a contraindication to the use of regional anesthesia. It can be started quickly and causes a rapid loss of consciousness. General anesthesia can be administered by IV injection, inhalation of anesthetic agents, or both. Commonly, thiopental, a short-acting barbiturate, is given IV to produce unconsciousness. This is followed by administration of a muscle relaxant. After the woman is intubated, nitrous oxide and oxygen are administered. A volatile halogenated agent may also be administered to produce amnesia (Hawkins et al., 2002).

All anesthetic agents cross the placenta and affect the fetus. The primary complication with general anesthesia is fetal depression, along with uterine relaxation and potential maternal vomiting and aspiration.

Although the anesthesiologist or nurse anesthetist administers the various general anesthesia agents, the nurse needs to be knowledgeable about the pharmacologic aspects of the drugs used and must be aware of airway management. Ensure that the woman is NPO and has a patent IV. In addition, administer a non-particulate (clear) oral antacid (e.g., Bicitra or sodium citrate) or a proton pump inhibitor (Protonix) as ordered to reduce gastric acidity. Assist with placement of a wedge under the woman's right hip to displace the gravid uterus and prevent vena cava compression in the supine position. Once the newborn has been removed from the uterus, assist the perinatal team in providing supportive care.

Nursing Management During Labor and Birth

A major focus of care for the woman during labor and birth is maintaining control over her pain, emotions, and actions while being an active participant. Nurses can help and support women to be actively involved in their childbirth experience by allowing time for discussion, offering companionship, listening to worries and concerns, paying attention to the woman's emotional needs, and actively helping and offering information to assist in her understanding of what is happening in each stage of labor.

Nursing Management During the First Stage of Labor

Depending on how far advanced the woman's labor is when she arrives at the facility, the nurse will determine assessment parameters of maternal-fetal status and plan care accordingly. The nurse will provide high-touch, low-tech supportive nursing care during the first stage of labor when admitting the woman and orienting her to the labor and birth suite. Nursing care during this stage will include taking an admission history (reviewing the prenatal record);

checking the results of routine laboratory tests and any special tests such as chorionic villi sampling, amniocentesis, genetic studies, and biophysical profile done during pregnancy; asking the woman about her childbirth preparation (birth plan, classes taken, coping skills); and completing a physical assessment of the woman to establish a baseline of values for future comparison.

Key nursing interventions include:

- Identifying the estimated date of birth from the client and the prenatal chart
- Validating the client's prenatal history to determine fetal risk status
- Determining fundal height to validate dates and fetal growth
- Performing Leopold's maneuvers to determine fetal position, lie, and presentation
- Checking FHR
- Performing a vaginal examination (as appropriate) to evaluate effacement and dilation progress
- Instructing the client and her partner about monitoring techniques and equipment
- Assessing fetal response and FHR to contractions and recovery time
- Interpreting fetal monitoring strips to provide optimal fetal care
- Checking FHR baseline for accelerations, variability, and decelerations
- Repositioning the client to obtain optimal FHR pattern
- Recognizing FHR problems and initiating corrective measures
- Checking amniotic fluid for meconium staining, odor, and amount
- Comforting client throughout testing period and labor
- Supporting client's decisions regarding intervention or avoidance of intervention
- Assessing client's support system and coping status frequently

In addition to these interventions to promote the optimal outcome for the mother and fetus, the nurse must document care accurately and in a timely fashion (Fig. 14-16). Accurate and timely documentation helps to decrease professional liability exposure and minimize the risk of preventable injuries to women and infants during labor and birth (Simpson & Knox, 2003). Guidelines for recording care include documenting:

- All care rendered, to prove that standards were met
- Conversations with all providers, including notification times
- Nursing interventions before and after notifying provider
- Use of the chain of command and response at each level
- All flow sheets and forms, to validate care given
- All education given to client and response to it
- Facts, not personal opinions
- Initial nursing assessment, all encounters, and discharge plan

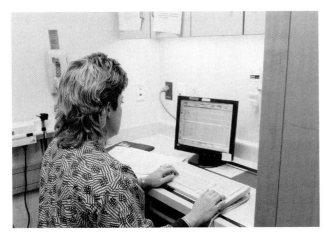

● Figure 14-16 The nurse documenting care.

• All telephone conversations (Greenwald & Mondor, 2003)

This standard of documentation is needed to prevent litigation, which is prevalent in the childbirth arena.

Assessment

After the admission assessment (see discussion earlier in the chapter) is complete, assessment continues for changes that would indicate that labor is progressing as expected. Assess the woman's knowledge, experience, and expectations of labor. Typically, blood pressure, pulse, and respirations are assessed every hour during the latent phase of labor unless the clinical situation dictates that vital signs be taken more frequently. During the active and transition phases, they are assessed every 30 minutes. The temperature is taken every 4 hours throughout the first stage of labor unless the clinical situation dictates it more frequently (maternal fever).

Vaginal examinations are performed periodically to track labor progress. This assessment information needs to be shared with the woman to reinforce that she is making progress toward the goal of birth. Uterine contractions are monitored for frequency, duration, and intensity every 30 to 60 minutes during the latent phase, every 15 to 30 minutes during the active phase, and every 15 minutes during transition. Note the changes in the character of the contractions as labor progresses, and inform the woman of her progress. Continually determine the woman's level of pain and her ability to cope and use relaxation techniques effectively.

When the fetal membranes rupture, spontaneously or artificially, assess the FHR and check the amniotic fluid for color, odor, and amount. Assess the FHR intermittently or continuously via electronic monitoring. During the latent phase of labor, assess the FHR every 30 to 60 minutes; in the active phase, assess FHR at least every 15 to 30 minutes. Also, be sure to assess the FHR before ambulation, prior to any procedure, and prior to administering analge-

sia or anesthesia to the mother. Table 14-3 summarizes assessments for the first stage of labor.

Nursing Interventions

Nursing interventions during the admission process should include:

• Asking about the client's expectations of the birthing process
• Providing information about labor, birth, pain-management options, and relaxation techniques
• Presenting information about fetal monitoring equipment and the procedures needed
• Monitoring FHR and identifying patterns that need further intervention
• Monitoring the mother's vital signs to obtain a baseline for later comparison
• Reassuring the client that her labor progress will be monitored closely and nursing care will focus on ensuring fetal and maternal well-being throughout

As the woman progresses through the first stage of labor, nursing interventions include:

• Encouraging the woman's partner to participate
• Keeping the woman and her partner up to date on the progress of the labor
• Orienting the woman and her partner to the labor and birth unit and explaining all of the birthing procedures
• Providing clear fluids (e.g., ice chips) as needed or requested
• Maintaining the woman's parenteral fluid intake at the prescribed rate if she has an IV
• Initiating or encouraging comfort measures, such as back rubs, cool cloths to the forehead, frequent position changes, ambulation, showers, slow dancing, leaning over a birth ball, side-lying, or counterpressure on lower back (Teaching Guidelines 14-1)
• Encouraging the partner's involvement with breathing techniques
• Assisting the woman and her partner to focus on breathing techniques
• Informing the woman that the discomfort will be intermittent and of limited duration; urging her to rest between contractions to preserve her strength; and encouraging her to use distracting activities to lessen the focus of uterine contractions
• Changing bed linens and gown as needed
• Keeping perineal area clean and dry
• Supporting the woman's decisions about pain management
• Monitoring maternal vital signs frequently and reporting any abnormal values
• Ensuring that the woman takes deep cleansing breaths before and after each contraction to enhance gas exchange and oxygen to the fetus
• Educating the woman and her partner about the need for rest and helping them plan strategies to conserve strength

Table 14-3 Summary of Assessments during the First Stage of Labor

Assessments*	Latent Phase (0–3 cm)	Active Phase (4–7 cm)	Transition (8–10 cm)
Vital signs (BP, pulse, respirations)	Every 30–60 min	Every 30 min	Every 15–30 min
Temperature	Every 4 hours	Every 4 hours	Every 4 hours
Contractions (frequency, duration, intensity)	Every 30–60 min by palpation or continuously if EFM	Every 15–30 min by palpation or continuously if EFM	Every 15 min by palpation or continuously if EFM
Fetal heart rate	Every hour by Doppler or continuously by EFM	Every 30 min by Doppler or continuously by EFM	Every 15–30 min by Doppler or continuously by EFM
Vaginal exam	Initially on admission to determine phase and as needed based on maternal cues to document labor progression	As needed to monitor labor progression	As needed to monitor labor progression
Behavior/psychosocial	With every client encounter: talkative, excited, anxious	With every client encounter: self-absorbed in labor; intense and quiet now	With every client encounter: discouraged, irritable, feels out of control, declining coping ability

*The frequency of assessments is dictated by the health status of the woman and fetus and can be altered if either one of their conditions changes.
EFM, electronic fetal monitoring.

- Monitoring FHR for baseline, accelerations, variability, and decelerations
- Checking on bladder status and encouraging voiding at least every 2 hours to make room for birth
- Repositioning the woman as needed to obtain optimal heart rate pattern
- Supporting requests from the woman and communicating them to appropriate personnel
- Respecting the woman's sense of privacy by covering her when appropriate
- Offering human presence (being physically present with the woman), not leaving her alone for long periods
- Exercising patience with the natural labor pattern to allow time for change
- Reporting any deviations from normal to the healthcare professional so that interventions can be initiated early to be effective (Simkin, 2002)

See Nursing Care Plan 14-1.

Nursing Management During the Second Stage of Labor

Nursing care during the second stage of labor focuses on supporting the woman and her partner in making active decisions about her care and labor management, imple-menting strategies to prolong the early passive phase of fetal descent, supporting involuntary bearing-down efforts, providing instruction and assistance, and using maternal positions that can enhance descent and reduce pain (Roberts, 2003). Research suggests that strong pushing during the second stage may be accompanied by a significant decline in fetal pH and may cause maternal muscle and nerve damage if done too early (Hansen et al., 2002). Shortening the phase of active pushing and lengthening the early phase of passive descent can be achieved by encouraging the woman not to push until she has a strong desire to do so and until the descent and rotation of the fetal head are well advanced. Effective pushing can be achieved by assisting the woman to assume a more upright or squatting position (Simkin & Ancheta, 2000).

Perineal lacerations or tears can occur during the second stage when the fetal head emerges through the vaginal introitus. The extent of the laceration is defined by depth: a first-degree laceration extends through the skin; a second-degree laceration extends through the muscles of the perineal body; a third-degree laceration continues through the anal sphincter muscle; and a fourth-degree laceration also involves the anterior rectal wall. Special attention needs to be paid to third- and fourth-degree lacerations to prevent future fecal incontinence (Ladewig, London, &

T E A C H I N G   G U I D E L I N E S   1 4 - 1

Teaching for Positioning During the
First Stage of Labor

Try using some of these positions during the first stage of labor:

- Walking with support from your partner (adds the force of gravity to contractions to promote fetal descent)
- Slow-dancing position with your partner holding you (adds the force of gravity to contractions and promotes support from and active participation of your partner)
- Side-lying with pillows between the knees for comfort (offers a restful position and improves oxygen flow to the uterus)
- Semi-sitting in bed or on a couch leaning against the partner (reduces back pain because fetus falls forward, away from the sacrum)
- Sitting in a chair with one foot on the floor and one on the chair (changes pelvic shape)
- Leaning forward by straddling a chair, a table, or a bed or kneeling over a birth ball (reduces back pain, adds the force of gravity to promote descent; possible pain relief if partner can apply sacral pressure)
- Sitting in a rocking chair or on a birth ball and shifting weight back and forth (provides comfort because rocking motion is soothing; uses the force of gravity to help fetal descent)
- Lunge by rocking weight back and forth with foot up on chair during contraction (uses force of gravity by being upright; enhances rotation of fetus through rocking)
- Open knee–chest position (helps to relieve back discomfort) (Simkin & Ancheta, 2000)

Davidson, 2006). Any lacerations should be repaired by the primary care provider during the third stage of labor.

An episiotomy is an incision made in the perineum to enlarge the vaginal outlet and theoretically to shorten the second stage of labor. Alternative measures such as warm compresses and continual massage with oil have been successful in stretching the perineal area to prevent cutting it. Further research needs to be done to validate the efficacy of natural measures versus the episiotomy. The midline episiotomy is the most common one used in the United States because it can be easily repaired and causes the least amount of pain (Lowdermilk & Perry, 2004). Figure 14-17 shows episiotomy locations.

Assessment

Assessment is continuous during the second stage of labor. Hospital policies dictate the specific type and timing of assessments, as well as the way in which they are documented. Figure 14-18 shows a sample form.

Assessment involves identifying the signs typical of the second stage of labor, including:

- Increase in apprehension or irritability
- Spontaneous rupture of membranes
- Sudden appearance of sweat on upper lip
- Increase in blood-tinged show
- Low grunting sounds from the woman
- Complaints of rectal and perineal pressure
- Beginning of involuntary bearing-down efforts

Other ongoing assessments include the contraction frequency, duration, and intensity; maternal vital signs every 5 to 15 minutes; fetal response to labor as indicated by FHR monitor strips; amniotic fluid for color, odor, and amount when membranes are ruptured; and the woman and her partner's coping status (Table 14-4).

Assessment also focuses on determining the progress of labor. Associated signs include bulging of the perineum, labial separation, advancing and retreating of the newborn's head during and between bearing-down efforts, and **crowning** (fetal head is visible at vaginal opening; Fig. 14-19).

A vaginal examination is completed to determine if it is appropriate for the woman to push. Pushing is appropriate if the cervix has fully dilated to 10 cm and the woman feels the urge to push.

Nursing Interventions

Nursing interventions during this stage focus on motivating the woman, encouraging her to put all her efforts to pushing this newborn to the outside world, and giving her feedback on her progress. If the woman is pushing and not making progress, the nurse can suggest she keep her eyes open during the contractions and look toward where the infant is coming out. Changing positions every 20 to 30 minutes will also help in making progress. Positioning a mirror so the woman can visualize the birthing process and how successful her pushing efforts are can help motivate her.

During the second stage of labor, an ideal position would be one that opens the pelvic outlet as wide as possible, provides a smooth pathway for the fetus to descend through the birth canal, uses the advantages of gravity to assist the fetus to descend, and gives the mother a sense of being safe and in control of the labor process (Gupta & Nikodem, 2003). Some suggestions for positions in the second stage include:

- Lithotomy with feet up in stirrups: most convenient position for caregivers
- Semi-sitting with pillows underneath knees, arms, and back
- Lateral/side-lying with curved back and upper leg supported by partner
- Sitting on birthing stool: opens pelvis, enhances the pull of gravity, and helps with pushing
- Squatting/supported squatting: gives the woman a sense of control

Nursing Care Plan 14-1

Overview of the Woman in the Active Phase of the First Stage of Labor

Candice, a 23-year-old gravida 1, para 0 (G1,P0) is admitted to the labor and birth suite at 39 weeks' gestation having contractions of moderate intensity every 5 to 6 minutes. A vaginal exam reveals her cervix is 80% effaced and 5 cm dilated. The presenting part (vertex) is at 0 station and her membranes ruptured spontaneously 4 hours ago at home. She is admitted and an IV is started for hydration and vascular access. An external fetal monitor is applied. FHR is 140 bpm and regular. Her partner is present at her bedside. Candice is now in the *active phase of the first stage of labor,* and her assessment findings are as follows: cervix dilated 7 cm, 80% effaced; moderate to strong contractions occurring regularly, every 3 to 5 minutes, lasting 45 to 60 seconds; at 0 station on pelvic exam; FHR auscultated loudest below umbilicus at 140 bpm; vaginal show—pink or bloody vaginal mucus; currently apprehensive, inwardly focused, with increased dependency; voicing concern about ability to cope with pain; limited ability to follow directions.

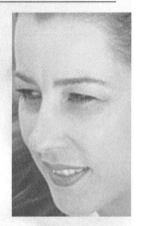

Nursing Diagnosis: Anxiety related to labor and birth process and fear of the unknown related to client's first experience

Outcome identification and *evaluation*	Interventions with *rationales*
Client will remain calm and in control *as evidenced by ability to make decisions and use positive coping strategies.*	Provide instruction regarding the labor process to allay anxiety. Reorient the woman to the physical environment and equipment as necessary *to keep client informed of events.* Encourage verbalization of feelings and concerns *to reduce anxiety.* Listen attentively to woman and partner *to demonstrate interest and concern.* Inform woman and partner of standard procedures/processes *to ensure adequate understanding of events and procedures.* Frequently update/inform woman of progress and labor status *to provide positive reinforcement for actions.* Reinforce relaxation techniques and provide instruction if needed *to aid in coping.* Encourage participation of the partner in the coaching role; role-model to facilitate partner participation in labor process *to provide support and encouragement to the client.* Provide a presence and remain with woman as much as possible *to provide comfort and support.*

Nursing Diagnosis: Pain related to effects of contractions and cervical dilatation and events of labor

Client will maintain a tolerable level of pain and discomfort *as evidenced by statements of pain relief, pain rating of 2 or less on pain rating scale, and absence of adverse effects in client and fetus from analgesia or anesthesia.*	Monitor vital signs, observe for signs of pain and have client rate pain on a scale of 0 to 10 *to provide baseline for comparison.* Encourage client to void every 1 to 2 hours *to decrease pressure from a full bladder.*

(continued)

Overview of the Woman in the Active Phase of the First Stage of Labor (continued)

Outcome identification and *evaluation*	Interventions with *rationales*
	Assist woman to change positions frequently *to increase comfort and promote labor progress.*
	Encourage use of distraction *to reduce focus on contraction pain.*
	Suggest pelvic rocking, massage, or counter back pressure *to reduce pain.*
	Assist with use of relaxation and breathing techniques *to promote relaxation.*
	Use touch appropriately (backrub) when desired by the woman *to promote comfort.*
	Integrate use of nonpharmacologic measures of pain relief, such as warm water, birthing ball, or other techniques *to facilitate pain relief.*
	Administer pharmacologic agents as ordered when requested *to control pain.*
	Provide reassurance and encouragement between contractions *to foster self-esteem and continued participation in labor process.*

Nursing Diagnosis: Risk of infection related to vaginal exams following rupture of membranes

Client will remain free of infection *as evidenced by absence of signs and symptoms of infection, vital signs and FHR within acceptable parameters, lab test results within normal limits, and clear amniotic fluid without odor.*	Monitor vital signs (every 1 to 2 hours after ROM) and FHR frequently as per protocol *to allow for early detection of problems;* report fetal tachycardia (early sign of maternal infection) *to ensure prompt treatment.*
	Provide frequent perineal care and pad changes *to maintain good perineal hygiene.*
	Change linens and woman's gown as needed *to maintain cleanliness.*
	Ensure that vaginal exams are performed only when needed *to prevent introducing pathogens into the vaginal vault.*
	Monitor lab test results such as white blood cell count *to assess for elevations indicating infection.*
	Use aseptic technique for all invasive procedures *to prevent infection transmission.*
	Carry out good handwashing techniques before and after procedures and use standard precautions as appropriate *to minimize risk of infection transmission.*
	Document amniotic fluid characteristics—color, odor—*to establish baseline for comparison.*

- Kneeling with hands on bed and knees comfortably apart

Other important nursing interventions during the second stage include:

- Providing continuous comfort measures such as mouth care, position changes, changing bed linen and underpads, and providing a quiet, focused environment

- Instructing the woman on the following bearing-down positions and techniques:
  - Pushing only when she feels an urge to push
  - Using abdominal muscles when bearing down
  - Using short pushes of 6 to 7 seconds
  - Focusing attention on the perineal area to visualize the newborn
  - Relaxing and conserving energy between contractions

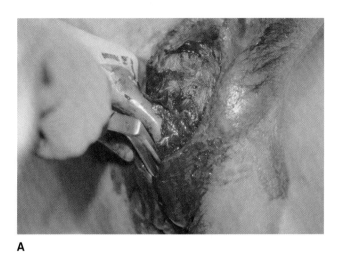

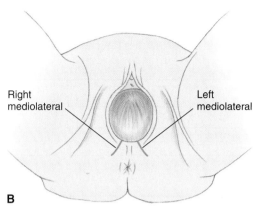

Right
mediolateral

Left
mediolateral

A

B

● Figure 14-17 Location of an episiotomy. (**A**) Midline episiotomy. (**B**) Right and left mediolateral episiotomies.

- Pushing several times with each contraction
- Pushing with an open glottis and slight exhalation (Roberts, 2003)
- Continuing to monitor contraction and FHR patterns to identify problems
- Providing brief, explicit directions throughout this stage
- Continuing to provide psychosocial support by re-assuring and coaching
- Facilitating the upright position to encourage the fetus to descend
- Continuing in assessment measurements: blood pressure, pulse, respirations, uterine contractions, bearing-down efforts, FHR, coping status of the client and her partner
- Providing pain management if needed
- Providing a continuous nursing presence
- Offering praise for the client's efforts
- Preparing for and assisting with delivery by:
  - Notifying the health care provider of the estimated timeframe for birth
  - Preparing the delivery bed and positioning client
  - Preparing the perineal area according to the facility's protocol
  - Offering a mirror and adjusting it so the woman can watch the birth
  - Explaining all procedures and equipment to the client and her partner
  - Setting up delivery instruments needed while maintaining sterility
  - Receiving newborn and transporting him or her to a warming environment, or covering the newborn with a warmed blanket on the woman's abdomen
  - Providing initial care and assessment of the newborn (see the Birth section that follows)

Birth

The second stage of labor ends with the birth of the newborn. The maternal position for birth varies from the standard lithotomy position to side-lying to squatting to standing or kneeling, depending on the birthing location, the woman's preference, and standard protocols. Once the woman is positioned for birth, the vulva and perineal area are cleansed. The primary healthcare provider then takes charge after donning protective eyewear, masks, gowns, and gloves and performing hand hygiene.

Once the fetal head has emerged, the primary care provider explores the fetal neck to see if the umbilical cord is wrapped around it. If it is, the cord is slipped over the head to facilitate delivery. As soon as the head emerges, the healthcare provider suctions the newborn's mouth and nares with a bulb syringe to prevent aspiration of mucus, amniotic fluid, or meconium (Fig. 14-20). The umbilical cord is double-clamped and cut between the clamps. With the first cries of the newborn, the second stage of labor ends.

Immediate Care of the Newborn

Once the infant is born, the nurse places the newborn under the radiant warmer, dries the newborn, assesses the newborn, wraps the newborn in warmed blankets, and places the newborn on the woman's abdomen for warmth and closeness. In some healthcare facilities, the newborn is placed on the woman's abdomen immediately after birth and covered with a warmed blanket. In either scenario, the stability of the newborn dictates the location of aftercare. The nurse can also assist with the first breastfeeding.

Assessment of the newborn begins at the moment of birth and continues until the newborn is discharged.

Labor Progress Chart
Maternal/Newborn Record System

	Admit date / /	Admit time	Blood type and Rh	Age	G	T	Pt	A	L	EDD___/___/___ LMP___/___/___	Membranes	☐ Intact ☐ Bulging	☐ Ruptured SROM AROM Date___/___/___ Time___

	Current date / /	Time →											
Vital signs	Temperature												
	Pulse												
	Respiration /O₂ saturation												
	Blood pressure												
Maternal	Deep tendon reflexes(L/R)	/	/	/	/	/	/	/	/	/	/	/	/
	Urine (protein/sugar)	/	/	/	/	/	/	/	/	/	/	/	/
	Vaginal bleeding												
	Pain												
	Edema (site, extent)												
Uterine activity	Monitor mode												
	Frequency												
	Duration												
	Peak IUP												
	Resting tone												
	Intensity												
	MVUs												
Fetal assessment	Monitor mode (Strip #____)												
	Baseline (FHR)												
	STV												
	LTV												
	Accelerations												
	Decelerations												
	Membranes/fluid												
	Scalp pH												
Intake/output (mLs/Hr)	IV												
	PO												
	Urine												
	Emesis												
Cont meds	Pitocin mU/min												
	Magnesium sulfate gms/hr												
Intervention	Treatments												
	Teaching/support												
	Touch												
	Position/activity												
	Physical care												
	Initials												

Abbreviations/key

Deep tendon reflexes	Vaginal bleeding	Pain	Uterine activity monitor mode	MVUs Montevideo units	Fetal monitor mode	STV short-term variability
0 = No response	NS = Normal show	0 = No pain	P = Palpation	The sum of the peak of each uterine contraction minus its resting tone, in a 10-minute period.	A = Auscultation (fetoscope)	+ = Present (roughness of tracing line present) ∅ = Absent (tracing line is smooth)
+1 = Sluggish	ABN = Frank vaginal bleeding	5 = Distressing pain	E = External		D = Doppler	**LTV long-term variability**
+2 = Normal		10 = Highest intensity	I = Internal		E = External	∅ = 0– 2 BPM = Absent
+3 = Hyperactive					I = Internal	↓ = 3– 5 BPM = Minimal
+4 = Brisk + hyperactive						+ = 6–25 BPM = Absent
C = Clonus						↑ = greater than 25 BPM = Marked

● Figure 14-18 A sample labor flow sheet. (Used with permission. Briggs Corporation, 2001.) *(continued)*

Labor Progress Chart
Maternal/Newborn Record System

| Current date / / | **Allergy/sensitivity** ☐ Other ___ | ☐ None | ☐ Latex | Chart ___ of ___ |

Accelerations
++ = 15 BPM ↑X 15 sec
+ = less than 15 BPM
↑+/or less than 15 sec
0 = None
Decelerations
N = None   L = Late
E = Early   P = Prolonged
V = Variable

Membranes
I = Intact
B = Bulging
R = Ruptured
Fluid
C = Clear
M = Meconium stained
B = Bloody
F = Foul odor
NF = No foul odor

Treatments
O₂ = O₂ L/min
IVB = IV bolus
SC = Straight catheterization
FC = Foley catheterization
ABD = Abdominal hair removal

Teaching/support
O = Orient to unit
SR = Safety review
LR = Labor review
F = Focusing
BRT = Breathing/relaxation techniques
PrO = PreOp.

Touch
E = Effleurage
B = Backrub
CP = Counterpressure
M = Massage

Position/activity
w = Walking
C = Chair
SQ = Squatting
JR = Jet hydrotherapy
SH = Shower
K = Kneeling
LS = Left side
RS = Right side
KC = Knee chest
T = Trendelenburg

Physical care
MC = Mouth care
SC = Superficial cold
SH = Superficial heat
PC = Peri care
BP = Bedpan

● Figure 14-18 (continued)

Labor Progress Chart
Maternal/Newborn Record System

TIME →											

Mark X ● 10

STATION		DILATATION	
	−4		9
	−3		8
	−2		7
	−1		6
	0		5
	+1		4
	+2		3
	+3		2

Effacement % and/or position

Examined by:

COMPOSITE NORMAL DILATATION CURVES

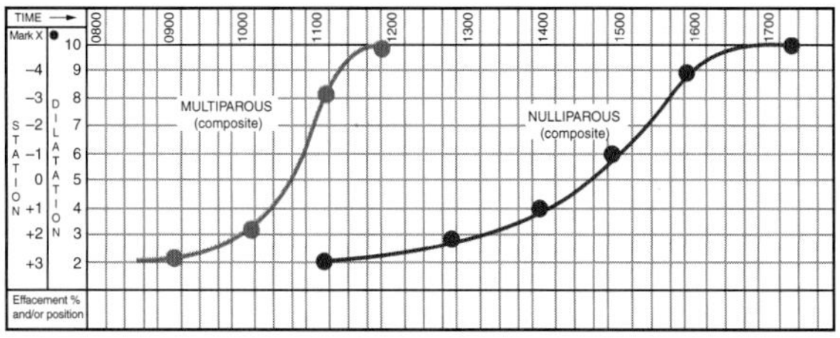

MULTIPAROUS (composite)

NULLIPAROUS (composite)

COMPOSITE CURVES OF ABNORMAL LABOR PROGRESS—MULTIPAROUS

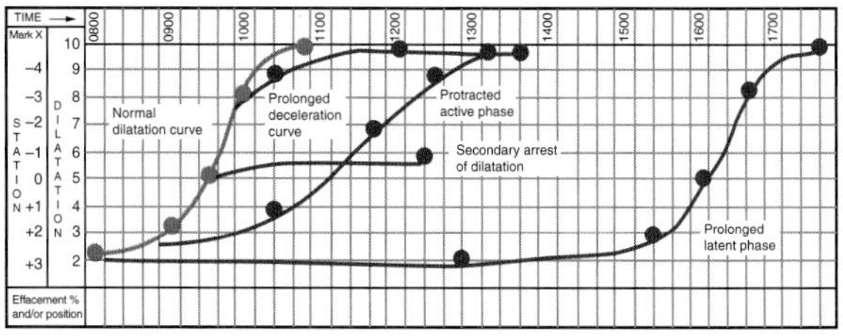

Normal dilatation curve

Prolonged deceleration curve

Protracted active phase

Secondary arrest of dilatation

Prolonged latent phase

Labor progress curves derived from the work of Emanuel A. Friedman, M.D.

IV Record

Start date	Time	Site	Solution	Amount (mL's)	Medication/dose added	Initials	Infused date	Time	Amount infused

Interval medications

Date, time	Medication/dose	Route	Site	Initials

Signature key

Initials	Signature

● Figure 14-18 (continued)

Table 14-4 Summary of Assessments During the Second, Third, and Fourth Stages of Labor

Assessments*	Second Stage of Labor (Birth of Neonate)	Third Stage of Labor (Placenta Expulsion)	Fourth Stage of Labor (Recovery)
Vital signs (BP, pulse, respirations)	Every 5–15 min	Every 15 min	Every 15 min
Fetal heart rate	Every 5–15 min by Doppler or continuously by EFM	Apgar scoring at 1 and 5 min	Newborn—complete head-to-toe assessment; vital signs every 15 min until stable
Contractions/uterus	Palpate every one	Observe for placental separation	Palpating for firmness and position every 15 min for first hr
Bearing down/ pushing	Assist with every effort Observe for signs of descent—bulging of perineum, crowning	None	None
Vaginal discharge		Assess bleeding after expulsion	Assess every 15 min with fundus firmness
Behavior/psychosocial	Observe every 15 min: cooperative, focus is on work of pushing newborn out	Observe every 15 min: often feelings of relief after hearing newborn crying; calmer	Observe every 15 min: usually excited, talkative, awake; needs to hold newborn, be close, and inspect body

*The frequency of assessments is dictated by the health status of the woman and fetus and can be altered if either one of their conditions changes.
EFM, electronic fetal monitoring.

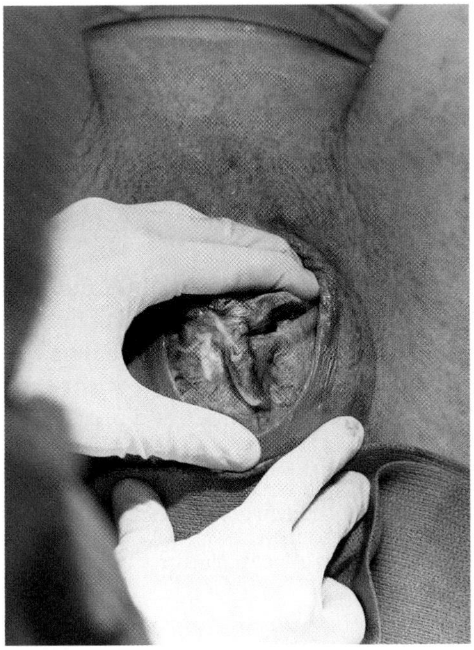

● Figure 14-19 Crowning.

Drying the newborn and providing warmth to prevent heat loss by evaporation is essential to help support thermoregulation and provide stimulation. Placing the newborn under a radiant heat source and putting on a stockinet cap will further reduce heat loss after drying.

The nurse assesses the newborn by assigning an Apgar score at 1 and 5 minutes. The Apgar score assesses five parameters—heart rate (absent, slow, or fast), respiratory effort (absent, weak cry, or good strong yell), muscle tone (limp, or lively and active), response to irritation stimulus, and color—that evaluate a newborn's cardiorespiratory adaptation after birth. The parameters are arranged from the most important (heart rate) to the least important (color). The newborn is assigned a score of 0 to 2 in each of the five parameters. The purpose of the Apgar assessment is to evaluate the functioning of the central nervous system; see Chapter 18 for additional information on Apgar scoring.

Two identification bands are secured on the newborn's wrist and ankle that match the band on the mother's wrist to ensure the newborn's identity. This identification process is completed in the birthing suite before anyone leaves the room. Some health care agencies also take an

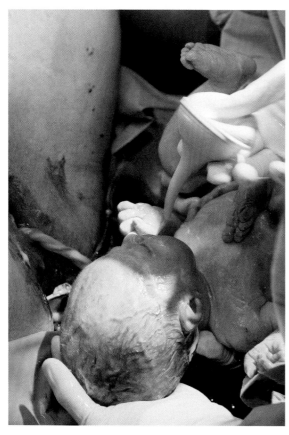

● Figure 14-20 Suctioning the newborn immediately after birth.

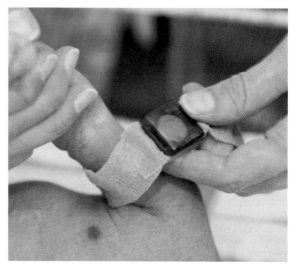

● Figure 14-21 An example of a security sensor applied to a newborn's arm.

early photo of the newborn for identification in the event of abduction (McKinney et al., 2005).

Other types of newborn security systems can also be used to prevent abduction. Some systems have sensors that are attached to the newborn's identification bracelet or cord clamp. An alarm is set off if the bracelet or clamp activates receivers near exits. Others have an alarm that is activated when the sensor is removed from the newborn (Fig. 14-21). Even with the use of electronic sensors, the parents, nursing staff, and security personnel are responsible for prevention strategies and ensuring the safety and protection of all newborns and their families (Shogan, 2002).

Nursing Management During the Third Stage of Labor

During the third stage of labor, strong uterine contractions continue at regular intervals under the continuing influence of oxytocin. The uterine muscle fibers shorten, or retract, with each contraction, leading to a gradual decrease in the size of the uterus, which helps shear the placenta away from its attachment site. The third stage is complete when the placenta is delivered. Nursing care during the third stage of labor primarily focuses on immediate newborn care and assessment and being available to

assist with the delivery of the placenta and inspecting it for intactness.

Three hormones play important roles in the third stage. During this stage the woman experiences peak levels of oxytocin and endorphins, while the high adrenaline levels that occurred during the second stage of labor to aid with pushing begin falling. The hormone oxytocin causes uterine contractions and helps the woman to enact instinctive mothering behaviors such as holding the newborn close to her body and cuddling the baby.

Skin-to-skin contact immediately after birth and the newborn's first attempt at breastfeeding further augment maternal oxytocin levels, strengthening the uterine contractions that will help the placenta to separate and the uterus to contract to prevent hemorrhage. Endorphins, the body's natural opiates, produce an altered state of consciousness and aid in blocking out pain. In addition, the drop in adrenaline level from the second stage, which had kept the mother and baby alert at first contact, causes most women to experience feelings of cold and shivering shortly after giving birth.

A crucial role for nurses during this time is to protect the natural hormonal process by ensuring unhurried and uninterrupted contact between mother and newborn after birth, providing warmed blankets to prevent shivering, and allowing skin-to-skin contact and breastfeeding.

Assessment

Assessment during the third stage of labor includes:

- Monitoring placental separation by looking for the following signs:
  - Firmly contracting uterus
  - Change in uterine shape from discoid to globular ovoid
  - Sudden gush of dark blood from vaginal opening
  - Lengthening of umbilical cord protruding from vagina

- Examining placenta and fetal membranes for intactness the second time (the health care provider assesses the placenta for intactness the first time) (Fig. 14-22)
- Assessing for any perineal trauma, such as the following, before allowing the birth attendant to leave:
  - Firm fundus with bright-red blood trickling: laceration
  - Boggy fundus with red blood flowing: uterine atony
  - Boggy fundus with dark blood and clots: retained placenta
- Inspecting the perineum for condition of episiotomy, if performed
- Assessing for perineal lacerations and ensuring repair by birth attendant

Nursing Interventions
Interventions during the third stage of labor include:

- Describing the process of placental separation to the couple
- Instructing the woman to push when signs of separation are apparent
- Administering an oxytocic if ordered and indicated after placental expulsion
- Providing support and information about episiotomy and/or laceration
- Cleaning and assisting client into a comfortable position after birth, making sure to lift both legs out of stirrups (if used) simultaneously to prevent strain
- Repositioning the birthing bed to serve as a recovery bed if applicable
- Assisting with transfer to the recovery area if applicable
- Providing warmth by replacing warmed blankets over the woman
- Applying an ice pack to the perineal area to provide comfort to episiotomy if indicated
- Explaining what assessments will be carried out over the next hour and offering positive reinforcement for actions
- Ascertaining any needs
- Monitoring maternal physical status by assessing:
  - Vaginal bleeding: amount, consistency, and color

- Vital signs: blood pressure, pulse, and respirations taken every 15 minutes
- Uterine fundus, which should be firm, in the midline, and at the level of the umbilicus
- Recording all birthing statistics and securing primary caregiver's signature
- Documenting birthing event in the birth book (official record of the facility that outlines every birth event), detailing any deviations

Nursing Management During the Fourth Stage of Labor

The fourth stage of labor begins after the placenta is expelled and lasts up to 4 hours after birth, during which time recovery takes place. This recovery period may take place in the same room where the woman gave birth, in a separate recovery area, or in her postpartum room. During this stage, the woman's body is beginning to undergo the many physiologic and psychological changes that occur after birth. The focus of nursing management during the fourth stage of labor involves frequent close observation for hemorrhage, provision of comfort measures, and promotion of family attachment.

Assessment
Assessments during the fourth stage center on the woman's vital signs, status of the uterine fundus and perineal area, comfort level, lochia amount, and bladder status. During the first hour after birth, vital signs are taken every 15 minutes, then every 30 minutes for the next hour if needed. The woman's blood pressure should remain stable and within normal range after giving birth. A decrease may indicate uterine hemorrhage; an elevation might suggest preeclampsia.

The pulse usually is typically slower (60 to 70 bpm) than during labor. This may be associated with a decrease in blood volume following placental separation. An elevated pulse rate may be an early sign of blood loss. The blood pressure usually returns to its prepregnancy level

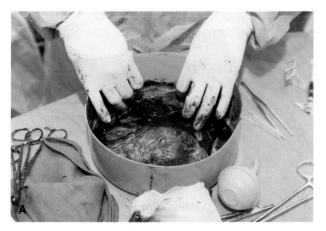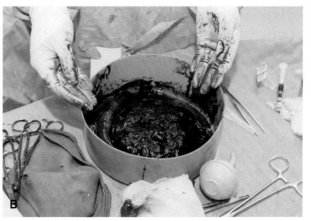

● Figure 14-22 Placenta. (**A**) Fetal side. (**B**) Maternal side.

and therefore is not a reliable early indicator of shock. Fever is indicative of dehydration (<100.4°F or 38°C) or infection (>101°F), which may involve the genitourinary tract. Respiratory rate is usually between 16 and 24 breaths per minute and regular. Respirations should be unlabored unless there is an underlying preexisting respiratory condition.

Assess fundal height, position, and firmness every 15 minutes during the first hour following birth. The fundus needs to remain firm to prevent excessive postpartum bleeding. The fundus should be firm (feels like the size and consistency of a grapefruit), located in the midline and below the umbilicus. If it is not firm (boggy), gently massage it until it is firm (see Nursing Procedure 22-1 for more information). Once firmness is obtained, stop massage. If the fundus is displaced to the right of the midline, suspect a full bladder as the cause.

The vagina and perineal areas are quite stretched and edematous following a vaginal birth. Assess the perineum, including the episiotomy if present, for possible hematoma formation. Suspect a hematoma if the woman reports excruciating pain or cannot void or if a mass is noted in the perineal area. Also assess for rectal hemorrhoids, which can cause discomfort.

Assess the woman's comfort level frequently to determine the need for analgesia. Ask the woman to rate her pain on a scale of 1 to 10; it should be less than 3. If it is higher, further evaluation is needed to make sure there aren't any deviations contributing to her discomfort.

Assess vaginal discharge (lochia) every 15 minutes for the first hour and every 30 minutes for the next hour. Palpate the fundus at the same time to ascertain its firmness and help to estimate the amount of vaginal discharge. In addition, palpate the bladder for fullness, since many women receiving an epidural block experience limited sensation in the bladder region. Voiding should produce large amounts of urine (diuresis) each time. Palpation of the woman's bladder after each voiding helps to ensure complete emptying. A full bladder will displace the uterus to either side of the midline and potentiate uterine hemorrhage secondary to bogginess.

Nursing Interventions

Nursing interventions during the fourth stage might include:

- Providing support and information to the woman regarding episiotomy repair and related pain-relief and self-care measures
- Applying an ice pack to the perineum to promote comfort and reduce swelling
- Assisting with hygiene and perineal care; teaching the woman how to use the perineal bottle after each pad change and voiding; helping the woman into a new gown
- Monitoring for return of sensation and ability to void (if regional anesthesia was used)

- Encouraging the woman to void by ambulating to bathroom, listening to running water, or pouring warm water over the perineal area with the peribottle
- Monitoring vital signs and fundal and lochia status every 15 minutes and documenting them
- Promoting comfort by offering analgesia for afterpains and warm blankets to reduce chilling
- Offering fluids and nourishment if desired
- Encouraging parent–infant attachment by providing privacy for the family
- Being knowledgeable and sensitive to typical cultural practices after birth
- Assisting the mother to nurse, if she chooses, during the recovery period to promote uterine firmness due to the release of oxytocin from the posterior pituitary gland, which stimulates uterine contractions
- Teaching the woman how to assess her fundus for firmness periodically and to massage it if it is boggy
- Describing the lochia flow and normal parameters to observe for postpartum
- Teaching safety techniques to prevent newborn abduction
- Demonstrating the use of the portable sitz bath as a comfort measure for her perineum if she had a laceration or an episiotomy repair
- Explain comfort/hygiene measures and when to use them
- Assisting with ambulation when getting out of bed for the first time
- Providing information about the routine on the mother–baby unit or nursery for her stay
- Observing for signs of early parent–infant attachment: fingertip touch to palm touch to enfolding of the infant (Murray et al., 2002)

KEY CONCEPTS

- A nurse provides physical and emotional support during the labor and birth process to assist a woman to achieve her goals.
- When a woman is admitted to the labor and birth area, the admitting nurse must assess and evaluate the risk status of this pregnancy and initiate appropriate interventions to provide optimal care for this client.
- Completing an admission assessment includes taking a maternal health history; performing physical assessment on the woman and fetus, including her emotional and psychosocial status; and obtaining the necessary laboratory studies.
- The nurse's role in fetal assessment for labor and birth includes determining fetal well-being and interpreting signs and symptoms of possible compromise. Determining the fetal heart rate (FHR) pattern and assessing amniotic fluid characteristics are key.
- FHR can be assessed intermittently or continuously. Although the intermittent method allows the client to move about during labor, the information

- obtained intermittently does not provide a complete picture of fetal well-being from moment to moment.
- Assessment parameters of the FHR are classified as baseline rate, baseline variability (long-term and short-term), and periodic changes in the rate (accelerations and decelerations).
- The nurse monitoring the laboring client needs to be knowledgeable about which parameters are reassuring, nonreassuring, and ominous so that appropriate interventions can be instituted.
- For a nonreassuring FHR pattern, the nurse should notify the healthcare provider about the pattern and obtain further orders, making sure to document all interventions and their effects on the FHR pattern.
- In addition to interpreting assessment findings and initiating appropriate inventions for the laboring client, accurate and timely documentation must be carried out continuously.
- Today's women have many safe nonpharmacologic and pharmacologic choices for the management of pain during childbirth. They may be used individually or in combination to complement one another.
- Nursing management for the woman during labor and birth includes comfort measures, emotional support, information and instruction, advocacy, and support for the partner.
- Nursing care during the first stage of labor includes taking an admission history (reviewing the prenatal record), checking the results of routine laboratory work and special tests done during pregnancy, asking the woman about her childbirth preparation (birth plan, classes taken, coping skills), and completing a physical assessment of the woman to establish a baseline of values for future comparison.
- Nursing care during the second stage of labor focuses on supporting the woman and her partner in making decisions about her care and labor management, implementing strategies to prolong the early passive phase of fetal descent, supporting involuntary bearing-down efforts, providing instruction and assistance, and encouraging the use of maternal positions that can enhance descent and reduce the pain.
- Nursing care during the third stage of labor primarily focuses on immediate newborn care and assessment and being available to assist with the delivery of the placenta and inspecting it for intactness.
- The focus of nursing management during the fourth stage of labor involves frequently observing the mother for hemorrhage, providing comfort measures, and promoting family attachment.

References

Albers, L. (2003). Commentary on "Impact of collaborative management and early admission in labor on method of delivery." *JOGNN, 32*(2), 158–160.

American College of Obstetricians and Gynecologists (ACOG). (2005). *Fetal heart rate patterns: monitoring, interpretation, and management* (Practice Bulletin Number 62). Washington, DC: Author.

American College of Obstetricians and Gynecologists (ACOG). (2002). *Obstetric analgesia and anesthesia* (Practice Bulletin Number 36). Washington, D.C: Author.

American Hospital Association. (2003). *Hospital statistics.* Chicago: Author.

Association of Women's Health, Obstetric and Neonatal Nurses (AWHONN). (2000). *Fetal assessment* (Clinical Position Statement). Washington, DC: Author.

Baird, S. M., & Ruth, D. J. (2002). Electronic fetal monitoring of the preterm fetus. *Journal of Perinatal and Neonatal Nursing, 16*(1), 12–24.

Breslin, E. T., & Lucas, V. A. (2003). *Women's health nursing: toward evidence-based practice.* St. Louis: Saunders.

Bricker, L., & Lavender, T. (2002). Parenteral opioids for labor pain relief: a systematic review. *American Journal of Obstetrics and Gynecology, 186*(5), S94–S109.

Buckley, S. (2001). A natural approach to the third stage of labor. *Midwifery Today, 59,* 33–37.

Campbell, G. (2004). Critical incident analysis of water immersion. *British Journal of Midwifery, 12*(1), 7–11.

Caton, D., Frolich, M. A., & Euliano, T. Y. (2002). Anesthesia for childbirth: controversy and change. *American Journal of Obstetrics & Gynecology, 186*(Suppl. 5), S25–30.

Chalk, A. (2004). Pushing in the second stage of labor: Part 1. *British Journal of Midwifery, 12*(8), 502–509.

Cypher, R., Adelsperger, D., & Torgersen, K. L. (2003). Interpretation of the fetal heart rate. In N. Feinstein, K. L. Torgersen, & J. L. Atterbury (Eds.), *Fetal heart monitoring principles and practices* (3rd ed., pp. 113–154). Dubuque, IA: Kendall-Hunt Publications.

Dillon, P. M. (2003). *Nursing health assessment: a critical thinking, case studies approach.* Philadelphia: F. A. Davis Company.

Duddridge, E. (2002). Using complementary therapies during the childbearing process. *British Journal of Midwifery, 10*(11), 699–704.

Eappen, S., & Robbins, D. (2002). Nonpharmacological means of pain relief for labor and delivery. *International Anesthesiology Clinics, 40*(4), 103–114.

Eltzschig, H., Lieberman, E., & Camann, W. (2003). Regional anesthesia and analgesia for labor and delivery. *New England Journal of Medicine, 348,* 319–332.

Engstrom, J. (2004). *Maternal-neonatal nursing made incredibly easy!* Philadelphia: Lippincott Williams & Wilkins.

Feinstein, N., Torgersen, K. L., & Atterbury, J. (2003). *AWHONN's fetal heart monitoring principles and practices* (3rd ed.). Dubuque, IA: Kendall-Hunt Publishing Company.

Florence, D. J., & Palmer, D. G. (2003). Therapeutic choices for the discomforts of labor. *Journal of Perinatal and Neonatal Nursing, 17*(4), 238–249.

Fontaine, P., Adam, P., & Svendsen, K. H. (2002). Should intrathecal narcotics be used as a sole labor analgesic? A prospective comparison of spinal opioids and epidural bupivacaine. *Journal of Family Practice, 51*(7), 630–635.

Garite, T. J. (2002). Intrapartum fetal evaluation. In S. G. Gabbe, J. R. Niebyl, & J. L. Simpson (Eds.), *Obstetrics: normal and problem pregnancies* (4th ed., pp. 395–429). New York: Churchill Livingstone.

Gilbert, E. S., & Harmon, J. S. (2003). *Manual of high risk pregnancy & delivery* (3rd ed.). St. Louis: Mosby.

Greenwald, L. M., & Mondon, M. (2003). Malpractice and the perinatal nurse. *Journal of Perinatal and Neonatal Nursing, 17*(2), 101–109.

Gupta, J. K., & Nikodem, V. C. (2003). Woman's position during second stage of labor. *The Cochrane Library,* Issue 4, Chichester, UK: John Wiley & Sons, Ltd.

Hansen, S., Clark, S., & Foster, J. (2002). Active pushing versus passive fetal descent in the second stage of labor: a randomized controlled trial. *Obstetrics & Gynecology, 99,* 29–34.

Hawkins, J., Chestnut, D., & Gibbs, C. (2002). Obstetric anesthesia. In S. Gabbe, J. Niebyl, & J. Simpson (Eds.), *Obstetrics: normal and problem pregnancies* (4th ed., pp. 431–472). Philadelphia: Churchill Livingstone.

Hodnett, E. D. (2002a). Pain and women's satisfaction with the experience of childbirth: a systematic review. *American Journal of Obstetrics & Gynecology, 186*(5 Pt. 2), 160–172.

Hodnett, E. D. (2002b). Caregiver support for women during childbirth. *Cochrane Database System Review* 2002; (1): CD000199.

Hunter, L. P. (2002). Being with woman: a guiding concept for the care of laboring woman. *JOGNN, 31*(6), 650–657.

Institute for Clinical Systems Improvement (ICSI). (2003). *ICSI Health Care Guidelines* (9th ed.). [Online] Available at: www.icsi.org

Iams, J. D., Newman, R. B., Thom, E. A., et al. (2002). Frequency of uterine contractions and the risk of preterm delivery. *New England Journal of Medicine, 346*(4), 250–255.

James, D. C., Simpson, K. R., & Knox, G. E. (2003). How do labor nurses view their role? *Journal of Obstetric, Gynecologic, and Neonatal Nursing, 32*, 814–823.

Kane, A. (2001). Focal point on childbirth education: hypnotic analgesic suggestion in childbirth. *International Journal of Childbirth Education, 16*(3), 20–22.

King, T. L., & Simpson, K. R. (2001). Fetal assessment during labor. In K. R. Simpson and P. Creehan (Eds.), *Perinatal nursing* (pp. 378–416). Philadelphia: Lippincott.

Landau, R. (2002). Combined spinal-epidural analgesia for labor: breakthrough or unjustified invasion. *Seminars in Perinatology, 26*, 109–121.

Ladewig, P. A., London, M. L., & Davidson, M. R. (2006). *Contemporary maternal-newborn nursing care* (6th ed.). Upper Saddle River, NJ: Pearson Prentice Hall.

Leeman, L., Fontaine, P., King, V., Klein, M. C., & Ratcliffe, S. (2003a). The nature and management of labor pain: Part I. Nonpharmacologic pain relief. *American Family Physician, 68*(6), 1109–1112.

Leeman, L., Fontaine, P., King, V., Klein, M. C., & Ratcliffe, S. (2003b). The nature and management of labor pain: Part II. Pharmacologic pain relief. *American Family Physician, 68*(6), 1115–1120.

Leonard, P. (2002). Childbirth education: a handbook for nurses. *Nursing Spectrum*, [Online] Available at: http://nsweb/nursingspectrum.com/ce/m350c.htm

Lieberman, E., & O'Donoghue, C. (2002). Unintended effects of epidural anesthesia during labor: a systematic review. *American Journal of Obstetrics and Gynecology, 186*, S31–68.

Littleton, L. Y., & Engebretson, J. C. (2005). *Maternity nursing care*. Clifton Park, NY: Thomson Delmar Learning.

Lowdermilk, D. L., & Perry, S. E. (2004). *Maternity & women's health care* (8th ed.). St. Louis: Mosby.

Mahlmeister, L. (2003). Nursing responsibilities in preventing, preparing for, and managing epidural emergencies. *Journal of Perinatal and Neonatal Nursing, 17*(1), 19–32.

Mainstone, A. (2004). The use of Doppler in fetal monitoring. *British Journal of Midwifery, 12*(2), 78–84.

Matthews, R., & Callister, L. C. (2004). Childbearing women's perceptions of nursing care that promotes dignity. *JOGNN, 33*(4), 498–507.

Mattson, S., & Smith, J. E. (2004). *Core curriculum for maternal-newborn nursing* (3rd ed.). St. Louis: Elsevier Saunders.

Mayberry, L., Clemmens, D., & De, A. (2002). Epidural analgesia side effects, co-interventions, and care of women during childbirth: a systematic review. *American Journal of Obstetrics and Gynecology, 186*(5), S81–S93.

McKinney, E. S., James, S. R., Murray, S. S., & Ashwill, J. W. (2005). *Maternal-child nursing* (2nd ed.). St. Louis: Elsevier Saunders.

Mitchell, J. (2002). Labor epidurals. *Advance for Nurses, 3*(23), 25–26.

Moore, M. L., & Moos, M. K. (2003). *Cultural competence in the care of childbearing families*. March of Dimes Nursing Module. White Plains, NY: March of Dimes Birth Defects Foundation Educational Services.

Moses, S. (2003). Fetal heart tracing. *Family Practice Notebook*. [Online] Available at: www.fpnotebook.com/OB45.htm

Murray, M. L. (2004). Maternal or fetal heart rate? Avoiding intrapartum misidentification. *JOGNN, 33*(1), 93–104.

Murray, S. S., McKinney, E. S., & Gorrie, T. M. (2002). *Foundations of maternal-newborn nursing*, 3rd ed. Philadelphia: W. B. Saunders.

Newman, R. B. (2003). Our unrequited love for simple explanation. *Journal of Perinatology, 23*, 504–506.

Olds, S. B., London, M. L., Ladewig, P. W., & Davidson, M. R. (2004). *Maternal-newborn nursing & women's health*. Upper Saddle River, NJ: Pearson Prentice Hall.

Paech, M. (2000). Client-controlled epidural analgesia. In D. Birnbach, S. Gatt, & S. Datta (Eds.), *Textbook of obstetric anesthesia* (pp. 189–202). New York: Churchill Livingstone.

Pillitteri, A. (2003). *Maternal & child health nursing: care of the childbearing and childrearing family* (4th ed.). Philadelphia: Lippincott Williams & Wilkins.

Pitter, C., & Preston, R. (2001). Modern pharmacologic methods in labor analgesia. *International Journal of Childbirth Education, 16*(2), 15–20.

Poole, J. H. (2003a). Neuraxial analgesia for labor and birth: implications for mother and fetus. *Journal of Perinatal and Neonatal Nursing, 17*(4), 252–267.

Poole, J. H. (2003b). Analgesia and anesthesia during labor and birth: implications for mother and fetus. *JOGNN, 32*(6), 780–793.

Priddy, K. D. (2004). Is there logic behind fetal monitoring? *JOGNN, 33*(5), 550–553.

Primeau, M. R, Lucey, K. A., & Crotty, P. M. (2003). Managing the pain of labor. *Advance for Nurses, 4*(12), 15–19.

Roberts, J. E. (2003). A new understanding of the second stage of labor: implications for nursing care. *JOGNN, 32*(6), 794–801.

Shogan, M. G. (2002). Emergency management plan for newborn abduction. *JOGNN, 31*(3), 340–346.

Simkin, P. (2002). Supportive care during labor: a guide for busy nurses. *JOGNN, 31*(6), 721–732.

Simkin, P. (2003). Maternal positions and pelves revisited. *Birth, 30*(2), 130–132.

Simkin, P., & Ancheta, R. (2000). *The labor progress handbook*. Oxford, UK: Blackwell Science.

Simkin, P., & O'Hara, M. (2002). Nonpharmacologic relief of pain during labor: systematic reviews of five methods. *American Journal of Obstetrics and Gynecology, 186*(5), S131–S159.

Simpson, K. R. (2003). Fetal pulse oximetry update. *AWHONN Lifelines, 7*(5), 411–412.

Simpson, K. R., & Knox, G. E. (2003). Common areas of litigation related to care during labor and birth. *Journal of Perinatal and Neonatal Nursing, 17*(2), 110–125.

Simpson, K. R., & Porter, M. L. (2001). Fetal oxygen saturation monitoring: using this new technology for fetal assessment during labor. *AWHONN Lifelines, 5*(2), 27–33.

Sisk, B. (2002). *Electronic fetal monitoring during labor*. [Online] Available at: http://enursesubscribe.com/fetal.htm

Skidmore-Roth, L. (2004). *Mosby's nursing drug reference*. St. Louis: Mosby.

Skilnand, E., Fossen, D., & Heiberg, E. (2002). Acupuncture in the management of pain in labor. *Acta Obstetricia et Gynecologica Scandinavica, 81*, 943–948.

Sloane, E. (2002). *Biology of women* (4th ed.). Albany, NY: Delmar.

Society of Obstetricians and Gynecologists of Canada (SOGC). (2002). Fetal health surveillance in labor (SOGC Clinical Practice Guidelines No. 112). *Journal of Obstetrics and Gynecology in Canada, 112*(March), 1–13.

Spratto, G. R., & Woods, A. L. (2004). *2004 edition PDR nurse's drug handbook*. Clifton Park, NY: Thomson Delmar Learning.

Stephens, K. C. (2003). An Appalachian perspective. In: M. L. Moore & M. K. Moos (Eds.), *Cultural competence in the care of childbearing families* (pp. 56–59). March of Dimes Nursing Module. White Plains, NY: March of Dimes Birth Defects Foundation Educational Services.

Thacker, S. B., & Stroup, D. F. (2003). Revisiting the use of the electronic fetal monitor. *Lancet, 361*(9356), 445–447.

Torgersen, K. L. (2004). Intrapartum fetal assessment. In: S. Mattson & J. E. Smith, *Core curriculum for maternal-newborn nursing* (3rd ed., pp. 303–368). St. Louis: Elsevier Saunders.

Trainor, C. L. (2002). Valuing labor support. *AWHONN Lifelines, 6*(5), 387–389.

Tucker, S. M. (2004). *Pocket guide to fetal monitoring and assessment* (5th ed.). St. Louis: Mosby.

U.S. Department of Health and Human Services. (2000). *Healthy people 2010: understanding and improving health* (2nd ed.). Chapter 16: Maternal, Infant, and Child Health. (DHHS Publication 017-001-00550-9). Washington, D.C.: Author.

Youngkin, E. Q., & Davis, M. S. (2004). *Women's health: a primary care clinical guide* (3rd ed.). Upper Saddle River, NJ: Prentice Hall.

Web Resources

Academy for Guided Imagery, Inc.: **www.interactiveimagery.com**
American College of Obstetricians and Gynecologists: **www.acog.org**
American Public Health Association: **www.apha.org**
Association of Labor Assistants and Childbirth Educators: **www.alace.org**
Association of Women's Health, Obstetric and Neonatal Nurses (AWHONN): **www.awhonn.org**
Birthworks: **www.birthworks.org**

BMJ Publication: Evidence-Based Nursing: **www.evidencebasednursing.com**
Child Find: **www.childfind.org**
Department of Health and Human Services: **www.4women.gov**
Diversity Rx: **www.diversityrx.org**
Doulas of North America (DONA): **www.dona.org**
Ethnomed: **http://ethnomed.org**
HypnoBirthing Institute: **www.hypnobirthing.com**
International Childbirth Education Association: **www.icea.org**
Lamaze International: **www.lamaze-childbirth.com**
National Center for Missing and Exploited Children: **www.missingkids.com**
Transcultural Health Links **www.iun.edu/~libemb/trannurs/trannurs.htm**

ChapterWORKSHEET

● MULTIPLE CHOICE QUESTIONS

1. When a client in labor is fully dilated, which instruction would be most effective to assist in encouraging effective pushing?

   a. Hold your breath and push through entire contraction.

   b. Use chest-breathing with the contraction.

   c. Pant and blow during each contraction.

   d. Push for 6 to 7 seconds several times during each contraction.

2. During the fourth stage of labor, the nurse palpates the uterus on the right side and sees a saturated perineal pad. What is the nurse's *first* action?

   a. Massage the uterus vigorously.

   b. Have the client void and reassess her.

   c. Notify the primary care provider.

   d. Document as a normal finding.

3. When managing a client's pain during labor, nurses should:

   a. Make sure the agents given don't prolong labor.

   b. Know that all pain-relief measures are similar.

   c. Support the client's decisions and requests.

   d. Not recommend nonpharmacologic methods.

4. When caring for a client during the active phase of labor without continuous electronic fetal monitoring, the nurse would intermittently assess FHR every:

   a. 15 minutes

   b. 5 minutes

   c. 30 minutes

   d. 60 minutes

5. The nurse notes the presence of transient fetal accelerations on the fetal monitoring strip. Which intervention would be most appropriate?

   a. Reposition the client on the left side.

   b. Begin 100% oxygen via face mask.

   c. Document this reassuring pattern.

   d. Call the healthcare provider immediately.

● CRITICAL THINKING EXERCISES

1. Carrie, a 20-year-old primigravida at term, comes to the birthing center in active labor (dilation 5 cm and 80% effaced, −1 station) with ruptured membranes. She states she wants an "all-natural" birth without medication. Her partner is with her and appears anxious but supportive. On the admission assessment, Carrie's prenatal history is unremarkable; vital signs are within normal limits; FHR via Doppler ranges between 140 and 144 bpm and is regular.

   a. Based on your assessment data and the woman's request not to have medication, what nonpharmacologic interventions could the nurse offer her?

   b. What positions might be suggested to help facilitate fetal descent?

2. Several hours later, Carrie complains of nausea and turns to her partner and angrily tells him to not touch her and to go away.

   a. What assessment needs to be done to determine what is happening?

   b. What explanation can you offer Carrie's partner regarding her change in behavior?

● STUDY ACTIVITIES

1. Interview a primigravida at a community maternity clinic in her last trimester of pregnancy about her birth plan for pain management and specific coping skills she will use for labor. Evaluate them in terms of effectiveness according to the literature, and share this information with the woman.

2. On the fetal heart monitor, the nurse notices an elevation of the fetal baseline with the onset of contractions. This elevation would describe _____.

3. Compare and contrast a local birthing center to a community hospital's birthing suite in terms of the pain management techniques and fetal monitoring used.

4. Select a childbirth website for expectant parents and critique the information provided in terms of its educational level and amount of advertising.

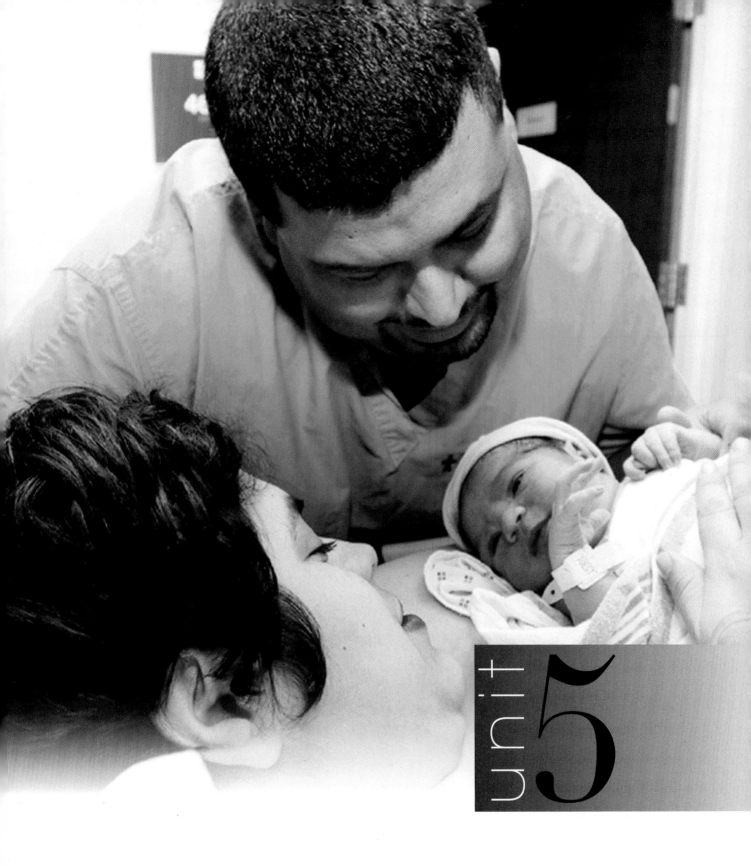

unit 5

Postpartum Period

chapter 15

Maternal Adaptation During the Postpartum Period

KeyTERMS

engorgement
engrossment
involution
lactation
letting-go phase
lochia
puerperium
taking-hold phase
taking-in phase
uterine atony

LearningOBJECTIVES

After studying the chapter content, the student should be able to accomplish the following:

1. Define the key terms.
2. Describe the systemic physiologic changes occurring in the woman after childbirth.
3. Identify the phases of maternal role adjustment as described by Reva Rubin.
4. Discuss the psychological adaptations occurring in the father after delivery.

The postpartum period covers a critical transitional time for a woman, her newborn, and her family on physiologic and psychological levels. The postpartum period begins after the delivery of the placenta and lasts for approximately 6 weeks.

This period, also known as the **puerperium,** generally encompasses the time after delivery as the woman's body begins to return to the prepregnant state until these changes resolve, generally by the sixth week after giving childbirth. However, the postpartum period can also be defined to include changes in all aspects of the mother's life that occur during the first year following the birth of her child. Some birth professionals feel the postpartum adjustment period lasts well into the first year, making the fourth phase of labor the longest.

This chapter describes the major physiologic and psychological changes that occur in a woman after childbirth. Various systemic adaptations take place throughout the woman's body systems. In addition, the mother and the family unit adjust to the new addition psychologically. The birth of a child changes the family structure and the roles of the family members. The adaptations are dynamic in nature and continue to evolve as physical changes occur and new roles emerge.

Maternal Physiologic Adaptations

During pregnancy, the woman's entire body system experienced changes to accommodate the needs of the growing fetus. After birth, the woman's body once again undergoes significant changes in all body systems to return her body to its prepregnant state.

Reproductive System Adaptations

The female reproductive system is unique in its capacity to remodel constantly throughout the woman's reproductive life. The events after birth, with the shedding of the placenta and subsequent uterine **involution,** involve substantial tissue destruction and subsequent repair and remodeling. For example, the woman's menstrual cycle, interrupted during pregnancy, will begin to return again several weeks after childbirth. The uterus, which has undergone tremendous expansion during pregnancy to accommodate progressive fetal growth, will now return to its prepregnant size over several weeks. In addition, the maternal breasts have grown to prepare for **lactation.** However, the breasts will not return to their prepregnant size as the uterus does.

The reproductive system goes through tremendous adaptations to return to the prepregnancy state. All organs and tissues of the reproductive system are involved.

Uterus

The uterus returns to its normal size through a gradual process of involution, which involves retrogressive changes that return it to its nonpregnant size and condition. Involution involves three retrogressive processes:

1. Contraction of muscle fibers to reduce those previously stretched during pregnancy
2. Catabolism, which reduces enlarged, individual myometrial cells
3. Regeneration of uterine epithelium from the lower layer of the decidua after the upper layers have been sloughed off and shed during **lochia** (Murray et al., 2006)

Uterine involution is fairly rapid. It requires massive remodeling of the extracellular matrix in association with cell proliferation as the uterus returns to the prepregnancy state. The uterus, which weighs approximately 1000 g (2.2 lb) soon after birth, undergoes physiologic involution in its return to its nonpregnant state. Approximately 1 week after birth, the uterus weights about 500 g (1 lb); at the end of six weeks, it weighs approximately 60 g (2 oz), about the weight before the pregnancy (Scoggin, 2004).

During the first 3 days postpartum, the endometrium is very thin with a variable amount of decidual tissue, which can be retained after labor. Within the first 2 weeks, a normal healing process appears to occur along with abundant shedding of lochia. From weeks 3 to 6, the endometrium appears to be inactive, resembling proliferative phase tissue and reflecting the completion of involution (Salamonsen, 2003).

During the first few days after birth, the uterus typically descends downward from the level of the umbilicus at a rate of 1 cm (1 finger breadth) each day. By the end of 10 days, the fundus of the uterus usually cannot be palpated because it descended into the true pelvis.

Within a week of birth, the uterus shrinks in size by 50%, and by 6 weeks has returned to its normal size (Lowdermilk & Perry, 2004; Fig. 15-1). If retrogressive changes do not occur as a result of retained placental fragments or infection, subinvolution results.

Factors that facilitate uterine involution include complete expulsion of amniotic membranes and placenta at birth, complication-free labor and birth process, breast-feeding, and early ambulation. Factors that inhibit involution include prolonged labor and difficult birth, incomplete expulsion of amniotic membranes and placenta, uterine infection, overdistension of uterine muscles

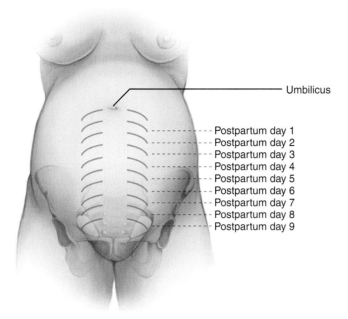

Umbilicus

Postpartum day 1
Postpartum day 2
Postpartum day 3
Postpartum day 4
Postpartum day 5
Postpartum day 6
Postpartum day 7
Postpartum day 8
Postpartum day 9

● Figure 15-1 Uterine involution.

(such as by multiple gestation, hydramnios, or large singleton fetus), full bladder (which displaces uterus and interferes with contractions), anesthesia (which relaxes uterine muscles), close childbirth spacing (frequent and repeated distention decreases tone and causes muscular relaxation), and anesthesia.

Lochia

Lochia refers to the discharge that occurs after birth. It results from involution, during which the superficial layer of the decidua basalis becomes necrotic and is sloughed off. Immediately after childbirth, lochia is bright red and consists mainly of blood, fibrinous products, decidual cells, and red and white blood cells. The lochia from the uterus is alkaline, but becomes acidic as it passes through the vagina. It could be equated with the amount occurring during a heavy menstrual period. The average amount of lochial discharge is 240 to 270 mL (8–9 oz)(Scoggin, 2004).

Women who have had cesarean births tend to have less flow because the uterine debris is removed manually along with delivery of the placenta. Lochia discharge is present in most women for at least 3 weeks after childbirth, but may persist in some women for as long as 6 weeks.

Lochia passes through three stages: lochia rubra, lochia serosa, and lochia alba. Lochia rubra is a deep-red mixture of mucus, tissue debris, and blood occurring for the first 3 to 4 days after birth. As uterine bleeding subsides, it becomes paler and more serous. Lochia serosa characterizes the second stage. It is pink to brown in color and is expelled 3 to 10 days postpartum. Lochia serosa primarily contains leukocytes, decidual tissue, RBCs, and serous fluid. Lochia alba is the final stage. The discharge is creamy white or light brown and consists of leukocytes,

decidual tissue, and reduced fluid content. It occurs from days 10 to 14, but can last 3 to 6 weeks postpartum in some women and still be considered normal. Lochia at any stage should have a fleshy smell; an offensive odor usually indicates an infection, such as endometritis. A danger signal is the reappearance of bright-red blood after lochia rubra has stopped. Reevaluation by the woman's healthcare professional is essential if this occurs.

Afterpains

Part of the involution process involves uterine contractions. Subsequently, many women are frequently bothered by painful uterine contractions termed *afterpains*. All women experience afterpains, but they are more acute in multiparous women secondary to repeated stretching of the uterine muscles. This repeated stretching reduces muscle tone, allowing for alternate uterine contraction and relaxation. The uterus of a primiparous woman tends to remain contracted after giving birth unless she is breastfeeding; has experienced a prolonged, difficult labor and birth; or had an overdistended uterus secondary to multiple gestation, hydramnios, or has retained blood clots or placental fragments.

Afterpains are usually stronger during breast-feeding because oxytocin released by the sucking reflex strengthens uterine contractions. Mild analgesics can reduce this discomfort.

Cervix

The cervix typically returns to its prepregnant state by week 6 of the postpartum period. The cervix gradually closes but never regains its prepregnant appearance. Immediately after childbirth, the cervix is shapeless and edematous, and is easily distensible for several days. The cervical os gradually closes and returns to normal by 2 weeks, whereas the external os widens and never appears the same after childbirth. The external cervical os is no longer shaped like a circle, but instead appears as a jagged slit-like opening, often described as a "fish mouth" (Fig. 15-2).

Vagina

Shortly after birth, the vaginal mucosa is edematous and thin with few rugae. As ovarian function returns and as

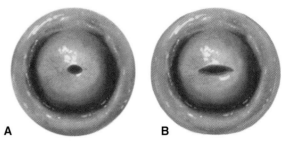

A   B

● Figure 15-2 Appearance of the cervical os. (**A**) Before the first pregnancy. (**B**) After pregnancy.

estrogen production resumes, the mucosa thickens and rugae return in approximately 3 weeks. The vagina gapes at the opening and is generally lax. The vagina returns to approximate prepregnant size by 6 to 8 weeks postpartum, but will always remain a bit larger than it had been before pregnancy. Normal mucus production and thickening of the vaginal mucosa usually returns with ovulation (Lowdermilk & Perry, 2004). Ovulation can return as early as a month after childbirth in non–breast-feeding women, with a mean time frame of 3 months. The mean time to ovulation in breast-feeding women is approximately 6 months, but can vary greatly depending on breast-feeding patterns (Bowes & Katz, 2002).

Localized dryness and coital discomfort (dyspareunia) usually plague most women until menstruation returns. Water-soluble lubricants can reduce discomfort during intercourse. Box 15-1 lists some commonly available water-soluble lubricants.

Perineum

The perineum is often edematous and bruised for the first day or two after birth. If the birth involved an episiotomy or laceration, complete healing may take as long as 4 to 6 months in the absence of complications at the site, such as hematoma or infection (Blackburn, 2003). Perineal lacerations may extend into the anus and cause considerable discomfort for the mother attempting to defecate or ambulate. The presence of swollen hemorrhoids may also heighten discomfort. Local comfort measures such as ice packs, warm water over the area via a peribottle, witch hazel pads, anesthetic sprays, and sitz baths can be helpful to relieve pain.

Supportive tissues of the pelvic floor are stretched during the childbirth process. Restoring their tone may require as long as 6 months. Pelvic relaxation can occur

---

BOX 15-1

WATER-SOLUBLE LUBRICANTS

- Astroglide
- Aqua Lube Personal
- Devine No 9
- Emerita
- Eros
- ID Glide sensual lubricant
- JO water-based lubricant
- K-Y personal lubricant
- LifeStyles personal lubricant
- Liquid Silk
- Nature's Dew
- Pre-Seed Intimate
- Replens
- Slippery Stuff

---

in any woman experiencing a vaginal birth. Nurses can encourage all women to practice Kegel exercises to improve pelvic floor tone, strengthen the perineal muscles, and promote healing. Not maintaining and restoring perineal muscular tone can lead to urinary incontinence later in life for many women.

Cardiovascular System Adaptations

The cardiovascular system undergoes dramatic changes after birth. During pregnancy, the heart is displaced slightly upward and to the left. This reverses as the uterus undergoes involution. Cardiac output remains high for the first few days postpartum and then gradually declines to nonpregnant values within 2 to 4 weeks of birth.

Blood volume, which has increased substantially during pregnancy, drops rapidly after birth and returns to normal within 4 weeks postpartum (Bridges et al., 2003). The decrease in both cardiac output and blood volume reflects the birth-related blood loss (an average of 500 mL with a vaginal birth and 1000 mL with a cesarean birth). Blood volume is further reduced through diuresis, which occurs during the early postpartum period (Bridges et al., 2003). Despite the decrease in blood volume, the hematocrit level remains relatively stable and may even increase, reflecting the predominant loss of plasma. Thus, an acute decrease in hematocrit is not an expected finding and may indicate hemorrhage.

Pulse and Blood Pressure

The increase in cardiac output during pregnancy begins to diminish after birth. This decrease in cardiac output is reflected in bradycardia (50–70 bpm) for the first two 2 weeks postpartum. This slowing of the heart rate is related to the increased blood that flows back to the heart and to the central circulation after it is no longer perfusing the placenta. This increase in central circulation brings about an increased stroke volume and allows a slower heart rate to provide ample maternal circulation. Gradually, cardiac output returns to prepregnant levels by 3 months after childbirth (Blackburn, 2003).

Tachycardia (>100 bpm) in the postpartum woman warrants further investigation. It may indicate hypovolemia, dehydration, or hemorrhage. However, because of the increased blood volume during pregnancy, a considerable loss may be well tolerated and not cause a compensatory cardiovascular response such as tachycardia. In most instances of postpartum hemorrhage, blood pressure and cardiac output remain increased because of the compensatory increase in heart rate. Thus, a decrease in blood pressure and cardiac output are not expected changes during the postpartum period. Early identification is essential to ensure prompt intervention.

Blood pressure values should be similar to those obtained during the labor process. In some women there may be a slight transient increase lasting for about a week after childbirth (Bowes & Katz, 2002). A significant increase accompanied by headache might indicate preeclampsia and requires further investigation. A decreased blood pressure may suggest orthostatic hypotension or uterine hemorrhage.

Coagulation

Clotting factors that increased during pregnancy tend to remain elevated during the early postpartum period. Giving birth stimulates this hypercoagulability state further. As a result, these coagulation factors remain elevated for 2 to 3 weeks postpartum (Littleton & Engebretson, 2005). This hypercoagulable state, combined with vessel damage during birth and immobility, places the woman at risk for thromboembolism (blood clots) in the lower extremities and the lungs.

Urinary System Adaptations

Pregnancy and birth can have profound affects on the urinary system. During pregnancy, the GFR and renal plasma flow increase significantly. Both usually normalize by 6 weeks after birth.

Many women have difficulty with feeling the sensation to void after giving birth if they have received an anesthetic block during labor (which inhibits neural functioning of the bladder), or if they received oxytocin to induce or augment their labor (antidiuretic effect). These women will be at risk for incomplete emptying, bladder distention, difficulty voiding, bladder distention and urinary retention. In addition, urination may be impeded by

- Perineal lacerations
- Generalized swelling and bruising of the perineum and tissues surrounding the urinary meatus
- Hematomas
- Decreased bladder tone as a result of regional anesthesia
- Diminished sensation of bladder pressure as a result of swelling, poor bladder tone, and numbing effects of regional anesthesia used during labor (McKinney et al., 2005)

Difficulty voiding can lead to urinary retention, bladder distention, and ultimately, urinary tract infection (UTI). Urinary retention and bladder distention can cause displacement of the uterus from the midline to the right and can inhibit the uterus from contracting properly, which increases the risk of postpartum hemorrhage. Urinary retention is a major cause of **uterine atony,** which allows excessive bleeding. Frequent voiding of small amounts (<150 mL) suggests urinary retention with overflow, and catheterization may be necessary to empty the bladder to restore tone.

Postpartum diuresis occurs as a result of several mechanisms: the large amounts of IV fluids given during labor, a decreasing antidiuretic effect of oxytocin as its level declines, the buildup and retention of extra fluids during pregnancy, and a decreasing production of aldosterone—the hormone that decreases sodium retention and increases urine production (Littleton & Engebretson, 2005). All these factors contribute to rapid filling of the bladder within 12 hours of birth. Diuresis begins within 12 hours after childbirth and continues throughout the first week postpartum. Normal function returns within a month after birth (Mattson & Smith, 2004).

An inability to void leads to bladder overfilling and distention. The uterus, in turn, is displaced and unable to contract effectively (uterine atony). As a result, the uterine blood vessels do not compress, placing the woman at risk for hemorrhage.

ConsiderTHIS!

Have you ever felt like a real idiot by not being able to complete a simple task in life? I had a beautiful baby boy after only 6 hours of labor. My epidural worked well and I actually felt very little discomfort throughout my labor. Because it was in the middle of the night when they brought me to my postpartum room, I felt a few hours of sleep would be all I needed to accomplish anything. During an assessment early the next morning, the nurse found my uterus had shifted to the right from my midline and I was instructed to empty my bladder. I didn't understand why the nurse was concerned about where my uterus was located and, besides, I didn't feel any sensation of a full bladder. But I did get up anyway and tried to comply. Despite all the nurse's tricks of faucet water running for sound effects, in addition to having warm water poured over my thighs via the peri-bottle, I was unable to urinate. How could I not accomplish one of life's simplest tasks?

Thoughts: Women who receive regional anesthesia frequently experience reduced sensation to their perineal area and do not feel a full bladder. The nursing assessment revealed a displaced uterus secondary to a full bladder. What additional "tricks" can be used to assist this woman to void? What explanation should be offered to her regarding why she is having difficulty urinating?

Gastrointestinal System Adaptations

The GI system quickly returns to normal because the gravid uterus is no longer encompassing the abdominal cavity and producing pressure on the abdominal organs. Progesterone levels, which caused relaxation of smooth muscle during pregnancy and diminished bowel tone, also are declining. Bowel tone remains slow for several days after birth. Subsequently constipation is a common problem during the postpartum period.

Regardless of the type of delivery, most women experience sluggish bowels for several days after birth. Decreased peristalsis occurs in response to analgesic pain management, surgery, diminished intraabdominal pressure, low-fiber diet and insufficient fluid intake, and diminished muscle tone. In addition, women with an episiotomy, perineal laceration, or hemorrhoids may fear pain or damage to the perineum with their first bowel movement, thereby attempting to delay it. A stool softener can be prescribed for this reason.

Most women are hungry and thirsty after childbirth, commonly related to restrictions imposed and energy expended during labor. Their appetite returns to normal immediately after giving birth. Anticipating the woman's need to replenish the body with food and fluids, and providing both soon after childbirth, are important.

Musculoskeletal System Adaptations

The effects of pregnancy on the muscles and joints vary widely. During pregnancy, the hormones relaxin, estrogen, and progesterone relax the joints. After birth, these hormones decline, resulting in a return of all joints to their prepregnant state, with the exception of the woman's feet. Parous women will note a permanent increase in their shoe size (Lowdermilk & Perry, 2004).

Woman commonly experience fatigue, activity intolerance, and have a distorted body image for weeks after birth secondary to declining relaxin and progesterone levels, which cause hip and joint pain that interferes with ambulation and exercise. Good body mechanics and correct position are important during this time to prevent low back pain and injury to the joints. Within 6 to 8 weeks after delivery, joints are completely stabilized and return to normal.

During pregnancy, stretching of the abdominal wall muscles occurs to accommodate the enlarging uterus. This stretching leads to a loss in muscle tone and possibly separation of the longitudinal muscles (rectus abdominis muscles) of the abdomen. Separation of the rectus abdominis muscles is called *diastasis recti* and is more common in women who have poor abdominal muscle tone before pregnancy. After birth, muscle tone is diminished and abdominal muscles are soft and flabby. Specific exercises are necessary to help the woman regain muscle tone. If rectus muscle tone is not regained through exercise, support may not be adequate during future pregnancies. Fortunately, diastasis responds well to exercise, and abdominal muscle tone can be improved (see Chapter 16 for more information about exercises to improve muscle tone).

Integumentary System Adaptations

Another system that experiences lasting effects of pregnancy is the integumentary system. As estrogen and progesterone levels decrease, the darkened pigmentation demonstrated on the abdomen (linea nigra), face (melasma), and nipples gradually fades. Some women experience hair loss during pregnancy and postpartum periods. Approximately 90% of hair is growing at any one time, with the other 10% entering a resting phase. Because of the high estrogen levels present during pregnancy, an increased number of hairs go into the resting phase, which is part of the normal hair loss cycle. The most common period of hair loss occurs within 3 months after birth, when estrogen returns to normal levels and more hair is allowed to fall out. This hair loss is temporary, and regrowth generally returns to normal levels in 6 to 12 months (Ladewig, London, & Davidson, 2006).

Striae gravidarum (stretch marks) developed during pregnancy on the breasts, abdomen, and hips gradually fade to silvery lines. However, these lines do not disappear completely. Although many products on the market claim to make stretch marks disappear, the actual effectiveness of these products is highly questionable.

The profuse diaphoresis (sweating) that is common during the early postpartum period is one of the most noticeable adaptations in the integumentary system. Many women will wake up drenched with perspiration during the puerperium. This postpartal diaphoresis is a mechanism to reduce the fluids retained during pregnancy and restore prepregnant body fluid levels. It can become profuse at times. It is common, especially at night during the first week after birth. Reassure the client that this is normal and encourage her to change her gown to prevent chilling.

Respiratory System Adaptations

Respirations usually remain within the normal adult range of 16 to 24 breaths per minute. As the abdominal organs resume their nonpregnant position, the diaphragm returns to its usual position. Anatomic changes in the thoracic cavity and rib cage caused by increasing uterine growth change quickly. As a result, discomforts such as shortness of breath and rib aching are relieved. Tidal volume, minute volume, vital capacity, and functional residual capacity return to prepregnant values, typically within 1 to 3 weeks of birth (Matteson, 2001).

Endocrine System Adaptations

The endocrine system undergoes several changes rapidly after birth. Levels of circulating estrogen and progesterone drop quickly with delivery of the placenta. Decreased estrogen levels are associated with breast **engorgement** and with the diuresis of excess extracellular fluid accumulated during pregnancy (Ladewig, London, & Davidson, 2006). Estrogen is at its lowest level a week after birth. For the nonbreast-feeding woman, estrogen levels begin to increase by 2 weeks after birth. For the breast-feeding woman, estrogen levels remain low until breast-feeding frequency decreases.

Other placental hormones (hCG, hPL, progesterone) decline rapidly after birth. hCG levels are nonexistent at the end of the first postpartum week and hPL is undetectable within 1 day after birth (Mattson & Smith, 2004). Progesterone levels are undetectable by 3 days after childbirth, and production is reestablished with the first menses. Prolactin levels decline within 2 weeks for the nonbreast-feeding mother and remain elevated for the lactating woman (McKinney et al., 2005).

Lactation

Lactation is the secretion of milk by the breasts. It is thought to be brought about by the interaction of progesterone, estrogen, prolactin, and oxytocin. Breast milk typically appears 3 days after childbirth.

During pregnancy, the breasts increase in size and functional ability in preparation for breast-feeding. Within the first month of gestation, the ducts of the mammary glands grow branches, forming more lobules and alveoli. These structural changes make the breasts larger, more tender, and heavy. Each breast gains nearly 1 lb in weight by term, the glandular cells fill with secretions, blood vessels increase in number, and there are increased amounts of connective tissue and fat cells (Sloane, 2002).

Prolactin from the anterior pituitary gland, secreted in increasing levels throughout pregnancy, triggers synthesis and secretion of milk after giving birth. During pregnancy, prolactin, estrogen, and progesterone cause synthesis and secretion of colostrum, which contains protein and carbohydrate, but no milk fat. It is only after birth takes place, when the high levels of estrogen and progesterone are abruptly withdrawn, that prolactin is able to stimulate the glandular cells to secrete milk instead of colostrum. This takes place within 2 to 3 days after giving birth. Oxytocin acts so that milk can be ejected from the alveoli to the nipple. Therefore, sucking by the newborn will release milk. Prolactin levels increase in response to nipple stimulation during feedings. Prolactin and oxytocin result in milk production if stimulated by sucking (Sloane, 2002)(Fig. 15-3). If the stimulus (sucking) is not present, as with a non–breast-feeding mother, breast engorgement and potential milk production will subside within 2 to 3 days postpartum.

Typically, during the first 2 days after birth, the breasts are soft and nontender. The woman also may report a tingling sensation occurring in both breasts. After this time, breast changes depend on whether the mother is breast-feeding or taking measures to prevent lactation.

Engorgement is the process of swelling of the breast tissue as a result of an increase in blood and lymph supply as a precursor to lactation (O'Toole, 2003). Breasts increase in vascularity and swell in response to prolactin 2 to 4 days after birth. If engorged, the breasts will be hard and tender to touch. They are temporarily full, tender, and very uncomfortable until the milk supply is ready. Frequent emptying of the breasts helps to minimize discomfort and resolve engorgement. Standing in a warm shower or applying warm compresses to the breasts may provide some relief. To maintain milk supply, the breasts need to be stimulated by a nursing infant, a breast pump, or manual expression of the milk (Fig. 15-4).

If the woman is not breast-feeding, relief measures include wearing a tight, supportive bra 24 hours daily,

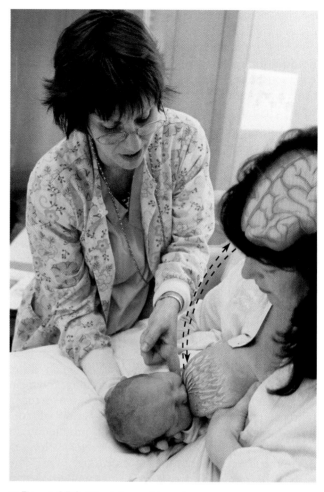

● Figure 15-3 **Physiology of lactation.**

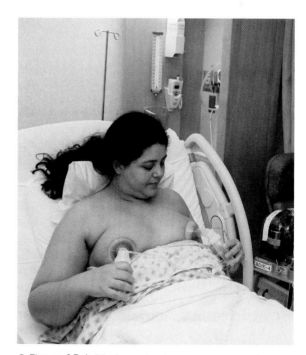

● Figure 15-4 Mother using breast pumps to stimulate milk production.

applying ice to her breasts for approximately 15 to 20 minutes every other hour, and not stimulating the breasts by squeezing or manually expressing milk from the nipples. In addition, avoiding exposing the breasts to warmth (e.g., hot shower water) will help relieve breast engorgement. Nonbreast-feeding engorgement typically subsides within 2 to 3 days with these measures.

Ovulation and Return of Menstruation

A series of changing hormone levels constantly interacts with one another to produce bodily changes. Four major hormones affect the postpartum period: estrogen, progesterone, prolactin, and oxytocin. Estrogen is the major female hormone during pregnancy, but it drops profoundly at birth and reaches its lowest level a week into the postpartum period. Progesterone quiets the uterus to prevent a preterm birth during pregnancy, and its increasing levels during pregnancy prevent lactation from starting before birth takes place. As with estrogen, progesterone levels decrease dramatically after birth and are undetected 72 hours after childbirth. Progesterone levels are reestablished with the first menstrual cycle (Behnke, 2003).

During the postpartum period, oxytocin stimulates the uterus to contract during the breast-feeding session and for as long as 20 minutes after each feeding. Oxytocin also acts on the breast by eliciting the milk let-down reflex during breast-feeding. Prolactin is also associated with the breast-feeding process by stimulating milk production. In women who breast-feed, prolactin levels remain elevated into the sixth week after birth (Bowes & Katz, 2002). The levels of the hormone increase and decrease in proportion to nipple stimulation. Prolactin levels decrease in nonlactating women, reaching the prepregnant levels by the third postpartum week (Bowes & Katz, 2002). High levels of prolactin have been found to delay ovulation by inhibiting ovarian response to FSH (Too, 2003).

Lactating and nonlactating women differ considerably in the timing of their first menses and ovulation after birth. For nonlactating women, menstruation usually resumes 7 to 9 weeks after giving birth, with the first cycle being anovulatory (Sloane, 2002). The return of menses in the lactating woman depends on breast-feeding frequency and duration. It can return anytime from 2 to 18 months after childbirth, depending on whether the breast-feeding mother is exclusively breast-feeding or supplementing with formula. The first postpartum menses may be heavier than prepregnant ones and are frequently anovulatory (Youngkin & Davis, 2004). However, ovulation may occur before menstruation; therefore, breast-feeding is not a reliable method of contraception. Other methods of family planning need to be used to control fertility (Alexander et al., 2004).

Psychological Adaptations

Mothers' and fathers' experiences of pregnancy are necessarily different, and this difference continues after childbirth as they both adjust to their new parenting roles. Parenting involves caring for infants physically and emotionally to foster the growth and development of responsible, caring adults. During the early months of parenthood, mothers experience more life changes and get more satisfaction from their new roles than fathers. However, fathers interact with their newborns much like mothers (Buist et al., 2003). Early parent–infant contact after birth improves attachment behaviors. Other members of the newborn's family unit, such as siblings and grandparents, also experience changes related to the birth of the newborn. Chapter 16 describes these changes.

Maternal Adaptations

The woman experiences a variety of responses as she adjusts to a new family member, postpartum discomforts, changes in her body image, and the reality of change within her life. In the early 1960s, Reva Rubin (1984) identified three phases that a mother goes through to adjust to her new maternal role. Rubin's maternal role framework can be used to monitor the client's progress as she "tries on" her new role as a mother. Absence of these processes or inability to progress through the phases satisfactorily may impede the appropriate development of the maternal role (Rubin, 1984). Although Rubin's maternal role development theories are of value, some of her observations regarding the length of each phase may not be completely relevant for the contemporary woman of the 21st century. Today, many women know their infant's gender, have "seen" their fetus in utero through four-dimensional ultrasound, and have a working knowledge of childbirth and child care. They are less passive than in years past and progress through the phases of attaining the maternal role at a much faster pace than Rubin would have imagined. Still, Rubin's framework is timeless for assessing and monitoring expected role behaviors when planning care and appropriate interventions.

Taking-In Phase

The **taking-in phase** is the time immediately after birth when the client needs sleep, depends on others to meet her needs, and relives the events surrounding the birth process. This phase is characterized by dependent behavior. During the first 24 to 48 hours after giving birth, mothers often assume a very passive role in meeting their own basic needs for food, fluids, and rest, allowing the nurse to make decisions for them concerning activities and care. They spend time recounting their labor experience to anyone who will listen. Such actions help the mother integrate the birth experience into reality—that is, the pregnancy is over and the newborn is now a unique individual, separate from herself. When interacting with the newborn, new mothers spend time claiming the newborn and touching them, commonly identifying specific features in the newborn, such as "he has my nose" or "his fingers are long like his father's" (Fig. 15-5). This phase

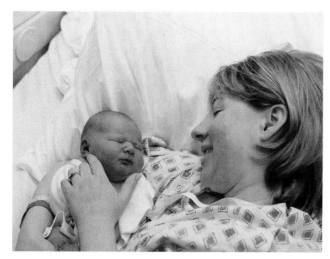

● Figure 15-5 Mother bonding with newborn during the taking-in phase.

typically lasts 1 to 2 days and may be the only phase observed by nurses in the hospital setting because shortened postpartum stays are the norm today.

Taking-Hold Phase
The **taking-hold phase** is the second phase of maternal adaptation, characterized by dependent and independent maternal behavior. This phase typically starts on the second to third day postpartum and may last several weeks.

As the client regains control over her bodily functions during the next few days, she will be *taking hold* and becoming preoccupied with the present. She will be particularly concerned about her health, the infant's condition, and her ability to care for him or her. She demonstrates increased autonomy and mastery of her own body's functioning, and a desire to take charge with support and help from others. She will show independence by caring for herself and learning to care for her newborn, but she still requires assurance that she is doing well as a mother. She expresses a strong interest in caring for the infant by herself.

Letting-Go Phase
The **letting-go phase** is the third phase of maternal adaptation, occurring later in the postpartum period when the woman reestablishes relationships with other people. She adapts to parenthood through her new role as a mother. She assumes the responsibility and care for the newborn with a bit more confidence now (Engstrom, 2004). The focus of this phase is to move forward by assuming the parental role and to separate herself from the symbiotic relationship that she and her newborn had during pregnancy. She establishes a lifestyle that includes the infant. The mother relinquishes the fantasy infant and accepts the real one.

Paternal Adaptations

For men, becoming a parent can be a perplexing time as well as a time for great social change. The transition to fatherhood is influenced by many factors, including participation in childbirth, relationships with significant others, competence in child care, the family role organization, the father's cultural background, and the method of infant feeding. Most research findings stress the importance of early contact for father and newborn, as well as participation in infant care activities to foster that relationship (Matteson, 2001). Infants have a powerful effect on their fathers, who become intensely involved with them (Fig. 15-6). The father's developing bond to his newborn—a time of intense absorption, preoccupation, and interest—is called **engrossment.** Engrossment is characterized by seven behaviors:

1. *Visual awareness of the newborn*—the father perceives the newborn as attractive, pretty, or beautiful
2. *Tactile awareness of the newborn*—the father has a desire to touch or hold the newborn and feels this activity as pleasurable to himself
3. *Perception of the newborn as perfect*—the father does not "see" any imperfections
4. *Strong attraction to the newborn*—the father focuses all attention on the newborn when he is in the room
5. *Awareness of distinct features of the newborn*—the father can distinguish his newborn from others in the nursery
6. *Extreme elation*—the father feels a "high" after the birth of his child
7. *Increased sense of self-esteem*—the father feels proud, bigger, more mature, and older after the birth of his child (Greenberg & Morris, 1974)

Similar to mothers, fathers also go through a predictable three-stage process during the first 3 weeks as

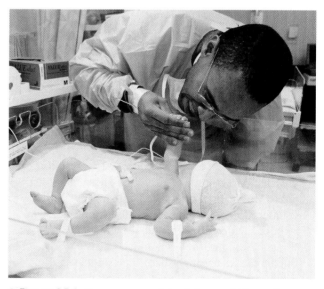

● Figure 15-6 Engrossment of the father and his newborn.

they too "try on" their roles as fathers. The three stages include expectations, reality, and transition to mastery (Henderson & Brouse, 1991).

Stage 1: Expectations

New fathers pass through stage 1 (expectations) with pre-conceptions about what home life will be like with a newborn. Many men may be unaware of the dramatic changes that can occur when this newborn comes home to live with them. For some, it is an "eye-opening" experience.

Stage 2: Reality

Stage 2 (reality) occurs when fathers realize that their expectations in stage 1 are not realistic. Their feelings change from those of elation to sadness, ambivalence, jealousy, and frustration. Many wish to be more involved in the newborn's care and yet do not feel prepared to do so. Some find parenting fun, but at the same time feel they are not fully prepared to take on that role.

Stage 3: Transition to Mastery

Stage 3 (transition to mastery) describes a father who makes a conscious decision to take control and be at the center of his newborn's life regardless of his preparedness. This adjustment period is similar to that of the mother's letting-go phase when she incorporates the newest member into the family unit.

Frequently, fathers are portrayed as well meaning, but bumbling, when caring for newborns. Fathers have their own unique way of relating to their newborns and can become as nurturing as mothers. A father's nurturing responses may be less automatic and slower to unfold than a mother's, but fathers are capable of a strong bonding attachment to their newborns (Sears, 2004). Encouraging fathers to express their feelings, by seeing, touching, and holding their son or daughter; and by cuddling, talking to, and feeding will help to cement this new relationship. Reinforcement of this engrossing behavior helps fathers to facilitate a positive attachment during this critical period.

KEY CONCEPTS

- The postpartum period or puerperium refers to the first 6 weeks after delivery. During this period, the mother experiences many physiologic and psychological adaptations to return her to the prepregnant state.
- Involution involves three processes: contraction of muscle fibers to reduce stretched ones, catabolism (which reduces enlarged, individual cells), and regeneration of uterine epithelium from the lower layer of the decidua after the upper layers have been sloughed off and shed in lochia.
- Lochia passes through three stages: lochia rubra, lochia serosa, and lochia alba during the postpartal period.

- Maternal blood volume decreases rapidly after birth and returns to normal within 4 weeks postpartum.
- Reva Rubin (1984) identified three phases the mother goes through to adjust to her new maternal role. The phases of maternal postpartum adjustment are taking in, taking hold, and letting go.
- The transition to fatherhood is influenced by many factors, including participation in childbirth, relationships with significant others, competence in child care, the family role organization, the father's cultural background, and the method of infant feeding.
- Similar to mothers, men go through a predictable three-stage process during the first 3 weeks as they too "try on" their roles as fathers. The three stages include expectations, reality, and transition to mastery.

References

Alexander, L. L., LaRosa, J. H., Bader, H., & Garfield, S. (2004). *New dimensions in women's health* (3rd ed.). Sudbury, MA: Jones and Bartlett Publishers.

Behnke, A. (2003). The physical and emotional effects of postpartum hormone levels. *International Journal of Childbirth Education, 18,* 11–14.

Blackburn, S. T. (2003). *Maternal, fetal, and neonatal physiology* (2nd ed.). Philadelphia: Saunders.

Bowes, W., & Katz, V. Postpartum care. (2002). In Gabbe, S., Niebyl, J., Simpson, J. (Eds.), *Obstetrics: normal and problem pregnancies* (4th ed.). New York: Churchill Livingstone.

Bridges, E. J., Womble, S., Wallace, M., & McCartney, J. (2003). Hemodynamic monitoring in high-risk obstetrics patients: expected hemodynamic changes in pregnancy. *Critical Care Nurse, 23,* 53–63.

Buist, A., Morse, C. A., & Durkin, S. (2003). Men's adjustment to fatherhood: implications for obstetric health care. *JOGNN, 32,* 172–180.

Engstrom, J. (2004). *Maternal–neonatal nursing made incredibly easy.* Philadelphia: Lippincott Williams & Wilkins.

Greenberg, M., & Morris, N. (1974). Engrossment: the newborn's impact upon the father. *American Journal of Orthopsychiatry, 44,* 520–531.

Henderson, A., & Brouse, A. (1991). The experiences of new fathers during the first three weeks of life. *Journal of Advanced Nursing, 16,* 293–298.

Ladewig, P. A., London, M. L., & Davidson, M. R. (2006). *Contemporary maternal-newborn nursing care* (6th ed.). Upper Saddle River, NJ: Pearson Prentice Hall.

Littleton, L. Y., & Engebretson, J. C. (2005). *Maternity nursing care.* Clifton Park, NY: Thomson Delmar Learning.

Lowdermilk, D. L., & Perry, S. E. (2004). *Maternity & women's health care* (8th ed.). St. Louis: Mosby.

Matteson, P. S. (2001). *Women's health during the childbearing years: a community-based approach.* St. Louis: Mosby.

Mattson, S., & Smith, J. E. (2004). *Core curriculum for maternal–newborn nursing* (3rd ed.). St. Louis: Elsevier Saunders.

McKinney, E. S., James, S. R., Murray, S. S., & Ashwill, J. W. (2005). *Maternal–child nursing* (2nd ed.). St. Louis: Elsevier Saunders.

Murray, S. S. & McKinney, E. S. (2006). *Foundations of maternal-newborn nursing* (4th ed.). St. Louis: Saunders Elsevier.

O'Toole, M. T. (2003). *Miller–Keane encyclopedia & dictionary of medicine, nursing, and allied health* (7th ed.). Philadelphia: Saunders.

Rubin, R. (1984). *Maternal identity and the maternal experience.* New York: Springer.

Salamonsen, L. A. (2003). Tissue injury and repair in the female reproductive tract. *Society of Reproduction and Fertility, 125,* 301–311.

Scoggin, J. (2004). Physical and psychologic changes. In Mattson, S., & Smith, J. E. (Eds.), *Core curriculum for maternal newborn nursing* (3rd ed., pp. 371–386). Philadelphia: WB Saunders.

Sears, W. (2004). Bonding with your baby. *Journal of Attachment and Parenting International.* [Online] Available at www. attachmentparenting.org/artbonding.shtml.

Sloane, E. (2002). *Biology of women* (4th ed.). Albany, NY: Delmar.

Too, S. (2003). Breastfeeding and contraception. *British Journal of Midwifery, 11,* 88–93.

Youngkin, E. Q., & Davis, M. S. (2004). *Women's health: a primary care clinical guide* (3rd ed.). Upper Saddle River, NJ: Prentice Hall.

Web Resources

American College of Nurse-Midwives, **www.midwife.org**

Association for Perinatal Psychology and Health, **www.birthpsychology.com**

Association of Maternal & Child Health Programs, **www.amchpl.org**

Center for Postpartum Health, **www.postpartumhealth.com**

Depression after Delivery, **www.depressionafterdelivery.com**

Home-Based Working Moms (HBWM), **www.hbwm.com**

International Lactation Consultants Association, **www.ilca.org**

La Leche League, **www.lalecheleague.org**

Midwifery Today, Inc., **www.midwiferytoday.com**

National Center for Fathering, **www.fathers.com**

National Parenting Center, **www.tnpc.com**

National Women's Health Information Center, **www.4women.gov**

Parenthood Web, **www.parenthoodweb.com**

Parenting Q & A, **www.parenting-qa.com**

Parents Anonymous, Inc., **www.parentsanonymous.org**

Parents Helping Parents, **www.php.com**

Postpartum Support International, **www.chss.iup.edu/postpartum/**

Chapter WORKSHEET

● MULTIPLE CHOICE QUESTIONS

1. The nurse understands that postpartal breast engorgement occurs 48 to 72 hours after giving birth as a result of an increase in

   a. Blood and lymph supply

   b. Estrogen and progesterone levels

   c. Colostrum production

   d. Fluid retention in the breasts

2. In the taking-in maternal role phase described by Rubin (1984), the nurse would expect the woman's behavior to be characterized as which of the following?

   a. Gaining self confidence

   b. Adjusting to her new relationships

   c. Being passive and dependent

   d. Resuming control over her life

3. The nurse is explaining to a postpartal woman that the afterpains she is experiencing are as a result of

   a. Manipulation of the uterus during labor

   b. A large infant weighing more than 8 lb

   c. Pregnancies that were too closely spaced

   d. Contractions of the uterus after birth

4. The nurse would expect a postpartal woman to demonstrate lochia in which sequence?

   a. Rubra, alba, serosa

   b. Rubra, serosa, alba

   c. Serosa, alba, rubra

   d. Alba, rubra, serosa

5. One of the mothers on the postpartum unit asks the nurse why she is sweating so much since giving birth to her baby. The nurse replies that profuse diaphoresis occurs because her body is

   a. Starting the lactation process

   b. Ridding her body of the pain medications

   c. Restoring her prepregnant fluid levels

   d. Signaling an infectious process

● CRITICAL THINKING EXERCISES

1. A new nurse assigned to the postpartum mother–baby unit makes a comment to the oncoming shift that Ms. Griffin, a 25-year-old primipara seems lazy and shows no initiative in taking care of herself or her baby. The nurse reported that Ms. Griffin talks excessively about her labor and birth experience, and seems preoccupied with herself and her needs, and not her newborn's care. She wonders if something is wrong with this mother because she seems so self-centered and has to be directed to do everything.

   a. Is there something "wrong" with the Ms. Griffin's behavior?

   b. What maternal role phase is being described by the new nurse?

   c. What role can the nurse play to support the mother through this phase?

2. Mrs. Lenhart, a primipara, gave birth to a healthy baby boy yesterday. Her husband John seemed elated at the birth, calling his friends and family on his cell phone minutes after the birth. He passed out cigars and praised his wife for her efforts. Today, when the nurse walked into their room, Mr. Lenhart seemed very anxious around his new son and called for the nurse whenever the baby cried or needed a diaper change. He seemed standoffish when asked to hold his son and he spent time talking to other fathers in the waiting room, leaving his wife alone in the room.

   a. Would you consider Mr. Lenhart's paternal behavior to be normal at this time?

   b. What might Mr. Lenhart be feeling at this time?

   c. How can the nurse help this new father adjust to his new role?

● STUDY ACTIVITIES

1. Find an Internet resource that discusses general postpartum care for new mothers who might have questions after discharge.

2. Prepare a teaching plan for new mothers outlining the various physiologic changes that will take place after discharge.

3. The term that describes the return of the uterus to its prepregnant state is _____.

4. A deviated fundus to the right side of the abdomen would indicate a _____.

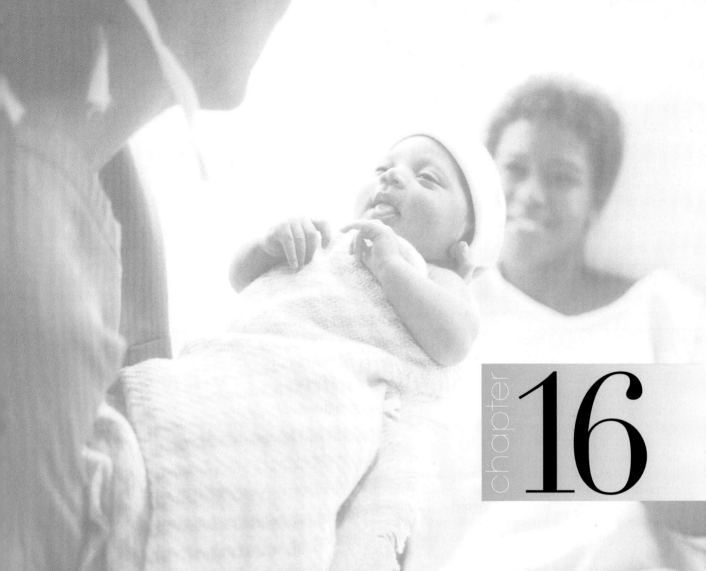

chapter 16

Nursing Management During the Postpartum Period

KeyTERMS

attachment
bonding
en face position
Kegel exercises
mastitis
peribottle
postpartum blues
sitz bath

LearningOBJECTIVES

After studying the chapter content, the student should be able to accomplish the following:

1. Define the key terms.
2. Describe the parameters requiring assessment during the postpartum period.
3. Discuss the bonding and attachment process.
4. Identify behaviors that enhance or inhibit the attachment process.
5. Outline nursing management for the woman and her family during the postpartum period.
6. Discuss the role of the nurse in promoting successful breast-feeding.
7. Identify areas of health education needed for discharge planning, home care, and follow-up.

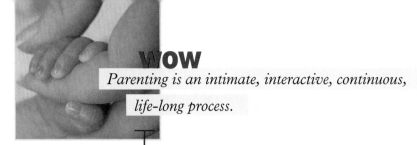

Parenting is an intimate, interactive, continuous, life-long process.

The postpartum period is a time of major adjustments and adaptations not just for the mother, but for all members of the family unit. It is during this time that parenting and a relationship with the newborn begins. A positive, loving relationship between parents and their newborn promotes the emotional well-being of all. This early-formed relationship endures through time and has profound effects on the child's growth and development.

Parenting is a skill that is often learned, to varying degrees of success, by trial and error. Successful parenting, a continuous and complex interactive process, requires the acquisition of new skills and the integration of the new member into the existing family unit.

Adapting to the role of a parent is not an easy process. The postpartum period is a "getting-to-know-you" time, when parents begin to integrate the newborn into their lives as they reconcile the fantasy child with the real one. This can be a very challenging period for families. Nurses play a major role in assisting families to adapt to the changes, thereby facilitating a smooth transition into parenthood. For established families with children, the addition of a new member may bring about role conflict and may present challenges to the entire family unit. Anticipatory guidance about other children's responses to the birth and new baby, increased emotional tension, child development, and meeting the multiple needs of their expanding family are key areas of discussion for the nurse. Although the multiparous woman has had previous experience with newborns, a nurse should not assume that it is current, accurate, and remembered, if it has been a while since the woman's last childbirth. Reinforcing previous instruction is important for all families.

As the face of America is changing with increasing diversity, nurses must be prepared to care for childbearing families from various cultures. For years, perinatal nurses have struggled with the issues surrounding the provision of optimal prenatal and postpartal care that meets the needs of women and their families from various cultures and ethnic groups. In many cultures, women and their families are cared for and nurtured by the community around them, sometimes for weeks, and possibly months, after the birth of a new family member. Box 16-1 highlights some of the major cultural influences during the postpartum period.

Sensitivity to how childbearing practices and beliefs vary for multicultural families is essential. Nurses need to understand how best to provide appropriate nursing care to meet their needs. Cultural practices may include the observance of certain dietary restrictions, clothing, or taboos for balancing the body; participation in certain activities for maintaining mental health; and the use of silence, prayer, or meditation for developing spiritual-

ity. Restoration of health may involve taking folk medicines or conferring with a tribe healer (Wong, Perry, & Hockenberry, 2002). The concept of family as paramount to beliefs surrounding health prevails among many ethnic cultures.

Nurses are responsible for providing culturally competent care in which the nurse must engage in ongoing cultural self-assessment and overcome any stereotyping that perpetuates prejudice or discrimination against any cultural group (Bowers, 2003). Implementing culturally competent nursing care during the postpartum period requires time, open-mindedness, and patience. Sensitivity to the woman's and family's culture, religion, and ethnic influences is essential in trying to promote positive health outcomes.

Strong social support is vital for positive integration of the newest member into the family unit. However, in today's mobile society, extended families do not live close by and may be unable to provide care for the new family. Subsequently, new parents turn to health care professionals for information as well as physical and emotional support during this adjustment period. Nurses provide a critical link and can be an invaluable resource by bridging the gap and providing mentoring, education about self-care measures and baby care basics, including feeding and the roles of the new family; and providing emotional support. Nurses can "mother" the new mother by offering physical, emotional, and informational support and practical help. The nurse's support and caring throughout this critical time can empower the parents and their families, increasing their confidence level and thereby providing them with a sense of accomplishment and feelings of success about their parenting skills.

One area of importance associated with the postpartum period is breast-feeding. Its importance is emphasized in Healthy People 2010 by the development of a specific goal for maternal, infant, and child health. This objective is presented in Healthy People 2010: National Health Goals Related to Breast-Feeding. Although the Department of Health and Human Services (DHHS) does not recommend universal breast-feeding for all women—such as those who use illicit drugs; who have active, untreated tuberculosis; or who test positive for HIV—the benefits of breast-feeding are well documented and thus are an important area to address.

This chapter describes the nursing management of the woman and her family during the postpartum period. It outlines physical assessment parameters necessary when caring for new mothers and their newborns. It also focuses on **bonding** and **attachment** behaviors of which nurses need to be aware so that appropriate interventions can be

BOX 16-1

CULTURAL INFLUENCES DURING THE POSTPARTUM PERIOD

African-American
- Mother may share care of the infant with extended family members.
- Experiences of older women within the family influence infant care.
- Mothers may protect their newborns from strangers for several weeks.
- Mothers may not bathe their newborns for the first week. Oils are applied to skin and hair to prevent dryness and cradle cap.
- Silver dollars may be taped over the infant's umbilicus in an attempt to flatten the slightly protruding umbilical stump.
- Sleeping with parents is a common practice (Thomas, 2003).

Amish
- Women consider childbearing their primary role in society.
- They generally oppose birth control or family planning practices.
- Pregnancy and childbirth are considered a private matter; they may conceal it from public knowledge.
- Women typically do not respond favorably when hurried to complete a self-care task. Nurses need to take cues from women indicating their readiness to complete morning self-care activities (Troyer & Troyer, 2003).

Appalachian
- Infant colic is treated by passing the newborn through a leather horse's collar or administering a weak catnip tea.
- An asafetida bag (a gum resin with a strong odor) is worn around the neck of the infant to keep away disease.
- Women may avoid eye contact with nurses and health-care providers.
- Women typically avoid asking questions even though they do not understand directions.
- The grandmother may rear the infant for the mother (Stephens, 2003).

Filipino-American
- Grandparents often assist in the care of their grandchildren.
- Breast-feeding is encouraged and some mothers will breast-feed their children for up to 2 years.
- Women have difficulty discussing birth control and sexual matters.
- Strong religious beliefs prevail and bedside prayer is common.
- Families are very close knit and numerous visitors can be expected to the hospital after childbirth (Anonas–Ternate, 2003).

Japanese-American
- Cleanliness and protection from cold are essential components of newborn care. Nurses are to give the daily bath to the infant.
- Newborns routinely are not taken outside the home because it is believed that newborns should not be exposed to outside or cold air. Infants should be kept in a quiet, clean, warm place for the first month of life.
- Breast-feeding is the primary method of feeding.
- Many women stay in their parents' home for 1 to 2 months after birth.
- Bathing the infant can be the center of family activity at home (Yeo, 2003).

Mexican-American
- The newborn's grandmother lives with the mother for several weeks after birth to help with housekeeping and child care.
- Most women will breast-feed more than 1 year. The infant is carried in a *rebozo* (shawl) that allows easy access to breast-feeding.
- Women may avoid eye contact and may not feel comfortable being touched by a stranger. Nurses need to respect this feeling.
- Some women may bring religious icons to the hospital and may want to display them in their postpartum room (Oria de Quinzanos, 2003).

Muslim
- Modesty is a primary concern; nurses need to protect their modesty.
- Most women will breast-feed, but religious events call for periods of fasting, which may increase the risk of dehydration or malnutrition.
- Women are exempt from obligatory prayer five times daily as long as lochia is present.
- Extended family is likely to be present throughout much of the woman's hospital stay and need an empty room to perform their prayers without having to leave the hospital (Badwan, 2003).

Native American
- Women are secretive about pregnancies and do not reveal them early.
- Touching is not a typical female behavior and eye contact is brief.
- They resent being hurried and need time for sitting and talking.
- Most mothers breast-feed and practice birth control (Plemmons, 2003).

National Health Goals Related to Breast-Feeding

Objective	Significance
Increase the proportion of mothers who breast-feed their babies. Increase in mothers who breast-feed during early postpartum from a baseline of 64% to 75%. Increase in mothers who breast-feed at 6 months from a baseline of 29% to 50%. Increase in mothers who breast-feed at 1 year from a baseline of 16% to 25%.	Will help to foster providing infants with the most complete form of nutrition, thereby affecting the infant's health, growth and development, and immunity Helpful in improving maternal health via breast-feeding's beneficial effects Will help increase the rate of breast-feeding, particularly among low-income and certain racial and ethnic populations less likely to begin breast-feeding in the hospital or to sustain it through the infant's first year

implemented to foster these behaviors. Interventions to address physiologic needs such as comfort, self-care, nutrition, and contraception are described. Additional information is discussed in helping the woman and her family adapt to the birth of the newborn (Fig. 16-1).

Nursing Management During the Postpartum Period

Nursing management during the postpartum period focuses on assessing the woman's ability to adapt to the physiologic and psychological changes occurring at this

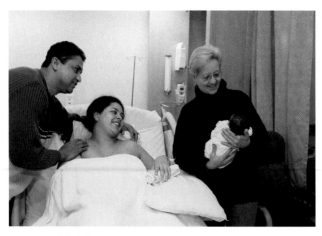

● Figure 16-1 Parents and grandmother interacting with the newborn.

time (see Chapter 15 for a detailed discussion of these adaptations). Family members are also assessed to determine their transition to this new stage. Based on assessment findings, the nurse plans and implements care to address the family's needs. Because of shortened lengths of stay, the nurse may be able to focus only on those needs considered priority and may be able arrange for follow-up in the home to ensure that all the family's needs are met.

Assessment

Comprehensive nursing assessment begins within an hour after the woman gives birth and continues through discharge. This assessment includes vital signs and physical and psychosocial assessments. Although the exact protocol may vary among facilities, postpartum assessment frequency typically is performed as follows:

- During the first hour: assessment every 15 minutes
- During the second hour: assessment every 30 minutes
- During the first 24 hours: assessment every 4 hours
- After 24 hours: assessment every 8 hours (Scoggin, 2004)

With each assessment, keep in mind possible risk factors that may lead to complications, such as infection or hemorrhage, during this recovery period (Box 16-2). Early identification is key to ensure prompt intervention.

As with any assessment, always review the woman's medical record for information related to her pregnancy,

---

BOX 16-2

FACTORS INCREASING THE WOMAN'S RISK FOR POSTPARTUM COMPLICATIONS

Risk Factors for Postpartum Infection
- Operative procedure (forceps, cesarean birth, vacuum extraction)
- History of diabetes, including gestational-onset diabetes
- Prolonged labor more than 24 hours
- Use of indwelling urinary catheter
- Anemia (hemoglobin < 10.5 mg/dL)
- Multiple vaginal examinations during labor
- Prolonged rupture of membranes more than 24 hours
- Manual extraction of placenta
- Compromised immune system (HIV positive)

Risk Factors for Postpartum Hemorrhage
- Precipitous labor less than 3 hours
- Uterine atony
- Placenta previa or abruption
- Labor induction or augmentation
- Operative procedures (vacuum extraction, forceps, cesarean birth)
- Retained placental fragments
- Prolonged third stage of labor more than 30 minutes
- Multiparity, more than three births closely spaced
- Uterine overdistention (large infant, twins, hydramnios)

labor, and birth. Note a history of any existing conditions or the development of problems or complications that may have occurred during pregnancy, labor, birth, and immediately afterward, along with any treatments initiated.

Postpartum assessment of the mother typically includes vital signs, pain level, and a systematic head-to-toe review of body systems. The acronym BUBBLE-HE—breasts, uterus, bladder, bowels, lochia, episiotomy/perineum, Homans' sign, emotional status—can be used as a guide to complete this head-to-toe review (Littleton & Engebretson, 2005).

While assessing the woman and her family during the postpartum period, be alert for findings that are considered danger signs (Box 16-3). Notify the primary health care provider immediately if any are noted.

Postpartum assessment also includes assessing the parents and other family members, such as siblings and grandparents, for attachment and bonding with the newborn.

Vital Signs

Obtain vital signs and compare them with the previous values, noting and reporting any deviations. Keep in mind that vital sign changes can be an early indicator of complications.

Temperature

Always assess temperature via the oral, axillary, or tympanic route to prevent the risk of perineal contamination via the rectal route. Typically, temperature during the first 24 hours postpartum is within the normal range. Some women experience a slight elevation in temperature, up to 38° C (100.4° F), during the first 24 hours. This elevation may be the result of dehydration because of fluid loss during labor. It should be normal after 24 hours. With replacement of fluids lost during labor and birth, temperature should stabilize and be within the normal range (Green & Wilkinson, 2004). A temperature greater than 38° C (100.4° F) at any time, or a subnormal temperature after the first 24 hours, may indicate infection and must

---

BOX 16-3

POSTPARTUM DANGER SIGNS

- Fever more than 38° C (100.4° F)
- Foul-smelling lochia or an unexpected change in color or amount
- Visual changes, such as blurred vision or spots, or headaches
- Calf pain experienced with dorsiflexion of the foot
- Swelling, redness, or discharge at the episiotomy site
- Dysuria, burning, or reports of incomplete emptying of the bladder
- Shortness of breath or difficulty breathing
- Depression or extreme mood swings

---

be reported. Abnormal temperature readings warrant continued monitoring until the presence of an infection can be ruled out through cultures or blood studies.

Pulse

As a result of the changes in blood volume and cardiac output after delivery, relative bradycardia may be noted. The woman's pulse rate may range from 50 to 70 bpm. Pulse usually stabilizes to prepregnancy levels within 10 days (Olds, London, Ladewig, & Davidson, 2004).

Tachycardia in the postpartum woman can suggest anxiety, excitement, fatigue, pain, excessive blood loss, infection, or underlying cardiac problems. Further investigation is warranted to rule out the possibility of complications.

Respirations

Respiratory rates in the postpartum woman should fall within the normal range of 16 to 20 breaths per minute. Any change in respiratory rate out of the normal range might be indicative of pulmonary edema, atelectasis, or pulmonary embolism and must be reported. Lungs should be clear on auscultation.

Blood Pressure

Blood pressure varies among individuals. Therefore, assess the woman's blood pressure and compare it with her usual range. Any deviation from this range must be reported. Elevations in blood pressure from the woman's baseline might suggest pregnancy-induced hypertension; decreases may suggest dehydration or excessive blood loss.

Blood pressure also may vary based on the woman's position, so be sure to assess blood pressure with the woman in the same position. Be alert for orthostatic hypotension, which can occur when the woman changes from a lying or sitting position to a standing one rapidly.

Pain Status

Pain, considered to be the fifth vital sign, is assessed along with the other four parameters. Question the woman about the type of pain, location, and severity. Have the woman rate the pain, such as with a numeric scale ranging from 0 to 10 points.

Many postpartum orders will have the nurse premedicate the woman routinely for afterbirth pains rather than wait for her to experience them first. The goal of pain management is to have the woman's pain scale rating maintained between 0 to 2 points at all times, especially after breast-feeding episodes. This can be accomplished by assessing the woman's pain level frequently and preventing pain by administering analgesics to keep the pain experienced at its lowest level (Fig. 16-2). If the woman complains of severe pain in the perineal region despite use of physical comfort measures, reexamine the area by inspection and palpation for the presence of a hematoma. If one

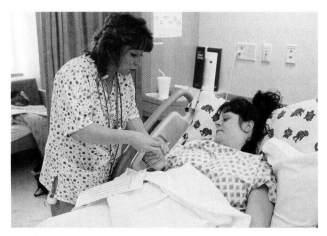

● Figure 16-2 Nurse administering analgesic to a postpartum woman.

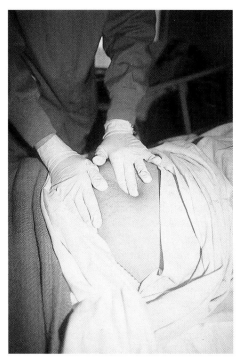

● Figure 16-3 Palpating the fundus.

is found, notify the health care provider immediately for corrective intervention.

Breasts

Inspect the breasts for size, contour, asymmetry, engorgement, or areas of erythema. Check the nipples for cracks, redness, fissures, or bleeding and note whether they are erect, flat, or inverted. Flat or inverted nipples can make breast-feeding challenging for both mother and infant. Cracked, blistered, fissured, bruised, or bleeding nipples in the breast-feeding woman are generally indications of improper positioning of the infant on the breast. Palpate the breasts to ascertain if they are soft, filling, or engorged, and document your findings. As milk is starting to come in, the breasts become firmer; this is charted as filling. Engorged breasts are hard, tender, and taut. Ask the woman if she is having any nipple discomfort. Also, palpate the breasts for any nodules, masses, or areas of warmth, which may indicate a plugged duct that may progress to **mastitis** if not treated promptly. Any discharge from the nipple should be described and documented if it is not colostrum (creamy yellow) or foremilk (bluish white).

Uterus

Assess the fundus (top portion of the uterus) to determine uterine involution. If possible, have the woman void to empty her bladder before assessing the fundus. Using a two-handed approach with the woman in the supine position and the bed in a flat position, palpate the abdomen gently, feeling for the top of the uterus while the other hand is placed on the lower segment of the uterus to stabilize it (Fig. 16-3).

The fundus should be midline and feel firm. A boggy or relaxed uterus is a sign of uterine atony. This can be the result of bladder distention, which displaces the uterus upward and to the right, or retained placental fragments. Either case predisposes the woman to hemorrhage.

Once the fundus is located, place your index finger on the woman's fundus and count the number of fingerbreadths between the fundus and the umbilicus (1 fingerbreadth is approximately equal to 1 cm). One to 2 hours after birth, the fundus typically is between the umbilicus and symphysis pubis. Approximately 6 to 12 hours after birth, the fundus usually is at the level of the umbilicus.

Normally, the fundus progresses downward at a rate of one fingerbreadth (or 1 cm) per day after childbirth (Cunningham et al., 2005). So on the first postpartum day, the top of the fundus is located 1 cm below the umbilicus and is recorded as U-1. Similarly, on the second postpartum day, the fundus would be 2 cm below the umbilicus and should be recorded as U-2, and so on.

If the fundus is not firm, gently massage the uterus using a circular motion until it becomes firm.

Bladder

Considerable diuresis—as much as 3000 mL—may follow for several days after childbirth, decreasing by the third day (Littleton & Engebretson, 2005). However, many women may not experience the sensation to void even if their bladder is full. Women who received regional anesthesia during labor are at risk for bladder distention and for difficulty voiding until sensation returns within several hours after birth.

Assess for potential voiding problems by asking the woman the following questions:

• Have you (passed your water, urinated, gone to the bathroom) yet?

- Have you noticed any burning or discomfort with urination?
- Do you have any difficulty passing your urine?
- Do you feel your bladder is empty when you finish urinating?
- Do you have any signs of infection such as urgency, frequency, or pain?
- Are you able to control the flow of urine by squeezing your muscles?
- Have you noticed any leakage of urine when you cough, laugh, or sneeze?

Assess the bladder for distention and adequate emptying after efforts to void. Palpate the area over the symphysis pubis. If empty, the bladder is not palpable. Palpation of a rounded mass suggests bladder distention. Also, percuss the area. A full bladder is dull to percussion. Also note the location and condition of the fundus, because a full bladder tends to displace the uterus up and to the right. Lochia drainage is more than normal because the uterus is not able to contract to suppress the bleeding.

After the woman voids, palpate and percuss the area again to determine adequate emptying of the bladder. If the bladder remains distended, the woman may be retaining residual urine in her bladder, and measures to initiate voiding should be instituted. Be alert for signs of infection, including infrequent or insufficient voiding (<200 mL), discomfort, burning, urgency, or foul-smelling urine (Condon, 2004). Document urine output.

Bowels

Spontaneous bowel movement may not occur for 2 to 3 days after giving birth because of a decrease in muscle tone in the intestines during labor. Normal patterns of bowel elimination usually return to normal within 8 to 14 days after birth (Blackburn, 2003).

Inspect the woman's abdomen for distention, auscultate for bowel sounds in all four quadrants, and palpate for tenderness. The abdomen typically is soft, nontender, and without distention. Bowel sounds are present in all four quadrants. Questioning the woman to see if she has had a bowel movement or has passed gas since giving birth is important, because constipation is a common problem during the postpartum period. Most women do not offer this information unless questioned about it. Finding active bowel sounds, verification of passing gas by the woman, and a nondistended abdomen are normal assessment results.

Lochia

Assess lochia according to its amount, color, and change with activity and time. To assess how much a woman is bleeding, ask her to identify how many perineal pads she has used in the past 1 to 2 hours. To determine the amount of lochia, observe the amount of lochia saturation on the perineal pad and relate it to time. A woman who saturates a perineal pad within 30 to 60 minutes is bleeding much

more than one who saturates a pad in 2 hours. Typically, describe the amount of lochia present by using the words *scant, light or small, moderate or heavy. Scant* would describe a 1 to 2-inch lochia stain on the perineal pad or an approximate 10-mL loss. *Light or small* would describe an approximate 4-inch stain or a 10- to 25-mL loss. *Moderate* lochia would describe a 4- to 6-inch stain with an estimated loss of 25 to 50 mL. A *large or heavy* lochia loss would describe a saturated pad within 1 hour after changing it (Scoggin, 2004). The total volume of lochia discharge is approximately 240 to 270 mL (8–9 oz) and it decreases daily (Blackburn, 2003).

Women who experience cesarean births will have less lochia discharge than those having a vaginal birth, but stages and color changes remain the same. Although the woman's abdomen is tender after surgery, it is important and necessary for the nurse to palpate the fundus and assess the lochia to make sure they are within the normal range and that there is no excessive bleeding.

Also ask the woman to state how much drainage was on each pad. For example, did she saturate the pad completely or was only half of the pad covered with drainage? Additionally, question the woman about the color of the drainage, odor, and the presence of any clots. Lochia has a definite musky scent, with an odor similar to that for menstrual flow without any large clots. However, foulsmelling lochia suggests an infection, and evidence of large clots suggests poor uterine involution, necessitating additional intervention.

Then inspect the perineal pad, noting the color, amount, and odor, and document your findings (Fig. 16-4). Keep in mind that lochia flow increases when the woman gets out of bed (resulting from pooling in the vagina and the uterus while she is lying down and when she breast-feeds as a result of the effect of oxytocin release causing uterine contractions). Report any abnormal find-

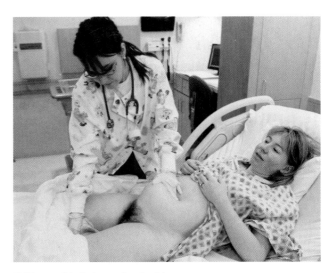

● Figure 16-4 Assessing lochia.

ings, which would include heavy, bright-red lochia with large tissue fragments or a foul odor.

Anticipatory guidance to give the woman at discharge should include information about lochia and the expected changes. Caution the woman to notify her health care provider if lochia rubra returns after serosa and alba lochia transitions have taken place. This is abnormal and may indicate subinvolution or that the woman is too active and needs to rest more.

Lochia is an excellent media for bacterial growth. Frequent changing of perineal pads and handwashing before and after pad changes are important infection control measures.

Episiotomy and Perineum

To assess the episiotomy and perineal area, position the woman on her side with her top leg flexed upward at the knee and drawn up toward her waist. If necessary, use a flashlight or a gooseneck lamp to provide adequate lighting during the assessment. Wearing gloves and standing at the woman's side with her back to you, gently lift the upper buttock to expose the perineum and anus (Fig. 16-5). Inspect the episiotomy for irritation, ecchymosis, tenderness, or hematomas. Also assess for hemorrhoids and their condition.

During the early postpartum period, the perineum tissue surrounding the episiotomy is typically edematous and slightly bruised. The normal episiotomy site should be without redness, discharge, or edema. The majority of healing takes place within the first 2 weeks, but it may take 4 to 6 months for the episiotomy to heal completely (Blackburn, 2003).

Lacerations to the perineal area sustained during the birthing process that were identified and repaired also need to be assessed to determine their healing status. Lacerations are classified based on their severity and tissue involvement as follows:

• First-degree laceration—involves only skin and superficial structures above muscle

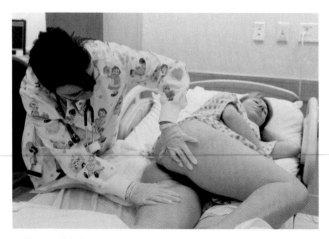

● Figure 16-5 Inspecting the perineum.

• Second-degree laceration—extends through perineal muscles
• Third-degree laceration—extends through the anal sphincter muscle
• Fourth-degree laceration—continues through anterior rectal wall

Assess the episiotomy and any lacerations at least every 8 hours to detect the presence of hematomas or signs of infection developing. Large areas of swollen, bluish skin with complaints of severe pain in the perineal area indicate pelvic or vulvar hematomas. Redness, swelling, increasing discomfort, or purulent drainage may indicate the presence of infection. Both discoveries warrant immediate reporting.

A white line the length of the episiotomy is a sign of infection, as is swelling or discharge. Severe, intractable pain; perineal discoloration; and ecchymosis indicate a perineal hematoma—a potentially dangerous condition. Report any unusual findings. Ice can be applied to relieve discomfort and reduce edema; **sitz baths** also can be helpful in promoting comfort and perineal healing.

Homans' Sign

Pregnancy is a state of hypercoagulability. This state coupled with stimulation of the coagulation process at birth increases the risk of thrombosis formation. In addition, the use of stirrups by some women during the birthing process impedes venous return and leads to blood stasis in the legs. Superficial or deep vein thrombophlebitis, a possible complication of childbirth, is caused by hypercoagulability of the blood during pregnancy, severe anemia, pelvic infection, traumatic birth, or obesity (Chalmers, Mangiaterra, & Porter, 2001). Elevations of clotting factors continue for several days or longer after childbirth, placing women at risk during the early postpartum period. It may take 3 to 4 weeks before the homeostasis returns to prepregnant levels (Blackburn, 2003). Women with a history of thrombophlebitis, varicose veins, or those who have had a cesarean birth are at special risk for this condition during the postpartum period and should be advised to wear antiembolism stockings or use sequential compression devices to reduce their risk of developing thrombophlebitis. Encouraging the client to ambulate after childbirth reduces the incidence of thrombophlebitis.

Assessing for Homans' sign may be helpful in identifying possible thrombosis. Position the woman's legs flat on the bed. Then place one hand under the leg near the back of the knee and gently flex her foot forward toward her ankle with the other hand. Repeat the test on the other leg (Fig. 16-6). If the woman experiences calf pain when you flex either foot, the Homans' sign is positive and further assessment is needed. A positive Homans' sign raises the suspicion for superficial thrombosis. Keep in mind that deep venous thrombosis may be silent, and thus does not produce pain on dorsiflexion. Note also the presence of foot or ankle edema, which normally diminishes during the first week postpartum.

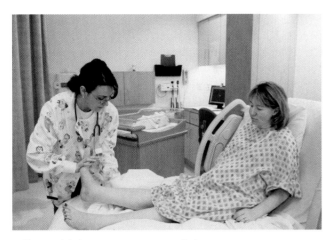

● Figure 16-6 Assessing Homans' sign.

Emotional Status

Asses the woman's emotional status by observing how she interacts with her family, her level of independence, energy levels, eye contact with her infant, body posture and comfort level while holding the newborn, and sleep and rest patterns. Be alert for mood swings, irritability, or any crying episodes.

Bonding and Attachment

Meeting the newborn for the first time after birth can be an exhilarating experience for parents. Although the mother has spent many hours dreaming of her unborn and how he or she will look, it is not until after birth that they meet face-to-face. They both need to get to know one another and to develop feelings for one another.

The development of a close emotional attraction to a newborn by the parents during the first 30 to 60 minutes after birth describes bonding. It is unidirectional, from parent to infant. It is thought that optimal bonding of the parents to a newborn requires a period of close contact within the first few minutes to a few hours after birth (Murray & McKinney, 2006). The mother initiates bonding when she caresses her infant and exhibits certain behaviors typical of a mother tending her child. The infant's responses to this, such as body and eye movements, are a necessary part of the process. During this initial period, the infant is in a quiet, alert state, looking directly at the holder. The length of time necessary for bonding depends on the health of the infant and mother, as well as the circumstances surrounding the labor and birth (Baradon, 2002).

The development of strong affectional ties between an infant and a significant other (mother, father, sibling, and caretaker) defines the process of attachment (O'Toole, 2003). This tie between two people is psychological, rather than biologic, and it does not occur overnight. The process of attachment follows a progressive or developmental course that changes over time. Attachment is not inclusive, but must be considered as an individualized and multi-

factorial process that is dependent on the health status of the newborn or infant, the mother, environmental circumstances, and the quality of care the infant receives (Tideman, Nilsson, Smith, & Stjernqvist, 2002). It occurs through mutually satisfying experiences. Maternal attachment begins during pregnancy as the result of fetal movement and maternal fantasies about the infant, and continues through the birth and postpartum periods. Attachment behaviors include seeking, maintaining close proximity to, and exchanging gratifying experiences with, the infant (Mercer & Ferketich, 1994). In a high-risk pregnancy, the attachment process may be complicated by lack of time to develop a parent–fetal relationship resulting from a premature birth, and by parental stress experienced in response to the fetal and/or maternal vulnerability.

Bonding is a vital component of the attachment process and is necessary in establishing parent–infant attachment and a healthy, loving relationship. During this early period of acquaintance, mothers touch their infants in a very characteristic manner. Mothers visually and physically "explore" their infants, initially using their fingertips on the infant's face and extremities, progressing to massaging and stroking the infant with their fingers. This is followed by palm contact on the trunk. Eventually, mothers draw their infant toward them and hold the infant. Mothers also interact with their infants through eye-to-eye contact in the **en face position** (Koulomzin et al., 2002) (Fig. 16-7).

Generally, research on attachment tends to demonstrate a similar process for fathers as for mothers, even though the pace may be different. Like mothers, fathers manifest attachment behaviors during pregnancy. Indeed, Ferketich and Mercer (1995) found that the best predictor of early postnatal attachment for fathers is fetal attachment. Developmentally, becoming a father requires a man to build on the experiences he has had throughout childhood and adolescence. Fathers develop an emotional tie

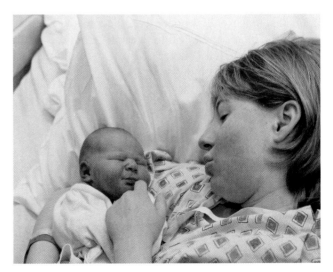

● Figure 16-7 En face position.

with their infants in a variety of ways. They seek and maintain closeness with the infant and are capable of recognizing particular characteristics of the infant. They feel a sense of responsibility for the infant's growth and development (Buist, Morse, & Durkin, 2003).

The attachment process is just that—a process. It does not occur instantaneously. Many parents believe in the romanticized version of parenthood, which happens right after birth. A delay or block in the attachment process can occur if a mother's physical and emotional states are adversely affected by exhaustion, pain, the absence of a support system, anesthesia, or an unwanted outcome (Littleton & Engebretson, 2005). Early research by Klaus and Kennel (1982) examined maternal attachment and found that the period when a mother falls in love with her infant was not easily identified. Researchers have not been able to pinpoint precisely the moment in time when attachment is complete. It can occur hours to months after birth or not at all.

The developmental task for the infant is learning to differentiate between trust and mistrust. If the mother or caretaker is consistently responsive to the infant's care, meeting physical and psychological needs, the infant will likely learn to trust his or her caretaker; view the world as a safe place; and grow up to be secure, self-reliant, trusting, cooperative, and helpful toward others. By contrast, if an infant grows up without his or her needs met, the risk of child abuse, developmental delays, and neglect increases (Tilokskulchai, Phatthanasiriwethin, Vichitsukon, & Serisathien, 2002).

Parental role attainment is an interactional and developmental process occurring over a period of time, during which the parents become attached to their infant and acquire competence in their roles as parents. Achieving this role of becoming parents may take 4 to 6 months. This transition to parenthood according to Mercer (1985) follows four stages:

1. Anticipatory stage—allows parents to seek out other role models
2. Formal stage—allows parents to become acquainted with the infant and begin to take cues from the infant
3. Informal stage—encourages parents to respond to the infant as a unique individual
4. Personal stage—attained when the parents feel a sense of harmony in their roles

Factors Affecting Attachment

Attachment behaviors are influenced by three major factors: *parent background,* includes the parent's care by his or her own mother, practices of the culture, relationship within the family, experience with previous pregnancies and planning and course of events during pregnancy; *infant,* which includes the infant's temperament and health status at birth; and *care practices,* the behaviors of physicians, midwives, nurses, and hospital personnel; care and support during labor; first day of life in separation of

mother and infant; and rules of the hospital or birthing center (Klaus & Kennel, 1982).

Attachment occurs more readily with the infant whose temperament, health status, appearance, and gender fit the parent's expectations. If the infant does not meet these expectations, attachment can be delayed or hampered (Koulomzin et al., 2002).

In addition, factors associated with the healthcare facility or birthing unit can influence attachment. These include

- Separation of infant and parents immediately after birth, and for long times during the day
- Policies that discourage or inhibit unwrapping and exploring infant, limiting parents' care taking
- Intensive care environment, restrictive visiting policies
- Staff indifference or lack of support for parent's caretaking attempts and abilities

Critical Attributes of Attachment

The terms *bonding* and *attachment* continue to be used interchangeably, even though they cover different time frames and interactions. A group of nursing researchers attempted to clarify attachment by outlining their critical attributes. According to Goulet and fellow researchers (1998), the attributes of parent–infant attachment include proximity, reciprocity, and commitment.

Proximity

Proximity refers to the physical and psychological experience of the parents being close to their infant. This attribute has three dimensions to it:

1. Contact—The sensory experiences of touching, holding, and gazing at the infant are found to be a part of proximity-seeking behavior.
2. Emotional state—The emotional state emerges from the affective experience of the new parents toward their infant and their parental role.
3. Individualization—Parents are also aware of the need to differentiate the infant's needs from themselves, to recognize and respond appropriately, making the attachment process also, in some way, one of detachment.

Reciprocity

Reciprocity is the process by which the infant's capabilities and behavioral characteristics elicit parental response. Reciprocity is described by two dimensions: complementary behavior and sensitivity. Complementary behavior recognizes taking turns and stopping when the other is not interested or becomes tired. An infant can coo and stare at the parent to elicit a similar parenteral response to complement their behavior. Parents who are sensitive and responsive to their infant's cues will promote their development and growth. Parents who develop sensitivity in recognizing the particular ways by which the infant communicates will respond appropriately by smiling, vocalizing, touching, and kissing.

Commitment

Commitment refers to the enduring nature of the attachment relationship. The components of this are twofold: centrality and parent role exploration. In centrality, parents place the infant at the center of their lives. They acknowledge and accept their responsibility to promote the infant's safety, growth, and development. Parent role exploration describes the ability of the parents to find their own way and integrate the parental identity into themselves and their life.

Positive and Negative Attachment Behaviors

Nurses can be very instrumental in facilitating attachment by assessing newborns and parents for attachment behaviors (positive and negative), ultimately intervening appropriately to promote and enhance attachment. Some signs of positive bonding behaviors include maintaining close physical contact; making eye-to-eye contact; speaking in soft, high-pitched tones; and touching and exploring the infant. Table 16-1 highlights typical positive and negative behaviors of attachment.

Nurses must be astute when assessing family units to identify any discord that might interfere with the attachment process. Cultural differences also must be considered because they can significantly influence the relationship between bonding and attachment behavior and affective perception. Recognize that mothers from different cultures may behave in ways that differ from what is expected in one's own culture. Negative labels may be inadvertently attached by health care providers to mothers who assume behavior that is different.

For example, Native American mothers tend to handle their newborns less often and use cradle boards to carry them. Native American mothers and many Asian-American mothers delay breast-feeding until their milk comes in, because colostrum is considered harmful for the newborn (Bowers, 2003). The culturally sensitive nurse needs to understand their sociocultural needs and not label different behavior as negative.

Nursing Interventions

In the health care arena today, "less is more," and this applies to hospital stays. If the woman had a vaginal delivery, she may receive up to 48 hours of continuous nursing care after birth before being discharged. If she experienced a cesarean birth, the woman may remain hospitalized from 72 to 96 hours. This shortened stay leaves little time for nurses to prepare the woman and her family for the many changes that are occurring and will occur as she returns home. Nurses need to use this limited time to address areas of pain and discomfort, immunizations, nutrition, activity and exercise, lactation, discharge teaching, sexuality and contraception, and follow-up (see Nursing Care Plan 16-1). Always adhere to standard precautions when providing direct care to reduce the risk of disease transmission.

Promoting Comfort

The postpartum woman may experience discomfort and pain from a variety of sources, such as an episiotomy,

Table 16-1 Positive and Negative Attachment Behaviors

	Positive Behaviors	**Negative Behaviors**
Infant	Smiles; is alert visually; demonstrates strong grasp reflex to hold parent finger; sucks well, feeds easily; enjoys being held close; makes eye-to-eye contact; follows parent's face; appears facially appealing; is consolable when crying	Feeds poorly, regurgitates often; cries for long periods, colicky and inconsolable; shows flat affect, rarely smiles even when prompted; resists holding and closeness; sleeps with eyes closed most of time; stiffens body when held; is unresponsive to parenting; shows inattention to parental faces
Parent	Makes direct eye contact; assumes en face position when holding infant; claims infant as family member, pointing out commonalities; expresses pride in infant; assigns meaning to infant's actions; smiles and gazes at infant; touches infant, progressing from fingertips to holding; names infant; requests to be close to infant as much as allowed; speaks positively about infant	Expresses disappointment or displeasure in infant; fails to "explore" visually or physically their infant; fails to "claim" infant into family unit; avoids caring for infant; finds excuses not to hold infant close; has negative self-concept; appears disinterested in having infant in room; requests frequently to have infant taken back to nursery to be cared for; assigns negative attributes to infant and calls infant inappropriate, negative names (e.g., frog, monkey, tadpole)

Sources: Ayers, 2003; Klaus & Kennel, 1982; Sameroff, McDonough, & Rosenblum, 2003; Sears & Sears, 2001.

Nursing Care Plan 16-1

Overview of the Postpartum Woman

Belinda, a 26-year-old gravida 2, para 2 (G2,P2) is a patient on the mother–baby unit after giving birth to a term 8-lb 12-oz baby boy yesterday. The night nurse reports that she has an episiotomy, complains of a pain rating of 7 points on a scale of 1 to 10 points, is having difficulty breast-feeding, and had heavy lochia most of the night. The nurse also reports that the patient seems focused on her own needs and not on her infant. Assessment this morning reveals the following:

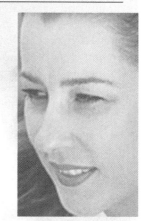

B: Breasts are soft with colostrum leaking; nipples cracked
U: Uterus is one finger breath below the umbilicus; deviated to right
B: Bladder is palpable; patient states she hasn't been up to void yet
B: Bowels have not moved; bowel sounds present; passing flatus
L: Lochia is moderate; peripad soaked from night accumulation
E: Episiotomy site intact; swollen, bruised; hemorrhoids present
—
H: Homans' sign negative; no edema over tibia
E: Emotional status is "distressed" as a result of discomfort and fatigue

Nursing Diagnosis: Impaired tissue integrity related to episiotomy

Outcome identification and *evaluation*	Interventions with *rationales*
The woman remains free of infection, *without any signs and symptoms of infection,* and exhibits evidence of progressive healing as demonstrated by clean, dry, intact episiotomy site.	Monitor episiotomy site *for redness, edema, and signs of infection.* Assess vital signs at least every 4 hours *to identify possible changes suggesting infection.* Apply ice pack to episiotomy site *to reduce swelling.* Instruct patient on use of sitz bath *to promote healing, hygiene, and comfort.* Encourage frequent perineal care and peripad changing *to prevent infection.* Recommend ambulation *to improve circulation and promote healing.* Instruct patient on positioning *to relieve pressure on perineal area.* Demonstrate use of anesthetic sprays *to numb perineal area.*

Nursing Diagnosis: Pain related to episiotomy, sore nipples and hemorrhoids

The woman experiences a decrease in pain, *reporting that her pain has diminished to a tolerable level, rating it as 2 points or less.*	Thoroughly visually inspect perineum *to rule out hematoma as cause of pain.* Administer analgesic medication as ordered as needed *to promote comfort.* Carry out comfort measures to episiotomy as outlined earlier *to help in reducing pain.* Offer an explanation of discomforts and reassure they are time limited *to assist in coping with pain.* Apply tucks to swollen hemorrhoids *to induce shrinkage and reduce pain.* Suggest use of sitz bath frequently *to assist in reducing hemorrhoid pain.* Administer stool softener and laxative *to prevent straining with first bowel movement.*

Overview of the Postpartum Woman (continued)

Outcome identification and *evaluation*	Interventions with *rationales*
	Observe positioning and latching-on technique while breast-feeding. Offer suggestions based on observation to correct positioning/latching *to minimize trauma to the breast.* Suggest air-drying of nipples after breast-feeding and use of plain water *to prevent nipple cracking.* Teach relaxation techniques when breast-feeding *to help reduce anxiety and discomfort level.*

Nursing Diagnosis: Risk for ineffective coping related to mood alteration and pain

The woman copes with mood alterations, *as evidenced by positive statements about newborn and participation in newborn care.*	Provide a supportive, nurturing environment and encourage the mother to vent her feelings and frustrations *to assist in relieving anxiety.* Provide opportunities for the mother to rest and sleep *to combat fatigue.* Encourage consumption of a well-balanced diet *to increase the mother's energy level.* Provide reassurance and explanations that mood alterations are common after birth secondary to waning hormones after pregnancy *to increase the mother's knowledge base.* Allow the mother relief from newborn care *to afford opportunity for self-care.* Discuss with partner expected behavior from mother and how additional support and help are needed during this stressful time *to promote partner participation in care.* Make appropriate community referral to continue mother–infant support *to ensure continuity of care.* Encourage frequent skin-to-skin contact and closeness between mother and infant *to facilitate bonding and attachment behaviors.* Encourage participation in infant care and provide instruction as needed *to foster a sense of independence and self-esteem.* Offer praise and reinforcement of positive mother–infant interactions *to enhance self-confidence in care.*

perineal lacerations, an edematous perineum, inflamed hemorrhoids, engorged breasts, and sore nipples if breast-feeding. Nonpharmacologic and pharmacologic measures can be used.

Applications of Cold and Heat

Commonly, an *ice pack* is the first measure used after a vaginal birth to provide perineal comfort from edema, an episiotomy, or laceration. It is applied during the fourth stage of labor and can be used for the first 24 hours to reduce perineal edema and to prevent hematoma formation, thus reducing pain and promoting healing. Ice packs are wrapped in a disposable covering or clean washcloth and are applied to the perineal area. Usually the ice pack is applied for 20 minutes and removed for 10 minutes. Many commercially prepared ice packs are available, but a latex glove filled with crushed ice and covered can also be used if the mother is not allergic to latex. Ensure that the ice pack is changed frequently to promote good hygiene and to allow for periodic assessments.

The **peribottle** is a plastic squeeze bottle filled with warm tap water that is sprayed over the perineal area after each voiding and before applying a new perineal pad. Usually the peribottle is introduced to the woman when she is assisted to the bathroom to freshen up and void for the first time—in most instances, once vital signs are stable after the first hour. Provide the woman with instructions on how and when to use the peribottle. Reinforce this practice each time she changes her pad, voids, or defecates, making sure that she understands to direct the flow of water from front to back. The peribottle will accompany the woman home to be used over the next several weeks until her lochia discharge stops. The peribottle is used by women who had vaginal and cesarean births to provide comfort and hygiene to the perineal area.

After the first 24 hours, a sitz bath with warm water may be prescribed and substituted for the ice pack to reduce local swelling and promote comfort for an episiotomy, perineal trauma, or inflamed hemorrhoids. The change from cold to warm therapy enhances vascular circulation and healing (Littleton & Engebretson, 2005). Prior to using a sitz bath, the woman should cleanse the perineum with a peribottle or take a shower using mild soap.

Most health care agencies use plastic disposable sitz baths that women can take home when they are discharged. The plastic sitz bath consists of a basin that fits on the commode with a bag filled with warm water hung on a hook connected via a tube onto the front of the basin (Fig. 16-8). Teaching Guidelines 16-1 highlights the steps for teaching a woman how to use a sitz bath.

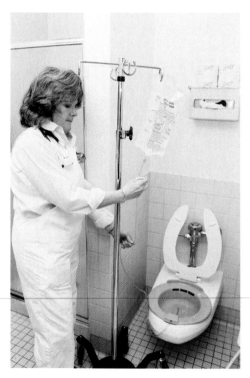

● Figure 16-8 Sitz bath set up.

 TEACHING GUIDELINES 16-1

Using a Sitz Bath

1. Close clamp on the tubing prior to filling bag with water to prevent leakage.
2. Fill the sitz bath basin and plastic bag with warm water (comfortable to touch).
3. Place the filled basin on the toilet with the seat raised and the overflow opening facing toward the back of the toilet.
4. Hang the filled plastic bag on a hook close to the toilet or an IV pole.
5. Attach the tubing into the opening on the basin.
6. Sit on the basin positioned on the toilet seat and release the clamp to allow warm water to irrigate the perineum.
7. Remain sitting atop the basin for approximately 15 to 20 minutes.
8. Stand up and pat the perineum area dry and then apply a clean peripad when finished.
9. Tip the basin to remove any remaining water in it and flush the toilet.
10. Wash the basin with warm water and soap, and dry in the sink after finishing.
11. Store basin and tubing in a clean, dry area until the next use.
12. Wash hands with soap and water when finished with the sitz bath.

Advise the woman to repeat this treatment several times daily to provide hygiene and comfort to the perineal area. Also, encourage the woman to continue this measure after discharge from the healthcare facility.

Some facilities have hygienic sitz baths called *Suri-Gators* in the bathroom that spray an antiseptic, water, or both onto the perineum. The woman sits on the toilet with legs apart so that the nozzle spray reaches her perineal area.

Keep in mind that tremendous hemodynamic changes are taking place within the mother during this early postpartum period and her safety must be a priority. Fatigue, blood loss, effects of medications, and lack of food may contribute to a woman's weakness when standing up. Assisting the woman to the bathroom to instruct her on how to use the peribottle and sitz bath is necessary to ensure her safety. Many women become lightheaded or dizzy on arising from their beds and need direct physical assistance to carry out their task. Staying in the woman's room, ensuring that the emergency call light is readily available, and being available if needed during this early period will ensure safety and prevent accidents and falls.

Topical Preparations

Several treatments may be applied topically for temporary relief of pain and discomfort. One such treatment used for temporary pain relief consists of local anesthetic sprays such as Dermoplast or Americaine. These agents numb the perineal area. They are used after cleansing the perineal area with water via the peribottle and/or a sitz bath.

For hemorrhoid discomfort, cool witch hazel pads, such as Tucks Pads, can be used. The pads are placed at the rectal area, between the hemorrhoids and the perineal pad. These pads cool the area, help relieve swelling, and minimize itching.

Analgesics

Analgesics such as acetaminophen (Tylenol) and oral nonsteroidal antiinflammatory drugs (NSAIDS) such as ibuprofen (Motrin) are prescribed to relieve mild postpartum discomfort. For moderate to more severe pain, a narcotic analgesic such as codeine or oxycodone in conjunction with aspirin or acetaminophen may be prescribed. Instruct the client about possible side effects of any medication prescribed. Common side effects of oral analgesics include dizziness, lightheadedness, nausea and vomiting, constipation, and sedation (Spratto & Woods, 2005).

Also, inform the client that the drugs are secreted in breast milk. Nearly all medications that the mother takes are passed into her breast milk; however, the mild analgesics (e.g., acetaminophen or ibuprofen) are considered relatively safe for breast-feeding mothers (American Academy of Pediatrics Committee on Drugs, 2001). Administering a mild analgesic approximately an hour before breast-feeding will usually promote comfort.

Assisting with Elimination

The bladder is edematous, hypotonic, and congested immediately postpartum. Consequently, bladder distention, incomplete emptying, and inability to void are common. A full bladder interferes with uterine contraction and may lead to hemorrhage, because it will displace the uterus out of the midline. Encourage the woman to void. Often, assisting her to assume the normal voiding position on the commode facilitates this. If the woman experiences difficulty with voiding, pouring warm water over the perineal area, hearing the sound of running tap water such as in the sink, blowing bubbles through a straw, standing in the shower with warm water turned on, drinking fluids, or placing her hand in a basin of warm water may be helpful to stimulate voiding. If these therapeutic actions are unsuccessful in stimulating urination within 4 to 6 hours after giving birth, catheterization may be needed. Palpate the bladder for distension and question the woman about voiding in small amounts (<100 mL) frequently (retention with overflow). If catheterization is necessary, be sure to use sterile technique during this procedure to reduce the risk of infection.

Intestinal motility can be affected by several factors, predisposing the woman to constipation. These factors may include decreased bowel motility during labor, high iron content in prenatal vitamins, postpartum fluid loss,

and side effects of pain medications and/or anesthesia. In addition, the woman may fear that bowel movements will cause pain or injury, especially if she has an episiotomy or has sustained a laceration that was repaired with sutures.

Usually a stool softener, such as docusate (Colace), with or without a laxative might prove helpful if the client experiences difficulty with bowel elimination. Other measures such as ambulating and increasing fluid and fiber intake may be helpful. Nutritional instruction might include increasing fruits and vegetables in diet; drinking plenty of fluids (8–12 cups) to keep the stool soft; drinking small amounts of prune juice and/or hot liquids to stimulate peristalsis; eating high-fiber foods such as bran cereals, whole grains, dried fruits, fresh fruits, and raw vegetables; and walking daily.

Promoting Activity, Rest, and Exercise

The postpartum period is an ideal time for nurses to promote the importance of physical fitness, help women incorporate exercise into their lifestyle, and encourage them to overcome barriers to exercise. Lifestyle changes that occur postpartum may affect a woman's health for decades. Early ambulation is encouraged to reduce the risk of thromboembolism and improve strengthening.

Many changes occur postpartum. Responsibility for a newborn alters eating and sleeping habits, work schedules, and time allocation. Postpartum fatigue is common during the early days after childbirth and it may continue for weeks or months (Troy, 2003). It affects the mother's relationships with significant others and her ability to fulfill household and child care responsibilities. Be sure that the mother recognizes her need for rest and sleep, and be realistic about her expectations. Some suggestions include the following:

- Nap when the infant is sleeping because uninterrupted sleep at night is altered.
- Reduce participation in outside activities and limit the number of visitors.
- Determine the infant's sleep–wake cycles and attempt to increase wakeful periods during the day so longer sleep stretches occur during the night hours.
- Stress the need for a balanced diet to promote healing and to increase energy levels.
- Encourage sharing household tasks to conserve the woman's energy.
- Request the father or other family members provide infant care during the night periodically to provide the mother an uninterrupted night of sleep.
- Review the family's daily routine to ascertain if clustering of activities might be helpful in conserving energy and promoting rest.

The demands of parenthood may reduce or prevent exercise in even the most committed person. Emphasize the benefits of a regular exercise program, which include

- Helping with loss of weight gained during the pregnancy
- Increasing energy level to help cope with new responsibilities
- Providing an outlet for stress
- Speeding the return to prepregnant size and shape (Ringdahl, 2002a)

More than one third of US women are overweight (CDC, 2003). Although the average gestational weight gain is small (approximately 25–35 lb), excess weight gain and failure to lose weight after pregnancy are important and identifiable predictors of long-term obesity. Breast-feeding and exercise may be beneficial to control long-term weight (Rooney & Schauberger, 2002).

Women who have not returned to their prepregnant weight by 6 months are likely to retain the extra weight long term (Ringdahl, 2002b). Encourage women to lose their pregnancy weight by 6 months postpartum, and refer those who fail to lose the weight they gained during pregnancy to community weight-loss programs.

The postpartum woman may face some obstacles to exercise for losing weight, including physical changes (ligament laxity), competing demands (newborn care), lack of information about weight retention (inactivity equates to weight gain), and stress incontinence (leaking of urine during activity).

A healthy woman with an uncomplicated vaginal birth can resume exercise in the immediate postpartum period. Advise the woman to start slowly and build the level of exercise over a period of several weeks as tolerated. Jogging strollers may be an option for some women, allowing them to exercise with their newborns. Also, exercise videos and home exercise equipment allow mothers to work out while the newborn naps.

To help facilitate the recovery process, women are encouraged to exercise after giving birth to promote feelings of well-being and to restore muscle tone lost during pregnancy. Routine exercise should be resumed gradually, beginning with **Kegel exercises** on the first postpartum day and, by the second week, progressing to abdominal, buttock, and thigh-toning exercises (Jeffreys & Nordahl, 2002). Walking is an excellent form of exercise as long as jarring and bouncing movements are avoided during this early period because joints do not stabilize until 6 to 8 weeks postpartum. Exercising too much too soon can cause the woman to bleed more and return her lochia color to bright red.

Recommended exercises for the first few weeks postpartum include abdominal breathing (expand the abdomen by inhaling through the nose and contract the abdominal muscles when exhaling slowly), head lifts (exhale while lifting the head off the floor onto the chest, hold for a few seconds and then relax), modified sit-ups (raise head and shoulders off the floor so that the hands reach the knees, while keeping waist on the floor), double knee roll (while lying flat on the floor with knees bent, roll knees to one side and then roll to the other side), and pelvic tilt (while lying on back, roll pelvis back by flattening the lower back on the floor; tighten buttocks and hold briefly). The number of exercises and their duration is gradually increased as strength is gained. Teaching Guidelines 16-2 highlights the steps for each of these exercises.

Be cognizant of the various cultures' attitudes regarding exercise, because some cultures (e.g., Haitian, Arab-American, and Mexican) have new mothers observe a specific period of bed rest or activity restriction; thus, active exercise would be inappropriate to discuss during the early postpartum period (Moore & Moos, 2003).

Fifty percent of all parous women develop some degree of pelvic prolapse in their lifetime that is associated with stress incontinence (McCrink, 2003). The more vaginal deliveries a woman has had, the more likely she is to have stress incontinence. Stress incontinence can occur with any activity that causes an increase in intraabdominal pressure. Postpartal women might consider alternate low-impact activities (such as walking, biking, swimming, or low-impact aerobics) so they can resume physical activity while strengthening the pelvic floor.

Kegel exercises help to strengthen the pelvic floor muscles if done with enough frequency or regularity. Kegel exercises were originally developed by Dr. Arnold Kegel as a method of controlling incontinence in women after childbirth. The principle behind these exercises is to strengthen the muscle of the pelvic floor, thus improving the urethral sphincter function. The success of Kegel exercises depends on proper technique and adherence to a regular exercise program (Gray, 2004).

Kegel exercises can be done inconspicuously. Therefore, advise women to perform these exercises, doing ten 5-second contractions, whenever they change diapers, talk on the phone, or watch TV. Teach the woman to perform Kegel's exercises properly and assist her to identify the correct muscles by trying to stop and start the flow of urine when sitting on the toilet (Teaching Guidelines 16-3). By doing these exercises frequently, many women can strengthen their pelvic floor muscles and prevent stress incontinence.

Use the opportunity during postpartum care to instruct women on primary prevention of stress incontinence by discussing the value and purpose of Kegel exercises. Approach the subject sensitively, avoiding the term *incontinent*. The terms *leakage, loss of urine*, or *bladder control issues* are more acceptable to most women. When properly performed, Kegel exercises have been effective in preventing or improving urinary continence (Shaw, 2004).

Assisting With Self-Care Measures

Demonstrate and discuss with the woman hygienic measures that prevent infection during the postpartum period. Because she may experience lochia drainage for as long as a month after childbirth, advising her of practices that

T E A C H I N G   G U I D E L I N E S   1 6 - 2

Exercising

Abdominal Breathing

1. While lying on a flat surface (floor or bed), take a deep breath through your nose and expand your abdominal muscles (they will rise up from your midsection).
2. Slowly exhale and tighten your abdominal muscles for 3 to 5 seconds.
3. Repeat this several times to build up progressively.

Head Lift

1. Lie on a flat surface with knees flexed and feet flat on the surface.
2. Lift your head off the flat surface, tuck it onto your chest, and hold for 3 to 5 seconds.
3. Relax your head and return to the starting position.
4. Repeat this several times, building up frequency slowly.

Modified Sit-Ups

1. Lie on a flat surface and raise your head and shoulders off of the flat surface (6 to 8 inches high) so that your outstretched hands reach your knees.
2. Keep your waist on the flat surface while performing this exercise.

3. Slowly return to the flat surface to the starting position.
4. Repeat this maneuver and increase in frequency as comfort level allows.

Double Knee Roll

1. Lie on a flat surface with your knees bent.
2. While keeping your shoulders flat, slowly roll your knees to your right side to touch the flat surface (floor or bed).
3. Roll knees back over your body to the left side until they touch the opposite side of the flat surface.
4. Return to the starting position on your back and rest.
5. Repeat this exercise several times, building up frequency progressively.

Pelvic Tilt

1. Lie on your back with your knees bent and your arms at your side on a flat surface.
2. Slowly contract your abdominal muscles while lifting your pelvis up toward the ceiling.
3. Hold for 3 to 5 seconds and slowly return to your starting position of lying flat.
4. Repeat this maneuver several times with progressive frequency over time.

---

will promote her well-being and healing also need to be stressed. These measures include

- Frequent changing of perineal pads, applying and removing them from front to back to prevent contamination from the rectal area to the genital area
- Avoiding the use of tampons after giving birth to decrease the risk of infection
- Showering once or twice daily using a mild soap, and avoiding soap on nipples
- Using a sitz bath after every bowel movement to cleanse the rectal area and provide relief from enlarged hemorrhoids
- Using the peribottle filled with warm water after urinating and prior to applying a new perineal pad
- Avoiding tub baths for 4 to 6 weeks to prevent falls until joints and balance are restored
- Washing hands prior to changing perineal pads, after disposing of previous lochia-soaked pad, and after voiding (Fong & Grant, 2005)

To reduce risk of infection at the episiotomy site, reinforce proper perineal care with the client, showing her how to rinse her perineum with the peribottle filled with water after she voids or defecates. Stress the importance of always wiping gently from front to back and washing hands thoroughly before and after perineal care. For hem-

orrhoids, have the client apply witch hazel-soaked pads (Tucks Pads), ice packs to relieve swelling, or hemorrhoidal cream or ointment if ordered.

Ensuring Safety

One of the safety concerns during the postpartum period is orthostatic hypotension. When the woman changes from a lying or sitting position to a standing one rapidly, her blood pressure can suddenly drop, causing her pulse rate to increase. Subsequently, she may experience dizziness and may faint. Be aware of this potential problem and initiate the following safeguards:

- Check blood pressure first before ambulating client.
- Elevate head of bed for a few minutes before ambulating client.
- Have the client sit on the side of the bed for a few moments before rising.
- Help the client to stand up and stay with her.
- Ambulate alongside the client and provide support.
- Frequently question the client about how her head feels.
- Stay close by to assist if she feels lightheaded suddenly.

Additional safety topics to address concern infant safety within the postpartum room. Instruct the woman to place the newborn back in the open crib on his/her back close to her bedside if she is feeling sleepy or tired.

T E A C H I N G   G U I D E L I N E S   1 6 - 3

Performing Kegel Exercises

1. Identify the correct pelvic floor muscles by contracting them to stop the flow of urine while sitting on the toilet.
2. Repeat this action of contraction several times to become familiar with it.
3. Start the exercises by emptying the bladder.
4. Tighten the pelvic floor muscles and hold for a count of 10 seconds.
5. Relax the muscle completely for a count of 10 seconds.
6. Perform 10 exercises at least three times daily and progressively increase.
7. Perform the exercises in different positions, such as standing, lying, and sitting.
8. Keep breathing during the exercises.
9. Don't contract the abdominal, thigh, leg, or buttocks muscles during these exercises.
10. Relax while doing Kegel exercises and concentrate on isolating the right muscles.
11. Attempt to tighten the pelvic muscles before sneezing, jumping, or laughing to protect them from additional laxness.
12. Be aware that you can perform Kegel exercises anywhere and in any place without anyone noticing.

Holding the infant and falling asleep might increase the risk of accidental falling from the bed. Providing for the infant's safety by placing him or her back in the open crib will ensure there are no injuries.

Counseling About Sexuality and Contraception

Sexuality is an important and integral part of every woman's life. Despite the importance of sexuality in their lives, many women find it difficult to talk to their healthcare provider about concerns. Questions and concerns about sexuality span a woman's entire lifetime.

During postpartum, many women experience fatigue, weakness, vaginal bleeding, perineal discomfort, hemorrhoids, sore breasts, decreased vaginal lubrication resulting from low estrogen levels, and dyspareunia. Women may be hesitant to resume sexual relations for a variety of factors. The physical demands made by the new infant and the stress of new parental roles, responsibilities, and fatigue place particular demands on the emotional reserves of couples. Men may feel they now have a secondary role within the family, and they may lack understanding of their partner's daily routine. These issues, combined with the woman's increased investment in the mothering role, can pose some difficulties with the sexual relationship. Parenthood, at times, allows limited privacy and

little rest, both of which are necessary for sexual pleasure (Fogel, 2003). Women want to get back to "normal" as soon as possible after giving birth. However, sexual relations cannot be isolated from the psychological and psychosocial adjustments that are needed by both partners.

Although couples are reluctant to ask, they often want to know when they can safely resume sexual intercourse after childbirth. Typically, sexual intercourse can be resumed once bright-red bleeding has stopped and the perineum is healed from an episiotomy or lacerations. This is usually by the third to the sixth week postpartum. However, there is not a set, prescribed time to resume sexual intercourse after childbirth. Each couple must set their own time frame when they feel it is appropriate to resume sexual intercourse.

When counseling the couple about sexuality, determine what knowledge and concerns the couple has about their sexual relationship. Initiate a discussion of the normality of fluctuations of sexual interest as part of discharge planning. Also inform the couple about what to expect when resuming sexual intercourse and how to prevent any discomfort. Precoital vaginal lubrication may be impaired during the postpartum period, especially in women who are breast-feeding. Use of water-based gel lubricants (KY jelly, Astroglide) can be helpful. Information on pelvic floor exercises to enhance sensation may be beneficial.

Contraceptive options are included in the discussions with the couple so that they can make an informed decision before resuming sexual activity. Many couples are overwhelmed with the amount of new information given to them during their brief hospitalization. Many are not ready for a lengthy discussion about contraceptives. Presenting a brief overview of the various options along with written literature may be appropriate. It may be suitable to ask them to think about contraceptive needs and preferences, and advise them to use a barrier method (condom with spermicidal gel or foam) until another form of contraceptive is chosen. This advice is especially important if the follow-up appointment will not occur for 4 to 6 weeks after childbirth. Many couples will resume sexual activity prior to their postpartum checkup appointment, and may become pregnant before the return of the woman's menses. In addition, some women ovulate before their menstrual period returns and thus need contraceptive protection to prevent pregnancy.

Open and effective communication is necessary for effective contraceptive counseling so that information is clearly understood. Provide clear, consistent information appropriate to the woman and her partner's language, culture, and educational level. Only then can the best contraceptive method to be selected (Niedrach & Foster, 2003).

Promoting Nutrition

For the new mother, the postpartum period may be quite stressful for a myriad reasons, such as the physical stress of pregnancy and birth, the required caregiving tasks associated with the newborn, meeting the needs of other family members, and fatigue. As a result, the new mother may ignore her own needs for health and nutrition. Whether breast-feeding or bottle feeding, encourage the new mother to take good care of herself and eat a healthy diet so that nutrients lost during pregnancy can be replaced and she can return to a healthy weight. In general, nutrition recommendations for the postpartum woman include the following:

- Eating a wide variety of foods with high nutrient density
- Using foods and recipes that require little or no preparation
- Avoiding high-fat fast foods
- Drinking plenty of fluids daily—at least 2500 mL (approximately 84 oz)
- Avoiding fad weight reduction diets and harmful substances such as alcohol, tobacco, and drugs
- Avoiding excessive intake of fat, salt, sugar, and caffeine
- Eating the recommended daily servings from each food group (Box 16-4)

Nutritional needs for mothers who choose to breast-feed are greater throughout pregnancy. Maternal diet and nutritional status influence the quantity and quality of breast milk. To meet the needs for milk production, the woman's nutritional needs increase as follows:

- Calories: +500 cal/day for the first and second 6 months of lactation
- Protein: +20 g/day, adding an extra 2 cups of skim milk
- Calcium: +400 mg daily—consumption of four or more servings of milk

---

BOX 16-4

NUTRITIONAL RECOMMENDATIONS FOR NUTRITION DURING THE POSTPARTUM PERIOD

General Dietary Guidelines for Americans From the Food Guide Pyramid
- Breads, grains, and cereals: 6 to 11 servings
- Fruits: 2 to 4 servings
- Vegetables: 3 to 5 servings
- Protein foods: 2 to 3 servings (3 servings for lactating women)
- Milk products: 2 to 3 servings
- Fats, oils, and sweets: use sparingly (USDA & USDHHS, 2005)

Recommendations for the Lactating Woman From the Food Guide Pyramid
- Fruits: 4 servings
- Vegetables: 4 servings
- Milk: 4 to 5 servings
- Bread, cereal, pasta: 12 or more servings
- Meat, poultry, fish, eggs: 7 servings
- Fats, oils, and sweets: 5 servings (Dudek, 2006)

- Fluid: +2 to 3 quarts of fluids daily (milk, juice or water); no sodas

Certain foods (usually gaseous or strong-flavored ones) eaten by the mother may affect the flavor of the breast milk or cause GI problems for the infant. Not all infants are affected by the same foods. If the particular food item seems to cause a problem, urge the mother to eliminate that food for a few days to determine whether the problem disappears.

During the woman's brief stay in the health care facility, she may demonstrate a healthy appetite and eat well. The nutritional concern usually starts at home when mothers need to make their own food selections and prepare their own meals. This is a crucial area to address on follow-up.

Support for Choice of Feeding Method

Many factors influence a woman's choice of feeding method such as culture, employment demands, support from significant other and family, and knowledge base. Although breast-feeding is encouraged, be sure that couples have the necessary information to make an informed decision. Whether a couple chooses to breast-feed or bottle feed the newborn, support and respect their choice.

Keep in mind that although breast-feeding is advocated for newborn and infant health, there are certain situations in which it should be avoided. These would include women taking drugs, such as antithyroid drugs, antineoplastic drugs, alcohol, or street drugs (amphetamines, cocaine, PCP, marijuana), that would enter the breast milk and harm the infant. Women who are HIV positive are cautioned not to breast-feed to prevent postnatal HIV transmission to their newborn. Other contraindications to breast-feeding would include a newborn with an inborn error of metabolism such as galactosemia or PKU and a current pregnancy or a serious mental health disorder that would preclude the mother from remembering to feed the infant consistently.

Feeding Assistance

First-time mothers often have many questions and concerns about feeding. Even women who have had experience with feeding, too, may have questions. Thus, regardless of whether the woman is breast-feeding or bottle feeding her newborn, the postpartum woman can benefit from instruction.

Education About Bottle Feeding

Nutritional needs of infants vary based on gestational age, metabolic state, and physiologic complications. Estimated energy requirements for full-term infants range from 100 to 115 kcal/kg/day at 1 month to approximately 85 to 95 kcal/kg/day from 6 to 9 months of age (Gregory, 2005). Commercial formulas and breast milk both typically provide 20 cal/oz. Commercial formulas are classified as milk based (SMA, Enfamil, Similac), elemental (for infants with protein allergies), or soy based (Isomil, Nursoy). Newborns need about 108 cal/kg or approximately 650 cal/day (Dudek, 2006). Commercial formulas can be purchased in various forms: powdered (must be mixed with water), condensed liquid (must be diluted with equal amounts of water), ready to use (poured directly into bottles), and prepackaged (ready to use in disposable bottles). Until about age 4 months, most infants need six feedings a day. After this period, the number of feedings declines to accommodate other foods (fruits, cereals, vegetables) introduced to the infant's diet (Engstrom, 2004). For more information on newborn nutrition, see Chapter 18.

Suggestions for mothers about bottle feeding are highlighted in Teaching Guidelines 16-4.

Education About Breast-Feeding

The American Academy of Pediatrics (AAP) advocates breast-feeding for all full-term newborns, maintaining that, ideally, breast milk should be the sole nutrient for the first 6 to 12 months of life (Sloane, 2002). Educating a mother about breast-feeding will increase the likelihood of a successful breast-feeding experience. At birth, all newborns should be quickly dried, assessed, and, if stable, placed immediately in uninterrupted skin-to-skin contact (kangaroo care) with their mother. This is good practice whether the mother is going to breast-feed or bottle feed her infant. Kangaroo care provides the newborn optimal physiologic stability, warmth, and opportunities for the first feed (Kirsten, Bergman, & Hann, 2001).

 T E A C H I N G   G U I D E L I N E S   1 6 - 4

Bottle Feeding

1. Make feeding a relaxing time—a time to provide both food and comfort to your newborn.
2. Always hold the newborn when feeding.
3. Use a comfortable position when feeding the newborn.
   a. Place the newborn in your dominant arm, which is supported by a pillow.
   b. Have the newborn in a semi-upright feeding position supported in the crook of your arm (this position reduces choking and the flow of milk into the middle ear).
4. Tilt the bottle so that the nipple and the neck of the bottle are always filled with formula. (This prevents the infant from taking in too much air.)
5. Refrigerate any formula combined with tap water once it is mixed.
6. Discard any formula not taken; do not keep it for future feedings.
7. Burp the infant frequently and place on back or side for sleeping.
8. Use only iron-fortified infant formula for first year (Youngkin et al., 2004).

The benefits of breast-feeding are clear (see Chapter 18). To promote breast-feeding, the Baby-Friendly Hospital Initiative, an international program of the World Health Organization and the United Nations Children's Fund, was started in 1991. Based on this program, the hospital or birth center must take steps to provide "an optimal environment for the promotion, protection, and support of breast-feeding." These steps are based on the program's Ten Steps to Successful Breast-feeding as follows:

1. Have a written breast-feeding policy that is communicated to all staff.
2. Educate all staff to implement this written policy.
3. Inform all women about the benefits and management of breast-feeding.
4. Show all mothers how to initiate breast-feeding within 30 minutes of birth.
5. Give no food or drink other than breast milk to all newborns.
6. Demonstrate to all mothers how to breast-feed and maintain it.
7. Encourage breast-feeding on demand.
8. Allow no pacifiers to be given to breast-feeding infants.
9. Establish breast-feeding support groups and refer mothers to them.
10. Practice rooming-in 24 hours daily (Yawman, 2003).

Thus the nurse is responsible for encouraging breast-feeding when appropriate. For the woman who chooses to breast-feed her infant, the nurse or lactation consultant will need to spend time instructing her how to do so successfully. Many women have the impression that breast-feeding is simple with the readily available equipment and supplies. Although it is a natural process, women may experience some difficulty in breast-feeding their newborns. Nurses can assist mothers in smoothing out this transition.

Assist and provide one-to-one instruction to breast-feeding mothers, especially first-time breast-feeding mothers to ensure correct technique:

- Offer a thorough explanation about the procedure involved.
- Instruct the mother to wash her hands prior to starting.
- Inform her that her afterpains will increase during breast-feeding.
- Show her different positions, such as cradle and football holds and side-lying positions (Fig. 16-9).
- Explain that breast-feeding is a learned skill for both parties.
- Make sure the mother is comfortable (pain free) and not hungry.
- Tell the mother to start the feeding with an awake and alert infant showing hunger signs.
- Assist the mother to position herself correctly for comfort.
- Urge the mother to relax to encourage the let-down reflex.

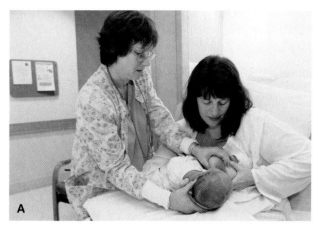
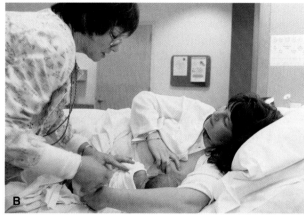

● Figure 16-9 Positions for breast-feeding. (**A**) Cradle hold; (**B**) lying down.

- Guide the mother's hand to form a "C" or "V" to access the nipple.
- Demonstrate stroking the infant's cheek to initiate sucking.
- Help her to elicit latching-on by inserting the nipple into infant's mouth.
- Show her how to check that the newborn's mouth position is correct and tell her to listen for a sucking noise.
- Demonstrate removal from the breast using a finder to break the suction.
- Instruct the mother on how to burp the infant between breasts.
- Reinforce and praise the mother for her efforts.
- Allow ample time to answer questions and address concerns.
- Refer the mother to support groups and community resources.

Reassuring mothers that some infants "latch on and catch on" right away, and some take more time and patience is important to help reduce their feelings of frustration and uncertainty about their ability. Tell them they need to believe in themselves and their ability to accomplish this task. Inform them not to panic if breast-feeding does not go smoothly at first; it takes time and practice.

Additional suggestions for mothers to help them relax and feel more comfortable breast-feeding, especially when the mother and newborn return home, include the following:

- Select a quiet corner or room where you won't be disturbed.
- Use of a rocking chair will soothe both you and your infant.
- Take long, slow deep breaths to help increase relaxation prior to nursing.
- Drink fluids during each breast-feeding session to replenish body fluids.
- Listen to soothing music during breast-feeding sessions.

- Cuddle and caress the infant during each breast-feeding time.
- Set out extra cloth diapers within reach to use as burping cloths.
- Allow sufficient time to enjoy each other in an unhurried atmosphere.
- Involve other family members in all aspects of the infant's care from the start.

Breast Care

Regardless of whether the mother is nursing, urge her to wear a very supportive, snug bra 24 hours a day to support enlarged breasts, prevent stretch marks, and promote comfort. A woman who is breast-feeding should wear a supportive bra throughout the lactation period. A nonnursing mother should wear it until engorgement ceases, and then should wear a less restrictive one. A supportive bra should fit the woman snugly, but still allow the mother to breathe without restriction.

Tell lactating and nonlactating mothers to use plain water to clean their breasts, especially the nipple area. Soap is drying and needs to be avoided.

Instruct the mother how to examine her breasts daily. Daily assessments of the breasts includes determining evidence of the mother's milk supply (breasts will feel full as the breasts are filling), condition of the nipples (red, bruised, fissured, or bleeding), and ascertaining how breast-feeding is going. The fullness of the breasts may progress to engorgement if feedings are delayed or breast-feeding is ineffective. Palpating both breasts will help the nurse identify whether the breasts are soft, filling, or engorged. A similar assessment of the breasts should be completed on the nonlactating mother to identify any problems such as engorgement and or mastitis.

Engorgement

Breast engorgement usually occurs during the first week postpartum. It is a common response of the breasts to the sudden change in hormones and the presence of an increased amount of milk. When this occurs, reassure the woman that this condition is temporary and usually resolves within 24 hours.

If the mother is breast-feeding, encourage frequent feedings, at least every 2 to 3 hours, with pumping just before feeding, to soften the breast so the newborn can latch on more effectively. Advise the mother to allow the newborn to feed on the first breast until it softens before switching to the other side.

Other tips to reduce engorgement include instructions such as the following:

- Take warm-to-hot showers to encourage milk release.
- Express some milk manually before breast-feeding.
- Wear a supportive nursing bra 24 hours daily to provide support.
- Feed the newborn in a variety of positions—sitting up and then lying down.
- Massage the breasts from under the axillary area down toward the nipple.
- Increase the frequency of feedings.
- Apply warm compresses to the breasts prior to nursing.
- Stay relaxed during the breast-feeding process.
- Use a breast pump if nursing or manual expression is not effective.
- Be aware that this condition is temporary and resolves quickly.

Lactation Suppression

In nonlactating women, breast engorgement is a self-limiting phenomenon that disappears as increasing estrogen levels suppress milk formation. Intervention consists of applying ice packs; wearing a snug, supportive bra 24 hours a day; and taking mild analgesics such as acetaminophen. Encourage the woman to avoid any stimulation to the breasts that might foster milk production, such as warm showers, pumping, or massaging the breasts. Medication is no longer given to hasten this process (see Teaching Guidelines 16-5).

Common Breast-Feeding Concerns

As much as every mother wants to progress through the breast-feeding process without incident, she may experience problems or concerns such as cracked nipples or mastitis. Breast-feeding should not cause the mother to verbalize pain. If the mother complains of sore, cracked nipples, the first step is to find the cause. If the infant is not positioned correctly, the mother takes the infant off the breast without first breaking the suction, the mother wears a bra too tight, or the infant does not latch on well, cracked or sore nipples result. Cracked nipples can increase the risk of lactating mothers for mastitis because a break in the skin may allow *Staphylococcus aureus* or other organisms to enter into the body. To prevent cracked nipples, instruct the mother to

- Apply warm water compresses over the nipple area
- Keep the nipples clean and dry

 TEACHING GUIDELINES 16-5

Suppressing Lactation

1. Wear a supportive, snugly fitting bra 24 hours daily, but not one that binds the breasts too tightly or interferes with your breathing.
2. Be aware that suppression may take 5 to 7 days to accomplish.
3. Take mild analgesics to reduce breast discomfort.
4. Let shower water flow over your back rather than your breasts.
5. Avoid any breast stimulation in the form of sucking or massage.
6. Drink to quench your thirst. Do not restrict your fluid intake, because this will not dry up your milk.
7. Reduce your salt intake to reduce your body's retention of fluids.
8. Use ice packs or cool compresses (for example, cool cabbage leaves) inside the bra to decrease local pain and swelling; change every 30 minutes (Moore & Catlin, 2003).

- Expose the nipples to air by pulling down the nursing bra flaps after each feeding
- Ensure the infant is positioned and latched on the nipple correctly

Sore nipples usually are caused by improper infant attachment on the nipple area, which traumatizes the tissue. First, rule out problems such as monilia, resulting from thrush in the newborn's mouth, and review techniques for proper positioning and latching on. Then recommend the following to the mother:

- Use only water, not soap, to clean the nipples to prevent dryness.
- Express some milk before feeding to stimulate the milk ejection reflex.
- Avoid breast pads with plastic liners, and change pads when they are wet.
- Wear a comfortable bra that is not too tight.
- Apply a few drops of breast milk to the nipples after feeding.
- Rotate positions when feeding the infant to promote complete breast emptying.
- Leave the nursing bra flaps down after feeding to allow nipples to air-dry.
- Inspect the nipples daily for redness or cracks (Edmondson, 2003).

To ease nipple pain and trauma, reinforce actions to ensure appropriate latching on and remind the woman about the need to break the suction at the breast prior to removing the newborn from the breast. Additional measures may include applying cold compresses over the area and massaging breast milk onto the nipple after feeding.

Mastitis, or inflammation of the breast, causes symptoms that include soreness, aching, swelling, redness occurring in the upper outer quadrant of the breast, and fever. This condition usually occurs in just one breast when a milk duct becomes blocked, causing inflammation, or through a cracked or damaged nipple, allowing bacteria to infect a portion of the breast. Treatment consists of rest, warm compresses, antibiotics, breast support, and continued breast-feeding (the infection will not pass into the breast milk). Explain to the mother that it is important to keep the milk flowing in the infected breast whether it is through nursing, manual expression, or with a breast pump.

Promoting Family Adjustment and Well-Being

The postpartum period involves extraordinary physiologic, psychological, and sociocultural changes in the life of a woman and her family. Appropriate and timely interventions can facilitate the process of adjustment to the role changes and attachment to the newborn.

Parental Roles

Parental roles develop and grow through interacting with their newborn (see Chapter 15 for additional information on maternal and paternal adaptation). The pleasure they derive from this interaction stimulates and reinforces this contact behavior. With repeated, continued contact with their newborn, parents learn to recognize cues and understand the newborn's behavior. This positive interaction contributes to family harmony.

Nurses need to be fully versed on the various phases and stages parents go through as they attempt to make their new parenting roles "fit" into their life experience. Be sure to assess the parents for attachment behaviors (normal and deviant), adjustment to the new parental role, family member adjustment, social support system, and educational needs. To facilitate parental role adaptation and parent–newborn attachment, include the following nursing interventions:

- Provide an opportunity for parents to interact with their newborn as much as possible. Encourage exploration, holding, and providing care.
- Model behaviors by holding the newborn close and speaking positively.
  - Always refer to the newborn by name in front of the parents.
  - Speak directly to newborn in a calm voice.
  - Encourage both parents to pick up and hold the newborn.
  - Point out the newborn's response to parental stimulation.
  - Point out the positive physical features of the newborn's appearance.

- Involve both parents in the newborn's care and praise them for their efforts.
- Evaluate family strengths and weaknesses, and parenting preparedness.
- Assess for risk factors such as lack of social support and presence of stressors.
- Observe the effect of culture on the family interaction to determine whether it is appropriate.
- Monitor parental attachment behaviors to determine whether alterations require referral.
  - Positive behaviors: holding the newborn closely or in an en face position, talking to or admiring the newborn, or demonstrating closeness
  - Negative behaviors: avoiding contact with newborn, calling it names, or showing a disinterest in caring for the newborn (see Table 16-1)
- Monitor the parental relationship to determine alterations that need intervention.
  - Coping behaviors: positive conversations between partners, both wanting to be involved with newborn care, or absence of arguments
  - Noncoping behaviors: signs of avoidance by not visiting, limited conversations or periods of silence, or heated arguments or conflict
- Identify a support system available to the new family and encourage help.
  - Ask direct questions about home or community support to ascertain availability and degree of assistance.
  - Make additional community resource referrals to meet family needs.
- Arrange for community home visits in high-risk families to provide positive reinforcement of parenting skills and nurturing behaviors with the newborn.
- Provide anticipatory guidance regarding the newborn before discharge to reduce frustration levels by not knowing what to expect:
  - Newborn sleep–wake cycles (warning they may be reversed)
  - Variations in newborn appearance to decrease fears of abnormalities
  - Infant developmental milestones (growth spurts)
  - Interpretation of crying cues (hunger, wet, discomfort)
  - Several comforting techniques to quiet crying infant (car ride)
  - Sensory enrichment/stimulation (colorful mobile)
  - Signs and symptoms of illness and how to assess for fever
  - Important phone numbers, follow-up care, and needed immunizations
  - Physical and emotional changes associated with the postpartum period that may impact her family relationships
  - Need for integrating siblings into care of the newborn with reassurance that sibling rivalry is normal, including ways to reduce it

• Allowance to make time for both parents as a couple
• Appropriate community referral resources

In addition, nurses can assist fathers to feel more competent in assuming their parental role by teaching and providing information (Fig. 16-10). Presenting the facts to them helps to displace any of their unrealistic expectations, ultimately helping them to cope more successfully with the demands of fatherhood and thereby fostering a nurturing family relationship.

Consider THIS!

I have always prided myself in being very organized and in control in most situations, but survival at home after childbirth wasn't one of them. I left the hospital 24 hours after giving birth to my son because my doctor said I could. The postpartum nurse encouraged me to stay longer, but wanting to be in control and sleeping in my own bed again won out. I thought my baby would be sleeping while I sent out birth announcements to my friends and family—*wrong!*

What happened instead was my son didn't sleep as I imagined and my nipples became sore after breastfeeding every few hours. I was weary and tired and wanted to sleep, but couldn't. Somehow I thought I would be getting a full night's sleep because I was up throughout the day, but that was a fantasy too. At two o'clock in the morning when you are up feeding your baby, you feel you are the only one in the world up at that time and feel very much alone. My feelings of being organized and in control all the time have changed dramatically since I left the hospital. I have learned to yield to the important needs of my son and derive satisfaction from being able to bring comfort to him and to let go of my control.

Thoughts: It is interesting to see how a newborn changed this woman's need to organize and control her environment. What "tips of survival" could the postpartum nurse offer this woman to help in her home transition? How can friends and family help when women arrive home from the hospital?

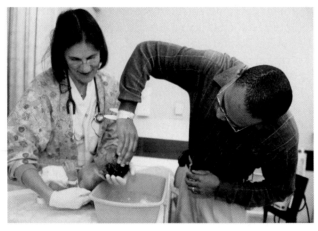

● Figure 16-10 Father participating in newborn care.

Sibling Roles

It can be overwhelming to a young child to have another family member introduced into their small, stable world. Although most parents try to prepare siblings for the arrival of their new little brother or sister, many young children experience stress. They may view the new infant as competition or fear that they will be replaced in the parent's affection. All siblings need extra attention from their parents and reassurance that they are loved and important. Many parents need reassurance that sibling rivalry is normal. Suggest the following to help parents minimize sibling rivalry:

• Expect and tolerate some regression (thumb sucking, bedwetting).
• Explain the childbirth in an appropriate way for the child's age.
• Encourage discussion about the new infant during relaxed family times.
• Encourage the sibling to participate in decisions, such as names, toys to buy.
• Take the sibling on the tour of the maternity suite to prepare him or her.
• Buy a t-shirt that says "I'm the [big brother or big sister]."
• Spend "special time" with the sibling
• Read with the sibling. Some suggested readings may include
  • *Things to Do with A New Baby* (Ormerod, 1984)
  • *Betsy's Baby Brother* (Wolde, 1975)
  • *The Berenstain Bear's New Baby* (Berenstain, 1974)
  • *Mommy's Lap* (Horowitz & Sorensen, 1993)
• Plan time for each child throughout the day.
• Role-play safe handling of a newborn with a doll. Give your preschooler or school-age child a doll to care for.
• Encourage older children to verbalize emotions about the newborn.
• Purchase a gift that can be given to the newborn by the sibling.
• Purchase a gift that can be given to the sibling by the newborn.
• Arrange for the sibling to come to the hospital to see the newborn (Fig. 16-11).
• Move the sibling from his or her crib to a youth bed months in advance of the birth of the newborn.
• Encourage grandparents to pay attention to the older child when visiting (Youngkin & Davis, 2004).

Grandparents' Role

The grandparents' role and involvement will depend on their proximity to the newborn and the nuclear family, their willingness to become involved, and cultural expectations of their role. Just as parents and siblings go through developmental changes, so too do grandparents. These changes can have a positive or negative effect on the relationship.

Newborn care, feeding, and childrearing have changed since grandparents raised the parents. New parents may

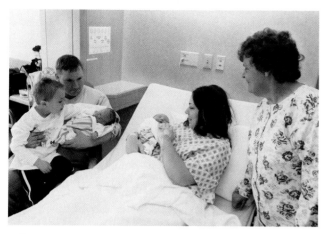

● Figure 16-11 Sibling visitation.

lack parenting skills, but want their parents' support without criticism. A grandparent's "take-charge approach" may not be welcome by new parents who are testing their own parenting roles. Thus, family conflict may ensue. Grandparents' involvement can enrich the lives of the entire family if accepted within the right context and dose by the family. Many grandparents realize their adult children's wishes for autonomy, respect these wishes, and remain resource people for them when requested.

Nurses can assist in the grandparents' role transition by assessing the communication skills, role expectations, and support skills of parents and grandparents during the prenatal period. Find out whether the grandparents are included in the couple's social support network and whether their support is wanted or helpful. If they are, and it is, then encourage the grandparents to learn about new parenting, feeding, and childrearing skills their children have learned in childbirth classes. This information is commonly found in "grandparenting" classes. These grandparenting classes may help them understand the new parenting concepts and bring them up-to-date on childbirth practices today. Grandparents can be a source of support and comfort to the new postpartum family if effective communication skills are used and roles are defined.

Postpartum Blues

The postpartum period is typically a happy yet stressful time, because the birth of an infant is accompanied by enormous physical, social, and emotional changes. The postpartum woman may report feelings of emotional lability, such as crying one minute and laughing the next. The blues symptoms (crying spells, sadness, confusion, insomnia, poor appetite, and anxiety) typically begin 3 to 4 days after childbirth and resolve by day 10 (Seyfried & Marcus, 2003). These mood swings may be confusing to new mothers but usually are self-limiting. **Postpartum blues** are transient emotional disturbances beginning within the first week after childbirth and are characterized by such feelings as anxiety, irritability, insomnia, crying, loss of appetite,

and sadness (Venis, 2002). Postpartum blues are thought to affect up to 75% of all new mothers; this condition is the mildest form of emotional disturbance associated with childbearing (Condon, 2004). The mother maintains contact with reality consistently and it tends to resolve spontaneously without therapy within 1 to 2 weeks. Postpartum blues have been regarded as brief, benign, and without clinical significance, but several studies have proposed a link between blues and subsequent depression in the 6 months following childbirth (Henshaw, Foreman, & Cox, 2004).

Postpartum blues requires no formal treatment, other than support and reassurance, because it does not usually interfere with the woman's ability to function and care for her infant. Further evaluation is necessary if symptoms persist more than 2 weeks (Nonacs, 2004). Nurses can ease a mother's distress by encouraging the woman to vent her feelings, and by demonstrating patience and understanding with her and her family. Suggesting that housework and infant outside help might assist her to feel less overwhelmed until the blues ease might be helpful during this time period. Providing supportive telephone numbers that she can call when she feels down during the day might also provide her with additional support during this very stressful time. Making women aware of this disorder while they are pregnant will also help increase their knowledge about this mood disturbance. Their knowledge about this mood disorder may lessen their embarrassment and increase their willingness to ask for and accept help.

The postpartum woman also is at risk for more long-term problems affecting her mental health. These problems include postpartum depression and postpartum psychosis. These conditions are discussed in greater depth in Chapter 22.

Preparing for Discharge

The AAP and the American College of Obstetricians and Gynecologists (ACOG) (2002) state that the length of stay in the facility should be individualized for each mother–baby dyad. If a shortened hospital stay is desired, the following criteria should be met:

- Mother is afebrile and vital signs are within normal range.
- Lochia is appropriate amount and color for stage of recovery.
- Hemoglobin and hematocrit values are within normal range.
- Uterine fundus is firm; urinary output is adequate.
- ABO blood groups and RhD status are known and, if indicated, anti-D immunoglobulin has been administered.
- Surgical wounds are healing and no signs of infection are present.
- Mother is able to ambulate without difficulty.
- Food and fluids are taken without difficulty.
- Self-care and infant care are understood and demonstrated.

- Family or other support system is available to care for both.
- Mother is aware of possible complications (AAP & ACOG, 2002)

Immunizations

Prior to discharge, check the immunity status for rubella for all mothers and give a subcutaneous injection of rubella vaccine if they are not serologically immune (titer < 1:10). Be sure that the client signs a consent form to receive the vaccine. Keep in mind that nursing mothers may be vaccinated because the live, attenuated rubella virus is not communicable. Inform all mothers requiring immunization about possible side effects (rash, joint symptoms, and a low-grade fever 5 to 21 days later) and the need to avoid pregnancy for at least 3 months after being vaccinated because of the risk of teratogenic effects (Lowdermilk & Perry, 2004).

If the client is Rh negative, check the Rh status of the newborn. Verify that the woman is Rh negative and has not been sensitized, that Coombs' test is negative, and that the newborn is Rh positive. Mothers who are Rh negative and have given birth to an infant who is Rh positive should receive an injection of Rh immunoglobulin within 72 hours after birth to prevent a sensitization reaction in the Rh-negative woman who received Rh-positive blood cells during the birthing process. The usual protocol is for the woman to receive two doses of Rh immunoglobulin (RhoGAM): one at 28 weeks' gestation and the second dose within 72 hours after childbirth. A signed consent form is needed after a thorough explanation is provided about the procedure, including the purpose, possible side effects, and effect on future pregnancies.

Ensuring Follow-Up Care

New mothers and their families need to be attended to over an extended period of time by nurses knowledgeable about mother care, infant feeding (breast-feeding and bottle feeding), infant care, and nutrition. Although continuous nursing care stops on discharge from the hospital or birthing center, extended episodic nursing care needs to follow the family home. The new family faces numerous challenges after discharge. These challenges are described in Box 16-5.

Many new mothers are reluctant to "cut the cord" after a brief stay in the facility and need expanded services within the community available to them. Early discharge from the hospital subjects a woman to certain risk factors: uterine involution, discomfort at an episiotomy or cesarean site, infection, fatigue, and maladjustment in her new role. Postpartum nursing care should include a range of family-focused care from telephone calls, outpatient clinics, and home visits. Typically, public health nurses, community and home health nurses, and health care provider office staff will carry on in the continuum of postpartum care after hospital discharge.

BOX 16-5

CURRENT CHALLENGES FACING FAMILIES AFTER DISCHARGE

- Lacking number of role models for breast-feeding and infant care today
- The decline in opportunities for family members to care for the newborn as extended families disintegrate
- Inability of many of the new mother's own mothers to provide support because they did not breast-feed
- Feelings of isolation and limited community ties for women working full time
- Feelings of being overwhelmed with learning and taking in all the information exposed to in the facility in 48 hours or less
- Focus of prenatal classes usually on the birthing event rather than skills needed to care for themselves and the newborn during the postpartum period
- Limited access to education and support systems addressing unique needs for many nontraditional families from diverse cultures
- Lack of nearby support system as a result of geographic dispersion and/or careers (Pease & Beigel, 2003)

Telephone Follow-Up

Telephone follow-up typically occurs during the first week after discharge to check on how things are going at home. Calls can be made by perinatal nurses within the agency as part of follow-up care or by the local health department nurses. A disadvantage to a phone call assessment is that the nurse cannot "see" the client and thus must rely on the mother or the family's observations. The experienced nurse needs to be able to cue in on distress and give appropriate advice and referral information if needed.

Outpatient Follow-Up

For mothers with established community health care providers such as private pediatricians and obstetricians, visits to their offices are arranged soon after discharge. For the woman with an uncomplicated vaginal birth, an office visit is usually scheduled for 4 to 6 weeks after childbirth. A woman who had a cesarean birth frequently is seen within 2 weeks after hospital discharge. The needed follow-up time frames are included in hospital discharge orders with the request to call their office to set up an appointment. Newborn examinations and further diagnostic lab studies are scheduled within the first week.

Outpatient clinics are available in many communities for referrals. If family members run into a problem they feel they need to address, the local clinic would be available for an assessment and validation or for assurance to the family. Clinic visits can be used to replace or supplement home visits. Unfortunately, the set daytime hours of operation and unfamiliarity of the staff with the family are disadvantages of this community resource. Still, it can be a valuable resource for the new family in need of consultation about a postpartal problem or concern.

Home Visit Follow-Up

Home visits are usually made within the first week of discharge to assess the mother and newborn. During the home visit, the nurse provides expertise in recognizing and managing common biomedical and psychosocial problems. In addition, the home nurse can offer understanding and guidance for the parents making the adjustment to a change in their lives. The postpartum home visit usually includes

- Maternal assessment: general well-being, vital signs, breast health and care; abdomen and musculoskeletal status; voiding status; fundus and lochia status; psychological and coping status; family relationships; proper feeding technique; environmental safety check; newborn care knowledge and health teaching needed identified during the assessment (see Fig. 16-12 for sample assessment forms)
- Infant assessment: physical examination, general appearance, and vital signs status; home safety check; child development status; and appropriate education needed for improvement of care-taking process.

The home care nurse must be prepared to support, advise, and educate the woman and her family. Common areas include

- Breast-feeding procedure
- Appropriate parenting behavior and problem solving
- Maternal/newborn physical, psychosocial, and culture–environmental needs
- Emotional needs of the new family, incorporating active listening skills as they deal with change
- Warning signs of problems and where to seek help to eliminate them
- Sexuality issues related to the postpartum period, including contraceptives and their proper use
- Immunization needs for both mother and infant
- Family dynamics for smooth transition
- Links to health care providers and community resources

KEY CONCEPTS

- The transitional adjustment period between birth and parenthood includes education about baby care basics, the role of the new family, emotional support, breast-feeding or bottle-feeding support, and maternal mentoring.
- Sensitivity to how childbearing practices and beliefs vary for multicultural families and how best to provide appropriate nursing care to meet their needs are important during the postpartum period.
- A thorough postpartum assessment is key to preventing complications.
- The postpartum assessment using the acronym BUBBLE-HE (breasts, uterus, bowel, bladder, lochia, episiotomy/perineum, Homans' sign, emotions) is a helpful guide in performing a systematic head-to-toe postpartum assessment.
- Lochia is assessed according to its amount, color, and change with activity and time. It proceeds from lochia rubra to serosa to alba.
- Because of shortened agency stays, nurses must use this brief time with the client to address areas of comfort, elimination, activity, rest and exercise, self-care, sexuality and contraception, nutrition, family adaptation, discharge, and follow-up.
- The AAP advocates breast-feeding for all full-term newborns, maintaining that, ideally, breast milk should be the sole nutrient for the first 6 to 12 months of life.
- Successful parenting is a continuous and complex interactive process that requires the acquisition of new skills and the integration of the new member into the existing family unit.
- Bonding is a vital component of the attachment process and is necessary in establishing parent–infant attachment and a healthy, loving relationship; attachment behaviors include seeking and maintaining close proximity to, and exchanging gratifying experiences with, the infant.
- Nurses can be instrumental in facilitating attachment by first understanding attachment behaviors (positive and negative) of newborns and parents, and intervening appropriately to promote and enhance attachment.
- New mothers and their families need to be attended to over an extended period of time by nurses knowledgeable about mother care, newborn feeding (breast-feeding and bottle feeding), newborn care, and nutrition.

Maternal Assessment
Maternal/Newborn Record System

Page 1 of 2

Date MO / DAY / YR Time begin: _____
                    Time end: _____   Date of delivery MO / DAY / YR

Medication allergy   ☐ None   Identify_____
Significant health history ☐ None   Identify_____

PHYSICAL

TEMP.	PULSE	RESP.	BP /

Breasts   ☐ Nursing   ☐ Non-nursing
Color   ☐ Normal   ☐ Reddened
Condition   ☐ Soft   ☐ Firm   ☐ Engorged   ☐ Blocked ducts
Secretion   ☐ Colostrum ☐ Milk   ☐ Other _____
Support bra   ☐ No   ☐ Yes, fit   ☐ Appropriate
                                          ☐ Inappropriate

Nipples (If nursing) ☐ Erect ☐ Flat   ☐ Inverted
  Condition ☐ Intact   ☐ Bruised   ☐ Blistered
             ☐ Fissured ☐ Bleeding ☐ Scabbed
  Care   ☐ Water only ☐ Soap   ☐ Air dry
             ☐ Topical agent (type/frequency) _____

             ☐ Other _____
Self-exam   ☐ Accurate ☐ Inaccurate/instructed

Abdomen
Diastasis recti ☐ Absent ☐ Present_____cm
                 ☐ Exercise taught
Incision   ☐ None
  Type   ☐ Transverse ☐ Vertical ☐ Umbilical
  Closure   ☐ Staples ☐ Sutures ☐ Steri-strips
  Condition ☐ Approximated   ☐ Open_____cm
            ☐ Redness _____
            ☐ Swelling _____
            ☐ Discharge _____
            ☐ Other _____

Reproductive Tract
Uterus   ☐ Firm ☐ Firm with massage ☐ Boggy
          Height_____ ☐ Midline ☐ Displaced L R
          ☐ Non tender   ☐ Tender ☐ With touch ☐ Constant
Lochia   ☐ Rubra ☐ Serosa ☐ Alba
          ☐ Clots (describe) _____
          ☐ Fleshy odor ☐ Foul odor
          Pads Type_____ Number/day_____

          Saturation %├────┼────┼────┼────┤
                       0   25   50   75 100

Perineum ☐ Intact ☐ Laceration
          ☐ Episiotormy Type_____ Extension_____
Condition ☐ Redness _____
          ☐ Edema _____
          ☐ Eccymosis _____
          ☐ Discharge _____
          ☐ Approximation _____
Care   ☐ Front-to-back cleansing ☐ Peri-bottle
          ☐ Soap/water
          ☐ Ice ☐ Sitz bath ☐ Warm ☐ Cool
          ☐ Topical agent (type/frequency) _____

          ☐ Other _____

Elimination
Urinary tract
  Voiding pattern   ☐ Normal   ☐ Incontinence
                      ☐ Bladder distention ☐ Catheter (type) _____
  Signs of infection ☐ None/reviewed ☐ Urgency ☐ Frequency
                      ☐ Dysuria ☐ CVA tenderness L R
Gastrointestinal tract
  Bowel pattern   ☐ Normal   ☐ No BM
                      ☐ Constipation ☐ Diarrhea
                      ☐ Meds/treatments (type, frequency, effect) _____

  Hemorrhoids   ☐ No ☐ Yes (describe) _____
                      ☐ Meds/treatments (type, frequency, effect) _____

Lower Extremities
Edema ☐ None ☐ Pedal ☐ Ankle ☐ Pretibial ☐ Thigh
       ☐ Pitting (describe) _____
Signs of thrombophlebitis   ☐ None

	L	R		L	R
Homan's sign	☐	☐	Redness	☐	☐
Pain	☐	☐	Warmth	☐	☐
Swelling	☐	☐			

Pain	**No**	**Yes**	
		Managed	Problematic
Abdominal incision	☐	☐	☐
Back	☐	☐	☐
Breasts	☐	☐	☐
Headache	☐	☐	☐
Hemorrhoid	☐	☐	☐
Nipple	☐	☐	☐
Perineum	☐	☐	☐
Uterine cramping	☐	☐	☐
Other _____	☐	☐	☐

Analgesic ☐ No
           ☐ Yes (type/dose/frequency) _____

Reportable danger signs ☐ Aware ☐ Unaware/instructed

TESTS ☐ None
           ☐ Urinalysis
           ☐ CBC
           ☐ _____

IDENTIFIED NEEDS

_____
_____
_____
_____
_____
_____
_____
_____
_____

Signature _____

● Figure 16-12 Sample postpartum home visit assessment form. (**A**) Maternal assessment.
(**B**) Newborn assessment. (Used with permission: Copyright Briggs Corporation. Professional
Nurse Associates.)

Maternal Assessment

Maternal/Newborn Record System

Page 2 of 2

PATIENT IDENTIFICATION

Record No. ______

Name ______

Home address ______ STREET

______ CITY STATE ZIP

ACTIVITIES OF DAILY LIVING - 24 HOUR HISTORY

Date MO / DAY / YR

Nutrition

Appetite ☐ Good ☐ Fair ☐ Poor

Usual pattern ☐ Yes ☐ No ______

Special diet ☐ No ☐ Yes ______

Food intolerance/allergy ☐ No ☐ Yes ______

Vitamin/mineral supplement ☐ No ☐ Yes ______

Fluid intake (type/amount) ______

BREAKFAST	LUNCH	DINNER	SNACKS
______	______	______	______
______	______	______	______
______	______	______	______

General Hygiene ☐ Adequate ☐ Inadequate (describe)

Sleep/Activity

Amount of Activity

Night, uninterrupted ______ hrs

Naps ☐ No ☐ Yes ______ hrs

Fatigue ☐ None ☐ Minimal ☐ Moderate ☐ Exhausted

Activities

Limitations ☐ None Identify ______

☐ Self-care ☐ Infant care

	Appropriate	Inappropriate/instructed
Stair climbing	☐	☐
Lifting	☐	☐
Household tasks	☐	☐
Outside home	☐	☐

Other ______

Exercise

☐ None

	Accurate	Inaccurate/instructed
Kegel	☐	☐
Postpartum	☐	☐

Other ______

PSYCHOLOGICAL

Review of Labor and Birth

Missing pieces ☐ No ☐ Yes

Unmet expectations ☐ No ☐ Yes

Unresolved feelings ☐ No ☐ Yes

Pertinent data ______

Postpartum Tmetable (Key on reverse side)

☐ Taking in ☐ Taking hold ☐ Letting go

Emotional Status ☐ Happy ☐ Ambivalent ☐ Anxious ☐ Sad ☐ Other ______

Postpartum-depression (Key on reverse side)

☐ 0 ☐ 1 ☐ 2 ☐ 3 ☐ 4

☐ Signs/Symptoms Reviewed

General Comments (body image, role changes, concerns) ______

SEXUALITY

	Aware	Unaware/instructed
Relationship with partner		
Adjustment	☐	☐
Expressions of affection	☐	☐
Resuming Intercourse		
Timing (lack of lochia, comfort)	☐	☐
Vaginal dryness	☐	☐
Milk ejection (if lactating)	☐	☐
Position variation	☐	☐
Libidinal changes	☐	☐
Return of Menses	☐	☐

Contraceptive Method

☐ None ☐ Undecided/aware of options

☐ Natural family planning

☐ Cervical cap

☐ Condom

☐ Diaphragm

☐ Hormones ☐ Pill ☐ Injection ☐ Implant

☐ IUD

☐ Spermicide

☐ Sterilization ☐ Female ☐ Male

☐ Other ______

Accurate use ☐ Yes ☐ No/instructed

IDENTIFIED NEEDS

______

Signature ______

● Figure 16-12 (continued)

Maternal Assessment
Maternal/Newborn Record System

Date MO / DAY / YR   Time begin: _____   Date of Birth MO / DAY / YR

Time end: _____

Significant history ☐ None   Identify _____

PHYSICAL

Temp _____ Pulse (rate/rhythm) _____ Resp _____
Weight _____ Birth weight _____ % Change _____
Length_____ Head _____ Chest _____

HEAD/NECK

1. Fontanels

	Level	Bulging	Depressed
Anterior	☐	☐	☐
Posterior	☐	☐	☐

   Sutures ☐ Open ☐ Closed ☐ Overriding
2. Variations ☐ Molding ☐ Caput ☐ Cephalhematoma

	NORMAL	ABNORMAL	DETAIL VARIATIONS/ ABNORMAL FINDINGS
3. Face (symmetry)	☐	☐	
4. Eyes (symmetry, conjunctiva, sciera, eyelids, PERL)	☐	☐	
5. Ears (shape, position, auditory response)	☐	☐	
6. Nose (patency)	☐	☐	
7. Mouth (lip, mucous membranes, tongue, palate)	☐	☐	

Chest

8. Neck (ROM, symmetry)	☐	☐	
9. Appearance (shape, breasts, nipples)	☐	☐	
10. Breath sounds	☐	☐	
11. Clavicles	☐	☐	

Cardiovascular

12. Heart sounds	☐	☐	
13. Brachial/femoral pulses (compare strength, equality)	☐	☐	

Abdomen

14. Appearance (shape, size)	☐	☐	
15. Cord (condition)	☐	☐	
16. Liver (less than or equal to 3 cm ↓ ®costal margin)	☐	☐	

Genitalia

17. Female (labia, introitus, discharge)	☐	☐	
18. Male (meatus, scrotum, testes)	☐	☐	
19. Circumcision ☐ No ☐ Yes	☐	☐	

Musculoskeletal

20. Muscle tone	☐	☐	
21. Extremities (symmetry, digits, ROM)	☐	☐	
22. Hips (symmetry, ROM)	☐	☐	
23. Spine (alignment, integrity)	☐	☐	

Neurologic

24. Reflexes (presence, symmetry)

Moro	☐	☐
Grasp	☐	☐
Babinski	☐	☐
25. Cry (presence, quality)	☐	☐

PHYSICAL (CONT'D)
Skin

Turgor ☐ Good ☐ Poor
Condition ☐ Smooth ☐ Dry, cracked ☐ Peeling
Color ☐ Pink ☐ Ruddy ☐ Cyanotic ☐ Pale
☐ Jaundice (note levels)
  ☐ Head (3 mg/dl)
  ☐ Head and upper chest (6 mg/dl)
  ☐ Head and entire chest (9 mg/dl)
  ☐ Head, chest and abdomen to umbilicus (12 mg/dl)
  ☐ Head, chest and entire abdomen (15 mg/dl)
  ☐ Head, chest, abdomen, legs and feet (18 mg/dl)
Variations (Rashes, lesions, birthmarks). _____

NUTRITION
Feeding

Reflexes ☐ Root ☐ Suck ☐ Swallow
Hunger cues identified ☐ Yes ☐ No/instructed

BREAST	FORMULA
Frequency___times in _____ hours	Type _____
Time per breast_____ min _____ min	Amount _____ oz.
Positioning ☐ Correct	Frequency _____
☐ Incorrect_____	Preparation ☐ Correct
Latch ☐ Correct	☐ Incorrect_____
☐ Incorrect	
Appropriate audible swallows	☐ Correct
☐ Yes ☐ No_____	☐

Satiation demonstrated ☐ Yes
   ☐ No (describe)_____
Regurgitation ☐ No ☐ Yes (describe)_____
Pacifier use ☐ No ☐ Yes (type/pattern)_____

Stool (number/day, color, consistency)_____
Urine (number/day, color)_____

BEHAVIOR
Sleep/Activity Pattern (24 hours)

Sleep (16–20 hrs)   ☐ Yes ☐ No (describe)_____

Awake-alert (2–3 hrs)   ☐ Yes ☐ No (describe)_____

Awake-crying (2–4 hrs)   ☐ Yes ☐ No (describe)_____

Consolability (Key on reverse) ☐ 0 ☐ 1 ☐ 2 ☐ 3 ☐ 4

TESTS ☐ None   Time
☐ Metabolic screen kit no. _____   _____
☐ Bilirubin   _____
☐ Hematocrit   _____
☐ _____   _____
☐ _____   _____

INENTIFIED NEEDS _____

_____

_____

_____

_____

Signature _____

● Figure 16-12 (continued)

References

American Academy of Pediatrics & American College of Obstetricians & Gynecologists. (2002). Postpartum and follow-up care. In *Guidelines for perinatal care* (5th ed., pp. 125–161, 187–283). Elk Grove Village, IL: AAP.

American Academy of Pediatrics Committee on Drugs. (2001). The transfer of drugs and other chemicals into human milk. *Pediatrics, 108,* 776–789.

Anonas–Ternate, A. (2003). A Filipino perspective. In M. L. Moore & M. K. Moos (Eds.), *March of Dimes nursing module: Cultural competence in the care of childbearing families.* White Plains, NY: March of Dimes Birth Defects Foundation Educational Services.

Ayers, M. (2003). *Mother–infant attachment and psychoanalysis: The eyes of shame.* Philadelphia: Brunner-Routledge Publishers.

Badwan, L. (2003). A Muslim perspective. In M. L. Moore & M. K. Moos (Eds.), *March of Dimes nursing module: Cultural competence in the care of childbearing families.* White Plains, NY: March of Dimes Birth Defects Foundation Educational Services.

Banks, J. W. (2003). Ka'nistenhsera Teiakotihsnie's: A native community rekindles the tradition of breast-feeding. *AWHONN Lifelines, 7,* 340–347.

Baradon, T. (2002). Psychotherapeutic work with parents and infants—psychoanalytic and attachment perspectives. *Attachment & Human Development, 4,* 25–38.

Blackburn, S. T. (2003). *Maternal, fetal, and neonatal physiology* (2nd ed.). Philadelphia: Saunders.

Bowers, P. (2003). *Cultural perspectives in childbearing.* [Online] Available at http://nsweb.nursingspectrum.com/ce/ce263.htm.

Buist, A., Morse, C. A., & Durkin, S. (2003). Men's adjustment to fatherhood: Implications for obstetric health care. *Journal of Obstetric, Gynecologic, and Neonatal Nursing, 32,* 172–180.

Center for Disease Control and Prevention, Office of Women's Health. (2003). *Overweight and obesity among U.S. adults.* [Online] Available at www.cdc.gov/od/spotlight/nwhw/pubs/overwght.htm.

Chalmers, B., Mangiaterra, V., & Porter, R. (2001). WHO principles of perinatal care: The essential antenatal, perinatal, and postpartum care course. *Birth, 28,* 202–207.

Condon, M. C. (2004). *Women's health: An integrated approach to wellness and illness.* Upper Saddle River, NJ: Prentice Hall.

Cunningham, F. G., Gant, N. F., Leveno, K. J., Gilstrap, L. C., Hauth, J. C., & Wenstrom, K. D. (2005). *Williams obstetrics* (22nd ed.). New York: Lippincott Williams & Wilkins.

Dudek, S. G. (2006). *Nutrition essentials for nursing practice* (5th ed.). Philadelphia: Lippincott Williams & Wilkins.

Edmondson, E. (2003). Breast care during breast-feeding. *Advance for Nurses, 5,* 29.

Engstrom, J. (2004). *Maternal–neonatal nursing made incredibly easy.* Philadelphia: Lippincott Williams & Wilkins.

Ferketich, S. L., & Mercer, R. T. (1995). Paternal–infant attachment of experienced and inexperienced fathers during infancy. *Nursing Research, 44,* 31–37.

Fogel, C. I. (2003). Female sexuality. In E. T. Breslin & V. A. Lucas (Eds.), *Women's health nursing: Toward evidence-based practice* (pp. 400–431.) St. Louis: Saunders.

Fong, W., & Grant, R. J. (2005). Postpartum perineal care. *eMedicine.* [Online] Available at www.emedicine.com/aaem/topic361.htm.

Goulet, C., Bell, L., St-Cyr Tribble, D., Paul, D., & Lang, A. (1998). A concept analysis of parent–infant attachment. *Journal of Advanced Nursing, 28,* 1071–1081.

Gray, M. (2004). Stress urinary incontinence in women. *Journal of the American Academy of Nurse Practitioners, 16,* 188–197.

Green, C. J., & Wilkinson, J. M. (2004). *Maternal–newborn nursing care plans.* St. Louis: Mosby.

Gregory, K. (2005). Update on nutrition for preterm and full-term infants. *Journal of Obstetric, Gynecologic, and Neonatal Nursing, 34,* 98–108.

Henshaw, C., Foreman, D., & Cox, J. (2004) Postnatal blues: A risk factor for postnatal depression. *Journal of Psychosomatic Obstetrics & Gynecology, 25,* 267–272.

Jeffreys, R., & Nordahl, K. (2002). Preconception, prenatal, and postpartum exercise. *Healthy Weight Journal,* May/June, 36–38.

Kirsten, G. F., Bergman, N. J., & Hann, F. M. (2001). Kangaroo mother care in the nursery. *Pediatric Clinics of North America, 48,* 443–452.

Klaus, M. H., & Kennel, J. H. (1982). *Parent–infant bonding* (2nd ed.) St. Louis: CV Mosby.

Koulomzin, M., Beebe, B., Anderson, S., Jaffe, J., Feldstein, S., & Crown, C. (2002). Infant gaze, head, face and self-touch at 4 months differentiate secure vs. avoidant attachment at 1 year: A microanalytic approach. *Attachment & Human Development, 4,* 3–24.

Littleton, L. Y., & Engebretson, J. C. (2005). *Maternity nursing care.* Clifton Park, NY: Thomson Delmar Learning.

Lowdermilk, D. L., & Perry, S. E. (2004). *Maternity & women's health care* (8th ed.). St. Louis: Mosby.

McCrink, A. (2003). Evaluating the female pelvic floor: Understanding and treating prolapse, incontinence in women. *AWHONN Lifelines, 7,* 516–522.

Mercer, R. T. (1985). The process of maternal role attainment. *Nursing Research, 34,* 198–204.

Mercer, R. T., & Ferketich, S. L. (1994). Maternal–infant attachment of experienced and inexperienced mothers during infancy. *Nursing Research, 43,* 344–351.

Moore, D. B., & Catlin, A. (2003). Lactation suppression: Forgotten aspect of care for the mother of a dying child. *Pediatric Nursing, 29,* 383–384.

Moore, M. L., & Moos, M. K. (2003). *March of Dimes nursing module: Cultural competence in the care of childbearing families.* White Plains, NY: March of Dimes Birth Defects Foundation Educational Services.

Murray, S. S. & McKinney, E. S. (2006). *Foundations of maternal–newborn nursing* (4th ed.). Philadelphia: WB Saunders.

Niedrach, M. K., & Foster, M. J. (2003). Contraceptive counseling for breast-feeding patients. [Online] Available at http://nsweb.nursingspectrum.com/ce/ce93.htm.

Nonacs, R. M. (2004). Postpartum depression. *eMedicine.* [Online] Available at www.emedicine.com/med/topic3408.htm.

Olds, S. B., London, M. L., Ladewig, P. A. W., & Davidson, M. R. (2004). *Maternal–newborn nursing & women's health care* (7th ed.). Upper Saddle River, NJ: Pearson Prentice Hall.

Oria de Quinzanos, G. (2003). A Mexican perspective. In M. L. Moore & M. K. Moos (Eds.), *March of Dimes nursing module: Cultural competence in the care of childbearing families.* White Plains, NY: March of Dimes Birth Defects Foundation Educational Services.

O'Toole, M. T. (2003). *Miller–Keane encyclopedia & dictionary of medicine, nursing, and allied health* (7th ed.). Philadelphia: Saunders.

Pease, S., & Beigel, H. (2003). In-home postpartum care: Much more than just good advice. *International Journal of Childbirth Education, 11,* 40–42.

Plemmons, N. (2003). A Cherokee perspective. In M. L. Moore & M. K. Moos (Eds.), *March of Dimes nursing module: Cultural competence in the care of childbearing families.* White Plains, NY: March of Dimes Birth Defects Foundation Educational Services.

Ringdahl, E. N. (2002a). Exercising after you have your baby. *Physician & Sports Medicine, 30,* 38.

Ringdahl, E. N. (2002b). Promoting postpartum exercise. *Physician & Sports Medicine, 30,* 31–36.

Rooney, B. L., & Schauberger, C. W. (2002). Excess pregnancy weight gain and long-term obesity: One decade later. *Obstetrics & Gynecology, 100,* 245–252.

Sameroff, A. J., McDonough, S. C., & Rosenblum, K. L. (2003). *Treating parent–infant relationship problems: Strategies for intervention.* New York: The Gilford Press.

Scoggin, J. (2004). Physical and psychological changes. In S. Mattson & J. E. Smith (Eds.), *Core curriculum for maternal newborn nursing* (3rd ed., pp. 371–386). Philadelphia: Elsevier Saunders.

Sears, W., & Sears, M. (2001). *The attachment parenting book: A commonsense guide to understanding and nurturing your baby.* Boston: Little, Brown & Company.

Seyfried, L. S., & Marcus, S. M. (2003). Postpartum mood disorders. *International Review of Psychiatry, 15,* 231–242.

Shaw, C. (2004). Stress urinary incontinence in women. *Primary Health Care, 14,* 27–31.

Sloane, E. (2002). *Biology of women* (4th ed.). Albany, NY: Delmar.

Spratto, G. R., & Woods, A. L. (2005). *PDR: Nurse's drug handbook.* Clifton Park, NY: Thomson Delmar Learning.

Stephens, K. C. (2003). An Appalachian perspective. In M. L. Moore & M. K. Moos (Eds.), *March of Dimes nursing module: Cultural competence in the care of childbearing families.* White Plains, NY: March of Dimes Birth Defects Foundation Educational Services.

Thomas, K. S. (2003). An African-American perspective. In M. L. Moore & M. K. Moos (Eds.), *March of Dimes nursing module: Cultural competence in the care of childbearing families.* White Plains, NY: March of Dimes Birth Defects Foundation Educational Services.

Tideman, E., Nilsson, A., Smith, G., & Stjernqvist, K. (2002). Longitudinal follow-up of children born preterm: The mother–child relationship in a 19-year perspective. *Journal of Reproductive and Infant Psychology, 20,* 43–56.

Tilokskulchai, F., Phatthanasiriwethin, S., Vichitsukon, K., & Serisathien, Y. (2002). Attachment behaviors in mothers of premature infants: A descriptive study in Thai mothers. *Journal of Perinatal and Neonatal Nursing, 16,* 69–83.

Troy, N. W. (2003). Is the significance of postpartum fatigue being overlooked in the lives of women? *American Journal of Maternal Child Nursing, 28,* 252–257.

Troyer, H., & Troyer, E. M. (2003). An Amish perspective. In M. L. Moore & M. K. Moos (Eds.), *March of Dimes nursing module: Cultural competence in the care of childbearing families.* White Plains, NY: March of Dimes Birth Defects Foundation Educational Services.

United States Department of Agriculture (USDA), United States Department of Health and Human Services (USDHHS). (2005). *Healthy eating pyramid. Center for nutrition policy and promotion.* [Online] Available at www.cnpp.usda.gov/pyramid-update/index.html.

United States Department of Health and Human Resources, Public Health Department. (2000). *Healthy people 2010.* [Online] Available at www.healthypeople.gov/document/HTML/Volume2/16MICH.htm.

Venis, J. A. (2002). Beyond the baby blues: Postpartum depression. *Nursing Spectrum.* [Online] Available at http://nsweb.nursingspectrum.com/ce/ce72.htm.

Wong, D. L., Perry, S. E., & Hockenberry, M. J. (2002). *Maternal–child nursing care* (2nd ed.). St. Louis: Mosby.

Yawman, D. (2003). Reflections on the Baby-Friendly Hospital Initiative. *Pediatric Annuals, 32,* 360–361.

Yeo, S. A. (2003). A Japanese perspective. In M. L. Moore & M. K. Moos (Eds.), *March of Dimes nursing module: Cultural competence in the care of childbearing families.* White Plains, NY: March of Dimes Birth Defects Foundation Educational Services.

Youngkin, E. Q., & Davis, M. S. (2004). *Women's health: A primary care clinical guide* (3rd ed.). Upper Saddle River, NJ: Prentice Hall.

Web Resources

American College of Nurse-Midwives, **www.midwife.org**
Association for Perinatal Psychology and Health, **www.birthpsychology.com**
Association of Maternal & Child Health Programs, **www.amchpl.org**
Baby-Friendly USA, **www.babyfriendlyusa.org**
Depression after Delivery, **www.depressionafterdelivery.com**
Home-Based Working Moms (HBWM), **www.hbwm.com**
International Lactation Consultants Association, **www.ilca.org**
La Leche League International, **www.lalecheleague.org**
Midwifery Today, Inc., **www.midwiferytoday.com**
National Alliance for Breast-feeding Advocacy, **www.naba-breast-feeding.org**
National Center for Fathering, **www.fathers.com**
National Women's Health Information Center, **www.4women.gov**
Parenthood Web, **www.parenthoodweb.com**
Parenting Q & A, **www.parenting-qa.com**
Parents Anonymous, Inc., **www.parentsanonymous.org**
Parents Helping Parents, **www.php.com**
The Center for Postpartum Health, **www.postpartumhealth.com**
The National Parenting Center, **www.tnpc.com**

ChapterWORKSHEET

● **MULTIPLE CHOICE QUESTIONS**

1. When assessing a postpartum woman, which of the following would lead the nurse to suspect postpartum blues?

   a. Panic attacks and suicidal thoughts

   b. Anger toward self and infant

   c. Periodic crying and insomnia

   d. Obsessive thoughts and hallucinations

2. Which of these activities would be most important for the postpartum nurse to ensure the provision of culturally sensitive care for the childbearing family?

   a. Taking a transcultural course

   b. Caring for only families of their cultural origin

   c. Teaching culturally diverse families Western beliefs

   d. Educating self about diverse cultural practices

3. Which of the following suggestions would be most appropriate to include in the teaching plan for a postpartum woman needing a greater focus on losing weight?

   a. Increase fluid intake and acid-producing food into her diet

   b. Avoid empty-calorie foods and increase exercise

   c. Start a high-protein diet and restrict fluids

   d. Completely avoid eating any snacks at all and carbohydrates

4. After teaching a group of breast-feeding women about nutritional needs, the nurse determines that the teaching was successful when the women state that they need to increase their intake of which nutrients?

   a. Carbohydrates and fiber

   b. Fats and vitamins

   c. Calories and protein

   d. Iron-rich foods and minerals

5. Which of the following would lead the nurse to suspect that a postpartum woman was developing a possible complication?

   a. Fatigue and irritability

   b. Perineal discomfort and pink discharge

   c. Pulse rate of 60 bpm

   d. Swollen, tender, hot area on breast

6. Which of the following would the nurse assess as indicating positive bonding between the parents and their newborn?

   a. Holding infant close to own body

   b. Having visitors hold infant

   c. Buying expensive infant clothes

   d. Requesting nurses care for infant

7. Which activity would the nurse include in the teaching plan for parents with a newborn and an older child to reduce the incidence of sibling rivalry when the newborn is brought home?

   a. Punishing child for bedwetting behavior

   b. Sending the sibling to grandparents' house

   c. Planning special time daily for the older sibling

   d. Allowing the sibling to share a room with the infant

● CRITICAL THINKING EXERCISES

1. As a nurse working on a postpartum unit, you enter the room of Ms. Jones, a 22-year-old primipara, and find her chatting on the phone while her newborn is crying loudly in the bassinette that has been pushed into the bathroom. You are assigned to this mother–newborn dyad and proceed to pick up and comfort the newborn. While holding the baby, you ask the client if she was aware her newborn was crying. Ms. Jones replies, "That is about all that monkey does since she was born!" You hand the newborn to her and she places the newborn on the bed away from her and continues her phone conversation.

   a. What is your nursing assessment of this encounter?

   b. What nursing interventions would be appropriate?

   c. What specific discharge interventions may be needed?

2. Jennifer Adamson, a 34-year-old single primipara, left the hospital after a 36-hour stay with her newborn son. She lives alone in a one-bedroom walk-up apartment. As the postpartum home health nurse visiting her 2 days later, you find the following:

   • Tearful client pacing the floor holding her crying son

   • Home environment cluttered and in disarray

   • Fundus firm and displaced to right of midline

   • Moderate lochia rubra; episiotomy site clean, dry, and intact

   • Vital signs within normal range; pain rating less than 3 points on scale of 1 to 10 points

   • Breasts engorged slightly; supportive bra on

   • Newborn assessment within normal limits

   • Distended bladder upon palpation; reporting frequency

   • Negative Homans' sign

   a. Which of these assessment findings warrants further investigation?

   b. What interventions are appropriate at this time and why?

   c. What health teaching is needed before you leave this home?

3. The nurse walks into the room of Lisa Drew, a 24-year-old primigravida. She asks the nurse to hand her the bottle sitting on the bedside table, stating, "I'm going to finish it off because my baby only ate half of it 3 hours ago when I fed him."

   a. What response by the nurse would be appropriate at this time?

   b. What action by the nurse should take place?

   c. What health teaching is needed for Lisa prior to discharge?

● STUDY ACTIVITIES

1. Identify three questions that a nurse would ask a postpartum woman to assess for postpartum blues.

2. Find an educational Internet Web site to which to refer new parents who may have questions about breast-feeding.

3. Outline instructions you would give to a new mother on how to use her peribottle.

4. Breast tissue swelling secondary to vascular congestion after childbirth and preceding lactation describes _____.

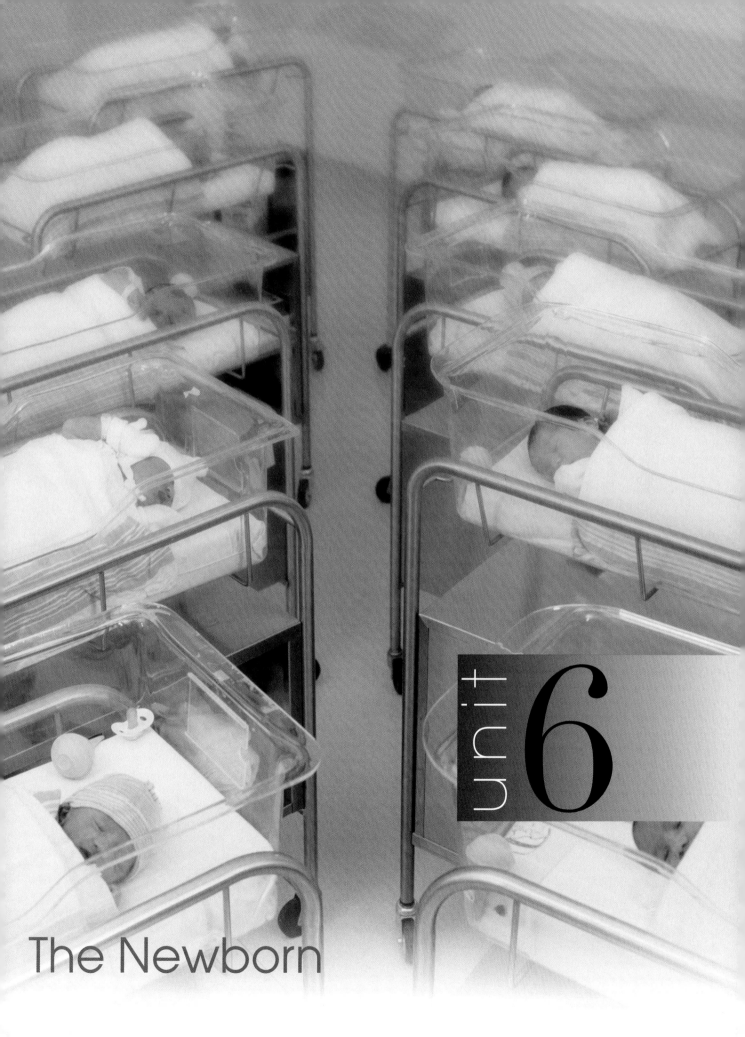

unit

6

The Newborn

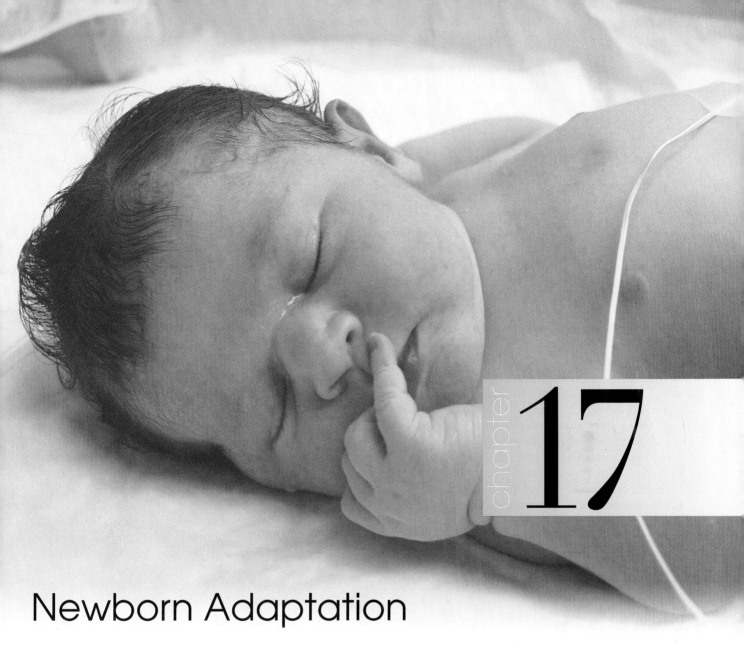

Newborn Adaptation

17

KeyTERMS

cold stress
jaundice
meconium
neonatal period
neurobehavioral response
neutral thermal
 environment (NTE)
periodic breathing
reflex
thermoregulation

LearningOBJECTIVES

After studying the chapter content, the student should be able to accomplish the following:

1. Define the key terms.
2. Identify the major changes in body systems that occur as the newborn adapts to extrauterine life.
3. Describe the primary challenges faced by the newborn during the adaptation to extrauterine life.
4. Explain the three behavioral patterns of newborn behavioral adaptation.
5. Identify the five typical behavioral responses of the newborn.

"Congratulations on the birth of your child" is a common expression heard by many parents after the labor and birth experience is over. Hearing their newborn's first cry typically ushers in feelings of relief and accomplishment for both parents. Although the exhaustion and stress of labor is over for the parents, the newborn now must begin the work of physiologically and behaviorally adapting to the new environment. The first 24 hours of life can be the most precarious (Verklan, 2002).

The **neonatal period** is defined as the first 28 days of life. After birth, the newborn is exposed to a whole new world of sounds, colors, smells, and sensations. The newborn, previously confined to a warm, dark, wet intra-uterine environment is now thrust upon an environment that is much brighter and cooler. As the newborn adapts to life after birth, numerous physiologic changes occur.

Awareness of these adaptations that are occurring forms the foundation for providing support to the newborn during this crucial time. Physiologic and behavioral changes occur quickly during this transition period. Being aware of any deviations from the norm is crucial to ensure early identification and prompt intervention.

This chapter describes the physiologic changes of the newborn's major body systems. It also discusses the behavioral adaptations, including behavioral patterns and the newborn's behavioral responses, occurring during this transition period.

Physiologic Adaptations

The mechanics of birth require an obligatory change in the newborn for successful survival outside the uterus. Immediately, respiratory gas exchange, along with circulatory modifications, must occur to sustain extrauterine life. During this time, as newborns strive to attain homeostasis, they also experience complex changes in major organ systems. Although the transition usually takes place within the first 6 to 10 hours of life, many adaptations may take weeks to attain full maturity.

Cardiovascular System Adaptations

During fetal life, the heart relies on certain unique structures that assist it in providing adequate perfusion of vital body parts. The *umbilical vein* carries oxygenated blood from the placenta to the fetus. The *ductus venosus* allows the majority of the umbilical vein blood to bypass the liver and merge with blood moving through the vena cava, bringing it to the heart sooner. The *foramen ovale* allows more than half the blood entering the right atrium to cross immediately to the left atrium, thereby passing the pulmonary circulation. The *ductus arteriosus* connects the pulmonary artery to the aorta, which allows bypassing of the pulmonary circuit. Only a small portion of blood passes through the pulmonary circuit for the main purpose of perfusion of the structure, rather than for oxygenation. The fetus depends on the placenta for providing oxygen and nutrients, and removing waste products.

At birth, the circulatory system must switch from fetal to newborn circulation and from placental to pulmonary gas exchange. The physical forces of the contractions of labor and birth, mild asphyxia, increased intracranial pressure as a result of cord compression and uterine contractions, as well as **cold stress** immediately experienced after birth lead to an increased release in catecholamines that is critical for the changes involved in the transition to extrauterine life. The increased levels of epinephrine and norepinephrine stimulate increased cardiac output and contractility, surfactant release, and promotion of pulmonary fluid clearance (Mercer & Skovgaard, 2002).

Fetal Structures

Changes in circulation occur immediately at birth as the fetus separates from the placenta. When the umbilical cord is clamped, the first breath is taken, and the lungs begin to function. As a result, systemic vascular resistance increases and blood return to the heart via the inferior cava decreases. Concurrently, with these changes, there is a rapid decrease in pulmonary vascular resistance and an increase in pulmonary blood flow (Asenjo, 2004). The foramen ovale functionally closes with a decrease in pulmonary vascular resistance, which leads to a decrease in right-side heart pressures. An increase in systemic pressure, after clamping of the cord, leads to an increase in left-side heart pressures. Ductus arteriosus, ductus venous, and umbilical vessels that were vital during fetal life are no longer needed. Over a period of months these fetal vessels form nonfunctional ligaments.

Before birth, the *foramen ovale* allowed most of the oxygenated blood entering the right atrium from the inferior vena cava to pass into the left atrium of the heart. With the newborn's first breath, air pushes into the newborn's lungs, triggering an increase in pulmonary blood flow and pulmonary venous return to the left side of the heart. As a result, the pressure in the left atrium becomes higher than in the right atrium. The increased left atrial pressure causes the foramen ovale to close, thus allowing the output from the right ventricle to flow entirely to the lungs. With closure of this fetal shunt, oxygenated blood is now separated from nonoxygenated blood. The subsequent increase in tissue oxygenation further promotes the increase in systemic blood pressure and continuing blood flow to the lungs. The foramen ovale normally closes functionally at birth when left atrial pressure increases and right atrial pressure decreases. Permanent anatomic closure, though, really occurs throughout the next several weeks.

During fetal life, the *ductus arteriosus*, located between the aorta and the pulmonary artery, protected the lungs against circulatory overload by shunting blood (right to left) into the descending aorta, bypassing the pulmonary circulation. Its patency during fetal life is promoted by continual production of prostaglandin E2 (PGE2) by the ductus (Neish, 2004). The ductus arteriosus becomes functionally closed within the first few hours after birth. Oxygen is the most important factor in controlling its closure. Closure depends on the high oxygen content of the aortic blood resulting from aeration of the lungs at birth. At birth, pulmonary vascular resistance decreases, allowing pulmonary blood flow to increase and oxygen exchange to occur in the lungs. It occurs secondary to an increase in PO_2 coincident with the first breath and umbilical cord occlusion when it is clamped.

The *ductus venosus* shunted blood from the left umbilical vein to the inferior vena cava during intrauterine life. It closes within a few days after birth, because this shunting is no longer needed as a result of activation of the liver, which now assumes the functions of the placenta (which has been expelled at birth). The ductus venosus becomes a ligament in extrauterine life.

The two umbilical arteries and one umbilical vein begin to constrict at birth, because with placental expulsion, blood flow ceases. In addition, peripheral circulation increases. Thus, the vessels are no longer needed and they too become ligaments.

Heart Rate

During the first few minutes after birth, the newborn's heart rate is approximately 120 to 180 bpm. Thereafter, it begins to decrease to an average of 120 to 130 bpm (Sherman et al., 2002). The newborn is highly dependent on heart rate for maintenance of cardiac output and blood pressure. Although the blood pressure is not taken routinely for the healthy term newborn, it is usually highest after birth and reaches a plateau within a week after birth. Transient functional cardiac murmurs may be heard during the neonatal period as a result of the changing dynamics of the cardiovascular system at birth (Hockenberry, 2005).

The fluctuations in both the heart rate and blood pressure tend to follow the changes in the newborn's behavioral state. An increase in activity, such as wakefulness, movement, or crying, corresponds to an increase in heart rate and blood pressure. In contrast, the compromised newborn demonstrates markedly less physiologic variability overall. Tachycardia may be found with volume depletion, cardiorespiratory disease, drug withdrawal, and hyperthyroidism. Bradycardia is often associated with apnea and is often seen with hypoxia.

Blood Volume

The blood volume of the newborn depends on the amount of blood transferred from the placenta at birth. It is usually estimated to be 80 to 85 mL/kg of body weight in the term infant (London et al., 2003). However, the volume may vary as much as 25 to 40%, depending on when clamping of the umbilical cord occurs. Early or late clamping of the umbilical cord changes circulatory dynamics during transition. Recent studies show the benefits of delayed cord clamping as improving the newborn's cardiopulmonary adaptation, preventing anemia, increasing blood pressures, improving oxygen transport, and increasing RBC flow (Mercer, 2001). However, concerns exist about volume overload and polycythemia (Mercer & Skovgaard, 2002). Further research is needed to explain the relationship among oxygen transport, RBC volume, and initiation of breathing, thereby indicating whether early or delayed cord clamping is beneficial.

Blood Components

Fetal RBCs are large, but few in number. After birth, the RBC count gradually increases as the cell size decreases, because they live in an environment with much higher PO_2. A newborn's RBCs have a life span of 80 to 100 days in comparison with an adult's RBC life span of 120 days.

Hemoglobin initially declines as a result of a decrease in neonatal red cell mass (physiologic anemia of infancy). Leukocytosis (elevated white blood cells) is present as a result of birth trauma soon after birth. The newborn's platelet count and aggregation ability are the same as adults.

The newborn's hematologic values are affected by the site of the blood sample (capillary blood has higher levels of hemoglobin and hematocrit compared with venous blood), placental transfusion (delayed cord clamping and normal shift of plasma to extravascular spaces, which causes higher levels of hemoglobin and hematocrit), and gestational age (increased age is associated with increased numbers of RBCs and hemoglobin) (Blackburn & Loper, 2002). See Table 17-1 for normal newborn blood values.

Table 17-1 Normal Newborn Blood Values

Lab Data	Normal Range
Hemoglobin	17–20 g/dL
Hematocrit	52–63%
Platelets	100,000–300,000/μL
RBCs	5.1–5.8 (1,000,000/μL)
WBCs	10–30,000/mm³

Respiratory System Adaptations

The first breath of life is a gasp that generates an increase in transpulmonary pressure and results in diaphragmatic descent. Hypercapnia, hypoxia, and acidosis resulting from normal labor become stimuli for initiating respirations. Inspiration of air and expansion of the lungs allow for an increase in tidal volume (amount of air brought into the lungs). Surfactant lining the alveoli enhances aeration of gas-free lungs, thus reducing surface tension and lowering the pressure required to open the alveoli. The newborn's first breath, in conjunction with surfactant, overcomes the surface forces to permit aeration of the lungs. In addition, vaginal births allow intermittent compression of the thorax, which facilitates removal of lung fluid.

The chest wall of the newborn is floppy because of the high cartilage content and poorly developed musculature. Thus, accessory muscles to help in breathing are ineffective.

One of the most crucial adaptations that the newborn makes at birth is adjusting from a fluid-filled intrauterine environment to a gaseous extrauterine environment. During fetal life, the lungs are expanded with an ultrafiltrate of the amniotic fluid. During and after birth, this fluid must be removed and replaced with air. Passage through the birth canal squeezes the thorax, which helps eliminate the fluid in the lungs. Pulmonary capillaries and the lymphatics remove the remaining fluid.

If fluid is removed too slowly or incompletely, such as what happens with decreased thoracic squeezing during birth or diminished respiratory effort, transient tachypnea (respiratory rate > 60 bpm) of the newborn occurs. Examples of situations involving decreased thoracic compression and diminished respiratory effort include cesarean birth and sedation in newborns (Askin, 2002).

Lungs

Before the newborn's lungs can maintain respiratory function, the following events must occur:

- Initiation of respiratory movement
- Expansion of the lungs
- Establishment of functional residual capacity (ability to retain some air in the lugs on expiration)
- Increased pulmonary blood flow
- Redistribution of cardiac output (Hockenberry, 2005)

Initial breathing is probably the result of a **reflex** triggered by pressure changes, noise, light, chilling, compression of the fetal chest during the delivery process, and high carbon dioxide and low oxygen concentrations of the newborn's blood. Many theories address the initiation of respiration in the newborn, but most are based on speculation from observations rather than on empirical research (Verklan, 2002). Research continues to search for answers to these questions.

Respirations

After respirations are established in the newborn, they are shallow and irregular, ranging from 30 to 60 breaths per minute, with short periods of apnea (<15 seconds). The newborn's respiratory rate varies according to its activity; the more active the newborn, the higher the respiratory rate, on average. Respirations should not be labored, and the chest movements should be symmetric. In some cases, **periodic breathing** may occur, which is the cessation of breathing that lasts 5 to 10 seconds without changes in color or heart rate (Murray et al., 2006). Periodic breathing may be observed in newborns within the first few days of life and requires close monitoring. Apneic periods lasting more than 15 seconds with cyanosis and heart rate changes require further evaluation (Hockenberry, 2005).

Body Temperature Regulation

Newborns are dependent on their environment for the maintenance of body temperature, much more immediately after birth than later in life. One of the most important elements in a newborn's survival is obtaining a stable body temperature to promote an optimal transition to extrauterine life.

Thermoregulation is the process of maintaining the balance between heat loss and heat production. It is a critical physiologic function that is closely related to the transition and survival of the newborn. An appropriate thermal environment is essential for maintaining a normal body temperature. Compared with adults, newborns tolerate a narrower range of environmental temperatures and are extremely vulnerable to both under- and overheating as well. Nurses play a key role in providing an appropriate environment to help newborns maintain thermal stability.

Heat Loss

Newborns have several characteristics that predispose them to heat loss:

- Thin skin with blood vessels close to the surface
- Lack of shivering ability to produce heat involuntarily
- Limited stores of metabolic substrates (glucose, glycogen, fat)
- Limited use of voluntary muscle activity or movement to produce heat
- Large body surface area relative to body weight
- Lack of subcutaneous fat, which provides insulation
- Little ability to conserve heat by changing posture (fetal position)
- No ability to adjust own their clothing or blankets to achieve warmth
- Inability to communicate that they are too cold or too warm

Every newborn struggles to maintain body temperature from the moment of birth, when the newborn's wet body is exposed to the much cooler environment of the birthing room. The amniotic fluid covering the newborn cools as it evaporates rapidly in the low humidity and air-conditioning of the room. During the period immediately after birth, the newborn's temperature may decrease 3° to 5° within minutes after leaving the warmth of the mother's uterus (99.6°F) (Thomas, 2003).

The transfer of heat depends on the temperature of the environment, air speed, and water vapor pressure or humidity. Heat exchange between the environment and the newborn involves the same mechanisms as those with any physical object and its environment. These mechanisms are conduction, convection, evaporation, and radiation. Prevention of heat loss is a key nursing intervention (Fig. 17-1).

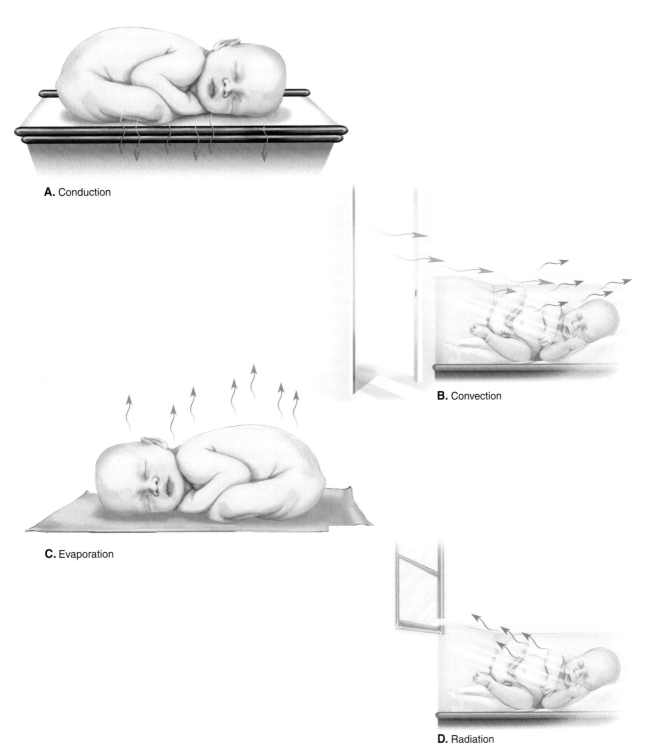

A. Conduction

B. Convection

C. Evaporation

D. Radiation

● Figure 17-1 The four mechanisms of heat loss in the newborn. (**A**) Conduction. (**B**) Convection. (**C**) Evaporation. (**D**) Radiation.

When I look down at my little miracle of life in my arms, I can't help but beam with pride at this great accomplishment. They seem so vulnerable and defenseless, and yet are equipped with everything they need to survive when they are born. When the nurse brought my daughter in for the first time after birth, I wanted to see and feel every part of her. Much to my dismay, she was wrapped up like a mummy in a blanket and she had a pink knit cap on her head. I asked the nurse why all the babies had to look like they were bound for the North Pole with all these layers on. Wasn't she aware it was summertime and probably at least 80° outside?

The nurse explained that newborns lose body heat easily and needed to be kept warm until their temperature stabilizes. Even though I wanted to get up close and personal with my baby, I decided to keep the pink polar bear outfit on her.

Thoughts: Newborns may be born with "everything they need to survive" on the outside, but they still experience temperature instability and lose heat through radiation, evaporation, convection, and conduction. Because the newborn's head is the largest body part, a great deal of heat can be lost if a cap is not kept on the head. What guidance can be given to this mother before discharge to stabilize her daughter's temperature while at home? What simple examples can be used to demonstrate your point?

Conduction

Conduction involves the transfer of heat from one object to another when the two objects are in direct contact with each other. Conduction refers to heat fluctuation between the newborn's body surface when in contact with other solid surfaces, such as a cold mattress, scale, or circumcision restraining board. Heat loss by conduction can also occur when touching a newborn with cold hands or when the newborn has direct contact with a colder object such as a metal scale. Using a warmed cloth diaper or blanket to cover any cold surface touching a newborn directly helps to prevent heat loss through conduction.

Convection

Convection involves the flow of heat from the body surface to cooler surrounding air or to air circulating over a body surface. An example of convection-related heat loss would be a cool breeze that flows over the newborn. To prevent heat loss by this mechanism, keep the newborn out of direct cool drafts (open doors, windows, fans, air conditioners) in the environment, work inside an isolette as much as possible and minimize opening portholes that allow cold air to flow inside, and warm any oxygen or humidified air that comes in contact with the newborn. Using clothing and blankets in isolettes is an effective means of reducing the newborn's exposed surface area

and providing external insulation. Also, transporting the newborn to the nursery in a warmed isolette, rather than carrying him or her, helps to maintain warmth and reduce exposure to the cool air.

Evaporation

Evaporation involves the loss of heat when a liquid is converted to a vapor. Evaporative loss may be insensible (such as from skin and respiration) or sensible (such as from sweating). Insensible loss occurs, but the individual isn't aware of it. Sensible loss is objective and can be noticed. It depends on air speed and the absolute humidity of the air. For example, when the newborn is born, the body is covered with amniotic fluid. The fluid evaporates into the air, leading to heat loss. Heat loss via evaporation also occurs when bathing a newborn. Drying newborns immediately after birth with warmed blankets and placing a cap on their head will help to prevent heat loss through evaporation. In addition, drying the newborn after bathing will help prevent heat loss through evaporation. Promptly changing wet linens, clothes, or diapers will also reduce heat loss and prevent chilling.

Radiation

Radiation involves loss of body heat to cooler, solid surfaces in close proximity, but not in direct contact with the newborn. The amount of heat loss is dependent on the size of the cold surface area, the surface temperature of the body, as well as the temperature of the receiving surface area. For example, when a newborn is placed in a single-wall isolette next to a cold window, heat loss from radiation occurs. Newborns will become cold even though they are in a heated isolette. To reduce heat loss by radiation, keep cribs and isolettes away from outside walls, cold windows, and air conditioners. Also, using radiant warmers for transporting newborns and when performing procedures that may expose the newborn to the cooler environment will help reduce heat loss.

A warmed transporter is an enclosed isolette on wheels. A radiant warmer is an open bed with a radiant heat source above. This type of environment allows healthcare professionals to reach the newborn to carry out procedures and treatments.

Overheating

The newborn is also prone to overheating. Large body surface area, limited insulation, and limited sweating ability can predispose any newborn to overheating. Control of body temperature is achieved via a complex negative feedback system that creates a balance between heat production, heat gain, and heat loss. The primary heat regulator is located in the hypothalamus and the central nervous system. The immaturity of the newborn's central nervous system makes it difficult to create and maintain this balance. Therefore, the newborn can become overheated easily. For example, an isolette that is too warm or one that is left too close to a sunny window may lead to hyperthermia. Although heat production can substantially increase in response to a cool environment, BMR and the resultant heat produced cannot be reduced. Overheating increases fluid loss, the respiratory rate, and the metabolic rate considerably.

Thermoregulation

Thermoregulation, the balance between heat loss and heat production, is related to the newborn's rate of metabolism and oxygen consumption. The newborn attempts to conserve heat and increase heat production in the following ways: increasing the metabolic rate, increasing muscular activity through movement, increasing peripheral vasoconstriction, and assuming a fetal position to hold in heat and minimize exposed body surface area.

An environment in which body temperature is maintained without an increase in metabolic rate or oxygen use is called a **neutral thermal environment (NTE).** Within an NTE, the rates of oxygen consumption and metabolism are minimal, and internal body temperature is maintained because of thermal balance (LeBlanc, 2002). Because newborns have difficulty in maintaining their body heat through shivering or other mechanisms, they need a higher environmental temperature to maintain an NTE. If the environmental temperature decreases, the newborn responds by consuming more oxygen. The respiratory rate increases (tachypnea) in response to the increased need for oxygen. As a result, the newborn's metabolic rate increases.

The newborn's primary method of heat production is through nonshivering thermogenesis, a process in which brown fat (adipose tissue) is oxidized in response to cold exposure. Brown fat is a special kind of highly vascular fat found only in newborns. The brown coloring is derived from the fat's rich supply of blood vessels and nerve endings. These fat deposits, which are capable of intense metabolic activity—and thus generate a great deal of heat—are found between scapulae, at the nape of the neck, in the mediastinum, and in areas surrounding the kidneys and adrenal glands. Brown fat makes up about 2 to 6% of body weight in the full-term newborn (Hockenberry, 2005). When the newborn experiences a cold environment, the release of norepinephrine increases, which in turn stimulates brown fat metabolism by the breakdown of triglycerides. Cardiac output increases, increasing blood flow through the brown fat tissue. Subsequently, this blood becomes warmed as a result of the increased metabolic activity of the brown fat.

Newborns can experience heat loss through all four mechanisms, ultimately resulting in cold stress. Cold stress is excessive heat loss that requires a newborn to use compensatory mechanisms (such as nonshivering thermogenesis and tachypnea) to maintain core body temperature (London et al., 2003). The consequences of cold stress can be quite severe. As the body temperature decreases, the newborn becomes less active, lethargic, hypotonic, and weaker. All newborns are at risk for cold stress, particularly within the first 12 hours of life. However, preterm newborns are at the greatest risk for cold stress and experience more profound effects than full-term newborns because they have less fat stores, poorer vasomotor responses, and less insulation to cope with a hypothermic event.

Cold stress in the newborn can lead to the following problems if not reversed: depleted brown fat stores, increased oxygen needs, respiratory distress, increased glucose consumption leading to hypoglycemia, metabolic acidosis, **jaundice,** hypoxia, and decreased surfactant production (Hockenberry, 2005).

To minimize the effects of cold stress and maintain an NTE, the following interventions are helpful:

- Prewarming the blankets and hats to reduce heat loss through conduction
- Keeping the infant transporter (warmed isolette) fully charged and heated at all times
- Drying the newborn completely after birth to prevent heat loss from evaporation
- Encouraging skin-to-skin contact with the mother if the newborn is stable
- Promoting early breast-feeding to provide fuels for nonshivering thermogenesis
- Using heated and humidified oxygen
- Always using radiant warmers and double-wall isolettes to prevent heat loss from radiation
- Deferring bathing until the newborn is medically stable and using a radiant heat source (Fig. 17-2)
- Avoiding the placement of a skin temperature probe over a bony area or one with brown fat because it does not give an accurate assessment of the whole body temperature (Most temperature probes are placed over the liver when the newborn is supine or side lying.)

Hepatic System Function

At birth, the newborn's liver assumes the functions that the placenta once handled during fetal life. These functions include iron storage, carbohydrate metabolism, blood coagulation, and conjugation of bilirubin.

Iron Storage

As RBCs are destroyed after birth, the iron is released and is stored by the liver until new RBCs need to be produced. Newborn iron stores are determined by total body hemoglobin content and length of gestation. At birth, the term newborn has iron stores sufficient to last approximately 4 to 6 months (Hockenberry, 2005).

Carbohydrate Metabolism

When the placenta is lost at birth, the maternal glucose supply is cut off. Initially, the newborn's serum glucose levels decline. Usually, a term newborn's blood glucose level is 70 to 80% of the maternal blood glucose level (Johnson, 2003).

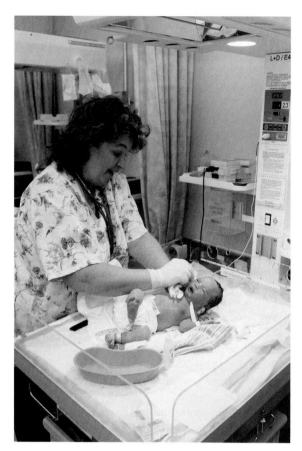

● Figure 17-2 Bathing a newborn under a radiant warmer to prevent heat loss.

Glucose is the main source of energy for the first several hours after birth. With the newborn's increased energy needs after birth, the liver releases glucose from glycogen stores for the first 24 hours. Initiating feedings helps to stabilize the newborn's blood glucose levels. Typically a newborn's blood glucose levels are assessed using a chemical reagent strip (such as a Chemstrip) on admission to the nursery and again in approximately 4 hours.

Bilirubin Conjugation

The liver is also responsible for the conjugation of bilirubin—a yellow to orange bile pigment produced by the breakdown of RBCs. In utero, elimination of bilirubin in the blood is handled by the placenta and the mother's liver. However, once the cord is cut, the newborn must now assume this function.

Bilirubin normally circulates in plasma, is taken up by liver cells, and is changed to a water-soluble pigment that is excreted in the bile. This conjugated form of bilirubin is excreted from liver cells as a constituent of bile.

The principal source of bilirubin in the newborn is the hemolysis of erythrocytes. This is a normal occurrence after birth, when fewer RBCs are needed to maintain extrauterine life.

When RBCs die after approximately 80 days of life, the heme in their hemoglobin is converted to bilirubin. Bilirubin is released in an *unconjugated* form called *indirect bilirubin,* which is fat soluble. Enzymes, proteins, and different cells in the reticuloendothelial system and liver process the unconjugated bilirubin into *conjugated bilirubin* or *direct bilirubin.* This form is water soluble and now enters the GI system via the bile and is eventually excreted through feces. A small amount is also excreted by the kidneys.

Newborns produce bilirubin at a rate of approximately 6 to 8 mg/kg/day. This is more than twice the production rate in adults, primarily because of relative polycythemia and increased RBC turnover. Bilirubin production typically declines to the adult level within 10 to 14 days after birth (Porter & Dennis, 2002). In addition, the metabolic pathways of the liver are relatively immature and thus are unable to conjugate bilirubin as fast as it needs to be.

Failure of the liver cells to break down and excrete bilirubin can cause an increased amount of bilirubin in the bloodstream, leading to jaundice (O'Toole, 2003). Bilirubin is toxic to the body and must be excreted. Blood tests ordered to determine bilirubin levels measure bilirubin in the serum. Total bilirubin is a combination of indirect (unconjugated) and direct (conjugated) bilirubin.

When unconjugated bilirubin pigment is deposited in the skin and mucous membranes, jaundice typically results. Jaundice, otherwise known as *icterus,* refers to the yellowing of the skin, sclera, and mucous membranes as a result of increased bilirubin blood levels. Visible jaundice as a result of increased blood bilirubin levels occurs in more than half of all healthy newborns. Even in healthy term newborns, extremely elevated blood levels of bilirubin during the first week of life can cause kernicterus, a permanent and devastating form of brain damage (Palmer et al., 2003).

Common risk factors for the development of jaundice include fetal–maternal blood group incompatibility, prematurity, breast-feeding, drugs (such as diazepam [Valium], oxytocin [Pitocin], sulfisoxazole/erythromycin [Pediazole], and chloramphenicol [Chloromycetin]), maternal gestational diabetes, infrequent feedings, male gender, trauma during birth resulting in cephalohematoma, cutaneous bruising, polycythemia, previous sibling with hyperbilirubinemia, infections such as TORCH (toxoplasmosis, other viruses, rubella, cytomegalovirus, herpes simplex viruses), and ethnicity such as Asian or Native American (Riskin et al., 2003).

The causes of newborn jaundice can be classified into three groups based on the mechanism of accumulation:

1. Bilirubin overproduction such as from blood incompatibility (Rh or ABO), drugs, trauma at birth, polycythemia, delayed cord clamping, and breast milk jaundice

2. Decreased bilirubin conjugation as seen in physiologic jaundice, hypothyroidism, and breast-feeding, for example

3. Impaired bilirubin excretion, as seen in biliary obstruction (biliary atresia, gallstones, neoplasm), sepsis, chromosomal abnormality (Turner syndrome, trisomy 18 and 21), and drugs (aspirin, acetaminophen, sulfa, alcohol, steroids, antibiotics) (Porter & Dennis, 2002)

Jaundice in the newborn is discussed in more detail in Chapter 24.

Gastrointestinal System Adaptations

The full-term newborn has the capacity to swallow, digest, metabolize, and absorb food taken in soon after birth. At birth, the pH of the stomach contents is mildly acidic, reflecting the pH of the amniotic fluid.

Mucosal Barrier Protection

An important adaptation of the GI system is the development of a mucosal barrier to prevent the penetration of harmful substances (bacteria, toxins, and antigens) present within the intestinal lumen. At birth, the newborn must be prepared to deal with bacterial colonization of the gut. Colonization is dependent on oral intake. It usually occurs by 4 to 6 days of age and is required for the production of vitamin K (Verklan & Walden, 2004). If harmful substances are allowed to penetrate the mucosal epithelial barrier under pathologic conditions, they can cause inflammatory and allergic reactions (Walker, 2001). Human milk provides a passive mechanism to protect the newborn against the dangers of a deficient intestinal defense system. It contains antibodies, viable leukocytes, and many other substances that can interfere with bacterial colonization and prevent harmful penetration.

Stomach and Digestion

The stomach of the newborn has a capacity ranging from 30 to 90 mL, with a variable emptying time of 2 to 4 hours. The cardiac sphincter and nervous control of the stomach is immature, which may lead to uncoordinated peristaltic activity and frequent regurgitation. Immaturity of the pharyngoesophageal sphincter and absence of lower esophageal peristaltic waves also contribute to the reflux of gastric contents. Avoiding overfeeding and stimulating frequent burping may help minimize regurgitation. Most digestive enzymes are available at birth, allowing newborns to digest simple carbohydrates and protein. However, they have limited ability to digest complex carbohydrates and fats, because amylase and lipase levels are low at birth. As a result, newborns excrete a fair amount of lipids, resulting in fatty stools.

Adequate digestion and absorption are essential for newborn growth and development. Normally, term newborns lose 5 to 10% of their birth weight as a result of insufficient caloric intake within the first week after birth, shifting of intracellular water to extracellular space, and insensible water loss. To gain weight, the term newborn requires an intake of 120 cal/kg/day (London et al., 2003).

Bowel Elimination

The frequency, consistency, and type of stool passed by newborns vary widely. The evolution of a stool pattern begins with a newborn's first stool, which is **meconium.** Meconium stool is composed of amniotic fluid, shed mucosal cells, intestinal secretions, and blood. It is greenish black, has a tarry consistency, and is usually passed within 12 to 24 hours of birth. The first meconium stool passed is sterile, but changes rapidly with ingestion of bacteria through feedings. After feedings are initiated, a transitional stool develops, which is greenish brown to yellowish brown, thinner in consistency, and seedy in appearance. Newborns who are fed early pass stools sooner, which helps to reduce bilirubin buildup.

The last development in the stool pattern is the milk stool. The characteristics differ in breast-fed and formula-fed newborns. The stools of the breast-fed newborn are described as yellow-gold, loose and stringy to pasty in consistency, and typically sour smelling. In comparison, the stool of the formula-fed newborn will vary depending on the type of formula ingested. It may be yellow, yellow-green, or greenish; loose, pasty, or formed in consistency; with an unpleasant odor.

Renal System Changes

The majority of term newborns void immediately after birth, indicating adequate renal function. Although the newborn's kidneys are able to produce urine, they are limited in their ability to concentrate it, until about 3 months of age, when the kidneys mature. Until that time, a newborn voids frequently and the urine has a low specific gravity (1.001–1.020). About 6 to 10 voidings daily is average for most newborns and indicative of adequate fluid intake (Ladewig, London, & Davidson, 2006).

The renal cortex is relatively underdeveloped at birth and does not reach maturity until 12 to 18 months of age. At birth, the GFR is approximately 30% of normal adult values, reaching approximately 50% of normal adult values by the 10th day of life and full adult values by the first year of life (Askin, 2002). The low GFR, and limited excretion and conservation capability of the kidney affect the newborn's ability to excrete for salt, water loads, and drugs. The possibility of fluid overload is increased and must be considered when administering IV therapy to a newborn.

Immune System Adaptations

Essential to the newborn's survival is an ability to respond effectively to hostile environmental forces. The developing newborn's immune system is initiated early in gestation, but many of the responses do not function adequately during the early neonatal period. The intrauterine environment usually protects the fetus from harmful micro-organisms and the necessity for defensive immunologic responses. With exposure to a wide variety of micro-organisms at birth, the newborn must develop a balance between its host defenses and the hostile environmental organisms to ensure a safe transition in the outside world.

Responses of the immune system serve three purposes: defense (protection from invading organisms), homeo-stasis (elimination of worn-out host cells), and surveil-lance (recognition and removal of enemy cells). The new-born's immune system response involves recognition of the pathogen or other foreign material, followed by activation of mechanisms to react against and eliminate it. All immune responses primarily involve leukocytes (white blood cells).

The immune system's responses can be divided into two categories: natural and acquired immunity. These mechanisms are interrelated and interdependent; both are required for immunocompetency.

Natural Immunity

Natural immunity includes responses or mechanisms that do not require previous exposure to the microorganism or antigen to operate efficiently. Physical barriers (such as intact skin and mucus membranes), chemical barriers (such as gastric acids and digestive enzymes), and resident nonpathologic organisms make up the newborn's natural immune system. Natural immunity involves the most basic host defense responses, that of ingestion and killing of microorganisms by phagocytic cells.

Acquired Immunity

Acquired immunity involves two primary processes: (1) the development of circulating antibodies or immunoglobulins capable of targeting specific invading agents (antigens) for destruction and (2) formation of activated lymphocytes designed to destroy foreign invaders. Acquired immunity is absent until after the first invasion by a foreign organism or toxin.

Immunoglobulins are subdivided into five classes: IgA, IgD, IgE, IgG, and IgM. The newborn depends largely on three immunoglobulins for defense mechanisms: IgG, IgA, and IgM.

IgG is the major immunoglobulin and the most abun-dant, comprising about 80% of all circulating antibodies (Schnell et al., 2003). It is found in serum and interstitial fluid. It is the only class able to cross the placenta, with active placental transfer beginning at approximately 20 to 22 weeks' gestation. IgG produces antibodies against bac-teria, bacterial toxins, and viral agents.

IgA is the second most abundant immunoglobulin in the serum. IgA does not cross the placenta, and maximum levels are reached during childhood. This immunoglobu-lin is believed to protect mucous membranes from viruses and bacteria. IgA is predominantly found in the GI and respiratory tracts, tears, saliva, colostrum, and breast milk. A major source of IgA is human breast milk, so breast-feeding is believed to have significant immunologic advan-tages over formula feeding (Madden et al., 2004).

IgM is found in blood and lymph fluid and is the first immunoglobulin to respond to infection. It does not cross the placenta, and levels are generally low at birth unless there is a congenital intrauterine infection. IgM offers a major source of protection from blood-borne infections. The predominant antibodies formed during neonatal or intrauterine infection are of this class.

Integumentary System

The most important function of the skin is to provide a protective barrier between the body and the environment. It limits the loss of water, prevents absorption of harmful agents, and protects against physical trauma. The epider-mal barrier begins to develop during mid-gestation and is fully formed by about 32 weeks' gestation. Although the neonatal and adult epidermis is similar in thickness and lipid composition, skin development is not complete at birth (Hoeger & Enzmann, 2002). Although the basic structure is the same as that of an adult, the less mature the newborn, the less mature the skin function. Fewer fibrils connect the dermis and epidermis in the newborn when compared with the adult. Also in a newborn, the risk of injury producing a break in the skin from tape, monitors, and handling is greater than that for an adult. In addition, sweat glands are present at birth, but full adult function-ing is not present until the second or third year of life (Mancini, 2001). Exposure to air after birth accelerates epidermal development in all newborns (Rutter, 2003).

Newborns vary greatly in appearance. Many of the variations are temporary and reflect the physiologic adap-tations that the newborn is experiencing. Skin coloring varies, depending on the newborn's age, race or ethnic group, temperature, and whether he or she is crying. Skin color changes with both the environment and health sta-tus. At birth, the newborn's skin is dark red to purple. As the newborn begins to breathe air, the skin color changes to red. This redness normally begins to fade the first day.

Neurologic System Adaptations

The nervous system consists of the brain, spinal cord, 12 cranial nerves, and a variety of spinal nerves that come from the spinal cord. Neurologic development follows cephalocaudal (head to toe) and proximal–distal (center to outside) patterns. Myelin develops early on in sensory impulse transmitters. Thus the newborn has an acute sense of hearing, smell, and taste. The newborn's sensory capabilities include

- Hearing—well developed at birth, responds to noise by turning to sound

- Taste—ability to distinguish between sweet and sour by 72 hours old
- Smell—ability to distinguish between mother's breast milk and breast milk from others
- Touch—sensitivity to pain, responds to tactile stimuli
- Vision—ability to focus on objects close by (10–12 in away), tracks objects in midline or beyond (Mattson & Smith, 2004).

Successful adaptations demonstrated by the respiratory, circulatory, thermoregulatory, and musculoskeletal systems indirectly indicate the central nervous system's successful transition from fetal to extrauterine life, because it plays a major role in all these adaptations. In the newborn, congenital reflexes are the hallmarks of maturity of the central nervous system, viability, and adaptation to extrauterine life.

The presence and strength of a reflex is an important indication of neurologic development and function. A reflex is an involuntary muscular response to a sensory stimulus. It is built into the nervous system and does not need the intervention of conscious thought to take effect (O'Toole, 2003). Many neonatal reflexes disappear with maturation, although some remain throughout adulthood.

The arcs of these reflexes end at different levels of the spine and brainstem, and reflect the function of the cranial nerves and motor systems. The way newborns blink, move their limbs, focus on a caretaker's face, turn toward sound, suck, swallow, and respond to the environment are all indications of their neurologic abilities. Congenital defects within the central nervous system are frequently not overt, but may be revealed in abnormalities in tone, posture, or behavior (Askin, 2002). Damage to the nervous system (birth trauma, perinatal hypoxia) during the birthing process can cause delays in the normal growth, development, and functioning of that newborn. Early identification may help to identify the cause and to start early intervention to decrease long-term complications or permanent sequelae.

Newborn reflexes are assessed to evaluate neurologic function and development. Absent or abnormal reflexes in a newborn, persistence of a reflex past the age when the reflex is normally lost, or redevelopment of an infantile reflex in an older child or adult may indicate neurologic pathology. (See Chapter 18 for a description of newborn reflex assessment.)

Behavioral Adaptations

In addition to adapting physiologically, the newborn also adapts behaviorally. All newborns progress through a specific pattern of events after birth, regardless of gestational age or type of birth they experienced.

Behavioral Patterns

The newborn usually demonstrates a predictable pattern of behavior during the first several hours after birth, char-

acterized by two periods of reactivity separated by a sleep phase. Behavioral adaptation is a defined progression of events triggered by stimuli from the extrauterine environment after birth.

First Period of Reactivity

The first period of reactivity begins at birth and lasts for the first 30 minutes after birth. The newborn is alert and moving, and may appear hungry. This period is characterized by myoclonic movements of the eyes, spontaneous Moro reflexes, sucking motions, chewing, rooting, and fine tremors of the extremities (Littleton & Engebretson, 2005). Respirations and heart rates are elevated and gradually begin to slow as the next period occurs.

This period of alertness allows parents to interact with their newborn and to enjoy close contact with their new baby (Fig. 17-3). The appearance of sucking and rooting behaviors provides a good opportunity for initiating breast-feeding. Many newborns latch on the nipple and suck well at this first experience.

Period of Deceased Responsiveness

At 30 to 120 minutes of age, the newborn enters the second stage of transition—that of sleep or a decrease in activity. This phase is referred to as a *period of decreased responsiveness.* Movements are less jerky and less frequent. Heart and respiratory rates decline as the newborn enters the sleep phase. The muscles become relaxed, and responsiveness to outside stimuli diminishes. During this phase, it is difficult to arouse or interact with the newborn. No interest in sucking is shown. This quiet time can be used for both mother and newborn to remain close and rest together after sustaining the laboring and birthing experience.

Second Period of Reactivity

The second period of reactivity begins as the newborn awakens and shows an interest in environmental stimuli. This period lasts 2 to 8 hours in the normal newborn (Thureen et al., 2005). Heart and respiratory rates

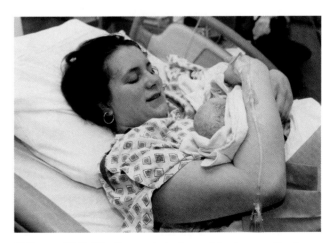

● Figure 17-3 The first period of reactivity is an optimal time for interaction.

increase. Peristalsis also increases. Thus, it is not uncommon for the newborn to pass meconium during this period. In addition, motor activity and muscle tone increase in conjunction with an increase in muscular coordination (Fig. 17-4).

Interaction between the mother and the newborn during this second period of reactivity is encouraged if the mother has rested and desires it. This period also provides a good opportunity for the parents to examine their newborn and ask questions about their observations. Teaching about feeding, positioning for feeding, and diaper-changing techniques can be reinforced during this time.

Newborn Behavioral Responses

Newborns demonstrate several predictable responses when interacting with their environment. How they react to the world around them is termed a **neurobehavioral response.** It comprises predictable periods that are probably triggered by stimuli from external stimuli.

Expected newborn behaviors include orientation, habituation, motor maturity, self-quieting ability, and social behaviors. Any deviation in behavioral responses requires further assessment, because it may indicate a complex neurobehavioral problem.

Orientation

The response of newborns to stimuli is called *orientation.* They become more alert when they sense a new stimulus in their environment. Orientation reflects newborns' response to auditory and visual stimuli, demonstrated by their movement of head and eyes to focus on that stimulus. Newborns prefer the human face and bright shiny objects. As the face or object comes into their line of vision, newborns respond by staring at the object intently. Newborns use this sensory capacity to become familiar with people and objects in their surroundings.

Habituation

Habituation is the newborn's ability to process and respond to visual and auditory stimuli—that is, how well and appropriately he or she responds to the environment. Habituation is the ability to block out external stimuli after the newborn has become used to the activity. During the first 24 hours after birth, newborns should increase their ability to habituate to environmental stimuli and sleep. Habituation provides a useful indicator of their neurobehavioral intactness.

Motor Maturity

Motor maturity depends on gestational age and involves evaluation of posture, tone, coordination, and movements. These activities enable newborns to control and coordinate movement. When stimulated, newborns with good motor organization demonstrate movements that are rhythmic and spontaneous. Bringing the hand up to the mouth is an example of good motor organization. As newborns adapt to their new environment, smoother movements should be observed. Such motor behavior is a good indicator of the newborn's ability to respond and adapt accordingly—that is, process stimuli appropriately by the central nervous system.

Self-Quieting Ability

Self-quieting ability refers to newborns' ability to quiet and comfort themselves. Newborns vary in their ability to console themselves or to be consoled. "Consolability" is how newborns are able to change from the crying state to an active alert, quiet alert, drowsy, or sleep state. They console themselves by hand-to-mouth movements, and sucking, alerting to external stimuli and motor activity (Hockenberry, 2005). Assisting parents to identify consoling behaviors to quiet their newborn if the newborn is not able to self-quiet is important. These behaviors include rocking, holding, gently patting, and softly singing to them.

Social Behaviors

Social behaviors include cuddling and snuggling into the arms of the parent when the newborn is held. Usually newborns are very sensitive to being touched, cuddled, and held. Cuddliness is very important to parents, because they frequently will gauge their ability to care for their newborn by the newborn's acceptance or positive repose to their actions. Specifically, it can be assessed by the degree to which the newborn nestles into the contours of the

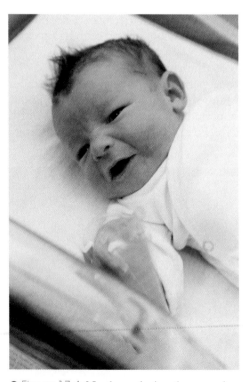

● Figure 17-4 Newborn during the second period of reactivity. Note the newborn's wide-eyed interest.

holder's arms. Most newborns cuddle, but some will resist. Assisting parents to assume comforting behaviors (e.g., by cooing while holding their newborn) and praising them for their efforts can help foster cuddling behaviors.

KEY CONCEPTS

- The neonatal period is defined as the first 28 days of life. As the newborn adapts to life after birth, numerous physiologic changes occur.
- At birth, the cardiopulmonary system must switch from fetal to neonatal circulation and from placental to pulmonary gas exchange.
- One of the most crucial adaptations that the newborn makes at birth is the adjustment of a fluid medium exchange from the placenta to the lungs and that of a gaseous environment.
- Neonatal RBCs have a life span of 80 to 100 days in comparison with the adult RBC life span of 120 days, which causes several adjustment problems.
- Thermoregulation is the maintenance of balance between heat loss and heat production. It is a critical physiologic function that is closely related to the transition and survival of the newborn.
- Heat loss in the newborn is the result of four mechanisms: conduction, convection, evaporation, and radiation.
- Responses of the immune system serve three purposes: defense (protection from invading organisms), homeostasis (elimination of worn-out host cells), and surveillance (recognition and removal of enemy cells).
- In the newborn, congenital reflexes are the hallmarks of maturity of the central nervous system, viability, and adaptation to extrauterine life.
- The newborn usually demonstrates a predictable pattern of behavior during the first several hours after birth, characterized by two periods of reactivity separated by a sleep phase.

References

Asenjo, M. (20034). *Transient tachypnea of the newborn.* [Online] Available at www.emedicine.com/radio/topic710.htm.

Askin, D. F. (2002). Complications in the transition from fetal to neonatal life. *JOGNN, 31,* 318–327.

Blackburn, S., & Loper, D. (2002). *Maternal fetal and neonatal physiology* (2nd ed.). Philadelphia: Saunders.

Engstrom, J. (2004). *Maternal–neonatal nursing made incredibly easy.* Springhouse, PA: Lippincott Williams & Wilkins.

Fuloria, M., & Kreiter, S. (2002a). The newborn examination: part I. Emergencies and common abnormalities involving the skin, head, neck, chest, and respiratory and cardiovascular systems. *American Family Physician, 65,* 61–68.

Fuloria, M., & Kreiter, S. (2002b). The newborn examination: part II. Emergencies and common abnormalities involving the abdomen, pelvis, extremities, genitalia, and spine. *American Family Physician, 65,* 265–270.

Hait, E. (2004). *Infantile reflexes.* [Online] Available at www.nim.nih.gov/medlineplus/ency/article/003292.htm.

Hockenberry, M. J. (2005). *Wong's essentials of pediatric nursing.* (7th ed.). St. Louis: Elsevier Mosby.

Hoeger, P. H., & Enzmann, C. C. (2002). Skin physiology of the newborn and young infant: a prospective study of functional skin parameters during early infancy. *Pediatric Dermatology, 19,* 256–262.

Johnson, T. S. (2003). Hypoglycemia and the full-term newborn: how well does birth weight for gestational age predict risk? *JOGNN, 32,* 48–57.

Ladewig, P. A., London, M. L. & Davidson, M. R. (2006). *Contemporary maternal-newborn nursing care* (6th ed.). Upper Saddle River, NJ: Pearson Prentice Hall.

LeBlanc, M. H. (2002). The physical environment. In Fanaroff, A. A., & Martin, R. J. (Eds.), *Neonatal–perinatal medicine* (7th ed., pp. 512–530). St. Louis: Mosby.

Littleton, L. Y. & Engebretson, J. C. (2005). *Maternity nursing care.* Clifton Park, NY: Thomson Delmar Learning.

London, M. L., Ladewig, P. W., Ball, J. W., & Bindler, R. C. (2003). *Maternal–newborn & child nursing: family-centered care.* Upper Saddle River, NJ: Pearson Education.

Lowdermilk, D. L., & Perry, S. E. (2004). *Maternity & women's health care* (8th ed.). St. Louis: Mosby.

Lumsden, H. (2002). Physical assessment of the newborn: a holistic approach. *British Journal of Midwifery, 10,* 205–209.

Madden, J. M., Soumerai, S. B., Lieu, T. A., Mandl, K. D., Zhang, F., & Ross–Degnan, D. (2004). Length-of-stay policies and ascertainment of postdischarge problems in newborns. *Pediatrics, 113,* 42–49.

Mancini, A. J. (2001). Structure and function of newborn skin. In Eichenfield, L. F., Freiden, I. J., & Esterly, N. B. (Eds.), *Textbook of neonatal dermatology* (pp. 18–32). Philadelphia: Saunders.

Mattson, S., & Smith, J. E. (2004). *Core curriculum for maternal–newborn nursing* (3rd ed.). St. Louis: Elsevier Saunders.

Mercer, J. S. (2001). Current best evidence: a review of the literature on umbilical cord clamping. *Journal of Midwifery and Womens Health, 46,* 402–414.

Mercer, J. S., & Skovgaard, R. L. (2002). Neonatal transitional physiology: a new paradigm. *Journal of Perinatal and Neonatal Nursing, 15,* 56–75.

Mitchell, M. (2003). Midwives conducting the neonatal examination: part 1. *British Journal of Midwifery, 11,* 16–21.

Murray, S. S. & McKinney, E. S. (2006). *Foundations of maternal–newborn nursing* (4th ed.). Philadelphia: WB Saunders.

Neish, S. (2004). Patent ductus arteriosus. *eMedicine.* [Online] Available at www.emedicine.com/ped/topic1747.htm.

O'Toole, M. T. (2003). *Miller–Keane encyclopedia and dictionary of medicine, nursing, and allied health* (7th ed.). Philadelphia: Saunders.

Palmer, R. H., Clanton, M., Ezhuthachan, S., Newman, C., Maisels, J., Plsek, P., & Salem–Schatz, S. (2003). Applying the "10 simple rules" of the Institute of Medicine to management of hyperbilirubinemia in newborns. *Pediatrics, 112,* 1388–1393.

Pillitteri, A. (2003). *Maternal & child nursing: care of the childbearing & childrearing family* (4th ed.). Philadelphia: Lippincott Williams & Wilkins.

Porter, M. L., & Dennis, B. L. (2002). Hyperbilirubinemia in the term newborn. *American Family Physician, 65,* 599–606.

Riskin, A., Abend–Weinger, M., & Bader, D. (2003). How accurate are neonatologists in identifying clinical jaundice in newborns? *Clinical Pediatrics, 42,* 153–158.

Rubaltelli, F. F. (1998). Current drug treatment options in neonatal hyperbilirubinemia and the prevention of kernicterus. *Drugs, 56,* 23–30.

Rutter, N. (2003). Applied physiology: the newborn skin. *Current Pediatrics,13,* 226–230.

Schnell, Z. B., Van Leeuwen, A. M., & Kranpitz, T. R. (2003). *Davis's comprehensive handbook of laboratory and diagnostic tests with nursing implications.* Philadelphia: FA Davis.

Sherman, J., Young, A., Sherman, M. P., Collazo, C., & Bernert, J. T. (2002). Prenatal smoking and alterations in newborn heart rate during transition. *Journal of Obstetrical, Gynecological, and Neonatal Nursing, 31,* 680–687.

Seidel, H. M., Rosenstein, B. J., & Pathak, A. (2001). *Primary care of the newborn* (3rd ed.). St. Louis: Mosby.

Thomas, K. A. (2003). Infant weight and gestational age effects on thermoneutrality in the home environment. *JOGNN, 32,* 745–752.

Thureen, P. J., Deacon, J., Hernandez, J. A., & Hall, D. M. (2005). *Assessment and care of the well newborn* (2nd ed.). St. Louis: Elsevier Saunders.

Verklan, M. T. (2002). Physiologic variability during transition to extrauterine life. *Critical Care Nursing Quarterly, 24,* 41–56.

Verklan, M. T., & Walden, M. (2004). *Core curriculum for neonatal intensive care nursing* (3rd ed.). St. Louis: Elsevier Saunders.

Walker, W. A. (2001). Absorption of protein and protein fragments in the developing intestines: role in immunologic/allergic reactions. *Pediatrics* (Suppl.), 67–171.

Wittmann–Price, R. A., & Pope, K. A. (2002). Universal newborn hearing screening. *American Journal of Nursing, 102,* 71–77.

Web Resources

Academy of Neonatal Nursing, **www.academyonline.org**
American Academy of Pediatrics, **www.aap.org**
National Association of Neonatal Nurses, **www.nann.org**
Neonatal Network, **www.neonatalnetwork.com**

Chapter WORKSHEET

● MULTIPLE CHOICE QUESTIONS

1. When assessing the term newborn, the following are observed: newborn is alert, heart and respiratory rates have stabilized, and meconium has been passed. The nurse determines that the newborn is exhibiting behaviors indicating

   a. Initial period of reactivity

   b. Second period of reactivity

   c. Decreased responsiveness period

   d. Period of sleep

2. When caring for a newborn, the nurse ensures that the doors of the nursery are closed and minimizes opening the portholes of the isolette to prevent heat loss via which mechanism?

   a. Conduction

   b. Evaporation

   c. Convection

   d. Radiation

3. After teaching a group of nursing students about thermoregulation and appropriate measures to prevent heat loss by evaporation, which of the following student behaviors would indicate successful teaching?

   a. Transporting the newborn in an isolette

   b. Maintaining a warm room temperature

   c. Placing the newborn on a warmed surface

   d. Drying the newborn immediately after birth

4. After birth, the nurse would expect which fetal structure to close as a result of increases in the pressure gradients on the left side of the heart?

   a. Foramen ovale

   b. Ductus arteriosus

   c. Ductus venosus

   d. Umbilical vein

● CRITICAL THINKING EXERCISE

1. As the nurse manager, you have been orienting a new nurse in the nursery for the past few weeks. Although she has been demonstrating adequacy with most procedures, today you observe her bathing several newborns without covering them, weighing them on the scale without a cover, leaving the storage door open with the transporter nearby, and leaving the newborns' head covers and blankets off after showing them to family and relatives through the nursery observation window.

   a. What is your impression of this observation?

   b. What principles concerning thermoregulation need to be reinforced?

   c. How will you evaluate your instruction after the in-service is presented?

● STUDY ACTIVITIES

1. While in the nursery clinical setting, identify the period of behavioral reactivity (first, inactivity, or second period) for two newborns born at different times. Share your findings in post conference that clinical day.

2. Obtain a set of vital signs (temperature, pulse, respiration) of a newborn on admission to the nursery. Repeat this procedure and compare changes in their values several hours later. Discuss what changes in the vital signs you would expect during this transitional period.

3. Find two Internet Web sites about transition to extrauterine life that can be shared with other nursing students as well as nursery nurses.

4. The most frequent mechanism of heat loss in the newborn is _____.

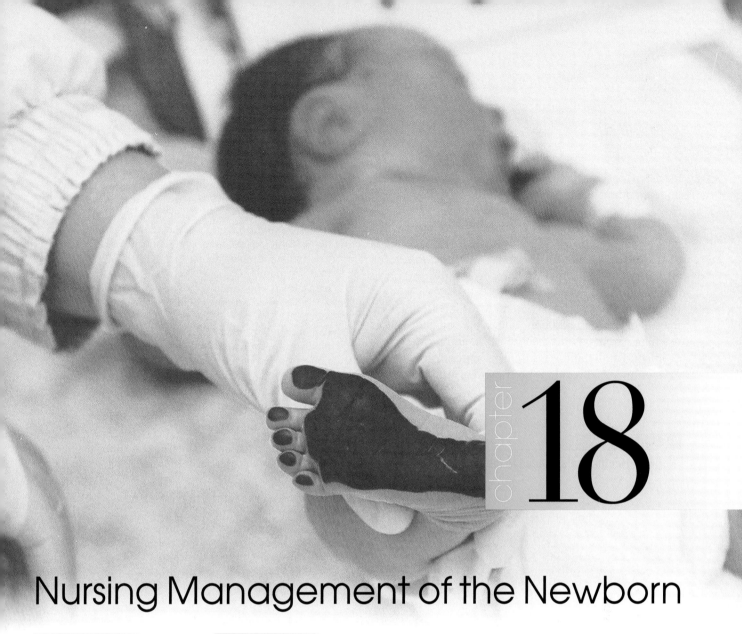

chapter 18

Nursing Management of the Newborn

KeyTERMS

acrocyanosis
Apgar score
caput succedaneum
cephalhematoma
circumcision
Epstein's pearls
erythema toxicum
gestational age
Harlequin sign
infant abduction
immunizations
milia
molding
mongolian spots
nevus flammeus
nevus vasculosus
ophthalmia neonatorum
pseudomenstruation
phototherapy
stork bites
vernix caseosa

LearningOBJECTIVES

After studying the chapter content, the student should be able to accomplish the following:

1. Define the key terms.
2. Discuss the assessments performed during the immediate newborn period.
3. Describe the interventions appropriate to meet the immediate needs of the term newborn.
4. Explain the components of a typical physical examination of a newborn.
5. Identify common variations that can be noted during a newborn's physical examination.
6. Identify common concerns of the newborn and appropriate interventions.
7. Explain the importance of the newborn screening tests.
8. Describe the common interventions appropriate during the early newborn period.
9. Delineate the nurse's role in meeting the newborn's nutritional needs.
10. Outline discharge planning content and education needed for the family with a newborn.

WOW

You can send a more powerful message with your actions and behavior than merely with words.

Immediately after the birth of a newborn, parents are faced with the task of learning and understanding as much as possible about caring for this new family member—a reality even for parents who are not experiencing childbirth for the first time. In their new or expanded role as parents, they will face many demands and challenges. For most, this is a wonderful, exciting time filled with many new discoveries and much information.

Parents learn as they watch nurses interacting with their newborns. In addition, nurses play a major role in teaching parents about their newborn and normal characteristics, and about ways to foster optimal growth and development. This role is even more crucial today as a

HEALTHY PEOPLE 2010

National Health Goals Related to the Newborn Period

Objective	Significance
Increase the proportion of mothers who breast-feed their babies during the early postpartum period from a baseline of 64% to 75%.	Will help to emphasize the importance of breast milk as the most complete form of nutrition for infants
Increase the proportion of mothers who breast-feed at 6 months from a baseline of 29% to 50%.	Will help to promote infant health, growth, immunity and development throughout the newborn and infant periods
Increase the proportion of mothers who breast-feed at 1 year from a baseline of 16% to 25%.	
Ensure appropriate newborn bloodspot screening, newborn hearing screening, follow-up testing, and referral services.	Will help to foster early detection and prompt treatment for conditions, thereby lessening the incidence of illness, disability, and death associated with these conditions and their overall effects on the newborn, infant, and family
Ensure that all newborns are screened at birth for conditions mandated by their state-sponsored newborn screening programs.	
Ensure that follow-up diagnostic testing for screening positives is performed within an appropriate time period.	

Source: U.S. DHHS, 2000.

result of the limited time spent by the mother and newborn in the health care facility.

The newborn has come from a dark, small, enclosed space within the mother's uterus into the bright, cold extrauterine environment. In day-to-day routines, nurses can easily forget that a small human being is experiencing his or her first taste of human interaction outside the uterus. The newborn period is an extremely important one. Subsequently, two specific National Health Goals have been developed to address this critical period (see Healthy People 2010: National Health Goals Related to the Newborn Period).

It is also easy to overlook the intensity with which that small human being's parents are watching nurses to learn how to care for their new family member, and easier still to be completely unaware of being observed by visitors, including siblings and other family members. Therefore, all nurses need to model nurturing care to all newborns. This chapter provides information about assessment and interventions in the period immediately following the birth of a newborn and during the early newborn period.

Nursing Management During the Immediate Newborn Period

The period of transition from intrauterine to extrauterine life occurs during the first several hours after birth. During this time, the newborn is undergoing numerous changes and adaptations, many of which are occurring simultaneously (see Chapter 17 for more information on the newborn's adaptation). It is a time of stabilization for the neonate's temperature, respiration, and cardiovascular dynamics. Close observation of the newborn's status is essential. Careful examination of the newborn at birth can detect anomalies, birth injuries, and disorders that can compromise successful adaptation to extrauterine life. Problems occurring during this critical time can dictate the quality of life for the newborn.

Assessment

The initial newborn assessment is completed in the birthing area to determine whether the newborn is stable enough to stay with the parents or whether resuscitation or immediate interventions are necessary. A second assessment is done within the first 2 to 4 hours when the newborn is admitted to the nursery. A third assessment is completed before discharge. The purpose of all three assessments is to confirm normality, to provide reassurance to the parents, and to identify apparent physical abnormalities (Lumsden, 2002).

During the initial newborn assessment, look for signs that might indicate a problem, including

- Nasal flaring
- Chest retractions
- Grunting on exhalation
- Labored breathing
- Generalized cyanosis
- Abnormal breath sounds: rhonchi, crackles (rales), wheezing, stridor
- Abnormal respiratory rates (tachypnea, > 60 breaths/minute; bradypnea, < 25 breaths/minute)
- Flaccid body posture
- Abnormal heart rates (tachycardia, > 160 bpm; bradycardia, < 100 bpm)
- Abnormal newborn size: small or large for **gestational age**

If any of these findings are noted, medical intervention may be necessary.

Apgar Scoring

The **Apgar score,** first proposed in 1952 by Dr. Virginia Apgar, is used to evaluate newborns at 1 minute and 5 minutes after birth. An additional Apgar assessment is done at 10 minutes if the 5-minute score is less than 7 points (Littleton & Engebretson, 2005). Assessment of the newborn at 1 minute provides data indicating the newborn's initial adaptation to extrauterine life. Assessment at 5 minutes provides a clearer indication of the newborn's overall central nervous system status.

Five parameters are assessed with Apgar scoring. A quick way to remember the parameters of Apgar scoring is as follows:

A = appearance (color)
P = pulse (heart rate)
G = grimace (reflex irritability)
A = activity (muscle tone)
R = respiratory (respiratory effort)

Each parameter is assigned a score ranging from 0 to 2 points, with 2 points being the maximum score. A score of 0 points indicates an absent or poor response; a score of 2 points indicates a normal response (Table 18-1). For a normal newborn, the score should be somewhere in the range of 8 to 10 points. The higher the score, the better the condition of the newborn. If the Apgar score is 8 points or higher, no intervention is needed other than supporting normal respiratory efforts and maintaining thermoregulation. Scores of 4 to 7 points signify moderate difficulty and scores of 0 to 3 points represent severe distress in adjusting to extrauterine life. The Apgar score is influenced by the presence of infection, congenital anomalies, physiologic immaturity, maternal sedation via medications, and neuromuscular disorders (Hockenberry, 2005).

When the newborn experiences depression, the Apgar score characteristics disappear in a predictable manner: First the pink coloration is lost, next the respiratory effort, and then the tone, followed by reflex irritability and, finally, heart rate (Verklan & Walden, 2004).

Although Apgar scoring is completed at 1 and 5 minutes, it also can be used as a guide during the immediate newborn period to evaluate the newborn's status for any changes because it focuses on critical parameters that must be assessed throughout the early transition period.

Length and Weight

Parents are anxious to know their newborn's size, such as length and weight. These measurements are taken soon after birth. A disposable tape measure or a built-in measurement board located on the side of the scale can be used. Length is measured from the head of the newborn to the heel with the newborn unclothed (Fig. 18-1). Because of the flexed position of the newborn after birth, it is essential to place the newborn in a supine position and extend the leg completely when measuring the length. The expected findings for length in full-term newborns usually ranges from 48 to 53 cm (19–21 inches). Molding can affect measurement (Dillon, 2003).

Most often, newborns are weighed using a digital scale that reads the weight in grams. Typically, in the

Table 18-1 Apgar Scoring for Newborns

Parameter (Assessment Technique)	0 Point	1 Point	2 Points
Heart rate (auscultation of apical heart rate for 1 full minute)	Absent	Slow (<100 bpm)	>100 bpm
Respiratory effort (observation of the volume and vigor of the newborn's cry; auscultation of depth and rate of respirations)	Apneic	Slow, irregular, shallow	Regular respirations (usually 30–60 breaths/minute), strong, good cry
Muscle tone (observation of extent of flexion in the newborn's extremities and newborn's resistance when the extremities are pulled away from the body)	Limp, flaccid	Some flexion, limited resistance to extension	Tight flexion, good resistance to extension with quick return to flexed position after extension
Reflex irritability (flicking of the soles of the feet or suctioning of the nose with a bulb syringe)	No response	Grimace or frown when irritated	Sneeze, cough, or vigorous cry
Skin color (inspection of trunk and extremities with the appropriate color (based on ethnicity) appearing within minutes after birth)	Cyanotic or pale	Body-appropriate ethnic color; blue extremities (acrocyanosis)	Completely appropriate color (pink on both trunk and extremities)

term newborn, weight ranges from 2700 to 4000 g (6–9 lb; Fig. 18-2). Birth weights less than 10% or more than 90% on a growth chart are outside the normal range and need further investigation. Subsequent weights taken at later times are compared with previous weights and are documented with regard to gain or loss on a nursing flow sheet. Newborns typically lose approximately 10% of their initial birth weight by 3 to 4 days of age secondary to loss of meconium, extracellular fluid, and limited food intake.

This weight loss is usually regained by the 10th day of life (Hockenberry, 2005).

Newborns can be classified by their birth weight regardless of their gestational age (AAP/ACOG, 2002) as follows:

- Low birth weight: <2500 g (<5.5 lb)
- Very low birth weight: <1500 g (<3.5 lb)
- Extremely low birth weight: <1000 g (<2.5 lb)

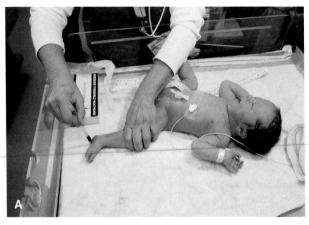
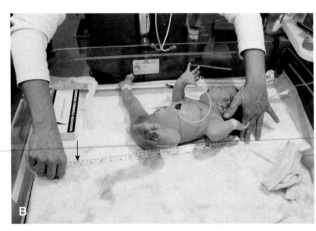

● Figure 18-1 Measuring a newborn's length. (**A**) The nurse extends the newborn's leg and marks the pad at the heel. (**B**) The nurse measures from the newborn's head to the heel mark.

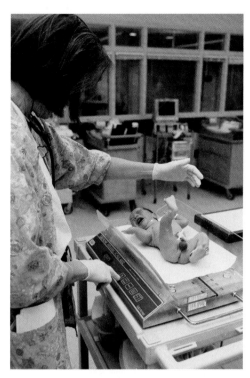

● Figure 18-2 **Weighing a newborn. Note how the nurse guards the newborn from above to prevent injury.**

Vital Signs

Heart rate and respiratory rate are assessed immediately after birth with Apgar scoring. Heart rate, obtained by taking an apical pulse for 1 full minute, typically ranges between 120 to 160 bpm. Newborns' respirations are assessed when they are quiet or sleeping. Place a stethoscope on the right side of the chest and count the breaths for 1 full minute to identify any irregularities. The newborn respiratory rate ranges from 30 to 60 breaths/minute with symmetric chest movement. Heart and respiratory rates are assessed every 30 minutes until stable for 2 hours after birth. Once stable, the heart rate and respiratory rate is checked every 8 hours (AAP/ACOG, 2002).

Axillary temperature is typically not assessed immediately after birth, but on admission to the nursery or when the initial newborn assessment is carried out (for example, LDR room). The normal axillary temperature range for a term newborn is 36.5 to 37.5°C (97.9–99.7°F). Rectal temperatures are no longer taken because of the risk of perforation (Blackburn, 2003). The thermometer or temperature probe is held in the midaxillary space according to manufacture's directions and hospital protocol. Temperature is reassessed every 30 minutes until it is stable for 2 hours, then every 8 hours until discharge (AAP/ACOG, 2002).

Measurement of a newborn's blood pressure is not usually assessed as part of a normal newborn examination unless there is a clinical indication or low Apgar scores. If assessed, an oscillometer (Dinamap) is used.

The typical range is between 50 to 75 mmHg (systolic) and 30 to 45 mmHg (diastolic). Crying, moving, and late clamping of the umbilical cord will increase systolic pressure (Dillon, 2003).

Gestational Age Assessment

To determine a newborn's gestational age (the stage of maturity), physical signs and neurologic characteristics are assessed. Typically, gestational age is determined by using a tool, most commonly the Dubowitz/Ballard or New Ballard Score system (Fig. 18-3). This scoring system provides an objective estimate of gestational age by scoring the specific parameters of physical and neuromuscular maturity. Points are given for each assessment parameter, with a low score of −1 point or −2 points for extreme immaturity to as high a score as 4 or 5 points for postmaturity. The scores from each section are added together to correspond to a specific gestational age in weeks.

The physical maturity section of the examination is done during the first 2 hours after birth. The physical maturity assessment section of the Ballard exam evaluates physical characteristics that appear different at different stages depending on a newborn's gestational maturity. Newborns who are physically mature have higher scores than those who are not. The areas assessed on the physical maturity exam are

- Skin texture—typically ranges from sticky and transparent to smooth, with varying degrees of peeling and cracking, to parchment-like or leathery with significant cracking and wrinkling
- Lanugo—soft downy hair on the newborn's body, which is absent in preterm newborns, appears with maturity, and then disappears again with postmaturity
- Plantar creases—creases on the soles of the feet, which range from absent to covering the entire foot, depending on maturity (the greater the number of creases, the greater the newborn's maturity)
- Breast tissue—the thickness and size of breast tissue and areola (the darkened ring around each nipple), which range from being imperceptible to full and budding
- Eyes and ears—eyelids can be fused or open and ear cartilage and stiffness determine the degree of maturity (the greater the amount of ear cartilage with stiffness, the greater the newborn's maturity)
- Genitals—in males, evidence of testicular descent and appearance of scrotum (which can range from smooth to covered with rugae) determine maturity; in females, appearance and size of clitoris and labia determine maturity (a prominent clitoris with flat labia suggests prematurity whereas a clitoris covered by labia suggests greater maturity)

The neuromuscular maturity section typically is completed within 24 hours after birth. Six activities or maneuvers that the newborn performs with various body parts are evaluated to determine the newborn's degree of maturity. These six maneuvers include

NEUROMUSCULAR MATURITY

NEUROMUSCULAR MATURITY SIGN	SCORE							RECORD SCORE HERE
	−1	0	1	2	3	4	5	
POSTURE								
SQUARE WINDOW (Wrist)	>90°	90°	60°	45°	30°	0°		
ARM RECOIL		180°	140°–180°	110°–140°	90°–110°	<90°		
POPLITEAL ANGLE	180°	160°	140°	120°	100°	90°	<90°	
SCARF SIGN								
HEEL TO EAR								
						TOTAL NEUROMUSCULAR MATURITY SCORE		

SCORE

Neuromuscular ____
Physical ____
Total ____

MATURITY RATING

Score	Weeks
−10	20
−5	22
0	24
5	26
10	28
15	30
20	32
25	34
30	36
35	38
40	40
45	42
50	44

PHYSICAL MATURITY

PHYSICAL MATURITY SIGN	SCORE							RECORD SCORE HERE
	−1	0	1	2	3	4	5	
SKIN	sticky, friable, transparent	gelatinous, red, translucent	smooth, pink, visible veins	superficial peeling and/or rash, few veins	cracking pale areas, rare veins	parchment, deep cracking, no vessels	leathery, cracked, wrinkled	
LANUGO	none	sparse	abundant	thinning	bald areas	mostly bald		
PLANTAR SURFACE	heel-toe 40–50 mm:−1 <40 mm:−2	>50 mm no crease	faint red marks	anterior transverse crease only	creases ant. 2/3	creases over entire sole		
BREAST	impercep- tible	barely perceptible	flat areola no bud	stippled areola 1–2 mm bud	raised areola 3–4 mm bud	full areola 5–10 mm bud		
EYE-EAR	lids fused loosely: −1 tightly: −2	lids open pinna flat stays folded	sl. curved pinna; soft; slow recoil	well-curved pinna; soft but ready recoil	formed and firm instant recoil	thick cartilage, ear stiff		
GENITALS (Male)	scrotum flat, smooth	scrotum empty, faint rugae	testes in upper canal, rare rugae	testes descending, few rugae	testes down, good rugae	testes pendulous, deep rugae		
GENITALS (Female)	clitoris prominent and labia flat	prominent clitoris and small labia minora	prominent clitoris and enlarging minora	majora and minora equally prominent	majora large, minora small	majora cover clitoris and minora		
						TOTAL PHYSICAL MATURITY SCORE		

● Figure 18-3 Gestational age assessment tool. (Ballard, J. L., Khoury, J. C., Wedig, K., et al. [1991]. New Ballard Score, expanded to include extremely premature infants. *Journal of Pediatrics, 119*[3], 417–423.)

1. Posture—How does the newborn hold his or her extremities in relation to the trunk? The greater the degree of flexion indicates greater maturity. For example, extension of arms and legs is scored as 0 point; full flexion of arms and legs is scored as 4 points.

2. Square window—How far can the newborn's hands can be flexed toward the wrist? The angle is measured and scored from more than 90 degrees to 0 degrees to determine maturity rating. As the angle decreases, the newborn's maturity increases. For example, an angle of

more than 90 degrees is scored as −1 point; an angle of 0 degrees is scored as 4 points.

3. Arm recoil—How far do the newborn's arms "spring back" to a flexed position? This measure evaluates the degree of arm flexion and the strength of recoil. The reaction of the arm is then scored from 0 to 4 points based on the degree of flexion as the arms are returned to their normal flexed position. The higher the points assigned, the greater the neuromuscular maturity (for example, recoil less than a 90-degree angle is scored as 4 points).

4. Popliteal angle—How far will the newborn's knees extend? The angle created when the knee is extended is measured. An angle less than 90 degrees indicates greater maturity. For example, an angle of 180 degrees is scored as −1 point; an angle of less than 90 degree is scored as 5 points.

5. Scarf sign—How far can the elbows be moved across the newborn's chest? An elbow that does not reach midline indicates greater maturity. For example, if the elbow reaches or nears the level of the opposite shoulder, this is scored as −1 point; if the elbow does not cross the proximate axillary line, it is scored as 4 points.

6. Heel to ear—How close can the newborn's feet be moved to the ears? This maneuver assesses hip flexibility, such that the lesser the flexibility, the greater the newborn's maturity. The heel-to-ear assessment is scored in the same manner as the scarf sign.

After the scoring is completed, the 12 scores are totaled and then compared with standardized values to determine the appropriate gestational age in weeks. Scores range from very low in preterm newborns to very high for mature and postmature newborns.

Typically newborns are also classified according to gestational age as

- Preterm or premature—born before 37 weeks' gestation, regardless of birth weight
- Term—born between 38 weeks and 42 weeks' gestation
- Postterm or postdate—born after completion of week 42 of gestation
- Postmature—born after 42 weeks and demonstrating signs of placental aging

Using the information about gestational age and then considering birth weight, newborns can also be classified as follows:

- Small for gestational age (SGA)—weight less than the 10th percentile on standard growth charts (usually < 5.5 lb)
- Appropriate for gestational age (AGA)—weight between 10th and 90th percentiles
- Large for gestational age (LGA)—weight more than the 90th percentile on standard growth charts (usually > 9 lb)

Chapter 23 describes these variations in birth weight and gestational age in greater detail.

Gestational age assessment is important because it allows the nurse to plot growth parameters, and to anticipate potential problems related to prematurity, postmaturity, and growth abnormalities such as SGA or LGA newborns.

Nursing Interventions

During the immediate newborn period, care focuses on facilitating the newborn's transition to extrauterine life. The nursing interventions include maintaining airway patency, ensuring proper identification, administering prescribed medications, and maintaining thermoregulation.

Maintaining Airway Patency

Immediately after birth, a newborn is suctioned to remove fluids and mucus from the mouth and nose. Typically, the newborn's mouth is suctioned first with a bulb syringe to remove debris. Then the nose is suctioned. Suctioning in this manner helps to prevent aspiration of fluid into the lungs by an unexpected gasp.

When suctioning a newborn with a bulb syringe, compress the bulb before placing it into the oral or nasal cavity. Release bulb compression slowly, making sure the tip is placed properly away from the mucous membranes to draw up the excess secretions. Remove the bulb syringe from the mouth or nose, and then, while holding the bulb syringe tip over an emesis basin lined with paper towel or tissue, compress the bulb to expel the secretions. Repeat the procedure several times until all secretions are removed. Always keep a bulb syringe near the newborn in case he or she develops sudden choking or a blockage in the nose.

Ensuring Proper Identification

Before the newborn and family leave the birthing area, be sure that agency policy dictating identification is followed. Typically, mother and newborn, and possibly father, receive matching identification (ID) bracelets. The newborn commonly receives two ID bracelets: one placed on a wrist and one placed on an ankle. The mother receives a matching one, usually placed on her wrist. The ID bands usually include name, gender, date and time of birth, and identification number. The imprinted identification number is identical to the other bracelet wearers.

These ID bracelets provide for the safety of the newborn and must be secured before the mother and newborn leave the birthing area. The ID bracelets are checked by all nurses to validate the correct newborn is brought to the right mother if they are separated for any period of time (Fig. 18-4). They also serve as the official newborn identification and are checked prior to initiating any procedure on that newborn and on discharge from the unit (Lowdermilk & Perry, 2004). Taking the newborn's picture within 2 hours after birth with a color camera or color video/digital image also assists in protecting against mixups and abduction. In some facilities, electronic devices

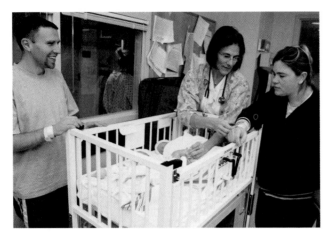

● Figure 18-4 The nurse checks the identification bands of the newborn with the mother.

may be used. These devices sound an alarm if the newborn is removed from the area.

Newborns are also footprinted by using a form that includes the mother's fingerprint, name, and date and time of the birth (Fig. 18-5). Some states require footprints of the newborn, although many studies point out that birthing room staff members do not take consistently legible footprints suitable for identification purposes (Kenner & Lott, 2004). Many states have stopped requiring newborn footprints, and thus other means of identification are needed, such as collecting cord blood at the time of birth for DNA testing and live scans to capture digital forensic-

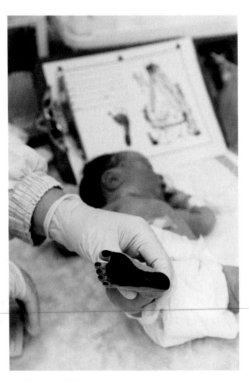

● Figure 18-5 The nurse obtains footprints on the newborn.

quality prints electronically that are suitable for identification purposes (Rabun, 2003).

Administering Prescribed Medications

During the immediate newborn period, two medications are commonly ordered to be given. These medications are vitamin K and eye prophylaxis with either erythromycin or tetracycline ophthalmic ointment (see Drug Guide 18-1).

Vitamin K

Vitamin K, a fat-soluble vitamin, promotes blood clotting by increasing the synthesis of prothrombin by the liver. A deficiency of this vitamin would delay clotting and might lead to hemorrhage.

Generally, the bacteria of the intestine produce vitamin K in quantities that are adequate. However, the newborn's bowel is sterile and thus vitamin K is not produced in the intestine until after microorganisms are introduced, such as with the first feeding. Usually, it takes about a week for the newborn to produce vitamin K in sufficient quantities to prevent vitamin K deficiency bleeding (VKDB) (Miller, 2003).

The efficacy of newborn vitamin K prophylaxis in the prevention of early VKDB is firmly established. It has been the standard of care since the AAP recommended it in the early 1960s. Their recommendation is for vitamin K to be administered to all newborns as a single intramuscular dose of 0.5 to 1 mg soon after birth (AAP, 2003d) (Fig. 18-6). They suggest that additional research is needed to validate the efficacy and safety of oral forms of vitamin K, which have been utilized in many parts of the world, but currently are not recommended in the United States.

Eye Prophylaxis

It is recommended that all newborns in the United States, whether delivered vaginally or by cesarean birth, receive an instillation of a prophylactic agent, such as erythromycin or tetracycline ophthalmic ointment, in their eyes within an hour or two of being born. This is mandated in all 50 states to prevent **ophthalmia neonatorum,** which can cause neonatal blindness (CDC, 2002).

Ophthalmia neonatorum is a hyperacute purulent conjunctivitis occurring during the first 10 days of life, usually contracted during birth from infected vaginal discharge of the mother (O'Toole, 2003). Most often both eyelids become swollen and red with purulent discharge.

Prophylactic agents that are currently recommended include erythromycin 0.5% ophthalmic ointment or tetracycline 1% ophthalmic ointment in a single application. Once recommended in the past, silver nitrate solution has little efficacy in preventing chlamydial eye disease (CDC, 2002).

Regardless of which agent is used, instillation should be accomplished as soon as possible after birth (Fig. 18-7). If instillation is delayed after birth to allow visualization and bonding, the nursery staff should make sure the agent

Drug Guide 18-1 Drugs for the Newborn

Drug	Action/Indication	Nursing Implications
Phytonadione (vitamin K (Aqua-MEPHYTON, Konakion, Mephyton))	Provides the newborn with vitamin K (necessary for production of adequate clotting factors II, VII, IX, and X by the liver) during the first week of birth until they can manufacture it themselves Prevents vitamin K deficiency bleeding (VKDB) of the newborn	Administer within 1 to 2 hours after birth. Give as an intramuscular injection at a 90-degree angle into the middle third of the vastus lateralis muscle. Use a 25-gauge, 5/8-in needle for injection. Hold the leg firmly and inject medication slowly after aspirating. Adhere to standard precautions. Assess for bleeding at injection site after administration.
Erythromycin ophthalmic ointment 0.5% or tetracycline ophthalmic ointment 1%	Provides bactericidal and bacteriostatic actions to prevent *Neisseria gonorrhoeae* and *Chlamydia trachomatis* conjunctivitis Prevents ophthalmia neonatorum	Be alert for possible chemical conjunctivitis for 1–2 days. Wear gloves, and open eyes by placing thumb and finger above and below the eye. Gently squeeze the tube or ampulla to apply medication into the conjunctival sac from the inner canthus to the outer canthus of each eye. Do not touch the tip to the eye. Close the eye to make sure the medication permeates. Wipe off excess ointment after 1 minute.

Sources: Hodgson & Kizior, 2004; Spratto & Woods, 2005.

is administered when the newborn reaches the nursery for observation and assessment.

Inform all parents about the eye treatment, including why the treatment is recommended, what advantages should be anticipated from the treatment, what problems may arise if the treatment is not given, and what side effects may arise from the treatment. Parents do have the right to refuse this treatment, but if the parents received adequate teaching about the treatment and understand the need for it, they usually will consent to it.

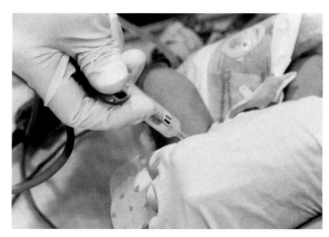

● Figure 18-6 The nurse administers vitamin K IM to the newborn.

Maintaining Thermoregulation

Newborns have temperature regulation problems, especially during the first few hours after birth (see Chapter 17 for a complete discussion). Therefore, maintaining body temperature is crucial.

Assess body temperature frequently during the immediate newborn period. It is recommended that the temperature be taken every 30 minutes for the first 2 hours or until stabilization is reached and then every 8 hours until discharge (AAP/ACOG, 2002).

Commonly, a thermistor probe (automatic sensor) is attached to the newborn to record body temperature on a monitoring device. The probe is taped to the newborn's abdomen, usually in the right upper quadrant, which allows for position changes without having to readjust the probe. The other end of the thermistor probe is inserted into the radiant heat control panel. Temperature parameters are set on an alarm system connected to the heat panel that will sound if the newborn's temperature falls out of the set range. Check the probe connection periodically to make sure that it remains secure. Be ever aware of the potential for heat loss in newborns, ensuring that all nursing interventions are performed to minimize heat loss and prevent hypothermia.

Frequent axillary temperatures can also be used to assess the newborn's body temperature. At one time, rectal thermometers were routinely used to monitor body temperature. However, their use is no longer recommended

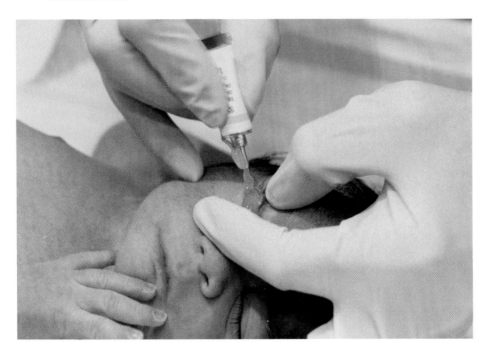

● Figure 18-7 The nurse administers eye prophylaxis.

because of the potential damage to the rectal lining on insertion (Blackburn, 2003). A newborn's temperature typically is maintained between 36.5 to 37.5°C (97.7 to 99.7°F) (Littleton & Engebretson, 2005).

Nursing interventions to help maintain body temperature include

- Drying newborns immediately after birth to prevent heat loss through evaporation
- Wrapping them in prewarmed blankets to reduce heat loss via convection
- Using warmed covers on scales to weigh unclothed newborn

- Warming stethoscopes and hands prior to examining or providing care
- Avoiding the placement of newborns in drafts or near air vents to prevent heat loss through convection
- Delaying the initial bath until temperature has stabilized to prevent heat loss through evaporation
- Avoiding crib placement near cold outer walls to prevent heat loss through radiation
- Putting a cap on the newborn's head after it is thoroughly dried after birth
- Placing a newborn under a temperature-controlled radiant warmer (Fig. 18-8)

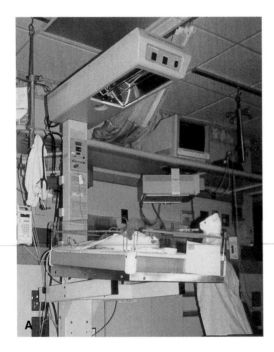
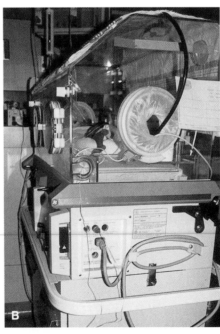

● Figure 18-8 Maintaining thermoregulation. (**A**) Radiant warmer. (**B**) Isolette.

Nursing Management During the Early Newborn Period

The early newborn period is a time of great adjustment for both the mother and the newborn, both of whom are adapting to many physiologic and psychological changes. In the past, mothers and newborns remained in the healthcare facility while these dramatic changes and phases of adjustment were taking place. Nursing and medical care providers were readily available to them. However, during the last decade, as a result of economics, healthcare facility stays have decreased significantly for mothers and their newborns, thus increasing the intensity of the experience. For example, the woman gives birth, experiences marked physiologic and psychological changes, adapts to her newborn, and learns the skills needed to care for herself and her newborn—all within a limited time frame. Subsequently, many new mothers are overwhelmed.

The nurse is challenged to assist the new mother and her newborn through this dramatic transition period. The newborn needs continued assessment to ensure health. The mother also needs to be prepared to care for the new addition to the family unit—all within 24 to 48 hours. When the day of discharge arrives, women may develop feelings of panic and insecurity about their role as primary caretaker. Thus, nurses play a major role in promoting the newborn's transition through ongoing assessment and care, and in promoting the woman's confidence through role modeling and teaching about proper newborn care.

Assessment

The newborn requires ongoing assessment after leaving the birthing area to ensure that his or her transition to extrauterine life is progressing without problems. The nurse uses the data gathered during the initial assessment as a baseline for comparison.

Perinatal History

Pertinent maternal and fetal data are vital to formulate a plan of care for the mother and her newborn. Historical information is obtained from the medical record and from interviewing the mother. Review the maternal history because it provides pertinent information, such as the presence of certain risk factors, that could affect the newborn. Keep in mind that a comprehensive maternal history may not be available, especially if the mother has had limited or no prenatal care.

Historical information usually includes the following:

- Mother's name, medical record number, blood type, serology result, rubella and hepatitis status, and history of substance abuse
- Other maternal tests that are relevant to the newborn and care, such as HIV and group B streptococcus status
- Intrapartum maternal antibiotic therapy (type, dose, and duration)

- Maternal illness potentially affecting the pregnancy, evidence of chorioamnionitis, maternal use of medications such as steroids
- Prenatal care, including timing of first visit and subsequent visits
- Risk for blood group incompatibility including Rh status and blood type
- Fetal distress or any nonreassuring fetal heart rate monitor patterns during labor
- Known inherited conditions such as sickle cell anemia, phenylketonuria (PKU)
- Birth weights of previous live-born children along with identification of any newborn problems
- Social history, including tobacco, alcohol, and recreational drug use
- History of depression or domestic violence
- Cultural factors, including primary language and educational level
- Pregnancy complications associated with abnormal fetal growth, fetal anomalies, or abnormal results from tests of fetal well-being
- Information regarding the labor and progress of labor, birth, labor complications, duration of ruptured membranes, and presence of meconium in the amniotic fluid
- Medications given during labor, at birth, and immediately after birth
- Time and method of delivery, including presentation and the use of any forceps or vacuum extractor
- Status of the newborn at birth, including Apgar scores at 1 and 5 minutes, the need for suctioning, weight, gestational age, vital signs, and umbilical cord status
- Medications administered to the newborn
- Postbirth maternal information, including placental findings, positive cultures, and presence of fever

Newborn Physical Examination

The initial newborn physical examination, which may demonstrate subtle differences related to the newborn's age, is carried out within the first 24 hours after birth. For example, a newborn that is 30 minutes old has not yet completed the normal transition from intrauterine to extrauterine life, and thus variability may exist in vital signs and in respiratory, neurologic, GI, skin, and cardiovascular systems. Therefore, it is ideal to perform a comprehensive examination after the newborn has completed transition.

In a quiet newborn, begin the examination with the least invasive and noxious elements of the exam (auscultation of heart and lungs). Then proceed to examining those areas most likely to irritate the newborn (for example, examining the hips and eliciting the Moro reflex). A general visual assessment provides an enormous amount of information regarding the well-being of a newborn. Initial observation gives an impression of healthy (stable) versus ill newborn and term versus preterm newborn.

The specific components of a typical physical newborn examination include a general survey of skin color, posture, state of alertness, head size, overall behavioral state, respiratory status, gender, and any obvious congenital anomalies. Check the overall appearance for anything unusual. Then complete the examination in a systematic fashion.

Anthropometric Measurements

Shortly after birth, after the gender of the child is revealed, most parents want to know the "vital statistics" of their newborn—length and weight to report to their interested family and friends. Additional measurements, including circumference of the newborn's head, chest, and abdomen, are also taken and recorded. Abdominal measurements are not routinely obtained unless there is a suspicion of pathology that causes abdominal distention. The newborn's progress from that point on will be validated based on these early measurements. These measurements will be compared with future serial measurements to determine growth patterns, which are plotted on growth charts to ascertain normalcy. Therefore, accuracy is key.

Length

The average length of most newborns is 50 cm (20 in), but can range from 45 to 55 cm (18–22 in). Measure length with the unclothed newborn lying on a warmed blanket placed on a flat surface with the knees held in an extended position. Then run a tape measure down the length of the newborn—from the head to the soles of the feet and record this measurement in the newborn's record.

Weight

The average newborn birth weight is 3400 g (7.5 lb), but it can range anywhere from 2700 to 4000 g (6–9 lb).

Newborns are weighed immediately after birth and then daily. Newborns usually lose up to 10% of their birth weight within the first few days of life, but regain it in approximately 10 days. Newborns are weighed on admission to the nursery or are taken to a digital scale to be weighed and returned to the mother's room.

First, balance the scale if it is not balanced. Place a protective, warmed cloth or paper as a barrier on the scale to prevent heat loss by conduction; recalibrate the scale to zero after applying the barrier. Next, place the newborn, unclothed, in the center of the scale. Be sure to keep a hand above the newborn to ensure safety (Fig. 18-2).

Weight is influenced by racial origin, maternal age, size of the parents, maternal nutrition, and placental perfusion (Fuloria & Kreiter, 2002b). Weight should be correlated with determination of gestational age. A newborn that is more than the normal weight values might be LGA or an infant of a diabetic mother (IDM). A newborn less than the normal weight range might be preterm, have a genetic syndrome, or be an SGA neonate. It is important to identify the cause for the deviation in size and monitor the newborn for complications common to that etiology.

Head Circumference

The average newborn head circumference is about 33 to 35 cm (13–14 in). Measure the circumference at the head's widest diameter: occipitofrontal circumference with a measuring tape. Use a flexible or paper measuring tape, wrap it snugly around the newborn's head, and record the measurement (Fig. 18-9A). Head circumference may need to be remeasured at a later time if the shape of the head is altered from birth.

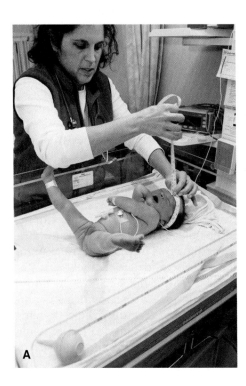 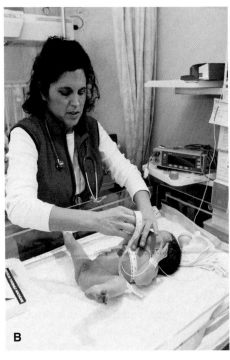

● Figure 18-9 (**A**) Measuring head circumference. (**B**) Measuring chest circumference.

The head is approximately one fourth of the newborn's length (McKinney, James, Murray, & Ashwill, 2005). A small-size head might indicate microcephaly caused by rubella, toxoplasmosis, or SGA status. An enlarged head circumference measurement might indicate hydrocephalus or increased intracranial pressure. In either case, both need to be documented and reported for further investigation.

Chest Circumference

The average chest circumference is about 30 to 33 cm (12–13 in). It is generally equal to or approximately 1 in less than the head circumference. Using a flexible or paper tape measure, place it around the unclothed newborn's chest at the nipple line without pulling it taut (Fig. 18-9B). The head and chest circumferences are usually equal by about one year of age.

Vital Signs

In the newborn, temperature, pulse, and respirations are monitored frequently and compared with baseline data obtained immediately after birth. General rules of thumb for monitoring vital signs (excluding blood pressure) are as follows:

- On admission to the nursery or in the LDR room after parents are allowed to hold and bond with their newborn
- Once every 30 minutes until the newborn has been stable for 2 hours
- Then once every 4 to 8 hours until discharge (AAP/ACOG, 2002)

Blood pressure is not routinely assessed in a normal newborn unless their clinical condition warrants it. This schedule can change depending on the health status of the newborn.

Obtain a newborn's temperature by placing an electronic temperature probe in the midaxillary area or by monitoring the electronic thermistor probe that has been taped to the abdominal skin (applied when the newborn was placed under a radiant heat source).

Monitor the newborn's temperature hourly for changes until it stabilizes. On average, a newborn's temperature ranges from 36.5 to 37.5°C (97.9–99.7°F). If the newborn's temperature is more than this range, adjust the environment, such as removing some clothing or blankets. If the temperature is less than this range, check the radiant warmer setting or add a warmed blanket if needed. Report any abnormalities to the primary healthcare provider if simple adjustments within the environment do not change temperature.

Obtain an apical pulse by placing the stethoscope over the fourth intercostal space on the chest. Listen for a full minute, noting rate, rhythm, and abnormal sounds such as murmurs. In the typical newborn, the heart rate ranges from 120 to 160 bpm, with wide fluctuations with activity and sleep. Sinus arrhythmia is a normal finding. Murmurs detected during the newborn period do not necessarily indicate congenital heart disease. They need to be assessed frequently over the next several months to validate their continued presence.

Also palpate the apical, femoral, and brachial pulses for presence and equality (Fig. 18-10). Report any abnormalities to the primary health care provider to ensure further evaluation.

Assess newborn respirations by observing the rising and falling of the chest for 1 full minute. Respirations should be symmetric, slightly irregular, shallow, and unlabored at a rate of 30 to 60 breaths/minute. The newborn's respirations are predominantly diaphragmatic, but

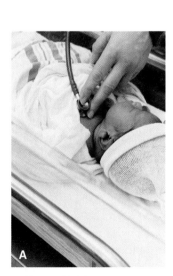 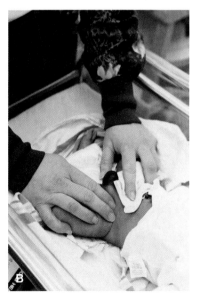 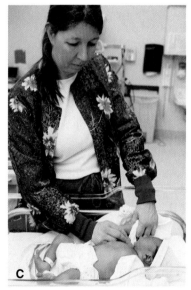

● Figure 18-10 Assessing the newborn's vital signs. (**A**) Assessing the apical pulse. (**B**) Palpating the femoral pulse. (**C**) Palpating the brachial pulse.

they are synchronous with abdominal movements. Also auscultate breath sounds. Note any abnormalities, such as tachypnea, bradypnea, grunting, gasping, periods of apnea lasting longer than 20 seconds, asymmetry or decreased chest expansion, abnormal breath sounds (rhonchi, crackles), or sternal retractions. Some variations might exist early in the period after birth, but if the abnormal pattern persists, notify the primary health care provider.

Skin

Observe the overall appearance of the skin, including color, texture, turgor, and integrity. The newborn's skin should be smooth and flexible, and the color should be consistent with genetic background. Check skin turgor by pinching a small area of skin over the chest or abdomen and note how quickly it returns to its original position. In a well-hydrated newborn, the skin should return to its normal position immediately. Skin that remains "tented" after being pinched is indicative of dehydration. A small amount of lanugo (fine downy hair) may be observed over the shoulders and on the sides of the face and upper back. There may be some cracking and peeling of the skin. It should be warm to the touch and intact.

The newborn's skin often appears blotchy or mottled, especially in the extremities. Persistent cyanosis of fingers, hands, toes, and feet with mottled blue or red discoloration and coldness describes **acrocyanosis.** It may be seen in newborns during the first few weeks of life in response to exposure to cold. Acrocyanosis is normal and intermittent.

Common Newborn Skin Variations

While assessing the skin, note any rashes, ecchymoses or petechiae, nevi, or dark pigmentation. Skin lesions may be present and can be congenital or transient; they may be a result of infection or may result from the mode of birth. If any are present, observe the anatomic location, arrangement, type, and color. Bruising may be a result of the use of devices such as a vacuum extractor during delivery. Petechiae may be the result of pressure on the skin during the birth process. Forceps marks may be observed over the cheeks and ears. A small puncture mark may be seen if internal fetal scalp electrode monitoring was used during labor.

Also be alert to common skin variations, which include **vernix caseosa, stork bites** or salmon patches, **milia, mongolian spots, erythema toxicum, harlequin sign, nevus flammeus,** and **nevus vasculosus** (Fig. 18-11).

Vernix caseosa is a thick white substance that provides a protective covering for the skin of the fetus. It is formed by secretions from the fetus' oil glands and is found during the first 2 or 3 days after birth in body creases and the hair. It does not need to be removed because it will be absorbed into the skin.

Stork bites or salmon patches are superficial vascular areas found on the nape of the neck, on the eyelids, and between the eyes and upper lip (Fig. 18-11A). The name comes from the marks on the back of the neck where, as myth goes, a stork may have picked up the baby. They are caused by a concentration of immature blood vessels and are most visible when the newborn is crying. They are considered a normal variant and most fade and disappear completely within the first year.

Milia are unopened sebaceous glands frequently found on a newborn's nose. They may also appear on the chin and forehead (Fig. 18-11B). They form from oil glands and disappear on their own within 2 to 4 weeks. When these occur in a newborn's mouth and gums, they are termed **Epstein's pearls.** They occur in approximately 60% of newborns (Weston, Lane, & Morelli, 2002).

Mongolian spots are blue or purple splotches that appear on the lower back and buttocks of newborns (Fig. 18-11C). They tend to occur in African-American, Asian, and Indian newborns, but can occur in dark-skin newborns of all races. The spots are caused by a concentration of pigmented cells and usually disappear within the first 4 years of life (Rutter, 2003).

Erythema toxicum (newborn rash) is a benign, idiopathic, very common, generalized, transient rash occurring in as many as 70% of all newborns during the first week of life. It consists of small papules or pustules on the skin resembling "flea bites." The rash is common on the face, chest, and back (Fig. 18-11D). One of the chief characteristics of this rash is its lack of pattern. It is caused by the newborn's eosinophils reacting to the environment as the immune system matures (Pillitteri, 2003). It does not require any treatment and it disappears in a few days.

Harlequin sign refers to the dilation of blood vessels on only one side of the body, giving the newborn the appearance of wearing a clown suit. It gives a distinct midline demarcation, which is described as pale on the nondependent side and red on the opposite, dependent side. It is as a result of immature autoregulation of blood flow and is commonly seen in LBW newborns when there is a positional change (Dillon, 2003). It is transit in nature, lasting as long as 20 minutes, and no intervention is needed.

Nevus flammeus, also called a *port wine stain,* commonly appears on the newborn's face or other body areas (Fig. 18-11E). It is a capillary angioma located directly below the dermis. It is flat with sharp demarcations and is purple–red in color. This skin lesion is made up of mature capillaries that are congested and dilated. It ranges in size from a few millimeters to large, occasionally involving as much as half the body surface. Although it does not progressively grow in area or size, it is permanent and will not fade. Port wine stains may be associated with structural malformations or bony or muscular overgrowth. Newborns with these lesions should be monitored with periodic eye examinations, neurologic imaging, and extremity measurements (Hockenberry, 2005). Pulsed dye laser surgery has

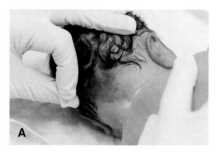

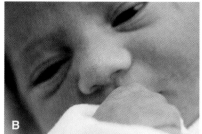

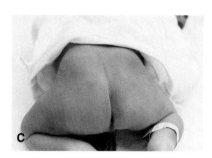

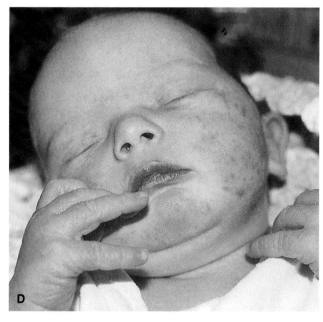

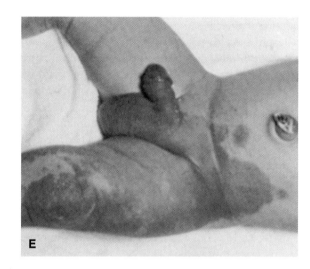

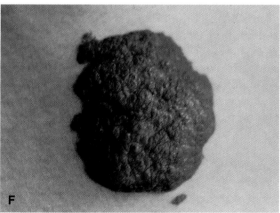

● Figure 18-11 Common skin variations. (**A**) Stork bite. (**B**) Milia. (**C**) Mongolian spots. (**D**) Erythema toxicum. (**E**) Nevus flammeus (port-wine stain). (**F**) Strawberry hemangioma.

been used to remove larger lesions with some success (O'Leary, 2004).

Nevus vasculosus, also call a *strawberry mark* or *strawberry hemangioma,* is a benign capillary hemangioma in the dermal and subdermal layers. It is raised, rough, dark-red, and sharply demarcated (Fig. 18-11F). It is commonly found in the head region within a few weeks after birth and can increase in size or number. Commonly seen in premature infants weighing less than 1500 g (Verklan & Walden, 2004), these hemangiomas tend to resolve by the age of 3 without any treatment.

Head

Head size varies with age, gender, and ethnicity, and has a general correlation with body size. Inspect a newborn's head from all angles. The head should appear symmetric and round. As many as 90% of the congenital malformations present at birth are visible on the head and neck, so careful assessment is very important (Verklan & Walden, 2004).

The newborn has two fontanels at the juncture of the cranial bones. The anterior fontanel is diamond shaped and closes by 18 to 24 months. Typically it measures 4 to

6 cm at the largest diameter (bone to bone). The posterior one is triangular in shape, smaller than the anterior fontanel, usually fingertip size or 0.5 to 1 cm, and closes by 6 to 12 weeks of age. Palpate both fontanels, which should be soft, flat, and open.

Then palpate the skull. It should feel smooth and fused, except at the area of the fontanels. Also assess the size of the head and the anterior and posterior fontanelles, and compare them with appropriate standards.

Common abnormalities in head or fontanel size that may indicate a potential problem include

- Microcephaly—a head circumference more than 2 SDs below average or less than 10% of normal parameters for gestational age caused by failure of brain development (Hockenberry, 2005). It can be familial, with autosomal dominant or recessive inheritance, and it may be associated with infections (cytomegalovirus) and syndromes such as trisomy 13 and 18, and fetal alcohol syndrome (Fuloria & Kreiter, 2002a).
- Macrocephaly—a head circumference more than 90% of normal measurement typically related to hydrocephalus (Dillon, 2003). It can be an isolated anomaly, is often familial (with autosomal dominant inheritance), and may be a manifestation of other anomalies, including hydrocephalus and skeletal disorders (achondroplasia).
- Large fontanelles—size more than 6 cm in the anterior diameter bone to bone or more than a 1-cm diameter in the posterior fontanelle possibly associated with malnutrition; hydrocephaly; congenital hypothyroidism; trisomies 13, 18, and 21; and various bone disorders such as osteogenesis imperfecta
- Small or closed fontanelles—less than the normal range measurements for anterior and posterior diameters or closed at birth associated with microcephaly or premature synostosis (union of two bones by osseous material) (O'Toole, 2003)

Variations in Head Size and Appearance

During inspection and palpation, be alert for common variations that may cause asymmetry. These include **caput succedaneum, cephalhematoma,** and molding.

Molding is the elongated shaping of the fetal head to accommodate passage through the birth canal (Fig. 18-12). It occurs with a vaginal birth from a vertex position in which elongation of the fetal head occurs with prominence of occiput and overriding sagittal suture line. It typically resolves within a week after birth without intervention.

Caput succedaneum describes localized edema on the scalp that occurs from the pressure of the birth process. It is commonly observed after prolonged labor. Clinically, it appears as a poorly demarcated soft tissue swelling that crosses suture lines. Pitting edema and overlying petechiae and ecchymosis are noted (Fig. 18-13A). The swelling, which crosses suture lines, will gradually dissipate in about

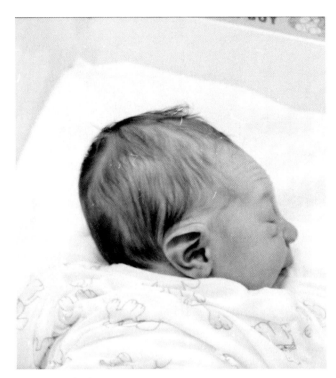

● Figure 18-12 Molding in a newborn's head.

3 days without any treatment. Newborns who were delivered via vacuum extraction usually have a caput in the area where the cup was used.

Cephalhematoma is a localized effusion of blood beneath the periosteum of the skull of the newborn. This condition is as a result of the disruption of the vessels during birth. It occurs after prolonged labor and use of obstetric instruments such as low-outlet forceps or vacuum extraction (a Silastic suction cup is applied to the presenting part and traction is exerted during pushing attempts). The clinical features include a well-demarcated, often fluctuant swelling with no overlying skin discoloration. The swelling does not cross suture lines and is firmer to the touch than an edematous area (Fig. 18-13B). Cephalhematoma usually appears on the second or third day after birth and disappears within weeks or months (Olds, London, Ladewig, & Davidson, 2004).

Face

Observe the newborn's face for fullness and symmetry. The face should have full cheeks and be symmetric when resting and crying. In an assisted birth, forceps blades lay over the fetal cheeks and parietal bones when traction is applied. After birth, the newborn may have bruising and reddened areas over both cheeks and parietal bones secondary to the pressure of the forceps blades. Reassure the parents that this resolves without treatment and be sure to point out improvement each day.

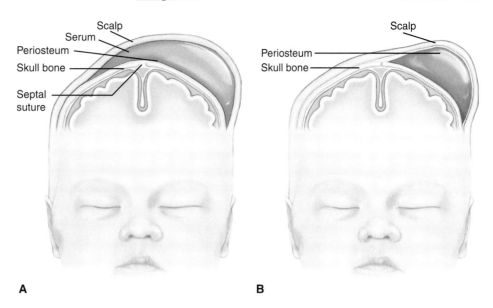

● Figure 18-13 Comparing caput succedaneum and cephalhematoma. (**A**) Caput succedaneum involves the collection of serous fluid and often crosses the suture line. (**B**) Cephalhematoma involves the collection of blood and does not cross the suture line.

Problems with the face can also involve facial nerve paralysis caused by trauma resulting from the use of forceps during the birthing process. Paralysis is usually apparent on the first or second day of life. Typically, the newborn will demonstrate asymmetry of the face with the inability to close the eye and move the lips on the affected side. Newborns with facial nerve paralysis have difficulty making a seal around the nipple and consequently exhibit drooling of milk or formula from the paralyzed side of the mouth. Most facial nerve palsies resolve spontaneously within days, although full recovery may require weeks to months. Attempt to determine the cause of the deviation from the newborn's history.

Nose

Inspect the nose for size, symmetry, position, and evidence of lesions. The newborn's nose is small and narrow. The nose should have a midline placement, patent nares, and an intact septum. The nostrils should be of equal size and patent. A slight mucus discharge may be present, but there should be no actual drainage. The newborn is a preferential nose breather and will use sneezing to clear the nose if needed. The newborn can smell after the nasal passages are cleared of amniotic fluid and mucus (Olds et al., 2004).

Mouth

Observe and inspect the newborn's mouth, lips, and interior structures. The lips should be intact with symmetric movement, positioned in the midline, and without any lesions. Inspect the lips for pink color, moisture, and cracking. The lips should encircle the examiner's finger to form a vacuum when inserted into the mouth orifice. Variations involving the lip might include cleft upper lip (separation extending up onto the nose) or thin upper lip associated with fetal alcohol syndrome.

Assess the inside of the mouth for alignment of the mandible, intact soft and hard palate, sucking pads inside the cheeks, a midline uvula, a free-moving tongue, and working gag, swallow, and sucking reflexes. The mucous membranes lining the oral cavity should be pink and moist with minimal saliva present.

Normal variations might include Epstein's pearls (small, white epidermal cysts on the gums and hard palate that disappear in weeks); erupted precocious teeth that may need to be removed to prevent aspiration; and thrush (white plaque inside the mouth caused by exposure to *Candida albicans* during birth), which cannot be wiped away with a cotton-tipped applicator.

Eyes

Inspect the external eye structures including the eyelids, lashes, conjunctiva, sclera, iris, and pupils for position, color, size, and movement. There may be marked edema of the eyelids and subconjunctival hemorrhages present from pressure occurring during birth. The eyes should be clear and symmetrically placed on the face. Test the blink reflex by bringing an object in close proximity to the eye. The newborn should respond quickly by blinking. Also test the newborn's papillary reflex. Pupils should be equal, round, and reactive to light bilaterally. Assess the newborn's gaze. The newborn should be able to track objects to the midline. Be aware that movement may be uncoordinated during the first few weeks of life. There is transient strabismus (deviation or wandering of eyes independently) and searching nystagmus (involuntary repetitive eye movement) in many newborns, which is caused by immature muscular control. These are normal for the first 3 to 6 months of age.

Examine the internal eye structures. A red reflex (luminous red appearance seen on the retina) should be seen bilaterally during retinoscopy. The red reflex normally shows no dullness or irregularities.

Chemical conjunctivitis is a common variation that usually occurs within 24 hours of instillation of eye prophylaxis after birth. There is lid edema with sterile discharge from both eyes. Usually it resolves within 48 hours without treatment.

Ears

Inspect the ears for size, shape, skin condition, placement, amount of cartilage, and patency of the auditory canal. The ears should be soft and pliable, and should recoil quickly and easily when folded and released. Ears should be aligned with the outer canthi of the eyes. Low-set ears are characteristic of many syndromes and genetic abnormalities such as trisomy 13 and 18, and internal organ abnormalities involving the renal system.

An otoscopic examination is not typically done because the newborn's ear canals are filled with amniotic fluid and vernix caseosa, which would make visualization of the tympanic membrane difficult.

Newborn hearing screening is required by law in a majority of states (discussed later in the chapter). Hearing loss is the most common birth defect in the United States. One in 1000 newborns is profoundly deaf and 2 to 3 in 1000 have partial hearing loss (Wittmann-Price & Pope, 2002). Delays in identification and intervention may affect the cognitive, verbal, behavioral, and emotional development of the child. Screening at birth has become commonplace in most states, has reduced the age at which newborns with hearing loss are identified, and has improved early intervention rates dramatically (AAP, 2003b). Prior to universal newborn screening, children were usually older than 2 years before significant congenital hearing loss was detected, already negatively affecting speech and language skills (Fligor & Neault, 2004).

To assess for hearing ability generally, observe the newborn's response to noises and conversations in close proximity. The newborn typically turns toward these noises and startles with loud ones.

Neck

Inspect the newborn's neck for movement and ability to support the head. The newborn's neck will appear almost nonexistent because it is so short. Creases are usually noted. The neck should move freely in all directions and be capable of holding the head in a midline position. There should be sufficient head control to hold it up briefly without support. Report any deviations such as restricted neck movement or absence of head control.

Also inspect the clavicles, which should be straight and intact. Clavicular fractures are the most common broken bones associated with newborns, especially large newborns. In most cases, the newborn is asymptomatic. However, decreased or absent movement and pain or tenderness on movement of the arm on the affected side may be noted (Fuloria & Kreiter, 2002a). Treatment is directed toward immobilization and minimizing pain.

Chest

Inspect the newborn's chest for size, shape, and symmetry. The newborn's chest should be round, symmetric, and 1 to 2 cm smaller than the head circumference. The xiphoid process may be prominent at birth; however, it usually becomes less apparent when adipose tissue accumulates. Nipples may be engorged and may secrete a white discharge. This discharge, which occurs in both male and female newborns, is as a result of their exposure to high levels of maternal estrogen while in utero. This enlargement and milky discharge usually dissipates within a few weeks. Some newborns may have extra nipples, called *supernumerary nipples*. They are typically small, raised, pigmented areas vertical to the main nipple line 5 to 6 cm below the normal nipple (Verklan & Walden, 2004). They tend to be familial and do not contain glandular tissue. Reassure parents the extra small nipples are harmless.

The newborn chest is usually barrel shaped with equal anteroposterior and lateral diameters, and symmetric. Auscultate the lungs bilaterally for equal breath sounds. Normal breath sounds should be heard with little differentiation between inspiration and expiration. Fine crackles can be heard on inspiration soon after birth as a result of clearing amniotic fluid from the lungs. Diminished breath sounds might indicate atelectasis, effusion, or poor respiratory effort (Colyar, 2003).

Auscultating the heart should be carried out when the newborn is quiet or sleeping to hear sounds effectively. S1 and S2 heart sounds are accentuated at birth. The point of maximal impulse (PMI) is a lateral to midclavicular line located at the fourth intercostal space. A displaced PMI may indicate tension pneumothorax or cardiomegaly. Murmurs are often heard and are usually benign, but if present after the first 12 hours of life should be evaluated to rule out a cardiac disorder (Haws, 2004).

Abdomen

Inspect the abdomen for shape and movement. Typically the newborn's abdominal contour is protuberant without appearing distended. This contour is as a result of the immaturity of the abdominal musculature. Abdominal movements are synchronous with respirations because newborns are, at times, abdominal breathers.

Next, auscultate bowel sounds in all four quadrants and then palpate the abdomen for consistency, masses, and tenderness. Perform auscultation and palpation systematically in a clockwise fashion until all four quadrants have been assessed. Palpate gently for liver enlargement, presence of kidneys, and presence of masses. The liver is normally palpable 1 to 3 cm below the costal margin in the midclavicular line. The kidneys are 1 to 2 cm above and to both sides of the umbilicus. Normal findings would include bowel sounds noted in all four quadrants, and no masses or tenderness elicited on palpation. Absent or hyperactive bowel sounds might indicate an intestinal obstruction. Abdominal distention present may indicate ascites, obstruction, infection, masses, or an enlarged abdominal organ (Furdon & Benjamin, 2004).

Inspect the umbilical cord area for the correct amount of blood vessels. The umbilical cord should contain three vessels: two arteries and one vein. The umbilical vein is larger than the two umbilical arteries. Evidence of only a single umbilical artery is associated with renal and GI anomalies. Be sure to count all vessels during the newborn assessment. Also inspect the umbilical area for signs of bleeding, infection, granuloma, or abnormal communication with the intraabdominal organs (Fuloria & Kreiter, 2002b).

Genitalia

Inspect the penis and scrotum in the male. For the circumcised male newborn, the glans should be smooth with the meatus centered at the tip of the penis. For the uncircumcised male, the foreskin should cover the glans. Inspect the position of the urinary meatus, which should be located in the midline at the glans tip. If it is located on the ventral surface of the penis, hypospadias is present; if it is located on the dorsal surface of the penis, it is termed *epispadias*. In either case, **circumcision** should be avoided until further evaluation.

Inspect the scrotum for size, symmetry, color, presence of rugae, and location of testes. The scrotum usually appears relatively large and should be pink in white neonates and dark brown in neonates of color. Rugae should be well formed and should cover the scrotal sac. Bulging, edema, or discoloration should be absent (Fig. 18-14A).

Palpate the scrotum for evidence of testes, which should be in the scrotal sac. The testes should feel firm and smooth, and of equal size on both sides of the scrotal sac in the term newborn. Undescended testes palpated in the inguinal canal are found in preterm infants. Undescended testes (cryptorchidism) can be unilateral or bilateral. If the testes are not palpable within the scrotal sac, further investigation is needed.

If the newborn is a female, inspect the external genitalia. By contrast, the female genitalia will be engorged; labia majora and minora may both be edematous. The labia majora is large and covers the labia minora. The clitoris is large and the hymen is thick. The urethral meatus is located below the clitoris in the midline (Dillon, 2003). All these findings are influenced by a withdrawal of the maternal hormones estrogen and progesterone (Fig. 18-14B). A vaginal discharge composed of mucus mixed with blood may also be present during the first few weeks of life. This discharge, called **pseudomenstruation,** requires no treatment. However, be sure to inform mothers of this finding so that they do not assume that something is wrong with their daughters.

Variations may include a labial bulge, which might indicate an inguinal hernia; ambiguous genitalia; rectovaginal fistula with feces present in the vagina; and an imperforate hymen.

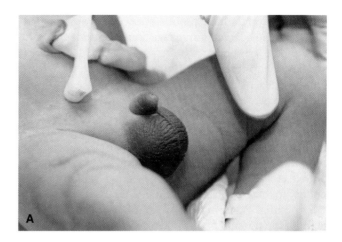

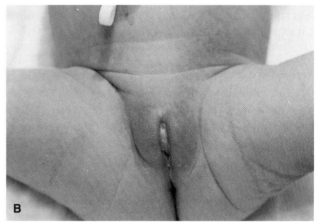

● Figure 18-14 Newborn genitalia. (**A**) Male genitalia. Note the darkened color of the scrotum. (**B**) Female genitalia.

Inspect the anus in both male and female newborns for position and patency. Passage of meconium ensures patency. A healthcare provider can insert a lubricated rectal thermometer or perform a digital examination to determine patency if meconium is not passed. Abnormal findings would include the presence of anal fissures or fistulas and no meconium passed within 24 hours after birth.

Extremities and Back

Inspect the newborn's upper extremities for appearance and movement. Inspect the hands for shape, number, and position of fingers, and presence of palmar creases. The newborn's arms and hands should be symmetric and move through range of motion without hesitation. Observe for spontaneous movement of the extremities. Each hand should have five digits. Note any extra digits (polydactyly) or fusing of two or more digits (syndactyly). Most newborns have three palmar creases of the hand. A single palmar crease, called a *simian line,* is frequently associated with Down syndrome.

A brachial plexus injury can occur during a difficult birth involving shoulder dystocia. Erb palsy is one injury resulting from damage to the upper plexus during birth. Clinically the affected arm hangs limp alongside the body. The affected shoulder and arm are adducted, extended, and internally rotated with a pronated wrist. The Moro reflex is absent on the affected side for brachial palsy. Complete recovery may take 3 to 6 months (Hockenberry, 2005).

Assess the lower extremities in the same manner as that for the upper extremities. The lower extremities should of equal length, with symmetric skin folds. Inspect both feet for a turning inward position (clubfoot) secondary to intrauterine positioning. This may be positional or structural. Perform Ortolani and Barlow maneuvers to identify the possibility of congenital hip dislocation, commonly termed *developmental dysplasia of the hip* (DDH). Nursing Procedure 18-1 highlights the steps for performing these maneuvers.

Inspect the back, including the spine. The spine should appear straight and flat, and should be easily flexed when held in a prone position. Observe for the presence of a tuft of hair, pilonidal dimple in the midline, cyst, or mass along the spine. These would be abnormal findings and need to be documented and reported to the primary health care provider (Table 18-2).

Neurologic Status

Assessment of the newborn's neurologic status involves assessing the newborn's state of alertness, posture, muscle tone, and reflexes. The newborn should be in an alert state and not one of persistent lethargy. The normal posture is one with hips abducted and partially flexed, and with knees flexed. Their arms are adducted and flexed at the elbow. The fists are often clenched, with fingers covering the thumb.

To assess for muscle tone, support the newborn with one hand under the chest. Observe how the neck muscles hold the head. The neck extensors should be able to hold the head in line briefly. Also, there should only be slight head lag when pulling the newborn from a supine position to a sitting one.

Newborn Reflexes

Assess the newborn's reflexes to evaluate neurologic function and development. Absent or abnormal reflexes in a newborn, persistence of a reflex past the age when the reflex is normally lost, or redevelopment of an infantile reflex in an older child or adult may indicate neurologic pathology (Table 18-3). Reflexes commonly assessed in the newborn include sucking reflex, Moro reflex, stepping, tonic neck, rooting, Babinski, and palmar grasp reflex. Spinal reflexes tested include truncal incurvation (Galant reflex) and anocutaneous reflex (anal wink).

The sucking reflex is elicited by gently stimulating the newborn's lips by touching them. The newborn will typically open their mouth and begin a sucking motion. Placing a gloved finger in the newborn's mouth will also educe a sucking motion of the finger (Fig. 18-15A).

The Moro reflex, also called the *embrace reflex,* occurs when the neonate is startled. To elicit this reflex, place the newborn on his back. Support the upper body weight of the supine newborn by the arms using a lifting motion without lifting the newborn off the surface. Then release the arms suddenly. The newborn will throw the arms outward and flex the knees; arms then return to the chest. The fingers also spread to form a C. The newborn initially appears startled, then relaxes to a normal resting position (Fig. 18-15B).

Assess the stepping reflex by holding the newborn upright and inclined forward with the soles of the feet touching a flat surface. Observe the neonate simulating a stepping motion or walking, alternating flexion and extension with the soles of their feet (Fig. 18-15C).

The tonic neck reflex resembles the stance of a fencer and is often called the *fencing reflex.* Test this reflex by having the newborn lie on his back. Then turn his head to one side. The arm toward which the neonate is facing extends straight away from the body with the hand partially open, whereas the arm on the side away from the face is flexed and the fist is clenched tightly. Reversing the direction in which the face is turned reverses the position (Fig. 18-15D).

Elicit the rooting reflex by stroking the newborn's cheek. The newborn will turn toward the side that was stoked and begin to make sucking movements with his mouth (Fig. 18-15E).

The Babinski reflex is present at birth and disappears at approximately 1 year of age. It is educed by stroking the lateral sole of the newborn's foot from the heel toward and across the ball of the foot. The toes should fan out. A diminished response is associated with a neurologic problem and needs follow-up evaluation (Fig. 18-15F).

The newborn exhibits two grasp reflexes: palmar grasp and plantar grasp. Elicit the palmar grasp reflex by placing a finger on the newborn's open palm. The newborn's hand will close around the finger. Attempting to remove the finger causes the grip to tighten. Newborns have strong grasps and can almost be lifted from a flat surface if both hands are used. The grasp should be equal bilaterally (Fig. 18-15G).

The plantar grasp is similar to the palmar grasp. Place a finger against the area just below the newborn's toes. The newborns' toes typically curl over the finger (Fig. 18-15H).

Blinking, sneezing, gagging, and coughing are all protective reflexes and are elicited when an object or light is brought close to the eye (blinking), something irritating is swallowed or a bulb syringe is used for suctioning (gagging and coughing), or an irritant is brought in close proximity to the nose (sneezing).

The truncal incurvation reflex (Galant reflex) is present at birth and disappears in a few days to 4 weeks. With the newborn in a prone position or held in ventral suspension, apply firm pressure and run a finger down either side of the spine. This stroking will cause the pelvis to flex toward the stimulated side. This indicates T2–S1

Nursing Procedure 18-1

Performing Ortolani and Barlow Maneuvers

Purpose: To Detect Possible Congenital Developmental Dysplasia of the Hip

Ortolani Maneuver

1. Place the newborn in the supine position and flex the hips and knees to 90 degrees at the hip.
2. Grasp the inner aspect of the thighs and abduct the hips (usually to approximately 180 degrees) while applying upward pressure.

Barlow Maneuver

1. With the newborn still lying supine and grasping the inner aspect of the thighs (as just mentioned), adduct the thighs while applying outward and downward pressure to the thighs.

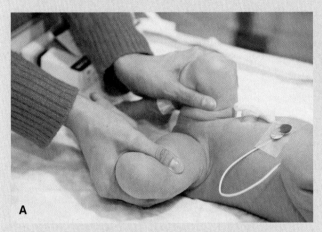

A

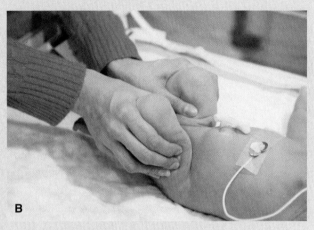

B

3. Listen for any sounds during the maneuver. There should be no "cluck" or "click" heard when the legs are abducted. Evidence of such a sound indicates the femoral head hitting the acetabulum as the head reenters the area. This suggests developmental hip dysplasia.

2. Feel for the femoral head slipping out of the acetabulum; also listen for a click (Haws, 2004).

innervation. An absent response would indicate a neurologic or spinal cord problem.

The anocutaneous reflex (anal wink) is elicited by stimulating the perianal skin close to the anus. The external sphincter will constrict (wink) immediately with stimulation. This indicates S4–5 innervation (Verklan & Walden, 2004).

Nursing Interventions

Becoming parents with the confidence to care for their newborn is challenging for most couples. It takes time and patience with a great deal of instruction provided by the nurse. "Showing and telling" parents about their newborn and all the necessary procedures (feeding, bathing, changing, handling) involved in daily care are key nursing interventions.

Providing General Newborn Care

Nurses role model appropriate care and provide teaching as necessary to meet the needs of the newborn. Generally,

newborn care involves bathing and hygiene, diaper care, cord care, circumcision care, use of appropriate clothing, environmental safety measures, and prevention of infection. Nurses can help families in these areas by role modeling appropriate and consistent interaction with newborns. Demonstration of respect for the newborn and his family is essential in fostering a positive atmosphere to promote the newborn's growth and development.

Bathing and Hygiene

Newborns are bathed primarily for aesthetic reasons. Such bathing is postponed until thermal and cardiorespiratory stability is ensured. The reasons cited for nurses bathing the newborn are to conduct a physical assessment, reduce the effect of hypothermia, and allow the mother to rest (Medves & O'Brien, 2004). Recent research suggests that nurses do not need to give the newborn an initial bath to reduce heat loss. Rather, the parents could be given this opportunity, supported by nurses. Heat loss was similar in newborns bathed by parents when com-

Table 18-2 Newborn Assessment Summary

Assessment	Usual Findings	Variations and Common Problems
Anthropometric measurements	Head circumference: 33–37 cm (13–14 in) Chest circumference: 30–33 cm (12–13 in) Weight: 2500–4000 g (5.5–8.5 lb) Length: 45–55 cm (19–21 in)	SGA, LGA, preterm, postterm
Vital signs	Temperature: 36.5–37.5°C (97–99°F) Apical pulse: 120–180 bpm Respirations: 30–60 breaths/minute	
Skin	Normal: smooth, flexible, good skin turgor, warm	Jaundice, acrocyanosis, milia, mongolian spots, stork bites
Head	Normal: varies with age, gender, and ethnicity	Microcephaly, macrocephaly, enlarged fontanelles
Face	Normal: full cheeks, facial features symmetric	Facial nerve paralysis, nevus flammeus, nevus vasculosus
Nose	Normal: small, placement in the midline and narrow, ability to smell	Malformation or blockage
Mouth	Normal: aligned in midline, symmetric, intact soft and hard palate	Epstein's pearls, erupted precocious teeth, thrush
Neck	Normal: short, creased, moves freely, holds head in midline	Restricted movement, clavicular fractures
Eyes	Normal: clear and symmetrically placed on face	Chemical conjunctivitis, subconjunctival hemorrhages
Ears	Normal: soft and pliable with quick recoil when folded and released	Low-set ears, hearing loss
Chest	Normal: round, symmetric, smaller than head	Nipple engorgement, whitish discharge
Abdomen	Normal: protuberant contour, soft, three vessels in umbilical cord	Distended, only two vessels in umbilical cord
Genitals	Normal male: smooth glans, meatus centered at tip of penis Normal female: swollen female genitals as a result of maternal estrogen	Edematous scrotum in males, vaginal discharge in females
Extremities and spine	Normal: extremities symmetric with free movement	Congenital hip dislocation; tuft or dimple on spine

pared with newborns who were bathed by nurses (Medves & O'Brien, 2004).

Wear gloves because of potential exposure to maternal blood on the newborn and perform the bath quickly, making sure to dry the newborn thoroughly to prevent heat loss by evaporation. Begin the bath, proceeding from the "cleanest" (eyes) to the most soiled area (diaper area) to prevent cross-contamination.

Use plain warm water on the face and eyes, adding a mild soap (such as Dove) to cleanse the remainder of the body. Instructing the parents to wash the face and neck gently after each feeding will help prevent rashes and prevent the odor that can develop when milk accumulates in the neck creases.

Washing the newborn's hair is best carried out close to a source of running water to afford thorough rinsing of the scalp. A mild shampoo or soap can be used to wash the hair and scalp. Wash both fontanel areas. Frequently parents choose to avoid these "soft spots" because they fear that they will "hurt their newborn's brain" if they rub too hard. Reassure parents that there is a strong membrane providing protection. Urge the parents to clean and rinse these areas well. If the anterior fontanelle is not rinsed well after shampooing, cradle cap—dry flakes on the scalp—can develop. Figure 18-16 shows the nurse demonstrating bathing a newborn while the father watches.

After bathing, place the newborn under the radiant warmer and wrap him securely in blankets to prevent

Table 18-3 Newborn Reflexes: Appearance and Disappearance

Reflex	Appearance	Disappearance
Blinking	Newborn	Persist into adulthood
Moro	Newborn	3–6 mo
Grasp	Newborn	3–4 mo
Stepping	Birth	1–2 mo
Tonic neck	Newborn	3–4 mo
Sneeze	Newborn	Persist into adulthood
Rooting	Birth	4–6 mo
Gag reflex	Newborn	Persist into adulthood
Cough reflex	Newborn	Persist into adulthood
Babinski sign	Newborn	12 mo

If the newborn has been circumcised, advise parents to wait until that area has also healed (usually 1–2 weeks). Clean the penis with mild soap and water and apply a small amount of Vaseline to the tip to prevent the diaper from adhering to the penis. Instruct parents to apply the diaper loosely and place the newly circumcised male infant on his side or back to prevent pressure and irritation on the penis.

Encourage the parents to gather items needed before starting the bath. These items include a soft, clean washcloth; two cotton balls to clean the eyes; mild, unscented soap and shampoo; towels or blankets; an infant tub with warm water; a clean diaper; and a change of clothes. Then provide the parents helpful guidelines for bathing their newborn (see Teaching Guidelines 18-1).

Elimination and Diaper Area Care

Newborn elimination patterns are highly individualized. Usually, urine is light amber in color, with newborns typically soaking 6 to 12 diapers per day, indicating adequate hydration. Stool characteristics change in color, texture, and frequency without signaling a problem. The normal progression of bowel movement changes include

1. Meconium—thick, tarry, sticky, dark green for the first 48 hours after birth
2. Transitional—thin, brown to green, typically appearing by day 3 after initiation of feeding; less sticky than meconium

Stool characteristics after transitional stool depend on whether the newborn is breast-fed or bottle-fed. Breast-fed newborns typically pass mustard-colored, soft stool with a seedy consistency; formula-fed newborns pass yellow to brown, formed stool with a pasty consistency. As long as the newborn seems content, is eating normally, and shows no signs of illness, the minor changes in bowel movements should not be a concern.

The newborn needs to be checked frequently to ascertain whether a diaper change is needed, especially after feeding. Be sure to adhere to standard precautions when providing diaper area care. Instruct parents to apply the new diaper top edge below the umbilical cord area to prevent irritation and to provide air to assist in drying the cord.

Meconium, the first stool passed by the newborn, can be difficult to remove from the skin. Use plain water or special cleansing wipes if necessary to clean the area.

Provide parents with instructions on how to clean the diaper area properly and how to prevent skin irritation. Encourage the avoidance of products such as powder and items with fragrance, which could promote irritation. Also discuss the pros and cons of using cloth diapers versus disposable diapers so that the parents can make informed decisions. Regardless of the type of diapers used, parents will need up to 10 diapers a day, or about

chilling. Check his temperature within an hour to validate it is within normal limits. If it is low, place the newborn under a radiant heat source.

The literature suggests that tub bathing, as opposed to sponge bathing, can be done without significantly lowering the newborn's temperature or increasing rates of cord infection in healthy term newborns (Bryanton, Walsh, Barrett, & Gaudet, 2004). Drying the newborn and removing blood may minimize the risk of infection caused by hepatitis B, herpes virus, and HIV. Specific benefits of this practice remain unclear currently. Until the newborn has been thoroughly bathed, standard precautions should be used when handling the newborn. Typically, a bath two or three times weekly is sufficient for the first year. More frequent bathing may be drying to the skin.

After the initial bath, the newborn may not receive another full one during the birthing unit stay. The diaper area will be cleansed at each diaper change, and any milk spilled will be cleaned. Clear water and a mild soap are appropriate to cleanse the diaper area. The use of lotions, baby oil, and powders is not encouraged because all can lead to skin irritation and potential rashes. If the parents desire to use them, have them apply a small amount onto their hand first, away from the newborn. Doing so helps to warm the lotion. Then instruct the parents to apply the lotion or oil sparingly.

The current recommendation is to advise parents not to immerse their newborns into water fully until the umbilical cord area is healed—about 2 weeks after birth. A sponge bath is encouraged until the umbilical cord falls off and the navel area is completely healed.

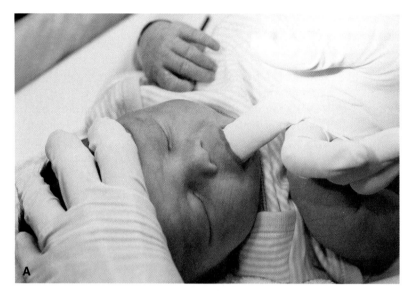

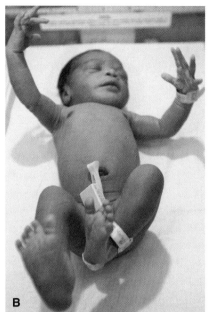

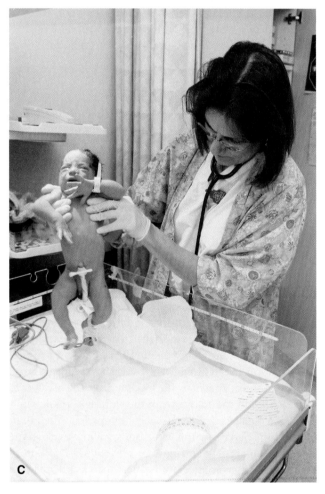

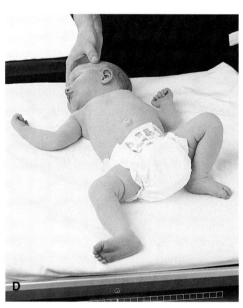

● Figure 18-15 Newborn reflexes. (**A**) Sucking reflex. (**B**) Moro reflex. (**C**) Stepping reflex. (**D**) Tonic neck reflex. (**E**) Rooting reflex. (**F**) Babinski reflex. (**G**) Palmar grasp. (**H**) Plantar grasp.

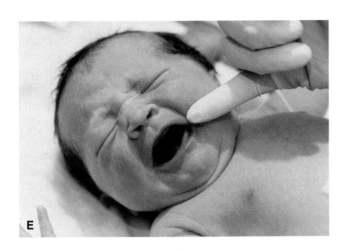

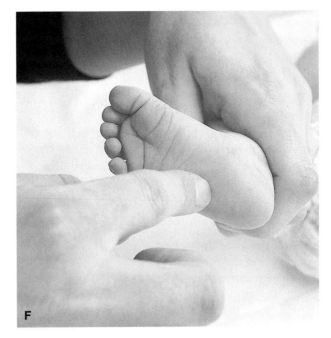

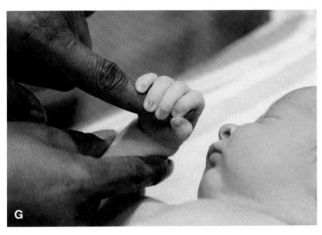

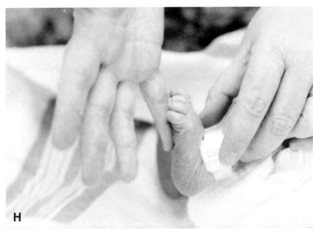

● Figure 18-15 (continued)

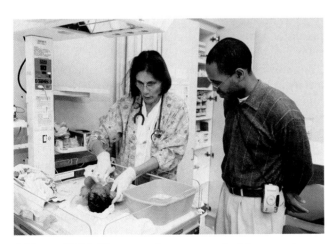

● Figure 18-16 The nurse demonstrates bathing a newborn while the father watches.

70 a week. Additional helpful information concerning diapering might include

- Before diapering, make sure all supplies are within reach, including clean diaper, cleaning agent or wipes, and ointment
- Lay the newborn on a changing table and remove the dirty diaper
- Use water and mild soap or wipes to gently wipe the genital area clean; wipe from front to back for girls to avoid a UTI
- Always wash hands thoroughly before and after changing diapers

While performing diaper area care, urge parents to observe the area closely for irritation or rash. Some helpful tips for preventing or healing a diaper rash include

TEACHING GUIDELINES 18-1

Bathing a Newborn

- Select a warm room with a flat surface at a comfortable working height.
- Before the bath, gather all supplies needed so they will be within reach.
- Never leave the newborn alone or unattended at any time during the bath.
- Undress the newborn down to his shirt and diaper.
- Always support the newborn's head and neck when moving or positioning him.
- Place a blanket or towel underneath the newborn for warmth and comfort.
- Follow this order, progressing from the cleanest to the dirtiest areas:
  - Wipe eyes with plain water either with cotton balls or a washcloth.
  - Wipe from the inner corner of the eyes to the outer with separate wipes.
  - Wash the rest of the face, including ears, with plain water.
  - Using baby shampoo, gently wash the head and rinse with water.
  - Pay special attention to body creases and dry thoroughly.
  - Wash extremities, trunk, and back: wash, rinse, dry, cover.
  - Wash diaper area last with soap and water and dry; observe for rash.
- Diaper and dress newborn at the conclusion of the bath.

- Changing diapers frequently, especially after bowel movements
- Applying a "barrier" cream, such as A & D ointment, after cleaning with mild soap and water
- Using dye and fragrance-free detergents for cloth diaper washing
- Avoiding the use of plastic pants because they tend to hold in moisture
- Exposing the newborn's bottom to air several times a day
- Placing the newborn's buttocks in warm water after having had a diaper on all night

Advise parents that if a rash does develop and persists for more than 3 days, the rash may be fungal in origin and may require additional treatment. Encourage the parents to notify the newborn's healthcare provider.

Cord Care

The umbilical cord begins drying within hours after birth and is shriveled and blackened by the second or third day. Within 7 to 10 days, it sloughs off and the umbilicus heals. During this transition, frequent assessments of the area are necessary to detect any bleeding or signs of infection. Cord bleeding is abnormal and may occur if the cord clamp is loosened. Any cord drainage is also abnormal and is generally caused by infection, which requires immediate treatment.

During each diaper change, apply the appropriate agent (such as triple dye, alcohol, or an antimicrobial agent), according to facility policy, to the cord stump to prevent any ascending infections. Single-use agents for cleaning are recommended to prevent cross-contamination with other newborns. Expect to remove the cord clamp approximately 24 hours after birth by using a cord-cutting clamp. However, if the cord is still moist, keep the clamp in place and ensure a referral to home health care so that the home care nurse can remove it after discharge. Always adhere to agency policies regarding cord care, being aware that changes may be necessary based on emerging research.

Because of the appearance of the cord site, many parents avoid contact with it to make sure they don't "bother" it. Advising them how to care for the cord site when they go home will hopefully prevent any complications from occurring (see Teaching Guidelines 18-2).

Circumcision Care

Circumcision is the surgical removal of all or part of the foreskin (prepuce) of the male penis (O'Toole, 2003). This has been traditionally done for hygienic and medical reasons and is the oldest known religious rite. In the Jewish faith, the circumcision is a ritual that is performed by a *mohel* (ordained circumciser) on the eighth day after birth if possible. The circumcision is then followed by a religious ceremony during which the newborn is also named.

During the circumcision procedure, part of the foreskin is removed by clamping and cutting with a scalpel (Gomco or Mogen clamp) or by using a plastic ring with a string tied around it to trim off the excess foreskin (Plastibell). Small sutures of pressure from the plastic ring are used to prevent bleeding and to promote wound closure (Littleton & Engebretson, 2005) (Fig. 18-17).

The debate over the practice of routine newborn circumcision remains alive and well in the United States. For many years, the purported benefits and harms of circumcision have been debated in the medical literature and society at large, with no clear consensus to date. Despite controversy about its indications, circumcision remains a procedure that is performed worldwide in large numbers. It is the most common surgical procedure performed on newborns, with almost two thirds of American male newborns being circumcised (Cunningham et al., 2005).

A policy statement by the AAP indicated that newborn circumcision has potential medical benefits and advantages as well as disadvantages and risks. For the first time in AAP circumcision policy history, the new recommendations also indicate that if parents decide to circumcise their newborn, it is essential that pain relief be provided. Research reports

TEACHING GUIDELINES 18-2

Umbilical Cord Care

- Apply alcohol or the recommended solution to the cord site at each diaper change to help dry it.
- Observe for any bleeding, redness, drainage, or foul odor from the cord stump and report it to your newborn's primary care provider immediately.
- Avoid tub baths until the cord has fallen off and the area has healed.
- Expose the cord stump to the air as much as possible throughout day.
- Fold diapers below the level of the cord to prevent contamination of the site and to promote air drying of the cord.
- Observe the cord stump, which will change color from yellow to brown to black. This is normal.
- Never pull the cord or attempt to loosen it; it will fall off naturally.

that newborns circumcised without analgesia experience pain and stress measured by changes in heart rate, blood pressure, oxygen saturation, and cortisol levels (Razmus, Dalton, & Wilson, 2004). Subsequently, the AAP policy recommends that analgesia be provided if the procedure is performed. Analgesic methods may include EMLA cream (a topical mixture of local anesthetics), a dorsal penile nerve block with buffered lidocaine, acetaminophen, sucrose pacifier, and swaddling (Cunningham et al., 2005). When being considered, the AAP recommends that parents be given accurate and unbiased information regarding the risks and benefits of the procedure.

The nurse's major responsibility is to inform the parents of the risks and benefits of the procedure and to address concerns so that the parents can reach a fully informed decision. Risks for the newborn include infection, hemorrhage, skin dehiscence, adhesions, potential urethral fistula, and pain. Benefits to the newborn include

decreased incidence of UTIs and sexually transmitted infections (STIs), and possible prevention of penile cancer:

- UTIs—slightly less common in circumcised boys; however, rates of UTI are low in both groups and are easily treated without long-term sequelae
- STIs—risk believed to be related more to behavioral factors than circumcision status except for HIV, which had a decrease in the risk of acquiring it of 50% (Kinkade & Meadows, 2005).
- Penile cancer—extremely rare in the United States. There appears to be a slightly lower rate of penile cancer in circumcised males; however, risk factors such as genital warts, infection with human papilloma virus (HPV), multiple sex partners, and cigarette smoking seem to play a much lager role in causing penile cancer than circumcision status (Dickey, 2002; Zepf, 2002).

Most studies are inconclusive concerning circumcision preventing STIs, cervical and penile cancer, and UTIs. The decision to circumcise the male newborn is often a social one made by parents, with the strongest factor associated with the decision being whether the newborn's father is himself circumcised (Bar-Yam, 2002).

The absence of compelling medical evidence in favor of or against newborn circumcision makes informed consent of parents paramount. The circumcision discussion involves cultural, religious, medical, and emotional considerations. Nurses may have difficulty remaining unbiased and unemotional as they present facts to the parents trying to make a decision. Nurses must remember that circumcision is a very personal decision for parents, involving medical, cultural, religious, and family considerations.

As with other newborn procedures, research on risks and benefits continues. Nurses must be informed about current medical research to help parents untangle the data to make truly informed decisions that are most comfortable for them.

Immediately after circumcision, the tip of the penis is usually covered with petroleum jelly-coated gauze to

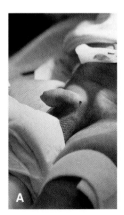 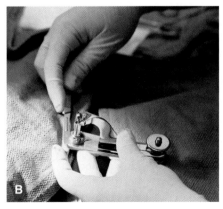 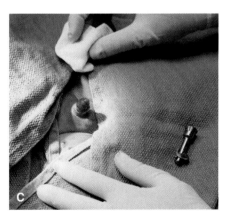

● Figure 18-17 Circumcision. (**A**) Before the procedure. (**B**) Clamp applied and foreskin removed. (**C**) Appearance after circumcision.

keep the wound from sticking to the diaper. Continued care of this site includes

- Squeezing soapy water over the area and then rinsing the area with warm water and patting dry daily
- Applying a small amount of petroleum jelly with every diaper change
- Fastening the diaper loosely over the penis and avoiding placing newborn on his abdomen to prevent friction

If a Plastibell has been used, it will fall off by itself in about a week. Inform parents of this and advise them never to pull it off sooner. Also instruct the parents to check daily for any foul-smelling drainage, bleeding, or unusual swelling.

If the newborn is uncircumcised, wash the penis with mild soap and water after each diaper change and refrain from forcing the foreskin back; it will retract normally over time.

Safety

Newborns are completely dependent on those around them to ensure their safety. Their safety must be ensured while in the health care facility and after they are discharged. Parental education is key, especially as the newborn grows and develops, and begins to respond to and explore his surroundings (see Teaching Guidelines 18-3).

Environmental Safety

People who enter any health care facility for treatment expect to be safe there until they return to their homes. Today, perhaps more than ever before, birthing centers and acute care hospitals face the daunting challenge of ensuring that all people have a safe environment while interacting within their facilities.

Consider this scenario: A woman dressed in nurse's clothing entered the hospital room of a new mother soon after she had given birth. This "nurse" told the mother she needed to take her newborn to the nursery to have him weighed. Sometime later, a staff nurse making her routine rounds realized something was wrong when she saw that the newborn's bassinet in the mother's room was empty and the mother was sound asleep in her bed. The staff nurse called security immediately because she suspected a newborn abduction had taken place.

This scenario represents a typical abduction that is repeated many times throughout the United States each year. An **infant abduction** is the taking of a child less than 1 year old by a nonfamily member (Burns, 2003). Infant abductions are extremely traumatic for the parents and affect the local community and beyond, possibly making national headlines. In addition, facilities may be faced with enormous insurance liability suits filed by the parents.

Unfortunately, research on infant abduction is limited. What is known about abductions is that they are usually carried out by women during daylight hours who are not

 TEACHING GUIDELINES 18-3

General Newborn Safety

- Have emergency telephone numbers readily available, such as those for emergency medical assistance and the poison control center.
- Keep small or sharp objects out of reach to prevent their aspiration.
- Put safety plugs in wall sockets within reach to prevent accidental electrocution.
- Do not leave the infant alone in any room without a portable intercom on.
- Always supervise a newborn in the tub, because she can drown in 2 in of water.
- Make sure the crib or changing table is sturdy, without any loose hardware, and is painted with lead-free paint.
- Avoid placing the crib or changing table near blinds or curtain cords.
- Provide a smoke-free environment for all infants.
- Place all infants on their backs to sleep to prevent SIDS.
- Prevent falls by not leaving a newborn alone on any elevated surface.
- Use sun shields on strollers and hats to avoid overexposing the newborn to the sun.
- Thoroughly wash hands before formula preparation to prevent infection.
- Thoroughly investigate any infant care facility before using (Brent & Weitzman, 2004)

criminally sophisticated. They may have experienced a pregnancy loss in the past and are often emotionally immature and compulsive, with low self-esteem. Most female abductors are able to play the role of a hospital employee convincingly and meet their objective of securing an infant (Shogan, 2002). Health care agencies are challenged to secure the newborn's safety with sound security practices and systems to prevent abduction (Rabun, 2003).

Preventative measures include

- Mandating that all newborns be transported in cribs and not carried
- Responding immediately to any security alarm that sounds on the unit
- Never leaving newborns unattended at any time, especially in hallways
- Ensuring that all staff wear appropriate identification at all times
- Being suspicious of visitors who do not seem to be visiting a specific mother
- Participating in checking the electronic security system to validate that it works
- Ensuring proper functioning and placement of any electronic sensors used on newborns

- Assessing parents' knowledge and providing education as necessary, such as
  - What infant abduction is
  - Why infant security is important
  - The facility's security policies and procedures
  - What they can do to protect their infant while they are there
  - Rules about visitor access while they are there
  - Which staff is allowed to handle the newborn
  - What a proper ID looks like

Providing a safe and secure environment in the birth center is a shared responsibility of the facility, staff, and parents. Only if all are educated about the rules and policies can safety be achieved and abductions stopped.

Car Safety

Every state requires the use of car seats for infants and children when riding in a car, because motor vehicle accidents are still the leading cause of unintentional injury and death in children under the age of five (AAP, 2005b). In more than half these deaths, the child was unrestrained, despite the known effectiveness of federally approved car seats in reducing morbidity and mortality in such crashes (AAP, 2005b).

The value of infant safety seats to prevent injury and death is well accepted. It has been shown that a lack of knowledge about them may contribute to under use and misuse of these devices (AAP, 2005b). It is imperative that nurses educate parents about this vital life-saving device and not release any newborn unless they have secured one for their first ride home (Fig. 18-18).

Prior to discharge from the hospital or birthing center, ascertain whether the parents have secured an infant car seat to transport their newborn home. If they cannot afford to purchase one, many community organizations will provide one for them. Make sure that both parents understand the importance of safely transporting their newborn in a federally approved safety car seat every time the infant rides in a car.

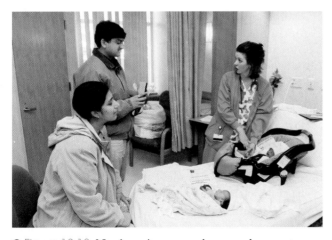

● Figure 18-18 Newborn in a properly secured car seat.

According to the AAP, no one car seat is considered to be the "safest" or the "best," but rather consistent and proper use will prevent injuries and deaths. Instruct parents in the following:

- Selecting a car seat that is appropriate for the newborn's size and weight, and using it correctly, including every time the newborn is in the car
- Using only rear-facing car seats for infants until they are at least 1 year old or weigh 20 lb
- Ensuring that the harness (most seats have a three to five-point harness) is in the slots at or below the shoulders

Infection Prevention

The nurse plays a major role in preventing infection within the newborn environment. The nurse needs to institute measures to control infection by minimizing exposure of newborns to organisms; washing hands before and after providing care; insisting that all personnel wash their hands before handling any newborn; not allowing ill staff or visitors to visit or handle newborns; monitoring umbilical cord stump and circumcision site for signs of infection; providing eye prophylaxis by instilling prescribed medication soon after birth; and educating parents about appropriate home measures that will prevent infections such as practicing good hand washing before and after diaper changes, keeping their newborn well hydrated, avoiding bringing their infant into public crowds (which may expose him or her to colds and flu viruses), observing for any early signs of symptoms of infection (elevated temperature, vomiting, loss of appetite, lethargy, labored breathing, green watery stools, drainage from umbilical cord site or eyes), and making sure to keep pediatrician appointments for routine **immunizations.**

Sleeping

Although many parents feel their newborns need them every minute of the day, they actually need sleep much of the day initially. Usually newborns sleep up to 15 hours daily, sleeping for periods of 2 to 4 hours at a time, but not sleeping through the night. This is because their stomach capacity is too small to go long periods of time without nourishment. All newborns develop their own sleep patterns and cycles, with parents possibly waiting several months before the newborn sleeps through the night.

Additional tips to share with parents would include placing the newborn on her back to sleep; removing all fluffy bedding, quilts, sheepskins, stuffed animals, and pillows from the crib to prevent potential suffocation; and avoiding bed sharing. Bringing a newborn into bed to nurse or quiet her down, and then falling asleep with the newborn is not a safe practice. Counsel parents about the potential risks. For example, infants who sleep in adult beds are up to 40 times more likely to suffocate than those who sleep in cribs (McGinnis, 2004). Suffocation also can occur when the infant gets entangled in bedding or caught under pillows, or slips between the bed and the wall or the headboard and mattress. It can also happen when someone accidentally rolls against or on top of them. Therefore, the safest sleeping location for all newborns is in their cribs without any movable objects close by. In addition, teach parents to avoid unsafe conditions for newborn sleeping, such as placing the newborn in the prone position, using a crib that does not meet federal safety guidelines, allowing window cords to hang loose and in close proximity to crib, or having the room temperature too high to cause overheating (Page-Goertz, 2004).

Enhancing Bonding

Encourage and enhance parent–newborn interaction by involving both parents with the new member of their family, and demonstrating and role modeling appropriate behaviors. To promote positive parent–newborn interactions, the following suggestions might help enhance the ways to model nurturing care:

- Say "hello" and introduce yourself to the newborn.
- Ask the parents permission to provide care and hold their newborn. This simple question assists parents in assimilating their new role of being responsible for their child and reminds nurses of their role.
- Show parents the power of a soothing voice to calm the newborn.
- Provide care to the newborn in the least stressful way for her.
- Demonstrate ways to wake the newborn up gently to feed better.
- Tell parents what you are doing, why you are doing it, and how they can duplicate what you are doing in their home environment.
- Offer the opportunity to perform care while you observe them. Affirm their efforts to soothe the newborn throughout the care process.
- Assist parents to understand the whole repertoire of "language" and communication cues the newborn uses to meet their needs.
- Point out the efforts the newborn is making to connect with the parents (e.g., alerting to the familiar voice, following the parents while they are speaking, quieting when held securely).

One of the most pleasurable aspects of newborn care is being close to them. Bonding begins soon after birth when parents cradle their newborn and gently stroke them with their fingers. Provide each parent with opportunities for "skin-to-skin" contact with their newborn, holding them against their own skin when feeding or cradling. Many newborns respond very positively to gentle massage. If necessary, recommend appropriate books and videos that cover the subject.

Newborns cry for a variety of reasons, because it is their only way to communicate that something is wrong.

Try to find out the reason *why* by making sure there is a dry diaper, the temperature of the room is not too hot or too cold, and checking for signs of discomfort such as a diaper rash or tight clothing. Suggest the following ways in which parents can soothe an upset newborn:

- Try feeding or burping to relieve air or stomach gas.
- Lightly rub the newborn's back and speak softly to her.
- Gently rock side to side by swaying or rock back and forth in a rocking chair.
- Talk with the newborn while making eye contact.
- Take the newborn for a walk in a stroller or carriage to get fresh air.
- Change the position from back to side or vice versa.
- Try singing, reciting poetry and nursery rhymes, or reading to her.
- Turn on a musical mobile above the newborn's head.
- Give more physical contact by walking, rocking, or patting the newborn.
- Swaddle the newborn to provide a sense of security and comfort. To do this
  1. Spread out a receiving blanket, with one corner folded slightly
  2. Lay the newborn face up with head at the folded corner.
  3. Wrap the left corner over her body and tuck it beneath her.
  4. Bring the bottom corner over her feet.
  5. Wrap the right corner around her, leaving only the head exposed.

Assisting With Screening Tests

Screening newborns for problems is important because some will be born with potentially life-threatening metabolic disease that may not be obvious at birth. Newborn screening tests that are required in most states for newborns before discharge from the birth facility evaluate certain genetic and inborn errors of metabolism and hearing. Early identification and initiation of treatment can prevent significant complications and can minimize the negative effects of untreated disease.

Genetic and Inborn Errors of Metabolism Screening

Although each state mandates which conditions must be tested, most commonly tests screen for PKU, hypothyroidism, galactosemia, sickle cell disease, as well as many other conditions.

The trend toward early discharge of newborns before 48 hours of age can influence the timing of screening and the accuracy of some test results. For example, the newborn needs to ingest enough breast milk or formula to elevate phenylalanine levels for the screening test to identify PKU accurately. Because of this needed time for the ingestion of protein, newborn screening for PKU testing should not be performed before 24 hours of age.

Screening tests for genetic and inborn errors of metabolism require a few drops of blood taken from the newborn's heel (Fig. 18-19). These tests are usually performed shortly before discharge. Newborns who are discharged prior to 24 hours of age need to have repeat tests done within a week in an outpatient healthcare facility. Selected conditions that are screened for in the newborn are summarized in Table 18-4.

Be aware of which conditions your state regularly screens for at birth to ensure that the families receive the necessary education about the tests and the importance of early treatment. Also be familiar with the optimal time frame for screening and conditions that could adversely influence results. Ensure that a satisfactory specimen has been obtained at the appropriate time and that circumstances that could cause false results have been minimized. Send out specimens and completed forms within 24 hours of collection to the appropriate laboratory (Spahis, 2003).

Hearing Screening

Universal screening programs have been implemented across the United States. Screening only those infants who

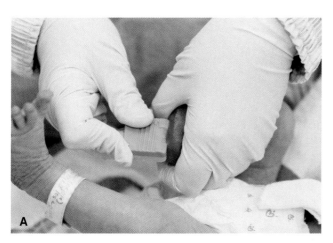

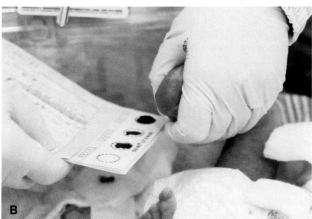

● Figure 18-19 Screening for PKU. (**A**) Performing a heel stick. (**B**) Applying the blood specimen to the required card for screening.

have a risk history is not enough, because as many as 50% of infants born with hearing loss have no known risk factors (De Michele & Ruth, 2005). Early identification and intervention can prevent severe psychosocial, educational, and language development delays.

Hearing loss is the most common birth disorder in the United States. Approximately three to five newborns of every 1000 have some degree of hearing loss. Unlike a physical deformity, hearing loss is not clinically detectable at birth and thus remains difficult to assess (De Michele & Ruth, 2005). Factors associated with an increased risk of hearing loss include

- Positive family history of childhood sensory hearing loss
- Congenital infections such as cytomegalovirus, rubella, toxoplasmosis, herpes
- Cranial facial anomalies involving the pinna or ear canal
- LBW of less than 1500 g
- Postnatal infections such as bacterial meningitis
- Head trauma
- Hyperbilirubinemia requiring an exchange transfusion
- Exposure to ototoxic drugs, especially aminoglycosides
- Perinatal asphyxia (De Michele & Ruth, 2005)

Delays in identification and intervention may affect language development, academic performance, and cognitive development in the older child. Detection before 3 months greatly improves outcomes. Because of this, auditory screening of all newborns is recommended by the AAP and is mandated by law in the majority of states. The current goals of Healthy People 2010 (see Healthy People 2010 display earlier in this chapter) are to screen all infants by 1 month of age, confirm hearing loss with audiologic examination by 3 months of age, and treat with comprehensive early intervention services before 6 months of age (Murray et al., 2004).

All newborns should be screened prior to discharge to ensure that any newborn with a hearing loss is not missed. Those with suspected hearing loss should be referred for follow-up assessment (see Box 18-1 for screening methods). In addition, nurses work to ensure that screening is accurate to facilitate early diagnosis and intervention services, and to optimize the newborn's developmental potential.

Promoting Nutrition

Several physiologic changes dictate the type and method of feeding throughout the newborn's first year. Some of these changes include the following:

- Stomach capacity is limited to about 90 mL at birth. The emptying time is short (2–3 hours) and peristalsis is rapid. Small, frequent feedings are needed early during the newborn and infancy period, with amounts progressively increasing with maturity.
- Immune system is immature at birth with a high risk for food allergies for the first 4 to 6 months of life.

Table 18-4 Selected Conditions Screened for in the Newborn

Condition	Description	Clinical Picture/ Effect If Not Treated	Treatment	Timing of Screening
PKU	Autosomal recessive inherited deficiency in one of the enzymes necessary for the metabolism of phenylalanine to tyrosine—essential amino acids found in most foods	Irritability, vomiting of protein feedings, and a musty odor to the skin or body secretions of the newborn; if not treated, mental and motor retardation, seizures, microcephaly, and poor growth and development	Lifetime diet of foods low in phenylalanine (low protein) and monitoring of blood levels (Spahis, 2003); special newborn formulas available: Phenex and Lofenalac	Universally screened for in the United States, testing done 24–48 hours after protein feeding (PKU)
Congenital hypothyroidism	Deficiency of thyroid hormone necessary for normal brain growth, calorie metabolism, and development; possibly resulting from maternal hypothyroidism	Increased risk for newborns with birth weight <2000 g or >4500 g, and those of Hispanic and Asian ethnic groups; feeding problems, growth and breathing problems; if not treated, irreversible brain damage and mental retardation	Lifelong thyroid replacement therapy (CMS, 2004).	Testing (measures thyroxin (T4) and TSH) done between fourth and sixth days of life
Galactosemia	Absence of the enzyme needed for the conversion of the milk sugar galactose to glucose	Poor weight gain, vomiting, jaundice, mood changes, loss of eyesight, seizures, and mental retardation; if untreated, galactose buildup causing permanent damage to the brain, eyes, liver, and eventually death	Elimination of milk from diet and substitute soy milk	First test done on discharge from the hospital with a follow-up test within 1 month
Sickle cell anemia	Recessively inherited abnormality in hemoglobin structure, most commonly found in African-American newborns	Anemia developing shortly after birth; increased risk for infection, growth restriction, vasoocclusive crisis	Maintenance of hydration and hemodilution, rest, electrolyte replacement, pain management, blood replacement, and antibiotics	Bloodspot obtained at same time of other newborn screening tests or prior to 3 months of age

---

BOX 18-1

NEWBORN HEARING SCREENING METHODS

A newborn's hearing can be screened one of two ways: otoacoustic emission (OAE) or automated auditory brainstem response (ABR). OAE technology requires placing an earphone in the infant's ear canal and measuring sounds produced by the newborn's inner ear in response to certain tones or clicks presented through the earphone. Preset parameters in the equipment decide whether the OAEs are sufficient for the newborn to pass or whether a referral is necessary for further evaluation.

ABR requires placing an earphone in the ear canal or an earmuff over the newborn's ear, through which a soft, rapid tapping noise is presented. Electrodes placed around the newborn's head, neck, and shoulders record neural activity from the infant's brainstem in response to the tapping noises. The ABR tests how well the ear and the nerves leading to the brain work. Like OAEs, automated ABR screening is sensitive to more than mild degrees of hearing loss, but a pass does not provide a guarantee of normal hearing (Fligor & Neault, 2004).

Introduction of solid foods prior to this time would only increase the risk of developing food allergies.

- Pancreatic enzymes and bile are in limited supply to assist in digestion of fat and starch until about 3 to 6 months if age. Infants are unable to digest cereal prior to this period, despite many parents adding it to their bottles.
- Kidneys are immature and not able to concentrate urine until about 4 to 6 weeks of age. Excess protein and mineral intake can place a strain on kidney function and can lead to dehydration. Infants need to consume more water per unit of body weight than adults do as a result of their high body weight from water.
- Immature muscular control at birth changes over time to assist in the feeding process by improving head and neck control, hand–eye coordination, swallowing, and ability to sit, grasp, and chew. At about 4 to 6 months, inborn reflexes disappear, head control develops, and the infant is able to sit to be fed, making spoon feeding possible (Dudek, 2006).

The newborn can be fed at any time during the transition period if assessments are normal and a desire is demonstrated. Before the newborn may be fed, determine the ability to suck and swallow. Clear any mucus present in the nares or mouth with a bulb syringe prior to initiating feeding. Auscultate bowel sounds, check for abdominal distention and inspect the anus for patency. After these feeding parameters are within in normal limits, newborn feeding may be started. Most newborns are on demand feeding schedules and are allowed to feed when they awaken. When they go home, mothers are encouraged to feed their newborns every 2 to 4 hours during the day and only when the newborn awakens during the night for the first few days after birth.

After deciding about whether to breast- or bottle-feed the newborn, parents often have many questions. Generally, it is recommended that newborns be fed on demand whenever they seem hungry. Most newborns will give clues about their hunger status by crying, placing their fingers or fist in their mouth, rooting around, and sucking.

Newborns differ in their feeding needs and preferences, but most breast-fed ones need to be fed every 2 to 3 hours and nurse 10 to 20 minutes on each breast. The length of feedings is up to the mother and her newborn. Encourage the mother to respond to cues from her infant, and not according to a standard or preset time schedule.

Formula-fed newborns usually feed every 3 to 4 hours, finishing a bottle in 30 minutes or less. Bottle-fed infants consume about 2 to 4 fl oz at first and double their intake within a few weeks of age (Meade Johnson, 2003). If the newborn seems satisfied, wets 6 to 12 diapers daily, produces several stools a day, sleeps well, and is gaining weight regularly, then they are probably receiving sufficient intake of breast milk or formula.

Newborns swallow air during feedings, which causes discomfort and fussiness. Parents can prevent this behavior by burping them frequently throughout the feeding. Helpful strategies to convey to parents about burping include

- Holding the newborn upright with her head on her parent's shoulder
- Supporting the head and neck while the parent gently pats or rubs the newborn's back
- Sitting with the newborn on a parent's lap, while supporting her chest and head
- Gently rubbing the newborn's back with the other hand while in the sitting position
- Laying the newborn on the parent's lap with her back facing up
- Supporting the newborn's head in the crook of the parent's arm and gently patting or rubbing the back (Tip: It is the upright position, not the strength of the patting or rubbing, that allows the newborn to release air accumulated in the stomach)

Figure 18-20 depicts a nurse demonstrating two proper burping techniques.

Stress to parents that feeding time is more than an opportunity to get nutrients into their newborn. It is a time for closeness and sharing. Their newborn's feedings are as much for her emotional pleasure as her physical well-being. Encourage parents to maintain eye contact with their newborn during the feeding, hold her comfortably close to them, and talk softly during the feeding to promote feelings of closeness and security.

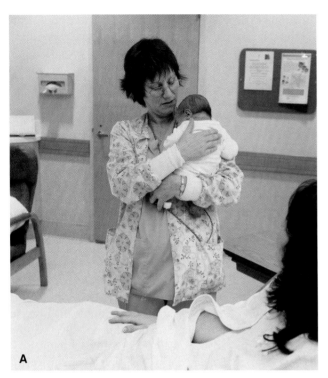

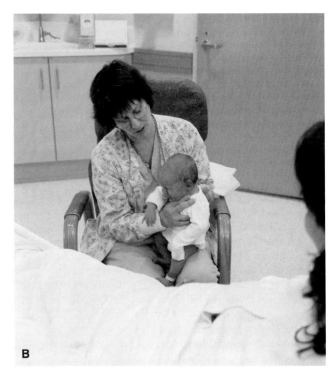

● Figure 18-20 The nurse demonstrates holding the newborn upright over the shoulder (**A**) and sitting the newborn upright, supporting the neck and chin (**B**).

Newborn Nutritional Needs

As newborns grow, energy and nutrient requirements change to meet their body's changing needs. During infancy, energy, protein, vitamin, and mineral requirements per pound of body weight are higher than at any other time during the life span. These high requirements are needed to sustain rapid growth and development during this stage of life. Generally, an infant's birth weight doubles in the first 4 to 6 months of life and triples within the first year (McCann, 2003).

A newborn infant's caloric needs range from 80 to 120 cal/kg body weight. For the first 3 months, the infant needs 110 cal/kg/day, decreasing to 100 cal/kg/day from 3 to 6 months (Lowdermilk & Perry, 2004). Breast milk and formulas contain approximately 20 cal/oz, which meets the caloric needs of young infants with several feedings throughout the day.

Fluid requirements for the newborn and infant range from 100 to 150 mL/kg daily. This requirement can be met through breast or bottle feedings. Additional water supplementation is not necessary. Adequate carbohydrates, fats, protein, and vitamins are achieved through consumption of breast milk or formula. The AAP recommends that bottle-fed infants be given iron supplementation, because iron levels are low in all types of formula milk. This can be achieved with iron fortification formula from birth. The breast-fed infant draws on iron reserves for the first 6 months and then needs iron-rich foods or supplementation added at

6 months of age. The AAP (AAP, 2003) also has recommended that all infants (breast- and bottle-fed) receive a daily supplement of vitamin D within the first 2 months of life to prevent rickets and vitamin D deficiency. It is also recommended that fluoride supplementation be given to infants not receiving fluoridated water after the age of 6 months (AAP, 2004a).

Feeding Methods

Parents typically decide about the method of feeding well before the infant is born. Prenatal and childbirth classes present information regarding breast-feeding versus bottle feeding and allow the parents to make up their minds which method is comfortable for them. Various factors can influence their decision, including socioeconomic status, culture, employment, levels of social support available, level of education, range of care interventions provided during pregnancy, childbirth and the early postpartum period, and especially partner support (RNAO, 2003). Nurses can be instrumental in providing further evidence-based practice information to assist the couple in making their decision. Regardless of which method is chosen, the nurse needs to respect and support the couple.

Breast-Feeding

There is consensus in the medical community that breast-feeding is considered optimal for all newborns. The AAP and the American Dietetic Association recommend breast feeding exclusively for the first 6 months of life, continuing it in conjunction with other food at least until the newborn's first birthday (AAP, 2004a). Box 18-2 highlights the advantages of breast-feeding for the mother and newborn. Keep in mind that during mild illnesses (colds, flu), breast-feeding can and should continue. In addition, mothers in the United States with HIV are advised not to breast-feed.

Breast milk composition changes over time: colostrum, transitional milk, and mature milk. *Colostrum* is a thick, yellowish substance secreted during the first few days after birth. It is high in protein, minerals, and fat-soluble vitamins. It is rich in immunoglobulins (IgA), which help protect the newborn's GI tract against infections. It is a natural laxative to help rid the intestinal tract of meconium quickly (McKinney et al., 2005).

Transitional milk occurs between colostrum and mature milk and contains all the nutrients in colostrum. It is thinner and less yellow than colostrum. This transitional milk is replaced by true or mature milk around day 10 after birth. *Mature milk* appears bluish in color and is not as thick as colostrum. It provides 20 cal/oz and contains

- Protein—Although the content is lower than formula, it is ideal to support growth and development for the newborn. The majority of protein is whey, which is easy to digest.
- Fat—Approximately 58% of total calories are fat, but they are easy to digest. Essential fatty acid content is high, as is cholesterol, which helps develop enzyme systems capable of handling cholesterol later in life.
- Carbohydrate—Approximately 35 to 40% of total calories are in the form of lactose, which stimulates growth of natural defense GI bacteria and promotes calcium absorption.
- Water—The major nutrient in breast milk comprises 85% to 95% of the total volume. Total milk volume varies with the age of the infant and demand.
- Minerals—Calcium, phosphorus, chlorine, potassium, and sodium with trace amounts of iron, copper, and manganese are provided. Iron absorption is about 50%, compared with about 4% of that in iron-fortified formulas.
- Vitamins—All vitamins are present in breast milk, with vitamin D being the lowest in amount. Discussion of the need of vitamin D supplementation is ongoing.
- Enzymes—Lipase and amylase are found in breast milk to assist with digestion (Dudek, 2006).

Formula Feeding

Despite the general acknowledgment that breast-feeding is the most desirable means of feeding infants, many mothers choose formula feeding. If approximately 60% of new mothers breast-feed, then the remaining 40% need information about how to formula-feed their newborns. Formula-fed infants grow more rapidly than breast-fed infants not only in weight but in length (Fomon, 2004).

Formula feeding requires more than opening, pouring, and feeding. Parents need information about the types of formula available, preparation and storage of formula, equipment, feeding positions, and the amount to feed their newborn. The nonbreast-feeding mother also needs information about measures to prevent lactation (see Chapter 16 for more information).

Commercially prepared formulas are regulated by the Food and Drug Administration (FDA) and are manufactured by one of three companies: Meade Johnson (Enfamil), Wyeth (SMA), and Ross Laboratories (Similac) in the United States. It is recommended that normal full-term infants receive conventional cow's milk-based formula, which is determined by the healthcare provider. If the infant shows signs of a reaction or a lactose intolerance, a switch to another formula type is recommended. The general recommendation is for all infants to receive iron-fortified formula until the age of

---

BOX 18-2

ADVANTAGES OF BREAST-FEEDING

Advantages for the Newborn
- Contributes to the development of a strong immune system
- Stimulates growth of positive bacteria in digestive tract
- Reduces incidence of stomach upset, diarrhea, and colic
- Begins the immunization process at birth by passive immunity
- Promotes optimal mother–infant bonding
- Reduces risk of newborn constipation
- Promotes greater developmental gains in preterm infants (O'Connor, 2003)
- Provides easily tolerated and digestible formula that is sterile, at proper temperature, and readily available with no artificial colorings, flavorings, or preservatives
- Is less likely to result in overfeeding, leading to obesity (Clifford, 2003)
- Promotes better tooth and jaw development as a result of sucking hard
- Provides protection against food allergies
- Is associated with avoidance of type 1 diabetes and heart disease

Advantages for the Mother
- Can facilitate a mother's loss of weight after birth
- Stimulates uterine contractions to control uterine bleeding
- Promotes uterine involution as a result of release of oxytocin
- Lowers risk against breast cancer and osteoporosis
- Affords some contraceptive protection, although it is not a reliable contraceptive method (Condon, 2004)

1 year. The latest generation of infant formulas includes some fortification with docosahexaenoic acid (DHA) and arachidonic acid (ARA), two natural components of breast milk. Researchers have found that formulas with DHA and ARA can enhance visual and cognitive development in children (Hatty, 2004).

Commercial formulas come in three forms: powder, concentrate, and easy to feed or ready to use. All are similar in terms of nutritional content, but differ in expense. Powdered formula is the least expensive, with concentrated formula the next most expensive. Both must be mixed with water before using. Ready-to-feed is the most expensive, but can be opened and poured into a bottle and fed directly to the infant.

Parents need important information about the equipment needed for formula feeding. Basic supplies needed will frequently consist of 4 to 6 4-oz bottles, 8 to 10 8-oz bottles, 8 to 10 nipple units, a bottle brush, and a nipple brush. A key area of instruction is assessing for flow of formula through the nipple and checking for any nipple damage. When the bottle is filled and turned upside down, the speed of flow from the nipple should be approximately one drop per second. If the parents are using bottles with disposable bags, instruct them to make sure they have a tight-fitting nipple to prevent leaks. Frequent observation of the flow rate from the nipple and the condition of the nipple will prevent choking and potential aspiration associated with too fast a rate of delivery. Request that parents fill a bottle with formula and then turn it upside down and observe the rate at which the formula drips from the bottle. If it is too fast (>1 drop/second), then the nipple should be replaced.

Formula preparation also is critical to the newborn's health and development. Many errors in dilution of formulas have been caused by a misunderstanding of proper preparation or improper measurement. Water safety in the preparation of formula always must be addressed with parents. If well water is used, advise the parents to sterilize the water by boiling it. Alternatively, bottled water can be used. Many health care providers still recommend that all water used in formula preparation be brought to a rolling boil for 1 to 2 minutes and be cooled to room temperature before using. Opened cans of ready-made or concentrated formula should be covered and refrigerated after being prepared for the day (24 hours). Instruct parents to discard any unused portions after 48 hours. Any formula left in the bottle after feeding should also be discarded, because the infant's saliva has been mixed with it.

To warm refrigerated formula, advise the parents to place the bottle in a pan of hot water and test the temperature by letting a few drops fall on the inside of the wrist. If it is comfortably warm to the mother, it is the correct temperature.

Breast-Feeding Assistance

If the mother has made the decision to breast-feed her newborn, this can be initiated immediately after birth. If the newborn is healthy and stable, wipe the newborn from head to toe with a dry cloth and place her skin-to-skin on the mother's abdomen. Then cover the newborn and mother with another warmed blanket to hold in the warmth. Immediate mother–newborn contact takes advantage of the newborn's natural alertness after a vaginal birth and fosters bonding. This immediate contact also reduces maternal bleeding and stabilizes the newborn's temperature, blood glucose level, and respiratory rate (AAP, 2004a).

Left alone on the mother's abdomen, a healthy newborn scoots upward, pushing with the feet, pulling with the arms, and bobbing the head until finding and latching on the mother's nipple. A newborn's sense of smell is highly developed, which also helps in finding the nipple. As the newborn moves to the nipple, the mother produces high levels of oxytocin, which contracts the uterus, thereby minimizing her bleeding. Oxytocin also causes her breasts to release colostrum when the newborn sucks on the nipple. Colostrum is rich in antibodies and thus provides the newborn with her "first immunization" against infection. Keys to successful breast-feeding include

- Initiating breast-feeding within the first hour of life if the newborn is stable
- Using the newborn's feeding schedule—8 to 12 times in 24 hours
- Allowing unrestricted length of breast-feeding
- Offering no supplement unless medically indicated
- Having a lactation consultant observe a feeding session
- Avoiding artificial nipples and pacifiers unless during painful procedure
- Encouraging breast-feeding from both breasts over each 24-hour period
- Instructing the mother regarding indicators of sufficient intake from infant
  - Six wet diapers daily
  - Waking up hungry 8 to 12 times in 24 hours
  - Acting content and falling asleep after feeding
- Keeping the newborn with her mother throughout the hospital stay

Assist with this task by positioning the newborn, so latching-on is effective and is not painful for the mother. Placing pillows or a folded blanket under the mother's head may help, or rolling her to one side and tucking the newborn next to her will facilitate breast-feeding initiation. Assess both the mother and newborn during this initial session to determine specific needs for assistance and additional areas for education. One tool used frequently in this assessment is the LATCH scoring tool (Table 18-5). The higher the score, the less nursing intervention is needed by this dyad.

Table 18-5 The LATCH Scoring Tool

Parameters	0 Point	1 Point	2 Points
L: latch	Sleepy infant, no sustained latch achieved	Must hold nipple in infant's mouth to sustain latch and suck; must stimulate infant to continue to suck	Grasps nipple; tongue down; rhythmic sucking
A: audible swallowing	None	A few observed with stimulation	Spontaneous and intermittent both < 24 hours old and afterward
T: type of nipple	Inverted (drawn inward into breast tissue)	Flat (not protruding)	Everted or protruding out after stimulation
C: comfort of nipple	Engorged, cracked, bleeding; severe discomfort	Filling; reddened, small blisters or bruises; mild to moderate discomfort	Soft, nontender
H: hold (positioning)	Nurse must hold infant to breast	Minimal assist; help with positioning, then mother takes over	No assistance needed by nurses

Modified from Jensen, D., Wallace, S., & Kelsey, P. (1994). LATCH: A breast-feeding charting system and documentation tool. *Journal of Obstetric and Gynecologic Neonatal Nursing, 23,* 27–32.

Breast-Feeding Positioning

The mother and infant must be in comfortable positions to ensure breast-feeding success. The four most common positions for breast-feeding are the football, cradle, across-the-lap, and side-lying holds. Each mother, on experimentation, can decide which positions feel most comfortable for her.

The football hold is achieved by holding the infant's back and shoulders in the palm of the mother's hand and tucking the infant under the mother's arm. Remind the mother to keep the infant's ear, shoulder, and hip in a straight line. Support the breast with the mother's hand and bring it to the infant's lips to latch on. Continue to support the breast until the infant begins to nurse. This position allows the mother to see the infant's mouth as she guides her infant to the nipple. This is another good choice for mothers who have had a cesarean birth to avoid pressure on the incision lines.

The cradling position is the most common one used. The newborn's head is held in the crook of the arm. The infant faces the mother, tummy to tummy. The opposite hand of the mother supports the breast. The across-the-lap position involves placing a pillow across the mother's lap with the infant facing the mother. The infant's back and shoulders are supported with the mother's palm. The mother supports her breast from underneath. After the infant is in position, the infant is pulled forward to latch on.

The fourth position is the side-lying position. The mother lies on her side with a pillow supporting her back and another pillow supporting the newborn in the front.

To start, the mother props herself up on an elbow and supports her newborn with that arm, while holding her breast with the opposite hand. Once nursing is started, the mother then lies down in a comfortable position.

To assist the mother in handling her breast to promote latching-on, instruct her to make a "C" or a "V" position with her fingers. In the C hold, the mother places her thumb well above the areola and the other four fingers below the areola and under the breast. In the V hold position, the mother places her index finger above the areola and her other three fingers below the areola and under the breast. Either method can be used as long as the mother's hand is well away from the nipple so the infant can latch on to the presenting breast.

Breast-Feeding Education

Breast-feeding is not an innate skill in human mothers. Almost all women have the potential to breast-feed successfully, but many fail because of inadequate knowledge. See Nursing Care Plan 18-1 for some typical nursing diagnoses, outcomes, and interventions. For many mothers and their newborns, breast-feeding goes smoothly from the start, whereas for others it is a struggle. Nurses can help throughout this experience by encouraging, demonstrating techniques, and offering praise for success. It is important to emphasize that the key to successful breast-feeding is correct positioning and latch-on.

Teaching by nurses has been shown to have a significant effect on both the ability to breast-feed successfully and the duration of lactation (Dudek, 2006). During the

Nursing Care Plan 18-1

Overview of the Mother and Newborn Having Some Difficulty with Breast-feeding

Baby boy James, weight 7 lb, 4 oz, was born to his mother, Jane, a 19-year-old gravida 1, para 1, who gave birth a few hours ago. He has Apgar scores of 9 points and 9 points at 1 and 5 minutes, respectively. Labor and birth events were unremarkable, and James was admitted to the nursery for assessment. After stabilization, James was brought to her mother, who had indicated she wished to breast-feed. The postpartum nurse assisted Jane with positioning and latching-on and left the room for a few minutes. On returning, Jane was upset, James was crying, and Jane stated she wanted a bottle of formula to feed him since she didn't have milk and her nipples hurt.

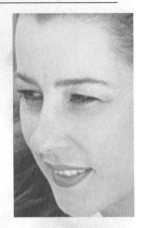

Assessment reveals a young, inexperienced mother placed in uncomfortable situation with limited knowledge of breast-feeding: positioning, latching-on. Anxiety from the mother transferred to James, resulting in crying. The mother, apprehensive about task of breast-feeding, needs additional help.

Nursing Diagnosis: Knowledge deficit related to skills involving breast-feeding

Outcome identification and *evaluation*	Interventions with *rationales*
Mother will demonstrate understanding of skills involved with breast-feeding *as evidenced by use of correct positioning and technique, and verbalization of appropriate information related to breast-feeding*	Instruct mother on proper positioning for breast-feeding; suggest use of football hold, side-lying position, modified cradle, and across-the-lap position *to ensure adequate comfort and to promote ease in breast-feeding* Review breast anatomy and milk let-down reflex for milk supply *to enhance mother's understanding of lactation* Observe newborn's ability to suck and latch on to the nipple *to determine adequate newborn ability* Monitor sucking and newborn swallowing for several minutes *to ensure adequate latching on and to assess intake* Reinforce nipple care with water and exposure to air *to maintain nipple integrity*

Nursing Diagnosis: Anxiety related to breast-feeding ability and irritable, crying newborn

Mother will verbalize increased comfort with breast-feeding *as evidenced by positive statements related to breast-feeding and verbalization of desire to continue to breast-feed newborn*	Ensure that the environment is calm and soothing without distractions *to promote maternal and newborn relaxation* Initiate correct latching-on technique *to enhance promotion of breast-feeding* Assist in calming newborn by holding and talking *to ensure that the newborn is relaxed prior to latching on* Reassure mother she can be successful at breast-feeding *to enhance her self-esteem and confidence* Encourage frequent trials and attempts *to enhance confidence* Support and encourage the mother to verbalize her anxiety/fears *to help reduce anxiety*

Overview of the Mother and Newborn Having Some Difficulty with Breast-feeding (continued)

Nursing Diagnosis: Pain related to breast-feeding and incorrect technique for latching-on

Outcome identification and *evaluation*	Interventions with *rationales*
Mother will experience a decrease in pain related to breast-feeding *as evidenced by statements of fewer complaints of nipple pain*	Suggest several alternate positions for breast-feeding *to increase comfort level* Demonstrate how to break suction to remove infant from breast *to minimize trauma to the nipple* Inspect nipple area *to promote early identification of trauma* Reinforce correct latching-on technique *to prevent nipple trauma* Administer pain medication if indicated *to aid in relief of pain* Instruct on nipple care between feedings *to maintain nipple integrity*

first few breast-feeding sessions, mothers want to know how often they should be nursing, whether breast-feeding is going well, if the newborn is getting enough nourishment, and what problems may ensue and how to cope with them. Education for the breast-feeding mother is highlighted in Teaching Guidelines 18-4.

Breast Milk Storage and Expression

If the breast-feeding mother becomes separated from the newborn for any reason (work, travel, illness), instruction on how to express and store milk safely is needed. Expressing milk can be done manually (hand compression of breast) or by using a breast pump. Manual or hand pumps are inexpensive and can be used by mothers who occasionally need an extra bottle if they are going out. The electric breast pumps are used for mothers who experience a lengthy separation from their infants and need to pump their breasts regularly (Fig. 18-21).

To ensure the safety of expressed breast milk, instruct the mother in the following:

- Washing hands before expressing milk or handling breast milk
- Using only clean containers to store expressed milk
- Using sealed and chilled milk within 24 hours
- Discarding any milk that is refrigerated more than 72 hours
- Using any frozen expressed milk within 3 months of obtaining
- Avoiding use of microwave ovens to warm chilled milk
- Discarding any used milk; never refreezing it
- Storing milk in quantities to be used for each feeding (2–4 oz)
- Thawing milk in warm water before using (AAP, 2004a)

Formula-Feeding Assistance

Feeding a newborn formula from a bottle should mirror breast-feeding as close as possible. Although nutrition is important, so are the emotional and interactive components of feeding. Encourage parents to cuddle their newborn closely and position her so that her head is in a comfortable position, not too far back or turned, which makes swallowing difficult. Also urge parents to communicate with their newborn during the feedings by talking and singing to her.

Although it may seem that bottle-feeding is not a difficult task to accomplish, many new parents may find it awkward. At first glance, holding an infant and a bottle to feed them appears simple enough, but getting the right position as well as the right angle to hold the bottle must be mastered to be successful.

Formula-Feeding Positions

Advise mothers to feed their newborns in a relaxed and quiet setting to create a calm feeling for themselves as well as their newborn. Make sure that comfort is a priority for both mother and newborn by having the mother's arm holding the newborn supported by a pillow in a comfortable chair. Have the mother cradle the newborn in a semi-upright position, supporting the newborn's head in the crook or bend of her arm. Holding the newborn close during feeding provides stimulation and helps prevent choking. Holding the newborn's head raised slightly will help prevent formula from washing backward into the eustachian tubes in the ears, which can lead to an ear infection.

Formula-Feeding Education

Parents of a newborn who is receiving formula require specific teaching related to preparation and storage of

T E A C H I N G   G U I D E L I N E S   1 8 - 4

Breast-Feeding

- Set aside a quiet place ahead of time where you can be relaxed and won't be disturbed. Relaxation promotes milk let-down.
- Sit in a comfortable chair, rocking chair, or lie on a bed to breast-feed. Try to make each feeding calm, quiet, and leisurely. Avoid distractions.
- Listen to soothing music and sip a nutritious drink during feedings.
- Initially, nurse the newborn every couple of hours to stimulate milk production. Remember that the supply of milk is equal to the demand—the more sucking, the more milk.
- Watch for signals from infant to indicate she is hungry, such as
  - Nuzzling against the mother's breasts
  - Demonstrating the rooting reflex by making sucking motions
  - Placing fist or hands in mouth to suck on
  - Crying and squirming around
  - Smacking of the lips
- Stimulate the rooting reflex by touching the newborn's cheek to initiate sucking.
- Look for signs indicating that the newborn has latched on correctly: wide-open mouth with the nipple and much of the areola in the mouth, lips rolled outward, and tongue over lower gum, visible jaw movement drawing milk out, rhythmic sucking with an audible swallowing (soft "ka" or "ah" sound indicates the infant is swallowing milk).
- Hold the newborn closely, facing the breast with the newborn's ear, shoulder, and hip in direct alignment.

- Nurse the infant on demand, not on a rigid schedule (for example, feeding every 2 to 3 hours within a 24-hour period; 8–12 feedings).
- Alternate between which breast is offered first; identify with a safety pin on bra.
- Vary your position for each feeding to empty breasts and reduce soreness.
- Look for signs that the newborn is getting enough milk:
  - At least six wet diapers and two to five loose yellow stools daily
  - Steady weight gain after the first week of age
  - Pale-yellow urine, not deep yellow or orange
  - Sleeping well, yet looks alert and healthy when awake (AAP, 2004a)
- Wake up the newborn if she has nursed less than 5 minutes by unwrapping her.
- Break the infant's suction before removing the nipple by inserting a finger.
- Burp the infant to release air when changing breasts and at the end of the breast-feeding session.
- Avoid supplemental formula feedings to prevent nipple confusion.
- Avoid pacifiers if possible because they are linked with reduced breast-feeding duration (Ullah & Griffiths, 2003).
- Do not take drugs or medications unless approved by the healthcare provider.
- Avoid drinking alcohol or caffeinated drinks because they pass through milk.
- Do not smoke while breast-feeding; it increases the risk of SIDS.
- Always wash hands before expressing or handling milk to store.
- Wear nursing bras and clothes that are easy to undo.

formula as well as the techniques for feeding. Formula feeding guidance tips for parents are highlighted in Teaching Guidelines 18-5.

Proper positioning makes bottle-feeding easier and more enjoyable for both mother and newborn, but frequent burping also is key. Advise the parent to hold the bottle so that formula fills the nipple, thereby allowing less air to enter. Infants get fussy when they swallow air during feedings and need to be relieved of it every 2 to 3 oz. Emphasize to parents that electrolyte imbalance can occur in infants who are fed formula that has been incorrectly mixed. Hypernatremia can result from formula mixed too thickly. The resulting concentration of sodium is too much for the immature kidneys to handle. As a result, sodium is excreted along with water, leading to dehydration. Mixing the formula with too much water in

an effort to save money can lead to failure to thrive and lack of weight gain (AAP, 2005a).

Weaning and Introduction of Solid Foods

Eventually, breast-feeding or formula feeding ends. The transitions from breast to bottle, from breast or bottle to cup, or from liquids to solids all describe weaning. Weaning from breast-feeding to cup has several advantages over weaning to a bottle because it eliminates the step of weaning first to a bottle and then to a cup. Another advantage is that the bottle does not become a security object that the infant does not want to give it up after it is introduced to her world.

Whether it is because the mother is returning to work and it is not feasible for her to continue to breast-feed or the infant is losing interest in breast-feeding and showing signs

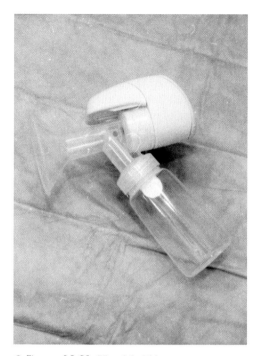

● Figure 18-21 Hand-held breast pump.

of independence, the weaning process is done gradually. There is no "right" time to wean; it depends on the desires of the mother and her infant. Either one can start the weaning process, but usually it occurs between 6 months and 1 year of age.

To begin weaning from the breast, instruct mothers to substitute breast-feeding with a cup or bottle. Often the midday feeding is the easiest feeding to start the weaning process. A trainer cup with two handles and a snap-on lid with a spout is appropriate and helps to minimize spilling. Because weaning is a process, it may take months to accomplish. Instruct parents to proceed gradually and let the infant's willingness and interest guide them.

Weaning from the bottle to the cup is also a process and needs to be timed appropriately for mother and infant. Weaning is a significant change in the way mother and infant interact with each other, and each mother must decide for herself when she and her infant are ready to take that step. Typically, the night bottle is the last to be given up, with cup drinking substituted throughout the daylight hours. Slowing diluting the formula with water over a week can help in this process with the final result—a water bottle. To prevent sucking on it during the night, remove it from the crib after the infant falls asleep.

When infants double their birth weight and weigh at least 13 lb, it is time to begin to consider introducing solid foods. Readiness cues include

- Consumption of 32 oz formula or breast milk daily (estimated)
- Ability to sit up with minimal support and turn head away to indicate fullness

 T E A C H I N G   G U I D E L I N E S   1 8 - 5

Formula-Feeding

- Wash hands with soap and water prior to preparing formula.
- Mix the formula and water amounts exactly as the label specifies.
- Always hold the newborn and bottle during feedings; never prop the bottle.
- Never freeze formula or warm it in the microwave.
- Place refrigerated formula in a pan of hot water for a few minutes to warm.
- Test the temperature of the formula by shaking a few drops on the wrist.
- Hold the bottle like a pencil, keeping it tipped to prevent air from entering, positioning the bottle so that the nipple remains filled with milk.
- Burp the infant after every few ounces to allow air swallowed to escape.
- Move the nipple around in the infant's mouth to stimulate sucking.
- Always keep a bulb syringe close by to use if choking occurs.
- Avoid putting the infant to bed with a bottle to prevent "baby bottle tooth decay."
- Feed the newborn approximately every 3 to 4 hours.
- Use an iron-fortified formula for the first year.
- Prepare enough formula for the next 24 hours.
- Check nipples regularly and discard any that are sticky, cracked, or leaking.
- Store unmixed, open liquid formula in the refrigerator for up to 48 hours.
- Throw away any formula left in the bottle after each feeding.

- Reduction of protrusion reflex so cereal can be propelled to back of throat
- Demonstration of interest in food others around them are eating
- Infant's ability to open mouth automatically when food approaches it

When introducing solid foods, certain principles apply:

- The order of food introduction is not important; however, introduction of just one new single-ingredient food (rice cereal or carrots) is recommended for several days to watch for allergies.
- Infants should be allowed to set the pace regarding how much they wish to consume.
- New foods are introduced one at a time so that any allergies or intolerances can be identified.
- New foods are introduced no more frequently than every 3 to 5 days.
- Fruits are added after cereals; then vegetables and meats are introduced; eggs are introduced last.

- A relaxed, unhurried, calm atmosphere for meals is important.
- A variety of foods are provided to ensure a balanced diet.
- Infants should never be force-fed (Krepcio, Foell, Folta, & Goldberg, 2004).

Nurses play an extremely important role in assisting new mothers to feed their infants by active listening to help a mother clarify her feelings and begin to problem solve with her. A warm, sincere manner and tone of voice will help put an anxious mother at ease. Giving accurate information, making suggestions, and presenting options will empower the mother to decide what is best for her and her infant. Within the context of this helping role, nurses need to be sensitive to the individual, family, and economic and cultural differences among mothers before offering suggestions for feeding practices that may not be appropriate.

Dealing With Common Concerns

During the newborn period of transition, certain conditions can develop that require intervention. These conditions, although not typically life-threatening, can be a source of anxiety for the parents. Common concerns include transient tachypnea of the newborn, physiologic jaundice, and hypoglycemia.

Transient Tachypnea of the Newborn

Transient tachypnea of the newborn appears soon after birth. It is accompanied by retractions, expiratory grunting, or cyanosis and is relieved by administration of low-dose oxygen therapy. A mild or moderate respiratory distress typically is present at birth or within 6 hours of birth. This condition usually resolves within 3 days.

Transient tachypnea of the newborn occurs when the fetal liquid in the lungs is removed slowly or incompletely, which correlates with decreased thoracic squeeze such as from cesarean birth, or diminished respiratory effort such as from sedation in the newborn secondary to maternal central nervous system depressant medication. Prolonged labor, macrosomia of the fetus, and maternal asthma also have been associated with a higher frequency of this condition (Asenjo, 2003).

Nursing interventions include providing supportive care such as giving the newborn oxygen, ensuring warmth, observing the newborn's respiratory status frequently, and allowing time for the pulmonary capillaries and the lymphatics to remove the remaining fluid. The clinical course is relatively benign, but any newborn respiratory issue can be very frightening to the parents. Provide a thorough explanation and reassurance that the condition will resolve over time.

Physiologic Jaundice

Physiologic jaundice is a very common condition in newborns, with the majority demonstrating yellowish skin, mucous membranes, and sclera within the first 3 days of life. In any given year, approximately 60% of the newborns in the United States will experience clinical jaundice (Holcomb, 2005). Jaundice is the visible manifestation of hyperbilirubinemia. It typically results from the deposition of unconjugated bilirubin pigment in the skin and mucous membranes of newborns.

The AAP has recently released guidelines to provide a framework for the prevention and management of hyperbilirubinemia in newborns, which includes

- Promotion and support of successful breast-feeding practices
- Completion of a systematic assessment before discharge for the risk of severe hyperbilirubinemia
- Provision of early and focused follow-up based on the risk assessment
- When indicated, treatment of newborns with **phototherapy** or exchange transfusion to prevent the development of kernicterus (AAP, 2004b)

Factors that contribute to the development of physiologic jaundice in the newborn include an increased bilirubin load because of relative polycythemia, a shortened erythrocyte life span (80 days compared with the adult 120 days), and immature hepatic uptake and conjugation processes (Dixon, 2004). Normally the liver removes bilirubin from the blood and changes it to a form in which it can be excreted. As the RBC breakdown continues at a fast pace, the newborn liver is unable to keep up with bilirubin removal. Thus, bilirubin accumulates in the blood, causing a yellowish discoloration on the skin.

Assess for jaundice in all newborns by pressing gently with a fingertip on the bridge of the nose, sternum, or forehead to ascertain the color of the blanched area. If jaundice is present, the blanched area will appear yellow before the capillary refill (Lowdermilk & Perry, 2004). If or when the levels of unconjugated serum bilirubin increase, phototherapy is used. Phototherapy involves treatment with exposure to light. Exposure of newborns to sunlight represents the first documented use of phototherapy in the medical literature. Sister J. Ward, a charge nurse in Essex, England, in 1956, recognized that when jaundiced newborns were exposed to the sun they became less yellow. This observation changed the entire treatment of jaundice in newborns (Ramer, 2005).

Phototherapy reduces bilirubin levels in the blood by breaking down unconjugated bilirubin into colorless compounds. These compounds can then be excreted in the bile. Phototherapy aims to curtail the increase in bilirubin blood levels, thereby preventing kernicterus, a condition in which unconjugated bilirubin enters the brain and, if not treated, can lead to brain damage and possibly death.

During the last several decades, phototherapy has generally been administered with either banks of fluorescent lights or spotlights. Factors that determine the dose of phototherapy include spectrum of light emitted, irradiance of light source, design of light unit, surface area of newborn exposed to the light, and distance of the newborn from the light source (Klein, 2004). For phototherapy to be effective, the rays must penetrate as much of the skin as possible. To accomplish this, the newborn must be naked and turned frequently to ensure maximum exposure of the skin. Several side effects of standard phototherapy have been identified: frequent loose stools, increased insensible water loss, transient rash, and potential retinal damage if the newborn's eyes are not covered sufficiently.

Recently, fiber optic pads (Biliblanket or Bilivest) have been developed that can be wrapped around newborns or on which newborns can lie. These pads consist of a light that is delivered from a tungsten–halogen bulb through a fiberoptic cable and is emitted from the sides and ends of the fibers inside a plastic pad (Ramer, 2005). They work on the premise that phototherapy can be improved by delivering higher-intensity therapeutic light to decrease bilirubin levels. The pads do not produce appreciable heat like the banks of lights or spotlights do, so insensible water loss is not increased. Eye patches also are not needed; thus, parents can feed and hold their newborns continuously to promote bonding.

Newborns undergoing phototherapy in the treatment of jaundice require close monitoring of their body temperature, fluid, and electrolyte balance; observation of skin integrity as a result of exposure to diarrhea and phototherapy lights; eye protection to prevent corneal injury related to phototherapy exposure; and encouragement of parents to participate in their newborn's care to prevent parent–infant separation. (See Chapter 24 for a more detailed discussion of hyperbilirubinemia.)

Hypoglycemia

Hypoglycemia, a problem experienced by newborns during the early postbirth period (6 hours after birth), affects as many as 40% of all full-term newborns (Johnson, 2003). It is defined as a blood glucose level of less than 35 mg/dL or as a plasma concentration of less than 40 mg/dL (Kenner & Lott, 2004). In newborns, blood glucose levels fall to a low point during the first few hours of life, because the source of maternal glucose is removed when the placenta is expelled. This period of transition is usually smooth, but certain newborns are at greater risk for development of hypoglycemia. These newborns include IDMs, preterm newborns, and newborns with IUGR, inadequate caloric intake, sepsis, asphyxia, hypothermia, polycythemia, glycogen storage disorders, and endocrine deficiencies (Johnson, 2003).

Most newborns experience transient hypoglycemia and are asymptomatic. The symptoms, when present, are nonspecific and include jitteriness, lethargy, cyanosis, apnea, seizures, high-pitched or weak cry, and poor feeding. If hypoglycemia is prolonged or is left untreated, serious, long-term adverse neurologic sequelae such as learning disabilities and mental retardation can occur

(Verklan & Walden, 2004). Subsequently, early diagnosis and appropriate intervention are essential for all newborns.

Nursing care directed toward the hypoglycemic newborn includes monitoring for signs and symptoms of hypoglycemia if present or identifying high-risk newborns prone to this disorder based on their perinatal history, physical examination, body measurements, and gestational age. Check the blood glucose level of all newborns within the first few hours after birth and every 4 hours thereafter. More frequent monitoring and early feeding may be necessary for newborns who are considered to be high risk. Prevent hypoglycemia for newborns at risk by initiating early feedings (breast milk or formula). If hypoglycemia persists despite feeding, notify the primary healthcare provider for orders such as IV therapy with dextrose solutions. Anticipate hypoglycemia in certain high-risk newborns and begin assessments immediately on nursery admission.

Preparing for Discharge

Preparing the parents for discharge is an essential task for the nurse. As a result of limited facility stays, the nurse must identify the major teaching topics for the parents and establish a climate that will facilitate learning. Nurses need to know where the parents place themselves within the context of the birth experience, and how best to meet their learning needs. Using the following principles helps to foster a learner-centered approach:

- Set a conducive environment for learning by encouraging clients to feel comfortable during this intense time by using support and praise.
- Share control of both the content and the process of learning by allowing the clients to make their own decisions about what they want and need to learn.
- Build self-esteem by confirming that their responses to the entire birthing process and aftercare are legitimate, and others have felt the same way.
- Ensure that what the parents learn applies to their home situation by integrating new information into their own situation and their day-to-day life.
- Encourage self-responsibility by reinforcing that their emotional and physical responses are within the normal range.
- Respect cultural beliefs and practices that are important to the family by teaching within their heritage and health beliefs regarding newborn care. Examples include placing a belly band over the newborn's navel by Hispanics and African-Americans, delaying naming their newborns by Asian-Americans and Haitians; and delaying breast-feeding by Native Americans because they regard colostrum as "bad" (D'Avanzo & Geissler, 2003).

Ensuring Follow-Up Care

Most newborns are scheduled for their first health follow-up appointment within 2 to 4 days after discharge to have additional lab work done as part of the newborn screening series, especially if they were discharged within 48 hours. After this first visit, the typical schedule of healthcare visits is as follows: 2 to 4 weeks of age; 2, 4, and 6 months of age for checkups and vaccines; 9 months of age for a checkup; 12 months for checkup and tuberculosis testing; 15 and 18 months for checkups and vaccines; and 2 years of age for a checkup. These appointments provide an opportunity for parents to ask questions and receive anticipatory guidance as their newborn grows and develops.

In addition to encouraging parents to keep follow-up appointments, advise parents to call their healthcare provider if they notice signs of illness in their newborn and which over-the-counter medicines would be important to keep on hand. Review the following warning signs of illness with parents:

- Temperature of 38.3°C (101°F) or higher
- Forceful, persistent vomiting, not just spitting up
- Refusal to take feedings
- Two or more green, watery diarrhea stools
- Infrequent wet diapers and changes in bowel movements from normal pattern
- Lethargy or excessive sleepiness
- Inconsolable crying and extreme fussiness
- Abdominal distention
- Difficult or labored breathing

Parents also need instructions about immunizations for their newborn. Immunization is the process of rendering an individual immune or of becoming immune to select communicable diseases (O'Toole, 2003). The purpose of the immune system is to identify unknown (nonself) substances in the body and develop a defense against these invaders. Disease prevention by immunization is a public health priority and one of the leading health indicators as part of Healthy People 2010. Despite many advances in vaccine delivery, the goal for universal immunization has not been reached (AAP, 2003). Nurses can help to meet this national goal by educating new parents about the importance of disease prevention through immunizations.

Immunity can be provided either passively or actively. *Passive immunity* is protection transferred via already formed antibodies from one person to another. Passive immunity includes transplacental passage of antibodies from a mother to her newborn, immunity passed through breast milk, and immunity from immunization from immunoglobulins. Passive immunity provides limited protection and decreases over a period of weeks or months (Dayton, 2004). Passive immunity is protection produced by an individual's own immune system. It can be obtained by having the actual disease or by receiving a vaccine in which there is an immunologic response by that person's body. Active immunity may be life-long either way.

Young infants and children are susceptible to various illnesses because their immune systems are not yet mature. Many of these illnesses can be prevented by following the recommended schedule of childhood immunizations. The schedule for immunizations should be reviewed with parents, stressing the importance of continual follow-up health care to preserve their infant's health.

The newborn's first immunization (hepatitis B) is received in the hospital soon after birth and prior to discharge. The first dose can also be given by age 2 months if the newborn's mother is HBsAg negative. If the newborn's mother is HbsAg positive, then the newborn should receive hepatitis B vaccine and hepatitis B immunoglobulin within 12 hours of birth (Cunningham et al., 2005). Education for the parents pertaining to immunizations should include risks and benefits for each vaccine, possible side effects, and information to answer their questions. Parents have the right to refuse based on religious beliefs and can sign a waiver noting their decision.

Federal legislation requires consent to be signed before administering a vaccine. The nurse administering the vaccine must document the date and time it was given, name and manufacturer, lot number and expiration date of the vaccine given, site and route of administration, and the name and title of the nurse who administered the vaccine (see Fig. 18-22 for the 2005 Childhood and Adolescent Immunization Schedule).

While in the hospital setting, women who give birth have continued assessment, support, and hands-on instruction regarding feeding and newborn care. When the new mother is discharged, this close supervision and support by nurses need not end abruptly when the newborn is placed in the car seat and the car door closes. Providing the new family with a "life-line" phone number of the mother–baby unit will help her through this stressful transitional period. Arming the new family with knowledge and offering backup support via the telephone will increase parenting success.

KEY CONCEPTS

- The period of transition from intrauterine to extrauterine life occurs during the first several hours after birth. It is a time of stabilization for the newborn's temperature, respiration, and cardiovascular dynamics.
- The newborn's bowel is sterile at birth. It usually takes about a week for the newborn to produce vitamin K in sufficient quantities to prevent VKDB.
- It is recommended that all newborns in the United States receive an instillation of a prophylactic agent (erythromycin or tetracycline ophthalmic ointment) in their eyes within an hour or two of being born.
- Nursing measures to maintain newborns' body temperature include drying them immediately after birth to prevent heat loss through evaporation, wrapping them in prewarmed blankets, putting a hat on their head, and placing them under a temperature-controlled radiant warmer.

RECOMMENDED CHILDHOOD AND ADOLESCENT IMMUNIZATION SCHEDULE—UNITED STATES, 2005

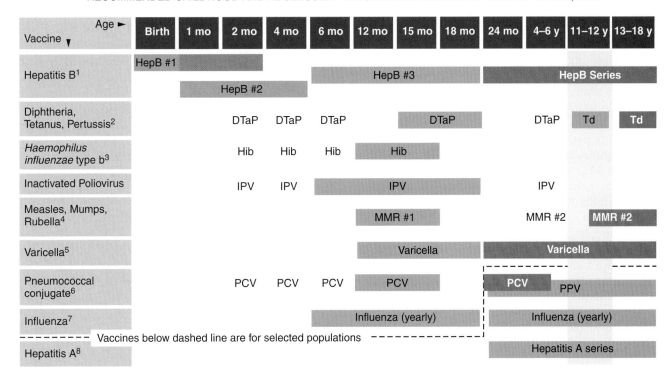

Vaccine ▼ / Age ►	Birth	1 mo	2 mo	4 mo	6 mo	12 mo	15 mo	18 mo	24 mo	4–6 y	11–12 y	13–18 y
Hepatitis B[1]	HepB #1	HepB #2				HepB #3				HepB Series		
Diphtheria, Tetanus, Pertussis[2]			DTaP	DTaP	DTaP		DTaP			DTaP	Td	Td
Haemophilus influenzae type b[3]			Hib	Hib	Hib	Hib						
Inactivated Poliovirus			IPV	IPV		IPV				IPV		
Measles, Mumps, Rubella[4]						MMR #1				MMR #2	MMR #2	
Varicella[5]						Varicella				Varicella		
Pneumococcal conjugate[6]			PCV	PCV	PCV	PCV				PCV	PPV	
Influenza[7]						Influenza (yearly)				Influenza (yearly)		

- - - - - - - Vaccines below dashed line are for selected populations - - - - - - - -

| Hepatitis A[8] | | | | | | | | | | Hepatitis A series | | |

This schedule indicates the recommended ages for routine administration of currently licensed childhood vaccines, as of December 1, 2004, for children through age 18 years. Any dose not administered at the recommended age should be administered at any subsequent visit when indicated and feasible.

Indicates age groups that warrant special effort to administer those vaccines not previously administered. Additional vaccines may be used whenever any components of the combination are indicated and other components of the vaccine are not contraindicated.

Providers should consult the manufacturers' package inserts for detailed recommendations. Clinically significant adverse events that follow immunization should be reported to the Vaccine Adverse Event Reporting System (VAERS). Guidance about how to obtain and complete a VAERS form is available at www.vaers.org or by telephone, 800-822-7967.

- Range of recommended ages
- Preadolescent assessment
- Only if mother HBsAg(−)
- Catch-up immunization

FOOTNOTES

1. Hepatitis B (HepB) vaccine. All infants should receive the first dose of HepB vaccine soon after birth and before hospital discharge; the first dose may also be administered by age 2 months if the mother is hepatitis B surface antigen (HBsAg)-negative. Only monovalent HepB may be used for the birth dose. Monovalent or combination vaccine containing HepB may be used to complete the series. Four doses of vaccine may be administered when a birth dose is given. The second dose should be given at least 4 weeks after the first dose, expect for combination vaccines which cannot be administered before age 6 weeks. The third dose should be given at least 16 weeks after the first dose and at least 8 weeks after the second dose. The last dose in the vaccination series (third or fourth dose) should not be administered before age 24 weeks.

Infants born to HBsAg-positive mothers should receive HepB and 0.5 mL of hepatitis B immune globulin (HBIG) at separate sites within 12 hours of birth. The second dose is recommended at age 1–2 months. The final dose in the immunization series should not be administered before age 24 weeks. These infants should be tested for HBsAg and antibody to HBsAg (anti-HBs) at age 9–15 months.

Infants born to mothers whose HBsAg status is unknown should receive the first dose of the HepB series within 12 hours of birth. Maternal blood should be drawn as soon as possible to determine the mother's HBsAg status; if the HBsAg test is positive, the infant should receive HBIG as soon as possible (no later than age 1 week). The second dose is recommended at age 1–2 months. The last dose in the immunization series should not be administered before age 24 weeks.

2. Diphtheria and tetanus toxoids and acellular pertussis (DTaP) vaccine. The fourth dose of DTaP may be administered as early as age 12 months, provided 6 months have elapsed since the third dose and the child is unlikely to return at age 15–18 months. The final dose in the series should be given at age ≥4 years. **Tetanus and diphtheria toxoids (Td)** is recommended at age 11–12 years if at least 5 years have elapsed since the last dose of tetanus and diphtheria toxoid-containing vaccine. Subsequent routine Td boosters are recommended every 10 years.

3. Haemophilus influenzae type b (Hib) conjugate vaccine. Three Hib conjugate vaccines are licensed for infant use. If PRP-OMP (PedvaxHIB® or ComVax® [Merck]) is administered at ages 2 and 4 months, a dose at age 6 months is not required. DTaP/Hib combination products should not be used for primary immunization in infants at ages 2, 4, or 6 months but can be used as boosters after any Hib vaccine. The final dose in the series should be administered at age ≥12 months.

4. Measles, mumps, and rubella vaccine (MMR). The second dose of MMR is recommended routinely at age 4–6 years but may be administered during any visit, provided at least 4 weeks have elapsed since the first dose and both doses are administered beginning at or after age 12 months. Those who have not previously received the second dose should complete the schedule by age 11–12 years.

5. Varicella vaccine. Varicella vaccine is recommended at any visit at or after age 12 months for susceptible children (i.e., those who lack a reliable history of chickenpox). Susceptible persons aged ≥13 years should receive 2 doses administered at least 4 weeks apart.

6. Pneumococcal vaccine. The heptavalent **pneumococcal conjugate vaccine (PCV)** is recommended for all children aged 2–23 months and for certain children aged 24–59 months. The final dose in the series should be given at age ≥12 months. **Pneumococcal polysaccharide vaccine (PPV)** is recommended in addition to PCV for certain high-risk groups. See *MMWR* 2000;49(RR-9):1-35.

7. Influenza vaccine. Influenza vaccine is recommended annually for children aged ≥6 months with certain risk factors (including, but not limited to, asthma, cardiac disease, sickle cell disease, human immunodeficiency virus [HIV], and diabetes), healthcare workers, and other persons (including household members) in close contact with persons in groups to high risk (see *MMWR* 2004;53[RR-6]:1-40). In addition, healthy children aged 6–23 months and close contacts of healthy children aged 0–23 months are recommended to receive influenza vaccine because children in this age group are at substantially increased risk for influenza-related hospitalization. For healthy persons aged 5–49 years, the intranasally administered, live, attenuated influenza vaccine (LAIV) is an acceptable alternative to the intramuscular trivalent inactivated influenza vaccine (TIV). See *MMWR* 2004;53(RR-6):1-40. Children receiving TIV should be administered a dosage appropriate for their age (0.25 mL if aged 6–35 months or 0.5 mL if aged ≥3 years). Children aged ≤8 years who are receiving influenza vaccine for the first time should receive 2 doses (separated by at least 4 weeks for TIV and at least 6 weeks for LAIV).

8. Hepatitis A vaccine. Hepatitis A vaccine is recommended for children and adolescents in selected states and regions and for certain high-risk groups; consult your local public health authority. Children and adolescents in these states, regions, and high-risk groups who have not been immunized against hepatitis A can begin the hepatitis A immunization series during any visit. The 2 doses in the series should be administered at least 6 months apart. See *MMWR* 1999;48(RR-12):1-37.

● Figure 18-22 Recommended childhood and adolescent immunization schedule.

- The specific components of a typical newborn examination include a general survey of skin color, posture, state of alertness, head size, overall behavioral state, respiratory status, gender, and any obvious congenital anomalies.

- Gestational age assessment is pertinent because it allows the nurse to plot growth parameters, and to anticipate potential problems related to prematurity/postmaturity and growth abnormalities such as SGA/LGA.

- After the newborn has passed the transitional period and stabilized, the nurse needs to complete ongoing assessments, vital signs, weight and measurements, cord care, hygiene measures, newborn screening tests, and various other tasks until the newborn is discharged home from the birthing unit.

- Important topics about which to educate parents include environmental safety, newborn characteristics, feeding and bathing, circumcision and cord care, sleep and elimination patterns of newborns, safe infant car seats, holding/positioning, and follow-up care.

- Newborn screening tests consist of hearing, and certain genetic and inborn errors of metabolism tests required in most states for newborns before discharge from the birth facility.

- The AAP and the American Dietetic Association recommend breast-feeding exclusively for the first 6 months of life and that it continue along with other food at least until their first birthday.

- Parents who choose not to breast-feed need to know what types of formula are available, preparation and storage of formula, equipment, feeding positions, and how much to feed their infant.

- Common problems associated with the newborn include transient tachypnea, physiologic jaundice, and hypoglycemia.

- Transient tachypnea of the newborn appears soon after birth and is accompanied by retractions, expiratory grunting, or cyanosis and is relieved by low-dose oxygen.

- Physiologic jaundice is a very common condition in newborns, with the majority demonstrating yellowish skin, mucous membranes, and sclera within the first 3 days of life. Newborns undergoing phototherapy in the treatment of jaundice require close monitoring of their body temperature, fluid, and electrolyte balance; observation of skin integrity; eye protection; and parental participation in their care.

- The newborn with hypoglycemia requires close monitoring for signs and symptoms of hypoglycemia if present. In addition, newborns at high risk need to be identified based on their perinatal history, physical examination, body measurements, and gestational age. Blood glucose levels of all newborns are checked within the first few hours after birth and every 4 hours thereafter.

- The schedule for immunizations should be reviewed with parents, stressing the importance of continual follow-up health care to preserve their infant's health.

References

American Academy of Pediatrics. (2003). Clinical report: Prevention of rickets and vitamin D deficiency: New guidelines for vitamin D intake. *Pediatrics 111*(4), 908–910.

American Academy of Pediatrics. (2003a). Committee on Injury, Violence, and Poison Prevention. Policy statement: Poison treatment in the home. *Pediatrics, 112*, 1182–1185.

American Academy of Pediatrics. (2003b). Hearing assessments in infants and children: Recommendations beyond neonatal screening, *Pediatrics, 111*, 436–440.

American Academy of Pediatrics. (2003c). Policy statement: Increasing immunization coverage. *Pediatrics, 112*, 993–996.

American Academy of Pediatrics. (2003d). Policy statement: Controversies concerning vitamin K and the newborn. *Pediatrics, 112*(1), 191–192.

American Academy of Pediatrics. (2004a). *A woman's guide to breast-feeding.* [Online] Available at www.aap.org/family/brstguid.htm.

American Academy of Pediatrics. (2004b). Clinical practice guideline: Management of hyperbilirubinemia in the newborn infant 35 or more weeks of gestation. *Pediatrics, 114*, 297–316.

American Academy of Pediatrics. (2004c). Management of hyperbilirubinemia in the newborn infant 35 or more weeks of gestation. Subcommittee on Hyperbilirubinemia. *Pediatrics, 114*, 297–316.

American Academy of Pediatrics. (2005a) Breast-feeding and the use of human milk. AAP policy statement. *Pediatrics, 115*, 496–506.

American Academy of Pediatrics. (2005b). Car safety seats: A guide for families. [Online] Available at www.aap.org/family/carseatguide.htm.

American Academy of Pediatrics & American College of Obstetricians and Gynecologists. (2002). *Guidelines for perinatal care* (5th ed.). Elk Village Grove, IL: AAP/ACOG.

Asenjo, M. (2003). Transient tachypnea of the newborn. *eMedicine.* [Online] Available at www.emedicine.com/radio/topic710.htm.

Ballard, J. L., Khoury, J. C., Wedig, K., et al. (1991). New Ballard score: Expanded to include extremely premature infants. *Journal of Pediatrics, 119*, 417–423.

Bar-Yam, N. B. (2002). The circumcision decision. *International Journal of Childbirth Education, 6*, 22–24.

Blackburn, S. T. (2003). Thermoregulation. In *Maternal, fetal, and neonatal physiology: A clinical perspective* (2nd ed., pp. 707–730). Philadelphia: WB Saunders.

Blackwell, J. T. (2003). Management of hyperbilirubinemia in the healthy term newborn. *Journal of the American Academy of Nurse Practitioners, 15*, 194–199.

Bryanton, J., Walsh, D., Barrett, M., & Gaudet, D. (2004). Tub bathing versus traditional sponge bathing for the newborn. *Journal of Obstetric, Gynecologic, and Neonatal Nursing, 33*, 704–712.

Burns, A. L. (2003). Protecting infants in healthcare facilities from abduction. *Journal of Perinatal and Neonatal Nursing, 17*, 139–147.

Centers for Disease Control and Prevention. (2002). *Sexually transmitted diseases treatment guidelines.* [Online] Available at www.cdc.gov/STD/treatment.

Children's Medical Services (CMS). (2004). *Florida's Newborn Screening Program: Screening for your baby's health.* Florida Department of Health.

Clifford, T. J. (2003). Breast-feeding and obesity. *British Medical Journal, 327*, 879–880.

Colyar, M. (2003). *Well-child assessment for primary care providers.* Philadelphia: FA Davis.

Condon, M. C. (2004). *Women's health: An integrated approach to wellness and illness.* Upper Saddle River, NJ: Prentice Hall.

Cunningham, F. G., Leveno, K. J., Bloom, S. L., Hauth, J. C., Gilstrap, L. C., & Wenstrom, K. D. (2005). *Williams obstetrics* (22nd ed.). New York: McGraw-Hill Medical Publishing Division.

D'Avanzo, C., & Geissler, E. (2003). *Pocket guide to cultural assessment* (3rd ed.). St. Louis: Mosby.

Dayton, L. V. (2004). Immunization update. *Advance for Nurses, 5*, 19–23.

De Michele, A. M., & Ruth, R. A. (2005). Newborn hearing screening. *eMedicine.* [Online] Available at www.emedicine.com/ent/topic576.htm.

Dickey, N. W. (2002). To circumcise or not to circumcise . . . Many parents are asking the question. *Medem.* [Online] Available at www.medem.com/MedLB/article_detailb.cfm?article_ID=ZZZG MO72B6D&sub_c.

Dillon, P. M. (2003). *Nursing health assessment: A critical thinking, case studies approach.* Philadelphia: FA Davis.

Dixon, K. T. (2004). Newborn jaundice and kernicterus. *Advance for Nurse Practitioners, 12,* 43–63.

Dudek, S. G. (2006). *Nutrition essentials for nursing practice* (5th ed.). Philadelphia: Lippincott Williams & Wilkins.

Engstrom, J. (2004). *Maternal–neonatal nursing made incredibly easy.* Springhouse: Lippincott Williams & Wilkins.

Fligor, B. J., & Neault, M. W. (2004). Newborn hearing screening. *Advance for Nurses, 6*(24); 19–36.

Fomon, S. J. (2004). Assessment of growth of formula-fed infants: Evolutionary considerations. *Pediatrics, 113*(2), 389–393.

Fuloria, M., Kreiter, S. (2002a). The newborn examination: part I. Emergencies and common abnormalities involving the skin, head, neck, chest, and respiratory and cardiovascular systems. *American Family Physician, 65,* 61–68.

Fuloria, M., & Kreiter, S. (2002b). The newborn examination: part II. Emergencies and common abnormalities involving the abdomen, pelvis, extremities, genitalia, and spine. *American Family Physician, 65,* 265–270.

Furdon, S. A., & Benjamin, K. (2004). Physical assessment. In M. T. Verklan & M. Walden (Eds.), *Core curriculum for neonatal intensive care nursing* (3rd ed., pp. 135–172). St. Louis: Elsevier Saunders.

Hatty, M. (2004). 15 new findings on caring for your baby. *USA Weekend,* January 9–11, 6–10.

Haws, P. S. (2004). *Care of the sick neonate: A quick reference for health care providers.* Philadelphia: Lippincott, Williams & Wilkins.

Hockenberry, M. J. (2005). *Wong's essentials of pediatric nursing* (7th ed.). St. Louis: Elsevier Mosby.

Hodgson, B. B., & Kizior, R. J. (2004). *Saunders nursing drug handbook.* St. Louis: Saunders.

Holcomb, S. S. (2005). Managing jaundice in full-term infants. *The Nurse Practitioner, 30,* 6–12.

Johnson, T. S. (2003). Hypoglycemia and the full-term newborn: How well does birth weight for gestational age predict risk? *JOGNN, 32*(1), 48–57.

Kenner, C., & Lott, J. W. (2004). *Neonatal nursing handbook.* St. Louis: Saunders.

Kinkade, S., & Meadows, S. (2005). Does neonatal circumcision decrease morbidity? *Journal of Family Practice, 54,* 81–82.

Klein, A. (2004). Management of hyperbilirubinemia in the healthy full-term infant. *Neonatology on the Web.* [Online] Available at www.neonatology.org/syllabus/bili.klein.html.

Krepcio, D., Foell, K., Folta, S. C., & Goldberg, J. P. (2004). Introduction to solid foods. *Nursing Spectrum, 14*(6), 16–18.

Littleton, L. Y., & Engebretson, J. C. (2005). *Maternity nursing care.* Clifton Park, NY: Thomson Delmar Learning.

Lowdermilk, D. L., & Perry, S. E. (2004). *Maternity & women's health care* (8th ed.). St. Louis: Mosby.

Mattson, S., & Smith, J. E. (2004). *Core curriculum for maternal–newborn nursing* (3rd ed.). St. Louis: Elsevier Saunders.

McGinnis, M. (2004). Bed sharing is risky. *Prevention, 56*(2), 125–127.

McKinney, E. S., James, S. R., Murray, S. S., & Ashwill, J. W. (2005). *Maternal–child nursing* (2nd ed.). St. Louis: Elsevier Saunders.

Meade Johnson. (2003). Caring for your new baby: Information for parents. Evansville, IN: Meade Johnson Nutritionals.

Medves, J. M. & O'Brien, B. (2004). The effect of bather and location of first bath on maintaining thermal stability in newborns. *JOGNN, 33*(2), 175–182.

Miller, C. A. (2003). Controversies concerning vitamin K and the newborn. *Pediatrics, 112,* 191–192.

Murray, G., Ormson, M. C., Lob, M. H. L., Ninan, B., Ninan, D., Dockery, L., & Fanaroff, A. A. (2004). Evaluation of the Natus ALGO 3 Newborn Hearing Screener. *Journal of Obstetric, Gynecologic, and Neonatal Nursing, 33,* 183–191.

O'Connor, D. (2003). Growth and development of preterm infants fed predominately human milk versus premature infant formula. *Journal of Pediatric Gastrointestinal Nutrition, 37,* 437–446.

Olds, S. B., London, M. L., Ladewig, P. A. W., & Davidson, M. R. (2004). *Maternal–newborn nursing & women's health care* (7th ed.). Upper Saddle River, NJ: Pearson Prentice Hall.

O'Leary, K. M. (2004). Skin and mucus membrane lesions. In P. S. Haws (Ed.), *Care of the sick neonate: A quick reference for health care providers* (pp. 255–265). Philadelphia: Lippincott Williams & Wilkins.

O'Toole, M. T. (2003). *Encyclopedia & dictionary of medicine, nursing and allied health* (7th ed.). Philadelphia: Saunders.

Page-Goertz, S. (2004). Leading families to breastfeeding success: Key principles of anticipatory guidance. *Advance for Nurse Practitioners, 12*(2), 23–34.

Pillitteri, A. (2003). *Maternal & child nursing: Care of the childbearing and childrearing family* (4th ed.). Philadelphia: Lippincott Williams & Wilkins.

Ramer, T. (2005). Breast milk jaundice. *eMedicine.* [Online] Available at www.emedicine.com/ped/topic282.htm.

Rabun, J. (2003). *For healthcare professionals: Guidelines on prevention of and response to infant abductions* (7th ed.). Alexandria, VA: National Center for Missing and Exploited Children.

Razmus, I. S., Dalton, M. E., & Wilson, D. (2004). Pain management for newborn circumcision. *Pediatric Nursing, 30,* 414–427.

Registered Nurses Association of Ontario (RNAO). (2003). *Breastfeeding best practice guidelines for nurses.* Toronto, Canada: Registered Nurses Association of Ontario (RNAO).

Rutter, N. (2003). Applied physiology: The newborn skin. *Current Pediatrics, 13,* 226–230.

Shogan, M. G. (2002). Emergency management plan for newborn abduction. *Journal of Obstetric, Gynecologic, and Neonatal Nursing, 31,* 340–346.

Spahis, J. (2003). Newborn screening: The nurse's role. *Nursing Spectrum.* [Online] Available at http://nsweb.nursingspectrum.com/ce/ce246.htm.

Spratto, G. R. & Woods, A. L. (2005). *PDR nurse's drug handbook.* Clifton Park, NY: Thomson Delmar Learning.

Ullah, S., & Griffiths, P. (2003). Does the use of pacifiers shorten breast-feeding duration in infants? *British Journal of Community Nursing, 8,* 458–463.

U.S. Department of Health and Human Services. (2000). *Healthy people 2010: Understanding and improving health* (2nd ed.). DHHS publication 017-001-00550-9. Washington, DC: Author.

Verklan, M. T., & Walden, M. (2004). *Core curriculum for neonatal intensive care nursing* (3rd ed.). St. Louis: Elsevier Saunders.

Weston, W. L., Lane, A. T., & Morelli, J. T. (2002). *Color textbook of pediatric dermatology* (3rd ed.) St. Louis: Mosby.

Wittmann–Price, R. A., & Pope, K. A. (2002). Universal newborn hearing screening. *American Journal of Nursing, 102,* 71–77.

Zepf, B. (2002). Does male cirumcision prevent cervical cancer in women? *American Family Physician, 66*(1), 147–149.

Web Resources

American Academy of Pediatrics: Newborn Screening Facts Sheets, **www.aap.org/policy/01565.html**
American Academy of Pediatrics: Breast-feeding and use of human milk, **www.aap.org/policy/re9729.html**
American Social Health Association, **www.vaccines.ashastd.org**
Baby Trend, **www.babytrend.com**
Breast-feeding information, **www.breastfeeding.com**
Bright Future Lactation Resource Center, **www.bflrc.com**
CDC's National Immunization Program, **www.cdc.gov/nip**
Graco/Century, **www.gracobaby.com**
Immunization Action Coalition, **www.immunize.org**
La Leche League International, **www.lalecheleague.org**
March of Dimes: Newborn Screening Tests, **www.marchofdimes.com/professionals/681_1200.asp**
National Center for Missing and Exploited Children, **www.missingkids.com**
National Healthy Mothers, Healthy Babies Coalition, **www.hmhb.org**
National Institute of Child Health and Human Development, **www.nih.gov**
National Newborn Screening and Genetics Resource Center, **http://genes-r-us.uthscsa.edu/resources/newborn/screstatus.htm**
Neonatal Network, **www.neonatalnetwork.com**
Safeline Corporation, **www.safelinekids.com**
The Vaccine Education Center, **www.vaccine.chop.edu**

Chapter WORKSHEET

● MULTIPLE CHOICE QUESTIONS

1. At birth, a newborn's assessment reveals the following: heart rate of 140 bpm, loud crying, some flexion of extremities, crying when bulb syringe is introduced into the nares, and a pink body with blue extremities. The nurse would document the newborn's Apgar score as

   a. 5 points

   b. 6 points

   c. 7 points

   d. 8 points

2. The nurse is explaining phototherapy to the parents of a newborn. The nurse would include which of the following as the purpose?

   a. Increase surfactant levels

   b. Stabilize the newborn's temperature

   c. Destroy Rh-negative antibodies

   d. Oxidize bilirubin on the skin

3. The nurse administers a single dose of vitamin K intramuscularly to a newborn after birth to promote

   a. Conjugation of bilirubin

   b. Blood clotting

   c. Foreman ovale closure

   d. Digestion of complex proteins

4. Instillation of a prophylactic agent is administered in both eyes of all newborns to prevent which of the following conditions?

   a. Gonorrhea and *Chlamydia*

   b. Thrush and *Enterobacter*

   c. *Staphylococcus* and syphilis

   d. Hepatitis B and herpes

5. The AAP recommends that all newborns be placed on their backs to sleep to reduce the risk of

   a. Respiratory distress syndrome

   b. Bottle mouth syndrome

   c. SIDS

   d. GI regurgitation syndrome

6. Which of the following immunizations is received by newborns before hospital discharge?

   a. Pneumococcus

   b. Varicella

   c. Hepatitis A

   d. Hepatitis B

7. Which condition would be missed if newborns are screened before they have tolerated protein feedings for at least 48 hours?

   a. Hypothyroidism

   b. Cystic fibrosis

   c. Phenylketonuria

   d. Sickle cell disease

● CRITICAL THINKING EXERCISES

1. Linda Scott, an African-American mother who delivered her first baby and is on the mother–baby unit, calls the nursery nurse into her room and appears upset about how her daughter looks. Ms. Scott tells the nurse that her baby's head looks like a "banana" and is mushy to touch, and she has white spots all over her nose. In addition, there appear to be big bluish bruises all over her baby's buttocks. She wants to know what is wrong with her baby's appearance and whether these problems go away.

   a. How should the nurse respond to Ms. Scott's questions?

   b. What additional newborn instruction might be appropriate at this time?

   c. What reassurance can be given to Ms. Scott regarding her daughter's appearance?

2. At approximately 12:30 AM on a Friday morning a woman entered a hospital through a busy emergency room. She was dressed in a white uniform and a lab coat with a stethoscope around her neck. She identified herself as a new nurse coming back to check on something she had left on the unit on a earlier shift. Subsequently, she entered a postpartum patient's room containing the patient's newborn infant, pushed the open crib down a hallway, and escaped through an exit. The security cameras weren't working at the time. The infant wasn't discovered missing until the 2 AM check by the nurse.

a. What impact does an infant abduction have on family and the hospital?

b. What security measure was the weak link in the chain of security?

c. What can hospitals do to prevent infant abduction from happening?

● STUDY ACTIVITIES

1. Interview a new mother on the postpartum unit on her second day about changes she has noticed in her newborn within the last 24 hours regarding his appearance and/or behavior. Discuss your interview findings at post conference.

2. Demonstrate a newborn bath to a new mother on a one-to-one basis in her room utilizing the principles of bathing from the cleanest to the dirtiest body part. Discuss the questions asked by the mother and her reaction to the bath demonstration in post conference.

3. Go to the La Leche League Web site (www.lalecheleague.org) and critique it for its information on breast-feeding and how helpful it would be to a new mother.

4. Debate the risks and benefits of neonatal circumcision within your nursing group at post conference. Did either side present a stronger position? What is your opinion and why?

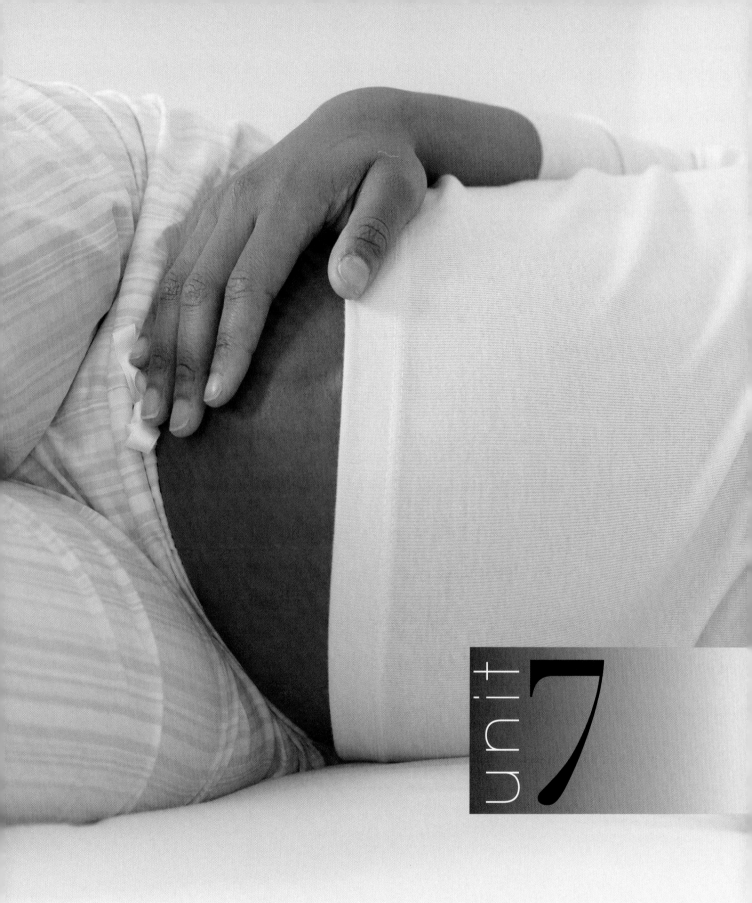

Childbearing at Risk

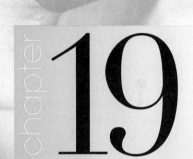

chapter 19

Nursing Management of Pregnancy at Risk: Pregnancy-Related Complications

KeyTERMS

abortion
abruptio placenta
clonus
ectopic pregnancy
eclampsia
gestational trophoblastic
    disease
gestational hypertension
high-risk pregnancy
hydramnios
hyperemesis gravidarum
oligohydramnios
multiple gestation
placenta previa
preeclampsia
preterm labor
premature rupture of
    membranes (or PROM)
tocolytic

LearningOBJECTIVES

After studying the chapter content, the student should be able to accomplish the following:

1. Define the key terms.
2. Identify common factors that might place a pregnancy at high risk.
3. Outline nursing management for the pregnant woman experiencing vaginal bleeding.
4. Describe the psychosocial impact of gestational diabetes and needed educational components for the woman and her family.
5. Summarize the management of preeclampsia, eclampsia, and HELLP syndrome.
6. Identify factors in a woman's prenatal history that place her at risk for preterm labor and/or premature rupture of membranes (PROM).
7. Explain the pathophysiology of hydramnios and subsequent management.
8. Formulate a teaching plan for maintenance of health for pregnant women experiencing a high-risk pregnancy.

Most individuals view pregnancy as a natural process with a positive outcome—that of the birth of a healthy newborn. Unfortunately, conditions can occur that possibly result in negative outcomes for the fetus, mother, or both. A **high-risk pregnancy** is one in which a condition exists that jeopardizes the health of the mother, her fetus, or both. The condition may be the sole result of the pregnancy or it may be a condition that existed before the woman became pregnant.

Approximately one in four pregnant women is diagnosed with complications or is considered high risk (Youngkin & Davis, 2004). Women who are considered high risk have a higher incidence of morbidity and mortality compared with mothers in the general population. In addition, the risk status of a woman and her fetus can change during the months of her pregnancy, with a number of problems occurring during labor, birth, or afterward, even in women without any known previous antepartal risk. Examples of high-risk conditions include gestational diabetes and ectopic pregnancy. These conditions are specifically addressed in Healthy People 2010 (see Healthy People 2010: National Health Goals Related to High-Risk Pregnancy). Early identification of the woman at risk is essential to ensure that appropriate interventions can be instituted promptly, increasing the opportunity to change the course of events and provide a positive outcome.

The term *risk* may mean different things to different groups. For example, healthcare professionals may focus on the disease processes and treatment to prevent complications. Nurses may focus on nursing care and on the psychosocial impact to the woman and her family. Insurance companies may concentrate on the economic issues related to the high-risk status, whereas the woman's attention may be focused on her own needs and those of her family. Together, working as a collaborative team, the ultimate goal of care is to ensure the best possible outcome for the woman, her fetus, and her family.

Risk assessment begins with the first antepartal visit and continues with each subsequent visit because additional factors may be identified in later visits that were not apparent during earlier visits. For example, as the nurse and client develop a trusting relationship, previously unidentified or unsuspected factors (such as drug abuse or intimate partner violence) may be revealed. Through education and support, the nurse can encourage the client to inform her healthcare provider of these concerns, and necessary interventions or referrals can be made.

Diverse factors must be considered when determining a woman's risk for adverse pregnancy outcomes (Gupton, Heaman, & Cheung, 2001). A comprehensive approach to high-risk pregnancy is needed, and the factors associated with them are grouped into broad categories based on threats to health and pregnancy outcome. Current categories of risk are biophysical, psychosocial, sociodemographic, and environmental (Gilbert & Harmon, 2003) (Box 19-1).

This chapter describes the major conditions related directly to the pregnancy that can complicate a pregnancy, possibly affecting maternal and fetal outcomes. These include bleeding during pregnancy (spontaneous abortion, ectopic pregnancy, gestational trophoblastic disease [GTD]), cervical insufficiency, placenta previa, and abruptio placenta), hyperemesis gravidarum, gestational hypertension, HELLP syndrome, gestational diabetes, blood incompatibility, hydramnios and oligohydramnios, multiple gestation, premature rupture of membranes (PROM), and preterm labor. Chapter 20 addresses preexisting conditions that can complicate a woman's pregnancy.

HEALTHY PEOPLE *2010*

National Health Goals Related to High-Risk Pregnancy

Objective	Significance
Decrease the proportion of pregnant women with gestational diabetes	Will help to promote proper prepregnant and pregnancy glycemic control; foster careful perinatal obstetric monitoring, thereby helping to reduce perinatal death and congenital abnormalities Will help to reinforce the importance of good nutrition during pregnancy as paramount in increasing better pregnancy outcomes
Reduce ectopic pregnancies	Will help to focus attention on the need for initiating prenatal care early and for continued monitoring throughout pregnancy, thus helping to decrease maternal mortality related to ectopic pregnancies through early detection

Source: U.S. DHHS, 2000.

Bleeding During Pregnancy

Bleeding any time during pregnancy is serious and potentially life-threatening. Bleeding can occur early or late in the pregnancy and may result from numerous conditions. Conditions commonly associated with early bleeding (first

---

BOX 19-1

FACTORS PLACING A WOMAN AT RISK DURING PREGNANCY

Biophysical Factors
- Genetic conditions
- Chromosomal abnormalities
- Multiple pregnancy
- Defective genes
- Inherited disorders
- ABO incompatibility
- Large fetal size
- Medical and obstetric conditions
- Preterm labor and birth
- Cardiovascular disease
- Chronic hypertension
- Incompetent cervix
- Placental abnormalities
- Infection
- Diabetes
- Maternal collagen diseases
- Pregnancy-induced hypertension
- Asthma
- Postterm pregnancy
- Hemoglobinopathies
- Nutritional status
- Inadequate dietary intake
- Food fads
- Excessive food intake
- Under- or overweight status
- Hematocrit value less than 33%
- Eating disorder

Psychosocial Factors
- Smoking
- Caffeine
- Alcohol
- Drugs
- Inadequate support system
- Situational crisis
- History of violence
- Emotional distress
- Unsafe cultural practices

Sociodemographic Factors
- Poverty status
- Lack of prenatal care
- Age younger than 15 years or older than 35 years
- Parity—all first pregnancies and more than five pregnancies
- Marital status—increased risk for unmarried
- Accessibility to health care
- Ethnicity—increased risk in nonwhite women

Environmental Factors
Exposure to
- Infections
- Radiation
- Pesticides
- Illicit drugs
- Industrial pollutants
- Secondhand cigarette smoke
- Personal stress (Gilbert & Harmon, 2003; Lee, 2003; Mattson & Smith, 2004; Verklan & Walden, 2004)

---

half of pregnancy) include spontaneous abortion, ectopic pregnancy, and GTD. Conditions associated with late bleeding include placenta previa and abruptio placenta, which usually occur after the 20th week of gestation.

Spontaneous Abortion

An **abortion** is the loss of an early pregnancy, usually before week 20 of gestation. Abortion can be spontaneous or induced. A spontaneous abortion refers to the loss of a fetus resulting from natural causes—that is, not elective or therapeutically induced by a procedure. The term *miscarriage* is often used by nonmedical people to denote an abortion that has occurred spontaneously. A miscarriage can occur during early pregnancy, and many women who miscarry may not even be aware that they are pregnant. About 80% of spontaneous abortions occur within the first trimester.

The overall rate for spontaneous abortion in the United States is reported as 15 to 20% of recognized pregnancies in the United States. However, with the development of highly sensitive assays for hCG levels that detect pregnancies prior to the expected next menses, the inci-

dence of pregnancy loss increases significantly—to about 60 to 70% (Puscheck & Pradhan, 2004).

Causes

The causes of spontaneous abortion are varied and often unknown. The most common cause for first trimester abortions is fetal genetic abnormalities, usually unrelated to the mother. Those occurring during the second trimester are more likely to have maternal causes, such as incompetent cervix, congenital or acquired anomaly of the uterine cavity, hypothyroidism, diabetes mellitus, chronic nephritis, use of crack cocaine, lupus, and acute infection such as rubella virus, cytomegalovirus, herpes simplex virus, bacterial vaginosis, and toxoplasmosis (Marchiano, 2004).

Spontaneous abortions may be classified into six categories based on the signs and symptoms exhibited. These categories include threatened abortion, inevitable abortion, incomplete abortion, complete abortion, missed abortion, and habitual abortion (Table 19-1).

Nursing Management

Nursing management of the woman with a spontaneous abortion focuses on psychological support for the family

Table 19-1 Categories of Abortion

Category	Assessment Findings	Diagnosis	Treatment
Threatened abortion	Vaginal bleeding (often slight) early in a pregnancy No cervical dilation or change in cervical consistency Mild abdominal cramping Closed cervical os No passage of fetal tissue	Vaginal ultrasound to confirm if sac is empty Declining maternal serum hCG and progesterone levels to provide additional information about viability of pregnancy	Conservative supportive treatment Possible reduction in activity in conjunction with nutritious diet and adequate hydration
Inevitable abortion	Vaginal bleeding (greater than that associated with threatened abortion) Rupture of membranes Cervical dilation Strong abdominal cramping Possible passage of products of conception	Ultrasound and hCG levels to indicate pregnancy loss	Vacuum curettage if products of conception are not passed, to reduce risk of excessive bleeding and infection Prostaglandin analogs such as misoprostol to empty uterus of retained tissue (only used if fragments are not completely passed)
Incomplete abortion (passage of some of the products of conception)	Intense abdominal cramping Heavy vaginal bleeding Cervical dilation	Ultrasound confirmation that products of conception still in uterus	Client stabilization Evacuation of uterus via dilation and curettage (D&C) or prostaglandin analog
Complete abortion (passage of all products of conception)	History of vaginal bleeding and abdominal pain Passage of tissue with subsequent decrease in pain and significant decrease in vaginal bleeding	Ultrasound demonstrating an empty uterus	No medical or surgical intervention necessary Follow-up appointment to discuss family planning
Missed abortion (nonviable embryo retained in utero for at least 6 weeks)	Absent uterine contractions Irregular spotting Possible progression to inevitable abortion	Ultrasound to identify products of conception in uterus	Evacuation of uterus (if inevitable abortion does not occur): suction curettage during first trimester, dilation and evacuation during second trimester Induction of labor with intravaginal PGE2 suppository to empty uterus without surgical intervention
Habitual abortion	History of three or more consecutive spontaneous abortions Not carrying the pregnancy to viability or term	Validation via client's history	Identification and treatment of underlying cause (possible causes such as genetic or chromosomal abnormalities, reproductive tract abnormalities, chronic diseases or immunologic problems) Cervical cerclage in second trimester if incompetent cervix is the cause

experiencing an acute loss and grief. In addition, women need reassurance that spontaneous abortions usually result from an abnormality and that their actions did not cause the abortion.

When a pregnant woman calls and reports vaginal bleeding, she must be seen as soon as possible by a health care professional to ascertain the etiology. Varying degrees of vaginal bleeding, low back pain, abdominal cramping, and passage of products of conception tissue may be reported. Ask the woman about the color of the vaginal bleeding (bright red is significant) and the amount—for example, question her about the frequency with which she is changing her peripads (saturation of one peripad hourly is significant). Also, obtain a description of any other signs and symptoms the woman may be experiencing, along with a description of their severity and duration. It is important to remain calm and listen to the woman's description.

Assessment

When the woman arrives and is admitted, the priorities are to assess her vital signs, amount and color of the bleeding, and current pain rating on a scale of 1 to 10 points. Also, evaluate the amount and intensity of the woman's abdominal cramping or contractions, and assess the woman's level of understanding about what is happening to her.

Nursing Interventions

Ongoing assessment is essential for the woman experiencing a spontaneous abortion. Nursing care focuses on monitoring the amount of vaginal bleeding through pad counts, observing for any passage of products of conception tissue, and providing pain management to address the cramping discomfort. In addition, the nurse plays a major role in providing emotional support to the woman and her family.

Keep in mind that the woman's emotional reaction may vary depending on her desire for this pregnancy and her available support network. Provide both physical and emotional support. In addition, prepare the woman and her family for the assessment process, and answer her ongoing questions regarding what is happening.

Offering a factual explanation about some of the causes of spontaneous abortions can assist the woman to understand what is happening and perhaps allay her fears and guilt that she did something to cause this pregnancy loss. Assist in preparing the woman for procedures and treatment such as surgery to evacuate the uterus or medications such as misoprostol or PGE2. If the woman is Rh negative and not sensitized, expect to administer RhoGAM within 72 hours after the abortion is complete. See Drug Guide 19-1 for more information about these medications.

Most women will experience an acute sense of loss and go through a grieving process with a spontaneous abortion. Providing sensitive listening, counseling, and anticipatory guidance to the woman and her family will allow them to verbalize their feelings and ask questions concerning future pregnancies.

The grieving period may last as long as 2 years after a pregnancy loss, with each person grieving in his or her own way. Encourage friends and family to be supportive, but give the couple space and time to work through their loss. Referral to a community support group for parents who have experienced a miscarriage can be very helpful during this grief process.

Ectopic Pregnancy

Normally, implantation of the fertilized ovum occurs in the uterus. An **ectopic pregnancy** is any pregnancy in which the fertilized ovum implants outside the uterine cavity. The most common site for implantation is the fallopian tubes, but some ova may implant in the cornua of the uterus, ovary, cervix, or abdominal cavity (Fig. 19-1) (Sepilian & Wood, 2004). Unfortunately, none of these anatomic sites can accommodate placental attachment or a growing embryo. Thus, the potential for rupture and hemorrhage exists. A ruptured ectopic pregnancy is a true medical emergency. It is a potentially life-threatening condition and involves pregnancy loss. It is the leading cause of maternal mortality in the first trimester and accounts for 10 to 15% of all pregnancy-related deaths (Sepilian & Wood, 2005).

Ectopic pregnancies occur from 1 in every 40 to 1 in every 100 pregnancies in the United States (Marchiano, 2004). Their incidence has increased dramatically in the past few decades as a result of improved diagnostic techniques, such as more sensitive beta-hCG assays and the availability of transvaginal ultrasound (Chen, 2004).

Causes

Ectopic pregnancies usually are caused by conditions that obstruct or slow the passage of the fertilized ovum through the fallopian tube to the uterus. This may be a physical blockage in the tube, or failure of the tubal epithelium to move the zygote (the cell formed after the egg is fertilized) down the tube into the uterus. In the general population, most cases are the result of tubal scarring secondary to pelvic inflammatory disease. Organisms such as *Neisseria gonorrhoeae* and *Chlamydia trachomatis* preferentially attack the fallopian tubes, producing silent infections. Even with early treatment, tubal damage can occur. Other contributing factors include

- Previous ectopic pregnancy
- History of STIs
- Endometriosis
- Previous tubal or pelvic surgery
- Infertility and infertility treatments, including use of fertility drugs
- Uterine abnormalities such as fibroids
- Presence of intrauterine device (IUD)
- Use of progestin-only mini pill (slows ovum transport)
- Postpartum or postabortion infection
- Increasing age older than 35 years
- Cigarette smoking (Owen, 2003)

Drug Guide 19-1 Medications Used With Spontaneous Abortions

Drug	Action	Indications	Nursing Implications
Misoprostol (RU 486; Cytotec)	Stimulates uterine contractions to terminate a pregnancy	Evacuate the uterus after abortion to ensure passage of all the products of conception	Monitor for side effects such as diarrhea, abdominal pain, nausea, vomiting, dyspepsia Assess vaginal bleeding and report any increased bleeding, pain, or fever Monitor for signs and symptoms of shock, such as tachycardia, hypotension, anxiety
PGE2, dinoprostone (Cervidil, Prepidil Gel, Prostin E2)	Stimulates uterine contractions, causing expulsion of uterine contents	Expel uterine contents in fetal death, missed abortion during second trimester, or to efface and dilate the cervix in pregnancy at term	Bring gel to room temperature before administering Avoid contact with skin Use sterile technique to administer Keep client supine 30 minutes after administering Document time of insertion and dosing intervals Remove insert with retrieval system after 12 hours or at the onset of labor Explain purpose and expected response to client
Rh (D) immunoglobulin (Gamulin, HydroRho-D, RhoGAM)	Suppresses immune response of nonsensitized Rh-negative patients who are exposed to Rh-positive blood	Prevent isoimmunization in Rh-negative women exposed to Rh-positive blood after abortions, miscarriages, and pregnancies	Administer intramuscularly in deltoid area Give only MICRhoGAM for abortions and miscarriages < 12 weeks unless fetus or father is Rh negative (unless patient is Rh positive, Rh antibodies are present) Educate woman that she will need this after subsequent deliveries if newborns are Rh positive; also check lab study results prior to administering the drug

Clinical Manifestations

Although onset may vary, clinical manifestations of an unruptured ectopic pregnancy usually begin at about the seventh or eighth week of gestation. A missed menses, adnexal fullness, and tenderness may indicate an unruptured tubal pregnancy. As the tube stretches, the pain increases. The hallmark of ectopic pregnancy is abdominal pain with spotting within 6 to 8 weeks after a missed menses. Other symptoms include breast tenderness, nausea, and low back pain. Pain may be unilateral, bilateral, or diffuse over the abdomen.

If rupture or hemorrhaging occurs before successfully treating the pregnancy, symptoms may worsen and include severe, sharp, and sudden pain in the lower abdomen as the tube tears open and the embryo is expelled into the pelvic cavity; feelings of faintness; referred pain to the shoulder area indicating bleeding into the abdomen caused by phrenic nerve irritation; hypotension; marked abdominal tenderness with distension; and hypovolemic shock.

The use of transvaginal ultrasound to visualize the misplaced pregnancy and low levels of serum beta-hCG assist in diagnosing an ectopic pregnancy. The ultrasound determines whether the pregnancy is intrauterine, assesses the size of the uterus, and provides evidence of fetus viability. Absence of an intrauterine gestational sac is diagnostic of ectopic pregnancy (Baines, 2003). In a normal intrauterine pregnancy, beta-hCG levels typically double every 2 to 4 days. Therefore, low beta-hCG levels are suggestive of an ectopic pregnancy or impending abortion. Other tests may be done to rule out other conditions such as spontaneous abortion, ruptured ovarian cyst, appendicitis, and salpingitis.

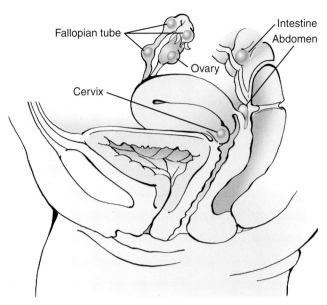

● Figure 19-1 Ectopic pregnancy: possible sites for implantation.

Treatment

The therapeutic management of ectopic pregnancy depends on whether the tube is intact or has ruptured. Historically, the treatment of ectopic pregnancy was limited to surgery, but medical therapy is currently available.

If the fallopian tube is still intact, medical management becomes an option. To be eligible for medical therapy, the client must be hemodynamically stable, with no signs of active bleeding in the peritoneal cavity, and the mass (which must measure less than 4 cm as determined by ultrasound) must be unruptured (Valley & Fly, 2005). The potential advantages include avoidance of surgery, the preservation of tubal patency and function, and a lower cost. Methotrexate, prostaglandins, misoprostol, and actinomycin have all been used in the medical (non-surgical) management of ectopic pregnancy (Youngkin & Davis, 2004).

Methotrexate, the agent most commonly used, is a folic acid antagonist that inhibits cell division in the developing embryo. It typically has been used as a chemotherapeutic agent in the treatment of leukemias, lymphomas, and carcinomas. It has been shown to produce results similar to that for surgical therapy, in terms of high success rate, low complication rate, and good reproductive potential (Simpson, 2002). Adverse effects associated with methotrexate include nausea, vomiting, stomatitis, diarrhea, gastric upset, increased abdominal pain, and dizziness. Prior to receiving the single-dose intramuscular injection to treat unruptured pregnancies, the woman should be counseled on the risks, benefits, adverse effects, and the possibility of failure of medical therapy, which would result in tubal rupture, necessitating surgery (Sepilian & Wood, 2005). The woman is then instructed to return weekly for follow-up lab studies for the next several weeks until beta-hCG titers decrease.

Surgical management for the unruptured fallopian tube might involve a linear salpingostomy to preserve the tube—an important consideration for the woman wanting to preserve her future fertility.

With a ruptured ectopic pregnancy, surgery is necessary as a result of possible uncontrolled hemorrhage. A laparotomy with a removal of the tube (salpingectomy) may be necessary. With earlier diagnosis and medial management, the focus has changed from prevention of maternal death to facilitating rapid recovery and preserving fertility.

Regardless of the treatment approach (medical or surgical), the woman's beta-hCG level is monitored until it is undetectable to ensure that any residual trophoblastic tissue that forms the placenta is gone. Also, all Rh-negative unsensitized clients are administered Rh immunoglobulin to prevent isoimmunization in future pregnancies.

Nursing Management

The woman with an ectopic pregnancy requires support throughout diagnosis, treatment, and aftercare. If surgery is needed, close assessment and monitoring of the client's vital signs, bleeding (peritoneal or vaginal), and pain status are critical to identify hypovolemic shock that may occur with tubal rupture. The client often experiences a great deal of pain. Administer analgesics as ordered to promote comfort and relieve discomfort from abdominal pain. If the woman is treated medically on an outpatient basis, it is important to outline the signs of ectopic rupture (severe, sharp, stabbing, unilateral abdominal pain; vertigo/fainting; hypotension; and increased pulse) and advise the woman to seek medical help immediately.

Prepare the client physiologically and psychologically for surgery or any procedure. Provide a clear explanation of the expected outcome. Astute vigilance and early referral will help reduce short- and long-term morbidity.

A woman's psychological reaction to an ectopic pregnancy is unpredictable. However, it is important to recognize she has experienced a pregnancy loss in addition to undergoing treatment for a potentially life-threatening condition. It can be difficult for the woman to comprehend what has happened to her because events occur so quickly. In the woman's mind, she had just started a pregnancy and now it has ended abruptly. Assist her with bringing this experience more into reality by encouraging the woman and her family to express their feelings and concerns openly, and validating that this is a loss of pregnancy and it is okay to grieve over the loss.

Provide emotional support, spiritual care, client education, and information about community support groups available (such as Resolve through Sharing) as the client grieves the loss of her unborn child and comes to terms with the medical complications of the situation. Acknowledge the client's pregnancy and allow her to discuss her feelings about what the pregnancy means. Also, stress the need for follow-up blood testing for several weeks to monitor hCG titers until they return to zero, indicating resolution of the ectopic pregnancy. Additionally, discuss her feelings and concerns about her future fertility and provide teaching about the need for using contraceptives at this time for at least three menstrual cycles to allow time for her reproductive tract to heal and tissue to be repaired. Include the woman's partner in this discussion to make sure there is understanding by both parties regarding what has happened, what intervention is needed, and what the future holds for both of them regarding childbearing.

Prevention of ectopic pregnancies through screening and client education is essential. Many can be prevented by avoiding those conditions that might cause scarring of the fallopian tubes. Such prevention education may include

- Reducing risk factors such as sexual intercourse with multiple partners or intercourse without a condom
- Avoiding contracting STIs that lead to pelvic inflammatory disease (PID)
- Obtaining early diagnosis and adequate treatment of STIs
- Avoiding the use of an IUD as a contraceptive method to reduce the risk of repeat ascending infections responsible for tubal scarring
- Using condoms to decrease the risk of infections that cause tubal scarring
- Seeking prenatal care early if pregnant to confirm location of pregnancy

Gestational Trophoblastic Disease

Gestational trophoblastic disease (GTD) comprises a spectrum of neoplastic disorders that originate in the human placenta. Gestational tissue is present, but the pregnancy is not viable. The incidence is about 1 in 1000 pregnancies (Cunningham, Gant, Leveno, Gilstrap, Hauth, & Wenstrom, 2005). The two most common types are hydatidiform mole (partial and complete) and choriocarcinoma.

The hydatidiform mole is a benign neoplasm of the chorion in which chorionic villi degenerate and become transparent vesicles containing clear, viscid fluid. Hydatiform mole is classified as complete or partial, distinguished by differences in clinical presentation, pathology, genetics, and epidemiology (Gerulath, 2002). The complete mole develops from an "empty egg," which is fertilized by a normal sperm (46 all-paternal chromosomes). The embryo dies early, no circulation is established, and no embryonic tissue is found. The complete mole is associated with the development of choriocarcinoma. The partial mole has a triploid karyotype (69 chromosomes), because two sperm have provided a double contribution by fertilizing the ovum (Fig. 19-2).

Having a molar pregnancy (partial or complete) results in the loss of the pregnancy and the possibility of developing choriocarcinoma, a chorionic malignancy from the trophoblastic tissue.

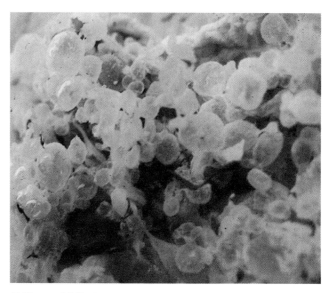

● Figure 19-2 Complete hydatidiform mole.

ConsiderTHIS!

We had lived across the dorm hall from each other during nursing school, but really didn't get to know each other except for a casual hello in passing. When we graduated, Rose went to work in the emergency room and I in OB. We saw each other occasionally in the employee cafeteria, but a quick hello was all that was usually exchanged. I heard she married one of the paramedics who worked in the ER and was soon pregnant. I finally got to say more than hello when she was admitted to the OB unit bleeding during her fourth month of pregnancy. What was discovered was gestational trophoblastic disease and not a normal pregnancy. I remember holding her in my arms as she wept. She was told she had a complete molar pregnancy after surgery, and she would need extensive follow-up for the next year. I lost track of her that summer as my life became busier. Around Thanksgiving time, I heard she had died from choriocarcinoma. I attended her funeral, finally, to get the time to say a final hello and good-bye, but this time with sadness and tears.

Thoughts: Rose was only 26 years old when she succumbed to this very virulent cancer. I think back and realize I missed knowing this brave young woman and wished that I had taken the time to say more than hello. Could her outcome have been different? Why wasn't it recognized earlier? Did she not follow up after her diagnosis? I can only speculate regarding the whom, what, and where. She lived a short but purposeful life, and hopefully continued research will change other women's outcomes in the future.

Causes

The exact cause of molar pregnancies is unknown, but recent research is looking into a genetic basis for it. Studies have revealed some remarkable features about molar pregnancies. They

- Have the ability to invade into the wall of the uterus
- Can metastasize to other organs
- Recur in subsequent pregnancies
- Can develop into choriocarcinoma, a virulent cancer
- Occur more in Asia (1 in 120 pregnancies) compared with the United States (1 in 1000 pregnancies)
- Are influenced by nutritional factors, such as protein deficiency
- Tend to affect older women more than younger women

Clinical Manifestations

Clinical manifestations of GTD are very similar to that of spontaneous abortion at about 12 weeks of pregnancy. Signs and symptoms of a molar pregnancy include

- Report of early signs of pregnancy, such as amenorrhea, breast tenderness, fatigue
- Brownish vaginal bleeding/spotting
- Anemia
- Severe morning sickness resulting from high hCG levels
- Fluid retention and swelling
- Larger size uterus when compared with that for pregnancy dates
- Expulsion of grapelike vesicles possibly occurring in some women
- Extremely high hCG levels present; no single value considered diagnostic
- Early development of **preeclampsia,** which usually is not present until after 24 weeks
- Absence of fetal heart rate or fetal activity
- Ultrasonic evidence of characteristic molar pattern

The diagnosis is made by visualizing the characteristic appearance of the vesicular molar pattern in the uterus via transvaginal ultrasound and high levels of hCG.

Treatment

Treatment consists of immediate evacuation of the uterine contents as soon as the diagnosis is made and long-term follow-up of the client to detect any remaining trophoblastic tissue that might become malignant. Dilation and suction curettage are used to empty the uterus. The tissue obtained is sent to the laboratory for analysis to evaluate for choriocarcinoma. Serial levels of hCG are used to detect residual trophoblastic tissue for 1 year. If any tissue remains, hCG levels will not regress. Because of this cancer risk, the client is advised to receive extensive follow-up therapy for the next 12 months. The follow-up protocol may include

- Baseline hCG level, chest radiograph, and pelvic ultrasound
- Weekly serum hCG levels until it drops to zero and remains at that level for 3 consecutive weeks, then

monthly for 6 months, then every 2 months for the remainder of the year
- Chest radiograph every 6 months to detect pulmonary metastasis
- Regular pelvic examinations to assess uterine and ovarian regression
- Systemic assessments for symptoms indicative of lung, brain, liver, or vaginal metastasis
- Strong recommendation to avoid pregnancy for 1 year because the pregnancy can interfere with the monitoring of hCG levels
- Use of reliable contraceptive (Gilbert & Harmon, 2003)

Nursing Management

Nursing management of the woman with GTD focuses on educating her about the potential risk of cancer that may develop after a molar pregnancy and the strict adherence needed for the follow-up program. The woman must understand the necessity for the continued follow-up care regimen to improve her chances of future pregnancies and to ensure her continued quality of life.

Assessment

The nurse plays a crucial role in identifying and bringing this condition to the attention of the health care provider based on sound knowledge of the typical clinical manifestations and through astute antepartal assessments. Assess the woman for potential clinical manifestations at each antepartal visit.

Nursing Interventions

After GTD is diagnosed, the nurse needs to educate the client about the condition and appropriate interventions that may be necessary to save her life. Explain each phase of treatment accurately and provide support for the woman and her family as they go through the grieving process. Prepare the woman physically and psychologically for D&C as indicated.

To aid the client and her family in coping with the loss of the pregnancy and the possibility of a cancer diagnosis, use the following interventions:

- Listen to their concerns and fears.
- Allow them time to grieve for their pregnancy loss.
- Acknowledge their loss and sad feelings (say you are sorry for their loss).
- Encourage them to express their grief; make it okay for them to cry.
- Provide them with as much factual information as possible to help them make sense of what is happening.
- Enlist support from additional family and friends as appropriate, and with the client's permission.

As with any facet of health care, the nurse needs to keep current on the latest research and new therapies. Inform the client about her follow up care, which will probably involve a close clinical surveillance for approximately 1 year, and reinforce its necessity in monitoring the client's condition. Serial serum beta-hCG levels are used to detect residual trophoblastic tissue. Continued high or increasing hCG titers are abnormal and need further evaluation.

Anticipate the use of chemotherapy, such as methotrexate, which may be started as prophylaxis. Inform the client about the need for using a reliable contraceptive to prevent pregnancy for 1 year. A positive pregnancy test would interfere with tracking of the serial beta-hCG levels used to identify a potential malignancy. Stress the need for client cooperation and adherence to the plan of therapy throughout this year-long follow-up.

Cervical Insufficiency

Cervical insufficiency describes a weak, structurally defective cervix that spontaneously dilates in the absence of contractions in the second trimester, resulting in the loss of the pregnancy. The incidence of cervical insufficiency is less than 1% and ranges in estimation from 1 in 500 to 1 in 2000 pregnancies, accounting for approximately 20 to 25% of midtrimester losses (Ahn & Hibbard, 2003).

Causes

Cervical insufficiency may result from an in utero exposure to diethylstilbestrol (DES), which was commonly used for the treatment of recurrent pregnancy loss until the mid-1970s; an acquired cause, such as trauma to the cervix from pervious gynecologic or obstetric procedures (cone biopsy, D&C); damage to the cervix from a previous difficult birth (cervical lacerations from forceps); increased uterine volume (multiple gestation, hydramnios); or unknown reasons (Creasy, Resnik, & Iams, 2004).

Clinical Manifestations

Commonly, with cervical insufficiency, the woman will report a pink-tinged vaginal discharge or an increase in pelvic pressure. History may reveal a previous loss of pregnancy around 20 weeks. Cervical dilation also occurs. Continuation leads to rupture of the membranes, release of amniotic fluid, and uterine contractions, subsequently resulting in delivery of the fetus, often before the time of viability.

Treatment

The diagnosis of cervical insufficiency remains difficult in many circumstances. The cornerstone of diagnosis is a history of midtrimester pregnancy loss associated with painless cervical dilatation without evidence of uterine activity. Close surveillance of cervical length with transvaginal ultrasound is typically started around 20 weeks' gestation. Regular evaluations are performed (particularly in women with pelvic pressure, backache, or increased mucoid discharge) every few days to avoid missing rapid changes in cervical dilation or until the trend in cervical length can be characterized (Ressel, 2004).

Cervical shortening occurs from the internal os outward and can be viewed on ultrasound as *funneling.* The amount of funneling can be determined on ultrasound by dividing funnel length by cervix length. A cervical length less than 25 mm is abnormal between 14 weeks and 24 weeks, and increases the risk of preterm labor. The most common time at which a short cervix or funneling develops is 18 to 22 weeks, so ultrasound screening should be performed during this interval (Berghella, 2004).

Management for cervical insufficiency has been treated in a variety of ways: bed rest; pelvic rest; avoidance of heavy lifting; or surgically, via a procedure of a cervical cerclage in the second trimester. Cervical cerclage involves using a heavy purse-string suture to secure and reinforce the internal os of the cervix (Fig. 19-3).

According to ACOG (2003a), if a short cervix is identified at or after 20 weeks with absence of infection (chorioamnionitis), the decision to proceed with cerclage should be made with caution; there have been limited numbers of well-designed randomized studies to support its efficacy. Suture displacement, rupture of membranes, and chorioamnionitis are the most common complications associated with cerclage placement, and incidence varies widely in relation to timing and indications for the cerclage (Ressel, 2004). The optimal timing for cerclage removal is unclear, according to ACOG (2003a).

Nursing Management

Nursing management related to women with cervical insufficiency involves taking a very thorough history to be alert to any risk factors that might have a bearing on this pregnancy—previous cervical trauma, preterm labor, fetal loss in second trimester, or previous surgeries or procedures involving the cervix. Monitor the woman very closely for signs of preterm labor: backache, increase in vaginal discharge, rupture of membranes, and uterine contractions. Provide emotional and educational support to allay the couple's anxiety about the well-being of their fetus. Continuing surveillance throughout the pregnancy is important to promote a positive outcome for the family.

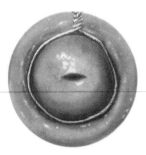

● Figure 19-3 Cervical cerclage.

Placenta Previa

Placenta previa is a bleeding condition that occurs during the last two trimesters of pregnancy. Placenta previa literally means "afterbirth first" and defines a condition in which the placenta implants over the cervical os. It may cause serious morbidity and mortality to fetus and mother. It complicates approximately 5 of 1000 births or 1 in every 200 pregnancies and is associated with potentially serious consequences from hemorrhage, abruption (separation) of the placenta, or emergency cesarean birth (Joy & Lyon, 2004).

Placenta previa is generally classified according to the degree of coverage or proximity to the internal os as follows (Fig. 19-4):

- Total placenta previa—occurs when the internal cervical os is completely covered by the placenta
- Partial placenta previa—occurs when the internal os is partially covered by the placenta
- Marginal placenta previa—occurs when the placenta is at the margin or edge of the internal os
- Low-lying placenta previa—occurs when the placenta is implanted in the lower uterine segment and is near the internal os but does not reach it

Causes

The exact etiology of placenta previa is unknown. Placenta previa is initiated by implantation of the embryo in the lower uterus. With placental attachment and growth, the cervical os may become covered by the developing placenta. Placental vascularization is defective, allowing the placenta to attach directly to the myometrium (accreta), invade the myometrium (increta), or penetrate the myometrium (percreta).

The condition may be multifactorial and is associated with the following risk factors:

- Advanced maternal age (more than 30 years old)
- Previous cesarean birth
- Multiparity
- Uterine insult or injury
- Cocaine use
- Prior placenta previa
- Male infants (Thompson, 2005)
- African-Americans and Asian cultural groups (Ko & Yoon, 2005)
- Multiple gestations
- Previous induced abortion
- Previous myomectomy to remove fibroids
- Smoking (Ko & Yoon, 2005)

Clinical Manifestations

The classical clinical presentation is painless, bright-red vaginal bleeding occurring during the second or third trimester. The initial bleeding is not usually profuse and it ceases spontaneously, only to recur again. The first episode of bleeding occurs (on average) at 27 to 32 weeks' gestation, and contractions may or may not occur with the bleeding. The bleeding is thought to arise secondary to the thinning of the lower uterine segment in preparation for the onset of labor. When the bleeding occurs at the implantation site in the lower uterus, the uterus is unable to contract adequately and stop the flow of blood from the open vessels. Typically with normal placental implantation in the upper uterus, minor disruptive placental attachment is not a problem, because there is a larger volume of myometrial tissue able to contract and constrict bleeding vessels. The client's uterus is soft and nontender on examination. Auscultation of fetal heart tones is within normal parameters, and fetal distress usually is not present unless a cord accident occurs or vaginal blood loss has been heavy enough to induce maternal shock or placenta abruption (Gaudier, 2003).

To validate the position of the placenta, a transvaginal ultrasound is done. In addition, MRI may be ordered in preparing for delivery because it allows identification of placenta accreta, increta, or percreta in addition to

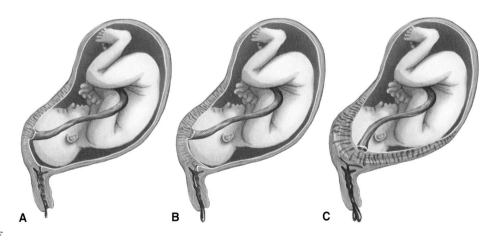

● Figure 19-4 Classification of placenta previa. (**A**) Marginal. (**B**) Partial. (**C**) Complete.

A

B

C

Marginal

Partial

Complete

placenta previa. These placental abnormalities, although rare, carry a very high morbidity and mortality rate, necessitating a possible hysterectomy at delivery.

Treatment

The treatment depends on the extent of bleeding, the amount of placenta over the cervical os, whether the fetus is developed enough to survive outside the uterus, the position of the fetus, the parity for the mother, and the presence or absence of labor (Gaudier, 2003).

If the mother and fetus are both stable, therapeutic management may involve expectant (or wait-and-see) care. This care can be carried out in the home or on an antepartal unit in the healthcare facility. If there is no active bleeding and the client has readily available access to reliable transportation, is able to maintain bed rest in the home setting, and has the ability to comprehend instructions, expectant care at home is appropriate. However, if the client requires continuous care and monitoring and is not able to comply with needed home care requirements, the antepartal unit is the best environment.

Nursing Management

Whether the care setting is in the client's home or in the healthcare facility setting, the nurse focuses on monitoring the maternal–fetal dyad status, assessing for signs and symptoms of vaginal bleeding and fetal distress, and providing support and education to the client and her family members, including what events and diagnostic studies are being performed. For the majority of women, a cesarean birth will be planned. See Nursing Care Plan 19-1 for application of the nursing process for the woman with placenta previa.

Assessment

Assessing the woman's degree of vaginal bleeding is paramount. Estimate and document the amount of bleeding. Perform a peripad count on an ongoing basis, making sure to report any changes in amount or frequency to the healthcare provider. If the woman is experiencing active bleeding, prepare for blood typing and crossmatching in the event a blood transfusion is needed.

Assess fetal heart rates via Doppler to detect fetal distress. Monitor the woman's cardiopulmonary status, reporting any difficulties in respirations, changes in skin color, or complaints of difficulty breathing. Have oxygen equipment readily available should fetal or maternal distress develop.

If the woman has an IV inserted, inspect the IV site frequently. Alternately, anticipate the insertion of an intermittent IV access device such as a saline lock, which can be used if quick access is needed for fluid restoration and infusion of blood products.

Assess the woman's level of understanding regarding the condition of placenta previa and associated procedures and treatment plan. Doing so is important to prevent confusion and gain the woman's cooperation. Provide information related to the condition and make sure that all information related is consistent with information from the primary care provider.

If the woman will require prolonged hospitalization or home bed rest, assess the physical and emotional impact that this may have on her. Evaluate the woman's coping mechanisms to aid in determining how well she will be able to adjust to and cooperate with the treatment plan. In addition to emotional impact with prolonged bed rest, thoroughly assess the woman's skin to prevent skin breakdown and to help alleviate the woman's discomfort secondary to limited physical activity.

Nursing Interventions

The following interventions would be appropriate for the woman with placenta previa regardless of the setting:

- Monitoring amount of blood loss, pain level, and uterine contractility
- Assessing maternal vital signs frequently
- Ascertaining the client's understanding and implications of this condition
- Monitoring the results of all laboratory testing, such as CBC, type and crossmatch, coagulation studies
- Providing emotional support and listening to her fears of the unknown
- Explaining assessments and treatment measures needed
- Assisting the client to remain on bed rest with bathroom privileges
- Counseling the client and family about all activities and interventions
- Providing opportunities for distraction—educational videos, arts and crafts, computer games, reading books
- Instructing the client to assess fetal activity via "kick counts" daily
- Acting as a client advocate in obtaining information for the family
- Monitoring the woman's coping ability to comply with activity restrictions
- Preventing any vaginal examinations from being performed, which might disrupt the placenta and cause hemorrhage
- Evaluating fetal heart rate via an external monitor or Doppler
- Encouraging a balanced, nutritious diet with plenty of fluid intake
- Administering Rh immunoglobulin if the client is Rh negative at 28 weeks' gestation
- Preparing the client for cesarean birth when necessary
- Informing the client and family of any status change that requires intervention
- Monitoring tocolytic medication if prevention of preterm labor is needed
- Educating the client regarding risk of reoccurrence of this condition

Nursing Care Plan 19-1

Overview of the Woman With Placenta Previa

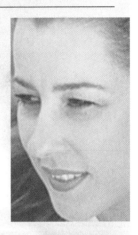

Sandy, a 39-year-old G5, P4, multigravida client at 32 weeks' gestation, was admitted to the labor and birth suite with sudden vaginal bleeding. Sandy had no further active bleeding and did not complain of any abdominal discomfort or tenderness. She did complain of occasional "tightening" in her stomach. Her abdomen palpated soft. Fetal heart rates were in the 140s with accelerations with movement. She was placed on bed rest with bathroom privileges. Ultrasound identified a low-lying placenta with a viable, normal-growth fetus. She was diagnosed with placenta previa and admitted for observation and surveillance of fetal well-being. Her history revealed two previous cesarean births, smoking half a pack of cigarettes per day, and endometritis infection after birth of her last newborn. Additional assessment findings included painless, bright-red vaginal bleeding with initial bleeding ceasing spontaneously; irregular, mild, and sporadic uterine contractions; fetal heart rate and maternal vital signs within normal range; fetus in transverse lie; anxiety related to the outcome of pregnancy; and expression of feelings of helplessness.

Nursing Diagnosis: Ineffective tissue perfusion (fetal and maternal) related to blood loss

Outcome identification and *evaluation*	Interventions with *rationales*
Client will maintain adequate tissue perfusion *as evidenced by stable vital signs, decreased blood loss, few or no uterine contractions, normal fetal heart rate patterns and variability, and positive fetal movement*	Establish intravenous access to allow for administration of fluids, blood, and medications as necessary Obtain type and crossmatch for at least 2 U blood products *to ensure availability should bleeding continue* Obtain specimens as ordered for blood studies, such as CBC and clotting studies *to establish a baseline and use for future comparison* Monitor output *to evaluate adequacy of renal perfusion* Administer IV fluid replacement therapy as ordered *to maintain blood pressure and blood volume* Palpate for abdominal tenderness and rigidity *to determine bleeding and evidence of uterine contractions* Institute bed rest *to reduce oxygen demands* Assess for rupture of membranes *to evaluate for possible onset of labor* Avoid vaginal examinations *to prevent further bleeding episodes* Complete an Rh titer *to identify need for RhoGAM* Avoid nipple stimulation *to prevent uterine contractions* Continuously monitor for contractions or PROM *to allow for prompt intervention* Administer tocolytic agents as ordered *to stall preterm labor* Monitor vital signs frequently *to identify possible hypovolemia and infection* Assess frequently for active vaginal bleeding *to minimize risk of hemorrhage* Continuously monitor fetal heart rate with electronic fetal monitor *to evaluate fetal status* Assist with fetal surveillance tests as ordered *to aid in determining fetal well-being*

(continued)

Overview of the Woman With Placenta Previa (continued)

Outcome identification and *evaluation*	Interventions with *rationales*
	Observe for abnormal fetal heart rate patterns, such as loss of variability, decelerations, tachycardia, *to identify fetal distress* Position patient in side-lying position with wedge for support *to maximize placental perfusion* Assess fetal movement *to evaluate for possible fetal hypoxia* Teach woman to monitor fetal movement *to evaluate well-being* Administer oxygen as ordered *to increase oxygenation to mother and fetus*

Nursing Diagnosis: Anxiety related to threats to self and fetus

Client will experience a decrease in anxiety *as evidenced by verbal reports of less anxiety, use of effective coping measures, and calm demeanor*	Provide factual information about diagnosis and treatment, and explain interventions and the rationale behind them *to provide client with understanding of her condition* Answer questions about health status honestly *to establish a trusting relationship* Speak calmly to patient and family members *to minimize environmental stress* Encourage the use of past effective techniques for coping *to promote relaxation and feelings of control* Acknowledge and facilitate the woman's spiritual needs *to promote effective coping* Involve the woman and family in the decision-making process *to foster self-confidence and control over situation* Maintain a presence during stressful periods *to allay anxiety* Use the sense of touch if appropriate to convey caring and concern Encourage talking *as a means to release tension*

Abruptio Placenta

Abruptio placenta refers to separation of a normally located placenta after the 20th week of gestation and prior to birth, producing hemorrhage. It is a significant cause of third trimester bleeding with a high mortality rate. It occurs in about 1% of all pregnancies throughout the world (Gaufberg, 2004). The overall fetal mortality rate for placenta abruption is 20% to 40%, depending on the extent of the abruption. This is caused by the insult of the abruption itself and by issues related to prematurity when early birth is required to alleviate maternal or fetal distress. Maternal mortality is approximately 6% in abruptio placenta and is related to cesarean birth and/or hemorrhage/coagulopathy (Deering & Satin, 2004).

Abruptio placenta is a major medical emergency. It requires rapid, effective interventions to prevent maternal and fetal morbidity and mortality.

Causes

The etiology of this condition is unknown. Several risk factors are associated with it, such as maternal smoking, extremes of age (<20 years or >35 years old), poor nutrition, multiple gestation, excessive intrauterine pressure caused by hydramnios, hypertension, prior abruption in a previous pregnancy, severe trauma (such as an auto accident or injury secondary to intimate partner violence), cocaine and methamphetamine abuse, alcohol ingestion, and multiparity (Chen, 2004). Other notable risk factors include male fetal gender, chorioamnionitis, prolonged premature ruptured membranes (>24 hours), oligohydramnios, preeclampsia, and low socioeconomic status (Deering & Satin, 2004).

Clinical Manifestations

Abruptio placenta is classified according to the extent of separation and the amount of blood loss from the maternal circulation. Classifications include

- Mild (grade 1)—minimal bleeding (<500 mL), marginal separation (10–20%), tender uterus, no coagulopathy, no signs of shock, no fetal distress
- Moderate (grade 2)—Moderate bleeding (1000–1500 mL), moderate separation (20–50%), continuous abdominal pain, mild shock
- Severe (grade 3)—absent to moderate bleeding (>1500 mL), severe separation (>50%), profound shock, agonizing abdominal pain, and development of disseminated intravascular coagulopathy (DIC) (Gilbert & Harmon, 2003)

Abruptio placenta also may be classified as partial or complete, depending on the degree of separation. Alternately, it can be classified as concealed or apparent, by the type of bleeding (Fig. 19-5).

As the placenta separates from the uterus, hemorrhage ensues. It can be apparent, appearing as vaginal bleeding, or it can be concealed. Classic manifestations include painful, dark-red vaginal bleeding (port wine color); "knifelike" abdominal pain; uterine tenderness; contractions; and decreased fetal movement. Vaginal bleeding is present in 80% of women diagnosed with abruptio placenta and may be significant enough to jeopardize both maternal and fetal health within a short time frame. The remaining 20% of abruptions are associated with a concealed hemorrhage and the absence of vaginal bleeding. Decreased fetal movement may be the presenting complaint resulting from fetal jeopardy or fetal death (Deering & Satin, 2004).

Laboratory and diagnostic tests may be helpful in diagnosing the condition and guiding management. These studies may include

- CBC—determines the current hemodynamic status; however, it is not reliable for estimating acute blood loss
- Fibrinogen levels—typically are increased in pregnancy (hyperfibrinogenemia); thus, a moderate dip in fibrinogen levels might suggest coagulopathy (DIC) and, if profuse bleeding occurs, the clotting cascade might be compromised
- Prothrombin time (PT)/activated partial thromboplastin time (aPTT)—determines the client's coagulation status, especially if surgery is planned
- Type and crossmatch—determines blood type if transfusion is needed
- Kleihauer–Betke test—detects fetal RBCs in the maternal circulation, determines the degree of fetal–maternal hemorrhage, helps calculate the appropriate dosage of RhoGAM to give for Rh-negative clients
- Ultrasound—helps to diagnose quickly the etiology of bleeding and visualize active or concealed hemorrhage, aids in identifying retroplacental hematoma
- Nonstress test—demonstrates findings of fetal jeopardy manifested by late decelerations or bradycardia
- Biophysical profile—used to evaluate clients with chronic abruption, provides information about possible fetal compromise by a low score (<6 points) (Cavanaugh, 2003)

Treatment

Treatment of abruptio placenta is designed to assess, control, and restore the amount of blood lost; to provide a positive outcome for both mother and newborn; and to prevent coagulation disorders, such as DIC (Box 19-2). Emergency measures include starting two large-bore IV lines with normal saline or lactated Ringer's solution to combat hypovolemia, obtaining blood specimens for evaluating hemodynamic status values and for typing and

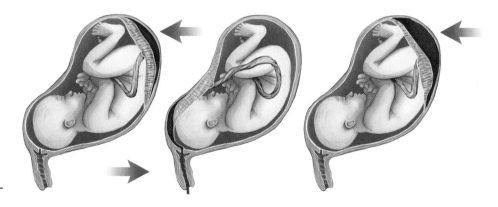

● Figure 19-5 Classifications of abruptio placenta. (**A**) Partial abruption with concealed hemorrhage. (**B**) Partial abruption with apparent hemorrhage. (**C**) Complete abruption with concealed hemorrhage.

A Partial abruption, concealed hemorrhage

B Partial abruption, apparent hemorrhage

C Partial abruption, concealed hemorrhage

BOX 19-2
DISSEMINATED INTRAVASCULAR COAGULATION

DIC is a bleeding disorder characterized by an abnormal reduction in the elements involved in blood clotting resulting from their widespread intravascular clotting (O'Toole, 2005). This disorder can occur secondary to abruptio placenta.

Simply, the clinical and pathologic manifestations of DIC can be described as a loss of balance between the clot-forming activity of thrombin and the clot-lysing activity of plasmin. Therefore, too much thrombin tips the balance toward the prothrombic state and the client develops clots. Alternately, too much clot lysis (fibrinolysis) results from plasmin formation and the client hemorrhages. Small clots form throughout the body, and eventually the blood-clotting factors are used up, rendering them unavailable to form clots at sites of tissue injury. Clot-dissolving mechanisms are also increased, which result in bleeding, which can be severe.

DIC can be stimulated by many factors including sepsis, malignancy, and obstetric conditions such as placenta abruption, missed abortion or retained dead fetus, amniotic fluid embolism, and eclampsia.

Laboratory studies assist in the diagnosis and include
- Decreased fibrinogen and platelets
- PT and aPTT times
- Positive D-dimer tests and fibrin (split) degradation products, which uncover objective evidence of the simultaneous formation of thrombin and plasmin (NANDA, 2005).

crossmatching, and frequently monitoring fetal and maternal well-being. After determining the severity of abruption, and appropriate blood and fluid replacement is given, cesarean birth is done immediately if fetal distress is evident. If the fetus is not in distress, close monitoring continues, with delivery planned at the earliest signs of fetal distress. Because of the possibility of fetal blood loss through the placenta, a critical care neonatal team should be available during the birth process to assess and treat the newborn immediately for shock, blood loss, and hypoxia.

If the woman develops DIC, treatment focuses on determining the underlying cause of DIC and correcting it. Replacement therapy of the coagulation factors is achieved by transfusion of fresh frozen plasma along with cryoprecipitate to maintain the circulating volume and provide oxygen to the cells of the body. Prompt identification and early intervention are essential for a woman with acute DIC associated with abruptio placenta to resolve DIC and possibly save the woman's life.

Nursing Management

Abruptio placenta warrants immediate care to provide the best outcome for both mother and fetus.

Assessment

The nurse's role in the assessment of the woman presenting with abdominal pain and/or experiencing vaginal bleeding is critical. An accurate assessment forms the basis of medical management and intervention, especially in a concealed hemorrhage in which the extent of bleeding is not recognized. Vital signs can be within normal range, even with significant blood loss, because a pregnant woman can lose up to 40% of her total blood volume without showing signs of shock (Gilbert & Harmon, 2003).

Nursing assessment includes

- Assessing all women for risk factors that might cause abruption of the placenta: hypertension, drug use, membrane status, smoking, etc.
- Assessing maternal level of consciousness and signs of shock
- Monitoring the fetal heart rate continuously electronically
- Assessing pain type, onset, and location
- Assessing for abdominal tenderness, pain, and rigidity
- Monitoring uterine contractions by frequent palpation

Nursing Interventions

When the woman arrives to the labor and birth suite, place the woman on strict bed rest and in a left lateral position to prevent pressure on the vena cava. This position provides uninterrupted perfusion to the fetus. Expect to administer oxygen therapy via nasal cannula to ensure adequate tissue perfusion.

Additional nursing interventions include

- Monitoring hourly intake and output after insertion of indwelling urinary (Foley) catheter
- Obtaining maternal blood pressure, pulse, respirations, and pulse rate; and assessing pain level every 15 to 60 minutes, depending on maternal stability and amount of blood loss
- Observing for changes in vital signs suggesting hypovolemic shock and reporting them immediately
- Observing and recording amount and time of bleeding every 30 minutes
- Initiating an IV line with a large-bore catheter and documenting fluid intake to prevent fluid overload
- Avoiding vaginal examinations until placenta previa is ruled out
- Administering pain medication as ordered
- Monitoring uterine contractions for increased rigidity and tenderness
- Monitoring the amount and nature (dark or bright red) of vaginal bleeding
- Evaluating the fundal height (increasing size would indicate bleeding)
- Observing for signs of DIC—bleeding gums, tachycardia, and petechiae—and administering blood products if DIC is apparent
- Observing for fetal distress and tetanic contractions on monitor

- Using pulse oximetry to monitor oxygen saturation levels of circulating blood
- Answering questions about fetal health status in an honest manner
- Acknowledging and facilitating the client's spiritual and cultural needs
- Communicating empathy and understanding of the client's experience, and providing emotional support throughout this frightening time
- Remaining with the couple and acknowledging their emotions and fears
- Providing the couple with factual information about projected management
- Explaining thoroughly the care needed so they will know what to expect
- Informing the client and family about diagnostic tests and surgery
- Preparing the client and family for the possibility of cesarean birth
- Reducing family anxiety by reassuring fetal well-being as appropriate based on test results
- Helping the family to deal with loss or with infant in the intensive care unit

Although abruptio placenta is not a preventable condition, client education is important to help reduce the risk for this condition. Educational topics would include encouraging the woman to avoid drinking, smoking, or using drugs during pregnancy, and to obtain rehabilitation services to eliminate drug abuse prior to the pregnancy; to seek early and continuous prenatal care; to recognize diabetes and hypertension early so that treatment can be started; to identify intimate partner abuse to prevent further abuse; and to receive prompt health care if any symptoms are present in the future.

Hyperemesis Gravidarum

Approximately 80% or more women experience nausea and vomiting during their pregnancy (Edelman & Logan, 2004). The term *morning sickness* is often used to describe this condition when symptoms are relatively mild. Such symptoms usually disappear after the first trimester. This mild form mostly impacts the quality of life of the woman and her family, whereas the severe form—hyperemesis gravidarum—results in dehydration, electrolyte imbalance, and the need for hospitalization (Koren & Maltepe, 2004).

Unlike morning sickness, **hyperemesis gravidarum** is a complication of pregnancy characterized by persistent, uncontrollable nausea and vomiting before the 20th week of gestation. This complication can lead to dehydration, acid–base imbalances, electrolyte imbalances, and weight loss. If it continues, it jeopardizes fetal well-being (Green & Wilkinson, 2004).

The incidence of hyperemesis is estimated to occur in approximately 1% of pregnant women. The prevalence increases in molar and multiple pregnancies. Its peak incidence occurs between 8 weeks and 12 weeks of pregnancy, usually resolving by week 16 (Garcia, 2003).

Causes

The cause of nausea and vomiting is unknown. Although theories abound, few studies have produced scientific evidence that determine the etiology of this condition. It is likely that multiple factors contribute to it.

Elevated levels of hCG are present in all pregnant women during early pregnancy, usually declining after 12 weeks. This corresponds to the usual duration of morning sickness. In hyperemesis gravidarum, the hCG levels are often higher and extend beyond the first trimester. Symptoms exacerbate the disease. Decreased fluid intake and prolonged vomiting cause dehydration; dehydration increases the serum concentration of hCG, which in turn exacerbates the nausea and vomiting—a vicious cycle. A few other theories that have been proposed to explain its etiology include

- Endocrine theory—high levels of hCG and estrogen during pregnancy
- Metabolic theory—vitamin B6 deficiency
- Psychological theory—psychological stress increasing the symptoms

Regardless of etiology, the client with hyperemesis gravidarum is extremely uncomfortable.

Risk factors associated with hyperemesis gravidarum include young age, nausea and vomiting with previous pregnancy, history of intolerance of oral contraceptives, multiple gestation, emotional or psychological stress, gastroesophageal reflux disease, primigravida status, obesity, hyperthyroidism, and *Helicobacter pylori* seropositivity (Swearingen, 2004).

Clinical Manifestations

Symptoms of hyperemesis gravidarum include, but are not limited to, disturbed nutrition, severe vomiting, electrolyte imbalance, ketosis, acetonuria, and weight loss greater than 5% of body mass. If it progresses untreated, it may cause neurologic disturbance, renal damage, retinal hemorrhage, or death (Christopher, 2003). In addition, it is exhausting and emotionally distressing.

Other common symptoms include ptyalism (excessive salivation), fatigue, weakness, and dizziness. Additionally, sleep disturbance, depression, anxiety, irritability, mood changes, and decreased ability to concentrate can add to the woman's emotional distress (Michelini, 2004).

The results of diagnostic studies may provide clues to the severity of the disorder: These may include

- Liver enzymes—elevations of aspartate aminotransferase (AST) and alanine aminotransferase (ALT) usually present

- CBC—elevated levels of RBCs and hematocrit denoting dehydration
- Urine ketones—positive when the body breaks down fat to provide energy in the absence of inadequate intake
- Blood, urea, nitrogen (BUN)—increased in the presence of salt and water depletion
- Urine specific gravity—greater than 1.025, possibly indicating concentrated urine linked to inadequate fluid intake or excessive fluid loss
- Serum electrolytes—decreased levels of potassium, sodium, and chloride resulting from excessive vomiting and loss of hydrochloric acid in stomach (Swearingen, 2004)

Treatment

Conservative management in the home is the first line of treatment for the woman with hyperemesis gravidarum. This usually focuses on dietary and lifestyle changes.

If conservative management fails to alleviate the client's symptoms, and nausea and vomiting continue, hospitalization is necessary to reverse the effects of severe nausea and vomiting.

On admission to the hospital baseline, blood tests are ordered to assess the severity of the client's dehydration, electrolyte imbalance, ketosis, and malnutrition. Parenteral fluid and drug therapy are ordered to rehydrate and reduce the symptoms. The first choice for fluid replacement is generally 5% dextrose in lactated Ringer's solution with vitamins and electrolytes added. Oral food and fluids are withheld for the first 24 to 36 hours to allow the GI tract to rest. Antiemetics may be administered orally, rectally, or intravenously to control the nausea and vomiting. Because the woman is initially considered "NPO," no food or fluids orally, her medication is administered parenterally or rectally until she is stabilized.

If the client does not improve after several days of bed rest, "gut rest," IV fluids, and antiemetics, total parenteral nutrition or percutaneous endoscopic gastrostomy tube feeding is instituted to prevent malnutrition.

The FDA has not approved any drugs for the treatment of nausea and vomiting in pregnancy, but the risk of administration must be balanced against the sequelae of prolonged starvation and dehydration. Finding a drug that works for any given client is largely a matter of trial and error. A client for whom one drug is ineffective may be helped by another class of drugs with a different mechanism of action. Promethazine (Phenergan) and prochlorperazine (Compazine) are among the older preparations usually tried first. If they fail to relieve symptoms, newer drugs such as ondansetron (Zofran) may be tried. Most drugs are given parenterally or rectally (Garcia, 2003) (see Drug Guide 19-2).

Drug Guide 19-2 Medications Used for Hyperemesis Gravidarum

Drug	Action	Indications	Nursing Implications
Promethazine (Phenergan)	Diminishes vestibular stimulation and acts on the chemoreceptor trigger zone (CTZ)	Symptomatic relief of nausea and vomiting, and motion sickness	Be alert for urinary retention, dizziness, hypotension, and involuntary movements Institute safety measures to prevent injury secondary to sedative effects Offer hard candy and frequent rinsing of mouth for dryness
Prochlorperazine (Compazine)	Acts centrally to inhibit dopamine receptors in the CTZ and peripherally to block vagus nerve stimulation in the GI tract	Controls severe nausea and vomiting	Be alert for abnormal movements and for neuroleptic malignant syndrome such as seizures, hyper-/hypotension, tachycardia, and dyspnea Assess mental status, intake/output Caution patient not to drive as a result of drowsiness or dizziness Advise to change position slowly to minimize effects of orthostatic hypotension
Odansetron (Zofran)	Blocks serotonin peripherally, centrally, and in the small intestine	Prevents nausea and vomiting	Monitor for possible side effects such as diarrhea, constipation, abdominal pain, headache, dizziness, drowsiness, and fatigue Monitor liver function studies as ordered

Sources: Skidmore-Roth, 2005; Spratto & Woods, 2005.

Few women receive complete relief of symptoms from any one therapy. Complementary treatments appeal to many to help supplement traditional ones. More popular therapies include acupressure, massage, therapeutic touch, ginger, and the wearing of seabands to prevent nausea and vomiting. Recent research has reported a positive effect of using acupressure over the Neiguan point on the wrist by Sea-bands to control nausea and vomiting associated with pregnancy (Steele et al., 2001).

Nursing Management

By the time clients are admitted to the hospital, many are exhausted, frustrated, and anxious. Nursing care focuses on providing comfort and emotional support to these distraught clients. Offer reassurance that all interventions are directed toward promoting positive pregnancy outcomes for both the woman and her fetus. Providing information about the expected plan of care may help to alleviate the client's anxiety. Attempting to provide the client a sense of control may help her overcome the feeling that she is "losing it" resulting from this condition.

Assessment

Nursing assessment related to hyperemesis gravidarum would begin with identifying the duration and course of the woman's nausea and vomiting, medications or treatments used and their efficacy, and specific signs and symptoms experienced. This information will help establish a baseline to make progressive comparisons of the current situation. Additional assessments will focus on identifying signs and symptoms of fluid and electrolyte imbalances and nutritional deficiencies by assessing the woman's mucus membranes for dryness, skin turgor for dehydration, low blood pressure, signs of weakness, and weight loss since this condition started. Additionally, assess for

- Anorexia, indigestion, abdominal pain or distension, and passage of blood or mucus rectally
- Daily weight, comparing prepregnancy weight with current weight to determine total loss
- Dietary intake by requesting a diet recall for past week
- Activity tolerance through job activities or daily exercise routine
- Knowledge of basic four food group and typical consumption patterns that may or may not trigger GI distress
- Intake and output for the previous 24 hours
- Type and amount of nutritional supplements taken
- Laboratory and diagnostic test results to validate dehydration and electrolyte imbalances
- Pain-precipitating factors the woman may be experiencing
- Client's perception of situation and future needs
- Support systems available to the client that can offer help

Nursing Interventions

Nursing interventions focus on controlling the woman's nausea and vomiting, promoting adequate nutrition,

improving the client's fluid and electrolyte balance, and providing comfort and support during this time. The following interventions may be included:

- Administer antiemetics as ordered and assess their effectiveness.
- Administer and maintain IV fluid and electrolyte replacements as ordered; monitor rate and sites of IV therapy to prevent complications.
- Monitor intake and output, including oral food and fluid intake when allowed.
- Evaluate the results of laboratory studies to determine effectiveness of treatment.
- Provide physical comfort measures, including environmental, hygiene (such as keeping the area free from pungent odors), and oral care.
- Reassure the client that treatment plan is in the best interest for the family unit.
- Encourage therapeutic lifestyle changes, such as avoiding stressors and fatigue that may trigger nausea and vomiting.
- Offer ongoing support and encouragement, empowering the client and her family with knowledge and choices.
- Involve the client and family in all decisions concerning care.
- Listen to concerns and feelings, and answer all questions asked honestly.
- Educate about the probable etiology of her condition and treatment options (see Teaching Guidelines 19-1).
- Refer the client to a spiritual leader or counseling as needed.

 TEACHING GUIDELINES 19-1

Teaching to Minimize Nausea and Vomiting

- Avoid noxious stimuli—such as strong flavors, perfumes, or strong odors such as frying bacon—that might trigger nausea and vomiting.
- Avoid tight waistbands to minimize pressure on abdomen.
- Eat small, frequent meals throughout the day—six small meals.
- Separate fluids from solids by consuming fluids in between meals.
- Avoid lying down or reclining for at least 2 hours after eating.
- Use high-protein supplement drinks.
- Avoid foods high in fat.
- Increase your intake of carbonated beverages.
- Increase your exposure to fresh air to improve symptoms.
- Eat when you are hungry, regardless of normal mealtimes.
- Drink herbal teas containing peppermint or ginger.
- Avoid fatigue and learn how to mange stress in life.
- Schedule daily rest periods to avoid becoming overtired.
- Eat foods that settle the stomach, such as dry crackers, toast, or soda

- Arrange for possible home care follow-up and reinforce home care on discharge to ensure understanding.
- Refer to local or national support organizations for additional information.
- Collaborate with community resources to ensure continuing care.

Gestational Hypertension

Gestational hypertension is characterized by hypertension without proteinuria after 20 weeks of gestation and a return of the blood pressure to normal postpartum. Previously, gestational hypertension was known as pregnancy-induced hypertension or toxemia of pregnancy, but these terms are no longer used. Gestational hypertension is clinically characterized by a blood pressure of 140/90 mmHg or more, on two occasions at least 6 hours apart (Youngkin & Davis, 2004). Gestational hypertension can be differentiated from *chronic hypertension,* which appears before the 20th week of gestation; or hypertension before the current pregnancy, which continues after giving birth.

Gestational hypertension is the leading cause of maternal death in the United States and the most common complication reported during pregnancy. Hypertension complicates 12 to 20% of pregnancies and has increased steadily, approximately 30 to 40% since 1990 for all ages, races, and ethnic groups (Martin et al., 2002). The highest rates of occurrence in women are those who are younger than 20 years and older than 40 years old (Mattson & Smith, 2004).

Classifications

The classification system used in the United States is based on reports from ACOG (2002) and the National High Blood Pressure Education Program (2000). Hypertension may be a preexisting condition (chronic hypertension) or it may present for the first time during pregnancy (gestational hypertension). Regardless of its onset, it jeopardizes the well-being of the mother as well as the fetus. The classification of hypertensive disorders in pregnancy currently consists of four categories, as described in Table 19-2.

Gestational hypertension can be classified as preeclampsia or **eclampsia.** Each is associated with specific criteria. Preeclampsia is clinically defined as a blood pressure greater than 140/90 mmHg after 20 weeks' gestation plus proteinuria (300 mg/24 hours or greater than 1+ protein on a dipstick sample of urine collected at random) (Bridges, Womble, Wallace, & McCartney, 2003). With *severe preeclampsia,* the blood pressure is higher than 160/110 mmHg on two occasions at least 6 hours apart. Proteinuria is greater than 500 mg in 24-hour urine collection, and oliguria (<500 mL in 24 hours) is present. Other symptoms that also present in severe preeclampsia include pulmonary edema or thrombocytopenia with or without liver damage, cerebral or visual disturbances, epigastric or right upper quadrant pain, and fetal growth restriction (Johnson, 2003). Eclampsia is the onset of seizure activity or coma in the woman diagnosed with preeclampsia, with no history of preexisting pathology, that can result in seizure activity (ACOG, 2002).

Causes

Gestational hypertension remains an enigma. The condition can be devastating to both the mother and her unborn child, and yet the etiology still remains a mystery to medical science, despite decades of research. Many different theories regarding it exist, but none have truly explained the widespread pathologic changes that result in pulmonary edema, oliguria, seizures, thrombocytopenia, and abnormal liver enzymes (Sibai, 2003). Despite the results of several research studies, the use of aspirin or supplementation

Table 19-2 Classification of Hypertensive Disorders

Type	Description
Gestational hypertension	Blood pressure elevation (140/90 mmHg) identified after midpregnancy without proteinuria
Preeclampsia	Pregnancy-specific syndrome occurring after 20 weeks' gestation with gestational hypertension plus proteinuria
Eclampsia	Seizure state in a woman with preeclampsia that cannot be attributed to any other cause
Chronic hypertension	Hypertension prior to the pregnancy or diagnosed before week 20 of gestation
Transient hypertension	Hypertension without preeclampsia at the time of birth, during labor, or within 24 hours postpartum; resolution within 12 weeks postpartum to normotensive blood pressure levels
Chronic hypertension with preeclampsia	Chronic hypertension with new proteinuria or exacerbation of previously controlled blood pressure, or proteinuria, thrombocytopenia, or elevated liver enzymes

Adapted from ACOG, 2002, and Blackburn, 2003.

with calcium, vitamins C and E, magnesium, zinc, or fish oils has not proved to prevent this destructive condition.

Factors associated with an increase risk for developing gestational hypertension have been identified and include

- Primigravida status
- History of preeclampsia in a previous pregnancy
- Excessive placental tissue, as is seen in women with GTD and multiple gestations
- Family history of preeclampsia (mother or sister)
- Lower socioeconomic group
- History of diabetes, hypertension, or renal disease
- Women with poor nutrition
- African-American ethnicity
- Age extremes of younger than 17 years or older than 35 years old
- Obesity (Green & Wilkinson, 2004)

Pathophysiologic Events

Vasospasm and hypoperfusion are the underlying mechanisms involved with this disorder. Several other changes are associated with gestational hypertension. Endothelial injury occurs, leading to subsequent platelet adherence, fibrin deposition, and the presence of schistocytes (fragment of an erythrocyte). Generalized vasospasm results in elevation of blood pressure and reduced blood flow to the brain, liver, kidneys, placenta, and lungs. Decreased liver perfusion leads to impaired liver function and subcapsular hemorrhage. This is demonstrated by epigastric pain and elevated liver enzymes in the maternal serum. Decreased brain perfusion leads to small cerebral hemorrhages and symptoms of arterial vasospasm such as headaches, visual disturbances, blurred vision, and hyperactive deep tendon reflexes (DTRs). A thromboxane/prostacyclin imbalance leads to increased thromboxane (potent vasoconstrictor and stimulator of platelet aggregation) and decreased prostacyclin (potent vasodilator and inhibitor of platelet aggregation), which contribute to the hypertensive state. Decreased kidney perfusion reduces GFR, resulting in decreased urine output and increased serum levels of sodium, BUN, uric acid, and creatinine, which further increases extracellular fluid and edema. Increased capillary permeability in the kidneys allows albumin to escape, which reduces plasma colloid osmotic pressure and moves more fluid into extracellular spaces, and leads to pulmonary edema and generalized edema. Poor placental perfusion resulting from prolonged vasoconstriction helps to contribute to intrauterine growth restriction, premature separation of the placenta (abruptio placenta), persistent fetal hypoxia, and acidosis. In addition, hemoconcentration (resulting from decreased intravascular volume) causes increased blood viscosity and elevated hematocrit (ACOG, 2002).

Clinical Manifestations

The significant signs of gestational hypertension—proteinuria and hypertension—occur without the woman's awareness. Unfortunately, by the time symptoms are noticed, gestational hypertension can be severe. The absolute blood pressure (value that validates elevation) of 140/90 mmHg should be obtained on two occasions 6 hours apart to be diagnostic of gestational hypertension.

Proteinuria develops later than hypertension and is defined as 300 mg or more of urinary protein per 24 hours or more than 1+ protein by chemical reagent strip or dipstick of at least two random urine samples collected at least 6 hours apart with no evidence of UTI (ACOG, 2002). Although edema is not a cardinal sign of preeclampsia, weight should be monitored frequently to identify sudden gains within a short time span. Current research relies less on the classic triad of symptoms (hypertension, proteinuria, and edema or weight gain) and more on decreased organ perfusion, endothelial dysfunction (capillary leaking and proteinuria), and elevated blood pressure as key indicators (Mattson & Smith, 2004).

Preeclampsia is characterized by generalized vasospasm, a decrease in circulating blood volume, and an activation of the coagulation system. Clinically, these changes present as hypertension and decreased perfusion to the placenta, kidneys, liver, and brain (National High Blood Pressure Education Program, 2000). The fetus can be severely affected by poor perfusion, especially to the uterus and thus the placenta.

Preeclampsia is categorized as mild or severe, or as complicated by the HELLP syndrome (discussed later in this chapter). In mild preeclampsia, the diastolic blood pressure is less than 100 mmHg, proteinuria is 1 or 2+ protein by dipstick, many women will demonstrate edema in the face and hands, and weight gain is noted. Mild preeclampsia can progress rapidly to the more severe form. Preeclampsia can place the woman at risk for eclampsia, abruptio placenta, DIC, liver and/or renal failure, pulmonary edema, and cerebral hemorrhage (Brooks, 2005). Women who have progressed to severe preeclampsia may present with any of the following:

- Diastolic blood pressure of 110 mmHg or higher
- Proteinuria less than 5 g protein excreted in a 24-hour specimen or a persistent greater than 2+ or 3+ on a dipstick measurement
- Increased hematocrit, creatinine, and uric acid levels
- Thrombocytopenia with a platelet count less than 100,000 platelets/mm^3
- Oliguria of less than 400 mL in 24 hours
- Epigastric or right upper quadrant pain linked to swelling of hepatic capsule
- Cerebral or visual disturbances—altered level of consciousness, headache, blurred vision, and scotomata (blind spots)
- Hyperreflexia of DTRs
- Markedly elevated liver enzymes
- Pulmonary edema with cyanosis
- Fetal growth restriction (ACOG, 2002; Sibai, 2003)

Table 19-3 compares mild and severe preeclampsia.

Table 19-3 Comparison of Clinical Manifestations: Mild vs. Severe Preeclampsia

Clinical Picture	Mild	Severe
Blood pressure, mmHg	140/90	160/110+
Urine for protein	2+	3+ to 4+
Urinary output, mL/hour	>30	<20
Pulmonary edema	Negative	Can be present
HELLP syndrome	Negative	Can be present

Eclampsia describes a condition during which a woman with preeclampsia develops seizures or goes into a coma. Its development is a major concern because maternal–fetal mortality or morbidity is very high. Signs and symptoms of eclampsia include tonic–clonic seizure activity, headache, hyperactive reflexes, marked proteinuria, generalized edema, visual disturbances, and right upper quadrant pain or epigastric pain. Twenty-five percent of eclampsia cases occur prenatally, 50% occur during labor, and 25% occur during the postpartal period (Fugate & Chow, 2004).

Eclampsia can lead to cerebral hemorrhage, pulmonary edema, and renal failure, and is associated with HELLP syndrome (Morgan, 2002). It develops after the 20th week of gestation and is considered a complication of severe preeclampsia. Eclampsia is a Greek word, meaning "bolt from the blue," which describes this condition well. The woman may have one or more seizures, generally lasting 60 to 75 seconds. The mechanisms leading to the development of seizures in women with eclampsia may include cerebral edema, ischemia, hemorrhage, or vasospasm. Severe headache and hyperreflexia are typically clinical precursors of eclamptic seizures (Longo, Dola, & Pridjian, 2003).

Although preeclampsia is not preventable, theoretically eclampsia should be preventable by identifying most cases of preeclampsia and swiftly delivering the newborn before seizures start.

Treatment

Antepartum Management

Conservative strategies for mild preeclampsia are used if the woman exhibits no signs of renal or hepatic dysfunctions or coagulopathy. A woman with mild elevations in blood pressure may be placed on rest at home. She is encouraged to rest as much as possible in the lateral recumbent position to improve uteroplacental blood flow, reduce her blood pressure, and promote diuresis. In addition, frequency of antepartal visits and diagnostic testing—such as CBC, clotting studies, liver enzymes, and platelet

levels—will increase. The woman will be asked to monitor her blood pressure daily (every 4–6 hours while awake) and report any increased readings, amount of protein found in urine using a dipstick, and weight gain. Daily fetal movement counts also are implemented. If there is any decrease in movement, the woman needs to be evaluated by her health care provider that day. A balanced, nutritional diet with no sodium restriction is advised. In addition, she is encouraged to drink six to eight 8-oz glasses of water daily.

If home management fails to reduce the blood pressure, admission to the hospital is warranted and the treatment strategy is individualized based on the severity of the condition and gestational age at the time of diagnosis. During the course of hospitalization, the woman with mild preeclampsia is monitored closely for signs and symptoms of severe preeclampsia or impending eclampsia (e.g., persistent headache, hyperreflexia). Blood pressure measurements are frequently recorded along with daily weights to detect excessive weight gain resulting from edema. Fetal surveillance is instituted in the form of daily fetal movement counts, nonstress testing, and serial ultrasounds to evaluate fetal growth and amniotic fluid volume to confirm fetal well-being. Expectant management usually continues until the pregnancy reaches term, the fetal lung maturity is documented, or complications develop that warrant immediate birth (Morley, 2004).

Severe preeclampsia may develop suddenly and bring with it high blood pressure of more than 160/110 mmHg, proteinuria of more than 5 g in 24 hours, oliguria of less than 400 mL in 24 hours, cerebral and visual symptoms, and rapid weight gain. This clinical picture signals severe preeclampsia, and immediate hospitalization is needed. After the woman is hospitalized for management of severe preeclampsia, the course of treatment is highly individualized and based on disease severity and fetal age. Birth of the infant is the only cure, because preeclampsia depends on the presence of trophoblastic tissue. Therefore, the exact age of the fetus is assessed to determine viability.

Severe preeclampsia is treated aggressively, because hypertension poses a serious threat to mother and fetus. The goal of care is to stabilize the mother–fetus dyad and prepare for birth. Therapy focuses on controlling hypertension, preventing seizures, preventing long-term morbidity, and preventing maternal, fetal, or newborn death (Mattson & Smith, 2004). Intense maternal and fetal surveillance starts when the mother enters the hospital and continues throughout her stay.

Eclamptic seizures are life-threatening emergencies and require immediate treatment to decrease maternal morbidity and mortality. In the woman who develops an eclamptic seizure, the convulsive activity begins with facial twitching followed by generalized muscle rigidity. Respirations cease for the duration of the seizure, resulting from muscle spasms, thus compromising fetal oxygenation. Coma usually follows the seizure activity with respiration resuming.

As with any seizure, the initial management is to clear the airway and administer adequate oxygenation. Positioning the woman on her left side and protecting her from injury during the seizure are key. Suction equipment must be readily available to remove secretions from her mouth after the seizure is over. IV fluids should be administered after the seizure at a rate to replace urine output and additional insensible losses. Fetal heart rate is monitored closely. Magnesium sulfate is administered intravenously to decrease and prevent further seizures from occurring. Hypertension is controlled with administration of antihypertensive medications. After the seizures are controlled, stability of the woman is assessed and birth via induction or cesarean birth is planned (Brooks, 2004).

Intrapartum Management

Intrapartal management of a woman with mild preeclampsia focuses on prevention of disease progression by frequent, consistent monitoring of blood pressure. On admission to the labor and birth suite, baseline vital signs, weight, DTRs, fetal heart rate, edema amount and location, proteinuria, and lung sounds are determined. Recent laboratory test results also are reviewed.

A quiet environment is important to minimize the risk of stimulation and to promote rest. IV magnesium sulfate is infused to prevent any seizure activity, along with antihypertensives if blood pressure values begin to elevate. Calcium gluconate is kept at the bedside in case the magnesium level becomes toxic. Continued close monitoring of neurologic status is warranted to detect any signs or symptoms of hypoxemia, impending seizure activity, or increased intracranial pressure. An indwelling urinary (Foley) catheter usually is inserted to allow for accurate measurement of urine output.

Intrapartum management of a woman with severe preeclampsia presents a challenge for the entire healthcare team. Oxytocin is used to stimulate uterine contractions, and magnesium sulfate is infused to prevent seizure activity. Oxytocin and magnesium sulfate can be given simultaneously via infusion pumps to ensure both are administered at the prescribed rate. The client is evaluated closely for magnesium toxicity. If at all possible, a vaginal delivery is preferable to a cesarean birth. PGE2 gel may be used to ripen the cervix. A cesarean birth may be performed if the client is seriously ill. A pediatrician/neonatologist must be available in the birthing room to care for the newborn. A newborn whose mother received high doses of magnesium sulfate needs to be monitored for respiratory depression, hypocalcemia, and hypotonia (Shennan, 2003).

Postpartum Management

Postpartum management of the client with preeclampsia or eclampsia continues until discharge. During this time, the woman is monitored as closely as before because her condition can still deteriorate. This risk can be enhanced by normal postpartum diuresis, which decreases the level of magnesium, subsequently leading to seizures. Usually the client improves rapidly, but still needs careful monitoring. Infusion of magnesium sulfate continues for at least 24 to 48 hours to prevent seizure activity. Frequent close surveillance of the client for signs of preeclampsia-eclampsia is continued in conjunction with routine postpartum assessments. Special attention should be paid to the fundal assessment because magnesium sulfate inhibits uterine tone, placing the client at risk for postpartum hemorrhage. Close surveillance after birth is critical because many complications, such as acute renal failure, pulmonary edema, seizures, liver failure, DIC, or cerebral hemorrhage, can occur. There is a direct correlation between severity of the disease and the length of time for recovery (Gilbert & Harmon, 2003).

Nursing Management

Assessment

Preventing hypertension-induced complications in pregnancy requires nurses to use their assessment, advocacy, and counseling skills. Assessment begins with the accurate measurement of the client's blood pressure at each encounter. In addition, nurses need to assess for subjective complaints that may indicate progression of the disease—visual changes, severe headaches, unusual bleeding or bruising, or epigastric pain (Peters & Flack, 2004).

Take a thorough history during the first antepartal visit to identify those women at risk for preeclampsia. In addition, complete a nutritional assessment that includes the woman's usual intake of protein, calcium, daily calories, and fluids. Women at risk for preeclampsia require more frequent prenatal visits throughout their pregnancy, and they require teaching about problems so that they can report them promptly.

At every antepartal visit, assess the fetal heart rate with a Doppler device, obtain maternal blood pressure, check a clean-catch urine specimen for protein using a dipstick, obtain the client's weight (noting gain since last visit and amount), and assess for amount and location of edema. Asking questions such as "Do your rings still fit on your fingers?" or "Is your face puffy when you get up in the morning?" will help to determine whether fluid retention is present or if the woman's status has changed since her last visit.

The supine pressor test, or *rollover test,* can be given between 28 weeks and 32 weeks' gestation. It is a screening tool to help identify asymptomatic clients who will likely develop preeclampsia. With this test, blood pressure is obtained at the brachial artery with the woman in the lateral recumbent position. She is then asked to roll over onto her back and her blood pressure is measured immediately and again in 5 minutes. An increase of 20 mmHg or greater in diastolic blood pressure is a positive indicator of potential preeclampsia (Harvey, 2004).

The *tolerance–hyperbaric test* (THT) is a more sensitive test that can detect gestational hypertension and preeclampsia risk at an earlier time than when clinical signs appear. This test can be done during the first trimester to identify a woman's risk for the development of preeclampsia, thus allowing for early intervention. The woman wears a portable blood pressure cuff and monitor, which records intermittent blood pressure readings during a 48-hour period. The THT compares actual recordings with the expected variation in blood pressure, allowing for detection of those women whose blood pressure is repeatedly outside the expected range (Hermida & Ayala, 2003).

In addition, blood pressures must be carefully and consistently measured to be meaningful. Obtain all measurements with the woman in the same position (blood pressure is highest in the sitting position and lowest in the side-lying position) and by using the same technique (automated vs. manual). This standardization in position and technique will yield the most accurate readings for determining treatment decisions (Bridges et al., 2003).

The woman with severe preeclampsia or who develops eclampsia is hospitalized. Nursing assessments are carried out frequently to monitor disease progress and the client's response to the therapy. These include assessing for edema, and evaluating the woman's overall health status, DTRs, and results of laboratory studies.

Assess edema for distribution, degree, and pitting. Document your findings and identify whether the edema is dependent or pitting. Dependent edema is present on the lower half of the body if the client is ambulatory, where hydrostatic pressure is greatest. It is usually observed in the feet and ankles or in the sacral area if the client is on bed rest.

Pitting edema is edema that leaves a small depression or pit after finger pressure is applied to a swollen area (Lowdermilk & Perry, 2004). Record the depth of pitting demonstrated when pressure is applied. Although subjective, the following is used to record relative degrees:

- 1+ pitting edema = 2-mm depression into skin; disappears rapidly
- 2+ pitting edema = 4-mm skin depression; disappears in 10 to 15 seconds
- 3+ pitting edema = 6-mm depression into skin; lasts more than 1 minute
- 4+ pitting edema = 8-mm depression into skin; lasts 2 to 3 minutes

If the client is receiving magnesium sulfate to suppress or control seizures, assess DTRs to determine the effectiveness of therapy. Clients with preeclampsia commonly present with hyperreflexia. Severe preeclampsia causes changes in the cortex, which disrupts the equilibrium of impulses between the cerebral cortex and the spinal cord. Brisk reflexes (hyperreflexia) are the result of an irritable cortex and indicate central nervous system involvement (Nick, 2003). Diminished or absent reflexes occur when the client develops magnesium toxicity. Because magnesium is a potent neuromuscular blockade, the afferent and efferent nerve pathways do not relay messages properly and hyporeflexia develops. Common sites used to assess DTRs are biceps reflex, triceps reflex, patellar reflex, Achilles reflex, and plantar reflex. Nursing Procedure 19-1 highlights the steps for assessing the patellar reflex.

The National Institute of Neurological Disorders and Stroke (NINDS), a division of the National Institutes

Nursing Procedure 19-1

Assessing the Patellar Reflex

Purpose: To Evaluate for Nervous System Irritability Related to Preeclampsia

1. Place the woman in the supine position (or sitting upright with the legs dangling freely over the side of the bed or examination table).
2. If lying supine, have the woman flex her knee slightly.
3. Place a hand under the knee to support the leg and locate the patellar tendon. It should be midline just below the knee cap.
4. Using a reflex hammer or the side of your hand, strike the area of the patellar tendon firmly and quickly.
5. Note the movement of the leg and foot. A patellar reflex occurs when the leg and foot move (documented as 2+).
6. Repeat the procedure on the opposite leg.

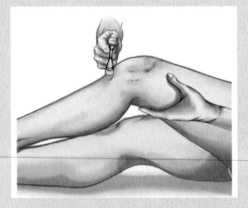

Table 19-4 Grading Deep Tendon Reflexes

Description of Finding	Grade
Reflex absent, no response detected	0
Hypoactive response, diminished	1
Reflex in lower half of normal range	2
Reflex in upper half of normal range	3
Hyperactive, brisk, clonus present	4

Sources: Dillon, 2003; Nick, 2003; and Seidel, Ball, Dains, & Benedict, 2003.

of Health, published a scale in the early 1990s that, although subjective, is used widely today. It grades reflexes from 0 to 4+. Grades 2+ and 3+ are considered normal whereas grades 0 and 4 may indicate pathology (Table 19-4). Because these are subjective assessments, to improve communication of reflex results it is recommended that condensed descriptor categories such as absent, average, brisk, or **clonus** be used, rather than numeric codes (Nick, 2003).

Clonus is the presence of rhythmic involuntary contractions, most often at the foot or ankle. Sustained clonus confirms central nervous system involvement. Nursing Procedure 19-2 highlights the steps when testing for ankle clonus.

Also assess the woman for signs and symptoms of pulmonary edema, such as crackles and wheezing heard on auscultation, dyspnea, decreased oxygen saturation levels, cough, neck vein distention, anxiety, and restlessness (Mattson & Smith, 2004).

Assess fetal well-being continuously via electronic fetal monitoring, noting trends in baseline rate and presence or absence of accelerations or decelerations.

Nursing Interventions for Preeclampsia

Preeclampsia can have a rapid onset and quick progression. Be sure that all women are taught the signs and symptoms of preeclampsia and know how to contact their healthcare professional for immediate evaluation.

Home care can be offered to many women if their condition is mild and they have a good understanding of the disease process, are stable, have no abnormal laboratory test results, and demonstrate good fetal movement (see Teaching Guidelines 19-2). The home care nurse makes frequent visits and follow-up phone calls to assess the woman's condition, to assist with scheduling periodic evaluations of the fetus (such as nonstress tests), and to evaluate any changes that might suggest a worsening of the woman's condition.

Early detection and management of mild preeclampsia is associated with the greatest success in reducing progression of this condition. As long as the client carries out the guidelines of care as outlined by the health care provider, and she remains stable, home care can continue to maintain the pregnancy until the fetus is mature. If disease progression occurs, hospitalization is required.

Nursing Interventions for Severe Preeclampsia

To achieve a safe outcome for the fetus, prepare the woman for possible testing to evaluate fetal status as preeclampsia progresses. These may include the nonstress test, serial ultrasounds to track fetal growth, amniocentesis to deter-

Nursing Procedure 19-2

Testing for Ankle Clonus

Purpose: To Evaluate for Nervous System Irritability Related to Preeclampsia

1. Place the woman in the supine position.
2. Dorsiflex the foot and then quickly release it.
3. Watch for the foot to rebound smoothly against your hand. If the movement is smooth, then clonus is not present; if the movement is jerky and rapid, clonus is present.
4. Repeat on the opposite side.

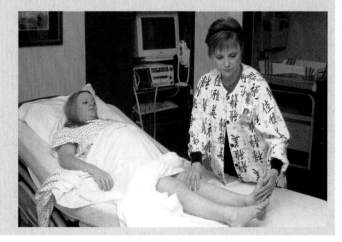

TEACHING GUIDELINES 19-2

Teaching for the Woman With Mild Preeclampsia

- Rest in a quiet environment to prevent cerebral disturbances.
- Drink 8 to 10 glasses of water daily.
- Consume a balanced, high-protein diet including high-fiber foods.
- Obtain intermittent bed rest to improve circulation to the heart and uterus.
- Limit your physical activity to promote urination and subsequent decreased in blood pressure.
- Enlist the aid of your family so that you can obtain appropriate rest time.
- Perform self-monitoring as instructed, including
  - Taking your own blood pressure twice daily
  - Checking and recording weight daily
  - Performing urine dipstick twice daily
  - Recording the number of fetal kicks daily
- Contact the home health nurse if any of the following occurs:
  - Increase in blood pressure
  - Protein present in urine
  - Gain of more than 1 lb in 1 week
  - Burning or frequency when urinating
  - Decrease in fetal activity or movement
  - Headache (forehead or posterior neck region)
  - Dizziness or visual disturbances
  - Increase in swelling in hands, feet, legs, and face
  - Stomach pain, excessive heartburn, or epigastric pain
  - Decreased or infrequent urination
  - Contractions or low back pain
  - Easy or excessive bruising
  - Sudden onset of abdominal pain
  - Nausea and vomiting

mine fetal lung maturity, Doppler velocimetry to screen for fetal compromise, and biophysical profile to evaluate ongoing fetal well-being (London, Ladewug, Ball, & Bindler, 2003).

Other laboratory tests may be performed to monitor the disease process and to determine if it is progressing into HELLP syndrome. These include liver enzymes such as lactic dehydrogenase (LDH), ALT, and AST; chemistry panel, such as creatinine, BUN, uric acid, and glucose; CBC, including platelet count; coagulation studies, such as PT, PTT, fibrinogen, and bleeding time; and a 24-hour urine collection for protein and creatinine clearance.

In addition, the following are appropriate when caring for the woman with severe preeclampsia:

- Maintain the client on complete bed rest in the left lateral lying position.
- Monitor intake and output every hour.

- Closely monitor for signs of labor.
- Administer fluid and electrolyte replacements as ordered based on laboratory test results.
- Give sedatives as ordered to encourage quiet bed rest.
- Offer a high-protein diet with 8 to 10 glasses of water daily.
- Administer glucocorticoid treatment as ordered to enhance fetal lung maturity
- Give parenteral magnesium sulfate as ordered to prevent seizures and lower blood pressure.
- Have calcium gluconate (antidote) readily available for magnesium toxicity.
- Administer antihypertensives as ordered to reduce blood pressure (see Drug Guide 19-3).
- Perform continuous electronic fetal monitoring to assess fetal well-being. Observe for signs of fetal distress and report immediately.
- Provide a quiet, darkened room to stabilize the client.
- Institute and maintain seizure precautions, such as padding the side rails and having oxygen, suction equipment, and call light readily available to protect the client from injury.
- Continue assessing edema and DTRs.
- Monitor vital signs, fetal heart rate, vision, and level of consciousness. Report any changes and any complaints of headache or visual disturbances.
- Prepare for labor induction if condition warrants.
- Keep client and family informed of condition and provide necessary education regarding course of treatment.
- Provide emotional support for the client and family.

With magnesium sulfate administration, the client is at risk for magnesium toxicity. Closely assess the client for signs and symptoms of toxicity, including absent or weak DTRs, respirations less than 12 breaths/minute, diminished level of consciousness, drowsiness, and urinary output of less than 30 mL/hour. Also monitor serum magnesium levels. Although exact levels may vary among agencies, serum magnesium levels ranging from 4 to 7 mEq/L are considered therapeutic, whereas levels more than 8 mg/dL are generally considered toxic. As levels increase, the woman is at risk for severe problems:

- 10 mEq/L, possible loss of DTRs
- 15 mEq/L, possible respiratory depression
- 25 mEq/L, possible cardiac arrest (Yankowitz, 2004)

Severe preeclampsia is very frightening for the client and her family, and most expectant mothers are very anxious about their own health status as well as that of the fetus. Use light touch to comfort and reassure her that the necessary actions are being completed to help allay anxiety. Actively listening to her concerns and fears, and communicating them to her health care provider is important in keeping lines of communication open. Offering praise for small accomplishments can provide positive reinforcement of behaviors to be continued.

Drug Guide 19-3 Medications Used With Preeclampsia and Eclampsia

Drug	Action	Indications	Nursing Implications
Magnesium sulfate	Blockage of neuromuscular transmission, vasodilation	Prevention and treatment of eclamptic seizures, reduction in blood pressure in preeclampsia and eclampsia	Administer IV loading dose of 4–6 g over 30 minutes, continue maintenance infusion of 2–4 g/hour as ordered Monitor serum magnesium levels closely Assess DTRs and check for ankle clonus Have calcium gluconate readily available in case of toxicity Monitor for signs and symptoms of toxicity, such as flushing, sweating, hypotension, and cardiac and central nervous system depression
Hydralazine hydrochloride (Apresoline)	Vascular smooth muscle relaxant, thus improving perfusion to renal, uterine, and cerebral areas	Reduction in blood pressure	Administer 5–10 mg by slow IV bolus every 20 minutes Use parenteral form immediately after opening ampule Withdraw drug slowly to prevent possible rebound hypertension Monitor for adverse effects such as palpitations, headache, tachycardia, anorexia, nausea, vomiting, and diarrhea
Labetalol hydrochloride (Normodyne)	Alpha 1 and beta blocker	Reduction in blood pressure	Be aware that drug lowers blood pressure without decreasing maternal heart rate or cardiac output Administer IV bolus dose of 10–20 mg and then administer IV infusion of 2 mg/minute until desired blood pressure value achieved Monitor for possible adverse effects such as gastric pain, flatulence, constipation, dizziness, vertigo, and fatigue
Nifedipine (Procardia)	Calcium channel blocker/dilation of coronary arteries, arterioles, and peripheral arterioles	Reduction in blood pressure, stoppage of preterm labor	Administer 10 mg orally for three doses and then every 4–8 hours Monitor for possible adverse effects such as dizziness, peripheral edema, angina, diarrhea, nasal congestions, cough
Sodium nitroprusside	Rapid vasodilation (arterial and venous)	Severe hypertension requiring rapid reduction in blood pressure	Administer via continuous IV infusion with dose titrated according to blood pressure levels Wrap IV infusion solution in foil or opaque material to protect from light Monitor for possible adverse effects, such as apprehension, restlessness, retrosternal pressure, palpitations, diaphoresis, abdominal pain
Furosemide (Lasix)	Diuretic action, inhibiting the reabsorption of sodium and chloride from the ascending loop of Henle	Pulmonary edema	Administer via slow IV bolus at a dose of 10–40 mg over 1–2 minutes Monitor urine output hourly Assess for possible adverse effects such as dizziness, vertigo, orthostatic hypotension, anorexia, vomiting, electrolyte imbalances, muscle cramps, and muscle spasms

Yankowitz, 2004.

Nursing Interventions for Eclampsia

Eclamptic seizures are generalized and typically start with facial twitching. The body then becomes rigid, in a state of tonic muscular contraction. The clonic phase of the seizure finds the client alternating contraction and relaxation of all body muscles. Respirations stop during seizure activity and resume shortly after it ends. Client safety is the primary concern during eclamptic seizures. If possible, turn the client to her side and remain with her. Make sure that the side rails are up and padded. Dim the lights and keep the room quiet. Box 19-3 presents a helpful acronym to use when intervening with a woman who is experiencing an eclamptic seizure.

Document the time and sequence of events as soon as possible. After the seizure activity has ceased, suction the nasopharynx as necessary and administer oxygen. Continue the magnesium sulfate infusion to prevent further seizures. Ensure continuous electronic fetal monitoring, evaluating fetal status for changes. Also assess the client for uterine contractions. After the client is stabilized, delivery should be planned as soon as possible to reduce the risk of perinatal mortality.

Nursing Interventions during the Postpartum Period

Postpartum management of the woman with gestational hypertension continues until discharge. Usually the client improves rapidly, but still needs careful monitoring. Continue assessing her for signs and symptoms of preeclampsia/eclampsia for at least 48 hours. Expect to continue to administer magnesium sulfate infusion for 24 hours to prevent possible seizure activity, and monitor serum magnesium levels for possible toxicity.

Assess vital signs at least every 4 hours along with routine postpartum assessments—fundus, lochia, breasts, bladder, bowels, and emotional state. Pay special attention when performing the fundal assessment and assessing lochia. Magnesium sulfate inhibits uterine tone, placing the client at risk for postpartum hemorrhage. Monitor urine output closely. Diuresis is a positive sign that, along with a decrease in proteinuria, signals resolution of the disease.

HELLP Syndrome

HELLP is an acronym for hemolysis, elevated liver enzymes, and low platelets. HELLP syndrome occurs in about 20% of pregnant women diagnosed with severe preeclampsia. Although it has been reported as early as 17 weeks' gestation, most of the time it is diagnosed between 22 weeks and 36 weeks' gestation (Kidner & Flanders–Stepans, 2004). This devastating maternal hypertensive complication results in multisystem changes that can rapidly cascade into organ failure and death.

Causes

The exact etiology of HELLP syndrome is unclear. The hemolysis that occurs is termed *microangiopathic hemolytic anemia*. It is thought to happen when RBCs become fragmented as they pass through small, damaged blood vessels. Elevated liver enzymes are the result of reduced blood flow to the liver secondary to obstruction from fibrin deposits. Hyperbilirubinemia and jaundice result from liver impairment. Low platelets result from vascular damage, which are the result of vasospasm, and platelets aggregate at sites of damage, resulting in thrombocytopenia in multiple sites (Murray & McKinney, 2006).

Clinical Manifestations

Signs and symptoms of HELLP syndrome include

- Nausea (with or without vomiting)
- Malaise
- Epigastric pain
- Upper right quadrant pain
- Demonstrable edema
- Hyperbilirubinemia
- Laboratory data
  - Low hematocrit that is not explained by any blood loss
  - Elevated LDH (liver impairment)
  - Elevated AST (liver impairment
  - Elevated ALT (liver impairment)
  - Elevated BUN
  - Elevated bilirubin level
  - Elevated uric acid and creatinine levels (renal involvement)
  - Low platelet count of less than 100,000 cells/mm^3

BOX 19-3

ACRONYM FOR INTERVENING IN ECLAMPSIA

Use the following acronym to help guide interventions for the woman with eclampsia:

S—Safety: Place client in lateral position with side rails up; remain with client throughout seizure activity.

E—Establish and maintain airway: Turn client's head to side; elevate head of bed 30°; provide 100% oxygen via facial mask

I—IV bolus: Administer ordered magnesium sulfate, 4- to 6-g loading dose over 15 minutes, followed by 2 to 3 g/hour; if seizure reoccurs, give 2 g over 3 to 5 minutes

Z—Zealous observation: Document seizure activity, auras, and responses

U—Uterine activity: Observe for signs of precipitous labor or placental abruption

R—Rapid resuscitation: Prepare client for further sedation and possible mechanical ventilation in face of continued seizure activity

E—Evaluate fetus: Monitor fetus for nonreassuring patterns and appropriately intervene (Curran, 2003)

A diagnosis of HELLP syndrome is made based on laboratory test results. HELLP syndrome leads to an increased maternal risk for developing liver hematoma or rupture, stoke, cardiac arrest, seizure, pulmonary edema, DIC, subendocardial hemorrhage, adult respiratory distress syndrome, renal damage, sepsis, hypoxic encephalopathy, and maternal or fetal death (Kidner & Flanders–Stepans, 2004).

Treatment

The treatment for HELLP syndrome is based on the severity of the disease, gestational age of the fetus, and the condition of the mother and fetus. The client should be admitted or transferred to a tertiary center with a neonatal intensive care unit available. In addition, additional treatments include magnesium sulfate, antihypertensives, and correction of the woman's coagulopathies that accompany HELLP syndrome. After this syndrome is diagnosed and the woman's condition is stable, birth of the infant is indicated.

Magnesium sulfate is used prophylactically to prevent seizures. Antihypertensives such as hydralazine or labetalol are given to control blood pressure. Blood component therapy—such as fresh frozen plasma, packed RBCs, or platelets—is transfused to address the microangiopathic hemolytic anemia. Delivery may be delayed up to 96 hours to administer dexamethasone (Decadron) to stimulate fetal lung maturation in the preterm fetus.

All women experiencing this syndrome need to be counseled about its high rate of reoccurrence (25%) in subsequent pregnancies (Harvey, 2004).

Nursing Management

Nursing management of the woman diagnosed with HELLP syndrome is the same as that for the woman with severe preeclampsia. Systematic assessments are important, with the frequency of assessments dictated by the woman's condition and response to therapy.

Gestational Diabetes

Gestational diabetes is a condition involving glucose intolerance that occurs during pregnancy. It is discussed in greater detail in Chapter 20.

Blood Incompatibility

Blood incompatibility most commonly involves blood type or the Rh factor. Blood type incompatibility, also known as *ABO incompatibility,* is not as severe a condition as Rh incompatibility, because most antibodies to A and B antigens are IgM antibodies, which do not cross the placenta. It rarely causes significant hemolysis, and antepartum treatment is not warranted. Usually, the mother is blood type O, with anti-A and anti-B antibodies in her serum; the infant is blood type A, B, or AB. The incompatibility arises as a result of the interaction of antibodies present in maternal serum and the antigen sites on the fetal RBCs. However, documentation of blood type (type O of the mother and type A or B of the father) at the first prenatal visit is important to note. After birth, the newborn will need careful evaluation and possible intervention for hyperbilirubinemia if the incompatibility manifests itself with jaundice.

Rh incompatibility is a condition that develops when a woman with Rh-negative blood type is exposed to Rh-positive blood cells and subsequently develops circulating titers of Rh antibodies. Individuals with Rh-positive blood type have the D antigen present on their RBCs, whereas individuals with an Rh-negative blood type do not. The presence or absence of the Rh antigen on the RBC membrane is genetically controlled.

In the United States, 15% of the population lack the Rh surface antigen on the erythrocyte and are considered Rh negative. The vast majority (85%) of individuals are considered Rh positive.

The most common cause of Rh incompatibility is exposure of an Rh-negative mother to Rh-positive fetal blood during pregnancy or birth, during which erythrocytes from the fetal circulation leak into the maternal circulation. After a significant exposure, alloimmunization or sensitization occurs. As a result, maternal antibodies are produced against the foreign Rh antigen. Rh sensitization occurs in approximately 1 in 1000 births to Rh-negative women (Hait, 2004).

Theoretically, fetal and maternal blood does not mix during pregnancy. In reality, however, small placental accidents (transplacental bleeds secondary to minor separation), abortions, ectopic pregnancy, abdominal trauma, trophoblastic disease, amniocentesis, placenta previa, or abruptio placenta allow fetal blood to enter the maternal circulation and initiate the production of antibodies to destroy Rh-positive blood. The amount of fetal blood necessary to produce Rh incompatibility varies. In one study, less than 1 mL Rh-positive blood was shown to result in sensitization of women who are Rh negative (Salem, 2005).

Once sensitized, it takes approximately a month for Rh antibodies in the maternal circulation to cross over into the fetal circulation. In 90% of cases, sensitization occurs during delivery (Neal, 2001). Thus, most firstborn infants with Rh-positive blood type are not affected because the short period from first exposure of Rh-positive fetal erythrocytes to the birth of the infant is insufficient to produce a significant maternal IgG antibody response.

The risk and severity of alloimmune response increases with each subsequent pregnancy involving a fetus with Rh-positive blood. A second pregnancy with an Rh-positive fetus often produces a mildly anemic infant, whereas succeeding pregnancies produce infants with more serious hemolytic anemia.

Nursing Management

At the first prenatal visit, all women should have their blood type and Rh status determined. While taking a history, note any reports of previous events involving hemorrhage to delineate risk for prior sensitization. When the client's history reveals an Rh-negative mother who may be pregnant with an Rh-positive fetus, an antibody screen (indirect Coombs test) is done to determine whether the woman has developed isoimmunity to the Rh antigen. This test detects unexpected circulating antibodies in a woman's serum that could be potentially harmful to the fetus (Schnell, Van Leeuwen, & Kranpitz, 2003). If the indirect Coombs test is negative (meaning no antibodies present), then the woman is a candidate for RhoGAM. If the test is positive, RhoGAM is of no value because isoimmunization has occurred. In this case, the fetus is carefully monitored for hemolytic disease.

The incidence of isoimmunization has declined dramatically as a result of prenatal and postnatal RhoGAM administration after any event in which blood transfer may occur. The standard dose is 300 µg, which is effective for 30 mL fetal blood. Rh immunoglobulin helps to destroy any fetal cells in the maternal circulation before sensitization occurs, thus inhibiting maternal antibody production. This provides temporary passive immunity, thereby preventing maternal sensitization. The current recommendation is that every Rh-negative nonimmunized woman receives RhoGAM at 28 weeks' gestation and again within 72 hours after giving birth. Other indications for RhoGAM include

- Ectopic pregnancy
- Chorionic villus sampling
- Amniocentesis
- Prenatal hemorrhage
- Molar pregnancy
- Maternal trauma
- Percutaneous umbilical sampling
- Therapeutic or spontaneous abortion
- Fetal death
- Fetal surgery (Youngkin & Davis, 2004)

Despite the availability of RhoGAM and laboratory tests to identify women and newborns at risk, isoimmunization cases remain a serious clinical reality that continues to contribute to perinatal and neonatal mortality. Nurses, as client advocates, are in a unique position to make sure test results are brought to the health care provider's attention so appropriate interventions can be initiated. In addition, nurses must stay abreast of current literature and research regarding isoimmunization and its management. Stress to all women that early prenatal care can help identify and prevent this condition. Nurses can make a tremendous impact to ensure positive outcomes for the greatest possible number of pregnancies through education.

Hydramnios

Amniotic fluid develops from several maternal and fetal structures, including the amnion, chorion, maternal blood, fetal lungs, GI tract, kidneys, and skin. Any alteration of one or more of the various sources will alter the amount of amniotic fluid. **Hydramnios**, also called *polyhydramnios*, is a condition in which there is too much amniotic fluid (>2000 mL) surrounding the fetus between 32 and 36 weeks. It occurs in approximately 3% to 4% of all pregnancies and is associated with fetal anomalies of development (Creasy et al., 2004). It is associated with poor fetal outcomes because of the increased incidence of preterm births, fetal malpresentation, and cord prolapse.

Causes

There are several causes of hydramnios. Generally, too much fluid is being produced, there is a problem with the fluid being taken up, or both. It can be associated with maternal disease and fetal anomalies, but it can also be idiopathic in nature. Common factors associated with hydramnios include

- Maternal diabetes
- Fetal esophageal atresia
- Fetal intestinal atresia
- Neural tube defects
- Multiple gestation
- Chromosomal deviations
- Fetal hydrops
- Central nervous defects
- Cardiovascular anomalies
- Hydrocephaly

Clinical Manifestations

With hydramnios, there is a discrepancy between fundal height and gestational age, or a rapid growth of the uterus is noted. The woman may complain of discomfort in her abdomen, such as being severely stretched and tight, and may also feel she is having uterine contractions resulting from overstretching of the uterus. She may experience shortness of breath resulting from pressure on her diaphragm and have edema in her lower extremities resulting from increased pressure on the vena cava. The fetal parts and heart rate are often difficult to obtain with the excess fluid present.

Diagnosis is made after a thorough history and physical examination with ultrasound by measuring pockets of amniotic fluid to estimate the total volume. In some cases, ultrasound is helpful in finding the etiology of hydramnios, such as multiple pregnancy or a fetal structural anomaly.

Treatment

Treatment may include close monitoring and frequent follow-up visits with the health care provider if the hydramnios is mild to moderate. In severe cases in which the woman is in pain and experiencing shortness of breath, an amniocentesis or artificial rupture of the membranes is done to reduce the fluid and the pressure. A noninvasive treatment may involve the use of a prostaglandin synthesis inhibitor (indomethacin) to decrease amniotic fluid volume by decreasing fetal urinary output (Cunningham et al., 2005).

Nursing Management

Nursing management related to hydramnios focuses on ongoing assessment and monitoring of the woman for symptoms of abdominal pain, dyspnea, uterine contractions, and edema of the lower extremities. Explain to the woman and her family that this condition can cause her uterus to become overdistended and may lead to preterm labor and PROM. Outline the signs and symptoms of both conditions with instructions for the woman to contact her health care provider if they do occur. If a therapeutic amniocentesis is performed, assist the health care provider and monitor maternal and fetal status throughout for any changes.

Oligohydramnios

Oligohydramnios is a decreased amount of amniotic fluid (<500 mL) between 32 weeks and 36 weeks' gestation. This condition predisposes the fetus to increased risk of perinatal morbidity and mortality (Creasy et al., 2004). Reduction in amniotic fluid reduces the ability of the fetus to move freely without risk of cord compression, which increases the risk for fetal death and intrapartal hypoxia.

Causes

Oligohydramnios may result from several causes. Any condition that prevents the fetus from making urine or blocks it from going into the amniotic sac can lead to oligohydramnios. Factors associated with oligohydramnios include

- Uteroplacental insufficiency
- PROM prior to labor onset
- Hypertension of pregnancy
- Maternal diabetes
- Intrauterine growth restriction
- Postterm pregnancy
- Fetal renal agenesis
- Polycystic kidneys
- Urinary tract obstructions

Clinical Manifestations

Clinical manifestations associated with oligohydramnios may include leaking of amniotic fluid from the woman's vagina when the cause is rupture of the amniotic sac or suspected when the uterus is small for expected dates of gestation. Typically, the reduced volume of amniotic fluid is identified on ultrasound because the woman may not present with any symptoms.

Treatment

The woman with oligohydramnios can be managed on an outpatient basis with serial ultrasounds and fetal surveillance through nonstress testing and biophysical profiles. As long as fetal well-being is demonstrated with frequent testing, no intervention is necessary. If fetal well-being is compromised, delivery is planned along with amnioinfusion (the transvaginal infusion of crystalloid fluid to compensate for the lost amniotic fluid). The infusion is administered in a controlled fashion to prevent overdistension of the uterus.

Nursing Management

Nursing management related to the woman with oligohydramnios involves continuous monitoring of fetal well-being during nonstress testing or during labor and birth by identifying nonreassuring patterns on the fetal monitor. Variable decelerations indicating cord compression is common. Changing the woman's position might be therapeutic in altering this fetal heart rate pattern. After the birth, evaluate the newborn for signs of postmaturity, congenital anomalies, and respiratory difficulty.

Multiple Gestation

Multiple gestation is defined as more than one fetus being born of a pregnant woman. This includes twins, triplets, and higher-order multiples such as quadruplets on up. In the past two decades, the number of multiple gestations in the United States has jumped dramatically because of the widespread use of fertility drugs, older women having babies, and assisted reproductive technologies to treat infertility. In the United States, the overall prevalence of twins is approximately 12 per 1000, and two thirds are dizygotic (Zach & Pramanik, 2005). The increasing number of multiple gestations is a concern because women who are expecting more than one infant are at high risk for preterm labor, hydramnios, hyperemesis gravidarum, anemia, preeclampsia, and antepartum hemorrhage. Fetal/newborn risks or complications include prematurity, respiratory distress syndrome, birth asphyxia/perinatal depression, congenital anomalies (central nervous system, cardiovascular, and GI defects), twin-to-twin transfusion syndrome (transfusion of blood from one twin [i.e., donor] to the other twin [i.e., recipient]), IUGR, and becoming conjoined twins (Zach & Pramanik, 2005).

The two types of twins are *monozygotic* and *dizygotic* (Fig. 19-6). Monozygotic twins develop when a single, fertilized ovum splits during the first 2 weeks after conception. Monozygotic twins also are called *identical twins*. Two sperm fertilizing two ova produce dizygotic twins, which are called *fraternal twins*. Separate amnions,

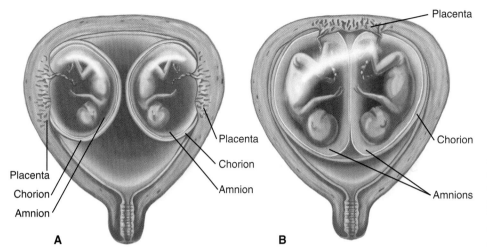

● Figure 19-6 Multiple gestation with twins. (**A**) Monozygotic twins where the fetuses share one placenta, two amnions, and one chorion. (**B**) Dizygotic twins, where each fetus has its own placenta, amnion, and chorion.

chorions, and placentas are formed in dizygotic twins. Triplets can be monozygotic, dizygotic, or trizygotic.

Clinical Manifestations

Typically, with a multiple gestation, the woman's uterus is larger than that associated with her estimated date of birth. Anemia, fatigue, and severe nausea and vomiting also may be present. The diagnosis of a multiple gestation is typically made on ultrasound early in the pregnancy.

Treatment

From the point of confirmation on, the woman is followed with serial ultrasounds to assess fetal growth patterns and development. Biophysical profiles along with nonstress tests are ordered to determine fetal well-being. Many women are hospitalized in late pregnancy to prevent preterm labor and receive closer surveillance. During intrapartum, the woman is closely monitored, with a perinatal team available to assist after birth. Operative delivery is frequently needed, resulting from fetal malpresentation.

Nursing Management

Nursing management during the prenatal period focuses on education and support of the woman in areas of nutrition, increased rest periods, and close observation for pregnancy complications—anemia, excessive weight gain, proteinuria, edema, vaginal bleeding, and hypertension. Instruct the woman to be alert for and report immediately any signs and symptoms of preterm labor—contractions, uterine cramping, low back ache, increase in vaginal discharge, loss of mucus plug, pelvic pain, and pressure.

When the woman with a multiple gestation is admitted for labor and birth, expect to monitor fetal heart rates continuously. Prepare the woman for an ultrasound to assess the presentation of each fetus to determine the best delivery approach. Ensure that extra nursing staff and the perinatal team are available for any birth or newborn com-

plications. After giving birth, closely assess the woman for hemorrhage by frequently assessing uterine involution. Palpate the uterine fundus and monitor the amount and characteristics of lochia. Throughout the entire pregnancy, birth, and hospital stay, inform and support the woman and her family regarding potential concerns that might occur. Encourage them to ask questions and verbalize any fears and concerns.

Premature Rupture of Membranes

Premature rupture of membranes (PROM) is defined as the rupture of the bag of waters prior to the onset of true labor. It carries a number of associated conditions and complications, such as infection, prolapsed cord, abruptio placenta, and preterm labor. This is the single most common diagnosis associated with preterm births (Moos, 2004).

The terminology pertaining to PROM can be confusing. PROM is rupture of the membranes prior to the onset of labor and is used appropriately when referring to a woman who is beyond 37 weeks' gestation, has presented with spontaneous rupture of the membranes, and is not in labor. Related terms include preterm premature rupture of membranes (PPROM), which is defined as rupture of membranes prior to the onset of labor in a woman who is less than 37 weeks of gestation. Perinatal risks associated with PPROM may stem from immaturity, including respiratory distress syndrome, intraventricular hemorrhage, patent ductus arteriosus, and necrotizing enterocolitis. Recent studies have shown clear benefits of antibiotics to decrease neonatal morbidity associated with PPROM (Wilkes & Galan, 2004).

The incidence of PROM is approximately 10% of pregnancies (Wilkes & Galan, 2004). Prolonged rupture of membranes consists of rupture of membranes for more than 24 hours, and women are at increasing risk for infection (chorioamnionitis, endometritis, sepsis, and neonatal infections) as the duration of rupture increases. The time interval from rupture of membranes to the onset of regular contractions is termed the *latent period*.

Cause

The exact mechanism of PROM is not known. However, various factors have been associated with the condition, including infection, increased uterine size (hydramnios, macrosomia, multifetal gestation), uterine and fetal anomalies, lower socioeconomic status, STIs, incompetent cervix, vaginal bleeding, and cigarette smoking during pregnancy. In many cases, however, PROM may occur in the absence of any recognized risk factors. Women who do not go into labor immediately are at increasing risk of infection as the duration of rupture increases. Chorioamnionitis, endometritis, sepsis, and neonatal infections are common sequelae.

Clinical Manifestations

The clinical picture presented by the woman with PROM may include labor symptoms (cramping, pelvic pressure, or back pain), history or symptoms of UTI (frequency, urgency, dysuria, or flank pain), history of or current symptoms of pelvic or vaginal infection (pain or vaginal discharge), and/or vital signs reflective of infection (temperature elevation and white blood cell elevation > 18,000 cells/mm^3) (Mattson & Smith, 2004).

To determine the diagnosis of PROM, several procedures may be used: the Nitrazine test, fern test, or ultrasound. After the insertion of a sterile speculum, a sample of the fluid found in the vaginal area is obtained. With a Nitrazine test, pH of the fluid is tested; amniotic fluid is more basic (7.0) compared with normal vaginal secretions (4.5). Nitrazine paper turns blue in the presence of amniotic fluid. Unfortunately, many false positives can occur if blood, urine, semen, or antiseptic chemicals are also present. All will increase the pH.

For the fern test, a sample of vaginal fluid is place on a slide to be viewed directly under a microscope. Amniotic fluid will develop a fern-like pattern when it dries, resulting from the amount of NaCl crystallization that occurs. If both previous tests are inconclusive, a transvaginal ultrasound can also be used to determine whether membranes have ruptured by demonstrating a decreased amount of amniotic fluid (oligohydramnios) in the uterus (Wilkes & Galan, 2004).

Treatment

Treatment of PROM typically depends on the gestational age. Under no circumstances is a digital cervical examination done until the woman enters active labor, to minimize infection exposure. If the fetal lungs are mature, induction of labor is initiated. PROM is not an indication, in and of itself, for surgical birth. If the fetal lungs are immature, expectant management is carried out with adequate hydration, reduced physical activity, pelvic rest, and close observation for possible infection, such as with frequent monitoring of vital signs and checking the results of laboratory tests (e.g., the white blood cell count). Corticosteroids may be given to enhance fetal lung maturity, although this remains controversial.

Nursing Management

Nursing management of PROM usually depends on the gestational age and presence or absence of an intraamniotic infection (chorioamnionitis). An accurate assessment of the gestational age and knowledge of the maternal, fetal, and neonatal risks are essential to appropriate evaluation, counseling, and management of women with PROM.

Assessment

After obtaining the woman's medical and obstetric history, set up and perform fetal heart rate monitoring to check for fetal well-being, assess the woman's labor status, and conduct a vaginal examination to ascertain the cervical status in PROM. If PPROM exists, a sterile speculum examination is done rather than a digital cervical examination because it may diminish latency (period of time from rupture of membranes to birth) and increase newborn morbidity (Cunningham et al., 2005). Key assessment areas are highlighted in Box 19-4.

Assessing the characteristics of the amniotic fluid is important. Abnormal findings would include presence

---

BOX 19-4

KEY ASSESSMENTS WITH PREMATURE RUPTURE OF MEMBRANES

For the woman with PROM, the following assessments are essential:

- Determining the date, time, and duration of membrane rupture by client interview
- Ascertaining gestational age of the fetus based on date of mother's LMP, fundal height, and ultrasound dating
- Questioning the woman about possible history of or recent UTI or vaginal infection that might have contributed to PROM
- Assessing for any associated labor symptoms, such as back pain or pelvic pressure
- Assisting with or performing diagnostic tests to validate leakage of fluid, such as Nitrazine test, "ferning" on slide, and ultrasound
- Continually assessing for signs of infection including
  - Elevation of maternal temperature and pulse rate
  - Abdominal/uterine tenderness
  - Fetal tachycardia more than 160 bpm
  - Elevated white blood cell count and C-reactive protein
  - Cloudy, foul-smelling amniotic fluid

of meconium, minimal amount, and a foul odor. When meconium is present in the amniotic fluid, it typically indicates fetal distress related to hypoxia. Meconium stains the fluid yellow to greenish brown, depending on the amount present. A decreased amount of amniotic fluid reduces the cushioning effect, thereby making cord compression a possibility. A foul odor of amniotic fluid indicates infection.

Nursing Interventions

Nursing interventions for the woman with PROM or PPROM focus on infection prevention and identification of preterm labor contractions. The risk for infection is great, resulting from the break in the amniotic fluid membrane and its close proximity to vaginal bacteria. Therefore, monitor maternal vital signs closely. Be alert for a temperature elevation or an increase in pulse, which would indicate infection. Also monitor fetal heart rate, reporting any fetal tachycardia, which could indicate a maternal infection. Evaluate the results of laboratory tests such as a CBC. An elevation in white blood cells would suggest infection.

Additional nursing interventions include

- Administering antibiotics if ordered
- Monitoring fetal heart rate patterns continuously, reporting any variable decelerations suggesting cord compression
- Assisting with amnioinfusion to alter variable deceleration pattern per orders or according to institutional protocol
- Educating the woman and her partner on the purpose of the protective membranes and implications related to early rupture
- Continually informing the woman and her partner of planned interventions, including potential complications and required therapy
- Encouraging the client and her partner to verbalize feelings and concerns
- Preparing the woman for induction or augmentation of labor as appropriate if the woman is near term

Client education is key, especially if the woman is to be discharged home. This may be the case for the woman with PPROM. Therefore, teach the couple about the signs and symptoms of infection if the client is to be discharged home, including who and when to call for problems or concerns (see Teaching Guidelines 19-3).

Preterm Labor

Preterm labor is defined as the occurrence of regular uterine contractions accompanied by cervical effacement and dilation before 37 weeks' gestation. It occurs between 20 weeks and 37 weeks' gestation. Preterm births remain one of the most problematic situations contributing to perinatal morbidity and mortality in the world. According to the March of Dimes (March of

 TEACHING GUIDELINES 19-3

Teaching for the Woman With PPROM

- Monitor your baby's activity by performing fetal kick counts daily.
- Check your temperature daily and report any temperature increases to your healthcare provider.
- Watch for signs related to the beginning of labor. Report any tightening of the abdomen or contractions.
- Avoid any touching or manipulating of your breasts, which could stimulate labor.
- Do not insert anything into your vagina or vaginal area.
- Maintain any specific activity restrictions as recommended.
- Wash your hands thoroughly after using the bathroom and make sure to wipe from front to back each time.
- Keep your perineal area clean and dry.
- Take your antibiotics as directed if your healthcare provider has prescribed them.
- Call your health care provider with changes in your condition, including fever, uterine tenderness, feeling like your heart is racing, and foul-smelling vaginal discharge.

Dimes, 2005), one in eight infants born in the United States is born prematurely.

Preterm birth is one of the most common obstetric complications, and its sequelae have a profound effect on the survival and health of about one in every eight infants born in the United States annually (March of Dimes, 2004). The rate of preterm births in the United States has increased 27% in the past 20 years. Preterm births account for 75% of neurodevelopmental disorders and other serious morbidities, as well as behavioral and social problems. In addition, up to $28 billion is spent on maternal and infant care related to prematurity (March of Dimes Birth Defects Foundation, 2003). Infants born prematurely also are at risk for serious sequelae such as respiratory distress syndrome, infections, congenital heart defects, thermoregulation problems that can lead to acidosis and weight loss, intraventricular hemorrhage, feeding difficulties resulting from diminished stomach capacity and underdeveloped suck reflex, and neurologic disorders related to hypoxia and trauma at birth (Newton, 2004). Although great strides have been made in neonatal intensive care, prematurity remains the leading cause of death within the first month of life and is the second leading cause of all infant deaths (March of Dimes, 2005).

Cause

The exact cause of preterm labor and birth is not known. Prevention is the goal. However, prevention of all preterm births is not possible because numerous risk factors exist.

Box 19-5 highlights some of the risk factors associated with preterm labor and birth.

Clinical Manifestations

Frequently, women are unaware that uterine contractions, effacement, and dilation are occurring, thus making early intervention and treatment ineffective in arresting preterm labor and preventing the birth of a premature infant. Recognizing preterm labor at an early stage requires that the expectant mother and her healthcare provider identify the subtle symptoms of preterm labor. These may include

- Change or increase in vaginal discharge
- Pelvic pressure (pushing down sensation)
- Low, dull backache
- Menstrual-like cramps
- Uterine contractions, with or without pain
- Intestinal cramping, with or without diarrhea (AAP & ACOG, 2003)

BOX 19-5

RISK FACTORS ASSOCIATED WITH PRETERM LABOR AND BIRTH

- African-American race (double the risk)
- Maternal age extremes less than 16 years and more than 40 years old
- Low socioeconomic status
- Alcohol or other drug use, especially cocaine
- Poor maternal nutrition
- Maternal periodontal disease
- Cigarette smoking
- Low level of education
- History of prior preterm birth (triples the risk)
- Uterine abnormalities, such as fibroids
- Low pregnancy weight for height
- Preexisting diabetes or hypertension
- Multiple gestation
- PROM
- Late or no prenatal care
- Short cervical length
- STIs: gonorrhea, *Chlamydia,* trichomoniasis
- Bacterial vaginosis (50% increased risk) (Newton, 2004)
- Chorioamnionitis
- Hydramnios
- Gestational hypertension
- Cervical insufficiency
- Short interpregnancy interval: less than 1 year between births
- Placental problems, such as placenta previa and abruption placenta
- Maternal anemia
- UTI
- Domestic violence
- Stress, acute and chronic (Moos, 2004)

Treatment

Predicting risk or preterm labor is only valuable if there is an available intervention that is likely to improve the situation and, according to ACOG, many factors should be considered before selecting an intervention. Many factors influence the decision to intervene when women present with symptoms of preterm labor, including the probability of progressive labor, gestational age, and the risks of treatment. ACOG (2003) recommends the following as guidelines:

- There are no clear "first-line" **tocolytic** drugs (drugs that promote uterine relaxation by interfering with uterine contraction) to manage preterm labor. Clinical circumstances and healthcare provider preference should dictate treatment.
- Antibiotics do not appear to prolong gestation and should be reserved for group B streptococcal prophylaxis in women in whom birth is imminent.
- Tocolytic drugs may prolong pregnancy for 2 to 7 days, which may allow for administration of steroids to improve fetal lung maturity and transporting the woman to a tertiary care center.

Despite the recommendations of ACOG (2003), health care providers continue to prescribe pharmacologic treatment for preterm labor at home and in the hospital setting. This treatment often includes oral or IV tocolytics and varying degrees of activity restriction. Antibiotics may also be prescribed to treat presumed or confirmed infections. Steroids may be given to enhance fetal lung maturity between 24 weeks and 34 weeks' gestation. Commonly used tocolytics include

- Beta-adrenergics, such as ritodrine (Yutopar) and terbutaline (Brethine)
- Calcium channel blockers, such as nifedipine (Procardia)
- Prostaglandin synthetase inhibitors, such as indomethacin (Indocin; not used after 32 weeks' gestation, because of its effects on the fetus)
- Magnesium sulfate, which reduces muscular ability to contract

Nursing Management

Nurses play a key role in reducing preterm labor and births to improve pregnancy outcomes for both mothers and their infants. Early detection of preterm labor is currently the best strategy to improve outcomes. Because of the numerous factors associated with preterm labor, it is challenging to identify and address all of them, especially when women experiencing contractions are frequently falsely reassured and not assessed thoroughly to determine the cause. This delay impedes initiation of interventions to reduce infant death and morbidity.

Preterm birth prevention programs for women at high risk have used self-monitoring of symptoms and patterns, weekly cervical examinations, telephone monitoring, home visiting, and home uterine activity monitoring, along or in combination, with mixed results (Weiss, Saks, & Harris, 2002).

Assessment

Signs and symptoms occurring between 20 weeks and 37 weeks of pregnancy that need to be assessed and evaluated further for preterm include

- Pelvic pressure (feels like the fetus is pushing down)
- Complaints of low, dull back pain
- Feelings of menstrual-like cramps
- Change or increase in vaginal discharge
- Heaviness or aching in the thighs
- Uterine contractions occurring every 10 minutes or more frequently
- Intestinal cramping, with or without diarrhea
- Fetal engagement into maternal pelvis
- Tachycardia (Freda & Patterson, 2004)

The diagnosis of preterm labor requires both uterine contractions and cervical change. The contractions must be persistent, such that four contractions occur every 20 minutes or eight contractions occur in 1 hour. Cervical effacement is 80% or greater and cervical dilation is greater than 1 cm (AAP & ACOG, 2003).

Diagnostic Methods

Currently, four tests are commonly used for preterm labor prediction: fetal fibronectin testing, cervical length evaluation by transvaginal ultrasound, salivary estriol, and home monitoring of uterine activity to recognize preterm contractions. Fetal fibronectin and cervical length examinations have a high negative predictive value and are thus better at predicting which pregnant women are unlikely to have a preterm birth as opposed to predicting those who will (Bernhardt & Dorman, 2004).

Other diagnostic testing used in preterm labor risk assessment include a CBC to detect the presence of infection, which may be a contributing factor to preterm labor; urinalysis to detect bacteria and nitrites, which are indicative of a UTI; and an amniotic fluid analysis to determine fetal lung maturity and presence of subclinical chorioamnionitis.

Fetal Fibronectin

Fetal fibronectin, a glycoprotein produced by the chorion, is found at the junction of the chorion and decidua (fetal membranes and uterus). It is present in cervicovaginal fluid prior to delivery, regardless of gestational age. It is not found in vaginal secretions unless there has been a disruption between the chorion and decidua. The test is a useful marker for impending membrane rupture within 7 to 14 days if the level increases to greater than 0.05 µg/mL. Conversely, if fetal fibronectin is not present, there is a 98% chance that the woman will not go into preterm (Schnell, Van Leeuwen, & Kranpitz, 2003).

A sterile applicator is used to collect a cervicovaginal sample during a speculum examination. The result is either positive (fetal fibronectin is present) or negative (fetal fibronectin is not present). Interpretation of fetal fibronectin results should always be used in conjunction with clinical findings and not used in isolation for preterm labor prediction.

Transvaginal Ultrasound

Transvaginal ultrasound of the cervix has been used as a tool to predict preterm labor in high-risk pregnancies and to differentiate between true and false preterm labor. Three parameters are evaluated during the transvaginal ultrasound: cervical length and width, funnel width and length, and percentage of funneling. Measurement of the closed portion of the cervix visualized during the transvaginal ultrasound is the single most reliable parameter for prediction of preterm delivery in high-risk women (Iams, 2003).

Cervical length varies during pregnancy. A cervical length of 3 cm or more indicates that delivery within 14 days is unlikely. Women with a short cervical length of 2.5 cm during the mid trimester have a substantially greater risk of preterm birth prior to 35 weeks' gestation (Iams & Creasy, 2004). As with fetal fibronectin testing, negative results can be reassuring and prevent unnecessary interventions (Abrahams & Katz, 2002).

Salivary Estriol

Salivary estriol is another biochemical marker that has been shown to increase before preterm labor. The woman can perform the test at home and send the sample to the lab. A value of estriol greater than 2.1 ng/mL is considered positive.

Observational studies have shown that maternal levels of estriol increase in their saliva and blood serum before the onset of spontaneous term and preterm labor. According to ACOG (2002), however, no current data support using salivary estriol screening as a strategy to identify or prevent preterm labor. The test carries a high percentage of false-positive results and has failed to establish its usefulness for anything more than investigational purposes (Ressel, 2004). Additional research is needed.

Home Uterine Activity Monitoring

Home monitoring of uterine activity can identify women in preterm labor at an early stage to reduce the rate of preterm birth (Moore, 2003). Home uterine activity monitoring does not prevent preterm labor or birth; it provides supplemental client education and clinical data for the healthcare provider in an effort to prolong gestation and maximize pregnancy outcomes through timely clinical interventions (Fig. 19-7). It involves client education, daily client assessment, data collection, data interpretation (Morrison et al., 2004).

The woman is asked to wear an ambulatory tocodynamometer and transmit data to the nurse or health-

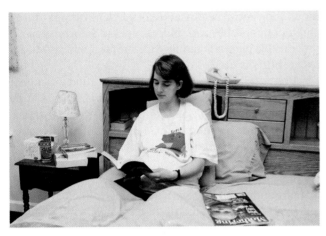

● Figure 19-7 The mother with preterm labor resting in bed at home.

care provider daily via telephone lines. Uterine and fetal activity data are transmitted to perinatal nurses who are available around-the-clock for detection of uterine contractions, in addition to picking up the fetal heart rate. Women are also asked to record uterine activity (uterine pressure, back pain, or cramps) they experience for an hour twice a day and then speak to a perinatal nurse who analyzes the results.

If the number of contractions exceeds a predetermined threshold, the woman drinks 8 to 12 oz of water, rests, empties her bladder, and then repeats uterine monitoring. This modality of screening remains somewhat controversial as to its real impact on preventing preterm birth.

Nursing Interventions

A reduction in the preterm birthrate cannot be achieved until there are effective strategies to predict risk for preterm birth as well as effective methods to prevent preterm births. Because the etiology is often multifactorial, an individualized approach is needed.

The signs or preterm labor are subtle and maybe disregarded by the client as well as the health care professional. Because risk assessment does not identify many women who will develop preterm labor, ensure that every pregnant woman receives basic education about preterm labor, including information about harmful lifestyles, the signs of genitourinary infections and preterm labor, and the appropriate response to these symptoms. Teach the client how to palpate for and time uterine contractions. Provide written materials to support this education at a level and in a language appropriate for the client. Also, educate clients about the importance of prenatal care, risk reduction, and recognizing the signs and symptoms of preterm labor. Teaching Guidelines 19-4 highlights important instructions related to preventing preterm labor.

Additional nursing interventions include the following activities:

 TEACHING GUIDELINES 19-4

Teaching to Prevent Preterm Labor

- Avoid traveling for long distances in cars, trains, planes, or buses.
- Avoid lifting heavy objects, such as laundry, groceries, or a young child.
- Avoid performing hard, physical work, such as yard work, moving of furniture, or construction.
- Visit a dentist in early pregnancy to evaluate and treat periodontal disease.
- Enroll in a smoking cessation program if you are unable to quit on your own.
- Curtail sexual activity until after 37 weeks if experiencing preterm labor symptoms.
- Consume a well-balanced nutritional diet to gain appropriate weight.
- Avoid the use of substances such as marijuana, cocaine, and heroin.
- Identify factors and areas of stress in your life, and use stress management techniques to reduce them.
- If you are experiencing intimate partner violence, seek resources to modify the situation.

Recognize the signs and symptoms of preterm labor and notify your birth attendant if any occur:
- Uterine contractions, cramping, or low back pain
- Feeling of pelvic pressure or fullness
- Increase in vaginal discharge
- Nausea, vomiting, and diarrhea
- Leaking of fluid from vagina
- If you are experiencing any of these signs or symptoms, do the following:
- Stop what you are doing and rest for 1 hour.
- Empty your bladder.
- Lie down on your side.
- Drink two to three glasses of water.
- Feel your abdomen and make note of the hardness of the contraction. Call your health care provider and describe the contraction as
  - Mild if it feels like the tip of the nose
  - Moderate if it feels like the tip of the chin
  - Strong if it feels like your forehead (Mattson & Smith, 2004)

- Assessing maternal and fetal vital signs frequently
- Stressing good hydration and consumption of a nutritious diet
- Advising against any activity, such as sexual activity or nipple stimulation, that might stimulate oxytocin release and initiate uterine contractions
- Encouraging clients to access their healthcare provider for reassurance
- Assessing stress levels of client and family, and making appropriate referrals

- Providing emotional support and client empowerment throughout
- Emphasizing the possible need more frequent supervision and office visits
- Raising public awareness of the problem of prematurity

Medication Administration

When preterm labor is identified because of PPROM or persistent uterine contractions accompanied by cervical change, treatment has commonly consisted of IV hydration, often accompanied by tocolytic therapy. Neither therapy has been shown to be effective for more than 48 hours. However, delaying birth for 48 hours allows time for the administration of corticosteroids to accelerate fetal lung maturity and client transfer to a medical facility where there is a neonatal intensive care unit (Newton, 2004).

Tocolytic Therapy

Tocolytics are agents that promote uterine relaxation by interfering with uterine contraction. Tocolytic therapy does not typically prevent preterm birth, but it may delay it. It is contraindicated for abruptio placenta, acute fetal distress or death, eclampsia or severe preeclampsia, active vaginal bleeding, dilation more than 6 cm, chorioamnionitis, and maternal hemodynamic instability (Harvey, 2003).

The decision to stop preterm labor is individualized, based on risk factors, extent of cervical dilation, membrane status, fetal gestational age, and presence or absence of infection. It is most likely ordered if preterm labor occurs before the 34th week of gestation, attempting to delay birth and thereby helping to reduce the severity of respiratory distress syndrome and other complications associated with prematurity. Medications most commonly used for tocolysis include magnesium sulfate, ritodrine (Yutopar), terbutaline (Brethine), indomethacin (Indocin), and nifedipine (Procardia). Ritodrine is the only FDA-approved agent for arresting preterm labor. The other drugs are used "off label." This means they are effective for this purpose, but have not been officially tested and developed for this purpose by the FDA (Lowdermilk & Perry, 2004). All these medications have serious side effects and warrant close supervision when being administered (see Drug Guide 19-4).

Corticosteroids

Corticosteroids given to the mother in preterm labor can help prevent or reduce the frequency and severity of respiratory distress syndrome in premature infants delivered between 24 weeks and 34 weeks' gestation. The beneficial effects of corticosteroids on fetal lung maturation have been reported within 48 hours of initial administration (Slattery & Morrison, 2002). These drugs require at least 24 hours to become effective, so timely administration is crucial.

Psychological Support

The birth of an preterm newborn can be a devastating event for family members, who may be faced with enormous long-term health and social implications during childhood, and beyond. Nurses are on the front lines to provide this high-risk family with support, education, and expert nursing care.

Preterm labor and birth present multifactorial challenges for everyone involved with this crisis event. If the woman is restricted in her activities, additional stresses may be placed on the family, contributing to the crisis. Every case of spontaneous preterm labor is unique, requiring individualization of care in light of the clinical circumstances, and the full and informed consent of the woman and her partner. Half of all women who ultimately give birth prematurely have no identifiable risk factors. Nurses need to take all women's complaints seriously and complete a thorough assessment to validate their etiology.

Work to ensure that all pregnant women have access to nurses who are sensitive to any complaint and are able to provide appropriate information and follow-up. Sensitivity to the subtle differences between normal pregnancy sensations and the prodromal symptoms of preterm labor is a key factor in ensuring timely access to care. Offer clarification and validation of their symptoms.

KEY CONCEPTS

- Identifying risk factors early on and ongoing throughout the pregnancy is important to ensure the best outcome for every pregnancy. Risk assessment should start with the first prenatal visit and continue with subsequent visits.
- The three most common causes of hemorrhage early in pregnancy (first half of pregnancy) are spontaneous abortion, ectopic pregnancy, and GTD.
- Ectopic pregnancies occur in about 1 in 50 pregnancies and have increased dramatically during the past few decades.
- Having a molar pregnancy results in the loss of the pregnancy and the possibility of developing choriocarcinoma, a chronic malignancy from the trophoblastic tissue.
- The classic clinical picture presentation for placenta previa is painless, bright-red vaginal bleeding occurring during the third trimester.
- Treatment of abruptio placenta is designed to assess, control, and restore the amount of blood lost; to provide a positive outcome for both mother and infant; and to prevent coagulation disorders.
- DIC can be described in simplest terms as a loss of balance between the clot-forming activity of thrombin and the clot-lysing activity of plasmin.
- Hyperemesis gravidarum is a complication of pregnancy characterized by persistent, uncontrollable nausea and vomiting before the 20th week of gestation.

Drug Guide 19-4 Medications Used With Preterm Labor

Drug	Action/Indication	Nursing Implications
Magnesium sulfate	Relaxes uterine muscles to stop irritability and contractions, to arrest uterine contractions for preterm labor (off-label use) Has aided in seizure prophylaxis and treatment of seizures in preeclamptic and eclamptic patients for almost 100 years (Rideout, 2005)	Administer intravenously with a loading dose of 4–6 g over 15–30 minutes initially, and then maintain infusion at 1–4 g per hour Assess vital signs and DTRs hourly; report any hypotension or depressed or absent DTRs Monitor level of consciousness; report any headache, blurred vision, dizziness, or altered level of consciousness Perform continuous electronic fetal monitoring; report any decreased fetal heart rate variability, hypotonia, or respiratory depression Monitor intake and output hourly; report any decrease in output (<30 mL/hour) Assess respiratory rate; report respiratory rate less than 12 breaths/minute; auscultate lung sounds for evidence of pulmonary edema Monitor for common maternal side effects including flushing, nausea and vomiting, drug mouth, lethargy, blurred vision, and headache Assess for complaints of nausea, vomiting, transient hypotension, lethargy Assess for signs and symptoms of magnesium toxicity, such as decreased level of consciousness, depressed respirations and DTRs, slurred speech, weakness, and respiratory and/or cardiac arrest Have calcium gluconate readily available at the bedside to reverse magnesium toxicity
Ritodrine (Yutopar)	Relaxes smooth muscles to calm the uterus, inhibits uterine activity to arrest preterm labor	Assess maternal vital signs frequently Monitor the woman for possible adverse effects including tachycardia, hypotension, palpitations, tremors, chest pain, hypokalemia, water retention, nausea, vomiting, diarrhea, hyperglycemia, decreased urinary output, and nervousness Monitor fetal status, being alert for tachycardia, heart failure, hyperglycemia, hypotension, and jaundice Be aware that side effects are dose related and will increase as dose is increased Perform cardiac assessment of woman to rule out preexisting cardiac disease and diabetes Perform continuous fetal monitoring Administer as IV infusion, at prescribed rate, increasing rate every 10–20 minutes as necessary; reduce rate gradually to lowest possible rate to stop contractions; maintain for 12–24 hours Expect to begin oral dose an hour before IV infusion is stopped; administer oral dose every 3–4 hours with meals Discontinue IV infusion if the following occur: maternal tachycardia >120 bpm, hypotension <90/60 mmHg, fetal heart rate >180 bpm, signs of maternal pulmonary edema Have propranolol (Inderal) available to reverse cardiac adverse effects

(continued)

Drug Guide 19-4 Medications Used With Preterm Labor (continued)

Drug	Action/Indication	Nursing Implications
Terbutaline sulfate (Brethine)	Relaxes smooth muscles to calm uterus, inhibits uterine activity to arrest preterm labor	Be aware that this drug is usually effective in delaying birth for up to 48 hours (Rideout, 2005) Monitor the mother for possible adverse effects such as tachycardia, hypotension, palpitations, tremors, chest pain, hypokalemia, water retention, nausea, vomiting, diarrhea, hyperglycemia, decreased urinary output, and nervousness Assess fetal well-being, noting any possible adverse effects such as tachycardia, heart failure, hyperglycemia, hypotension, newborn jaundice Be aware that adverse effects are dose related and will increase as dose is increased Perform cardiac assessment of woman to rule out preexisting cardiac disease and diabetes Institute continuous fetal monitoring Assess vital signs frequently for changes Discontinue drug for the following: maternal tachycardia >120 bpm, hypotension <90/60 mmHg, fetal heart rate >180 bpm, signs of maternal pulmonary edema Have propranolol (Inderal) available to reverse cardiac adverse effects
Indomethacin (Indocin)	Inhibits prostaglandins, which stimulate contractions; inhibits uterine activity to arrest preterm labor	Continuously assess vital signs, uterine activity, and fetal heart rate Administer oral form with food to reduce GI irritation Do not give to women with peptic ulcer disease Schedule ultrasound to assess amniotic fluid volume and function of ductus arteriosus before initiation of therapy; monitor for signs of maternal hemorrhage Be alert for possible maternal adverse effects such as nausea, vomiting, heartburn, rash, prolonged bleeding time, oligohydramnios, and hypertension Monitor for possible fetal adverse effects including constriction of ductus arteriosus, premature ductus closure, necrotizing enterocolitis, oligohydramnios, and pulmonary hypertension
Nifedipine (Procardia)	Blocks calcium movement into to muscle cells, inhibits uterine activity to arrest preterm labor	Use caution if giving this drug with magnesium sulfate because of increased risk for hypotension Monitor blood pressure hourly if giving with magnesium sulfate; report a pulse rate >110 bpm Monitor for possible fetal effects such as decreased uteroplacental blood flow and fetal bradycardia, which can lead to fetal hypoxia Monitor for possible adverse effects, such as flushing of the skin, headache, transient tachycardia, palpitations, postural hypertension, peripheral edema, and transient fetal tachycardia
Betamethasone (Celestone)	Promotes fetal lung maturity by stimulating surfactant production, prevents or reduces risk of respiratory distress syndrome and intraventricular hemorrhage in the preterm neonate less than 34 weeks' gestation	Administer two doses intramuscularly 24 hours apart Monitor for possible maternal infection or pulmonary edema Educate parents about potential benefits of drug to preterm infant Assess maternal lung sounds and monitor for signs of infection

- Gestational hypertension is the leading cause of maternal death in the United States and the most common complication reported during pregnancy.

- HELLP is an acronym for hemolysis, elevated liver enzymes, and low platelets.

- Rh incompatibility is a condition that develops when a woman of Rh-negative blood type is exposed to Rh-positive fetal blood cells and subsequently develops circulating titers of Rh antibodies.

- Hydramnios occurs in approximately 3 to 4% of all pregnancies and is associated with fetal anomalies of development.

- Nursing care related to the woman with oligohydramnios involves continuous monitoring of fetal well-being during nonstress testing or during labor and birth by identifying nonreassuring patterns on the fetal monitor.

- The increasing number of multiple gestations is a concern because women who are expecting more than one infant are at high risk for preterm labor, hydramnios, hyperemesis gravidarum, anemia, preeclampsia, and antepartum hemorrhage.

- Nursing care related to PROM centers around infection prevention and identification of preterm labor contractions.

- Early identification of preterm labor would allow for appropriate interventions that may prolong the pregnancy, such as transferring the woman to a facility with a neonatal intensive care unit for prenatal care, administering glucocorticoids to the mother to promote fetal lung maturity, and giving appropriate antibiotics to treat infections to arrest the labor process.

- It is essential that nurses teach all pregnant women how to detect the early symptoms of preterm labor and what to do if they experience contractions or cramping that does not go away.

References

Abrahams, C. & Katz, M. (2002). A perspective on the diagnosis of preterm labor. *Journal of Perinatal and Neonatal Nursing, 16*(1), 1–11.

Ahn, J. T., Hibbard, J. U. (2003). The short cervix in pregnancy: Which therapy reduces preterm birth? *OBG Management.* [Online] Available at www.obgmanagement.com/content/obg_featurexml.asp?file=203/08/obg_0803_00.

American Academy of Pediatrics, American College of Obstetricians and Gynecologists. (2003). *Guidelines for perinatal care* (5th ed.). Washington, DC: Author.

American College of Obstetricians and Gynecologists. (2002). *ACOG practice bulletin: Diagnosis and management of preeclampsia and eclampsia.* Number 33. Washington, DC: Author.

American College of Obstetricians and Gynecologists. (2003a). ACOG practice bulletin: Cervical insufficiency. *Obstetrics and Gynecology, 102,* 1091–1099.

American College of Obstetricians and Gynecologists. (2003b). ACOG practice bulletin: Management of preterm labor. *Obstetrics and Gynecology, 101,* 1039–1047.

Baines, E. (2003). A test for ectopic pregnancy. *GP: General Practitioner,* February, 74–76.

Berghella, V. (2004). Grand rounds: The short and funneled cervix: What do I do now? *Contemporary OB/GYN, 49,* 26–34.

Bernhardt, J. & Dorman, K. F. (2004). Pre-term birth risk assessment tools: Exploring fetal fibronectin and cervical length for validating risk. *JOGNN, 8*(1), 38–44.

Blackburn, S. (2003). *Maternal, fetal, & neonatal physiology: A clinical perspective* (2nd ed.). St. Louis: WB Saunders.

Bridges, E. J., Womble, S., Wallace, M., & McCartney, J. (2003). Hemodynamic monitoring in high-risk obstetrics patients II: Pregnancy-induced hypertension and preeclampsia. *Critical Care Nurse, 23,* 52–56.

Brooks, M. B. (2005). Pregnancy, preeclampsia. *eMedicine.* [Online] Available at http://emedicine.com/emerg/topic480.htm.

Brooks, M. B. (2004). Pregnancy, eclampsia. *eMedicine.* [Online] Available at http://emedicine.com/emerg/topic796.htm.

Cavanaugh, B. M. (2003). *Nurse's manual of laboratory and diagnostic tests* (4th ed.). Philadelphia: FA Davis.

Chen, P. (2004). Ectopic pregnancy. *Medline Plus.* [Online] Available at www.nlm.nih.gov/medlineplus/ency/article/000895.htm.

Chen, P. (2004). Placenta abruptio. *Medline Plus.* [Online] Available at www.nlm.nih.gov/medlineplus/ency/article/000901.htm.

Christopher, K. L. (2003). Hyperemesis gravidarum. *Journal of Obstetric, Gynecologic, and Neonatal Nursing, 32,* 435–436.

Creasy, R., Resnik, R., & Iams, J. (Eds.), (2004). *Maternal fetal medicine* (5th ed.). Philadelphia: WB Saunders.

Cunningham, F. G., Gant, N. F., Leveno, K. J., Gilstrap, L. C., Hauth, J. C., & Wenstrom, K. D. (2005). *Williams' obstetrics* (22nd ed.). New York: McGraw-Hill.

Curran, C. A. (2003). Intrapartum emergencies. *Journal of Obstetric, Gynecologic, and Neonatal Nursing, 32,* 802–813.

Deering, S. H., & Satin, A. (2004). Abruptio placenta. *eMedicine.* [Online] Available at www.emedicine.com/med/topic6.htm.

Dillon, P. M. (2003). *Nursing health assessment: A critical thinking, case studies approach.* Philadelphia: FA Davis.

Edelman, A. & Logan, J. R. (2004). Pregnancy, hyperemesis gravidarum. *eMedicine.* [Online] Available at www.emedicine.com/emerg/topic479.htm.

Freda, M. C., & Patterson, E. T. (2004). Preterm labor: Prevention and nursing management. In *March of Dimes nursing module.* White Plains, NY: March of Dimes Education and Health Promotion.

Fugate, S. R., & Chow, G. E. (2004). Eclampsia. *eMedicine.* [Online] Available at www.emedicine.com/med/topic633.htm.

Garcia, R. (2003). Hyperemesis gravidarum: More than morning sickness. *Nursing Spectrum.* [Online] Available at http://nsweb.nursingspectrum.com/ce/ce273.htm.

Gaudier, F. L. (2003). Placenta previa. *Medline Plus.* [Online] Available at www.nlm.nih.gov/medlineplus/ency/article/000900.htm.

Gaufberg, S. V. (2004). Abruptio placenta. *eMedicine.* [Online] Available at www.emedicine.com/emerg/topic12.htm.

Gerulath, A. H. (2002). Gestational trophoblastic disease. *Journal of Obstetric & Gynecology of Canada, 24,* 434–439.

Gilbert, E., & Harmon, J. (2003). *Manual of high-risk pregnancy and delivery* (3rd ed.). Saint Louis: Mosby.

Goldenberg, R. L. (2002). The management of preterm labor. *Obstetrics and Gynecology, 100,* 1020–1037.

Green, C. J., & Wilkinson, J. M. (2004). *Maternal newborn nursing care plans.* St. Louis: Mosby.

Gupton, A., Heaman, M., & Cheung, L. W. (2001). Complicated and uncomplicated pregnancies: Women's perception of risk. *Journal of Obstetric, Gynecologic, and Neonatal Nursing, 30,* 192–201.

Hail, E. (2004). Infantile reflexes. *Medline Plus.* [Online] Available at: http://www.nim.nih.gov/medlineplus/ency/article/003292.htm.

Harvey, E. A. (2004). Hypertensive disorders of pregnancy: Pathophysiology, symptoms and treatment. *Nursing Spectrum.* [Online] Available at http://nsweb.nursingspectrum.com/ce/m23c-1.htm.

Hermida, R. C., & Ayala, D. E. (2003). Sampling requirements for ambulatory blood pressure monitoring in the diagnosis of hypertension in pregnancy. *Hypertension, 42,* 619–626.

Iams, J. D. (2003). Prediction and early detection of preterm labor. *Obstetrics and Gynecology, 101,* 402–412.

Iams, J. D. & Creasy, R. K. (2004). Preterm labor and delivery. In R. K. Creasy, R. Resnik & J. D. Iams (Eds.), *Maternal-fetal medicine:*

Principles and practice (5th ed., pp. 623–661). Philadelphia: Saunders.

Johnson, K. D. (2003). Preeclampsia and eclampsia. *Medical Library Home.* [Online] Available at www.medical-library.org/journals/secure/01110/preeclampsiaeclampsia.htm.

Joy, S., & Lyon, D. (2004). Placenta previa. *eMedicine.* [Online] Available at www.emedicine.com/med/topics3271.htm.

Kidner, M. C., & Flanders–Stepans, B. (2004). A model for the HELLP syndrome: The maternal experience. *Journal of Obstetric, Gynecologic, and Neonatal Nursing, 33,* 44–53.

Ko, P., & Yoon, Y. (2005). Placenta previa. *eMedicine.* [Online] Available at www.emedicine.com/emerg/topic427.htm.

Koren, G., & Maltepe, C. (2004). Preemptive therapy for severe nausea and vomiting of pregnancy and hyperemesis gravidarum. *Journal of Obstetrics and Gynecology, 24,* 530–533.

Lee, R. V. (2003). What maternal mortality statistics tell us: High-risk pregnancy, a consequence of medical progress. *Journal of Obstetrics and Gynecology, 23,* 532–534.

London, M. L., Ladewug, P. W., Ball, J. W., & Bindler, R. C. (2003). *Maternal–newborn & child nursing.* Upper Saddle River, NJ: Prentice Hall.

Longo, S. A., Dola, C. P., & Pridjian, G. (2003). Preeclampsia and eclampsia revisited. *Southern Medical Journal, 96,* 891–899.

Lowdermilk, D. L., & Perry, S. E. (2004). *Maternity and women's health care* (8th ed.). St. Louis: Mosby.

March of Dimes (MOD). (2005). Preterm birth. [Online] Available at: http://www.marchofdimes.com/prematurity/5196_5799.asp.

March of Dimes Birth Defects Foundation. (2003). Taking action against prematurity. *Contemporary Obstetrics and Gynecology, 48,* 92–104.

Marchiano, D. (2004). Ectopic pregnancy. *Medline Plus.* [Online] Available at www.nlm.nih.gov/medlineplus/ency/article/000895.htm.

Martin, J. A., Hamilton, B. E., Ventura, S. J., Menacker, F., Park, M. M., & Sutton, P. (2002). Births: Final data for 2001. *National Vital Statistics Report, 50,* 1–104.

Mattson, S., & Smith, J. E. (2004). *Core curriculum for maternal–newborn nursing* (3rd ed.). St. Louis: Elsevier Saunders.

Michelini, G. A. (2004). Hyperemesis gravidarum. *eMedicine.* [Online] Available at www.emedicine.com/med/topic1075.htm.

Moore, M. L. (2003). Preterm labor and birth: What have we learned in the past two decades? *JOGNN, 32*(5), 638–649.

Moos, M. (2004). Understanding prematurity: Sorting fact from fiction. *AWHONN Lifelines, 8*(1), 32–37.

Morgan, E. (2002). Action stat: Eclampsia. *Nursing 2002, 32,* 104.

Morley, A. (2004). Pre-eclampsia: Pathophysiology and its management. *British Journal of Midwifery, 12*(1), 30–37.

Morrison, J. C., Roberts, W. E., Jones, J. S., Istwan, N., Rhea, D., & Stanziano, G. (2004). Frequency of nursing, physician and hospital interventions in women at risk for preterm delivery. *Journal of Maternal–Fetal and Neonatal Medicine, 16,* 102–105.

Murray, S. S. & McKinney, E. S. (2006). *Foundations of maternal–newborn nursing* (4th ed.). Philadelphia: WB Saunders.

National High Blood Pressure Education Program. (2000). Working Group in High Blood Pressure in Pregnancy report. *American Journal of Obstetrics and Gynecology, 183,* S1–S22.

Neal, J. L. (2001). RhD isoimmunization and current management modalities. *Journal of Obstetric, Gynecologic, and Neonatal Nursing, 30,* 589–606.

Newton, E. R. (2004). Preterm labor. *eMedicine.* [Online] Available at: http://www.emedicine.com/med/topic3245.htm.

Nick, J. M. (2003). Deep tendon reflexes: The what, why, where, and how of tapping. *Journal of Obstetric, Gynecologic, and Neonatal Nursing, 32,* 297–306.

O'Toole, M. T. (2005). *Miller–Keane encyclopedia and dictionary of medicine, nursing and allied health* (7th ed.). Philadelphia: Saunders.

Owen, P. (2003). Management options in ectopic pregnancy. *Clinical Pulse,* June, 68–71.

Peters, R. M., & Flack, J. M. (2004). Hypertensive disorders of pregnancy. *Journal of Obstetric, Gynecologic, and Neonatal Nursing, 33,* 209–220.

Puscheck, E., & and Pradhan, A. (2004). *Complete abortion.* [Online] Available at www.emedicine.com/med/topic3310.htm.

Ressel, G. W. (2004). Practice guidelines: ACOG releases bulletin on managing cervical insufficiency. *American Family Physician.* [Online] Available at www.aafp.org/afp/20040115/practice.html.

Rideout, S. L. (2005). Tocolytics for preterm labor: What nurses need to know. *AWHONN Lifelines, 9*(1), 56–61.

Salem, L. (2005). Rh incompatibility. *eMedicine.* [Online] Available at www.emedicine.com/emerg/topic507.htm.

Schmaier, A. H. (2003). Disseminated intravascular coagulation. *eMedicine.* [Online] Available at www.emedicine.com/med/topic577.htm.

Schnell, Z. B., Van Leeuwen, A. M., & Kranpitz, T. R. (2003). *Davis's comprehensive handbook of laboratory and diagnostic tests with nursing implications.* Philadelphia: FA Davis.

Seidel, H. M., Ball, J. W., Dains, J. E., & Benedict, G. W. (2003). *Mosby's guide to physical examination* (5th ed.). St. Louis: Mosby.

Sepilian, V., & Wood, E. (2005). Ectopic pregnancy. *eMedicine.* [Online] Available at www.emedicine.com/med/topic3212.htm.

Shennan, A. H. (2003). Recent developments in obstetrics. *British Medical Journal, 327,* 604–609.

Sibai, B. M. (2003). Diagnosis and management of gestational hypertension and preeclampsia. *Obstetrics and Gynecology, 102,* 181–192.

Simpson, J. (2002). Fetal wastage. In S. Gabbe, J. Niebyl, & J. Simpson (Eds.), *Obstetrics: Normal and problem pregnancies* (4th ed.). New York: Churchill Livingstone.

Skidmore–Roth, L. (2005). *Mosby's 2005 nursing drug reference.* St. Louis: Mosby.

Slattery, M. M. & Morrison, J. J. (2002). Review: Preterm delivery. *Lancet, 360*(9344), 1489–1497.

Spratto, G. R., & Woods, A. L. (2005). *PDR nurse's drug handbook.* Clifton Park, NY: Delmar Learning.

Steele, N. M., French, J., Gatherer–Boyles, J., Newman, S., Leclaire, S. (2001). Effect of acupressure by sea-bands on nausea and vomiting of pregnancy. *Journal of Obstetric, Gynecologic, and Neonatal Nursing, 30,* 61–70.

Swearingen, P. L. (2004). *All-in-one care planning resource.* St. Louis: Mosby.

Thompson, S. R. (2005). Placenta previa. *Medline Plus.* [Online] Available at: http://www.nlm.nih.gov/medlineplus/ency/article/000900.htm.

US Department of Health and Human Services. (2000). *Healthy people 2010* (conference edition, in two volumes). Washington, DC: Author.

Valley, V. T., & Fly, C. A. (2005). Ectopic pregnancy. *eMedicine.* [Online] Available at www.emedicine.com/EMERG/topic478.htm.

Verklan, M. T., & Walden, M. (2004). *Core curriculum for neonatal intensive care nursing* (3rd ed.). St. Louis: Elsevier Saunders.

Weiss, M. E., Saks, N. P. & Harris, S. (2002). Resolving the uncertainty of preterm symptoms: Women's experiences with the onset of preterm labor. *JOGNN, 31,* 66–76.

Wilkes, P. T., & Galan, H. (2004). Premature rupture of membranes. *eMedicine.* [Online] Available at: http://www.emedicine.com/med/topic3246.htm.

Yankowitz, J. (2004). Pharmacologic treatment of hypertensive disorders during pregnancy. *Journal of Perinatal and Neonatal Nursing, 18,* 230–240.

Youngkin, E. Q., & Davis, M. S. (2004). *Women's health: A primary care clinical guide* (3rd ed.). Upper Saddle River, NJ: Pearson Prentice Hall.

Zach, T., & Pramanik, A. (2005). Multiple births. *eMedicine.* [Online] Available at www.emedicine.com/ped/topic2599.htm.

Web Resources

American Academy of Pediatrics, **www.aap.org**
American College of Obstetricians and Gynecologists, **www.acog.org**
Association of Women's Health, Obstetric & Neonatal Nurses, **www.awhonn.org**
March of Dimes, **www.modimes.org**
Resolve through Sharing, **www.ectopicpregnancy.com**
Sidelines High-Risk Pregnancy Support Office, **www.sidelines.org**

ChapterWORKSHEET

● MULTIPLE CHOICE QUESTIONS

1. The nurse understands that the purpose of administering magnesium sulfate to a client with preeclampsia is to

   a. Reduce central nervous system irritability to prevent seizures

   b. Provide supplementation of an important mineral she needs

   c. Prevent constipation during and after the birthing process

   d. Decrease musculoskeletal tone to augment labor

2. Which of the following women would the nurse identify as being at the greatest risk for preterm labor?

   a. A woman who had twins in a previous pregnancy

   b. A woman who lives in a big metropolitan city

   c. A woman who works full-time as a computer programmer

   d. A woman who has a history of preterm birth

3. The signs and symptoms of abruptio placenta depend on the amount of placental separation and type of abruption. Which of the following would the nurse assess as a classic symptom?

   a. Painless, bright-red bleeding

   b. "Knife-like" abdominal pain

   c. Excessive nausea and vomiting

   d. Hypertension and headache

4. Which of the following medications would the nurse expect the physician to order for tocolysis?

   a. Diazepam (Valium)

   b. Phenobarbital

   c. Nifedipine (Procardia)

   d. Butorphanol (Stadol)

5. RhoGAM is given to Rh-negative women to prevent maternal sensitization from occurring. The nurse is aware that in addition to pregnancy, Rh-negative women would also receive this medication after which of the following?

   a. Therapeutic or spontaneous abortion

   b. Head injury from a car accident

   c. Blood transfusion after a hemorrhage

   d. Unsuccessful artificial insemination procedure

● CRITICAL THINKING EXERCISES

1. Suzanne, a 16-year-old primigravida, presents to the maternity clinic complaining of continual nausea and vomiting for the past 3 days. She states she is approximately 15 weeks pregnant and she has been unable to hold anything down or take any fluids in without throwing up for the past 3 days. She reports she is dizzy and weak. On examination, Suzanne appears pale, anxious, mucus membranes are dry, skin turgor is poor, and her lips are dry and cracked.

   a. What is your impression of this condition?

   b. What risk factors does Suzanne have?

   c. What intervention is appropriate for this woman?

2. Betty, a 20-year-old African-American primigravida client, comes to the prenatal clinic for her first visit. She is 4 months pregnant based on dates. As the nurse assigned to her, you interview her and start to record her history as follows:

   • Is single, unmarried, lives with father of child

   • Smokes 1.5 packs of cigarettes a day

   • Works as a laborer in a nursery 12 hours daily

   • Quit high school in the ninth grade and has no plans to get GED

   • Eats poorly, is underweight for height, and is anemic

   • Reports she has frequent UTIs

   a. Based on her history, what might this client be at risk for? Why?

   b. What client education is needed at this visit?

   c. What specific nursing interventions might help reduce her risk?

● STUDY ACTIVITIES

1. Identify a woman hospitalized on bed rest with preterm labor. Ask her about her experience associated with the hospitalization and how nurses could be helpful to her throughout her experience.

2. Ask a public health maternity nurse how the signs and symptoms of preterm labor are taught, and how effective they have been in reducing the incidence in their area.

3. Search the Internet for a Web site to help parents who have suffered a pregnancy loss and critique it for current information and audience level.

4. A pregnancy in which the blastocyst implants outside the uterus describes an _____ pregnancy.

5. The gravest complication of hydatidiform mole is the development of _____ afterward.

6. Discuss various activities a woman with a multiple gestation could engage in to help pass the time when ordered to be on bed rest at home for 2 months.

7. The type of medication used to stop preterm labor is called _____.

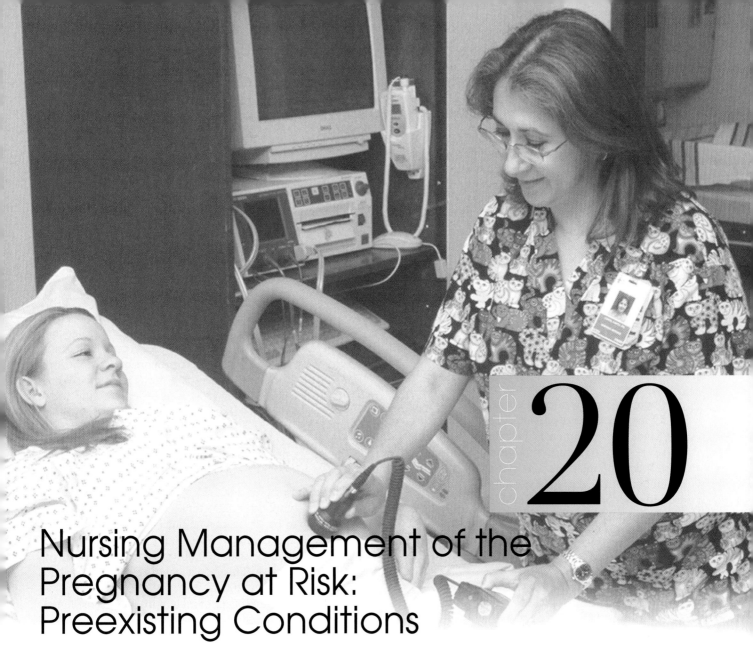

chapter 20

Nursing Management of the Pregnancy at Risk: Preexisting Conditions

KeyTERMS

acquired immunodeficiency
  syndrome (AIDS)
adolescence
anemia
fetal alcohol spectrum
  disorder
gestational diabetes mellitus
glycosylated hemoglobin
  (HbA1C) level
human immunodeficiency
  virus (HIV)
impaired fasting glucose
impaired glucose tolerance
neonatal abstinence
  syndrome
perinatal drug abuse
pica
teratogen
Type 1 diabetes
Type 2 diabetes

LearningOBJECTIVES

After studying the chapter content, the student should be able to:

1. Define the key terms.
2. Identify at least two preexisting conditions that can affect a pregnancy.
3. Analyze the physiologic and psychological impact of a preexisting condition on a pregnancy.
4. Describe the nursing management for a pregnant woman with diabetes.
5. Explain the effects, treatment, and nursing management of heart disease and respiratory conditions during pregnancy.
6. Outline appropriate assessment and interventions for the client experiencing violence during her pregnancy.
7. Differentiate among the types of anemia in terms of prevention and management.
8. Identify the infections that can jeopardize a pregnancy.
9. Describe the nurse's role in the prevention and management of adolescent pregnancy.
10. Discuss the importance of continued prenatal care for high-risk women.
11. Identify the effects, treatment, and nursing management of HIV/AIDS and substance abuse during pregnancy.
12. Delineate the role of the nurse in assessing, managing care, and referring high-risk clients to appropriate community services and resources.

Pregnancy and childbirth are exciting yet complex facets within the continuum of women's health. Ideally the pregnant woman is free of any pre-existing conditions, but in reality many women enter pregnancy with a multitude of medical or psychosocial issues that can have a negative impact on the outcome.

Most pregnant women express the wish, "I hope my baby is born healthy." Nurses can be instrumental in helping this to become a reality by educating women before they become pregnant. In addition, medical conditions such as diabetes, cardiac and respiratory disorders, anemias, and specific infections can frequently be controlled so that their impact on pregnancy is minimized through close prenatal management. Pregnancy-prevention strategies are helpful when counseling teenagers. Meeting the developmental needs of pregnant adolescents is challenging for many healthcare providers. Finally, lifestyle choices can place many women at risk during pregnancy and nurses need to remain nonjudgmental in working with these special populations. Lifestyle choices such as use of alcohol, nicotine, and illicit substances during pregnancy are addressed in a National Health goal.

Chapter 19 described pregnancy-related conditions that place the woman at risk. This chapter addresses the most common conditions that are present before pregnancy that can have a negative effect on the pregnancy and outlines appropriate nursing assessments and interventions for each. The unique skills of nurses, in conjunction with the other members of the healthcare team, can increase the potential for a positive outcome in many high-risk pregnancies.

Diabetes Mellitus

Diabetes mellitus is a chronic disease characterized by a relative lack of insulin or absence of the hormone, which is necessary for glucose metabolism. The prevalence of diabetes in the United States is increasing at an alarming rate, already reaching epidemic proportions. A contributing factor to these increasing rates is the incidence of obesity. It is a common endocrine disorder affecting 1% to 14% of all pregnancies (American Diabetes Association [ADA], 2004).

Diabetes in pregnancy is categorized into two groups: preexisting diabetes, which includes women with type 1 or type 2 disease, and gestational diabetes, which develops in women during pregnancy (Kendrick, 2004). Pregestational diabetes complicates 0.2% to 0.3% of all pregnancies and affects up to 14,000 women annually. Gestational diabetes occurs in approximately 7% of all pregnant women and complicates more than 200,000 pregnancies annually in the United States. This type accounts for 90% of diabetic pregnancies (ADA, 2004).

Before the discovery of insulin in 1922, most female diabetics were infertile or experienced spontaneous abortion (Kendrick, 2004). Over the past several decades, great strides have been made in improving the outcomes of pregnant women with diabetes, but this chronic metabolic disorder remains a high-risk condition during pregnancy. A favorable outcome requires commitment on the woman's part to comply with frequent prenatal visits, dietary restrictions, self-monitoring of blood glucose levels, frequent laboratory tests, intensive fetal surveillance, and perhaps hospitalization.

Classification of Diabetes

Some form of diabetes mellitus complicates up to 14% of all pregnancies. The classification system commonly used is based on disease etiology (Expert Committee, 2003). It includes four groups (Box 20-1). The vast majority of women (88%) have gestational diabetes; the remainder have pregestational diabetes (Samson & Ferguson, 2004).

Attempting to classify women as having pregestational or gestational diabetes is problematic because many women are not aware they have a problem before their pregnancy. Many women with type 2 diabetes have gone

BOX 20-1
CLASSIFICATION OF DIABETES MELLITUS

- **Type 1 diabetes**—absolute insulin deficiency (due to an autoimmune process); usually appears before the age of 30 years; approximately 10% of those diagnosed have type 1 diabetes (Wallerstedt & Clokey, 2004)
- **Type 2 diabetes**—insulin resistance or deficiency (related to obesity, sedentary lifestyle); diagnosed primarily in adults older than 30 years of age, but is now being seen in children; accounts for 90% of all diagnosed cases.
- **Impaired fasting glucose and impaired glucose tolerance**—characterized by hyperglycemia at a level lower than what qualifies as a diagnosis of diabetes; symptoms of diabetes are absent; newborns are at risk for being large for gestational age (LGA) (Wallerstedt & Clokey, 2004).
- **Gestational diabetes mellitus**—glucose intolerance due to pregnancy

Thoughts: This woman is typical of a gestational diabetic in that she was older and found it difficult to change her old dietary habits. Perhaps her blood glucose levels had been out of control throughout the pregnancy, or maybe just recently. It is difficult to pinpoint the how and whys of such a tragedy, but it remains a reality even today. What went wrong? How can you help this family to cope with this loss?

Effects of Diabetes on Pregnancy

Pregnancy produces profound metabolic alterations that are necessary to support the growth and development of the fetus. Maternal metabolism is directed toward supplying adequate nutrition for the fetus. In pregnancy, placental hormones cause insulin resistance at a level that tends to parallel the growth of the fetoplacental unit. As the placenta grows, more placental hormones are secreted. Human placental lactogen (hPL) and growth hormone (somatotropin) increase in direct correlation with the growth of placental tissue, rising throughout the last 20 weeks of pregnancy and causing insulin resistance. Subsequently, insulin secretion increases to overcome the resistance of these two hormones. In the nondiabetic pregnant woman, the pancreas can respond to the demands for increased insulin production to maintain normal glucose levels throughout the pregnancy (Ryan, 2003). However, the woman with glucose intolerance or diabetes during pregnancy cannot cope with changes in metabolism resulting from insufficient insulin to meet the needs during gestation.

Over the course of pregnancy, insulin resistance changes. It peaks in the last trimester to provide more nutrients to the fetus. The insulin resistance typically results in postprandial hyperglycemia, although some women also have an elevated fasting blood glucose level (Turok et al., 2003). With this increased demand on the pancreas in late pregnancy, women with diabetes or glucose intolerance cannot accommodate the increased insulin demand.

The pregnancy of a woman with diabetes carries risk factors such as perinatal mortality and congenital anomalies. Tight metabolic control reduces this risk, but still many problems remain for her and her fetus. Major effects of hyperglycemia on a pregnancy include:

- Hydramnios due to fetal diuresis caused by hyperglycemia
- Gestational hypertension due to an unknown etiology
- Ketoacidosis due to uncontrolled hyperglycemia
- Preterm labor secondary to premature membrane rupture
- Cord prolapse secondary to hydramnios and abnormal fetal presentation
- Stillbirth in pregnancies complicated by ketoacidosis and poor glucose control

undiagnosed; only when they are screened at a prenatal visit is the diabetes discovered. Although the classifications seem clear-cut, many women have glucose intolerance long before they become pregnant, but it has not been diagnosed. Preconceptual counseling might help to identify women who have not been diagnosed so that measures can be taken to achieve glucose control, thereby helping to prevent congenital anomalies during the embryonic stage of development.

Consider THIS!

Scott and I had been busy all day setting up the new crib and nursery, and we finally sat down to rest. I was due any day, and we had been putting this off until we had a long weekend to complete the task. I was excited to think about all the frilly pinks that decorated her room. I was sure that my new daughter would love it as much as I loved her already. A few days later I barely noticed any fetal movement, but I thought that she must be as tired as I was by this point.

That night I went into labor and kept looking at the worried faces of the nurses and the midwife in attendance. I had been diagnosed with gestational diabetes a few months ago and had tried to follow the instructions regarding diet and exercise, but old habits are hard to change when you are 38 years old. I was finally told after a short time in the labor unit that they couldn't pick up a fetal heartbeat and an ultrasound was to be done—still no heartbeat was detected. Scott and I were finally told that our daughter was a stillborn. All I could think about was that she would never get to see all the pink colors in the nursery. . . . .

- Hypoglycemia as glucose is diverted to the fetus (occurring in first trimester)
- Urinary tract infections resulting from excess glucose in the urine (glucosuria), which promotes bacterial growth
- Chronic monilial vaginitis due to glucosuria, which promotes growth of yeast
- Difficult labor, cesarean birth, postpartum hemorrhage secondary to an overdistended uterus to accommodate a macrosomic infant

In addition, fetal-neonatal risks include:

- Congenital anomaly due to hyperglycemia in the first trimester (cardiac problems, neural tube defects, skeletal deformities, and genitourinary problems)
- Macrosomia resulting from hyperinsulinemia stimulated by fetal hyperglycemia
- Birth trauma due to increased size of fetus, which complicates the birthing process (shoulder dystocia)
- Preterm birth secondary to hydramnios and an aging placenta, which places the fetus in jeopardy if the pregnancy continues
- Perinatal death due to poor placental perfusion and hypoxia
- Fetal asphyxia secondary to fetal hyperglycemia and hyperinsulinemia
- Respiratory distress syndrome (RDS) resulting from poor surfactant production secondary to hyperinsulinemia inhibiting the production of phospholipids, which make up surfactant
- Polycythemia due to excessive red blood cell (RBC) production in response to hypoxia
- Intrauterine growth restriction (IUGR) secondary to maternal vascular impairment and decreased placental perfusion, which restricts growth
- Hyperbilirubinemia due to excessive RBC breakdown from hypoxia and an immature liver unable to break down bilirubin
- Neonatal hypoglycemia resulting from ongoing hyperinsulinemia after the placenta is removed
- Subsequent childhood obesity and carbohydrate intolerance (Messner, 2004)

Pregestational Diabetes

Pregestational diabetes exists when an alteration in carbohydrate metabolism is identified before conception. The client's diabetes may be long standing or of short duration. As with most chronic disorders, a stable disease state before conception will produce the best pregnancy outcome. Excellent control of blood glucose, as evidenced by normal fasting blood glucose levels and a **glycosylated hemoglobin (HbA1C) level** (an average measurement of the glucose levels over the past 100 to 120 days), is a key factor to address in preconception counseling. A glycosylated hemoglobin level of 7% to 10% indicates good control; a value of more than 15%

indicates that the diabetes is out of control and warrants notification of the healthcare provider (Samson & Ferguson, 2004).

Infants born to diabetic mothers are at risk for congenital malformations. The most common ones associated with diabetes occur in the renal, cardiac, skeletal, and central nervous systems. Since these defects occur by the eighth week of gestation, the need for preconception counseling is critical. The rate of congenital anomalies in women with pregestational diabetes can be reduced if excellent glycemic control is achieved at the time of conception (Feig & Palda, 2003). This information needs to be stressed with all diabetic women contemplating a pregnancy (Nursing Care Plan 20-1).

Treatment

In addition to preconception counseling, the woman needs to be evaluated for complications of diabetes. This evaluation should be part of baseline screening and continuing assessment during pregnancy. These women need comprehensive prenatal care. The primary goals of care are to maintain glycemic control and minimize the risks of the disease on the fetus. Key aspects of treatment include dietary management, insulin regimens, and close maternal and fetal surveillance.

Dietary Management

Dietary management may be sufficient to control the woman's glucose levels and ideally is handled by a nutritionist. Nutritional recommendations include:

- Adhere to the same nutrient requirements and recommendations for weight gain as the nondiabetic woman.
- Avoid weight loss and dieting during pregnancy.
- Ensure food intake is adequate to prevent ketone formation and promote weight gain.
- Eat three meals a day plus three snacks to promote glycemic control.
- Include complex carbohydrates, fiber, and limited fat and sugar in the diet.
- Continue dietary consultation throughout pregnancy (Dudek, 2006).

Insulin Regimens

At present, insulin remains the medication of choice for glycemic control in pregnant and lactating women with any type of diabetes (Turok et al., 2003). Insulin is required when diet alone is ineffective in maintaining normal glucose control. Oral hypoglycemic agents are not usually prescribed to control blood glucose levels because of their potential teratogenic effect. However, they may be an option in the future after additional research has been completed. Glyburide is one alternative to insulin that does not cross the placenta. Diabetes can be controlled in many women with this agent, and it has a low risk of producing maternal hypoglycemia (Barbour, 2003).

Nursing Care Plan 20-1

Overview of the Pregnant Woman with Type 1 Diabetes

Donna, a 30-year-old type 1 diabetic, presents to the maternity clinic for preconception care. She has been a diabetic for 8 years and takes insulin twice daily by injection. She does blood glucose self-monitoring four times daily. She reports that her disease is fairly well controlled but worries about how her diabetes will affect a pregnancy. She is concerned about what changes she will have to make in her regimen and what the pregnancy outcome will be. She reports that she recently had a foot infection and needed to go to the emergency room because it led to an episode of ketoacidosis. She states that her last glycosylated hemoglobin A1c test results were abnormal.

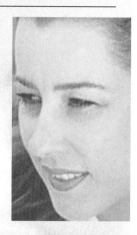

Nursing Diagnosis: Deficient knowledge related to type 1 diabetes, blood glucose control, and effects of condition on pregnancy

Outcome identification and *evaluation*	Interventions with *rationales*
Client will demonstrate increased knowledge of type 1 diabetes and effects on pregnancy *as evidenced by proper techniques for blood glucose monitoring and insulin administration, ability to modify insulin doses and dietary intake to achieve control, and verbalization of need for glycemic control prior to pregnancy, with blood glucose levels remaining within normal range.*	Assess client's knowledge of diabetes and pregnancy. Review the underlying problems associated with diabetes and how pregnancy affects glucose control *to provide client with a firm knowledge base for decision making.* Review signs and symptoms of hypoglycemia and hyperglycemia and prevention and management measures *to ensure client can deal with them should they occur.* Provide written materials describing diabetes and care needed for control *to provide opportunity for client's review and promote retention of learning.* Observe client administering insulin and self-glucose testing for technique and offer suggestions for improvement if needed *to ensure adequate self-care ability.* Discuss proper foot care *to prevent future infections.* Teach home treatment for symptomatic hypoglycemia *to minimize risk to client and fetus.* Outline acute and chronic diabetic complications *to reinforce the importance of glucose control.* Discuss use of contraceptives until blood glucose levels can be optimized before conception occurs *to promote best possible health status before conception.* Discuss the rationale for good glucose control and the importance of achieving excellent glycemic control before pregnancy *to promote a positive pregnancy outcome.* Review self-care practices—blood glucose monitoring and frequency of testing; insulin administration; adjustment of insulin dosages based on blood glucose levels—*to foster independence in self-care and feelings of control over the situation.*

(continued)

Overview of the Pregnant Woman with Type 1 Diabetes (continued)

Outcome identification and *evaluation*	Interventions with *rationales*
	Refer client for dietary counseling *to ensure optimal diet for glycemic control.*
	Outline obstetric management and fetal surveillance needed for pregnancy *to provide client with information on what to expect.*
	Discuss strategies for maintaining optimal glycemic control during pregnancy *to minimize risks to client and fetus.*

Nursing Diagnosis: Anxiety related to future pregnancy and its outcome secondary to underlying diabetes

Client will express her feelings related to her diabetes and pregnancy *as evidenced by statements of feeling better about her pre-existing condition and pregnancy outlook, and statements of understanding related to future childbearing by linking good glucose control with positive outcomes for both herself and offspring.*	Review the need for a physical examination *to evaluate for any effects of diabetes on the client's health status.*
	Explain the rationale for assessing client's blood pressure, vision, and peripheral pulses at each visit *to provide information related to possible effects of diabetes on health status.*
	Identify any alterations in present diabetic condition that need intervention *to aid in minimizing risks that may potentiate client's anxiety level.*
	Review potential effects of diabetes on pregnancy *to promote client understanding of risks and ways to control or minimize them.*
	Encourage active participation in decision making and planning pregnancy *to promote feelings of control over the situation and foster self-confidence.*
	Provide positive reinforcement for healthy behaviors and actions *to foster continued use and enhancement of self-esteem.*
	Discuss feelings about future childbearing and managing pregnancy *to help reduce anxiety related to uncertainties.*
	Encourage client to ask questions or voice concerns *to help decrease anxiety related to the unknown.*

Glyburide is not yet approved by the U.S. Food and Drug Administration (FDA) for the treatment of gestational diabetes. Studies of the use of these agents during pregnancy are in their infancy, but they may hold great promise for reducing the long-term metabolic effects on women and their offspring (Kendrick, 2004).

Insulin requirements may drop slightly in the first trimester before increasing significantly during the latter half of the pregnancy. Changes in diet and activity level add to the changes in insulin dosages throughout pregnancy.

Insulin regimens vary, and controversy remains over the best strategy for insulin delivery in pregnancy. Many healthcare providers use a split-dose therapy with morning and evening doses. Others advocate the use of an insulin pump to deliver a continuous subcutaneous insulin infusion. Regardless of which protocol is used, frequent blood glucose measurements are necessary, and the insulin dosage is adjusted on the basis of daily glucose levels.

Maternal and Fetal Surveillance

Frequent laboratory studies are done during pregnancy to monitor the woman's diabetic status. These studies might include:

- Fingerstick blood glucose levels at every prenatal visit to evaluate the accuracy of the self-monitoring documentation brought in by the woman
- Urine check for protein (may indicate the need for further evaluation for preeclampsia) and for nitrates and leukocyte esterase (may indicate a urinary tract infection)
- Urine check for ketones (may indicate the need for evaluation of eating habits)
- Kidney function evaluation every trimester for creatinine clearance and protein levels
- Eye examination in the first trimester to evaluate the retina for vascular changes
- HbA1c every 4 to 6 weeks to monitor glucose trends (Gilbert & Harmon, 2003)

Fetal surveillance is essential during the pregnancy to evaluate the fetal well-being and assist in determining the best time for birth. The evaluation may include:

- Ultrasound to provide information about fetal growth, activity, and amniotic fluid volume and to validate gestational age
- Alpha-fetoprotein levels to detect an open neural tube or ventral wall defects of omphalocele or gastroschisis
- Fetal echocardiogram to rule out cardiac anomalies
- Daily fetal movements to monitor fetal well-being
- Biophysical profile to monitor fetal well-being and uteroplacental profusion
- Nonstress tests weekly after 28 weeks to determine fetal well-being
- Amniocentesis to determine the lecithin/sphingomyelin (L/S) ratio and the presence of phosphatidyl glycerol (PG) to evaluate whether the fetal lung is mature enough for birth (Gilbert & Harmon, 2003)

Gestational Diabetes

One of the biggest challenges nurses and other healthcare providers face is the growing number of women developing gestational diabetes as the obesity epidemic escalates. The increasing development of gestational diabetes in the mother and glucose intolerance in the offspring set the stage for a perpetuating cycle that must be addressed with effective primary prevention strategies and more effective antepartum interventions (Barbour, 2003).

Gestational diabetes mellitus is defined as glucose intolerance with its onset during pregnancy (or first detected during pregnancy). Major risk factors for developing gestation diabetes include maternal age older than 30 years, being obese or overweight, a family history of diabetes, a history of diabetes in a prior pregnancy, a history of poor obstetric outcome (such as a large-for-gestational age [LGA] infant or stillbirth), and African-American, Hispanic, or Native American ethnicity (U.S. Preventive Services Task Force, 2003).

Women with gestational diabetes mellitus are at increased risk for preeclampsia and glucose control-related complications such as hypoglycemia, hyperglycemia, and ketoacidosis. Gestational diabetes of any severity increases the risk of fetal macrosomia. It is also associated with an increased frequency of maternal hypertensive disorders and the need for an operative birth. This may be the result of fetal growth disorders (ADA, 2004). Even though gestational diabetes is diagnosed during pregnancy, the woman may have had glucose intolerance before the pregnancy.

Screening

The American College of Obstetricians and Gynecologists (ACOG) currently recommends routine screening of all pregnant women at 24 to 28 weeks, or earlier if risk factors are present, although this is controversial. Published data indicate that universal screening is not cost-effective (Samson & Ferguson, 2004). The ADA recommends selective screening based on the woman's risk factors. High-risk women include those with a prior history of gestational diabetes, a strong family history of type 2 diabetes, marked obesity, multiple pregnancy, glycosuria, advanced maternal age, non-white ethnicity, history of polycystic ovary syndrome, hydramnios, recurrent vaginal or urinary infections, prior infant with macrosomia, or prior poor obstetric outcome. Women at high risk should be screened earlier than 24 weeks. If the initial screening is negative, rescreening should take place between 24 and 28 weeks. A woman with abnormal early results may have had diabetes before the pregnancy, and her fetus is a great risk for congenital anomalies. An elevated glycosylated hemoglobin supports the likelihood of gestational diabetes (Gabbe & Graves, 2003).

There is little consensus regarding the value of screening for gestational diabetes and the appropriate screening method. Typically, screening is based on a 50-g 1-hour glucose challenge test, usually performed between week 24 and 28 of gestation (U.S. Preventive Services Task Force, 2003). A 50-g oral glucose load is given, without regard to the timing or content of the last meal. Blood glucose is measured 1 hour later; a level above 140 mg/dL is abnormal. If the result is abnormal, a 3-hour glucose tolerance test is done. A diagnosis of gestational diabetes can be made only after an abnormal result on the glucose tolerance test. Normal values are:

- Fasting blood glucose level: less than 105 mg/dL
- At 1 hour: less than 190 mg/dL
- At 2 hours: less than 165 mg/dL
- At 3 hours: less than 145 mg/dL

Two or more abnormal values confirm a diagnosis of gestational diabetes (ADA, 2004).

Treatment

Women with gestational diabetes may be asymptomatic throughout the pregnancy or they may exhibit subtle signs. Early identification is important to facilitate prompt intervention. Controlling maternal hyperglycemia with diet alone or diet and insulin can reduce the risk of inappropriate accelerated fetal growth. Once the diagnosis of gestational diabetes is made, the management is similar to treatment for pregestational diabetes.

Nursing Management

The ultimate goal of nursing management when caring for the woman with pregestational or gestational diabetes is to minimize risks and complications. Education and patient cooperation are key in achieving this goal. The ideal outcome of every pregnancy is a healthy newborn and mother, and nurses can be pivotal in realizing this positive outcome.

Nursing management of the woman with pregestational diabetes or gestational diabetes is the same. Careful, frequent antepartum care visits are necessary. The nurse must take time to counsel and educate the women about the changes needed in diet, possible need for insulin or increased insulin dosages, and lifestyle changes. Since the diabetic client is at high risk, the prenatal visits will be more frequent (every 2 weeks up to 28 weeks and then twice a week until birth).

Assessment

Nursing assessment should begin at the first prenatal visit. For the woman with pregestational diabetes, obtain a thorough history of the woman's preexisting diabetic condition. Ask about her duration of disease, management of glucose levels (insulin injections, insulin pump, or oral hypoglycemic agents), dietary adjustments, presence of vascular complications and current vascular status, current insulin regimen, and technique used for glucose testing. The nurse should have a working knowledge of the nutritional requirements of diabetics and should be able to assess the adequacy and pattern of the woman's dietary intake. Assess the woman's blood glucose self-monitoring in terms of frequency and her ability to adjust the insulin dose based on the changing patterns. Ask about the frequency of episodes of hypoglycemia or hyperglycemia to ascertain the woman's ability to recognize and treat them.

During antepartum visits, assess the client's knowledge about her disease, including the signs and symptoms of hypoglycemia, hyperglycemia, and diabetic ketoacidosis, insulin administration techniques, and impact of pregnancy on her chronic condition. Although the client may have had diabetes for some time, do not assume that she has a firm knowledge base about her disease process or management of it (Fig. 20-1).

Risk assessment for gestational diabetes also is undertaken at the first prenatal visit. Women with clinical characteristics consistent with a high risk for gestational diabetes should undergo glucose testing as soon as feasible. These risk factors include:

- Previous infant with congenital anomaly (skeletal, renal, central nervous system [CNS], cardiac)

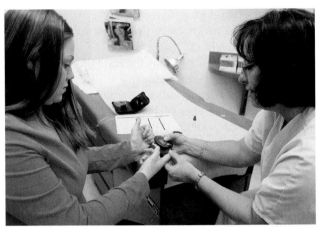

● Figure 20-1 The nurse is demonstrating the technique for self-blood glucose monitoring with a pregnant client.

- History of gestational diabetes or hydramnios in a previous pregnancy
- Family history of diabetes
- Age 35 or older
- Previous infant weighing more than 9 pounds (4,000 g)
- Previous unexplained fetal demise or neonatal death
- Maternal obesity (Body Mass Index [BMI] > 30)
- Hypertension
- Hispanic, Native American, or African-American ethnicity
- Recurrent *Monilia* infections that don't respond to treatment
- Signs and symptoms of glucose intolerance (polyuria, polyphagia, polydipsia, fatigue)
- Presence of glycosuria or proteinuria (Mattson & Smith, 2004)

Assessment of the woman's psychosocial adaptation to her condition is critical to gain her cooperation for a change in regimen or the addition of a new regimen throughout pregnancy. Identify her support systems and note any financial constraints, as she will need more intense monitoring and frequent fetal surveillance. Laboratory studies may include a glycosylated hemoglobin to determine the mean blood glucose levels for the previous few months, urine testing for glucose and protein, and cardiovascular assessment.

Nursing Interventions

Nursing interventions include counseling and education about the need for strict glucose monitoring, diet and exercise, and signs and symptoms of complications. Encourage the client and her family to make any lifestyle changes needed to maximize the pregnancy outcome. Providing dietary education and lifestyle advice that extends beyond pregnancy may have the potential to lessen the risk of gestational diabetes in subsequent pregnancies as well as type 2 diabetes in the mother (Dornhorst & Frost, 2002).

At each visit reinforce the importance of performing blood glucose screening and documenting the results. With proper instruction, the client and her family will be able to cope with all the changes in her body during pregnancy (Teaching Guidelines 20-1).

During the antepartum period, nursing interventions typically include:

- Monitoring weight, urine glucose, protein, and ketone levels
- Obtaining blood pressure measurements at each visit
- Teaching the mother how to assess fetal activity to evaluate fetal well-being
- Assisting with serial ultrasounds to monitor fetal growth and with assessments of fetal well-being through non-stress tests and biophysical profiles
- Anticipating complications and planning appropriate interventions or referrals
- Discussing dietary measures related to blood glucose control (Fig. 20-2); initiating referrals for nutritional counseling to individualize the dietary plan
- Encouraging the client to participate in an exercise program that includes at least three sessions lasting longer than 15 minutes per week (exercise may lessen the need for insulin or dosage adjustments)
- Assessing for signs and symptoms of preeclampsia and hydramnios
- Assisting with and teaching about insulin therapy, including any changes needed if glucose levels are not controlled
- Urging the woman to perform blood glucose screening (usually four times a day, before meals and at bedtime)
- Reviewing discussions about the timing of birth and the rationale
- Counseling the client about the possibility of cesarean birth for an LGA infant or informing the woman who will be giving birth vaginally of the possible need for augmentation with oxytocin (Pitocin)
- Establishing fetal lung maturity prior to birth
- Encouraging breastfeeding to normalize blood glucose levels
- Teaching the woman that her insulin needs after birth will drastically decrease
- Discussing future childbearing plans and contraception after birth
- Informing the client that she will need a repeat glucose challenge test at a postpartum visit (ADA, 2004)

Nursing Interventions During the Intrapartum Period

In the woman with well-controlled diabetes, birth is typically not induced before term unless there are complications, such as preeclampsia or fetal compromise. An early delivery date might be set for the woman with poorly controlled diabetes who is having complications. During labor, intravenous saline is given and blood

 TEACHING GUIDELINES 20-1

Teaching for the Pregnant Woman With Diabetes

- Be sure to keep your appointments for frequent prenatal visits and tests for fetal well-being.
- Perform blood glucose self-monitoring as directed, usually before each meal and at bedtime. Keep a record of your results and call your healthcare provider with any levels outside the established range. Bring your results to each prenatal visit.
- Perform daily "fetal kick counts." Document them and report any decrease in activity.
- Drink 8 to 10 8-ounce glasses of water each day to prevent bladder infections and maintain hydration.
- Wear proper, well-fitted footwear when walking to prevent injury.
- Engage in a regular exercise program such as walking to aid in glucose control, but avoid exercising in temperature extremes.
- Consider breastfeeding your infant to lower your blood glucose levels.
- If you are taking insulin:
  - Administer the correct dose of insulin at the correct time every day.
  - Eat breakfast within 30 minutes after injecting regular insulin to prevent a reaction.
  - Plan meals at a fixed time and snacks to prevent extremes in glucose levels.
- Avoid simple sugars (cake, candy, cookies), which raise blood glucose levels.
- Know the signs and symptoms of hypoglycemia and treatment needed:
  - Sweating, tremors, cold, clammy skin, headache
  - Feeling hungry, blurred vision, disorientation, irritability
  - Treatment: Drink 8 ounces of milk and eat two crackers or glucose tablets
- Carry "glucose boosters" (such as Life Savers) to prevent hypoglycemia.
- Know the signs and symptoms of hyperglycemia and treatment needed:
  - Dry mouth, frequent urination, excessive thirst, rapid breathing
  - Feeling tired, flushed, hot skin, headache, drowsiness
  - Treatment: Notify health care provider, since hospitalization may be needed
- Wear a diabetic identification bracelet at all times.
- Wash your hands frequently to prevent infections.
- Report any signs and symptoms of illness, infection, and dehydration to your health care provider, because these can affect blood glucose control.

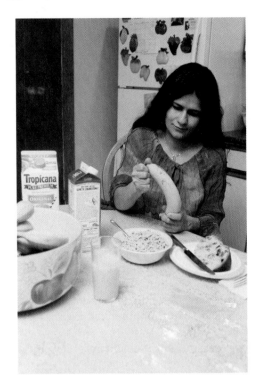

● Figure 20-2 The pregnant client eating a nutritious meal to ensure adequate glucose control.

glucose levels are monitored every 1 to 2 hours. Glucose levels should be kept below 110 mg/dL throughout labor. If necessary, an infusion of regular insulin may be given to sustain this level (Messner, 2004).

When caring for the laboring woman with diabetes, adjust the IV rate and the rate of supplemental regular insulin based on the blood glucose levels as ordered. Keep a syringe with 50% dextrose solution available at the bedside to treat profound hypoglycemia. Monitor fetal heart rate patterns throughout labor to detect reassuring or nonreassuring patterns. Assess maternal vital signs every hour, in addition to assessing the woman's urinary output with an indwelling catheter. If a cesarean birth is scheduled, monitor the woman's blood glucose levels hourly and administer short-acting insulin or glucose based on the blood glucose levels as ordered. After birth, monitor blood glucose levels every 2 to 4 hours and continue IV fluid administration as ordered.

Nursing Interventions During the Postpartum Period

Nursing care should focus on monitoring blood glucose levels during this period. Maternal control of glucose is essential in the first few weeks postpartum, and breast-feeding should be encouraged to assist in maintaining good control. For the pregestational diabetic, no insulin may be needed due to the sudden drop in human placental lactogen (hPL) after the delivery of the placenta.

For the woman with gestational diabetes, the focus is on lifestyle education. Women with gestational diabetes have a greater than 50% increased risk of developing type 2 diabetes (ADA, 2004). Screening should be done at the postpartum follow-up appointment in 6 weeks. Women with normal results at that visit should be screened every 3 years thereafter (ADA, 2004). The woman should maintain an optimal weight to reduce her risk of developing diabetes. A referral to a dietitian can be helpful in outlining a balanced nutritious diet for the woman to achieve this goal.

Cardiovascular Disorders

Every minute, an American woman dies of cardiovascular disease (Wenger, 2004). Cardiovascular disease is the leading cause of death for men and women in the United States. It kills nearly 500,000 women each year (Katz, 2004). Despite the prominent reduction in cardiovascular mortality among men, it has not declined for women. Cardiovascular disease has killed more women then men since 1984 (American Heart Association, 2003). In addition to being the number-one killer of women, on diagnosis, women have both a poorer overall prognosis and a higher risk of death than men diagnosed with heart disease (Peddicord, 2005).

Approximately 1% of pregnant women have cardiac disease, which can be dangerous to maternal well-being (Cunningham et al., 2001). Rheumatic heart disease used to represent the majority of cardiac conditions during pregnancy, but congenital heart disease now constitutes nearly half of all cases of heart disease encountered during pregnancy. Management of heart disease during pregnancy has improved, and most women can continue the pregnancy successfully (Kuczkowski, 2004). Few women with heart disease die during pregnancy, but they are at risk for other complications such as heart failure, arrhythmias, and stroke. Their offspring are also at risk of complications such as premature birth, low birthweight for gestational age, respiratory distress syndrome, intraventricular hemorrhage, and death (Siu & Colman, 2004).

Effects of Heart Disease on Pregnancy

To understand the consequences of heart disease during pregnancy, it is important to review the hemodynamic changes that occur in all pregnant women. First, blood volume increases by approximately 50%, starting in early pregnancy and rising rapidly by the third trimester. Proportionately, plasma volume increases much more than erythrocyte mass, which can lead to physiologic anemia. These changes usually raise the maternal heart rate by 10 beats per minute (Prasad & Ventura, 2001).

Similarly, cardiac output increases steadily during pregnancy by 30% to 50% over prepregnancy levels. The increase is due to both the expansion in blood volume and the augmentation of stroke volume and heart rate. Other hemodynamic changes associated with pregnancy include a decrease in both the systemic vascular resistance and pulmonary vascular resistance, thereby lowering the systolic and diastolic blood pressure. In addition, the hypercoagulability associated with pregnancy might increase the risk of arterial thrombosis and embolization. These normal physiologic changes may increase the risks of pregnancy for women with underlying cardiovascular disease (Samson & Ferguson, 2004) (Table 20-1).

Classification of Heart Disease

How a woman is able to function during her pregnancy is often more important than the diagnosis of cardiovascular disease. The following is a functional classification system developed by the Criteria Committee of the New York Heart Association (1994) based on past and present disability and physical signs:

- **Class I:** asymptomatic with no limitation of physical activity
- **Class II:** symptomatic (dyspnea, chest pain) with increased activity
- **Class III:** symptomatic (fatigue, palpitations) with normal activity
- **Class IV:** symptomatic at rest or with any physical activity

The classification may change as the pregnancy progresses due to the expanding stress on the cardiovascular system. Typically, a woman with class I or II cardiac disease can go through a pregnancy without major complications. A woman with class III disease usually has to maintain bed rest during pregnancy. A woman with class IV disease should avoid pregnancy (McCann, 2004). Many pregnant women progress through all the func-

Table 20-1 Expected Cardiovascular Changes in Pregnancy

Measurement	Prepregnancy	Pregnancy
Heart rate	72 (±10 bpm)	+10–20%
Cardiac output	4.3 (±0.9 L/min)	+30% to 50%
Blood volume	5 L	+20% to 50%
Stroke volume	73.3 (±9 mL)	+30%
Systemic vascular resistance	1,530 (±520 dyne/cm/sec)	–20%
Oxygen consumption	250 mL/minute	+20–30%

Sources: Martin and Foley, 2002; Mattson and Smith, 2004; Blackburn, 2003; Harvey, 2004.

tional classes as they cope with the numerous physiologic changes taking place. Women with cardiac disease may benefit from preconception counseling so that they know the risks before deciding to become pregnant.

Maternal mortality varies directly with the functional class at pregnancy onset. ACOG has adopted a three-tiered classification according to risks for death during pregnancy.

Group I (minimal risk) has a mortality rate of 1% and comprises women with:

- Patent ductus arteriosus
- Tetralogy of Fallot, corrected
- Atrial septal defect
- Ventricular septal defect
- Mitral stenosis, class I and II

Group II (moderate risk) has a mortality rate of 5% to 15% and comprises women with:

- Tetralogy of Fallot, uncorrected
- Mitral stenosis with atrial fibrillation
- Aortic stenosis, class III and IV
- Aortic coarctation without valvular involvement
- Artificial valve replacement

Group III (major risk) has a 25% to 50% mortality rate and comprises women with:

- Pulmonary hypertension
- Complicated aortic coarctation
- Previous myocardial infarction (Gilbert & Harmon, 2003)

Clinical Manifestations

The clinical picture varies with the type of cardiac disorder. Symptoms such as fatigue, dyspnea, palpitations, lightheadedness, and swollen feet may mimic many common complaints of pregnancy, making clinical assessment of the underlying cardiac disease challenging.

Congenital Heart Conditions

Pregnancy in women with congenital heart disease is a relatively new field, since until recently women with congenital heart defects didn't live long enough to bear children. Today, due to new surgical techniques to correct these defects, many of these women can bear children. Table 20-2 highlights some of these congenital conditions.

In some congenital heart conditions, women should be advised to avoid pregnancy: uncorrected tetralogy of Fallot or transposition of the great arteries, and Eisenmenger's syndrome, a defect with both cyanosis and pulmonary hypertension (Martin & Foley, 2002). In most other congenital heart conditions, pregnancy can be attempted, although close monitoring is needed.

Pregnancy is considered safe for many women once congenital defects are corrected. However, a cardiologist

Table 20-2 Selected Heart Conditions Affecting Pregnancy

Condition	Description	Management
Tetralogy of Fallot	Four structural anomalies: obstruction to pulmonary flow; ventricular septal defect (abnormal opening between the right and left ventricles); dextroposition of the aorta (aortic opening overriding the septum and receiving blood from both ventricles); and right ventricular hypertrophy (increase in volume of the myocardium of the right ventricle) (O'Toole, 2003)	Hospitalization and bed rest possible after the 20th week with hemodynamic monitoring via a pulmonary artery catheter to monitor volume status Oxygen therapy may be necessary during labor and birth
Atrial septal defect (ASD)	Congenital heart defect involving a communication or opening between the atria with left-to-right shunting due to greater left-sided pressure Arrhythmias present in some women	Treatment with atrioventricular nodal blocking agents, and at times with electrical cardioversion (Wolbretta, 2003)
Ventricular septal defect (VSD)	Congenital heart defect involving an opening in the ventricular septum (normal in the fetus) persisting after birth, permitting blood flow from the left to the right ventricle, resulting in bypassing of the pulmonary circulation. Complications include arrhythmias, heart failure, and pulmonary hypertension (Lowdermilk & Perry, 2004).	Rest with limited activity if symptomatic
Patent ductus arteriosus (PDA)	Abnormal persistence of an open lumen in the ductus arteriosus between the aorta and the pulmonary artery after birth (O'Toole, 2003)	Surgical ligation of the open ductus during early childhood; subsequent problems minimal after surgical correction
Mitral valve prolapse	Very common in the general population, occurring most often in younger women Leaflets of the mitral valve prolapse into the left atrium during ventricular contraction The most common cause of mitral valve regurgitation if present during pregnancy (Martin & Foley, 2002) Usually improvement in mitral valve function due to increased blood volume and decreased systemic vascular resistance of pregnancy; most women are able to tolerate pregnancy well.	Most women are asymptomatic; diagnosis is made incidentally Occasional palpations, chest pain, or arrhythmias in some women, possibly requiring beta-blockers Usually no special precautions are necessary during pregnancy
Mitral valve stenosis	Most common chronic rheumatic valvular lesion in pregnancy Causes obstruction of blood flow from the atria to the ventricle, thereby decreasing ventricular filling and causing a fixed cardiac output Resultant pulmonary edema, pulmonary hypertension, and right ventricular failure (Goswami & Ong, 2005) Most pregnant women with this condition can be managed medically.	General symptomatic improvement with medical management involving diuretics, beta-blockers, and anticoagulant therapy Activity restriction, reduction in sodium, and potentially bed rest if condition severe

Table 20-2 Selected Heart Conditions Affecting Pregnancy (continued)

Condition	Description	Management
Aortic stenosis	Narrowing of the opening of the aortic valve, leading to an obstruction to left ventricular ejection (Lowdermilk & Perry, 2004) Women with mild disease can tolerate hypervolemia of pregnancy; with progressive narrowing of the opening, cardiac output becomes fixed. Diagnosis can be confirmed with echocardiography. Most women can be managed with medical therapy, bed rest, and close monitoring.	Diagnosis confirmed with echocardiography Pharmacologic treatment with beta-blockers and/or antiarrhythmic agents to reduce risk of heart failure and/or dysrhythmias Bed rest/limiting activity and close monitoring
Peripartum cardiomyopathy	Rare congestive cardiomyopathy that may arise during pregnancy. Multiparity, age, multiple fetuses, hypertension, an infectious agent, autoimmune disease, or cocaine use may contributing to its presence (Siu & Colman, 2004). Development of heart failure in the last month of pregnancy or within 5 months of giving birth without any preexisting heart disease or any identifiable cause	Preload reduction with diuretic therapy Afterload reduction with vasodilators Improvement in contractility with inotropic agents Nonpharmcologic approaches include salt restriction and daily exercise such as walking or biking The question of whether another pregnancy should be attempted is controversial due to the high risk of repeat complications
Myocardial infarction (MI)	Rare during pregnancy but incidence is expected to increase as older women are becoming pregnant and the risk factors for coronary artery disease become more prevalent. Factors contributing to MI include family history, stress, smoking, age, obesity, multiple fetuses, hypercholesterolemia, and cocaine use (Wolbretta, 2003). Increased plasma volume and cardiac output during pregnancy increase the cardiac workload as well as the myocardial oxygen demands; imbalance in supply and demand may contribute to myocardial ischemia.	Incorporation of usual treatment modalities for any acute MI along with consideration for the fetus Anticoagulant therapy, rest, and lifestyle changes to preserve the health of both parties

Sources: Goswami and Ong, 2005; Sui and Colman, 2004; Lowdermilk and Perry, 2004; Martin and Foley, 2002; O'Toole, 2005; Wolbretta, 2003.

should be consulted and should play a role in preconception counseling so that risks can be discussed.

Acquired Heart Disease

Acquired heart disease is typically rheumatic in origin (see Table 20-2). The incidence of rheumatic heart disease has declined dramatically in the past several decades because of prompt identification of streptococcal throat infections and treatment with antibiotics. When the heart is involved, valvular lesions such as mitral stenosis, prolapse, or aortic stenosis are common.

In addition, many women are postponing childbearing until the fourth or fifth decade of life. With advancing maternal age, underlying medical conditions such as hypertension, diabetes, and hypercholesterolemia contributing to ischemic heart disease become more common and increase the incidence of acquired heart disease complicating pregnancy. Coronary artery disease and myocardial infarction may result.

Treatment

The woman with known cardiac disease should consult her health care provider before becoming pregnant so that she can determine the advisability and optimal time for a pregnancy, the need for and timing of diagnostic procedures, and any medical management changes needed. If the woman presents for care after she has become pregnant, prenatal counseling should focus on the signs and symptoms of cardiac compromise, dietary and lifestyle changes needed, and the impact of the hemodynamic changes of pregnancy. More frequent prenatal visits (every 2 weeks until the last month and then weekly) are usually needed to ensure the health and safety of the mother and fetus.

Nursing Management

Nursing management of the pregnant woman with heart disease focuses on assisting with measures to stabilize the mother's hemodynamic status, because a decrease in maternal blood pressure or volume will cause blood to be shunted away from the uterus, thus reducing placental perfusion. Collaboration between the cardiologist, obstetrician, perinatologist, and nurse is needed to promote stabilization.

Assessment

Risk assessment should be completed before a woman becomes pregnant. The data needed for risk assessment can be acquired from a thorough cardiovascular history and examination, a 12-lead electrocardiogram (ECG), and evaluation of oxygen saturation levels by pulse oximetry. When possible, any surgical procedures, such as valve replacement, should be done before pregnancy to improve fetal and maternal outcomes (Goswami & Ong, 2005).

Frequent and thorough assessments are crucial during the antepartum period to ensure early detection and prompt intervention should the woman experience cardiac decompensation. Monitor the woman closely for changes in vital signs, and auscultate heart sounds for abnormalities, including murmurs. Check the client's weight, reporting any weight gain outside recommended parameters. Evaluate for edema and note any pitting.

Assess the fetal heart rate and review serial ultrasound results to monitor fetal growth. Ask the woman about fetal activity, and report any changes such as a decrease in fetal movements. Ask the woman about any symptoms of preterm labor, such as low back pain, uterine contractions, and increased pelvic pressure and vaginal discharge, and report them immediately. Assess the client's lifestyle patterns and suggest realistic modifications. As the client's pregnancy advances, expect her functional class to be revised based on her level of disability.

In addition, the nurse plays a major role in recognizing the signs and symptoms of cardiac decompensation. This is vital because the mother's hemodynamic status determines the health of the fetus. These signs and symptoms include:

- Shortness of breath on exertion
- Cyanosis of lips and nail beds
- Swelling of face, hands, and feet
- Rapid respirations
- Abnormal heartbeats, racing heart, or palpitations
- Chest pain
- Syncope
- Increasing fatigue
- Moist, frequent cough

Nursing Interventions

Nursing interventions for the woman with heart disease include ongoing assessment of the mother and fetus to ensure the best outcome. Additional nursing interventions include:

- Review the client's prescribed cardiac medications; reinforce their use and explain about their potential side effects.
- Outline the diagnostic tests that may be used, including ECG and echocardiogram.
- Advise the client to make time for rest periods in the side-lying position.
- Teach the woman to assess fetal activity daily and report any changes.
- Stress the importance of frequent prenatal visits; reinforce the need for close medical supervision throughout pregnancy.
- Promote good prenatal nutrition, with a possible referral to a nutritionist.
- Discuss the need to limit dietary sodium if indicated to reduce fluid retention.
- Help the client to prioritize household chores and childcare.
- Teach the client about signs and symptoms of cardiac decompensation; instruct her to notify the health care provider should any occur.
- Explain the need for serial nonstress testing at about 32 weeks.
- Stress the need to notify the health care professional of any infection exposure.
- Instruct the client about the need to consume a high-fiber diet to prevent straining or constipation.
- Prepare the client and family for labor and birth and the options available.
- Identify support systems available to the client and her family; encourage their use.

During labor, anticipate the need for invasive hemodynamic monitoring, and make sure the woman has been prepared for this beforehand. Monitor her fluid volume carefully to prevent overload. Anticipate the use of epidural anesthesia if a vaginal birth is planned. After birth, assess the client for possible fluid overload as peripheral fluids mobilize. This fluid shift from the periphery to the central circulation taxes the heart, and signs of heart failure such as cough, progressive dyspnea, edema, palpitations, and crackles in the lung bases may ensue before postpartum diuresis begins. Because hemodynamics do not return to baseline for several days after childbirth, women at intermediate or high risk require monitoring for at least 72 hours postpartum (Siu & Colman, 2004).

Women with a high-risk pregnancy involving cardiac disease need assistance in reducing risks that would lead to complications or further cardiac compromise. Counseling and education are key. Assess the client's understanding of her condition and what restrictions and lifestyle changes may be needed to provide the best outcome for both her and her fetus. Ensuring a healthy infant and mother at the end of pregnancy is the ultimate goal.

Chronic Hypertension

Chronic hypertension exists when the woman has high blood pressure before pregnancy or before the 20th week of gestation, or when hypertension persists for more than 12 weeks postpartum (London et al., 2003). The Seventh Report of the Joint National Committee on Prevention, Detection, Evaluation, and Treatment of High Blood Pressure (JNC, 2003) has classified blood pressure as follows:

- Normal: systolic less than 120 mm Hg, diastolic less than 80 mmHg
- Prehypertensive: systolic 120 to 139 mm Hg, diastolic 80 to 89 mmHg
- Mild hypertension: systolic 140 to 159 mm Hg, diastolic 90 to 99 mmHg
- Severe hypertension: systolic 160 mm Hg or higher, diastolic 100 mm Hg or higher

Chronic hypertension is typically seen in older, obese women with glucose intolerance. The most common complication is preeclampsia, which is seen in approximately 20% of women who enter the pregnancy with hypertension. This preexisting condition places the woman at greater risk for developing preeclampsia (see Chapter 19) and fetal growth restriction during pregnancy.

Treatment

Preconception counseling is important in fostering positive outcomes. Typically, it involves lifestyle changes involving diet, exercise, weight loss, and smoking cessation to modify this condition.

Treatment for women with chronic hypertension focuses on maintaining normal blood pressure, preventing superimposed preeclampsia/eclampsia, and ensuring normal fetal development. Once the woman is pregnant, antihypertensive agents are typically reserved for severe hypertension (150 to 160 mm Hg/100 to 110 mm Hg). Methyldopa (Aldomet) is a commonly prescribed agent because of its safety record during pregnancy. Methyldopa (Aldomet), a slow-acting antihypertensive agent, helps to improve uterine perfusion. Typically 1 g is given orally, followed by a regimen of 1 to 2 g daily.

Other antihypertensive agents that can be use include labetalol (Transdate), atenolol (Tenorium), and nifedipine (Procardia) (Goswami & Ong, 2005). Lifestyle changes are needed and should continue throughout gestation. The woman with chronic hypertension will be seen more frequently prenatally (every 2 weeks until 28 weeks and then weekly until birth) to monitor her blood pressure and to assess for any signs of preeclampsia. At approximately 24 weeks' gestation, the woman will be instructed to document fetal movement. At this same time, serial ultrasounds will be ordered to monitor fetal growth and amniotic fluid volume. Additional tests will be included if the client's status changes.

Nursing Management

Preconception counseling is the ideal time to discuss lifestyle changes to prevent or control hypertension. One area to cover during this visit would be the Dietary Approaches to Stop Hypertension (DASH) diet, which contains an adequate intake of potassium, magnesium, and calcium. Sodium is usually limited to 2.4 g. Suggest aerobic exercise until the woman becomes pregnant, although she should cease it once the pregnancy is confirmed. Encourage smoking cessation and avoidance of alcohol. If the woman is overweight, encourage her to lose weight before becoming pregnant, not during the pregnancy (Dudek, 2006). Stressing the positive benefits of a healthy lifestyle might help motivate the woman to make the modifications and change unhealthy habits.

Encourage women with chronic hypertension to use home blood pressure monitoring devices to document values; any elevations should be reported. Scheduling appointments for antepartum fetal assessment (28 to 30 weeks) and explaining the rationale for the need to monitor fetal growth are important to gain the woman's cooperation in the planned regimen. Also carefully monitor the woman for abruptio placentae (abdominal pain, rigid abdomen, vaginal bleeding), as well as superimposed preeclampsia (elevation in blood pressure, weight gain, edema, proteinuria). Alerting the woman to these potential risks is critical to early identification of these complications and prompt intervention.

In addition, stress the importance of daily periods of rest (1 hour) in the left lateral recumbent position to maximize placental perfusion. Instruct the woman and her family how to take and record a daily blood pressure, and reinforce the need for her to take her medications as prescribed to control her blood pressure as well as to ensure the well-being of her unborn child. Praising her for her efforts at each prenatal visit may help motivate her to continue the regimen throughout her pregnancy.

Respiratory Conditions

During pregnancy, the respiratory system is affected by hormonal changes, mechanical changes, and prior respiratory conditions. These changes can cause a woman with a history of compromised respiration to decompensate during pregnancy. While upper respiratory infections are typically self-limiting, chronic respiratory conditions, such as asthma or tuberculosis, can have a negative effect on the growing fetus when alterations in oxygenation occur in the mother. The outcome of pregnancy in a woman with a respiratory condition depends on the severity of the oxygen alteration as well as the degree and duration of hypoxia on the fetus.

Asthma

Asthma is the most common respiratory disease complicating pregnancy, affecting approximately 7% of childbearing women in the United States (Kazzi & Marachelian, 2004). Asthma affects 20 million Americans and is one of the most common potentially serious medical conditions to complicate pregnancy.

Effects of Asthma on Pregnancy

Maternal asthma is associated with an increased risk of infant death, preeclampsia, IUGR, preterm birth, and low birthweight. These risks are linked to the severity of asthma: more severe asthma increases the risk (NAEPP, 2005). Asthma is also known as reactive airway disease because the bronchioles constrict in response to allergens, irritants, and infections. In addition to bronchoconstriction, inflammation of the airways produces thick mucus that further limits the movement of air and makes breathing difficult.

The normal physiologic changes of pregnancy affect the respiratory system. While the respiratory rate does not change, hyperventilation increases at term by 48% due to high progesterone levels. Diaphragmatic elevation and a decrease in functional lung residual capacity occur late in pregnancy, which may reduce the woman's ability to inspire deeply to take in more oxygen. Oxygen consumption and the metabolic rate both increase, placing additional stress on the woman's respiratory system (Beckmann, 2002).

A pregnant woman with asthma has a one-in-three chance of the asthma changing, but the effect of pregnancy on asthma is unpredictable. Studies have shown that in one third of pregnancies the asthma will get better; in one third it will get worse, and in the remaining third it will remain the same. The greatest increase in asthma attacks usually occurs between 24 and 36 weeks' gestation; flare-ups are rare during the last 4 weeks of pregnancy and during labor (Blaiss, 2004).

Both the woman and her fetus are at risk if asthma is not well managed during pregnancy. When a pregnant woman has trouble breathing, her fetus also has trouble getting the oxygen it needs for adequate growth and development. Severe persistent asthma has been linked to the development of maternal hypertension, preeclampsia, placenta previa, uterine hemorrhage, and oligohydramnios. Women whose asthma is poorly controlled during pregnancy are at increased risk of preterm birth, low birthweight, and stillbirth (Beckmann, 2003).

Treatment

Successful management of asthma in pregnancy involves drug therapy, client education, and the elimination of environmental triggers. Triggers provoke an exacerbation and need to be identified and controlled. Some common asthma triggers are listed in Box 20-2.

Asthma should be treated as aggressively in pregnant women as in nonpregnant women because the benefits of averting an asthma attack outweigh the risks of medications. The two major classifications of drugs used to treat asthma are bronchodilators, such as albuterol (Proventil), pirbuterol acetate (Maxair), and salmeterol (Serevent), and corticosteroids, such as prednisone (Deltasone), beclomethasone (Beclovent), and fluticasone propionate (Flovent). Clients with asthma typically receive these medications by inhalation.

Nursing Management

Complete a thorough assessment of asthma triggers and recommend strategies to reduce exposure to them, review the client's medication therapy, and educate her about controlling asthma symptoms.

Assessment

Obtain a thorough history of the disease. Auscultate the lungs and assess respiratory and heart rates. The physical examination should include rate, rhythm, and depth of respirations; skin color; blood pressure and pulse rate; and evaluation for signs of fatigue. Women experiencing an acute asthma attack often present with wheezing, chest

---

BOX 20-2

COMMON ASTHMA TRIGGERS

- Smoke and chemical irritants
- Air pollution
- Dust mites
- Animal dander
- Seasonal changes with pollen, molds, and spores
- Upper respiratory infections
- Esophageal reflux
- Medications, such as aspirin and nonsteroidal anti-inflammatory drugs (NSAIDs)
- Exercise
- Cold air
- Emotional stress (Kazzi & Marachelian, 2004)

tightness, tachypnea, nonproductive coughing, shortness of breath, and dyspnea. Lung auscultation findings might include diffuse wheezes and rhonchi, bronchovesicular sounds, and a more prominent expiratory phase of respiration compared to the inspiratory phase (Blaiss, 2004). If the pregnancy is far enough along, the fetal heart rate is measured and routine prenatal assessments (weight, blood pressure, fundal height, urine for protein) are completed.

Laboratory studies usually ordered include a complete blood count with differential (to assess the degree of nonspecific inflammation and identify anemia) and pulmonary function tests (to assess the severity of an attack and to provide a baseline to determine the client's response to treatment).

Nursing Interventions

Nursing interventions focus on client education to promote adherence to the treatment regimen, thereby fostering the optimal environment for fetal growth and development. Provide the client with suggestions on how to control her environment (Teaching Guidelines 20-2).

Client education is essential to ensure that the woman understands drug actions and interactions, the uses and potential abuses of asthma medications, and the symptoms that require medical evaluation. Reviewing potential perinatal complications with the woman is helpful in motivating her to adhere to the prescribed regimen. At each antepartum visit, reassess the efficacy of the treatment plan to determine whether adjustments are needed.

Taking control of asthma in pregnancy is the responsibility of the client along with her health care team. Providing the client with the knowledge and tools to monitor her condition, control triggers, and use medications to prevent acute exacerbations assists the client in taking control. Facilitating this partnership with the woman will improve perinatal outcomes.

When teaching the pregnant woman with asthma, cover the following topics:

- Signs and symptoms of asthma progression and exacerbation
- Importance and safety of medication to fetus and to herself
- Warning signs that indicate the need to contact the healthcare provider
- Potential harm to fetus and self by undertreatment or delay in seeking help
- Prevention and avoidance of known triggers
- Home use of metered-dose inhalers
- Adverse effects of medications

During labor, nursing interventions focus on monitoring the client's oxygenation saturation by pulse oximetry and providing pain management through epidural analgesia to reduce stress, which may trigger an acute attack. Continuously monitor the fetus for distress during labor and assess fetal heart rate patterns for indications of hypoxia. Assess the newborn for signs and symptoms of hypoxia. Asthma medications can be used throughout the pregnancy and labor and during the postpartum period to control symptoms.

Tuberculosis

Tuberculosis (TB) is a disease that has been around for years but never seems to go away completely. It remains the most common respiratory disease in the world (Herchline & Amorosa, 2005). Although it is not prevalent in the United States, a resurgence was noted starting in the mid-1980s secondary to the acquired immunodeficiency syndrome (AIDS) epidemic and immigration. Therefore, all nurses must be skilled in screening for and managing this condition.

Women at risk for TB are those who are immunocompromised, homeless, or using injectable drugs. Women emigrating from developing countries such as Latin America, Asia, China, Mexico, Haiti, and Africa with high rates of TB also are at risk.

The lung is the major site of involvement. A person becomes infected by breathing in the infectious organism, *Mycobacterium tuberculosis,* carried on a droplet nuclei and spread by airborne transmission. Clients can remain asymptomatic for long periods of time as the organism may lie dormant.

Treatment

Treatment of TB during pregnancy is essentially the same as that for the general population. Medications are the cornerstone of treatment to prevent infection progression.

 T E A C H I N G   G U I D E L I N E S   2 0 - 2

Teaching to Control Environmental Triggers

- Remove any carpeting in the house, especially the bedroom, to reduce dust mites.
- Use allergen-proof encasing on the mattress, box spring, and pillows.
- Wash all bedding in hot water.
- Remove dust collectors in house, such as stuffed animals, books, knick-knacks.
- Avoid pets in the house to reduce exposure to pet dander.
- Use a high-efficiency particulate air-filtering system in the bedroom.
- Do not smoke, and avoid places where you can be exposed to passive cigarette smoke from others.
- Stay indoors and use air conditioning when the pollen or mold count is high or air quality is poor.
- Wear a covering over your nose and mouth when going outside in the cold weather.
- Avoid exposure to persons with colds, flu, or viruses.

The medical therapy for pregnant women is a combination of medications such as isoniazid, rifampin, and ethambutol, taken daily for up to 9 months. These anti-TB agents appear to have minimal risks for the development of congenital anomalies and may be started as soon as the diagnosis of TB is made. However, extensive research has not been done to determine the definitive safety of these drugs (Herchline & Amorosa, 2005).

Nursing Management

Educating the client and her family about the correct administration of medications and potential side effects is necessary. Nursing management focuses on infection control measures and client and family education. Nurses play a major role in TB prevention by teaching family members how the disease is transmitted so they can protect the newborn and other family members from airborne organisms (McKinney et al., 2005).

Assessment

At antepartum visits, be alert for clinical manifestations of TB, including fatigue, fever or night sweats, nonproductive cough, slow weight loss, anemia, hemoptysis, and anorexia (Lake, 2001). If TB is suspected or the woman is at risk for developing TB, anticipate screening with the tuberculin skin test. Screening is recommended for pregnant women who fall into a high-risk group: born in a country with a high incidence of TB, alcohol abuse, injectable drug use, HIV infection, and immunosuppression.

Screening is done with the tuberculin skin test using purified protein derivative (PPD), which is given by intradermal injection. If the client has been exposed to TB, a reddened induration will appear within 72 hours. A follow-up chest x-ray with lead shielding over the abdomen and sputum cultures will confirm the diagnosis.

Nursing Interventions

Compliance with the multidrug therapy is critical to protect the woman and her fetus from progression of TB. Nurses can assist by first identifying high-risk women for screening and then educating them about the disease process, mode of transmission, prevention, potential complications, and the importance of adherence to the treatment regimen.

Stressing the importance of health-promotion activities throughout the pregnancy is important. Some suggestions might include avoiding crowded living conditions, avoiding sick people, maintaining adequate hydration, eating a nutritious, well-balanced diet, keeping all prenatal appointments to evaluate fetal growth and well-being, and getting plenty of fresh air by going outside frequently. Determining the woman's understanding of her condition and treatment plan is important for compliance. A language interpreter may be needed to validate and reinforce her understanding if she does not speak English.

Breastfeeding is not contraindicated during the medication regimen and should in fact be encouraged. Management of the newborn of a mother with TB involves preventing transmission by teaching the parents not to cough, sneeze, or talk directly into the newborn's face. Nurses should keep up to date with new therapies and screening techniques to treat this centuries-old disease.

Hematologic Conditions

Anemia, a reduction in red blood cell volume, is measured by hematocrit (Hct) or a decrease in the concentration of hemoglobin (Hgb) in the peripheral blood. This results in reduced capacity of the blood to carry oxygen to the vital organs of the mother and fetus. Anemia is a sign of an underlying problem but does not indicate its origin.

In women, Hgb below 12 g/100 mL or Hct below 37% indicates anemia (Youngkin & Davis, 2004). During pregnancy, anemia increases the risk of preterm birth, infections, and delayed healing.

Iron Deficiency Anemia

Iron deficiency anemia affects one in four pregnancies and is usually caused by inadequate dietary intake of iron (McCann, 2004). It is a very common state in pregnant women and can be caused by a variety of factors, including poor nutrition, hemolysis, **pica** (consuming non-food substances), multiple gestation, limited intervals between pregnancies, and blood loss. Anemia at term increases the perinatal risk for both the mother and newborn. The risks of hemorrhage (impaired platelet function) and infection during and after birth also are increased. Anemia during the early part of pregnancy can increase the likelihood of preterm birth, low birthweight, and perinatal mortality (Blackburn, 2003).

The effects of maternal iron deficiency on the fetus and newborn have not been substantiated. Even with significant maternal iron depletion, the fetus will receive adequate stores, but at the cost to the mother (McKinney et al., 2005).

Clinical Manifestations

Typically, the woman with iron deficiency anemia presents with fatigue, weakness, malaise, anorexia, susceptibility to infection (frequent colds), pale mucus membranes, tachycardia, and pallor. Laboratory studies usually reveal low Hgb (<11 g/dL), low Hct (<35%), low serum iron level (<30 ug/dL), microcytic and hypochromic cells, and low serum ferritin level (<100 mg/dL).

Treatment

The goals of treatment for iron deficiency anemia in pregnancy are to eliminate symptoms, correct the deficiency, and replenish iron stores. Early and daily administration of prenatal vitamins and iron is recommended, because fulfilling maternal iron requirements solely through diet in the face of diminished iron stores is difficult.

Nursing Management

Since the treatment of iron deficiency anemia is pharmacologic and dietary in nature, the nurse's role is to encourage compliance with drug therapy and provide dietary instruction about the intake of foods high in iron. Although iron constitutes a minimal percentage of the body's total weight, it has several major roles: it assists in the transport of oxygen and carbon dioxide throughout the body, it aids in the production of red blood cells, and it plays a role in the body's immune response.

Stress the importance of taking the prenatal vitamin and iron supplement consistently. Taking iron on an empty stomach improves its absorption, but many women cannot tolerate the gastrointestinal discomfort it causes. In such cases, taking it with meals is advised. Adverse effects are predominantly gastrointestinal and include gastric discomfort, nausea, vomiting, anorexia, diarrhea, metallic taste, and constipation. Taking the iron supplement with meals and increasing intake of fiber and fluids will typically overcome the most common side effects.

Dietary counseling includes assessing the woman's dietary intake as well as the quantity and timing of ingestion of substances that interfere with iron absorption, such as tea, coffee, chocolate, and high-fiber foods. Foods high in iron to recommend include dried fruits, whole grains, green leafy vegetables, meats, peanut butter, and iron-fortified cereals (Dudek, 2006). A referral to a dietitian might be in order. Teaching Guidelines 20-3 highlights the instructions for the pregnant woman with iron deficiency anemia.

 TEACHING GUIDELINES 20-3

Teaching for the Woman with
Iron Deficiency Anemia

- Take your prenatal vitamin daily; if you miss a dose, take it as soon as you remember.
- For best absorption, take iron supplement between meals.
- Avoid taking iron supplement with coffee, tea, chocolate, and high-fiber food.
- Eat foods rich in iron, such as:
  ○ Meats, green leafy vegetables, legumes, dried fruits, whole grains
  ○ Peanut butter, bean dip, whole-wheat fortified breads and cereals
- For best iron absorption from foods, consume the food along with a food high in vitamin C.
- Increase your exercise, fluids, and high-fiber foods to reduce constipation.
- Plan frequent rest periods during the day.

Thalassemia

Thalassemia is a group of hereditary anemias in which synthesis of one or both chains of the hemoglobin molecule (alpha and beta) is defective. A low Hgb and a microcytic, hypochromic anemia result (Youngkin & Davis, 2004). The prevalence and severity of thalassemia depend on the population, with the type of thalassemia seen dependent on racial background: persons of Mediterranean, Asian, Italian, or Greek heritage and African-Americans are most frequently affected. Beta-thalassemia is the most common form found in the United States (McKinney et al., 2005).

Thalassemia occurs in two forms: minor and major. Thalassemia minor, the heterozygous form, results from the inheritance of one abnormal gene from either parent, placing the offspring in a carrier trait state. These women have little or no hematologic disease and are clinically asymptomatic (silent carrier state). Thalassemia major is the form involving inheritance of the gene from both parents. Thalassemia major can be very severe. Genetic counseling might be necessary when decisions about childbearing are being made.

Thalassemia minor has little effect on the pregnancy, although the woman will have mild, persistent anemia. This anemia does not respond to iron therapy, and iron supplements should not be prescribed. Women with thalassemia major do not usually become pregnant because of lifelong severe hemolysis, anemia, and premature death (Poole, 2003).

Diagnostic studies typically used to diagnose thalassemia include a complete blood count, bone marrow examination, peripheral blood smear, iron studies, and Hgb (Blackburn, 2003).

Management of thalassemia during pregnancy depends on the severity of the disease. Identification and screening are important to plan care. The woman's ethnic background, medical history, and blood studies are analyzed. If the woman is determined to be a carrier, screening of the father of the child is indicated. Knowledge of the carrier state of each parent provides the genetic counselor with knowledge about the risk that the fetus will be a carrier or will have the disease (Poole, 2003). Mild anemia may be present, and instructions to rest and avoid infections are helpful. Nurses should provide supportive care and expectant management throughout the pregnancy.

Sickle Cell Anemia

Sickle cell anemia is an autosomal recessive inherited condition that results from a defective hemoglobin molecule (hemoglobin S). It is found most commonly in African-Americans, Southeast Asians, and Middle Eastern populations. About 1 in 10 African-Americans are carriers of the trait, while approximately 3 in 800 are affected with the disease (McCann, 2004). People with only one gene for the trait (heterozygous) will have sickle cell trait without obvious symptoms of the disease and with little effect on the pregnancy.

In the human body, the hemoglobin molecule serves as the oxygen-carrying component of the red blood cells. Most people have several types of circulation hemoglobin (HbA and HbA2) that make up the majority of their circulatory system. In sickle cell disease, the abnormal hemoglobin S (HbS) replaces HbA and HbA2. This abnormal hemoglobin (HbS) becomes sickle-shaped when it isn't fully saturated with oxygen. Subsequently, it begins to build up in the capillaries and smaller blood vessels, making blood more viscous. These sickle cells clump together, clogging the small blood vessels. As a result, hypoxia occurs and leads to a crisis. In addition, sickle cells have a shorter life span (10 to 20 days) than the normal red blood cell (120 days). The combination of clumped red cells, fragile cells, and shortened lifespan contribute to the severe anemia (Samson & Ferguson, 2004).

Sickle cell anemia during pregnancy is associated with more severe anemia and frequent vaso-occlusive crises, with increased maternal and perinatal morbidity and mortality (Mattson & Smith, 2004).

Clinical Manifestations

Women with sickle cell anemia present with anorexia, dyspnea, malaise, and pallor. If in sickle cell crisis, the woman will report severe abdominal pain, muscle spasms, leg pains, joint pain, fever, stiff neck, nausea and vomiting, and seizures (McCann, 2004).

Treatment

Ideally, women with hemoglobinopathies are screened before conception and are made aware of the risks of sickle cell anemia to themselves and to the fetus. A blood Hgb electrophoresis is done for all women from high-risk ancestry at their first prenatal visit to determine the types and percentages of Hgb present. This information should help them in making future reproductive decisions.

Treatment depends on the health status of the woman. During pregnancy, only supportive therapy is used: blood transfusions for severe anemia, analgesics for pain, and antibiotics for infection.

Nursing Management

Clients require emotional support, education, and follow-up care to deal with this chronic condition, which has a great impact on them and their families. Nursing care of women with sickle cell anemia includes:

- Educate the client to avoid infection exposure, cigarette smoking, alcohol consumption, and temperature extremes.
- Monitor laboratory test results.

- Assess hydration status at each visit and urge the client to drink 8 to 10 glasses of fluid daily to prevent dehydration.
- Monitor vital signs, fetal heart rate, weight gain, and fetal growth.
- Assess for early signs of crisis.
- Schedule frequent fetal well-being assessments, such as biophysical profiles, nonstress tests, and contraction stress tests.
- Encourage rest and pain management during labor.
- Prevent infection during the postpartum period by meticulous handwashing.
- Discuss family planning options to control fertility.

Infections

A wide variety of infections can affect the progression of pregnancy, possibly having a negative impact on the outcome. The effect of the infection depends on the timing of the infection, the body systems involved, and the severity of the infection. Common viral infections include cytomegalovirus (CMV), rubella, herpes simplex, hepatitis B, varicella, parvovirus B19, and several sexually transmitted infections (Table 20-3). Toxoplasmosis and group B *Streptococcus* are common nonviral infections. Only the most common infections will be discussed here.

Cytomegalovirus

Cytomegalovirus (CMV) is the most common congenital and perinatal viral infection in the world, possibly affecting up to 3% of all newborns (Damato & Winnen, 2002). Pregnant women acquire active disease primarily from sexual contact, blood transfusions, kissing, and contact with children in daycare centers. The virus can be found in virtually all body fluids. Prevalence rates in women in the United States range from 50% to 85% (Damato & Winnen, 2002). CMV infection during pregnancy may result in abortion, stillbirth, low birthweight, IUGR, microcephaly, deafness, blindness, mental retardation, jaundice, or congenital or neonatal infection. If the first or primary infection occurs during pregnancy, the fetus has a 40% to 50% chance of being infected. Primary CMV is the most dangerous to the fetus (Gibbs et al., 2004).

Nursing Management

Most women are asymptomatic and don't know they have been exposed to CMV. Symptoms of CMV in the fetus and newborn include IUGR, microcephaly, hearing loss, chorioretinitis, and mental retardation (London et al., 2003). Since no therapy prevents or treats CMV infections, nurses have a responsibility for educating and supporting childbearing women at risk for CMV infection

Table 20-3 Sexually Transmitted Infections Affecting Pregnancy

Infection/Organism	Effect on Pregnancy and Fetus/Newborn	Implications
Syphilis (*Treponema pallidum*)	Maternal infection increases risk of premature labor and birth. Newborn may be born with congenital syphilis—jaundice, rhinitis, anemia, IUGR, and CNS involvement.	All pregnant women should be screened for this STI and treated with benzathine penicillin G 2.4 million units IM to prevent placental transmission.
Gonorrhea (*Neisseria gonorrhoeae*)	Majority of women are asymptomatic. It causes ophthalmia neonatorum in the newborn from birth through infected birth canal.	All pregnant women should be screened at first prenatal visit, with repeat screening in the third trimester. All newborns receive mandatory eye prophylaxis with tetracycline or erythromycin within the first hour of life. Mother is treated with ceftriaxone (Rocephin) 125 mg IM in single dose before going home.
Chlamydia (*Chlamydia trachomatis*)	Majority of women are asymptomatic. Infection is associated with infertility and ectopic pregnancy, spontaneous abortions, preterm labor, premature rupture of membranes, low birthweight, stillbirth, and neonatal mortality. Infection is transmitted to newborn through vaginal birth. Neonate may develop conjunctivitis or pneumonia.	All pregnant women should be screened at first prenatal visit and treated with erythromycin.
Human papillomavirus (HPV)	Infection causes warts in the anogenital area, known as condylomata acuminata. These warts may grow large enough to block a vaginal birth. Fetal exposure to HPV during birth is associated with laryngeal papillomas.	Warts are treated with trichlorocetic acid, liquid nitrogen, or laser therapy under colposcopy.
Trichomonas (*Trichomonas Vaginalis*)	Infection produces itching and burning, dysuria, strawberry patches on cervix, and vaginal discharge. Infection is associated with premature rupture of membranes and preterm birth.	Treatment is with a single 2-g dose of metronidazole (Flagyl).

Sources: London et al, 2003; O'Toole, 2005; Youngkin and Davis, 2004; Tiller, 2002.

during the perinatal period. Stressing the importance of good handwashing and use of sound hygiene practices can help to reduce transmission of the virus to a woman who could pass the virus on to her fetus.

Rubella

Rubella, commonly called German measles, is spread by droplets or through direct contact with a contaminated object. The risk of a pregnant woman transmitting this virus through the placenta to her fetus increases the earlier her exposure to the virus. When infections occurs within the first month after conception, 50% of fetuses show signs of infection; in the second month following conception, 25% of fetuses will be infected; and in the third month, 10% of fetuses will be affected (Youngkin & Davis, 2004).

Nursing Management

Ideally, all women have been vaccinated and have adequate immunity against rubella. However, all women are still screened at their first prenatal visit to determine their status. If her rubella antibody titer is 1:8 or greater, this proves evidence of immunity. Women who are not immune should be vaccinated during the immediate postpartum period so they will be immune before becoming pregnant again (CDC, 2003). Nurses need to check the rubella immune status of all new mothers and should make sure all mothers with a titer of less than 1:8 are immunized prior to discharge.

Herpes Simplex Virus

Approximately 45 million people are infected with genital herpes in the United States, and 500,000 new cases are diagnosed annually. Despite strategies designed to prevent perinatal transmission, the number of cases of newborn herpes simplex virus (HSV) continues to rise, mirroring the rising prevalence of genital herpes infection in women of childbearing age (Fischer, 2004).

HSV is a DNA virus with two subtypes: HSV-1 and HSV-2. HSV-1 infections were traditionally associated with oral lesions (fever blisters), whereas HSV-2 infections occurred in the genital region. Currently, either type can be found in either location (Fischer, 2004).

Infection occurs by direct contact of the skin or mucous membranes with an active lesion. HSV is associated with infections of the genital tract that when acquired during pregnancy can result in severe systemic symptoms in the mother and significant morbidity and mortality in the newborn (Donahue, 2002). Once the virus enters the body, it never leaves.

Infants born to mothers with a primary HSV infection have a 30% to 50% risk of acquiring the infection via perinatal transmission near or during birth. Recurrent genital herpes simplex infections carry a 1% to 3% risk of neonatal infection if the recurrence occurs around the time of vaginal birth (Donahue, 2002). HSV can be vertically transmitted to the fetus or newborn during the prenatal, intrapartum, or postpartum periods. Most infants infected by perinatal transmission are born to mothers with no evidence of genital herpes lesions, so prevention is a challenge.

Nursing Management

Nursing management for the woman with genital herpes in pregnancy should address the care of the pregnant woman as well as reducing the risk of newborn herpes. Since the majority of newborn herpes results from perinatal transmission of the virus during vaginal birth, and because transmission can result in severe neurologic impairment or death, treatment of the mother with an antiviral agent such as acyclovir must be started as soon as the culture comes back positive. Universal screening for herpes is not economically sound, so nurses need to remain knowledgeable about current practice to be able to provide accurate and sensitive care to all women.

Hepatitis B Virus

Hepatitis B virus (HBV) is one of the most prevalent chronic diseases in the world. HBV can be transmitted through contaminated blood, illicit drug use, blood products, and sexual contact. The virus is 100 times more infectious than HIV and, unlike HIV, it can live outside the body in dried blood for more than a week (Lin & Kirchner, 2004).

Sexual transmission accounts for most adult HBV infections in the United States. Acutely infected women develop hepatitis with anorexia, nausea, vomiting, fever, abdominal pain, and jaundice. In women with acute hepatitis B, vertical transmission occurs in approximately 10% of newborns when infection occurs in the first trimester and in 80% to 90% of newborns when acute infection occurs in the third trimester (Landon, 2004).

Women at greatest risk for contracting HBV infection include those with:

- A history of sexually transmitted infections
- Household contacts of HBV-infected persons
- Jobs as healthcare workers
- Intravenous drug abuse
- Multiple sexual partners
- Chinese, Southeast Asian, or African heritage
- Partners who are HBV infected (CDC, 2005)

Women who work as prostitutes or are foreign-born also are at high risk for contracting HBV (CDC, 2005).

Hepatitis B infection during pregnancy is associated with an increased risk of preterm birth, low birthweight, and neonatal death. Newborns infected with HBV are likely to become chronic carriers of the virus, becoming reservoirs for continued infection in the population (CDC, 2005). The fetus is at risk primarily at birth because of the possible contact with contaminated blood at this time.

Nursing Management

Screen for hepatitis B surface antigen (HbsAg) via blood studies in all pregnant women at their first prenatal visit. Repeat this screening later in pregnancy for women in high-risk groups (Youngkin & Davis, 2004). If positive, expect to administer HBV immune globulin (HBIG, Hep-B-Gammagee) followed by HBV vaccine (Recombivax-HB, Engerix-B) to the newborn within 12 hours of birth. The second and third doses of the vaccine are given at 1 month and 6 months of age (CDC, 2005). The CDC recommends routine vaccination of all newborns.

Women who are HbsAg negative may be vaccinated safely during pregnancy. No current research supports the use of surgical births to reduce vertical transmission of HBV. In addition, breastfeeding by mothers with chronic HBV infection does not increase the risk of viral transmission to their newborns (Lin & Kirchner, 2004).

HBV can be prevented through safer sex practices, good handwashing technique, and the use of standard precautions with all body fluid contact. Client education is essential (Teaching Guidelines 20-4). Protection can be afforded with the highly effective hepatitis B vaccine.

Treatment for hepatitis B rarely produces permanent remission of the disease. Therefore, the goals of therapy are long-term suppression of viral replication and prevention of end-stage liver disease. Urge the woman to consume a high-protein diet and avoid fatigue. A healthy lifestyle can help delay disease progression. Initiate an open discussion about the modes of transmission and use of condoms to prevent spread.

Varicella Zoster virus

Varicella zoster virus (VZV) is a member of the herpesvirus family and is the virus that causes both varicella (chickenpox) and herpes zoster (shingles). Pregnant women are at risk for developing varicella when they come in close contact with children who have active infection. Maternal varicella can be transmitted to the fetus through the placenta, leading to congenital varicella, via an ascending infection during birth, or by direct contact with infectious lesions, leading to infection after birth. Varicella occurs in approximately 1 to 7 of 10,000 pregnancies (Anderson & Safdar, 2005).

Congenital varicella syndrome can occur among newborns of mothers infected during early pregnancy. It is characterized by low birthweight, spontaneous abortion, chorioretinitis, cataracts, cutaneous scarring, limb hypoplasia, microcephaly, ocular abnormalities, mental retardation, and early death (Laartz & Gompf, 2004).

Nursing Management

Nursing management focuses on prevention of this condition through preconception counseling. This counsel-

 TEACHING GUIDELINES 20-4

Teaching to Prevent Hepatitis B Virus

- Abstain from alcohol.
- Avoid intravenous drug exposure or sharing of needles.
- Encourage all household contacts and sexual partners to be vaccinated.
- Receive immediate treatment for any sexually transmitted infection.
- Know that your newborn will receive the hepatitis B vaccine soon after birth.
- Use good handwashing techniques at all times.
- Avoid contact with blood or body fluids.
- Use barrier methods such as condoms during sexual intercourse.
- Avoid sharing any personal items, such as razors, toothbrushes, or eating utensils.

ing also should include determining the woman's varicella immunity; the vaccine is administered if needed. Alert women in occupations that increase the risk of exposure to the virus: daycare workers, teachers of young children, and staff caring for children in institutional settings.

Parvovirus B19

Parvovirus B19 is a common, self-limiting benign childhood virus that causes erythema infectiosum, also known as fifth disease (McCarter-Spaulding, 2002). The prevalence of this virus among pregnant women and fetuses is not known. The infection is spread transplacentally, by the oropharyngeal route in casual contact, and through infected blood. Approximately 50% to 65% of women of reproductive age have developed immunity to parvovirus B19.

Acute infection in pregnancy can cause B19 infection in the fetus, leading to nonimmune fetal hydrops secondary to severe anemia or fetal loss, depending on the gestational age at the time of infection. The risk to the fetus is greatest when the woman is exposed and infected in the first 20 weeks of gestation. In addition to hydrops, other fetal effects of parvovirus include spontaneous abortion, congenital anomalies (CNS, craniofacial, and eye), and long-term effects such as hepatic insufficiency, myocarditis, and learning disabilities (Cunningham & Rennels, 2004).

Clinical Manifestations

The characteristic rash starts on the face with a "slapped-cheeks" appearance. The rash is followed by a generalized maculopapular rash. Fever, arthralgia, and generalized malaise are usually present in the mother.

Treatment

Generally, diagnosis of parvovirus is based on clinical symptoms and serologic antibody testing for parvovirus immunoglobulin G and parvovirus immunoglobulin M (IgM). Schoolteachers, daycare workers, and women living with school-aged children are at highest risk for being seropositive for parvovirus B19, especially if a recent outbreak has occurred in those settings. Pregnant women who have been exposed to or who develop symptoms of parvovirus B19 require assessment to determine whether they are susceptible to infection (nonimmune). If the woman is immune, she can be reassured that she will not develop infection and that the virus will not adversely affect her pregnancy. If she is nonimmune, then referral to a perinatologist is recommended and counseling regarding the risks of fetal transmission, fetal loss, and hydrops is necessary. The likelihood of a healthy outcome is very high after parvovirus B19 infection in pregnancy. Because most pregnant women who become infected are asymptomatic, it is difficult to determine the risk of fetal infection. The infected newborn is assessed for any anomaly and followed for up to 6 years to identify any sequelae (Cunningham & Rennels, 2004).

Nursing Management

Prevention is the best strategy. Stress the need for hand-washing after handling children; cleaning toys and surfaces that children have been in contact with; and avoiding the sharing of food and drinks (McCarter-Spaulding, 2002).

Group B *Streptococcus*

Group B *Streptococcus* is a naturally occurring bacterium found in the human body that can cause sepsis in newborns. It is rarely serious in adults but can be life-threatening to newborns. It colonizes in the rectum, vagina, urethra, and cervix of women. Genital tract colonization poses the most threat to the newborn because of exposure during birth and to the mother because of ascending infection after the membranes rupture.

Group B *Streptococcus* affects about 1 in every 2,000 newborns in the United States (March of Dimes, 2004). If a pregnant woman carries the bacterium in her vagina or rectum during labor, there is a 1-in-100 chance that her newborn will become ill from a group B streptococcal infection. The risk rises to 4% if the woman has a preterm birth, prolonged rupture of membranes (>18 hours), or fever (100.4°F or higher) during labor. It is thought that newborns who become ill with group B streptococcal infection take the bacterium into their bodies by ingesting infected amniotic fluid or vaginal fluids during birth (Narayanan & Ossiani, 2004).

Clinical Manifestations

Most often, women with group B streptococcal infection are asymptomatic. However, many present with urinary tract infections, uterine infections, and chorioamnionitis. Newborns with early-onset (within a week after birth) group B streptococcal infections may have pneumonia or sepsis, whereas late-onset (after the first week) infections often manifest with meningitis (CDC, 2002).

Treatment

Antibiotic therapy usually is effective in treating women with infections of the urinary tract or uterus, or chorioamnionitis without any sequelae. According to the 2002 CDC guidelines, all pregnant women should be screened for group B *Streptococcus* at 35 to 37 weeks' gestation. The recommendation resulted from ACOG's review of the latest data, which compared a risk-based versus a screening approach. Vaginal and rectal specimens are cultured for the presence of the bacterium. If positive, the woman should be treated with intravenous antibiotics during labor. A recent CDC study (2002) suggested that this approach may prevent nearly 90% of early-onset group B streptococcal infections.

Treatment of group B streptococcal infection includes penicillin G because of its narrow spectrum, with alternative antibiotics prescribed for clients with a penicillin allergy. The drug is usually administered intravenously at least 4 hours before birth so that it can reach adequate levels in the serum and amniotic fluid to reduce the risk of newborn colonization. Close monitoring is required during the administration of intravenous antibiotics because severe allergic reactions can occur rapidly.

Nursing Management

Nurses can assume the role of educator and advocate for all women and newborns to reduce group B streptococcal infections. When obtaining the woman's prenatal history, ask about any previous infection, and document this information to help prevent vertical transmission to the newborn. All women with a previous group B streptococcal infection during pregnancy should be treated with intravenous antibiotics during labor. Also ensure that pregnant women between 35 and 37 weeks' gestation are screened for group B streptococcal infection during their prenatal visit. Record the results and notify the birth attendant that the woman has tested positive for group B *Streptococcus*.

Toxoplasmosis

Toxoplasmosis is a relatively widespread parasitic infection caused by a one-celled organism, *Toxoplasma gondii*. When a pregnant woman is exposed to this protozoan, the infection can pose serious risks to her fetus. Between 1 in 1,000 and 8,000 newborns are born infected with toxoplasmosis in the United States (Gibbs et al., 2004). It is transferred by hand to mouth after touching cat feces while changing the cat litter box or through gardening in contaminated soil. Consuming undercooked meat, such as pork, lamb, or venison, can also transmit this organism.

A pregnant woman who contracts toxoplasmosis for the first time has approximately a 40% chance of passing the infection to her fetus (March of Dimes, 2005). Although the woman typically remains asymptomatic, transmission to her fetus can occur throughout pregnancy, the most severe being prior to the third trimester. A fetus who contracts congenital toxoplasmosis typically has a low birthweight, enlarged liver and spleen, chorioretinitis, jaundice, neurologic damage, and anemia (London et al., 2003).

Treatment of the woman during pregnancy to reduce the risk of congenital infection is a combination of pyrimethamine and sulfadiazine. Treatment with sulfonamides during pregnancy has been shown to reduce the risk of congenital infection.

Nursing Management

Prevention is the key to managing this infection. Nurses play a key role in educating the woman in measures to prevent toxoplasmosis (Teaching Guidelines 20-5).

T E A C H I N G G U I D E L I N E S 2 0 - 5

Teaching to Prevent Toxoplasmosis

- Avoid eating raw or undercooked meat, especially lamb or pork. Cook all meat to an internal temperature of 160°F throughout.
- Clean cutting boards, work surfaces, and utensils with hot soapy water after contact with raw meat or unwashed fruits and vegetables.
- Peel or thoroughly wash all raw fruits and vegetables before eating them.
- Wash hands thoroughly with warm water and soap after handling raw meat.
- Avoid feeding the cat raw or undercooked meats.
- Avoid emptying or cleaning the cat's litter box. Have someone else do it daily.
- Keep the cat indoors to prevent it from hunting and eating birds or rodents.
- Avoid uncooked eggs and unpasteurized milk.
- Wear gardening gloves when in contact with outdoor soil.
- Avoid contact with children's sandboxes, because cats can use them as litter boxes.

Special Populations at Risk

Every year there are an estimated 210 million pregnancies worldwide, with about 6 million of them in the United States (Alan Guttmacher Institute, 2004). Each pregnancy runs the risk of an adverse outcome for the mother and the baby. Risks are dramatically increased for certain populations: adolescents, women who are HIV positive, older women, and substance abusers. While risks cannot be totally eliminated once pregnancy has begun, they can be reduced through appropriate and timely interventions.

Every woman's experience with pregnancy is unique and personal. The circumstances each one faces and what pregnancy means to her involve emotions and experiences that belong solely to her. Many women in these special population groups go through this experience in confusion and isolation, feeling desperately in need of help but not knowing where to go. Although all pregnant women experience these emotions to a certain extent, they are heightened in women who have numerous psychosocial issues. Pregnancy is a stressful time. Pregnant women face wide-ranging changes in their lives, relationships, and bodies as they move toward parenthood. These changes can be challenging for a woman without any additional stresses but are even more so in the face of age extremes, illness, or substance abuse.

Skilled nursing interventions are essential to promote the best outcome for the client and her baby. Timely support and appropriate interventions during the perinatal

period can have long-standing implications for the mother and her newborn, ultimately with the goal of stability and integration of the family as a unit.

Pregnant Adolescent

Adolescence spans the time frame from the onset of puberty to the cessation of physical growth, roughly from 11 to 19 years of age. Adolescents vacillate between being children and being adults. They need to adjust to the physiologic changes their bodies are undergoing and establish a sexual identity during this time. They search for personal identity and desire freedom and independence of thought and action. However, they continue to have a strong dependence on their parents (O'Toole, 2005).

Developmental Tasks of Adolescence

Certain developmental tasks need to be accomplished during this period before an adolescent can advance to the next stage of maturity. The developmental tasks of adolescents include:

- Seeking economic and social stability
- Developing a personal value system
- Building meaningful relationships with others (Fig. 20-3)
- Becoming comfortable with their changing bodies
- Working to become independent from their parents
- Learning to verbalize conceptually (Bayley, 2003)

Adolescents have special needs related to their lifestyle to accomplish their developmental tasks in making a smooth transition to young adulthood. One of the biggest areas of need is sexual health. Adolescents commonly lack the information, skills, and services necessary to make informed choices related to their sexual and reproductive health. As a result of these issues, unplanned pregnancies occur. When they do, achievement of their developmental tasks, especially identity, often is interrupted as the adolescent attempts to integrate the tasks of pregnancy,

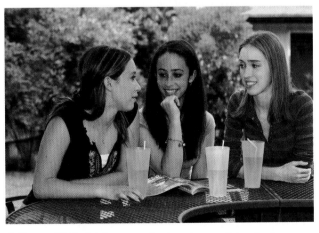

● Figure 20-3 Adolescents sharing time and developing relationships.

bonding, and preparing to care for another with the tasks of developing self-identity and independence. The process of learning how to separate from the parents while learning how to bond and attach to a newborn brings conflict and stress.

Adolescents have difficulty coping with and accomplishing their developmental tasks of identity formation and autonomy. Developmentally, adolescents are trying to figure out who they are and how they fit into society. As they mature, parents become less influential and peers become increasingly influential. Peer pressure and the desire to please their peers can influence adolescents to participate in behaviors in which they might normally not be involved. In addition, the onset of sexual maturation and the adolescent's belief that "it won't happen to me" contribute to high-risk behaviors.

The younger the adolescent is at the time of the first pregnancy, the more likely it is that she will have another pregnancy during her teens (Montgomery, 2003). In addition, a pregnancy can exacerbate an adolescent's feeling of loss of control (Youngkin & Davis, 2004). Healthcare providers must be able to communicate with adolescents in a manner they can understand, and respect them as unique individuals.

Incidence of Adolescent Pregnancy

The incidence of teenage pregnancy has steadily declined since the early 1990s, but it is still higher in the United States than in any other industrialized country (Green & Wilkinson, 2004). Even this reduced incidence represents what is considered an unacceptably high level of pregnancy in an age group that is likely to suffer the social consequences of early pregnancy most. Subsequently, adolescent pregnancy is considered a major health problem and is addressed in Healthy People 2010.

HEALTHY PEOPLE *2010*

National Health Goals Related to Adolescent Pregnancy

Objective	Significance
Reduce pregnancy among adolescent females from a baseline of 68 pregnancies per 1,000 adolescent girls to 43 pregnancies per 1,000 adolescent girls	Will help to foster a continued decline in adolescent pregnancy rates by focusing on interventions related to pregnancy prevention, including safe sex practices and teaching about the complications associated with adolescent pregnancy

USDHHS, 2000.

Each year in the United States, approximately 1 million adolescents, or 10% of girls between the ages of 15 to 19 years, become pregnant. These pregnancies, which account for 13% of all births, are typically unintended and occur outside of marriage (Alan Guttmacher Institute, 2004). In addition, about half of all teen pregnancies occur within 6 months of first having sexual intercourse. Of girls who become pregnant, one in six will have a repeat pregnancy within 1 year. Most of these girls are unmarried, and many are not ready for the emotional, psychological, and financial responsibilities of parenthood (Lowdermilk & Perry, 2004). Adolescent pregnancy is further complicated by the adolescent's lack of financial resources: the income of teen mothers is half that for women who have given birth in their 20s (Farrington, 2003).

Impact of Pregnancy on Adolescents

Adolescent pregnancy is a complex issue. Risk factors that contribute to adolescent pregnancy might include:

- Early menarche
- Peer pressure to become sexually active
- Sexual or other abuse as a child
- Lack of accurate contraceptive information
- Fear of telling parents of sexual activity
- Feelings of invulnerability
- Poverty (85% of births occur in poor families)
- Culture or ethnicity (high incidence in Hispanic and African-American girls)
- Unprotected sex
- Low self-esteem and inability to negotiate
- Lack of appropriate role models
- Strong need for someone to love
- Drug use, truancy from school, or other behavioral problems
- Wish to escape a bad home situation
- Early dating without supervision (Koshar, 2001)

Adolescent pregnancy has a negative impact in terms of both health and social consequences. For example, seven out of ten adolescents will drop out of school. More than 75% will receive public assistance within 5 years of having their first child. In addition, children of adolescent mothers are at greater risk of preterm birth, low birthweight, child abuse, neglect, poverty, and death (As-Sanie et al., 2004). The psychosocial risks associated with early childbearing often have an even greater impact on mothers, families, and society than the obstetric or medical risks (Pollard, 2003).

Pregnant adolescents also experience higher rates of domestic violence and substance abuse. Those experiencing abuse are more likely to abuse substances, receive inadequate prenatal care, and have lower pregnancy weight compared with those who are not (Harner, 2004). Moreover, substance abuse (cigarettes, alcohol, or illicit drugs) can contribute to low birthweight, IUGR, preterm births, newborn addiction, and sepsis (Montgomery, 2003).

Although early childbearing (12 to 19 years of age) occurs in all socioeconomic groups, it is more prevalent among poor women and those from minority backgrounds, who face more obstetric and newborn risks than their more affluent counterparts (Koniak-Griffin & Turner-Pluta, 2001). Poverty often contributes to delayed prenatal care and medical complications related to poor nutrition, such as anemia.

The financial burden of adolescent pregnancy is high and costs taxpayers an estimated $7 billion to $15 billion annually in the United States (McKinney et al., 2005). Much of the expense stems from Medicaid, food stamps, state health department maternity clinics, Aid to Families and Children, and direct payments to healthcare providers. However, this amount does not address the potential costs to society in terms of the loss of human resources and the far-reaching intergenerational effects of adolescent parenting.

For some adolescents, pregnancy may be seen as a hopeless situation: a grim story of poverty and lost dreams, of being trapped in a life that was never wanted. Health-related behaviors, such as smoking, eating habits, sexual behavior, and help-seeking behaviors, developed during adolescence often endure into later life (Bayley, 2003). Additionally, the consequences associated with an adolescent's less-than-optimal health status at this age due to pregnancy can ultimately affect her long-term health and that of her children. However, some adolescents can create a happy, stable life for themselves and their children by facing their challenges and working hard to beat the odds.

Nursing Management

Dealing with the complicated issues of adolescent pregnancy can be an emotionally charged situation, laden with ethical dilemmas and decisions. Topics such as abstinence, safer sex, abortion, and the decision to have a child are sensitive issues. Adolescent pregnancy is an area when a nurse's moral convictions may influence the care provided to clients. Nurses need to examine their own beliefs about teen sexuality to identify personal assumptions and discuss them. Putting aside one's moral convictions may be difficult, but it is necessary when working with adolescents who might be making decisions about their pregnancies.

Assessment

Assessment of the pregnant adolescent parallels that for any pregnant woman. However, the nurse also needs to address specific areas when dealing with pregnant teens. Areas to assess include:

- How does the girl see herself in the future?
- Are realistic role models available to her?
- How much does she know about child development?
- What financial resources are available to her?
- Does she work? Does she go to school?

- What emotional support is available to her?
- Can she resolve conflicts and manage anger?
- What does she know about health and nutrition for herself and her child?
- Will she need help dealing with the challenges of the new parenting role?
- Does she need information about community resources?

Having an honest regard for adolescents requires getting to know them and being able to appreciate the important aspects of their life. Doing so forms a basis for the nurse's clinical judgment and promotes care that takes into account the concerns and practical circumstances of the teen and her family. Skillful practice includes knowing how and when to advise a teen and when to listen and refrain from giving advice. Giving advice can be misinterpreted as "preaching," and the adolescent will probably ignore the information. The nurse must be perceptive, flexible, and sensitive and must work to establish a therapeutic relationship.

Nursing Interventions

For adolescents, as for all women, pregnancy can be a physically, emotionally, and socially stressful time. The pregnancy is often both the result of and cause of social problems and stressors that can be overwhelming to them. Nurses must support them during the transition from childhood into adulthood, which is complicated by their emergence into motherhood. Stress that the girl's physical well-being is significant for both her and her developing fetus, which depends on her for its own health-related needs. Monitor weight gain, sleep and rest patterns, and nutritional status to promote positive outcomes for both. Having a healthy newborn eases the transition to motherhood somewhat, rather than having to deal with the added stress of caring for an unhealthy baby (Harner, 2004).

Help the adolescent identify the options for this pregnancy, such as abortion, self-parenting of the child, temporary foster care for the baby or herself, or placement of the child for adoption. Explore with the adolescent why she became pregnant. Awareness of why she decided to have a child is necessary to help with the development of the adolescent and her ability to parent. Identify barriers to seeking prenatal care such as lack of transportation, too many problems at home, financial concerns, the long wait for an appointment, and lack of sensitivity on the part of the healthcare system.

Key nursing activities appropriate when caring for pregnant adolescents include:

- Provide appropriate teaching based on the adolescent's developmental level.
- Encourage the girl to return to school and further education.
- Make a referral for career or job counseling.

- Identify and support family and friends who want to become involved.
- Assist with arranging foster care, including stress management and self-care.
- Stress the importance of attending prenatal education classes.
- Monitor maternal and fetal well-being throughout pregnancy and labor (Fig. 20-4)
- Stress the importance of continued prenatal and follow-up care
- Encourage the girl to set goals and work toward them for the future.

Nurses can also play a major role in preventing adolescent pregnancies, perhaps by volunteering to talk to teen groups. Box 20-3 highlights the key areas for teaching adolescents about pregnancy prevention.

Tackling the many issues surrounding adolescent pregnancy is difficult. Making connections with clients is crucial regardless of how complex their situation is. The future challenges nurses to find solutions to teenage pregnancies. Nurses must take proactive positions while working with adolescents, parents, schools, and communities to reduce the problems associated with early childbearing.

The Pregnant Woman Over Age 35

The term "elderly primip" is used to describe women ages 35 or older who are pregnant for the first time. A few decades ago, a woman having a baby after the age of 35 probably was giving birth to the last of several children, but today she may be having her first. With advances in technology and the tendency of women to seek career advancement prior to childbearing, the dramatic increase in women having first pregnancies after the age of 35 will likely continue.

Whether childbearing is delayed by choice or by chance, starting a family at age 35 is different and not without risks. Women in this age group may already have chronic health conditions that may put the pregnancy at

---

BOX 20-3

TOPICS FOR TEACHING ADOLESCENTS TO PREVENT PREGNANCY

- High-risk behaviors that lead to pregnancy
- Involvement in programs such as Free Teens, Teen Advisors, or Postponing Sexual Involvement
- Planning and goal setting to visualize their futures in terms of career, college, travel, and education
- Choice of abstinence or taking a step back to become a "second-time virgin"
- Discussions about sexuality with a wiser adult—someone they respect can help put things in perspective
- Protection against sexually transmitted infections and pregnancy if they choose to remain sexually active
- Critical observation and review of peers and friends to make sure they are creating the right atmosphere for friendship
- Empowerment to make choices that will shape their life for years to come, including getting control of their own lives now
- Appropriate use of recreational time, such as sports, drama, volunteer work, music, jobs, church activities, and school clubs (Farrington, 2003)

---

risk. In addition, numerous studies have shown that increasing maternal age is a risk factor for infertility and spontaneous abortions, gestational diabetes, chronic hypertension, preeclampsia, preterm labor and birth, multiple pregnancy, genetic disorders and chromosomal abnormalities, placenta previa, IUGR, low Apgar scores, and surgical births (Neumann & Graf, 2003). However, even though increased age implies increased complications, most women today who become pregnant after age 35 have healthy pregnancies and healthy newborns (March of Dimes, 2004).

Nursing Management

In a woman of this age, a preconception visit is important to identify chronic health problems that might affect the pregnancy and also to address lifestyle issues that may take time to modify, such as cigarette smoking, poor nutrition, overweight or underweight, alcohol use, or illicit drug use. This visit provides the opportunity to educate the woman about risk factors and provide information on how to modify lifestyle habits to improve the pregnancy outcome.

During routine prenatal visits, the nurse can play a key role in promoting a healthy pregnancy. Social, genetic, and environmental factors that are unique to the older pregnant women need to be considered and assessed, with appropriate interventions planned. Although research has shown increases in preterm labor and births, low-birth-weight newborns, and operative interventions for older

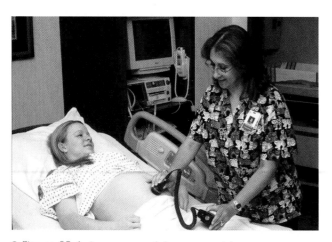

● Figure 20-4 A pregnant adolescent receiving care during labor.

women, many carry their pregnancies to term without incident (Neumann & Graf, 2003).

Encourage the older woman to plan for the pregnancy by seeing her healthcare provider before getting pregnant to discuss preexisting medical conditions, medications, and lifestyle choices. Also assist the woman with lifestyle changes so that she can begin pregnancy in an optimal state of health. For example, if the woman is overweight, educate her about weight loss so that she can start the pregnancy at a healthy weight. If the woman smokes, encourage smoking cessation to reduce the effects of nicotine on herself and her fetus. Additional teaching topics for the older woman to reduce her risks include:

• Get early and regular prenatal care to ensure the best possible outcomes.
• Take a multivitamin containing 400 micrograms of folic acid daily.
• Eat a variety of nutritious foods, especially fortified cereals, enriched grain products, and fresh fruits and vegetables, and drink at least six to eight glasses of water daily.
• Avoid alcohol intake during pregnancy.
• Avoid exposure to secondhand smoke.
• Take no drugs unless they are prescribed.

Women Who Are HIV Positive

Human immunodeficiency virus (HIV) is a retrovirus that is transmitted by blood and body fluids. The three recognized modes of HIV transmission are unprotected sexual intercourse with an infected partner, contact with infected blood or blood products, and perinatal transmission. HIV is not transmitted by doorknobs, faucets, toilets, dirty dishes, mosquitoes, wet towels, coughing or sneezing, shaking hands, or being hugged or by any other indirect method. The number of people living with HIV infection in 2004 was estimated at nearly 38 million, including approximately 20 million women of childbearing age and 2.5 million children, most of whom acquired HIV from mother-to-child transmission (Mirochnick & Capparelli, 2004).

The virus attacks the T4 cells, decreases the CD4 cell count, and disables the immune system. The HIV condition can progress to a severe immunosuppressed state termed **acquired immunodeficiency syndrome (AIDS).** AIDS is a progressive, debilitating disease that suppresses cellular immunity, predisposing the infected person to opportunistic infections and malignancies. The CDC defines AIDS as an HIV-infected person with a specific opportunistic infection or a CD4 count of less than 200 (Katz, 2003). Eventually, death occurs (Green & Wilkinson, 2004). The time from infection with HIV to development of AIDS is a median of 11 years but varies depending on whether the patient is taking current antiretroviral therapy (McKinney et al., 2005). Research indicates that pregnancy does not accelerate the progression of HIV to AIDS or death (Public Health Service Task Force, 2002).

Incidence and Prevalence

Despite the revolutionary strides that have been made in treatment and detection and recent clinical advances and cautious optimism associated with combination therapies and potential vaccines, the number of individuals who are HIV positive continues to climb worldwide. Intensive efforts notwithstanding, there still remains no real "cure" on the horizon (Penny, 2003).

Historically, HIV/AIDS was associated with the male homosexual community and intravenous drug users, but currently the prevalence of HIV/AIDS is now increasing more rapidly among women than men (PHSTF, 2002). Women are the fastest-growing segment of persons becoming infected with HIV; transmission in women occurs most frequently from sexual contact (64%) and from intravenous drug use (33%) (Koniak-Griffin et al., 2003). Most women, a large number of whom are mothers, have acquired the disease through heterosexual contact. The risk of acquiring HIV through heterosexual contact is greater for women due to exposure to the higher viral concentration in semen. In addition, sexual intercourse may cause breaks in the vaginal lining, increasing the chances that the virus will enter the woman's body. Fifty percent of all the HIV/AIDS cases worldwide occur in women. AIDS is the third leading cause of death among all U.S. women aged 25 to 44 years and the leading cause of death among African-American women in this age group (CDC, 2002).

Stages of Infection

Once infected with HIV, the woman develops antibodies that can be detected with the enzyme-linked immunosorbent assay (ELISA) and confirmed with the Western blot test. Antibodies develop within 6 to 12 weeks after exposure, although this latent period is much longer in some women. Table 20-4 highlights the four stages of HIV infection according to the CDC (2002).

Perinatal Transmission

Cases of perinatal transmission (mother to fetus or child) of HIV have decreased in the past several years in the United States, primarily due to the use of zidovudine (ZDV) therapy in pregnant women infected with HIV. This has not been the case in poor countries without similar resources. The Joint United Nations programs on HIV/AIDS (UNAIDS) estimates that over 600,000 new infections due to mother-to-child transmission occur annually. This number is expected to increase rapidly as prevalence rises in Southeast Asia (McIntyre & Gray, 2002). Perinatal transmission rates are as high as 35% when there is no intervention (antiretroviral therapy) and below 5% when antiretroviral treatment and appropriate care are available.

Table 20-4 Stages of HIV Infection Outlined by the CDC

Stages	Description	Clinical Picture
I	Acute infection	Early stage with pervasive viral production Flu-like symptoms 2–4 weeks after exposure Signs and symptoms: weight loss, low-grade fever, fatigue, sore throat, night sweats, and myalgia
II	Asymptomatic infection	Viral replication continues within lymphatics Usually free of symptoms; lymphadenopathy
III	Persistent generalized lymphadenopathy	Possibly remaining in this stage for years; AIDS develops in most within 7–10 years Opportunistic infections occur
IV	End-stage disease (AIDS)	Severe immune deficiency High viral load and low CD4 counts Signs and symptoms: bacterial, viral, or fungal opportunistic infections, fever, wasting syndrome, fatigue, neoplasms, and cognitive changes

With perinatal transmission, approximately 25% to 50% of children manifest AIDS within the first year of life, and about 80% have clinical symptoms of the disease within 3 to 5 years (Penny, 2003). Breastfeeding is a major contributing factor for mother-to-child transmission, and the infected mother must be informed about this (Bartlett & Anderson, 2001). Given the devastating effects of HIV infection on children, preventing its transmission is critical (Littleton & Engebretson, 2005).

Maternal and Fetal/Newborn Risks

When a woman who is infected with HIV becomes pregnant, the risks to herself, her fetus, and the newborn are great. The risks are compounded by problems such as drug abuse, lack of access to prenatal care, poverty, poor nutrition, and high-risk behaviors such as unsafe sex practices and multiple sex partners, which can predispose the woman to additional sexually transmitted infections such as herpes, syphilis, or human papillomavirus (HPV). Subsequently, pregnant women who are HIV positive are at risk for preterm delivery, premature rupture of membranes, intrapartal or postpartum hemorrhage, postpartum infection, poor wound healing, and genitourinary tract infections (London et al., 2003).

The fetus and newborn also are at risk for prematurity, IUGR, low birthweight, and infection. Prompt treatment with antiretroviral medications for the HIV-infected infant may slow the progression of the disease.

Screening and Diagnosis

Screening only women that are identified as high risk based on their histories is inadequate due to the prolonged latency period that can exist after exposure. Also, research indicating that treatment with antiretroviral agents could reduce vertical transmission from the infected mother to the newborn has dramatically increased the importance of HIV antibody screening in pregnancy. As a result, the U.S. Public Health Service (USPHS) has recommended that all pregnant women be offered HIV antibody testing, regardless of their risk of infection, and that testing be done during the initial prenatal evaluation (Bartlett & Anderson, 2001). Testing is essential because treatments are available that can reduce the likelihood of perinatal transmission and maintain the health of the woman.

All women who are pregnant or planning a pregnancy should be offered HIV testing using ELISA. Reactive screening tests must be confirmed by an additional test, such as the Western blot or an immunofluorescence assay. The Western blot is the confirmatory diagnostic test. A positive antibody test confirmed by a supplemental test indicates that the woman has been infected with HIV and can pass it on to others. HIV antibodies are detectable in at least 95% of women within 3 months after infection (Lowdermilk & Perry, 2004).

Treatment

Women who are seropositive for HIV should be counseled about the risk of perinatal transmission and the potential for obstetric complications. The risk of perinatal transmission directly correlates with viral load (Minkoff, 2003). A discussion of the options on continuing the pregnancy, medication therapy, risks, perinatal outcomes, and treatment is warranted. Women who elect to continue with the pregnancy should be treated with antiretroviral therapy regardless of their CD4 count or viral load.

Treatment for pregnant women infected with HIV focuses on reducing the risk of perinatal transmission by drug therapy. The standard treatment is oral antiretroviral drugs given twice daily from 14 weeks' gestation until giving birth, intravenous administration during labor, and oral syrup for the newborn in the first 6 weeks of life (Katz, 2003). The goal of therapy is to reduce the viral load as much as possible, which reduces the risk of transmission to the fetus.

Decisions about the birthing method to be used are made on an individual basis based on several factors involving the woman's health status. Some reports suggest that cesarean birth may reduce the risk of HIV infection (PHSTF, 2002). Efforts to reduce instrumentation, such as avoiding the use of an episiotomy, fetal scalp electrodes, and scalp pH, will assist in reducing the newborn's exposure to bodily fluids. The Public Health Service recommends that women who are HIV positive should avoid breastfeeding to prevent HIV transmission to the newborn.

With access to appropriate therapies, the prognosis for pregnant women with HIV infection has improved significantly. In addition, the newborns of women with HIV infection who have received treatment usually do not become infected.

Unfortunately, therapy is complicated and medications are expensive. Moreover, the medications are associated with numerous adverse effects and possible toxic reactions. These therapies offer a dual purpose: reduce the likelihood of mother-to-infant transmission, and provide optimal suppression of the viral load in the mother. The core goal of all medical therapy is to bring the client's viral load to an undetectable level, thus minimizing the risk of transmission to the fetus and newborn.

Nursing Management

Women infected with HIV should have comprehensive prenatal care, which starts with pretest and posttest counseling. In pretest counseling, the client completes a risk assessment survey and the nurse explains the meaning of positive versus negative test results, obtains informed consent for HIV testing, and educates the woman on how to prevent HIV infection by changing lifestyle behaviors if needed. Posttest counseling includes informing the client of the test results, reviewing the meaning of the results again, and reinforcing safer sex guidelines. All pretest and posttest counseling should be documented in the client's chart.

Assessment

The usual screening tests done in normal pregnancy should be completed, but with an emphasis on sexually transmitted infections. Women infected with HIV have high rates of sexually transmitted infections, especially HPV, vulvovaginal candidiasis, bacterial vaginosis, syphilis, HSV, chancroid, CMV, gonorrhea, chlamydia, and hepatitis B (Williams, 2003). If there is no history of hepatitis B, the woman should receive the hepatitis vaccine, as well as the pneumococcal vaccine. Close follow-up of suspicious Pap smear results is prudent because of the increased risk of cervical changes associated with HPV and HIV (Dole, 2001).

Nursing Interventions

Pregnant clients are dealing with many issues at their first prenatal visit. The confirmation of pregnancy may be accompanied by feelings of joy, anxiety, depression, or other emotions. Simultaneously, the client is given many pamphlets and receives advice and counseling about many important health issues (e.g., nutrition, prenatal development, appointment schedules). This health teaching may be done while the woman feels excited, tired, and anxious. To expect women to understand detailed explanations of a complex disease entity (HIV/AIDS) too may be unrealistic. Determine the client's readiness for this discussion.

When providing direct care, follow standard precautions. Identify the client's individual needs for teaching, emotional support, and physical care. Approach education and counseling of HIV-positive pregnant women in a caring, sensitive manner. Address the following information:

- Infection control issues at home
- Safer sex precautions
- Stages of the HIV disease process
- Treatment modalities for each stage
- Preventive drug therapies for her unborn infant
- Symptoms of opportunistic infections
- Avoidance of breastfeeding
- Referrals to community counseling and financial aid
- Client's support system and potential caretaker
- Importance of continual prenatal care
- Well-balanced diet
- Measures to reduce exposure to infections

Be aware of the psychosocial sequelae of HIV/AIDS. A diagnosis of HIV can put a woman into an emotional tailspin, where she is worried about her own health and that of her unborn infant. She may experience grief, fear, or anxiety about the future of her children. Along with the medications that are so important to her health maintenance, a woman's mental health needs, family dynamics, capacity to work, and social concerns also must be addressed.

Nurses can help women face the reality of the diagnosis and the treatment options by first examining their own beliefs and attitudes toward women who are HIV positive or have AIDS. Empathy, understanding, caring, and assistance are key to helping the client and her family.

Nurses also need to be informed about HIV infection and how HIV is transmitted; to share the knowledge they have with all women; and to work to influence legislators, public health officials, and the entire health establishment toward policies to address the HIV epidemic. Research toward treatment and cure is tremendously important, but the major key to prevention of the spread of the virus is education. Nurses play a major role in this education.

Current evidence suggests that cesarean birth performed before the onset of labor and before the rupture of membranes significantly reduces the rate of perinatal transmission. ACOG recommends that women with HIV be offered elective cesarean birth to reduce the rate of transmission beyond that which may be achieved through antiretroviral therapy. They further suggest that operative births be performed at 38 weeks' gestation and that amniocentesis be avoided to prevent contamination of the amniotic fluid with maternal blood. Decisions concerning the method of delivery should be based on the woman's viral load, the duration of ruptured membranes, the progress of labor, and other pertinent clinical factors (USPHSTF, 2004).

After the birth of the newborn, the motivation for taking antiretroviral medications may be lower, thus affecting the woman's compliance with therapy. Encourage the woman to continue therapy for her own sake as well as that of the newborn. Nurses can make a difference in helping women to adhere to their complex drug regimens.

Reinforce family planning methods during this time, incorporating a realistic view of her disease status. The use of oral contraceptives with concurrent use of condoms is recommended (Katz, 2003). Advise the woman that breastfeeding is not recommended. Instruct the HIV-positive woman in self-care measures, including the proper method for disposing of perineal pads to reduce the risk of exposing others to infected body fluids. Adhere to standard precautions when providing direct client care. Finally, teach the HIV-positive woman the signs and symptoms of infection in newborns and infants, encouraging her to report any to the healthcare provider.

The Pregnant Woman With Substance Abuse

The incidence of substance abuse during pregnancy is highly variable because most pregnant women are reluctant to reveal the extent of their use. **Perinatal drug abuse** is the use of alcohol and other drugs among pregnant women. The National Institute on Drug Abuse estimates that 6% of the women in the United States have used illicit drugs while pregnant, including cocaine, marijuana, heroin, and psychotherapeutic drugs that were not prescribed by a healthcare professional. More than 18% used alcohol and 21% smoked cigarettes during their pregnancy (Carter, 2002).

The use of drugs, legal or not, increases the risk of medical complications in the mother and poor birth outcomes in the newborn. The placenta acts as an active transport mechanism, not as a barrier, and thus substances pass from a mother to her fetus through the placenta, directly affecting its growth and development.

A woman who claims to have taken no drugs while pregnant may be unaware that substances such as hair dye, diet cola, paint, or over-the-counter (OTC) medications for colds or headaches are still considered drugs. Thus, it is very difficult to get a true picture of the real use of drugs by pregnant women.

Many drugs are considered to have a teratogenic effect on growing fetuses. A **teratogen** is any environmental substance that can cause physical defects in the developing embryo and fetus. Pregnant women with substance abuse commonly present with polysubstance abuse, which is likely to be more damaging than the use of any single substance. Thus, it is inherently difficult to ascribe a specific perinatal effect to any one substance (Shieh & Kravitz, 2002).

Maternal and Fetal Effects

Substance abuse during pregnancy, particularly in the first trimester, has a negative effect on the health of the mother and the growth and development of the fetus. The fetus experiences the same systemic effects as the mother, but often more severely. The fetus cannot metabolize drugs as efficiently as the expectant mother and will experience the effects long after the drugs have left the women's system. Substance abuse during pregnancy is associated with preterm labor, abortion, low birthweight, CNS and fetal anomalies, and long-term childhood developmental consequences (Littleton & Engebretson, 2005). Table 20-5 summarizes the effects of selected drugs during pregnancy.

Impact of Addiction

Addiction is a multifaceted process that is affected by environmental, psychological, family, and physical factors. Women who use drugs, alcohol, or tobacco come from all socioeconomic backgrounds, cultures, and lifestyles. Risk factors associated with substance abuse during a pregnancy may include low self-esteem, inadequate support systems, low self-expectations, high levels of anxiety, socioeconomic barriers, involvement in abusive relationships, chaotic familial and social systems, and a history of psychiatric illness or depression (Lowdermilk & Perry, 2004). Women often become substance abusers to relieve their anxieties, depression, and feelings of worthlessness (Green & Wilkinson, 2004).

Societal attitudes regarding women and substance abuse may prohibit them from admitting the problem and seeking treatment. Society sanctions women for failing to live up to expectations of how a pregnant woman "should" behave, thereby possibly driving them further away from the treatment they so desperately need. For many reasons, pregnant women who abuse substances feel unwelcome in prenatal clinics or medical settings. Often they seek prenatal care late or not at all. They may fear being shamed or reported to legal or child protection authorities. A non-judgmental atmosphere and unbiased teaching to all pregnant women regardless of their lifestyle is crucial. A caring, concerned manner is critical to help these women feel "safe" and respond honestly to assessment questions.

Pregnancy can be a motivator for some who want to try treatment. The goal of therapy is to help the client deal

Table 20-5 Effects of Selected Drugs on Pregnancy

Substance	Effect on Pregnancy
Alcohol	Spontaneous abortion, inadequate weight gain, IUGR, fetal alcohol spectrum disorder, the leading cause of mental retardation
Caffeine	Vasoconstriction and mild diuresis in mother; fetal stimulation, but teratogenic effects not documented via research
Nicotine	Vasoconstriction, reduced uteroplacental blood flow, decreased birthweight, abortion, prematurity, abruptio placentae, fetal demise
Cocaine	Vasoconstriction, gestational hypertension, abruptio placentae, abortion, "snow baby syndrome," CNS defects, IUGR
Marijuana	Anemia, inadequate weight gain, "amotivational syndrome," hyperactive startle reflex, newborn tremors, prematurity, IUGR
Narcotics	Maternal and fetal withdrawal, abruptio placentae, preterm labor, premature rupture of membranes, perinatal asphyxia, newborn sepsis and death, intellectual impairment, malnutrition
Sedatives	CNS depression, newborn withdrawal, maternal seizures in labor, newborn abstinence syndrome, delayed lung maturity

Sources: Youngkin and Davis, 2004; McKinney et al., 2005; London et al., 2003.

with pregnancy by developing a trusting relationship. Providing a full spectrum of medical, social, and emotional care is needed.

Common Substances Abused During Pregnancy

Alcohol

Alcohol abuse is a major public health issue in the United States. Alcohol is a teratogen, a substance known to be toxic to human development. Approximately 10% of pregnant women report alcohol consumption (CDC, 2004). Theoretically, no mother would give a glass of wine, beer, or hard liquor to her newborn, but when she drinks, her embryo or fetus is exposed to the same blood alcohol concentration as she is. The teratogenic effects of heavy maternal drinking have been recognized since 1973, when fetal

alcohol syndrome was first described. Fetal alcohol syndrome is now a classification under the broader term of **fetal alcohol spectrum disorder;** this disorder includes the full range of birth defects, such as structural anomalies and behavioral and neurocognitive disabilities caused by prenatal exposure to alcohol (Eustace et al., 2003; Hoyme et al., 2005). Fetal alcohol spectrum disorder is completely preventable and is the leading cause of mental retardation (CDC, 2004).

Not every woman who drinks during pregnancy will give birth to an affected child. Based on the best research available, the following is known about alcohol consumption during pregnancy:

- Intake increases the risk of alcohol-related birth defects, including growth deficiencies, facial abnormalities, CNS impairment, behavioral disorders, and intellectual development.
- No amount of alcohol consumption is considered safe during pregnancy.
- Damage to the fetus can occur at any stage of pregnancy, even before a woman knows she is pregnant.
- Cognitive defects and behavioral problems resulting from prenatal exposure are lifelong.
- Alcohol-related birth defects are completely preventable (USDHHS, 2005).

Risk factors for giving birth to an alcohol-affected newborn include maternal age, socioeconomic status, ethnicity, genetic factors, depression, family disorganization, unplanned pregnancy, and maternal metabolism (Mattson & Smith, 2004). Identification of risk factors strongly associated with alcohol-related birth outcomes could help identify high-risk pregnancies requiring intervention.

Characteristics of fetal alcohol spectrum disorder include craniofacial dysmorphia, IUGR, microcephaly, and congenital anomalies such as limb abnormalities and cardiac defects. Long-term sequelae include postnatal growth restriction, attention deficits, delayed reaction time, and poor scholastic performance (NoFAS, 2003). The complex neurobehavioral problems typically manifest themselves insidiously. Common cognitive and behavioral problems are listed in Box 20-4.

The child with fetal alcohol spectrum disorder presents with characteristic facial features (Fig. 20-5) that include a small head circumference, short palpebral fissures, and small eye openings, a thin upper lip, a receding jaw, a short nose, a low nasal bridge, a groove between the nose and the upper lip, skin folds at the corner of the eye (epicanthal folds), and a small, flat midface area. Minor ear abnormalities also may be noted (Hoyme et al., 2005).

One of the biggest challenges in determining the true prevalence of fetal alcohol spectrum disorder is how to recognize the syndrome, which depends in part on the age and physical features of the person being assessed. Difficulty in identifying alcohol abuse is due to the client's denial of alcohol use, unwillingness to report alcohol

BOX 20-4

COMMON COGNITIVE AND BEHAVIORAL PROBLEMS ASSOCIATED WITH FETAL ALCOHOL SPECTRUM DISORDER

- Attention-deficit/hyperactivity disorder (ADHD)
- Inability to foresee consequences
- Inability to learn from previous experience
- Lack of organization
- Learning difficulties
- Poor abstract thinking
- Poor impulse control
- Speech and language problems
- Poor judgment

consumption, underreporting, and limited ability to recollect the frequency, quantity, and type of alcohol consumed. This makes it difficult to identify women who are drinking during pregnancy, institute preventive measures, or refer them for treatment.

Women who drink excessively while pregnant are at high risk for giving birth to children with birth defects. Thus, to prevent these defects, women should stop drinking during all phases of a pregnancy. Unfortunately, many women continue to drink during their pregnancy despite warnings from professionals.

Currently, it is not known whether there is a minimal amount of alcohol safe to drink during pregnancy; an occasional glass of wine might be harmless or might not be. Therefore, eliminating alcohol consumption during pregnancy is the ultimate goal to prevent fetal alcohol spectrum disorder. Most women know they shouldn't drink during pregnancy, but the "window of vulnerability"—the time lag between conception and the discovery of pregnancy—may put substantial numbers of children at risk. A multidisciplinary approach is key.

A key challenge in screening pregnant women for alcohol use arises from the fact that traditional alcohol-

screening questionnaires, such as the Michigan Alcoholism Screening Test (MAST) and the CAGE Questionnaire, are not sensitive enough to detect low levels of alcohol consumption among women. Several challenges remain for the future in preventing birth defects due to alcohol consumption:

- Ways to improve clinical recognition of high-risk women who drink alcohol
- Ways to intervene more effectively to modify drinking behaviors
- In utero approaches to prevent or minimize fetal injury
- Strategies to address the neurodevelopmental problems of children affected by maternal alcohol ingestion

Caffeine

Caffeine is a CNS stimulant and is present in varying amounts in such common products as coffee, tea, colas, and chocolate. It is also in cold remedies and analgesics. Birth defects have not been linked to caffeine consumption, but maternal coffee consumption decreases iron absorption and may increase the risk of anemia during pregnancy. The FDA recommends that pregnant women eliminate or limit their consumption of caffeine to less than 300 mg/day (three cups of coffee or cola) (Lowdermilk & Perry, 2004).

Nicotine

Nicotine, found in cigarettes, is another substance that is harmful to the pregnant women and her fetus. Nicotine, which causes vasoconstriction, transfers across the placenta and reduces blood flow to the fetus, contributing to fetal hypoxia. When compared with alcohol, marijuana, and other illicit drug use, tobacco use is less likely to decline as the pregnancy progresses (Wang, 2004).

Women who smoke during the pregnancy also continue to smoke after giving birth, and thus the infant will be exposed to nicotine after birth. This environmental or passive exposure has an impact on the child's development and increases the risk of childhood respiratory disorders.

Smoking increases the risk of spontaneous abortion, preterm labor and birth, maternal hypertension, placenta previa, and abruptio placentae. The perinatal death rate among infants of smoking mothers is 20% to 35% higher (Gabbe et al., 2002). It has also been considered an important risk factor for low birthweight; sudden infant death syndrome (SIDS); and cognitive deficits, especially in language, reading, and vocabulary, as well as poorer performances on tests of reasoning and memory. Researchers have also reported behavior problems, such as increased activity, inattention, impulsivity, opposition, and aggression (Wang, 2004).

Cocaine

Cocaine use is second only to marijuana in women who abuse drugs during pregnancy. The incidence of cocaine

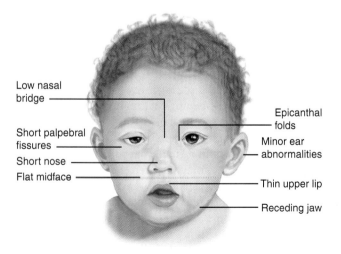

Low nasal bridge

Short palpebral fissures

Short nose

Flat midface

Epicanthal folds

Minor ear abnormalities

Thin upper lip

Receding jaw

● Figure 20-5 Facial characteristics in a newborn with FASD.

exposure in utero is 1 to 10 per 1,000 live births (Weekes & Lee, 2004).

Cocaine is a psychoactive drug derived from the leaves of the coca plant, which grows in the Andes Mountains of Peru, Ecuador, and Bolivia. The freebase form, called "crack" because of the cracking or popping noise made in its preparation, is less expensive, easily made, and smokable. Cocaine is a powerful vasoconstrictor. When sniffed into the mucous membranes of the nose, it produces an intense "rush" that some have compared to an orgasmic experience (Sloane, 2002). Smoked crack is absorbed rapidly by the pulmonary vasculature and reaches the brain's circulation in 6 to 8 seconds (Weekes & Lee, 2004).

Cocaine use produces vasoconstriction, tachycardia, and hypertension in both the mother and the fetus (Weekes & Lee, 2004). Uteroplacental insufficiency may result from reduced blood flow and placental perfusion. Chronic use can result in low birthweight, the most common effect of cocaine use in pregnancy (Littleton & Engebretson, 2005).

Studies suggest that perinatal cocaine use increases the risk of preterm labor, abortion, abruptio placentae, IUGR, intrauterine fetal distress and demise, seizures, withdrawal, and cerebral infarcts. Cocaine may increase the risk of uterine rupture and congenital anomalies (London et al., 2003). Some infants exposed to cocaine in utero show increased irritability and are difficult to calm and soothe to sleep.

Other fetal anomalies associated with cocaine use in early pregnancy involve neurologic problems such as neural tube defects and microcephaly; cardiovascular anomalies such as congenital heart defects; genitourinary conditions such as prune belly syndrome, hydronephrosis, and ambiguous genitalia; and gastrointestinal system problems such as necrotizing enterocolitis (Mattson & Smith, 2004).

Marijuana

Marijuana is the most commonly used illicit drug in America, with about 83 million people having tried it at least once. It is often called pot, reefer, grass, weed, herb, Mary Jane, or MJ (Mattson & Smith, 2004). Marijuana is a preparation of the leaves and flowering tops of *Cannabis sativa*, the hemp plant, which contains a number of pharmacologically active agents. Tetrahydrocannabinol (THC) is the most active ingredient of marijuana. With heavy smoking, THC narrows the bronchi and bronchioles and produces inflammation of the mucous membranes. Smoking marijuana causes tachycardia and a reduction in blood pressure, resulting in orthostatic hypotension.

Marijuana is not considered teratogenic, but many newborns display altered responses to visual stimuli, increased tremulousness, and a high-pitched cry, which might indicate CNS insults (Wang, 2004). The effects of marijuana smoking on pregnancy are not yet fully understood because there are very few studies on its long-term effects on child development. One can speculate that the effects of marijuana on the immature nervous system may be subtle and not detected until more complex functions are required, usually in a formal educational setting. There is some evidence that marijuana increases the risk of spontaneous abortion and preterm delivery (O'Toole, 2003). Use of marijuana is highly correlated with use of alcohol and cigarettes.

Opiates and Narcotics

Opiates and narcotics include opium, heroin (known as horse, junk, smack, downtown), morphine, codeine, hydromorphone (Dilaudid; little D), oxycodone (Percodan, perkies), meperidine (Demerol, demise), and methadone (meth, dollies). These drugs are CNS depressants that soothe and lull. They may be used medically for pain, but all have a high potential for abuse. Most cause an intense addiction in both mother and newborn.

Narcotic dependence is particularly problematic in pregnant women. It leads to medical, nutritional, and social neglect by the woman due to the long-term risks of physical dependence, malnutrition, compromised immunity, hepatitis, and fatal overdose (Alexander et al., 2004). Taking opiates or narcotics during pregnancy places the woman at increased risk for preterm labor, IUGR, and preeclampsia (Wang, 2004).

Heroin is the most common illicitly used opioid. It is derived from the seeds of the poppy plant and can be sniffed, smoked, or injected. It crosses the placenta via simple diffusion within 1 hour of maternal consumption (Moran, 2004). Use of heroin during pregnancy is believed to affect the developing brain of the fetus and may cause behavioral abnormalities in childhood (Alexander et al., 2004).

The most common harmful effect of heroin on newborns is withdrawal, or **neonatal abstinence syndrome** (see Chapter 24). This collection of symptoms may include irritability, hypertonicity, a high-pitched cry, vomiting, diarrhea, respiratory distress, disturbed sleeping, sneezing, diaphoresis, fever, poor sucking, tremors, and seizures (Littleton & Engebretson, 2005).

Withdrawal from opiates during pregnancy is extremely dangerous for the fetus, so a prescribed oral methadone maintenance program combined with psychotherapy is recommended. This closely supervised treatment program reduces withdrawal symptoms and exposure to HIV and other sexually transmitted infections because she is no longer injecting drugs. However, methadone has the same withdrawal consequences for women and newborns as heroin does.

Sedatives

Sedatives relax the CNS and are used medically for inducing relaxation and sleep, relieving tension, and treating seizures. Sedatives easily cross the placenta and cause birth defects and behavioral problems. Infants born to mothers who abuse sedatives during pregnancy may be physically dependent on the drugs themselves and are more prone to respiratory problems, feeding difficulties, disturbed sleep, sweating, irritability, and fever (Alexander et al., 2004)

Nursing Management

Substance abuse during pregnancy remains a huge problem in our society. The maternal and fetal consequences are still underestimated and more research is needed to validate its impact. Nursing management emphasizes screening and prevention to reduce the high incidence of obstetric and medical complications among users, as well as the morbidity and mortality among their passively addicted infants.

Assessment

Substance abuse screening in pregnancy is done to detect the use of any substance known or suspected to exert a deleterious effect on the client or her fetus. Routinely ask about substance abuse with all women of childbearing age, inform them of the risks involved, and advise them against continuing. Screening questionnaires are helpful in identifying potential users, may reduce the stigma of asking clients about substance abuse, and result in a more accurate and consistent evaluation. The questions in Box 20-5 may help assess a client who is at risk for substance abuse during pregnancy. Using accepting terminology may encourage honest answers without fear of reproach.

A urine toxicology screen may also be helpful in determining drug use, although a urine screen identifies only recent or heavy use of drugs. The length of time a drug is present in urine is as follows:

- Cocaine: 24 to 48 hours in an adult, 72 to 96 hours in an infant
- Heroin: 24 hours in an adult, 24 to 48 hours in an infant
- Marijuana: 1 week to 1 month in an adult, up to a month or longer in an infant
- Methadone: up to 10 days in an infant (Wang, 2004)

A positive drug screen in a newborn warrants an investigation by the state protection agency. In the interim, the newborn's comfort is paramount; environmental control will help reduce the stress and stimuli (see Chapter 24 for a more in-depth discussion).

A positive screen is an opportunity for the nurse and the client to discuss prenatal exposure to substances that may be harmful. The discussion may lead the nurse to refer the client for a diagnostic assessment or identify an intervention such as counseling that may be helpful. Being nonjudgmental is a key to success; a client is more apt to trust and reveal patterns of abuse if the nurse does not judge the client and her lifestyle choices.

Nursing Interventions

Nursing interventions must be provided in a supportive, proactive, and accepting fashion. Assure women with substance abuse problems that sharing information of a confidential nature with healthcare providers will not render them liable to criminal prosecution. Perform counseling and education, emphasizing the following:

- Education about the effects of substance exposure on the fetus
- Interventions to improve mother–child attachment and improve parenting
- Psychosocial support if treatment is needed to reduce substance abuse
- Referral to outreach programs to improve access to treatment facilities
- Hazardous legal substances to avoid during pregnancy
- Follow-up of children born to substance-dependent mothers
- Dietary counseling to improve the pregnancy outcome for both mother and child
- Drug screening to identify all drugs a client is using
- More frequent prenatal visits to monitor fetal well-being
- Maternal and fetal benefits of remaining drug-free
- Cultural sensitivity
- Coping skills, support systems, and vocational assistance

Substance abuse is a complex problem that requires sensitivity to each woman's unique situation and contributing factors. Be sure to address individual psychological and sociocultural factors to help the woman to regain control of her life. Treatment must combine different approaches and provide ongoing support for women learning to live drug-free. Developing personal strengths,

---

BOX 20-5

SAMPLE QUESTIONS FOR ASSESSING SUBSTANCE USE

- Have you ever used recreational drugs? If so, when and what?
- Have you ever taken a prescription drug other than as intended?
- What are your feelings about drug use during pregnancy?
- How often do you smoke cigarettes? How many per day?
- How often do you drink alcohol?

If the assessment reveals substance use, obtain additional information by using the RAFFT questions, which are a sensitive screening instrument for identifying substance abuse (Weekes & Lee, 2004):

R: Do you drink or take drugs to **R**elax, improve your self-image, or fit in?

A: Do you ever drink or take drugs while **A**lone?

F: Do you have any close **F**riends who drink or take drugs?

F: Does a close **F**amily member have a problem with alcohol or drugs?

T: Have you ever gotten in **T**rouble from drinking or taking drugs?

such as communication skills and assertiveness, and self-confidence will help the woman to resist drugs. Encourage the use of appropriate coping skills. Enhancing self-esteem also helps provide a foundation to avoid drugs.

KEY CONCEPTS

● Preconception counseling for the woman with diabetes is helpful in promoting blood glucose control to prevent congenital anomalies.

● The classification system for diabetes commonly used is based on disease etiology and not pharmacology management; the classification includes type 1 diabetes, type 2 diabetes, gestational diabetes, and impaired fasting glucose and impaired glucose tolerance.

● A functional classification for heart disease during pregnancy is based on past and present disability: class I, asymptomatic with no limitation of physical activity; class II, symptomatic (dyspnea, chest pain) with increased activity; class III, symptomatic (fatigue, palpitation) with normal activity; and class IV, symptomatic at rest or with any physical activity.

● Chronic hypertension exists when the woman has a blood pressure of 140/90 mm Hg or higher before pregnancy or before the 20th week of gestation or when hypertension persists for more than 12 weeks postpartum.

● Successful management of asthma in pregnancy involves elimination of environmental triggers, drug therapy, and client education.

● Ideally, women with hematologic conditions are screened before conception and are made aware of the risks to themselves and to a pregnancy.

● A wide variety of infections, such as rubella, herpes simplex, hepatitis B, varicella, parvovirus B19, and many sexually transmitted infections can affect the pregnancy, having a negative impact on its outcome.

● The younger the adolescent is at the time of the first pregnancy, the more likely it is that she will have another pregnancy during her teens. About 1 million teenagers between the ages of 15 and 19 become pregnant each year; about half give birth and keep their infants.

● The nurse's role in caring for the pregnant adolescent is to assist her in identifying the options for this pregnancy, including abortion, self-parenting of the child, temporary foster care for the baby or herself, or placement for adoption.

● The prevalence of HIV/AIDS is increasing more rapidly among women then men: half of all the HIV/AIDS cases worldwide now occur in women. There are only three recognized modes of HIV transmission: unprotected sexual intercourse with an infected partner, contact with infected blood or blood products, and perinatal transmission.

Breastfeeding is a major contributing factor in mother-to-child transmission of HIV.

● Cases of perinatal AIDS have decreased in the past several years in the United States, primarily because of the use of zidovudine (ZDV) therapy in pregnant women with HIV. The U.S. Public Health Service recommends that all pregnant women should be offered HIV antibody testing regardless of their risk of infection, and that testing should be done during the initial prenatal evaluation.

● Pregnant women with substance abuse problems commonly abuse several substance, making it difficult to ascribe a specific perinatal effect to any one substance. Societal attitudes regarding pregnant women and substance abuse may prohibit them from admitting the problem and seeking treatment.

● Substance abuse during pregnancy is associated with preterm labor, abortion, low birthweight, CNS and fetal anomalies, and long-term childhood developmental consequences.

● Fetal alcohol spectrum disorder is a lifelong yet completely preventable set of physical, mental, and neurobehavioral birth defects; it is the leading cause of mental retardation in the United States.

● Nursing management for the woman with substance abuse focuses on screening and preventing substance abuse to reduce the high incidence of obstetric and medical complications as well as the morbidity and mortality among passively addicted newborns.

References

Alan Guttmacher Institute (2004). *In the know about pregnancy, contraception and abortion.* [Online] Available at: http://www.guttmacher.org/in-the-know/pregnancy.html

Alexander, L. L., LaRosa, J. H., Bader, H., & Garfield, S. (2004). *New dimensions in women's health* (3rd ed.). Sudbury: Jones & Bartlett Publishers.

American Diabetes Association (ADA) (2004). Gestational diabetes mellitus. *Diabetes Care, 27,* S88–S90.

American Heart Association (2003). *Heart disease and stroke statistics, 2003 update.* Dallas: American Heart Association.

Anderson, W. E., & Safdar, A. (2005). Varicella-zoster virus. EMedicine. [Online] Available at: http://emedicine.com/med/topic2361.htm.

As-Sanie, S., Gantt, A., & Rosenthal, M. S. (2004) Pregnancy prevention in adolescents. *American Family Physician, 70*(8), 1517–1524.

Barbour, L. A. (2003) New concepts in insulin resistance of pregnancy and gestational diabetes: long-term implications for mother and offspring. *Journal of Obstetrics and Gynecology, 23*(5), 545–549.

Bartlett, J. G., & Anderson, J. R. (2001). Updated guidelines for managing HIV in pregnancy for the USPHS Task Force. The Hopkins HIV Report [Online]. Available at: http://www.hopkins-aids.edu/publications/report/may01_1.html

Bayley, O. (2003). Improvement of sexual and reproductive health requires focusing on adolescents. *Lancet, 362*(9386), 830–832.

Beckmann, C. A. (2002). Women's perceptions of their asthma during pregnancy. *MCN, 27*(2), 98–102.

Beckmann, C. A. (2003). The effects of asthma on pregnancy and perinatal outcomes. *Journal of Asthma, 40*(2), 171–180.

Blackburn, S. T. (2003). *Maternal, fetal, & neonatal physiology: a clinical perspective.* Philadelphia: Saunders.

Blaiss, M. S. (2004). Managing asthma during pregnancy. *Postgraduate Medicine, 115*(5), 55–63.

Carter, C. S. (2002). Perinatal care for women who are addicted: implications for empowerment. *Health and Social Work, 27*(3), 166–175.

CDC (2002). Semiannual HIV/AIDS surveillance report, 13(2) [Online]. Available at: www.cdc.gov/hiv/stats/htm

CDC (2002). Prevention of perinatal group B streptococcal disease: revised guidelines from CDC. *Morbidity and Mortality Weekly Report, 51*(RR-11), 1–28.

CDC (2003). *Rubella* [Online] Available at: www.cdc.gov/nip/publications/pink/rubella.pdf

CDC (2004). Alcohol consumption among women who are pregnant or who might become pregnant, United States, 2002. *Morbidity and Mortality Weekly Report, 53*(50), 1178–1181.

CDC (2005). *Fact sheet: viral hepatitis B.* [Online] Available at: http://www.cdc.gov/ncidod/diseases/hepatitis/b/fact.htm

Criteria Committee of the New York Heart Association (1994). *Nomenclature and criteria for diagnosis of diseases of the heart and great vessels* (9th ed.). Dallas: American Heart Association.

Cunningham, D., & Rennels, M. B. (2004). Parvovirus B19 infection. *eMedicine.* [Online] Available at: http://www.emedicine.com/ped/topic192.htm

Cunningham, F. G., Gant, N. F., Leveno, K. J., et al. (2001). *Williams obstetrics* (21st ed.). New York: McGraw-Hill.

Damato, E. G., & Winnen, C. W. (2002). Cytomegalovirus infection: perinatal implications. *JOGNN, 31*(1), 86–92.

Dole, P. J. (2001). Primary care of HPV management in HIV-infected women. *Nurse Practitioner Forum, 12*(4), 214–222.

Donahue, D. B. (2002). Diagnosis and treatment of herpes simplex infection during pregnancy. *JOGNN, 31*(1), 99–106.

Dornhorst, A., & Frost, G. (2002). The principles of dietary management of gestational diabetes: reflection on current evidence. *Journal of Human Nutrition & Dietetics, 15*, 145–156.

Dudek, S. G. (2006). *Nutrition essentials for nursing practice* (5th ed.). Philadelphia: Lippincott Williams & Wilkins.

Eustace, L. W., Kang, D. H., & Coombs, D. (2003). Fetal alcohol syndrome: a growing concern for health care professionals. *JOGNN, 32*(2), 215–221.

Expert Committee on the Diagnosis and Classification of Diabetes Mellitus (2003). Report of the Expert Committee on the Diagnosis and Classification of Diabetes Mellitus. *Diabetes Care, 26*(suppl 1), S5–S20.

Farrington, J. (2003). The realities of teen parenting. *Current Health 2* (Human Sexuality Supplement), *29*(7), 1–5.

Feig, D. S., & Palda, V. A. (2003). Type 2 diabetes in pregnancy: a growing concern. *Lancet, 359*, 1690–1692.

Fischer, R. (2004). Genital herpes in pregnancy. *EMedicine.* [Online] Available at: http://www.emedicine.com/med/topic3554.htm

Gabbe, S. G., & Graves, C. R. (2003). Management of diabetes mellitus complicating pregnancy. *Obstetrics and Gynecology, 102*, 857–868.

Gabbe, S., Niebyl, J., & Simpson, J. (2002). *Obstetrics: normal and problem pregnancies.* Philadelphia: Churchill Livingstone.

Gibbs, R. S., Sweet, R. L., & Duff, W. P. (2004). Maternal and infectious diseases. In R. K. Creasy, R. Resnik, & J. D. Iams (Eds.), *Maternal-fetal medicine: principles and practice* (5th ed., pp. 741–801). Philadelphia: Saunders.

Gilbert, E., & Harmon, J. (2003) *Manual of high-risk pregnancy and delivery* (3rd ed.). St. Louis: Mosby.

Goswami, G., & Ong, K. (2005). Cardiovascular disease and pregnancy. *EMedicine.* [Online] Available at: http://www.emedicine.com/med/topic3251.htm

Green, C. J., & Wilkinson, J. M. (2004). *Maternal newborn nursing care plans.* St. Louis: Mosby.

Harner, H. M. (2004). Domestic violence and trauma care in teenage pregnancy: does paternal age make a difference? *JOGNN, 33*(3), 312–319.

Harvey, E. A. (2004). Hypertensive disorders or pregnancy: pathophysiology, symptoms and treatment. *Nursing Spectrum.* [Online] Available at http://nsweb.nursingspectrum.com/ce/m23c-1.htm.

Herchline, T., & Amorosa, J. K. (2005) Tuberculosis. *EMedicine.* [Online] Available at: http://www.emedicine.com/MED/topic2324.htm

Hoyme, H. E., May, P. A., Kalberg, W. O., et al. (2005). A practical clinical approach to diagnosis of fetal alcohol spectrum disorders:

clarification of 1996 Institute of Medicine Criteria. *Pediatrics, 115*(1), 39–47.

Joint National Committee (JNC). *Seventh Report of the Joint National Committee on Prevention, Detection, Evaluation, and Treatment of High Blood Pressure.* (2003). National Institutes of Health (NIH), National Heart, Lung, and Blood Institute. NIH Publication No. 035233. Washington, D.C.: NIH.

Katz, A. (2003). The evolving art of caring for pregnant women with HIV infection. *JOGNN, 32*(1), 102–108.

Katz, A. (2004). Preventing heart disease in women: new guidelines take personal approach to preventing cardiovascular disease. *AWHONN Lifelines, 8*(2), 119–120.

Kazzi, A. A., & Marachelian, A. (2004). Pregnancy, asthma. *EMedicine.* [Online] Available at: http://www.emedicine.com/emerg/topic476.htm

Kendrick, J. M. (2004). Diabetes in pregnancy. *March of Dimes Nursing Module.* White Plains, NY: March of Dimes Education and Health Promotion.

Koniak-Griffin, D., Lesser, J., Uman, G., Stein, J. A., & Cumberland, W. G. (2003). Project CHARM: an HIV prevention program for adolescent mothers. *Family and Community Health, 26*(2), 94–107.

Koniak-Griffin, D., & Turner-Pluta, C. (2001). Health risks and psychosocial outcomes of early childbearing: a review of the literature. *Journal of Perinatal and Neonatal Nursing, 15*(2), 1–17.

Koren, G., Nulman, I., Chudley, A. E., & Loocke, C. (2003). Fetal alcohol spectrum disorder. *Journal of the Canadian Medical Association, 169*(11), 1181–1185.

Koshar, J. H. (2001). Teen pregnancy 2001: still no easy answers. *Pediatric Nursing, 27*(5), 505–509.

Kuczkowski, K. M. (2004). Labor analgesia for the parturient with cardiac disease: what does the obstetrician need to know? *Acta Obstetrics and Gynecology Scandinavica, 83*, 223–233.

Laartz, B., & Gompf, S. G. (2004). Viral infections and pregnancy. *EMedicine.* [Online] Available at: http://www.emedicine.com/med/topic3270.htm

Lake, M. F. (2001). Tuberculosis in pregnancy. *AWHONN Lifelines, 5*(5), 35–40.

Landon, M. B. (2004) Diseases of the liver, biliary system, and pancreas. In R. K. Creasy, R. Resnik, & J. D. Iams (Eds.), *Maternal-fetal medicine: principles and practice* (5th ed., pp. 1127–1145), Philadelphia: Saunders.

Lin, K. W., & Kirchner, J. T. (2004). Hepatitis B. *American Family Physician, 69*(1), 75–86.

Littleton, L. Y., & Engebretson, J. C. (2005). *Maternity nursing care.* Clifton Park, NY: Thomson Delmar Learning.

London, M. L., Ladewug, P. W., Ball, J. W., & Bindler, R. C. (2003). *Maternal-newborn & child nursing.* Upper Saddle River, NJ: Prentice-Hall.

Lowdermilk, D. L., & Perry, S. E. (2004). *Maternity & women's health care* (8th ed.). Philadelphia: Mosby.

March of Dimes (2004). *Pregnancy after 35: Quick reference and fact sheet.* [Online] Available at: http://www.modimes.org/professionals/681_1155.asp

March of Dimes (2004). Group B strep infection. *March of Dimes Birth Defects Foundation.* [Online] Available at: http://www.marchofdimes.com/professionals/681_1205.asp

March of Dimes (2005). Toxoplasmosis. *March of Dimes Birth Defects Foundation.* [Online] Available at: http://www.marchofdimes.com/printableArticles/681_1228.asp?printable=true

Martin, J., et al. (2002). Births: final data for 2000. *National Vital Statistics Report, 50*(5), 1–104.

Martin, S. R., & Foley, M. R. (2002). Adult-onset heart disease in pregnancy. *Contemporary OB/GYN, 47*(11), 74–92.

Mattson, S., & Smith, J. E. (2004). *Core curriculum for maternal-newborn nursing* (3rd ed.). St. Louis: Elsevier Saunders.

McCann, J. A. S. (2004). *Maternal-neonatal nursing made incredibly easy.* Philadelphia: Lippincott Williams & Wilkins.

McCarter-Spaulding, D. E. (2002). Parvovirus B19 in pregnancy. *JOGNN, 31*(1), 107–112.

McIntyre, J., & Gray, G. (2002). What can we do to reduce mother to child transmission of HIV? *British Medical Journal, 324*(7331), 218–222.

Messner, M. G. (2004). Managing women with gestational diabetes. *Clinical Advisor, 7*(11), 32–35.

Minkoff, H. (2003). Human immunodeficiency virus infection in pregnancy. *Obstetrics & Gynecology, 101*(4), 797–811.

McKinney, E. S., James, S. R., Murray, S. S., & Ashwill, J. W. (2005). *Maternal-child nursing* (2nd ed.). St. Louis: Elsevier Saunders.

Mirochnick, M., & Capparelli, E. (2004). Pharmacokinetics of anti-retrovirals in pregnant women. *Clinical Pharmacokinetics, 43*(15), 1071–1087.

Montgomery, K. S. (2003). Nursing care for pregnant adolescents. *JOGNN, 32*(2), 249–257.

Moran, B. A. (2004). Substance abuse in pregnancy. In S. Mattson & J. E. Smith, *Core curriculum for maternal-newborn nursing* (3rd ed., pp. 750–770). St. Louis: Elsevier Saunders.

Murray, S. S. & McKinney, E. S. (2006). *Foundations of maternal-newborn nursing* (4th ed.) Philadelphia: W. B. Saunders.

Narayanan, S. K., & Ossiani, M. (2004). Streptococcus group B infections. *eMedicine.* [Online] Available at: http://www.emedicine.com/med/topic2185.htm

National Asthma Education and Prevention Program (NAEPP) (2005). NAEPP Expert Panel Report: managing asthma during pregnancy. *Journal of Allergy & Clinical Immunology, 115*, 36–46.

Neumann, M., & Graf, C. (2003). Pregnancy after age 35. *AWHONN Lifelines, 7*(5), 423–430.

NoFAS (2003). What is fetal alcohol syndrome? [Online]. Available at: http://www.nofas.org/main/what_is_FAS.htm

O'Toole, M. T. (2005). *Encyclopedia & dictionary of medicine, nursing, & allied health,* 7th ed. Philadelphia: Saunders.

Peddicord, K. (2005). Healthy hearts for women. *AWHONN Lifelines, 9*(1), 35–38.

Penny, J. (2003). HIV/AIDS—2003 update. *Vital Signs, 8*(3), 15–19.

Pollard, T. (2003). Teenage pregnancy still a challenge for all. *British Journal of Community Health, 8*(3), 102.

Poole, J. H. (2003). Thalassemia and pregnancy. *Journal of Perinatal and Neonatal Nursing, 17*(3), 196–208.

Prasad, A. K., & Ventura, H. O. (2001). Valvular heart disease and pregnancy. *Postgraduate Medicine, 110*(2), 69–79.

Public Health Service Task Force (PHSTF) (Feb. 4, 2002). *Recommendations for use of antiretroviral drugs in pregnant HIV-infected women for maternal health and interventions to reduce perinatal HIV-transmission in the United States.* Washington, D.C.: Author.

Ryan, E. A. (2003). Hormones and insulin resistance during pregnancy. *Lancet, 362,* 1777–1778.

Samson, L., & Ferguson, H. W. (2004). Chronic medical conditions and pregnancy, part I. *Nursing Spectrum.* [Online] Available at: http://nsweb.nursingspectrum.com/ce/m23a-1.htm

Shieh, C., & Kravitz, M. (2002). Maternal-fetal attachment in pregnant women who use illicit drugs. *JOGNN, 31*(2), 156–164.

Siu, S., & Colman, J. M. (2004). Cardiovascular problems and pregnancy: an approach to management. *Cleveland Clinic Journal of Medicine, 71*(12), 977–985.

Sloane, E. (2002). *Biology of women* (4th ed.). New York: Delmar.

SmithBattle, L. (2003). Displacing the "Rule Book" in caring for teen mothers. *Public Health Nursing, 20*(5), 369–376.

Tiller, C. M. (2002) Chlamydia during pregnancy: implications and impact on neonatal outcomes. *JOGNN, 31*(1), 93–98.

Turok, D. K., Ratcliffe, S. D., & Baxley, E. G. (2003). Management of gestational diabetes mellitus. *American Family Physician, 68*(9), 1767–1772.

U.S. Department of Health and Human Services (USDHHS) (2000) *Healthy people 2010* (Conference Edition, vol. 1). Washington, D.C.

U.S. Department of Health and Human Services (USDHHS) (2005) *U.S. Surgeon General releases advisory on alcohol use in pregnancy.* HHS Office of the Surgeon General. [Online] Available at: http://hhs.gov/surgeongeneral/pressreleases/sg02222005.html

U.S. Preventive Services Task Force (USPSTF) (2003). Screening for gestational diabetes mellitus: recommendation and rationale. *American Family Physician, 68*(2), 331–336.

U.S. Preventive Services Task Force (USPSTF) (2004). *Updated USPHSTF recommendations for the use of antiretroviral drugs in pregnant HIV-1-infected women for maternal health and interventions to reduce perinatal HIV-1 transmission in the United States.* [Online] Available at: http://aidsinfo.nih.gov

Wallerstedt, C., & Clokey, D. E. (2004). Endocrine and metabolic disorders. In S. Mattson & J. E. Smith, *Core curriculum for maternal-newborn nursing* (3rd ed., pp. 660–702). St. Louis: Elsevier Saunders.

Wang, M. (2004). Perinatal drug abuse and neonatal withdrawal. *eMedicine.* [Online] Available at: http://www.emedicine.com/ped/topic2631.htm

Weekes, A. J., & Lee, D. S. (2004). Substance abuse: cocaine. *eMedicine.* [Online] Available at: http://www.emedicine.com/ped/topic2666.htm

Wenger, N. K. (2004). Cardiovascular disease in women: new guidelines stress prevention. *Consultant, 44*(4), 660–663.

Williams, A. (2003). Gynecologic care for women with HIV infection. *JOGNN, 32*(1), 87–93.

Wolbretta, D. (2003). Treatment of arrhythmias during pregnancy. *Current Women's Health Reports, 3,* 135–139.

Youngkin, E. Q., & Davis, M. S. (2004). *Women's health: a primary care clinical guide* (3rd ed.). Upper Saddle River, NJ: Pearson Prentice Hall.

Web Resources

Alan Guttmacher Institute: **http://www.agi-usa.org**
Alcoholics Anonymous: **www.alcoholics-anonymous.org**
American Academy of Pediatrics: **www.aap.org**
American College of Obstetricians and Gynecologists: **www.acog.org**
American Diabetes Association: **www.diabetes.org**
American Lung Association: **www.lungusa.org**
American Medical Association HIV/AIDS Resource Center: **www.ama-assn.org/special/hiv**
American Society of Addiction Medicine: **www.asam.org**
Association of Women's Health, Obstetric & Neonatal Nurses: **www.awhonn.org**
Association of Nurses in AIDS Care: **www.anacnet.org**
Asthma and Allergy Foundation of America: **www.aafa.org**
Allergy & Asthma Network of Mothers of Asthmatics: **www.breatherville.org**
CDC National Prevention Information Network: 1-800-458-5231, **www.cdcnpin.org**
HIV websites: www.hivinsite.ucsf.edu, **www.hivatis.org**
International Nurses Society on Addictions: **www.intnsa.org**
March of Dimes: **www.modimes.org**
Narcotics Anonymous: **www.na.org**
National Campaign to Prevent Teen Pregnancy: **www.teenpregnancy.org**
National Clearinghouse for Alcohol and Drug Abuse Information: **www.health.org**
National Heart, Lung and Blood Institute of NIH: **www.nhlbi.nih.gov**
National Institute on Drug Abuse: **www.nida.nih.gov**
National Organization for Fetal Alcohol Syndrome: **www.nofas.org**
Planned Parenthood: **wwwplannedparenthood.org**
Sex Information and Education Council of United States: **www.siecus.org**
Sidelines High Risk Pregnancy Support Office: **www.sidelines.org**
Tobacco Information and Prevention Source (TIPS): **www.cdc.gov/tobacco**
Women for Sobriety Support Group: **www.womenforsobriety.org**

Chapter WORKSHEET

● MULTIPLE CHOICE QUESTIONS

1. Which of the following would the nurse include when describing the pathophysiology of gestational diabetes?

   a. Pregnancy fosters the development of carbohydrate cravings.

   b. There is progressive resistance to the effects of insulin.

   c. Hypoinsulinemia develops early in the first trimester.

   d. Glucose levels decrease to accommodate fetal growth.

2. When providing prenatal education to a pregnant woman with asthma, which of the following would be important for the nurse to do?

   a. Explain that she should avoid steroids during her pregnancy.

   b. Demonstrate how to assess her blood glucose levels.

   c. Teach correct administration of subcutaneous bronchodilators.

   d. Ensure she seeks treatment for any acute exacerbation.

3. Which of the following conditions would cause an insulin-dependent diabetic client the most difficulty during her pregnancy?

   a. Placenta previa

   b. Hyperemesis gravidarum

   c. Abruptio placentae

   d. Rh incompatibility

4. Women who drink alcohol during pregnancy:

   a. Often produce more alcohol dehydrogenase

   b. Usually become intoxicated faster than before

   c. Can give birth to an infant with fetal alcohol spectrum disorder

   d. Gain fewer pounds throughout the gestation

5. Transmission of HIV from an infected individual to another person occurs:

   a. Only if there is a large viral load in the blood

   b. Most commonly as a result of sexual contact

   c. In all infants born to women with HIV infection

   d. Most frequently in nurses with needlesticks

● CRITICAL THINKING EXERCISES

1. A client at 26 weeks' gestation came to the clinic to follow up on her previous 1-hour glucose screening. Her results had come back outside the accepted screening range, and a 3-hour glucose tolerance test (GTT) had been ordered. It resulted in three abnormal values, confirming a diagnosis of gestational diabetes. As the nurse in the prenatal clinic you are seeing her for the first time.

   a. What additional information will you need to provide care for her?

   b. What education will she need to address this new diagnosis?

   c. How will you evaluate the effectiveness of your interventions?

2. A 14-year-old white girl comes to the public health clinic with her mother. The mother tells you that her daughter has been "out messing around and has got herself pregnant." The girl is crying quietly in the corner and avoids eye contact with you. The mother reports that her daughter "must be following in my footsteps" because she herself became pregnant when she was only 15 years old. The client's mother goes back out into the waiting room and leaves the client with you.

   a. What is your first approach with the client to gain her trust?

   b. List the client's educational needs during this pregnancy.

   c. What prevention strategies are needed to prevent a second pregnancy?

3. Linda, a 27-year-old G3, P2 is admitted to the labor and birth suite because of preterm rupture of membranes at an estimated 35 weeks' gestation. She has received no prenatal care and reports this was an unplanned pregnancy. Linda appears distracted and very thin. She reports that her two previous children have been in foster care since birth because the child welfare authorities "didn't think I was an adequate mother." She denies any recent use of alcohol or drugs but offers no further explanation. She has a spontaneous vaginal birth a few hours later, producing a 4-lb boy with Apgar scores of 8 at one minute and 9 at 5 minutes.

   a. What aspects of this woman's history make you concerned that this infant is at risk for fetal alcohol spectrum disorder?

b. What additional screening or laboratory tests might validate your suspicion?

c. What physical and neurodevelopmental deficits might present later in life if the infant has fetal alcohol spectrum disorder?

● STUDY ACTIVITIES

1. In the maternity clinic or hospital setting, interview a pregnant woman with a preexisting medical condition (e.g., diabetes, asthma, sickle cell anemia) and find out how this condition affects her life and this pregnancy, especially her lifestyle choices.

2. You have a close friend who has a problem with drugs or alcohol but doesn't think she has a problem. How would you handle this situation?

3. Should marijuana be legalized in the United States? What impact might your view (pro or con) have on pregnant women and their offspring?

4. Outline a discussion you might have with an HIV-positive pregnant woman who doesn't see the need to take antiretroviral agents to prevent perinatal transmission.

5. Which of the following conditions would not preclude a woman from breastfeeding? Select all that apply:

a. Hepatitis B

b. Parvovirus B19

c. Herpesvirus type 2

d. HIV-positive status

e. Cytomegalovirus

f. Varicella-zoster virus

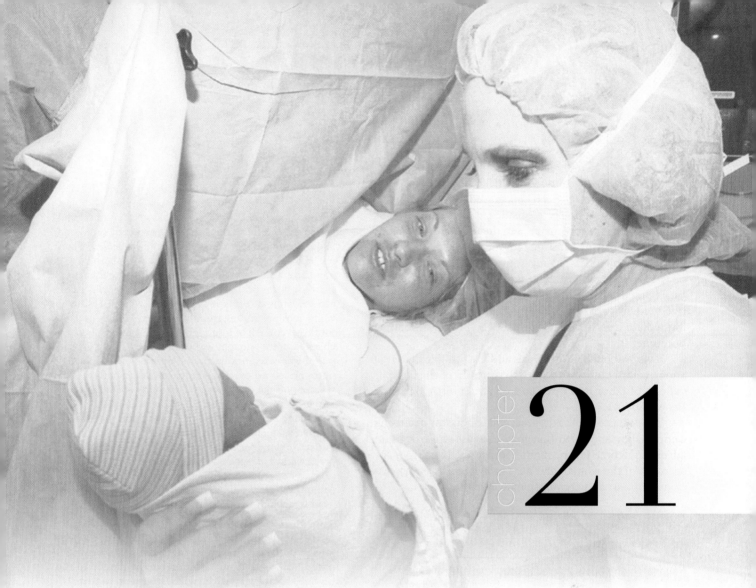

chapter 21

Nursing Management of Labor and Birth at Risk

KeyTERMS

amnioinfusion
cesarean birth
dystocia
hypertonic uterine
    dysfunction
hypotonic uterine
    dysfunction
forceps
labor induction
postterm pregnancy
umbilical cord prolapse
vacuum extractor
vaginal birth after
    cesarean (VBAC)

LearningOBJECTIVES

After studying the chapter content, the student should be able to accomplish the following:

1. Define the key terms.
2. Identify dysfunctional labor patterns and appropriate interventions to promote maternal and fetal well-being.
3. Discuss the care needed for a woman experiencing a postterm pregnancy.
4. Describe obstetric emergency situations, including appropriate management.
5. Explain nursing management for the woman undergoing labor induction/augmentation, forceps- and vacuum-assisted birth, cesarean birth and vaginal birth after cesarean (VBAC).

In face of a crisis or a potentially bad outcome, add a mixture of warmth and serenity to your technical abilities.

Most women describe pregnancy as an exciting time in their life, but the development of an unexpected problem can suddenly change this description dramatically. Consider the woman who has had a problem-free pregnancy and then suddenly develops a condition during labor, changing a routine situation into a possible crisis. Many complications give little or no warning and present challenges for the perinatal healthcare team as well as the family. The nurse plays a major role in identifying the problem quickly and coordinating immediate intervention, ultimately achieving a positive outcome.

Two National Health Goals address positive maternal and newborn outcomes related to issues involving complications of labor and birth and cesarean birth (Healthy People 2010).

This chapter will address several conditions occurring during labor and birth that may increase the risk of an adverse outcome for the mother and fetus. Nursing management of the woman and her family focuses on professional support and compassionate care.

HEALTHY PEOPLE 2010

National Health Goals Related to Labor and Birth at Risk

Objective	Significance
Reduce maternal illness and complications due to pregnancy	Will help to focus attention on the need for close antepartum surveillance and identification of risk factors for maternal illness and complications, particularly those most likely to be associated with maternal death
Reduce maternal complications during hospitalized labor and delivery from a baseline of 31.2/100 deliveries to a target of 24/100 deliveries	
Reduce cesarean births among low-risk (full term, singleton, vertex presentation) women	Will help to promote development of specific guidelines for trials of labor and labor management, continual labor support, and practice patterns, while helping to ensure positive maternal and newborn outcomes
Reduce the number of cesarean births in women giving birth for the first time from a baseline of 18% to 15%	
Reduce the number of cesarean births in women with prior cesarean birth from 72% to 63%	

USDHHS, 2000.

Consider THIS!

I attended all the natural childbirth classes and felt like I would be prepared for anything concerning labor and birth. I had purchased several books on the subject and surfed the Internet extensively for anything I could find about birthing. I was truly "up for the challenge" when my labor pains started. My partner was ready to be a good coach and help me through this life experience, until my water broke spontaneously and the baby's cord came floating down too. There I was, with this glistening white cord protruding from my vagina. I didn't prepare for this event! All of a sudden the whole atmosphere changed, from one that was calm to, now, a big production. I was asked to turn myself upside down while the nurse placed a gloved hand into my raised bottom to take pressure off the cord as we sailed to the operating room in this position for an immediate cesarean birth.

Looking back over that experience, I was glad for everyone's quick response, which saved my child's life, but at the same time it taught me a life lesson—You can prepare for the expected childbirth events, but you really need to be prepared for the unexpected ones that occur without warning! I am grateful for the nurses, who knew what to do, and I appreciate their quick actions.

Thoughts: No one has a crystal ball to see what the future holds for any of us, and certainly not a prolapsed cord. It is an event that rarely can be anticipated, although many women can be placed in the high-risk category with twins, malpresentation, hydramnios, or preterm infants. Despite not being in a high-risk category, this woman still experienced this unexpected event. Nurses always need to be prepared for any emergency, even if risk factors are absent. What important assessment is needed when membranes rupture? What instructions should the woman be given should this occur?

Dysfunctional Labor

Dystocia, defined as abnormal or difficult labor, can be influenced by a vast number of maternal and fetal factors. Dystocia is said to exist when the progress of labor deviates from normal and is characterized by a slow and abnormal progression of labor. It occurs in approximately 8% to 11% of all labors and is the leading indicator for primary cesarean birth in the United States (Ressel, 2004).

To characterize a labor as abnormal, a basic understanding of normal labor is essential. Normal labor starts with regular uterine contractions that are strong enough to result in cervical effacement and dilation. Early in labor, uterine contractions are irregular and cervical effacement and dilation are gradual. When cervical dilation reaches 4 cm and uterine contractions become more powerful, the active phase of labor begins. It is usually during the active phase that dystocia becomes apparent. Because dystocia cannot be predicted or diagnosed with certainty, the term "failure to progress" is often used. This term includes lack of progressive cervical dilation, lack of descent of the fetal head, or both. An adequate trial of labor is needed to declare with confidence that dystocia or "failure to progress" exists.

Early identification of and prompt interventions for dystocia are essential to minimize risk to the woman and fetus. According to American College of Obstetrics and Gynecology (ACOG), factors associated with an increased risk for dystocia include epidural analgesia, excessive analgesia, multiple gestation, hydramnios, maternal exhaustion, ineffective maternal pushing technique, occiput posterior position, longer first stage of labor, nulliparity, short maternal stature (<5′), fetal birth weight (>8.8 lb), shoulder dystocia, abnormal fetal presentation or position (breech), fetal anomalies (hydrocephalus), maternal age older than 35 years, gestational age more than 41 weeks, chorioamnionitis, ineffective uterine contractions, and high fetal station at complete cervical dilation (Ressel, 2004).

Dystocia can result from problems or abnormalities involving the expulsive forces (known as the "powers"); presentation, position, and fetal development (the "passenger"); the maternal bony pelvis or birth canal (the "passageway"); and maternal stress (the "psyche").

Problems With the Powers

When expulsive forces of the uterus become dysfunctional, the uterus may either never fully relax (hypertonic contractions), placing the fetus in jeopardy, or relax too much (hypotonic contractions), causing ineffective contractions. Still another dysfunction can occur when the uterus contracts so frequently and with such intensity that a very rapid birth will take place (precipitous labor).

Hypertonic Uterine Dysfunction
Hypertonic uterine dysfunction occurs when the uterus never fully relaxes between contractions. Subsequently, contractions are erratic and poorly coordinated because more than one uterine pacemaker is sending signals for contraction. Placental perfusion becomes compromised, thereby reducing oxygen to the fetus. These hypertonic contractions exhaust the mother, who is experiencing frequent, intense, and painful contractions with little progression. This dysfunctional pattern occurs in early labor and affects nulliparous women more than multiparous women (Smith, 2004).

These contractions occur in the latent phase of the first stage of labor (cervical dilation of <4 cm) and are uncoordinated. Typically, the force of the contractions occurs in the midsection of uterus at the junction of the active upper and passive lower segments of the uterus rather than in the fundus. Thus, the downward pressure to push the presenting part against the cervix is lost (Gilbert & Harmon, 2003). Commonly, the woman becomes discouraged due to her lack of progress and has increased pain secondary to uterine anoxia.

Diagnosis
The diagnosis of a hypertonic labor pattern is based on the characteristic hypertonicity of the contractions and the lack of labor progress.

Treatment
Treatment of this dysfunctional labor pattern involves therapeutic rest with the use of sedatives to promote relaxation and stop the abnormal activity of the uterus. Any factors that might be contributing to this abnormal labor pattern are identified and addressed. Because high resting tone and persistent pain are also seen in abruptio placentae, this complication needs to be ruled out prior to making treatment decisions. After a 4- to 6-hour rest period, many women will awaken and begin a normal labor pattern (Condon, 2004).

Hypotonic Uterine Dysfunction
Hypotonic uterine dysfunction occurs during active labor (dilation >4 cm) when contractions become poor in quality and lack sufficient intensity to dilate and efface the cervix. This dysfunction is often termed secondary uterine inertia because the labor begins normally and then the frequency and intensity of contractions decrease (Joy & Lyon, 2005). Common factors associated with this dysfunctional labor pattern include an overdistended uterus with a multifetal pregnancy or a large single fetus; too much pain medicine given too early in labor; fetal malposition; and regional anesthesia (Bonilla & Forouzan, 2004). The major risk with this complication is hemorrhage after giving birth because the uterus cannot contract effectively to compress blood vessels.

Diagnosis
Diagnosis of this dysfunctional labor pattern includes evaluation of the woman's labor to confirm that the woman is having hypotonic active labor rather than a long latent phase. The maternal pelvis and fetal presentation and position are also evaluated to ensure that they are not contributing to the prolonged labor without noticeable progress.

Treatment
Treatment of this dysfunctional labor pattern involves identifying the causes of inefficient uterine action, which might include a malpositioned fetus, a maternal pelvis that is too small, or overdistention of the uterus with fluid or a macrosomic fetus. If all of the causes that might contribute to dysfunction are ruled out, then rupture of the amniotic sac (amniotomy) usually is performed. In addition, labor augmentation with oxytocin (Pitocin) may be used to stimulate effective uterine contractions. If neither of these interventions evokes a change in progress, a cesarean birth is needed.

Precipitous Labor

Precipitous labor is one that is completed in less than 3 hours. This pattern is characterized by an abrupt onset of higher-intensity contractions occurring in a shorter period of time instead of the more gradual increase in frequency, duration, and intensity that typifies most spontaneous labors. Women experiencing precipitous labor typically have soft perineal tissues that stretch readily, permitting the fetus to pass through the pelvis quickly and easily. Maternal complications are rare if the maternal pelvis is adequate and the soft tissues yield to a fast fetal descent.

Diagnosis

Diagnosis of this rapid labor pattern is based on the rapidity of progress through the stages of labor. Potential fetal complications may include head trauma, such as intracranial hemorrhage or nerve damage, and hypoxia due to the rapid progression of labor (Kennelly et al., 2003).

Treatment

Typically, the fetus is delivered vaginally if the maternal pelvis is adequate.

Problems With the Passenger

Any presentation other than occiput anterior or a slight variation of the fetal position or size increases the probability of dystocia. These variations can affect the contractions or fetal descent through the maternal pelvis. Common problems involving the fetus include occiput posterior position, breech presentation, multifetal pregnancy, excessive size (macrosomia) as it relates to cephalopelvic disproportion (CPD), and structural anomalies.

Persistent Occiput Posterior Position

Persistent occiput posterior is the most common malposition, occurring in about 15% of laboring women. The fetal head engages in the left or right occipito-transverse position and the occiput rotates posteriorly rather than into the more favorable occiput anterior position. In effect, the fetus will be born facing upward instead of the normal downward position (Bonilla & Forouzan, 2004).

The reasons for this malrotation are often unclear. This position presents slightly larger diameters to the maternal pelvis, thus slowing the progress of fetal descent. A fetal head that is poorly flexed may be responsible. In addition, poor uterine contractions may not push the fetal head down into the pelvic floor to the extent that the fetal occiput sinks into it rather than being pushed to rotate in an anterior direction. The labor is usually much longer and more uncomfortable (causing increased back pain during labor) if the fetus remains in this position.

Diagnosis

The diagnosis is made clinically by vaginal examination in conjunction with the mother's complaints of severe back pain, because the back of the fetal head is pressing on her sacrum and coccyx. The fetus may experience extensive caput succedaneum and molding from the sustained occiput posterior position.

Treatment

The best management is to allow the labor to proceed, preparing the woman for a long labor. Many malpositions resolve themselves without intervention. Comfort measures and maternal position changes can help promote fetal head rotation.

Effective pain relief is crucial to help the woman to tolerate the back discomfort. Low back counterpressure during contractions helps to ease the discomfort. Other helpful measures to attempt to rotate the fetal head include lateral abdominal stroking in the direction that the fetal head should rotate; assisting the client into a hands-and-knees position (all fours); and squatting, pelvic rocking, stair climbing, assuming a side-lying position toward the side that the fetus should rotate, and side lunges (Lowdermilk & Perry, 2004). In addition, anxiety reduction, continuous reinforcement of the woman's progress, and education about measures to facilitate fetal head rotation are essential.

Face and Brow Presentations

Face and brow presentations are rare and are associated with fetal abnormalities (anencephaly), pelvic contractures, high parity, placenta previa, hydramnios, low birthweight, or a large fetus (Olds et al., 2004). If there is a complete extension of the fetal head, the face will present for delivery.

In a brow presentation, the fetal head stays between full extension and full flexion so that the largest fetal skull diameter presents to the pelvis. This condition can be diagnosed only once labor is well established.

Diagnosis

Diagnosis is made clinically by a vaginal examination. Typically, the examiner can feel the facial features as the presenting part rather than the fetal head.

Treatment

With a face presentation, labor will be longer, but if the pelvis is adequate and the head rotates, a vaginal birth is possible. If the head rotates backward, a cesarean birth is necessary. With a brow presentation, unless the head flexes, a vaginal birth is not possible.

The birth attendant needs to explain fetal malpositions to the woman and her partner. In addition, close observation for any signs of fetal hypoxia, as evidenced by late decelerations on the fetal monitor, is important.

Breech Presentation

Breech presentation, which occurs in 3% to 4% of labors, is frequently associated with multifetal pregnancies, grand multiparity (more than five births), advanced maternal age, placenta previa, hydramnios, preterm births, and fetal anomalies such as hydrocephaly (London et al., 2003). In this malpresentation the fetal buttocks, or breech, presents first rather than the head. Perinatal mortality is increased 2- to 4-fold with a breech presentation, regardless of the mode of delivery (Molkenboer et al., 2004).

Diagnosis

Vaginal examination determines a breech presentation. "Breech babies" can present in three different attitudes:

- *Frank breech:* The buttocks is the presenting part, with hips flexed and legs and knees extended upward.
- *Complete breech (or full breech):* The buttocks is the presenting part, with hips flexed and knees flexed in a "cannonball" position.
- *Footling or incomplete breech:* One or two feet are the presenting part, with one or both hips extended (see Fig. 13-7).

Treatment

The optimal method of birth for a breech presentation is controversial. Some health care providers consider any type of breech presentation as an indication for cesarean birth unless the fetus is small and the mother has a large pelvis. Others believe that a vaginal birth is appropriate for a breech presentation, with each occurrence treated individually and labor monitored very closely.

Regardless of the birth method selected, the risk for maternal and fetal trauma remains high due to the abnormal presentation. When a vaginal delivery is determined to be safe, the fetus will be allowed to spontaneously deliver up to the umbilicus. Then, maneuvers will be initiated to assist in the delivery of the remainder of the body, arms, and head. Fetal membranes typically are left intact as long as possible to act as a dilating wedge and to prevent cord prolapse. An anesthesiologist and a pediatrician are present for all vaginal breech deliveries because of the increased risk to mother and fetus.

Breech presentation also places a fetus at increased risk. The outcome for the baby is improved with a planned caesarean birth compared with current medical practice for planned vaginal birth. External cephalic version (turning the fetus to the vertex position by external manipulation) attempts to reduce the chance of breech presentation at birth, thus reducing the adverse effects of cesarean birth. However, this technique is not always successful.

External cephalic version is the transabdominal manual manipulation of the fetus into a vertex presentation. It is attempted after the 36th week of gestation but before the start of labor, because some fetuses spontaneously turn to a cephalic presentation on their own toward term, and some will return to the breech presentation if external cephalic version is attempted too early (Fischer, 2005). Success rates vary and risks include fractured bones, ruptured viscera, abruptio placentae, fetomaternal hemorrhage, and umbilical cord entanglement (Fischer, 2005). Tocolytic drugs to relax the uterus, as well as other methods, have been used in an attempt to facilitate external cephalic version at term (Hofmeyr & Gyte, 2004). After the procedure, RhoGAM is administered to the Rh-negative woman to prevent a sensitization reaction from occurring if trauma has occurred and the potential for mixing of blood exists (Gilbert & Harmon, 2003). Each woman must be evaluated individually for all factors before any interventions are initiated.

Shoulder Dystocia

Shoulder dystocia is defined as the obstruction of fetal descent and birth by the axis of the fetal shoulders after the fetal head has been delivered. The fetal head delivers but the neck does not appear and the chin retracts against the perineum, much like a turtle's head going back into his shell. The shoulders remain wedged behind the mother's pubic bone, causing a difficult birth with potential for injury to both mother and baby. If the shoulders are still above the brim at this stage, no advance occurs. The newborn's chest is trapped within the vaginal vault. Although the nose and mouth are outside, the chest cannot expand with respiration. When shoulder dystocia occurs, umbilical cord compression between the fetal body and the maternal pelvis is a risk due to impending fetal acidosis.

Shoulder dystocia is an emergency, an often unexpected complication that can result in significant neonatal and maternal morbidity. It is one of the most anxiety-provoking emergencies encountered in labor. Failure of the shoulders to deliver spontaneously places both the woman and the fetus at risk for injury. Fetal risks include asphyxia, nerve damage, clavicle fracture, central nervous system (CNS) injury or dysfunction, and death. Poor maternal outcomes may include postpartum hemorrhage, extensive lacerations, uterine rupture, infection, fistulas, bladder injury, and psychological trauma (Connors, 2004).

Diagnosis

The diagnosis is made when the newborn's head delivers but the neck and remaining body structures do not. History may reveal primary risk factors such as suspected infant macrosomia (weight >4,500 g), presence of diabetes mellitus in the mother, excessive maternal weight gain, abnormal maternal pelvic anatomy, post-dates pregnancy, short stature, a history of previous shoulder dystocia, and use of epidural analgesia (Baxley & Gobbo, 2004). If shoulder dystocia is anticipated on the basis of these risk factors, preparatory tasks can be accomplished before the birth: key personnel can be alerted, the woman and her family can be educated about the steps that will be taken in the event of a difficult birth, and the woman's bladder is emptied to allow additional room for possible maneuvers needed for the birth.

Treatment

Once shoulder dystocia is identified, the health care provider usually initiates manual maneuvers to facilitate birth (Fig. 21-1). In McRobert's maneuver, the mother's thighs are flexed and abducted as much as possible, which straightens the pelvic curve. Another method used to relieve shoulder dystocia is suprapubic pressure: pressure is applied just above the pubic bone, pushing the fetal anterior shoulder downward to displace it from above the mother's symphysis pubis. The newborn's head is depressed toward the maternal anus while suprapubic pressure is applied. These actions offer additional space and a better maternal position for birth. The combination of the McRoberts maneuver with suprapubic pressure may relieve more than 50% of cases of shoulder dystocia (Baxley & Gobbo, 2004).

The neonatal resuscitation team should be readily available in case of potential newborn injury, asphyxia, or both. The room must be cleared of unnecessary clutter to make room for additional personnel and equipment (Curran, 2003). After the birth, the newborn should be assessed for crepitus, deformity, or bruising, which might suggest that a fracture is present (McKinney et al., 2005).

Multiple Gestation

Multiple gestation refers to twins, triplets, or more infants within a single pregnancy (Box 21-1). The incidence is increasing, primarily as a result of infertility treatment (both ovarian stimulation and in vitro fertilization) and an increased number of women giving birth at older ages (Damato et al., 2005). The incidence of twins is approxi-mately 1 in 30 conceptions, with about two thirds of them due to the fertilization of two ova (dizygotic or fraternal) and about one third occurring from the splitting of one fertilized ovum (monozygotic or identical twins). One in approximately 8,100 pregnancies results in triplets (Green & Wilkinson, 2004).

Multiple gestations may result in dysfunctional labor or dystocia due to uterine overdistention, which may lead to hypotonic contractions, and abnormal presentations of the fetuses. In addition, fetal hypoxia during labor is a significant threat because the placenta must provide oxygen and nutrients to more than one fetus. The most common maternal complication is postpartum hemorrhage resulting from uterine atony.

Diagnosis

Nearly all multiple gestations are now diagnosed early by ultrasound. In addition, most women with a multiple gestation go into labor earlier than 37 weeks.

Treatment

A woman with a multiple gestation who goes into labor should be admitted to a hospital with a specialized care unit to handle any newborn problems after birth. With no complicating factors, the mother can go into spontaneous labor provided the first fetus is lying longitudinally. Fetal presentations can be vertex, breech, or a combination. Labor may proceed rapidly if each fetus is small and mal-presentation is not an issue.

Throughout labor and birth, each fetal heart rate is monitored separately. Once the first fetus is delivered,

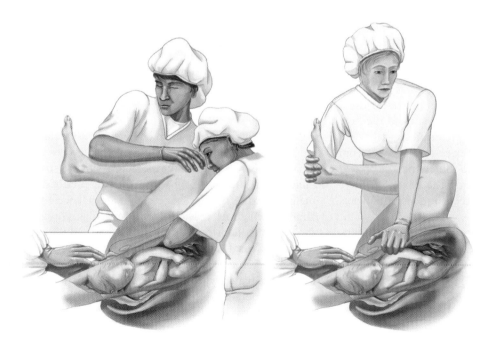

● Figure 21-1 Maneuvers to relieve shoulder dystocia. (**A**) McRobert's maneuver. (**B**) Suprapubic pressure.

A   B

MULTIPLE GESTATION

As the name implies, multiple gestation involves more than one fetus. These fetuses can result from fertilization of a single ovum or multiple ova. Twin pregnancies that are single-ovum conceptions (monozygotic twins) share one chorion (membrane closest to the uterus), and each twin has his or her own amnion (membrane surrounding the amniotic fluid). One fertilized ovum splits into two separate individuals who are said to be natural clones. They have separate amniotic sacs and placentas, are identical in appearance, and are always the same gender. Twin pregnancies that are multiple-ova conceptions (dizygotic twins) result from two ova fertilized by two sperm. Genetically, dizygotic twins are as alike (or unlike) as any other pair or siblings.

The fetuses of a twin gestation, whether monozygotic or dizygotic, are slightly "squashed" because two fetuses develop in a space usually occupied by one. This compression is reflected in the slowing of weight gain in both twins compared to that for singletons (Hall, 2003).

Multiple births other than twins can be of the identical type, the fraternal type, or combinations of the two. Triplets can occur from the division of one zygote into two, with one dividing again, producing identical triplets, or they can come from two zygotes, one dividing into a set of identical twins, and the second zygote developing as a single fraternal sibling, or from three separate zygotes. Triplets are said to occur once in 7,000 births and quadruplets once in 660,000 births (Sloane, 2002). In recent years, fertility drugs used to induce ovulation have resulted in a greater frequency of quadruplets, quintuplets, sextuplets, and even octuplets.

the cord is clamped and the lie of the second twin is assessed carefully. External cephalic version may be necessary to assist in providing a longitudinal lie. In addition, the second and subsequent fetuses are at greater risk for birth-related complications, such as umbilical cord prolapse, malpresentation, and abruptio placentae (Leonard, 2002). If risk factors are high, a cesarean birth is done.

Excessive Fetal Size and Abnormalities

Excessive fetal size and abnormalities can also contribute to labor and birth dysfunctions. Complications associated with dystocia related to excessive fetal size and anomalies include an increased risk for postpartum hemorrhage, dysfunctional labor, fetopelvic disproportion, soft tissue laceration during vaginal birth, fetal injuries or fractures, and asphyxia (Joy & Lyon, 2005).

Although vaginal births are possible, much of the time vacuum-assisted or low forceps are needed to assist in the birthing process.

A macrosomic newborn weighs 4,000 to 4,500 g (8.13 to 9.15 lb) or more at birth. Macrosomia complicates approximately 10% of all pregnancies (Jazayeri & Contreras, 2005). This excessive size can cause fetopelvic disproportion, in which the fetus cannot fit through the maternal pelvis to be born vaginally. When the uterus is overdistended by a large fetus, contraction strength is reduced, leading to a prolonged labor and the potential for birth injury and trauma. Fetal abnormalities such as hydrocephalus, ascites, or a large mass on the neck or head may interfere with fetal descent, causing labor to be prolonged and birth to be difficult.

Diagnosis

A diagnosis of fetal macrosomia can be confirmed by measuring the birthweight after birth. Macrosomia can be suspected based on the findings of an ultrasound examination before labor begins. When a woman is admitted to the labor and birth unit, Leopold's maneuvers are used to estimate fetal weight and position. If macrosomia is suspected, such as with maternal diabetes mellitus or obesity, fetal weight may be estimated using ultrasound.

Treatment

If the diagnosis was made before the onset of labor, a cesarean birth might be scheduled to reduce the risk of injury to both the newborn and the mother. If identified by Leopold's maneuvers, some healthcare providers allow a trial labor to evaluate progress. However, many opt to proceed with a cesarean birth in a primigravida with a macrosomic fetus (Jazayeri & Contreras, 2005).

Problems With the Passageway

Problems with the passageway (pelvis and birth canal) are related to a contraction of one or more of the three planes of the maternal pelvis: inlet, midpelvis, and outlet.

The female pelvis can be classified into four types based on the shape of the pelvic inlet, which is bounded anteriorly by the posterior border of the symphysis pubis, posteriorly by the sacral promontory, and laterally by the linea terminalis. The four basic types are gynecoid, anthropoid, android, and platypelloid (see Chapter 12 for additional information). Women with gynecoid and anthropoid types have a good prognosis for vaginal births, while those with android and platypelloid types have a poorer prognosis.

Contraction of the midpelvis is more common than inlet contraction and typically causes an arrest of fetal descent. It is difficult to diagnose in advance. The outlet of the pelvis can be assessed in early pregnancy to determine whether it can accommodate a normal-sized fetus.

Obstructions in the maternal birth canal, termed soft tissue dystocia, are factors that impede labor progression outside the maternal bony pelvis. Examples of obstructions include placenta previa that partially or completely obstructs the internal os of the cervix; fibroids in the lower uterine segment; a full bladder or rectum; an edematous cervix caused by premature bearing-down efforts; and human papillomavirus (HPV) warts.

Problems With Psyche

Many women experience an array of emotions during labor, which may include fear, anxiety, helplessness, being alone, and weariness. These emotions can lead to psychological stress, which indirectly can cause dystocia. Dystocia occurs due to the release of stress-related hormones (catecholamines, cortisol, epinephrine, beta-endorphin), which act on smooth muscle (uterus) and reduce uterine contractility. Excessive release of catecholamines and other stress-related hormones is not therapeutic. In addition to leading to dystocia, their release can also result in decreased uteroplacental perfusion and increase the risk of poor newborn adjustment (Gilbert & Harmon, 2003).

Ongoing encouragement to minimize the woman's stress is helpful in assisting her to cope with labor and to promote a positive, timely outcome. Assisting her to relax and providing for her comfort will help her body work more effectively with the forces of labor.

Nursing Management

Nursing management of dystocia, regardless of the etiology, requires patience and the provision of physical and emotional support to the client and her family. The final outcome of any labor depends on the size and shape of the maternal pelvis, the quality of the uterine contractions, and the size, presentation, and position of the fetus. Thus, dystocia is diagnosed not at the start of labor, but rather after it has progressed for a time. The nurse monitors cervical dilation, effacement, and fetal descent and documents that all assessed parameters are progressing. If a dysfunctional labor occurs, contractions will slow or fail to advance in frequency, duration, or intensity; the cervix will fail to respond to uterine contractions by dilating and effacing; and the fetus will fail to descend. Table 21-1 summarizes the management of dystocia based on the underlying problem.

Assessment

Assessment starts at admission by reviewing the client's history to look for risk factors for dystocia. Include in the assessment the mother's frame of mind to identify fear, anxiety, stress, lack of support, and pain, which can hinder uterine contractions and impede labor progress. Helping the woman to relax will promote normal labor progress. Additional assessments include:

- Monitor maternal vital signs for signs of infection or hypovolemia.
- Assess for abnormal uterine contractions (hypotonic versus hypertonic).
- Monitor the fetal heart rate to identify abnormal patterns indicating hypoxia.

- Review laboratory test results for signs contributing to dystocia.
- Assess for emotional factors that might impede labor progress or affect the woman's level of coping.
- Assess for a full bladder every 2 hours and encourage bladder emptying.
- Assess the mother's level of fatigue throughout labor, such as:
  - Verbal expressions of feeling exhausted
  - Inability to cope in early labor
  - Inability to rest or calm down between contractions
- Monitor hydration level and correlating it with intake and output.
- Assess fetal position via Leopold's maneuvers to identify any deviations; report any deviations found during vaginal examinations.
- Assess for signs of infection, such as fever or foul-smelling amniotic fluid.
- Assess the woman's level of pain and degree of distress using a 1-to-10 scale.
- Monitor bowel status to prevent obstruction of fetal descent.
- Assess for cervical edema or excessive fetal caput.
- Observe for visible cord prolapse when membranes rupture.
- Observe for visible cord and/or variable decelerations if breech.

Nursing Interventions

During labor, assessments are ongoing to evaluate fetal descent, cervical effacement and dilation, and characteristics of the contractions. These are paramount to determine progress or lack of progress. Additional nursing interventions include:

- Provide labor support: emotional, educational, physical, and advocacy.
- Provide an environment conducive to rest so the woman can conserve her energy:
  - Lower the lights and reduce external noise by closing the hallway door.
  - Offer a warm shower to promote relaxation (if not contraindicated).
  - Support the woman in a comfortable position with pillows.
  - Change the woman's position every 30 minutes to reduce tension and to enhance uterine activity/efficiency.
  - Offer a backrub to reduce muscle tension.
  - Offer fluids/food to moisten the woman's mouth and replenish her energy (Fig. 21-2).
  - Encourage the woman to visualize the descent and birth of the fetus.
  - Praise the woman and her partner for their efforts.
- Use physical comfort measures to promote relaxation and reduce stress.
- Perform vaginal examinations to determine dilation and effacement and progression.

Table 21-1 Management of Dystocia

Problems with the Powers	
Hypertonic labor contractions	Bed rest and sedation to promote relaxation and reduce pain
	Measures to rule out fetopelvic disproportion and fetal malpresentation
	Evaluate of fetal tolerance to labor pattern, such as monitoring of FHR patterns
	Assess for signs of maternal infection
	Adequate hydration through IV therapy
	Pain management through epidural or IV analgesics
	Administration of intravenous oxytocin (Pitocin) to promote normal labor pattern
	Amniotomy to augment labor
	Explanations to woman and family of dysfunctional pattern
	Planning for operative birth if normal labor pattern is not achieved
Hypotonic labor contractions	Oxytocin augmentation probable after fetopelvic disproportion is ruled out
	Amniotomy if membranes are intact
	Continuous electronic fetal monitoring
	Ongoing monitoring of vital signs, contractions, and cervix
	Assessment for signs of maternal and fetal infection
	Explanations to woman and family of dysfunctional pattern
	Planning for surgical birth if normal labor pattern is not achieved or fetal distress occurs
Precipitous labor	Close monitoring of woman with previous history of this
	Use of scheduled induction to control labor rate
	Pharmacologic agents, such as tocolytics, to slow labor
	Constant attendance to monitor progress
Problems with the Passenger	
Persistent occiput-posterior position	Assessment for complaints of intense back pain in first stage of labor
	Possible use of forceps to rotate to anterior position at birth
	Manual rotation to anterior position at end of second stage
	Assessment for prolonged second stage of labor with arrest of descent (common with this malposition)
	Maternal position changes to promote fetal head rotation: hands and knees and rocking pelvis back and forth; side-lying position; side lunges during contractions; sitting, kneeing, or standing while leaning forward; squatting position to give birth and enlarge pelvic outlet
	Possible cesarean birth if rotation is not achieved
Face and brow presentations	Palpation of fetal forehead or face as presenting part
	Evaluation for fetopelvic disproportion
	Cesarean birth if vertex position is not achieved
Breech presentation	Assessment for possible associated conditions such as placenta previa, hydramnios, fetal anomalies, and multiple gestation
	Ultrasound to confirm fetal presentation
	External cephalic version possible at 37 weeks
	Tocolytics to assist with external cephalic version
	Trial labor for 4 to 6 hours to evaluate progress if version is unsuccessful
	Planning for cesarean birth if no progress is seen or fetal distress occurs
Shoulder dystocia	Urgent intervention necessary due to cord compression
	McRobert's maneuver and application of suprapubic pressure
	Squatting position, hands and knees position, or lateral recumbent position for birth to free shoulders
	Cesarean birth if no success in dislodging shoulders

(continued)

Table 21-1 Management of Dystocia (continued)

Multiple gestation	Assessment for hypotonic labor pattern due to overdistention Evaluation of fetal presentation, maternal pelvic size, and gestational age to determine mode of delivery Presence of neonatal team for birth of multiples Cesarean births common in multiple gestations
Excessive fetal size and abnormalities	Assessment for inability of fetus to descend Difficulty in ascertaining true fetal size prior to birth Vacuum and forceps-assisted births are very common Cesarean birth is possible if maternal parameters are not adequate to give birth to large fetus
Problems with the Passageway	Assessment for poor contractions, slow dilation, prolonged labor Evaluation of bowel and bladder status to reduce soft tissue obstruction and allow increased pelvic space Trial of labor; if no labor progression after an adequate trial, plan for cesarean birth
Problems with the Psyche	Provide comfortable environment—dim lighting, music Encourage partner to participate Pain management measures to reduce anxiety and stress Continuous presence of staff to allay anxiety Frequent updates concerning fetal status and progress

- Be prepared to administer a labor stimulant such as oxytocin (Pitocin) in hypotonic labor.
- Keep the birth attendant informed of the progress or lack thereof.
- Be prepared to assist with manipulations if shoulder dystocia is diagnosed.
- Make sure the woman avoids supine positions, which cause vena cava compression.
- Provide backrubs and counterpressure if the baby is in the occiput posterior position.
- Encourage upright positions to facilitate fetal rotation and descent.
- Evaluate progress in active labor by using the simple rule of 1 cm/hour.
- Prepare the woman and family for the possibility of a cesarean birth if there is no progress.
- Educate the client and family about dysfunctional labor and its causes and therapies.
- Administer needed analgesics according to protocol or the provider's order.
- Assist the client to assume different positions to encourage fetal rotation.
- Remain with the client to demonstrate caring.
- Prepare the woman for any therapeutic intervention to assist the labor process.
- Keep the woman and her partner informed of progress.
- Provide empathetic listening to increase the client's coping ability.

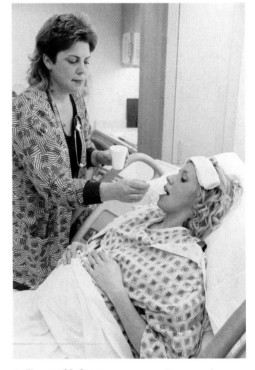

● Figure 21-2 The nurse applies a cool, moist washcloth and offers ice chips to combat thirst and provide comfort for the woman with dystocia.

- Encourage the client and her partner to participate in decision-making before any interventions.
- Encourage the woman to express her fears and anxieties.
- Provide encouragement to help the woman to maintain control.
- Support and encourage the client and her partner in their coping efforts.
- Coach the woman not to push until the cervix is completely dilated.
- Document the timing of events, the maneuvers used, and the care given.

Postterm Labor and Birth

Usually a term pregnancy lasts 38 to 42 weeks. A **postterm pregnancy** is one that continues past the end of the 42nd week of gestation, or 294 days, from the first day of the last menstrual period. Postterm pregnancies account for about 10% of births (Wilkes & Galan, 2004). Incorrect dates account for the majority of these cases: many women have irregular menses and thus cannot identify the date of their last menstrual period accurately.

The exact etiology of a postterm pregnancy is unknown because the mechanism for the initiation of labor is not completely understood. Theories suggest there may be a deficiency of estrogen and continued secretion of progesterone that prohibits the uterus from contracting, but no evidence has validated this. A woman who has one postterm pregnancy is at greater risk for another in subsequent pregnancies.

Postterm pregnancies may adversely affect both the mother and fetus or newborn. Maternal risk is related to the large size of the fetus at birth, which increases the chances that a cesarean birth will be needed. Other issues might include dystocia, birth trauma, postpartum hemorrhage, and infection. Mechanical or artificial interventions such as forceps or vacuum-assisted birth and labor induction with oxytocin may be necessary. In addition, maternal exhaustion and feelings of despair over this prolonged gestation can add to the woman's anxiety level and reduce her coping ability.

Fetal risks associated with a postterm pregnancy include macrosomia, shoulder dystocia, brachial plexus injuries, and cephalopelvic disproportion. All of these conditions predispose this fetus to birth trauma or a surgical birth. The perinatal mortality rate at more than 42 weeks of gestation is twice that at term and increases sixfold and higher at 43 weeks of gestation and beyond. Uteroplacental insufficiency, meconium aspiration, and intrauterine infection contribute to the increased rate of perinatal deaths (ACOG, 2004). As the placenta ages, its perfusion decreases and it becomes less efficient at delivering oxygen and nutrients to the fetus. Amniotic fluid volume also begins to decline by 40 weeks of gestation, possibly leading to oligohydramnios, subsequently resulting in fetal

hypoxia and an increased risk of cord compression because the cushioning effect offered by adequate fluid is no longer present. Hypoxia and oligohydramnios predispose the fetus to aspiration of meconium, which is released by the fetus in response to a hypoxic insult (Sanchez-Ramos et al., 2003). All of these issues can compromise fetal well-being and lead to fetal distress.

Nursing Management

Many women are unsure of the date of their last menstrual period, so the date given may be unreliable. Despite numerous methods used to date pregnancies, many are still misdated. Accurate gestational dating via ultrasound is key.

Once the dates are established and postdate status is confirmed, monitoring fetal well-being becomes critical. When determining the plan of care for a woman with a postterm pregnancy, the first decision is whether to deliver the baby or wait. If the decision is to wait, then fetal surveillance is key. If the decision is to have the woman deliver, labor induction is initiated. Both decisions remain controversial, and there is no clear answer about which option is more appropriate. Therefore, the plan must be individualized.

Assessment

Antepartum assessment for a postterm pregnancy typically includes daily fetal movement counts done by the woman, nonstress tests done twice weekly, amniotic fluid assessments as part of the biophysical profile, and weekly cervical examinations to evaluate for ripening. This intense surveillance is time-consuming and intrusive, adding to the anxiety and worry already being experienced by the woman about her overdue status. Be alert to the woman's anxiety and allow her to discuss her feelings. Provide reassurance about the expected time range for birth and the well-being of the fetus based on the assessment tests. Validating the woman's stressful state due to the prolonged pregnancy provides an opportunity for her to verbalize her feelings openly. Key areas of assessment include:

- Pregnancy date to ascertain the most accurate one
- Client's understanding of the various fetal well-being tests
- Client's stress and anxiety concerning her lateness
- Client's coping ability and support network

During the intrapartum period, continuous assessment and monitoring of the fetal heart rate (FHR) is needed to identify potential fetal distress early (e.g., late or variable decelerations) so that interventions can be initiated. Assessment of the woman's hydration status is important to maximize placental perfusion. Assessment of the amniotic fluid characteristics (color, amount, and odor) is vital to identify previous fetal hypoxia and prepare for prevention of meconium aspiration. Assessment of the woman's labor pattern is essential because dysfunctional patterns are common (Gilbert & Harmon, 2003).

Nursing Interventions

Nursing care for the postterm client is similar to that for any client at term. However, the following interventions are key:

- Educate the woman and family about the purpose and findings of each test.
- Prepare the woman for the possibility of induction if her labor isn't spontaneous or a surgical delivery if fetal distress occurs.
- Discuss the cervical ripening methods that may be used for induction.
- Inform the woman about potential complications of postterm pregnancies.
- Encourage the woman to verbalize her feelings and concerns; answer all questions.
- Keep the woman well hydrated to increase placental perfusion for the fetus.
- Provide continuous electronic fetal monitoring throughout labor.
- Provide support, presence, information, and encouragement throughout.
- Explain that amnioinfusion may be used to minimize the risk of meconium aspiration by diluting meconium in amniotic fluid expelled by the hypoxic fetus.
- Report meconium-stained amniotic fluid when the membranes rupture.
- Support the client and family throughout the experience (Gilbert, 2004).

Women Requiring Induction and Augmentation of Labor

Ideally, all pregnancies go to term, with labor beginning spontaneously. However, many women need help to initiate or sustain the labor process. **Labor induction** involves the stimulation of uterine contractions by medical or surgical means to produce delivery before the onset of spontaneous labor. The labor induction rate is at an all-time high in the United States. The widespread use of artificial induction of labor for convenience has contributed to the recent increase in the number of cesarean births. Evidence is compelling that elective induction of labor significantly increases the risk of cesarean birth, instrumented delivery, use of epidural analgesia, and neonatal intensive care unit admission, especially for nulliparous women (Simpson & Atterbury, 2003).

Labor induction is not an isolated event: it brings about a cascade of other interventions that may or may not produce a favorable outcome. Labor induction also involves intravenous therapy, bed rest, continuous electronic fetal monitoring, significant discomfort from stimulating uterine contractions, epidural analgesia/anesthesia, and a prolonged stay on the labor unit (Simpson & Atterbury, 2003).

Labor augmentation enhances ineffective contractions after labor has begun. Continuous electronic FHR monitoring is necessary.

There are multiple medical and obstetric reasons for inducing labor, the most common being postterm gestation. Other indications for inductions include prolonged premature rupture of membranes, gestational hypertension, renal disease, chorioamnionitis, dystocia, intrauterine fetal demise, isoimmunization, and diabetes (Baxley, 2003). Contraindications to labor induction include complete placenta previa, abruptio placentae, transverse fetal lie, prolapsed umbilical cord, a prior classic uterine incision that entered the uterine cavity, pelvic structure abnormality, previous myomectomy, vaginal bleeding with unknown cause, invasive cervical cancer, active genital herpes infection, and abnormal FHR patterns (Littleton & Engebretson, 2005). In general, labor induction is indicated when the benefits of birth outweigh the risks to the mother or fetus for continuing the pregnancy. However, the balance between risk and benefit remains controversial.

Considerations for Induction

The decision to induce labor is based on a thorough assessment of maternal and fetal status. Typically, this includes an ultrasound to evaluate fetal size, position, and gestational age and to locate the placenta; pelvimetry to rule out fetopelvic disproportion; a nonstress test to evaluate fetal well-being; a phosphatidylglycerol (PG) level to assess fetal lung maturity; Nitrazine paper and/or fern test to confirm ruptured membranes; complete blood count and urinalysis to rule out infection; and a vaginal examination to evaluate the cervix for inducibility (Green & Wilkinson, 2004). Accurate dating of the pregnancy also is essential before cervical ripening and induction are initiated to prevent a preterm birth.

Cervical Ripeness and Labor Induction

There has been increasing awareness that if the cervix is unfavorable or unripe, a successful vaginal birth is unlikely. Cervical ripeness is an important variable when labor induction is being considered. A ripe cervix is shortened, centered (anterior), softened, and partially dilated. An unripe cervix is long, closed, posterior, and firm. Cervical ripening usually begins prior to the onset of labor contractions and is necessary for cervical dilatation and the passage of the fetus.

Various scoring systems to assess cervical ripeness have been introduced, but the Bishop score is most commonly used today. The Bishop score helps identify women who would be most likely to achieve a successful induction (Table 21-2). The duration of labor is inversely correlated with the Bishop score: a score over eight indicates a successful vaginal birth. Bishop scores of less than six usually indicate that a cervical ripening method should be used prior to induction (Tenore, 2003).

Nonpharmacologic Methods

Nonpharmacologic methods are less used today, but nurses need to be aware of them and question clients about their

Table 21-2 Bishop Scoring System

Score	Dilation (cm)	Effacement (%)	Station	Cervical Consistency	Position of Cervix
0	Closed	0–30%	–3	Firm	Posterior
1	1–2 cm	40–50%	–2	Medium	Midposition
2	3–4 cm	60–70%	–1 or 0	Soft	Anterior
3	5–6 cm	80%	+1 or +2	Very soft	Anterior

Modified from Bishop, E. H. (1964). Pelvic scoring for elective induction. *Obstetrics & Gynecology, 24*(2), 267.

use. Methods may include herbal agents such as evening primrose oil, black haw, black and blue cohosh, and red raspberry leaves. In addition, castor oil, hot baths, and enemas are used for cervical ripening and labor induction. The risks and benefits of these agents are unknown.

Another nonpharmacologic method suggested for labor induction is sexual intercourse along with breast stimulation. This promotes the release of oxytocin, which stimulates uterine contractions. In addition, human semen is a biological source of prostaglandins used for cervical ripening. According to a Cochrane Review, sexual intercourse with breast stimulation would appear beneficial, but safety issues have not been fully evaluated, nor can this activity be standardized (Kavanagh & Kelly, 2005). Therefore, its use as a method for labor induction is not validated by research.

Mechanical Methods

Mechanical methods are used to open the cervix and move labor along. All share a similar mechanism of action—application of local pressure stimulates the release of prostaglandins to ripen the cervix. The risks associated with these methods include infection, bleeding, membrane rupture, and placental disruption (Simpson, 2002).

For example, an indwelling (Foley) catheter (e.g., 26 French) can be inserted into the endocervical canal to ripen and dilate the cervix. The catheter is placed in the uterus, and the balloon is filled. Direct pressure is then applied to the lower segment of the uterus and the cervix. This direct pressure causes stress in the lower uterine segment and probably the local production of prostaglandins (Rai & Schreiber, 2005).

Hygroscopic dilators absorb endocervical and local tissue fluids; as they enlarge they expand the endocervix and provide controlled mechanical pressure. The products available include natural osmotic dilators (laminaria, a type of dried seaweed) and synthetic dilators containing magnesium sulfate (Lamicel, Dilapan). Hygroscopic dilators are advantageous because they can be inserted on an outpatient basis and no fetal monitoring is needed. As many dilators are inserted in the cervix as will fit, and they expand over 12 to 24 hours as they absorb water.

Absorption of water leads to expansion of the dilators and opening of the cervix. They are a reliable alternative when prostaglandins are contraindicated or unavailable (Lowdermilk & Perry, 2004).

Surgical Methods

Surgical methods used to ripen the cervix and induce labor include stripping of the membranes and performing an amniotomy. Stripping of the membranes is accomplished by inserting a finger through the internal cervical os and moving it in a circular direction. This motion causes the membranes to detach. Manual separation of the amniotic membranes from the cervix is thought to induce cervical ripening and the onset of labor (Rai & Schreiber, 2005).

An amniotomy involves inserting a cervical hook (Amniohook) through the cervical os to rupture the membranes. This promotes pressure of the presenting part on the cervix and stimulates an increase in the activity of prostaglandins locally. Risks associated with these procedures include umbilical cord prolapse or compression, maternal or neonatal infection, FHR deceleration, bleeding, and client discomfort (Tenore, 2003).

When either of these techniques is used, amniotic fluid characteristics (such as whether it is clear or bloody, or meconium is present) and the FHR pattern must be monitored closely.

Pharmacologic Agents

The use of pharmacologic agents has revolutionized cervical ripening. The use of prostaglandins to attain cervical ripening has been found to be highly effective in producing cervical changes independent of uterine contractions (Baxley, 2003). In some cases, women will go into labor, requiring no additional stimulants for induction. Induction of labor with prostaglandins offers the advantage of promoting both cervical ripening and uterine contractility. A drawback of prostaglandins is their ability to induce excessive uterine contractions, which can increase maternal and perinatal morbidity (Sanchez-Ramos & Hsieh, 2003). Currently, three prostaglandin analogs are used for the purpose of cervical ripening: dinoprostone gel (Prepidil), dinoprostone inserts (Cervidil), and misoprostol (Cytotec).

Misoprostol (Cytotec), a synthetic PGE1 analog, is a gastric cytoprotective agent used in the treatment and prevention of peptic ulcers. It can be administered intravaginally or orally to ripen the cervix or induce labor. It is available in 100-mcg or 200-mcg tablets, but doses of 25 to 50 g are typically used. However, it is not approved by the FDA for cervical ripening (Drug Guide 21-1).

Oxytocin (Pitocin) is one of the most commonly used drugs for labor induction and augmentation in the United States. It is produced naturally by the posterior pituitary gland and stimulates contractions of the uterus. For women with low Bishop scores, cervical ripening is typically initiated before oxytocin is used. Once the cervix is ripe, oxytocin is the most popular pharmacologic agent used for inducing or augmenting labor. Frequently a woman with an unfavorable cervix is admitted the evening before induction to ripen her cervix with one of the prostaglandin agents. Then induction begins with Pitocin the next morning if she has not already gone into labor. Doing so markedly enhances the induction success. Response to oxytocin varies widely: some women are very sensitive to even small amounts. The most common adverse effect of oxytocin is uterine hyperstimulation, leading to fetal compromise and impaired oxygenation (Breslin & Lucas, 2003). Close attention must be paid to the uterine response throughout labor so that the oxytocin infusion can be titrated appropriately. In addition, oxytocin has an antidiuretic effect, resulting in decreased urine flow that may lead to water intoxication. Symptoms to watch for include headache and vomiting.

Oxytocin is administered via an IV infusion pump piggybacked into the main IV line at the port most proxi-

Drug Guide 21-1 Drugs Used for Cervical Ripening and Labor Induction

Drug	Action/Indication	Nursing Implications
Dinoprostone (Cervidil insert; Prepidil gel)	Directly softens and dilates the cervix/to ripen cervix and induce labor	Provide emotional support. Administer pain medications as needed. Frequently assess degree of effacement and dilation. Monitor uterine contractions for frequency, duration, and strength. Assess maternal vital signs and FHR pattern frequently. Monitor woman for possible adverse effects such as headache, nausea and vomiting, and diarrhea.
Misoprostol (Cytotec)	Ripens cervix/to induce labor	Instruct client about purpose and possible adverse effects of medication. Ensure informed consent is signed per hospital policy. Assess vital signs and FHR patterns frequently. Monitor client's reaction to drug. Initiate oxytocin for labor induction at least 4 hours after last dose was administered. Monitor for possible adverse effects such as nausea and vomiting, diarrhea, uterine hyperstimulation, and nonreassuring FHR pattern.
Oxytocin (Pitocin)	Acts on uterine myofibrils to contract/to initiate or reinforce labor	Administer as an IV infusion via pump, increasing dose based on protocol until adequate labor progress is achieved. Assess baseline vital signs and FHR and then frequently after initiating oxytocin infusion. Determine frequency, duration, and strength of contractions frequently. Notify health care provider of any uterine hypertonicity or abnormal FHR patterns. Maintain careful I & O, being alert for water intoxication. Keep client informed of labor progress. Monitor for possible adverse effects such as hyperstimulation of the uterus, impaired uterine blood flow leading to fetal hypoxia, rapid labor leading to cervical lacerations or uterine rupture, water intoxication (if oxytocin is given in electrolyte-free solution or at a rate exceeding 20 mU/min), and hypotension.

mal to the venous site. Usually 10 units of Pitocin is added to 1 L of isotonic solution to achieve an infusion rate of 1 mU/min = 6 mL/hr. The dose is titrated according to protocol to achieve stable contractions every 2 to 3 minutes lasting 40 to 60 seconds (London et al., 2003). The uterus should relax between contractions. If the resting uterine tone remains above 20 mm Hg, utero-placental insufficiency and fetal hypoxia can result. This outcome underscores the importance of continuous FHR monitoring.

Oxytocin has many advantages: it is potent and easy to titrate, it has a short half-life (1 to 5 minutes), and it is generally well tolerated. However, induction using oxytocin has side effects, but because the drug does not cross the placental barrier, no direct fetal problems have been observed (Simpson & Atterbury, 2003) (Fig. 21-3).

Nursing Management

Nurses working with women in labor play an important role acting as the "eyes" and "ears" for the healthcare provider because they remain at the client's bedside throughout the entire experience. Close, frequent assessment and follow-up interventions are essential to ensure the safety of the mother and her unborn child during cervical ripening and labor induction or augmentation.

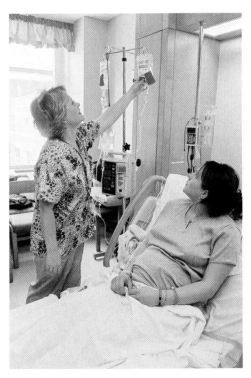

● Figure 21-3 The nurse monitors an intravenous infusion of oxytocin being administered to a woman in labor. Note the use of an infusion pump to regulate the flow of the oxytocin, which has been piggybacked into the main IV line.

Nursing Care Plan 21-1 presents an overview of nursing care for a woman undergoing labor induction.

Assessment

Assessment of the woman undergoing labor induction or augmentation includes:

- Assess cervical status, including cervical dilatation and effacement, and station via vaginal examination before cervical ripening or induction is started.
- Assess fetal well-being to validate the client's and fetus's ability to withstand labor contractions.
- Review relative indications for induction or augmentation, such as diabetes, hypertension, postterm status, dysfunctional labor pattern, prolonged ruptured membranes, maternal or fetal infection, and contraindications such as placenta previa, overdistended uterus, active genital herpes, fetopelvic disproportion, fetal malposition, or severe fetal distress.
- Determine the gestational age of the fetus to prevent a preterm birth.
- Assess contractions for frequency, duration, and intensity and resting tone.
- Evaluate for any contraindications to prostaglandin use, such as infection or bleeding.
- Assess the need for pain management and provide comfort measures.
- Determine Bishop score to determine probable success of induction.

Nursing Interventions

Explain to the woman and her partner about the induction or augmentation procedure clearly, using simple terms (Teaching Guidelines 21-1). Ensure that an informed consent has been signed after the client and her partner have received complete information about the procedure, including its advantages, disadvantages, and potential risks. Determine the cervical Bishop score before proceeding.

Prepare the oxytocin infusion by diluting 10 units of oxytocin in 1,000 mL of lactated Ringer's solution. Use an infusion pump on a secondary line connected to the primary infusion. Start the oxytocin infusion in mU/min or milliliters per hour as ordered. Typically, the initial dose is 0.5 to 1 mU/min; anticipate increasing the rate in increments of 1 to 2 mU/min every 30 to 60 minutes. Maintain the rate once the desired contraction frequency has been reached. To ensure adequate maternal and fetal surveillance during induction or augmentation, the nurse-to-client ratio should not exceed 1:2 (Smith, 2004).

During induction or augmentation, monitoring of the maternal and fetal status is essential. Apply an external electronic fetal monitor or assist with placement of an internal device. Obtain the mother's vital signs and the FHR every 15 minutes during the first stage. Evaluate the contractions for frequency, duration, and intensity, and

(text continues on page 602)

Nursing Care Plan 21-1

Overview of the Woman Undergoing Labor Induction

Rose, a 29-year-old primipara, is admitted to the labor and birth suite at 40 weeks' gestation for induction of labor. Assessment reveals that her cervix is ripe and 80% effaced, and she is 2 cm dilated. Rose tells the nurse she is very anxious about being induced and is afraid of the pain associated with the medication used to start contractions. She consents to being induced but wants reassurance that this procedure won't harm the baby. Upon examination the fetus is engaged and in a cephalic presentation, with the vertex as the presenting part. Her partner is at her side.

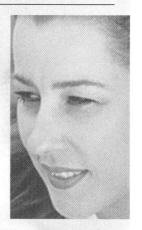

Nursing Diagnosis: Anxiety related to induction of labor and lack of experience with labor

Outcome identification and *evaluation*	Interventions with *rationales*
Client will experience decrease in anxiety *as evidenced by ability to verbalize understanding of procedures involved and use coping skills to reduce anxious state.*	Provide a clear explanation of the labor induction process *to provide client and partner with a knowledge base.* Maintain continuous physical presence *to provide physical and emotional support and demonstrate concern for maternal and fetal well-being.* Explain each procedure before carrying it out and field questions *to promote understanding of procedure and rationale for use.* Encourage use of coping strategies used in the past *to aid in controlling anxiety.* Instruct client's partner in helpful measures to assist client in coping and encourage their use *to foster joint participation in the process and provide support to the client.* Offer frequent reassurance of fetal status and labor progress *to help alleviate client's concerns and foster continued participation in the labor process.*

Nursing Diagnosis: Pain related to uterine contractions

Client will report a decrease in pain as evidenced *by statements of increased comfort and pain rating of 3 or less on numerical pain rating scale.*	Explain to the client that she will experience discomfort sooner than with naturally occurring labor *to promote client awareness of events and prepare client for the experience.* Frequently assess client's pain using a pain rating scale *to quantify client's level of pain and evaluate effectiveness of pain-relief measures.* Provide comfort measures, such as hygiene, backrubs, music, and distraction and encourage the use of breathing and relaxation techniques *to help promote relaxation.*

Overview of the Woman Undergoing Labor Induction (continued)

Outcome identification and *evaluation*	Interventions with *rationales*
	Provide support for her partner *to aid in alleviating stress and concerns.* Employ nonpharmacologic methods, such as position changes, birthing ball, hydrotherapy, visual imagery, and effleurage, *to help in managing pain.* Administer analgesia or anesthesia as appropriate and ordered *to control pain.* Evaluate pain-management techniques used *to determine their effectiveness.*

Nursing Diagnosis: Risk for injury (maternal or fetal) related to induction procedure

Clients will remain free of complications associated with induction as evidenced by *progression of labor as expected, delivery of healthy newborn, and absence of signs and symptoms of maternal and fetal adverse effects.*	Follow agency's protocol for medication use and infusion rate *to ensure accurate, safe drug administration.* Set up oxytocin IV infusion to piggyback into the primary IV bag *to allow for prompt discontinuation should adverse effects occur.* Use an infusion pump *to deliver accurate dose as ordered.* Gradually increase oxytocin dose in increments of 1 to 2 mU/min every 30 to 60 minutes based on assessment findings and protocol *to promote effective uterine contractions.* Maintain oxytocin rate once desired frequency has been reached *to ensure continued progress in labor.* Accurately monitor contractions for frequency, duration, and intensity and resting tone *to prevent development of hypertonic contractions.* Maintain a nurse–client ratio of 1:2 *to ensure maternal and fetal safety.* Monitor FHR via an electronic fetal monitoring during induction and constantly observe the FHR response to titrated medication rate *to ensure fetal well-being and identify adverse effects immediately.* Obtain maternal vital signs every 1 to 2 hours or as indicated by agency's protocol, reporting any deviations, *to promote maternal well-being and allow for prompt detection of problems.* Communicate with birth attendant frequently concerning progress *to ensure continuity of care.* Discontinue oxytocin infusion if tetanic contraction (>90 seconds), uterine hyperstimulation (<2 minutes apart), elevated uterine resting tone, or a nonreassuring FHR pattern occurs *to minimize risk of drug's adverse effects.* Provide frequent reassurance of maternal and fetal status *to alleviate anxiety.*

T E A C H I N G G U I D E L I N E S 2 1 - 1

Teaching in Preparation for Labor Induction

• Your health care provider may recommend that you have your labor induced. This may be necessary for a variety of reasons, such as elevated blood pressure, a medical condition, prolonged pregnancy over 41 weeks, or problems with fetal heart rate patterns or fetal growth.

• Your health care provider may use one or more methods to induce labor, such as stripping the membranes, breaking the amniotic sac to release the fluid, administering medication close to or in the cervix to soften it, or administering a medication called oxytocin (Pitocin) to stimulate contractions.

• Labor induction is associated with some risks and disadvantages, such as overactivity of the uterus; nausea, vomiting, or diarrhea; and changes in fetal heart rate.

• Prior to inducing your labor, your health care provider may perform a procedure to ripen your cervix to help ensure a successful induction.

• Medication may be placed around cervix the day before you are scheduled to be induced.

• During the induction, your contractions may feel stronger than normal. However, the length of your labor may be reduced with induction.

• Medications for pain relief and comfort measures will be readily available.

• Health care staff will be present throughout labor.

resting tone and make rate adjustments to the oxytocin infusion accordingly. Monitor the characteristics of the FHR, including baseline rate, baseline variability, and decelerations to determine whether the oxytocin rate needs adjustment. Discontinue the oxytocin and notify the birth attendant if uterine hyperstimulation or a nonreassuring FHR pattern occurs. Perform or assist with periodic vaginal examinations to determine cervical dilation and fetal descent: cervical dilation of 1 cm/hour typically indicates satisfactory progress.

Continue to monitor the FHR continuously and document it every 15 minutes during the active phase of labor and every 5 minutes during the second stage. Assist with pushing efforts during the second stage.

Provide pain management as needed by asking the woman frequently about her pain level. Monitor her need for comfort measures as contractions increase. Measure and record intake and output to prevent excess fluid volume. Encourage the client to empty her bladder every 2 hours to prevent soft tissue obstruction.

Throughout induction and augmentation, frequently reassure the woman and her partner about the fetal status and labor progress. Assess the woman's ability to cope with stronger contractions (Simpson, 2002). Note her reaction to any medication given, and document its effect.

Intrauterine Fetal Demise

When an unborn life suddenly ends with fetal demise or stillbirth, the family members are profoundly affected. The sudden loss of an expected child is tragic and the family's grief can be very intense, can last for years, and can cause extreme psychological stress and emotional problems (Lindsey & Hernandez, 2004). History and physical examination are of limited value in the diagnosis of fetal death, since the only history tends to be recent absence of fetal movement. An inability to obtain fetal heart sounds on examination suggests fetal demise, but an ultrasound is necessary to confirm the absence of fetal cardiac activity. Once fetal demise is confirmed, induction of labor is indicated.

The cause of fetal death can be due to numerous conditions, such as prolonged pregnancy, infection, hypertension, advanced maternal age, Rh disease, uterine rupture, diabetes, congenital anomalies, cord accident, abruption, premature rupture of membranes, or hemorrhage; it may be unexplained (Gilbert & Harmon, 2003). Early pregnancy loss may be through a spontaneous abortion (miscarriage), an induced abortion (therapeutic abortion), or a ruptured ectopic pregnancy. A wide spectrum of feelings may be expressed, from relief to sadness and despair. A stillbirth can occur at any gestational age, and typically there is little or no warning other than reduced fetal movement.

The period following a fetal death is extremely difficult for the family. For many women, emotional healing takes much longer than physical healing. The feelings of loss can be intense. The grief response in some women may be so great that their relationships become strained, and healing can become hampered unless appropriate interventions and support are provided.

Fetal death also affects the healthcare staff. Despite the trauma that the loss of a fetus causes, some staff members avoid dealing with the bereaved family, never talking about or acknowledging their grief. This seems to imply that not discussing the problem will allow the grief to dissolve and vanish. This is unreasonable and merely makes the bereaved family members feel that they are alone and their needs are unrecognized. Failing to keep the lines of communication open with a bereaved client and her family closes off some of the channels to recovery and healing that may be desperately needed.

Nursing Management

The nurse can play a major role in assisting the grieving family. With skillful intervention, the bereaved family may be better prepared to resolve their grief and move forward. To assist families in the grieving process, use the following interventions:

• Provide accurate, understandable information to the family.

- Encourage discussion of the loss and venting of feelings of grief and guilt.
- Provide the family with baby mementos and pictures to validate the reality of death.
- Allow unlimited time with the stillborn infant after birth to validate the death; provide time for the family members to be together and grieve; offer the family the opportunity to see, touch, and hold the infant.
- Use appropriate touch, such as holding a hand or touching a shoulder.
- Inform the chaplain or the religious leader of the family's denomination about the death and request his or her presence.
- Assist the parents with the funeral arrangements or disposition of the body.
- Provide the parents with brochures offering advice about how to talk to other siblings about the loss.
- Refer the family to the support group SHARE Pregnancy and Infant Loss Support, Inc., which is designed for those who have lost an infant through abortion, miscarriage, fetal death, stillbirth, or other tragic circumstances.
- Make community referrals to promote a continuum of care on discharge.

Obstetric Emergencies

Obstetric emergencies are challenging to all labor and birth personnel because of the increased risk of adverse outcomes for the mother and fetus. Quick clinical judgment and good critical decision-making will increase the odds of a positive outcome for both mother and fetus. This chapter will discuss a few of these emergencies: umbilical cord prolapse, placental abruption, uterine rupture, and amniotic fluid embolism.

Umbilical Cord Prolapse

An **umbilical cord prolapse,** although rare, requires prompt recognition and intervention for a positive out-

come. The condition is defined as the protrusion of the umbilical cord alongside (occult) or ahead of the presenting part of the fetus (Fig. 21-4). It occurs in 1 out of every 300 births (March of Dimes, 2005). With a 50% perinatal mortality rate, it is one of the most catastrophic events in the intrapartum period (Gabbe et al., 2002). Although rare in a full-term fetus with a cephalic presentation, cord prolapse is more common in pregnancies involving malpresentation, growth restriction, prematurity, ruptured membranes with a fetus at a high station, hydramnios, grandmultiparity, and multifetal gestation (Poole & White, 2003).

Prolapse usually leads to total or partial occlusion of the cord. Since this is the fetus's only lifeline, fetal perfusion deteriorates rapidly. Complete occlusion renders the fetus helpless and oxygen-deprived. Without quick intervention to relieve cord compression, the fetus will die.

Nursing Management

Prevention is the key to managing cord prolapse by identifying clients at risk for this condition. When the presenting part does not fully occupy the pelvic inlet, prolapse is more likely to occur. Nurses can be instrumental in promoting positive perinatal outcomes for women in this situation.

Assessment

Carefully assess each client to help predict her risk status. Ensure continuous assessment of the client and fetus to detect changes and to evaluate the effectiveness of any interventions performed. Provide emotional support and explanations as to what is going on to allay the woman's fears and anxiety.

Nursing Interventions

Prompt recognition of a prolapsed cord is essential to reduce the risk of fetal hypoxia resulting from prolonged cord compression. When membranes are artificially

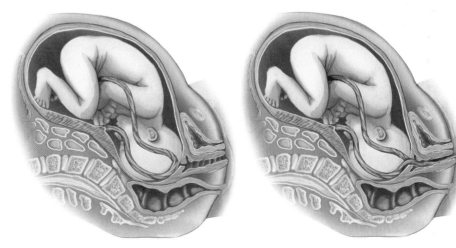

● Figure 21-4 Prolapsed cord.
(**A**) Prolapse within the uterus.
(**B**) Prolapse with the cord visible at the vulva.

A

B

ruptured, assist with verifying that the presenting part is well applied to the cervix and engaged into the pelvis. If pressure or compression of the cord occurs, assist with measures to relieve the compression. Typically, the examiner places a sterile gloved hand into the vagina and holds the presenting part off the umbilical cord. Changing the woman's position to a modified Sims, Trendelenburg, or knee–chest position also helps relieve cord pressure. An emergency cesarean birth is typically done to save the fetus's life if the mother's cervix is not fully dilated.

Placental Abruption

Placental abruption refers to premature separation of a normally implanted placenta from the maternal myometrium. Risk factors include preeclampsia, gestational hypertension, seizure activity, uterine rupture, trauma, smoking, cocaine use, coagulation defects, previous history of abruption, domestic violence, and placental pathology. These conditions may force blood into the underlayer of the placenta and cause it to detach (Curran, 2003).

Management of placental abruption depends on the gestational age, the extent of the hemorrhage, and maternal–fetal oxygenation perfusion/reserve status (see Chapter 19 for additional information on abruptio placentae). Treatment should be individualized depending on the circumstances. Typically once the diagnosis is established, the focus is on maintaining the cardiovascular status of the mother and developing a plan to deliver the fetus quickly. A cesarean birth takes place if the fetus is still alive. A vaginal birth may take place if there is fetal demise.

Uterine Rupture

Uterine rupture is a catastrophic tearing of the uterus at the site of a previous scar into the abdominal cavity. Its onset is often marked only by sudden fetal bradycardia, and treatment requires rapid surgical attention for good outcomes. Among the many clinical conditions associated with uterine rupture are uterine scars, prior cesarean births, prior rupture, trauma, prior invasive molar pregnancy, history of placenta percreta or increta, malpresentation, labor induction with excessive uterine stimulation, and crack cocaine use (Toppenberg & Block, 2002).

Nursing Management

Timely management of uterine rupture depends on prompt detection. Because many women desire a trial of labor after a previous cesarean birth, the nurse must be familiar with the signs and symptoms of uterine rupture. It is difficult to prevent uterine rupture or to predict which women will experience rupture, so constant preparedness is necessary.

Assessment

Generally, the first and most reliable symptom of uterine rupture is sudden fetal distress. Other signs may include acute and continuous abdominal pain with or without an epidural, vaginal bleeding, hematuria, irregular abdominal wall contour, loss of station in the fetal presenting part, and hypovolemic shock in the woman, fetus, or both (Curran, 2003). Screening all women with previous uterine surgical scars is important, and continuous electronic fetal monitoring should be used during labor because this may provide the only indication of an impending rupture. Reviewing a client's history for risk factors might prove to be life-saving for both mother and fetus.

Nursing Interventions

Because the presenting signs may be nonspecific, the initial management will be the same as that for any other cause of acute fetal distress. Urgent delivery by cesarean birth is indicated. The life-threatening nature of uterine rupture is underscored by the fact that the maternal circulatory system delivers approximately 500 mL of blood to the term uterus every minute (Toppenberg & Block, 2002). Maternal death is a real possibility without rapid intervention.

Newborn outcome after rupture depends largely on the speed with which surgical rescue is carried out. Monitor maternal vital signs and observe for hypotension and tachycardia, which might indicate hypovolemic shock. Assist in preparing for an emergency cesarean birth by alerting the operating room staff, anesthesia provider, and neonatal team. Insert an indwelling urinary (Foley) catheter if one isn't in place already. Inform the woman of the seriousness of this event and remind her that the healthcare staff will be working quickly to ensure her health and that of her fetus. Remain calm and provide reassurance that everything is being done to ensure a safe outcome for both.

Amniotic Fluid Embolism

Amniotic fluid embolism is a rare and often fatal event characterized by the sudden onset of hypotension, hypoxia, and coagulopathy. Amniotic fluid containing particles of debris (e.g., hair, skin, vernix, or meconium) enters the maternal circulation and obstructs the pulmonary vessels, causing respiratory distress and circulatory collapse (Lowdermilk & Perry, 2004). The incidence is approximately 1 case per 8,000 to 30,000 pregnancies (Moore & Ware, 2004).

Normally, amniotic fluid does not enter the maternal circulation because it is contained within the uterus, sealed off by the amniotic sac. An embolus occurs when the barrier between the maternal circulation and the amniotic fluid is broken and amniotic fluid enters the maternal venous system via the endocervical veins, the placental site (if the placenta is separated), or a site of uterine trauma (Perozzi & Englert, 2004). This condition has a high mortality rate: as many as 60% of women die within the first hour after the onset of symptoms, and a large percentage of survivors have permanent hypoxia-induced neurologic damage (Perozzi & Englert, 2004).

Although medical science has supplied many answers to questions about this condition, health care providers remain largely unable to predict or prevent an amniotic fluid embolism or to decrease its mortality rate.

Nursing Management

Immediate recognition and diagnosis of this condition are essential to improve maternal and fetal outcomes. Until recently, the diagnosis could be made only after an autopsy of the mother revealed squamous cells, lanugo hair, or other fetal and amniotic material in the pulmonary arterial vasculature (Gilbert, 2004).

Assessment

The clinical appearance is varied, but most women report difficulty breathing. Other symptoms include hypotension, cyanosis, seizures, tachycardia, coagulation failure, disseminated intravascular coagulation pulmonary edema, uterine atony with subsequent hemorrhage, adult respiratory distress syndrome, and cardiac arrest (Mitchell, 2002). Amniotic fluid embolism should be suspected in any pregnant women with an acute onset of dyspnea, hypotension, and disseminated intravascular coagulation.

Nursing Interventions

Once the signs and symptoms are recognized, supportive measures should be implemented: oxygenation (resuscitation and 100% oxygen), circulation (IV fluids, inotropic agents to maintain cardiac output and blood pressure), control of hemorrhage and coagulopathy (oxytocic agents to control uterine atony and bleeding), and administration of steroids (Solu-Cortef) to control the inflammatory response (Moore & Ware, 2004).

Care is largely supportive and aimed at maintaining oxygenation and hemodynamic function and correcting coagulopathy. There is no specific therapy that is lifesaving once this condition starts. Adequate oxygenation is necessary, with endotracheal intubation and mechanical ventilation for most women. Vasopressors are used to maintain hemodynamic stability. Management of disseminated intravascular coagulation may involve replacement with packed red blood cells or fresh-frozen plasma as necessary. Oxytocin infusions and prostaglandin analogs can be used to address uterine atony.

Explain to the client and family what is happening and what therapies are being instituted. The woman is usually transferred to a critical care unit for intensive observation and care. Assist the family to express their feelings and provide support as needed.

Women Requiring Birth-Related Procedures

Most women can give birth without the need for operative obstetric interventions. Most will expect to have a "natural" birth experience and don't anticipate the need for medical intervention. However, in some situations interventions are necessary to safeguard the health of the mother and fetus. The most common birth-related procedures are amnioinfusion, episiotomy (see Chapter 14), forceps-assisted or vacuum-assisted birth, cesarean birth, and vaginal birth following a previous cesarean birth. Nurses play a major role in helping the couple to cope with any unanticipated procedures by offering thorough explanations of the procedure, its anticipated benefits and risks, and any other options available.

Amnioinfusion

Amnioinfusion is a technique in which a volume of warmed, sterile, normal saline or Ringer's lactate solution is introduced into the uterus through an intrauterine pressure catheter to increase the volume of fluid when oligohydramnios is present (Olds et al., 2004). It is used to change the relationship of the uterus, placenta, cord, and fetus to improve placental and fetal oxygenation. Instilling an isotonic glucose-free solution into the uterus helps to cushion the umbilical cord or dilute thick meconium (Littleton & Engebretson, 2005). This procedure is commonly indicated for severe variable decelerations due to cord compression, oligohydramnios due to placental insufficiency, postmaturity or rupture of membranes, preterm labor with premature rupture of membranes, and thick meconium fluid. Contraindications to amnioinfusion include vaginal bleeding of unknown origin, umbilical cord prolapse, amnionitis, uterine hypertonicity, and severe fetal distress (Green & Wilkinson, 2004).

There is no standard protocol for amnioinfusion. After obtaining informed consent, a vaginal examination is performed to evaluate for cord prolapse, establish dilation, and confirm presentation. Next, 250 to 500 mL of warmed normal saline or lactated Ringer's solution is administered using an infusion pump over 20 to 30 minutes. Overdistention of the uterus is a risk, so the amount of fluid infused must be monitored closely (Lowdermilk & Perry, 2004).

Nursing Management

Nursing management during this procedure includes:

- Explain the need for the procedure, what it involves, and how it may solve the problem.
- Inform the mother that she will need to remain on bed rest during the procedure.
- Assess the duration and intensity of uterine contractions frequently to identify overdistention or increased uterine tone.
- Monitor the mother's vital signs and associated discomfort level.
- Maintain adequate intake and output records.
- Stay alert to the FHR pattern to determine whether the amnioinfusion is improving the fetal status.

• Prepare the mother for a possible cesarean birth if the FHR does not improve after the amnioinfusion.

Forceps- or Vacuum-Assisted Birth

Forceps or a vacuum extractor may be used to apply traction to the fetal head or to provide a method of rotating the fetal head during birth. **Forceps** are stainless-steel instruments, similar to tongs, with rounded edges that fit around the fetus's head. Some forceps have open blades and some have solid blades. Outlet forceps are used when the fetal head is crowning and low forceps are used when the fetal head is at a +2 station or lower but not yet crowning. The forceps are applied to the sides of the fetal head. The type of forceps used is determined by the birth attendant. All forceps have a locking mechanism that prevents the blades from compressing the fetal skull (Fig. 21-5).

A **vacuum extractor** is a cup-shaped instrument attached to a suction pump used for extraction of the fetal head (Fig. 21-6). The suction cup is placed against the occiput of the fetal head. The pump is used to create negative pressure (suction) of approximately 50 to 60 mm Hg. The birth attendant then applies traction until the fetal head emerges from the vagina.

The indications for the use of either method are similar and include a prolonged second stage of labor, a nonreassuring FHR pattern, failure of the presenting part to fully rotate and descend in the pelvis, limited sensation and inability to push effectively due to the effects of regional anesthesia, maternal heart disease, acute pulmonary edema, intrapartum infection, maternal fatigue, or infection (Olds et al., 2004).

The use of forceps or a vacuum extractor poses the risk of tissue trauma to the mother and the newborn. Maternal trauma may include lacerations of the cervix, vagina, or perineum; hematoma; extension of the episiotomy incision into the anus; hemorrhage; and infection. Potential newborn trauma includes ecchymoses, facial and scalp lacerations, facial nerve injury, cephalhematoma, and caput succedaneum (Smith, 2004).

Nursing Management

Nursing management for either forceps or vacuum extraction involves preventive measures to reduce the need for either procedure. These measures include frequently changing the client's position, encouraging ambulation if permitted, frequently reminding the client to empty her bladder to allow maximum space for birth, and providing adequate hydration throughout labor. Additional nursing measures include assessing maternal vital signs, the contraction pattern, the fetal status, and the maternal response to the procedure. Provide a thorough explanation of the procedure and the rationale for its use. Reassure the mother that any marks or swelling on the newborn's head or face will disappear without treatment within 2 to 3 days. Alert the postpartum nursing staff about the use of the technique so that they can observe for any bleeding or infection related to genital lacerations.

Cesarean Birth

A **cesarean birth** is the delivery of the fetus through an incision in the abdomen and uterus. A classic (vertical) or low transverse incision may be used; today, the low transverse incision is more common (Fig. 21-7).

The number of cesarean births has steadily risen in the United States: today approximately one in five births occurs this way (Mackenzie et al., 2003). Although there has been some decline in rates since the 1980s, the United States still has a way to go to reduce its surgical birth rates (USDHHS, 2000).

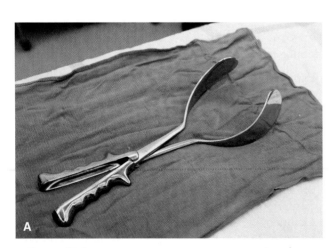

A

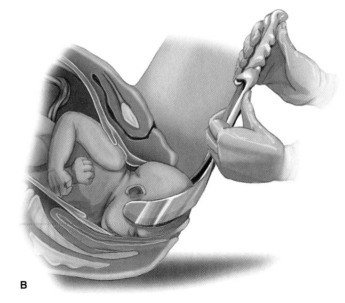

B

● Figure 21-5 Forceps delivery. (**A**) Example of forceps. (**B**) Forceps applied to the fetus.

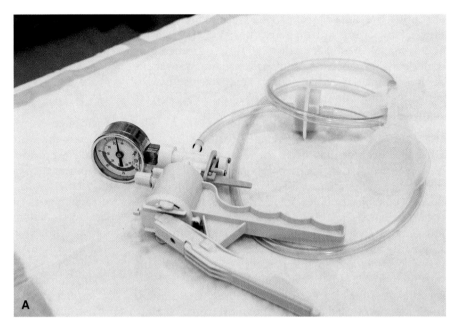

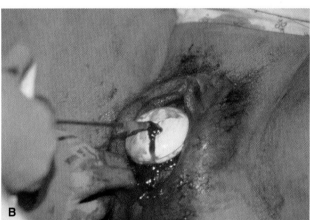

● Figure 21-6 Vacuum extractor for delivery. (**A**) Example of a vacuum extractor. (**B**) Vacuum extractor applied to the fetal head to assist in delivery.

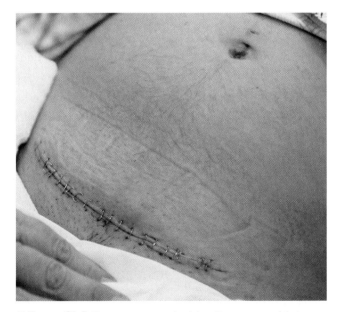

● Figure 21-7 Low transverse incision for cesarean birth.

Several factors may explain this increased incidence of cesarean deliveries: the use of electronic fetal monitoring, which identifies fetal distress early; the reduced number of forceps-assisted births; older maternal age and reduced parity, with more nulliparous women having infants; convenience to the client and doctor; and a increase in malpractice suits (Youngkin & Davis, 2004).

Cesarean birth is a major surgical procedure with increased risks compared to a vaginal birth. The client is at risk for complications such as infection, hemorrhage, aspiration, pulmonary embolism, urinary tract trauma, thrombophlebitis, paralytic ileus, and atelectasis. Fetal injury and transient tachypnea of the newborn also may occur (Green & Wilkinson, 2004).

Any condition that prevents the safe passage of the fetus through the birth canal or that seriously compromises maternal or fetal well-being may be an indication for a cesarean birth. Examples include active genital herpes, fetal macrosomia, fetopelvic disproportion, prolapsed umbilical cord, placental abnormality (previa or abruptio), previous classic uterine incision or scar, gestational hypertension, diabetes, positive HIV status, and dystocia (Breslin & Lucas, 2003). Fetal indications include malpresentation (nonvertex presentation), congenital anomalies (fetal neural tube defects, hydrocephalus, abdominal wall defects), and fetal distress (Sehdev, 2005).

Preoperative Nursing Management

Once the decision has been made to proceed with a cesarean birth, extensive preparation is needed. Several diagnostic studies are usually ordered to ensure the well-being of both parties. These may include a complete blood count; urinalysis to rule out infection; blood type and cross-match so that blood is available for transfusion if needed; an ultrasound to determine fetal position and placental location; and an amniocentesis to determine fetal lung maturity if needed. Spinal, epidural, or general anesthesia is used for cesarean births. Epidural anesthesia is most commonly used today because most women wish to be awake and aware of the birth expe-rience. The healthcare provider usually discusses the need for the cesarean birth and the risks and obtains a signed informed consent. Client preparation varies depending on whether the cesarean birth is planned or unplanned.

The nurse's role before surgery includes the following:

- Assess maternal and fetal status frequently.
- Determine the time of last oral intake and document what was eaten.
- Ascertain the client's and family's understanding of the surgical procedure.
- Allow discussion of fears and expectations if the surgery is unplanned.
- Schedule all diagnostic tests ordered and monitor the results.
- Reinforce the reasons for surgery given by the surgeon.
- Outline the procedure and expectations of the surgical experience.
- Provide teaching about interventions to reduce postoperative complications.
- Demonstrate the use of the incentive spirometer and deep-breathing exercises.
- Prepare the surgical site as ordered.
- Start an IV infusion for fluid replacement therapy as ordered.
- Insert an indwelling (Foley) catheter and inform the client about how long it will remain in place (usually 24 hours).
- Administer any preoperative medications as ordered; document the time administered and the client's reaction.
- Reassure the client that pain management will be provided throughout the procedure and afterward.
- Explain what to expect postoperatively to allay anxiety.
- Help transport the client and her partner to the operative area.
- Maintain a calm, confident manner in all interactions with the client and family.

Postoperative Nursing Management

Postoperative care for the mother who has had a cesarean birth is similar to that for one who has had a vaginal birth, with a few additional measures:

- Assess vital signs and lochia flow every 15 minutes for the first hour, then every 30 minutes for the next hour, and then every 4 hours if stable.
- Assess the woman's level of consciousness if sedative drugs were administered.
- Monitor the return of sensation to the legs if a regional anesthetic was used.
- Encourage the woman to cough, perform deep-breathing exercises, and use the incentive spirometer every 2 hours.
- Inspect the abdominal dressing and document description of drainage.
- Assess uterine tone to determine fundal firmness.
- Monitor urinary output and check for flow within the catheter system.
- Instruct the client on perineal hygiene.
- Administer pain medication as ordered and provide comfort measures.
- Assist the client to move in bed and turn side to side to improve circulation.
- Check the patency of the IV line, make sure the infusion is flowing at the correct rate, and inspect the infusion site frequently for redness.
- Monitor intake and output as per orders.
- Encourage early touching and holding of the newborn to promote bonding.
- Assist with breastfeeding initiation and offer continued support.
- Complete a complete head-to-toe assessment daily and document.
- Assess for evidence of abdominal distention and auscultate bowel sounds.
- Assist with early ambulation to prevent respiratory and cardiovascular problems.
- Assess the couple's perception of the surgical birth experience.
- Provide discharge teaching such as adequate rest, signs of infection, lifting restrictions.

Although the nurse's role in a cesarean birth can be very technical and skill-oriented at times, the focus must remain on the woman, not the equipment surrounding the bed. Care should be centered on the family, not the surgery. Provide education and minimize separation of the mother, father, and newborn. Remember that the client is anxious and concerned about her welfare as well as that of her child. Use touch, eye contact, therapeutic communication, and genuine caring to provide couples with a positive birth experience, regardless of the type of delivery.

Vaginal Birth After Cesarean

Vaginal birth after cesarean (VBAC) describes a woman who gives birth vaginally after having at least one previous cesarean birth. The old expression "once a cesarean, always a cesarean" is still largely true today. Despite evidence that some women who have had a cesarean birth are suitable candidates for vaginal birth, most women who have had a cesarean birth once undergo another for subsequent pregnancies (Dauphinee, 2004). The choice of a vaginal or a repeat cesarean birth can be offered to women who had a lower abdominal incision. However, controversy remains. The argument against VBAC focuses on the risk of uterine rupture and hemorrhage. Although the risk of uterine rupture is relatively low, concerns over malpractice issues have resulted in an increased incidence of repeat cesarean births.

Contraindications to VBAC include a prior classic uterine incision, prior transfundal uterine surgery (myomectomy), uterine scar other than low-transverse cesarean scar, contracted pelvis, and inadequate staff or facility if a cesarean birth is required (Caughey, 2004). Most women go through a trial of labor to see how they progress, but this must be performed in an environment capable of handling the acute emergency of uterine rupture. The use of cervical ripening agents increases the risk of uterine rupture and thus is contraindicated in VBAC clients. The woman considering induction of labor after a previous cesarean birth needs to be informed of the increased risk of uterine rupture with an induction than with spontaneous labor (Dauphinee, 2004).

Women are the primary decision-makers about the choice of birth method, but they need education about VBAC during their prenatal course.

Nursing Management

Nursing management is similar for any women experiencing labor, but certain areas require special focus:

- *Consent:* Fully informed consent is essential for the woman who wants to have a trial of labor after cesarean birth. The client must be advised about the risks as well as the benefits. She must understand the ramifications of uterine rupture, even though the risk is small.
- *Documentation:* Record-keeping is an important component of safe client care. If and when an emergency occurs, it is imperative to take care of the client, but also to keep track of the plan of care, interventions and their timing, and the client's response. Events and activities can be written right on the fetal monitoring tracing to correlate with the change in fetal status.
- *Surveillance:* A nonreassuring fetal monitor tracing in a women undergoing a trial of labor after a cesarean birth should alert the nurse to the possibility of uterine rupture. Terminal bradycardia must be considered an emergency situation, and the nurse should prepare the team for an emergency delivery.
- *Readiness for emergency:* According to ACOG criteria for a safe trial of labor for a woman who has had a previous cesarean birth, the physician, anesthesia provider, and

operating room team must be immediately available. Anything less would place the women and fetus at risk (Dauphinee, 2004).

Nurses must act as advocates, giving input on the appropriate selection of women who wish to undergo VBAC. Nurses also need to become experts at reading fetal monitoring tracings to identify a nonreassuring pattern and set in motion an emergency delivery. Including all these nursing strategies will make VBAC safer for all.

KEY CONCEPTS

- Risk factors for dystocia include epidural analgesia, occiput posterior position, longer first stage of labor, nulliparity, short maternal stature (<5'), high birth weight, maternal age older than 35 years, gestational age more than 41 weeks, chorioamnionitis, pelvic contractions, macrosomia, and high station at complete cervical dilation.
- Dystocia may result from problems in the powers, passenger, passageway, or psyche.
- Problems involving the powers that lead to dystocia include hypertonic uterine dysfunction, hypotonic uterine dysfunction, and precipitous labor.
- Management of hypertonic labor pattern involves therapeutic rest with the use of sedatives to promote relaxation and stop the abnormal activity of the uterus.
- Any presentation other than occiput or a slight variation of the fetal position or size increases the probability of dystocia.
- Multiple gestation may result in dysfunctional labor due to uterine overdistention, which may lead to hypotonic dystocia, and abnormal presentations of the fetuses.
- During labor, evaluation of fetal descent, cervical effacement and dilation, and characteristics of uterine contractions are paramount to determine progress or lack thereof.
- Antepartum assessment for a postterm pregnancy typically include daily fetal movement counts done by the woman, nonstress tests done twice weekly, amniotic fluid assessments as part of the biophysical profile, and weekly cervical examinations to check for ripening for induction.
- Once the cervix is ripe, oxytocin is the most popular pharmacologic agent used for inducing or augmenting labor.
- Generally, the first and most reliable symptom of uterine rupture is fetal distress.
- Amniotic fluid embolism is a rare but often fatal event characterized by the sudden onset of hypotension, hypoxia, and coagulopathy.
- Cesarean births have steadily risen in the United States; today, approximately one in five births occurs this way. Cesarean birth is a major surgical procedure and has increased risks over vaginal birth.

References

Abrahams, C., & Katz, M. (2002). A perspective on the diagnosis of preterm labor. *Journal of Perinatal & Neonatal Nursing, 16*(1), 1–11.

American Academy of Pediatrics (AAP) and American College of Obstetricians and Gynecologists (ACOG) (2003). *Guidelines for perinatal care* (5th ed.). Washington, D.C.: Author.

American College of Obstetricians and Gynecologists (ACOG) (2002). *Diagnosis and management of preeclampsia and eclampsia* (Practice Bulletin No. 33). Washington, D.C.: Author.

American College of Obstetricians and Gynecologists (ACOG) (2004). Management of postterm pregnancy (Practice Bulletin #55). *Obstetrics and Gynecology, 194*, 639–646.

Baxley, E. G. (2003). Labor induction: a decade of change. *American Family Physician, 67*(10), 2076–2080.

Baxley, E. G., & Gobbo, R. W. (2004). Shoulder dystocia. *American Family Physician, 69*(7), 1707–1714.

Bernhardt, J., & Dorman, K. (2004). Pre-term birth risk: assessment tools. *AWHONN Lifelines, 8*(1), 38–44.

Bonilla, M. M., & Forouzan, I. (2004). Dystocia. *eMedicine.* [Online] Available at: http://www.eMedicine.com/med/topic3280.htm

Breslin, E. T., & Lucas, V. A. (2003). *Women's health nursing: toward evidence-based practice.* St. Louis: Saunders.

Caughey, A. B. (2004). Vaginal birth after cesarean delivery. *eMedicine.* [Online] Available at: http://www.emedicine.com/med/topic3434.htm

Church-Balin, C., & Damus, K. (2003). Preventing prematurity. *AWHONN Lifelines, 17*(2), 97–101.

Cockey, C. D. (2004). Prematurity hits record high: more babies born at risk for lifetime disabilities. *AWHONN Lifelines, 8*(2), 104–107.

Condon, M. C. (2004). *Women's health: an integrated approach to wellness and illness.* Upper Saddle River, NJ: Prentice Hall.

Connors, P. (2004). Not a second to spare when managing shoulder dystocia. *Nursing Spectrum,* [Online] Available at: http://community.nursingspectrum.com/MagazineArticles/article.cfm?AID=11289

Curran, C. A. (2003). Intrapartum emergencies. *JOGNN, 32*(6), 802–813.

Damato, E. G., Dowling, D. A., Madigan, E. A., & Thanattherakul, C. (2005). Duration of breastfeeding for mothers of twins. *JOGNN, 34*(2), 201–209.

Dauphinee, J. D. (2004). VBAC: safety for the patient and the nurse. *JOGNN, 33*, 105–115.

Fischer, R. (2005). Breech presentation. *eMedicine.* [Online] Available at: http://www.emedicine.com/med/topic3272.htm

Freda, M. C., & Patterson, E. T. (2004). *Pre-term labor: prevention and nursing management* (3rd ed.). March of Dimes Nursing Module Series. White Plains, NY: March of Dimes.

Gabbe, S., Niebyl, J., & Simpson, J. (Eds.) (2002). *Obstetrics: normal and problem pregnancies* (4th ed.). New York: Churchill Livingstone.

Gilbert, E. (2004). Labor and delivery at risk. In S. Mattson & J. E. Smith, *Core curriculum for maternal-newborn nursing* (3rd ed., pp. 818–849). St. Louis: Elsevier Saunders.

Gilbert, E., & Harmon, J. (2003). *Manual of high-risk pregnancy and delivery* (3rd ed.). St. Louis: Mosby.

Green, C. J., & Wilkinson, J. M. (2004). *Maternal newborn nursing care plans.* St. Louis: Mosby, Inc.

Hall, J. G. (2003). Twinning. *Lancet, 362*, 735–743.

Harvey, E. A. (2003). Managing preterm labor with home uterine monitoring and tocolytics. *Nursing Spectrum.* [Online] Available at: http://nsweb.nursingspectrum.com/ce/ce162.htm

Hodgson, B. B., & Kizior, R. J. (2004). *Saunders nursing drug handbook.* St. Louis: Saunders.

Hofmeyr, G. J., & Gyte, G. (2004). Interventions to help external cephalic version for breech presentation at term. *The Cochrane Database Systematic Reviews 2004,* 1(CD000184.pub2). DOI: 1002/14651858.CD000184.pub2.

Iams, J. D. (2003). Prediction and early detection of pre-term labor. *Obstetrics and Gynecology, 101*, 402–412.

Iams, J. D., & Creasy, R. K. (2004). Preterm labor and delivery. In R. K. Creasy & R. Resnik (Eds.), *Maternal-fetal medicine: principles and practice* (5th ed., pp. 498–531). Philadelphia: Saunders.

Jazayeri, A., & Contreras, D. (2005). Macrosomia. *EMedicine.* [Online] Available at: http://emedicine.com/med/topic3279.htm

Joy, S., & Lyon, D. (2005). Diagnosis of abnormal labor. *EMedicine.* [Online] Available at: http://www.emedicine.com/med/topic3488.html

Kavanagh, J., & Kelly, A. J. (2005). Sexual intercourse for cervical ripening and induction of labor. *The Cochrane Database of Systematic Reviews.* Issue No.: CD003093. DOI: 10.1002/14651858. CD003093.

Kavanagh, J., Kelly, A. J., & Thomas, J. (2005). Breast stimulation for cervical ripening and induction of labor. *The Cochrane Database of Systematic Reviews.* Issue No.: CD003392. DOI: 10.1002/14651858. CD003392.

Kennelly, M. M., Anjum, R., Lyons, S., & Burke, G. (2003). Postpartum fetal head circumference and its influence on labor duration in nullipara. *Journal of Obstetrics and Gynecology, 23*(5), 496–499.

Leonard, L. G. (2002). Prenatal behavior of multiples: implications for families and nurses. *JOGNN, 31*(3), 248–255.

Lewis, D. F. (2005). PPROM: new strategies for expectant management. *OBG Management.* [Online] Available: http://www.obgmanagement.com/content/obg_featurexml.asp?file=2004/10obg_1004_00

Lindsey, J. L., & Hernandez, G. (2004) Evaluation of fetal death. *eMedicine.* [Online] Available: http://www.emedicine.com/med/topic3235.htm

Littleton, L. Y., & Engebretson, J. C. (2005). *Maternity nursing care.* Clifton Park, NY: Thomson Delmar Learning.

London, M. L., Ladewig, P. W., Ball, J. W., & Bindler, R. C. (2003). *Maternal-newborn & child nursing: family-centered care.* Upper Saddle River, NJ: Prentice Hall.

Lowdermilk, D. L., & Perry, S. E. (2004). *Maternity & women's health care* (8th ed.) St. Louis: Mosby.

Mackenzie, I. Z., Cooke, I., & Annan, B. (2003). Indications for cesarean section in a consultant obstetric unit over three decades. *Journal of Obstetrics and Gynecology, 23*(3), 233–338.

March of Dimes (2005). Preterm labor and birth: a serious pregnancy complication. *March of Dimes Birth Defects Foundation.* [Online] Available at: http://www.marchofdimes.com/printableArticles/240_1080.asp?printable=true

March of Dimes (2005). Umbilical cord abnormalities. *March of Dimes Birth Defects Foundation.* [Online] Available at: http://www.marchofdimes.com/professionals/681_4546.asp

Mattson, S., & Smith, J. E. (2004). *Core curriculum for maternal-newborn nursing* (3rd ed.). St. Louis: Elsevier Saunders.

McKinney, E. S., James, S. R., Murray, S. S., & Ashwill, J. W. (2005). *Maternal-child nursing* (2nd ed.). St. Louis: Elsevier Saunders.

Mills, L. W., & Moses, D. T. (2002). Oral health during pregnancy. *MCN, 27*(5), 275–281.

Mitchell, L. (2002). Amniotic fluid embolism. *Topics in Emergency Medicine, 24*(4), 21–25.

Molkenboer, J. F. M., Reijners, E. P. J., Nijhuis, J. G., & Roumen, F. J. M. E. (2004). Moderate neonatal morbidity after vaginal delivery. *Journal of Maternal-Fetal and Neonatal Medicine, 16*, 357–361.

Moore, L. E., & Ware, D. (2004). Amniotic fluid embolism. *eMedicine.* [Online] Available at: http://emedicine.com/med/topic122.htm

Moore, M. L. (2003). Preterm labor and birth: what have we learned in the past two decades? *JOGNN, 32*(5), 638–649.

Moos, M. K. (2004). Understanding prematurity: sorting fact from fiction. *AWHONN, 8*(1), 32–37.

Morantz, C., & Torrey, B. (2003). ACOG recommendations on preterm labor. *American Family Physician, 68*(4), 763–764.

Morrison, J. C., Roberts, W. E., Jones, J. S., Istwan, N., Rhea, D., & Stanziano, G. (2004). Frequency of nursing, physician, and hospital interventions in women at risk for preterm delivery. *Journal of Maternal-Fetal and Neonatal Medicine, 16*, 102–105.

Newton, E. R. (2004). Preterm labor. *eMedicine.* [Online] Available at: http://www.emedicine.com/med/topic3245.htm

Olds, S. B., London, M. L., Ladewig, P. W., & Davidson, M. R. (2004). *Maternal-newborn nursing & women's health care* (7th ed.). Upper Saddle River, NJ: Pearson Prentice Hall.

Olds, S. B., London, M. L., Ladewig, P. W., & Davidson, M. R. (2004). *Clinical handbook for maternal-newborn nursing & women's health care* (7th ed.). Upper Saddle River, NJ: Pearson Prentice Hall.

Perozzi, K. J., & Englert, N. C. (2004). Amniotic fluid embolism: an obstetric emergency. *Critical Care Nurse, 24*(4), 54–61.

Poole, J., & White, D. (2003) *March of Dimes nursing modules: obstetrical emergencies for the perinatal nurse.* White Plains, NY: March of Dimes Birth Defects Foundation.

Rai, J., & Schreiber, J. R. (2005). Cervical ripening. *eMedicine.* [Online] Available at: http://www.emedicine.com/med/topic3282.htm

Ressel, G. W. (2002). ACOG issues recommendations on assessment of risk factors for preterm birth. *American Family Physician.* [Online] Available at: http://www.aafp.org/afp/20020201/practice.html

Ressel, G. W. (2004). ACOG releases report on dystocia and augmentation of labor. *American Family Physician, 69*(5), 1290–1291.

Rideout, S. L. (2005). Tocolytics for the pre-term labor: what nurses need to know. *AWHONN Lifelines, 9*(1), 56–61.

Sanchez-Ramos, L., & Hsieh, E. (2003) Pharmacologic methods for cervical ripening and labor induction. *Current Women's Health Reports, 3*(1), 55–60.

Sanchez-Ramos, L., Oliver, F., Delke, I., & Kaunitz, A. M. (2003). Labor induction verses expectant management for postterm pregnancies: a systematic review with meta-analysis. *Obstetrics & Gynecology, 101*(6), 1312–1318.

Schnell, Z. B., Van Leeuwen, A. M., & Kranpitz, T. R. (2003). *Davis's comprehensive laboratory and diagnostic test handbook—with nursing implications.* Philadelphia: F. A. Davis.

Sehdev, H. M. (2005). Cesarean delivery. *eMedicine.* [Online] Available at: http://www.emedicine.com/med/topic3283.htm

Simpson, K. (2002). *Cervical ripening and induction and augmentation of labor* (2nd ed.) Washington, D.C.: AWHONN.

Simpson, K. R., & Atterbury, J. (2003). Trends and issues in labor induction in the United States: implications for clinical practice. *JOGNN, 32*(6), 767–779.

Slattery, M. M., & Morrison, J. J. (2002). Preterm delivery. *Lancet, 360*, 1489–1497.

Sloane, E. (2002). *Biology of women* (4th ed.). Albany, NY: Delmar Thomson Learning.

Smith, K. V. (2004). Normal childbirth. In S. Mattson & J. E. Smith, *Core curriculum for maternal-newborn nursing* (3rd ed., pp. 271–302). St. Louis: Elsevier Saunders.

Tenore, J. L. (2003). Methods for cervical ripening and induction of labor. *American Family Physician, 67*(10), 2123–2128.

Toppenberg, K. S., & Block, W. A. (2002). Uterine rupture: what family physicians need to know. *American Family Physician, 66*(5), 823–829.

U.S. Department of Health and Human Services (USDHHS), Public Health Service. (2000). *Healthy people 2010* (conference edition, in two volumes). U.S. Department of Health and Human Services. Washington, D.C.: U.S. Government Printing Office.

Webb, D. A., & Culhane, J. (2002). Hospital variation in episiotomy use and the risk of perinatal trauma during childbirth. *Birth, 29*(2), 132–136.

Weiss, M. E., Saks, N. P., & Harris, S. (2002). Resolving the uncertainty of preterm symptoms: women's experiences with the onset of preterm labor. *JOGNN, 31*(1), 66–75.

Wilkes, P. T., & Galan, H. (2002). Postdate pregnancy. *eMedicine.* [Online] Available at: http://www.emedicine.com/med/topic3248.htm

Wilkes, P. T., & Galan, H. (2004). Premature rupture of membranes. *eMedicine.* [Online] Available at: http://www.emedicine.com/med/topic3246.htm

Witcher, P. S. (2002). Treatment of preterm labor. *Journal of Perinatal & Neonatal Nursing, 16*(1), 25–46.

Youngkin, E. Q., & Davis, M. S. (2004). *Women's health: a primary care clinical guide* (3rd ed.). Upper Saddle River, NJ: Pearson Prentice Hall.

Web Resources

American Society of Reproductive Medicine: **www.asrm.org**
American Academy of Pediatrics: **www.app.org**
American College of Obstetricians and Gynecologists: **www.acog.org**
Association of Women's Health, Obstetric and Neonatal Nurses: **www.awhonn.org**
Birthrites: Healing after Cesarean, Inc.: **www.birthrites.org**
Department of Health and Human Services: **www.4women.gov**
International Cesarean Awareness Network: **www.ican-online.org**
March of Dimes: **www.modimes.org**
Mothers of Super Twins: **www.mostonline.org**
National Perinatal Association: **www.nationalperinatal.org**
SHARE Parents support group: **www.nationalshareoffice.com/**
Sidelines: High Risk Pregnancy Support Group: **www.sidelines.org**
Smoke-free Families: **www.smokefreefamilies.org**
VBAC: **www.vbac.com**

Chapter WORKSHEET

● MULTIPLE CHOICE QUESTIONS

1. The medical record of a client reveals a condition in which the fetus cannot physically pass through the maternal pelvis. The nurse interprets this as:

   a. Cervical insufficiency

   b. Contracted pelvis

   c. Maternal disproportion

   d. Fetopelvic disproportion

2. The nurse would anticipate a cesarean birth for a client who has which infection present at the onset of labor?

   a. Hepatitis

   b. Herpes simplex virus

   c. Toxoplasmosis

   d. Human papillomavirus

3. After a vaginal examination, the nurse determines that the client's fetus is in an occiput posterior position. The nurse would anticipate that the client will have:

   a. Intense back pain

   b. Frequent leg cramps

   c. Nausea and vomiting

   d. A precipitous birth

4. The rationale for using a prostaglandin gel for a client prior to the induction of labor is to:

   a. Stimulate uterine contractions

   b. Numb cervical pain receptors

   c. Prevent cervical lacerations

   d. Soften and efface the cervix

5. A client in active labor and dilated 4 cm suddenly has no progress and her contractions weaken in intensity and frequency. The nurse interprets this as a sign of:

   a. Hypertonic labor

   b. Precipitous labor

   c. Hypotonic labor

   d. Dysfunctional labor

● CRITICAL THINKING EXERCISES

1. Marsha, a 26-year-old multipara, is admitted to the labor and birth suite in active labor. After a few hours, the nurse notices a change in her contraction pattern—poor contraction intensity and no progression of cervical dilatation beyond 5 cm. Marsha keeps asking about her labor progress and appears anxious about "how long this labor is taking."

   a. Based on the nurse's findings, what might you suspect is going on?

   b. How can the nurse address Marsha's anxiety?

   c. What are the appropriate interventions to change this labor pattern?

2. Marsha activates her call light and states, "I feel increased wetness down below."

   a. What new development might be occurring?

   b. How will the nurse confirm her suspicions?

   c. What interventions are appropriate for this finding?

● STUDY ACTIVITIES

1. Visit the SHARE Pregnancy and Infant Loss Support, Inc. website (http://www.nationalshareoffice.com/) and critique it as to its helpfulness to parents and resources available to assist them locally.

2. Outline the fetal and maternal risks associated with a postterm pregnancy.

3. An abnormal or difficult labor describes
   _____.

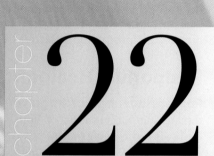

Nursing Management of the Postpartum Woman at Risk

KeyTERMS

mastitis
metritis
postpartum depression
postpartum hemorrhage
subinvolution
thrombophlebitis
uterine atony
uterine inversion

LearningOBJECTIVES

After studying the chapter content, the student should be able to accomplish the following:

1. Define the key terms.
2. Discuss the risk factors, clinical manifestations, preventive measures, and management of common postpartum complications.
3. Describe at least two affective disorders that can occur in women after birth and specific therapeutic management to address them.
4. Differentiate the causes of postpartum hemorrhage and list appropriate assessments and interventions.
5. Outline the role of the nurse in assessing and managing care of women with selected postpartum complications.

After holding their breath during the childbirth experience, nurses shouldn't let it out fully and relax until discharge.

ypically, recovery from childbirth proceeds normally in both physiologic and psychological aspects. It is a time filled with many changes and wide-ranging emotions, and the new mother commonly experiences a great sense of accomplishment. However, the woman can experience deviations from the norm, developing a postpartum condition that places her at risk. The development of a high-risk condition or complication can become a life-threatening event, and Healthy People 2010 addresses these risks in two National Health Goals (Healthy People 2010).

This chapter will address the nursing management of the most common conditions that place the postpartum woman at risk: hemorrhage, infection, thromboembolic disease, and postpartum affective disorders.

Postpartum Hemorrhage

Postpartum hemorrhage is a potentially life-threatening complication of both vaginal and cesarean births. It is the leading cause of maternal mortality in the United States (Smith & Brennan, 2004). Roughly one third of maternal deaths are related to postpartum hemorrhage, and it occurs in 4% of deliveries (Scott et al., 2003).

Postpartum hemorrhage is defined as a blood loss greater than 500 mL after vaginal birth or more than 1,000 mL after a cesarean birth. Blood loss that occurs within 24 hours of birth is termed early postpartum hemorrhage; blood loss that occurs 24 hours to 6 weeks after birth is termed late postpartum hemorrhage. However, this definition is arbitrary, because estimates of blood loss at birth are subjective and generally inaccurate. Studies have suggested that health care providers consistently underestimate actual blood loss (Wainscott, 2004). A more objective definition of postpartum hemorrhage would be any amount of bleeding that places the mother in hemodynamic jeopardy.

Factors that place a woman at risk for postpartum hemorrhage are listed in Box 22-1.

Etiology

Excessive bleeding can occur at any time between the separation of the placenta and its expulsion or removal. The most common cause of postpartum hemorrhage is **uterine atony,** failure of the uterus to contract and retract after birth. The uterus must remain contracted after birth to control bleeding from the placental site. Any factor that causes the uterus to relax after birth will cause bleeding—even a full bladder that displaces the uterus.

Over the course of a pregnancy, maternal blood volume increases by approximately 50% (from 4 to 6 L). The plasma volume increases somewhat more than the total red blood cell volume, leading to a fall in the hemoglobin and hematocrit. The increase in blood volume meets the perfusion demands of the low-resistance uteroplacental unit and provides a reserve for the blood loss that occurs at delivery (Cunningham, 2005). Given this increase, the typical signs of hemorrhage (e.g., falling blood pressure, increasing pulse rate, and decreasing urinary output) do not appear until as much as 1,800 to 2,100 mL has been lost (Gilbert & Harmon, 2003). In addition, accurate determination of actual blood loss is difficult because of pooling inside the uterus, on peripads, mattresses, and the floor. Because no universal clinical standard exists, nurses must be vigilant of risk factors, checking clients carefully before letting the birth attendant leave.

Other causes of postpartum hemorrhage include lacerations of the genital tract, episiotomy, retained placental fragments, uterine inversion, coagulation disorders, and hematomas of the vulva, vagina, or subperitoneal areas (London et al., 2003). A helpful way to remember the causes of postpartum hemorrhage is the "4 Ts": *tone, tissue, trauma,* and *thrombosis* (Society of Obstetricians and Gynecologists of Canada, 2002).

BOX 22-1

FACTORS PLACING A WOMAN AT RISK FOR POSTPARTUM HEMORRHAGE

- Prolonged first, second, or third stage of labor
- Previous history of postpartum hemorrhage
- Multiple gestation
- Uterine infection
- Manual extraction of placenta
- Arrest of descent
- Maternal exhaustion, malnutrition, or anemia
- Mediolateral episiotomy
- Preeclampsia
- Precipitous birth
- Maternal hypotension
- Previous placenta previa
- Coagulation abnormalities
- Birth canal lacerations
- Operative birth (forceps or vacuum)
- Augmented labor with medication
- Coagulation abnormalities
- Grand multiparity
- Hydramnios (Higgins, 2004)

Tone

Altered uterine muscle tone most commonly results from overdistention of the uterus. Overdistention can be caused by multifetal gestation, fetal macrosomia, hydramnios, fetal abnormality, or placental fragments. Other causes might include prolonged or rapid, forceful labor, especially if stimulated; bacterial toxins (e.g., chorioamnionitis, endomyometritis, septicemia); use of anesthesia, especially halothane; and magnesium sulfate used in the treatment of preeclampsia (Youngkin & Davis, 2004). Overdistention of the uterus is a major risk factor for uterine atony, the most common cause of early postpartum hemorrhage, which can lead to hypovolemic shock.

Tissue

Uterine contraction and retraction lead to detachment and expulsion of the placenta after birth. Complete detachment and expulsion of the placenta permit continued contraction and optimal occlusion of blood vessels. Failure of complete separation of the placenta and expulsion does not allow the uterus to contract fully, since retained fragments occupy space and prevent the uterus from contracting fully to clamp down on blood vessels; this can lead to hemorrhage. After the placenta is expelled, a thorough inspection is necessary to confirm its intactness; tears or fragments left inside may indicate an accessory lobe or placenta accreta. Placenta accreta is an uncommon condition in which the chorionic villi adhere to the myometrium. This causes the placenta to adhere abnormally to the uterus and not separate and spontaneously deliver. Profuse hemorrhage results because the uterus cannot contract fully.

A prolapse of the uterine fundus to or through the cervix so that the uterus is turned inside out after birth is called **uterine inversion.** This condition is associated with abnormal adherence of the placenta, excessive traction on the umbilical cord, vigorous fundal pressure, precipitous labor, or vigorous manual removal of the placenta. Acute postpartum uterine inversion is rare, with an estimated incidence of 1 in 2,000 births (Pope & O'Grady, 2003). Prompt recognition and rapid treatment to replace the inverted uterus will avoid morbidity and mortality for this serious complication (McKinney et al., 2005).

Subinvolution refers to the incomplete involution of the uterus or failure to return to its normal size and condition after birth (O'Toole, 2005). Complications of subinvolution include hemorrhage, pelvic peritonitis, salpingitis, and abscess formation (Youngkin & Davis, 2004). Causes of subinvolution include retained placental fragments, distended bladder, uterine myoma, and infection. The clinical picture includes a postpartum fundal height that is higher than expected, with a boggy uterus; the lochia fails to change colors from red to serosa to alba within a few weeks. This condition is usually identified at the woman's postpartum examination 4 to 6 weeks after birth with a bimanual vaginal examination or ultrasound. Treatment is directed toward stimulating the uterus to expel fragments with a uterine stimulant, and antibiotics are given to prevent infection.

Trauma

Damage to the genital tract may occur spontaneously or through the manipulations used during birth. For example, a cesarean birth results in more blood loss than a vaginal birth. The amount of blood loss depends on suturing, vasospasm, and clotting for hemostasis. Uterine rupture is more common in women with previous cesarean scars or those who had undergone any procedure resulting in disruption of the uterine wall, including myomectomy, uteroplasty for a congenital anomaly, perforation of the uterus during a dilation and curettage (D&C), biopsy, or intrauterine device (IUD) insertion (Smith & Brennan, 2004).

Trauma can also occur after prolonged or vigorous labor, especially if the uterus has been stimulated with oxytocin or prostaglandins. Trauma can also occur after extrauterine or intrauterine manipulation of the fetus.

Cervical lacerations commonly occur during a forceps delivery or in mothers who have not been able to resist bearing down before the cervix is fully dilated. Vaginal sidewall lacerations are associated with operative vaginal births but may occur spontaneously, especially if the fetal hand presents with the head. Lacerations can arise during manipulations to resolve shoulder dystocia. Lacerations should always be suspected in the face of a contracted uterus with bright-red blood continuing to trickle out of the vagina.

Thrombosis

Thrombosis (blood clots) helps to prevent postpartum hemorrhage immediately after birth by providing a homeostasis in the woman's circulatory system. As long as there is a normal clotting mechanism that is activated, postpartum bleeding will not be exacerbated. Disorders of the coagulation system do not always appear in the immediate postpartum period due to the efficiency of stimulating uterine contractions through medications to prevent hemorrhage. Fibrin deposits and clots in supplying vessels play a significant role in the hours and days after birth. Coagulopathies should be suspected when postpartum bleeding persists without any identifiable cause (Benedetti, 2002).

Ideally, the client's coagulation status is determined during pregnancy. However, if she received no prenatal care, coagulation studies should be ordered immediately to determine her status. Abnormal results typically include decreased platelet and fibrinogen levels, increased prothrombin time, partial thromboplastin time, and fibrin degradation products, and a prolonged bleeding time (Lowdermilk & Perry, 2004). Conditions associated with coagulopathies in the postpartum client include idiopathic thrombocytopenic purpura (ITP), von Willebrand disease (vWD), and disseminated intravascular coagulation (DIC).

Idiopathic Thrombocytopenia Purpura

ITP is a disorder of increased platelet destruction caused by the development of autoantibodies to platelet-membrane antigens. The incidence of ITP in adults is approximately 66 cases per 1 million per year (Silverman, 2005). Thrombocytopenia, capillary fragility, and increased bleeding time define the disorder. Clinical manifestations include easy bruising, bleeding from mucous membranes, menorrhagia, epistaxis, bleeding gums, hematomas, and severe hemorrhage after a cesarean birth or lacerations (Blackwell & Goolsby, 2003). Glucocorticoids and immune globulin are the mainstays of medical therapy.

von Willebrand Disease

von Willebrand disease (vWD) is a congenital bleeding disorder, inherited as an autosomal dominant trait, that is characterized by a prolonged bleeding time, a deficiency of von Willebrand factor, and impairment of platelet adhesion (O'Toole, 2005). In the United States, it is estimated to affect fewer than 3% of the population (Geil, 2004). Most cases remain undiagnosed from lack of awareness, difficulty in diagnosis, a tendency to attribute bleeding to other causes, and variable symptoms (Paper, 2003). Symptoms include excessive bruising, prolonged nosebleeds, and prolonged oozing from wounds after surgery and after childbirth. The goal of therapy is to correct the defect in platelet adhesiveness by raising the level of von Willebrand factor with medications (Bjoring & Baxi, 2004).

Disseminated Intravascular Coagulation

DIC is a life-threatening, acquired pathologic process in which the clotting system is abnormally activated, resulting in widespread clot formation in the small vessels throughout the body (London et al., 2003). It can cause postpartum hemorrhage by altering the blood clotting mechanism. DIC is always a secondary diagnosis that occurs as a complication of abruptio placentae, amniotic fluid embolism, intrauterine fetal death with prolonged retention of the fetus, severe preeclampsia, septicemia, and hemorrhage. Clinical features include petechiae, ecchymoses, bleeding gums, tachycardia, uncontrolled bleeding during birth, and acute renal failure (Higgins, 2004). Treatment goals are to maintain tissue perfusion through aggressive administration of fluid therapy, oxygen, and blood products.

Nursing Management

Pregnancy and childbirth involve significant health risks, even for women with no preexisting health problems. There are an estimated 14 million cases of pregnancy-related hemorrhage every year, with some of these women bleeding to death. Most of these deaths occur within 4 hours of giving birth and are a result of problems during the third stage of labor (MacMullen et al., 2005). The period after the birth and the first hours postpartum are crucial times for the prevention, assessment, and management of bleeding. Compared with other maternal risks such as infection, bleeding can rapidly become life-threatening, and nurses, along with other health care providers, need to identify this condition quickly and intervene appropriately.

Assessment

Since the most common cause of immediate severe postpartum hemorrhage is uterine atony (failure of the uterus to properly contract after birth), assessing uterine tone after birth by palpating the fundus for firmness and location is essential. A soft, boggy fundus indicates uterine atony. A soft, boggy uterus that deviates from the midline suggests a full bladder interfering with uterine involution. If the uterus is not in correct position (midline), it will not be able to contract to control bleeding.

Assess the amount of bleeding. If bleeding continues even though there are no lacerations, suspect retained placental fragments. The uterus remains large with painless dark-red blood mixed with clots. This cause of hemorrhage can be prevented by carefully inspecting the placenta for intactness.

If trauma is suspected, attempt to identify the source and document it. Typically, the uterus will be firm with a steady stream or trickle of unclotted bright-red blood noted in the perineum. Most deaths from postpartum hemorrhage are not due to gross bleeding, but rather to inadequate management of slow, steady blood loss (Olds et al., 2004).

Assessment for a suspected hematoma would reveal a firm uterus with bright-red bleeding. Observe for a localized bluish bulging area just under the skin surface in the perineal area (Fig. 22-1). Often, the woman will report severe perineal or pelvic pain and will have difficulty voiding. In addition, she will have hypotension, tachycardia, and anemia (Higgins, 2004).

Assessment for coagulopathies as a cause of postpartum hemorrhage would reveal prolonged bleeding from the gums and venipuncture sites, petechiae on the skin, and ecchymotic areas. The amount of lochia would be much greater also. Urinary output would be diminished, with signs of acute renal failure. Vital signs would show an increase in pulse rate and a decrease in level of consciousness. Signs of shock do not appear until hemorrhage is far advanced due to the increased fluid and blood volume of pregnancy.

Nursing Interventions

Massage the uterus if uterine atony is noted. The uterine muscles are sensitive to touch; massage aids in stimulating the muscle fibers to contract. Massage the boggy uterus while supporting the lower uterine segment to stimulate contractions and expression of any accumulated blood clots. As blood pools in the vagina, stasis of blood causes clots to form; they need to be expelled as pressure is placed on the fundus. Overly forceful massage can tire the uterine muscles, resulting in further uterine atony and increased pain. See Nursing Procedure 22-1 for the steps in massaging the fundus.

If repeated fundal massage and expression of clots fail, medication is probably needed to contract the uterus to control bleeding from the placental site. The injection

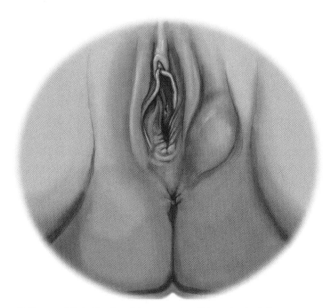

● Figure 22-1 Perineal hematoma. Note the bulging, swollen mass.

of a uterotonic drug immediately after birth is an important intervention used to prevent postpartum hemorrhage. Oxytocin (Pitocin); methylergonovine maleate (Methergine); ergonovine maleate (Ergotrate); a synthetic analog of prostaglandin E1 misoprostol (Cytotec); and prostaglandin (PGF2a, Prostin/15m, Hemabate) are drugs used to manage postpartum hemorrhage (Drug Guide 22-1). The choice of which uterotonic drug to use for management of bleeding depends on the clinical judgment of the health care provider, the availability of drugs, and the risks and benefits of the drug.

Maintain the primary IV infusion and be prepared to start a second infusion at another site in case blood transfusions are necessary. Draw blood for type and crossmatch and send it to the laboratory. Administer oxytocics as ordered, correlating and titrating the IV medication infusion rate to assessment findings of uterine firmness and lochia. Assess for visible vaginal bleeding, and count or weigh perineal pads: 1 g of pad weight is equivalent to 1 mL of blood loss (Green & Wilkinson, 2004).

Check vital signs every 15 to 30 minutes, depending on the acuity of the mother's health status. Monitor her complete blood count to identify any deficit or assess the adequacy of replacement. In addition, assess the woman's level of consciousness to determine changes that may result from inadequate cerebral perfusion.

If a full bladder is present, assist the woman to empty her bladder to reduce displacement of the uterus. If the woman cannot void, anticipate the need to catheterize her to relieve bladder distention.

Retained placental fragments usually are manually separated and removed by the birth attendant. Be sure that the birth attendant remains long enough after birth to assess the bleeding status of the woman and determine the etiology. Assist the birth attendant with suturing any lacerations immediately to control hemorrhage and repair the tissue.

For the woman who develops ITP, glucocorticoids, intravenous immunoglobulin, intravenous anti-Rho D, and platelet transfusions may be administered. A splenectomy may be needed if the bleeding tissues do not respond to medical management.

In vWD, there is a decrease in von Willebrand factor, which is necessary for platelet adhesion and aggregation. It binds to and stabilizes factor VIII of the coagulation cascade (Bjoring & Baxi, 2004). Desmopressin, a synthetic form of vasopressin (antidiuretic hormone), may be used to treat vWD. This drug stimulates the release of stored factor VIII and von Willebrand factor from the lining of blood vessels, which increases platelet adhesiveness and shortens bleeding time. Other treatments that may be ordered include clotting factor concentrates, replacement of von Willebrand factor and factor VIII (Alphanate, Humate-P); antifibrinolytics (Amicar); and nonsteroidal anti-inflammatory drugs (NSAIDs) that do not cause platelet dysfunction (Bextra) (Paper, 2003).

Nursing Procedure 22-1

Massaging the Fundus

Purpose: To Promote Uterine Contraction

1. After explaining the procedure to the woman, place one gloved hand (usually the dominant hand) on the fundus.
2. Place the other gloved hand on the area above the symphysis pubis (this helps to support the lower uterine segment).
3. With the hand on the fundus, gently massage the fundus in a circular manner. Be careful not to overmassage the fundus, which could lead to muscle fatigue and uterine relaxation.
4. Assess for uterine firmness (uterine tissue responds quickly to touch).
5. If firm, apply gentle yet firm pressure in a downward motion toward the vagina to express any clots that may have accumulated.
6. Do not attempt to express clots until the fundus is firm because the application of firm pressure on an uncontracted uterus could cause uterine inversion, leading to massive hemorrhage.
7. Assist the woman with perineal care and applying a new perineal pad.
8. Remove gloves and wash hands.

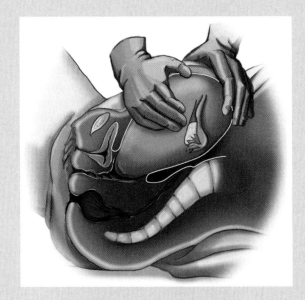

Be alert for women with abnormal bleeding tendencies, ensuring that they receive proper diagnosis and treatment. Teach them how to prevent severe hemorrhage by learning how to feel for and massage their fundus when boggy, assisting the nurse to keep track of the number of and amount of bleeding on perineal pads, and avoiding any medications with antiplatelet activity such as aspirin, antihistamines, or NSAIDs.

If the woman develops DIC, institute emergency measures to control bleeding and impending shock and prepare to transfer her to the intensive care unit. Identification of the underlying condition and elimination of the causative factor are essential to correct the coagulation problem. Be ready to replace fluid volume, administer blood component therapy, and optimize the mother's oxygenation and perfusion status to ensure adequate cardiac output and end-organ perfusion. Continually reassess the woman's coagulation status via laboratory studies.

Monitor vital signs closely, being alert for changes that signal an increase in bleeding or impending shock. Observe for signs of bleeding, including spontaneous bleeding from gums or nose, petechiae, excessive bleeding from the cesarean incision site, hematuria, and blood in the stool. These findings correlate with decreased blood volume,

decreased organ and peripheral tissue perfusion, and clots in the microcirculation (Green & Wilkinson, 2004).

Institute measures to avoid tissue trauma or injury, such as giving injections and drawing blood. Also provide emotional support to the client and her family throughout this critical time by being readily available and providing explanations and reassurance.

Thromboembolic Conditions

A thrombosis (blood clot within a blood vessel) can cause an inflammation of the blood vessel lining (**thrombophlebitis**) which in turn can lead to a possible thromboembolism (obstruction of a blood vessel by a blood clot carried by the circulation from the site of origin). Thrombi can involve the superficial or deep veins in the legs or pelvis. Superficial venous thrombosis usually involves the saphenous venous system and is confined to the lower leg. Superficial thrombophlebitis may be caused by the use of the lithotomy position in some women during birth. Deep venous thrombosis can involve deep veins from the foot to the calf, to the thighs, or pelvis. In both locations, thrombi can dislodge and migrate to the lungs, causing a pulmonary embolism.

Drug Guide 22-1 Drugs Used to Control Postpartum Hemorrhage

Drug	Action/Indication	Nursing Implications
Oxytocin (Pitocin)	Stimulates the uterus to contract/ to contract the uterus to control bleeding from the placental site	Assess fundus for evidence of contraction and compare amount of bleeding every 15 minutes or according to orders. Monitor vital signs every 15 minutes. Monitor uterine tone to prevent hyperstimulation. Reassure client about the need for uterine contraction and administer analgesics for comfort. Offer explanation to client and family about what is happening and the purpose of the medication. Provide nonpharmacologic comfort measures to assist with pain management. Set up the IV infusion to be piggybacked into a primary IV line. This ensures that the medication can be discontinued readily if hyperstimulation or adverse effects occur while maintaining the IV site and primary infusion.
Methylergonovine maleate (Methergine)	Stimulates the uterus/to prevent and treat postpartum hemorrhage due to atony or subinvolution	Assess baseline bleeding, uterine tone, and vital signs every 15 minutes or according to protocol. Offer explanation to client and family about what is happening and the purpose of the medication. Monitor for possible adverse effects, such as hypertension, seizures, uterine cramping, nausea, vomiting, and palpitations. Report any complaints of chest pain promptly.
Ergonovine maleate (Ergotrate)	Stimulates uterine contractions/ to control postpartum or post-abortion hemorrhage	Assess baseline bleeding, uterine tone, and vital signs every 15 minutes or according to protocol. Offer explanation to client and family about what is happening and the purpose of the medication. Monitor for possible adverse effects, such as nausea, vomiting, weakness, muscular pain, headache, or dizziness.
Prostaglandin (PGF-2a, Prostin/15m, Hemabate)	Stimulates uterine contractions/ to treat postpartum hemorrhage due to uterine atony when not controlled by other methods	Assess vital signs, uterine contractions, client's comfort level, and bleeding status as per protocol. Offer explanation to client and family about what is happening and the purpose of the medication. Monitor for possible adverse effects, such as fever, chills, headache, nausea, vomiting, diarrhea, flushing, and bronchospasm.

Pulmonary embolism is a potentially fatal condition that occurs when the pulmonary artery is obstructed by a blood clot that has traveled from another vein into the lungs, causing an obstruction and infarction. When the clot is large enough to block one or more of the pulmonary vessels that supply the lungs, it can result in sudden death. Pulmonary embolism is the second leading cause of pregnancy-related deaths in the United States (Green & Wilkinson, 2004). In the United States, more women die of it each year than from car accidents, breast cancer, or AIDS (Goldhaber, 2003). Many of these deaths can be prevented by the routine use of simple measures:

- Developing public awareness about risk factors, symptoms, and preventive measures
- Preventing venous stasis by encouraging activity that causes leg muscles to contract and promotes venous return (leg exercises and walking)
- Using intermittent sequential compression devices to produce passive leg muscle contractions until the woman is ambulatory
- Elevating the woman's legs above her heart level to promote venous return
- Stopping smoking to reduce or prevent vascular vasoconstriction
- Applying compression stockings and removing them daily for inspection of legs
- Performing passive range-of-motion exercises while in bed
- Using postoperative deep-breathing exercises to improve venous return by relieving the negative thoracic pressure on leg veins
- Reducing hypercoagulability with the use of warfarin, aspirin, and heparin
- Preventing venous pooling by avoiding pillows under knees, not crossing legs for long periods, and not leaving legs up in stirrups for long periods
- Padding stirrups to reduce pressure against the popliteal angle
- Avoiding sitting or standing in one position for prolonged periods
- Using a bed cradle to keep linens and blankets off extremities
- Avoiding trauma to legs to prevent injury to the vein wall
- Increasing fluid intake to prevent dehydration
- Avoiding the use of oral contraceptives

Etiology

The major causes of a thrombus formation (blood clot) are venous stasis, injury to the innermost layer of the blood vessel, and hypercoagulation. Venous stasis and hypercoagulation are both common in the postpartum period. Other factors that place women at risk for thrombosis include prolonged bed rest, diabetes, obesity, cesarean birth, smoking, progesterone-induced distensibility of the veins of the lower legs during pregnancy, severe anemia, his-

tory of previous thrombosis, varicose veins, diabetes mellitus, advanced maternal age (>35), multiparity, and use of oral contraceptives before pregnancy (Trizna & Goldman, 2005).

Nursing Management

The three most common thromboembolic conditions occurring during the postpartum period are superficial venous thrombosis, deep venous thrombosis, and pulmonary embolism. Although thromboembolic disorders occur in less than 1% of all postpartum women, pulmonary embolus can be fatal if a clot obstructs the lung circulation; thus, early identification and treatment are paramount.

Prevention of thrombotic conditions is an essential aspect of nursing management. In women at risk, early ambulation is the easiest and most cost-effective method. Use of elastic compression stockings (TED hose or Jobst stockings) decrease distal calf vein thrombosis by decreasing venous stasis and augmenting venous return (McKinney et al., 2005). Women who are at a high risk for thromboembolic disease based on risk factors or previous history of deep vein thrombosis or pulmonary embolism may be placed on prophylactic heparin therapy during pregnancy. Standard heparin or a low-molecular-weight heparin such as enoxaparin (Lovenox) can be given, since neither one crosses the placenta. It is typically discontinued during labor and birth and then restarted during the postpartum period.

Assessment

Assess the woman closely for risk factors and signs and symptoms of thrombophlebitis. Look for risk factors in the woman's history such as use of oral contraceptives before the pregnancy, employment that necessitates prolonged standing, history of thrombophlebitis or endometritis, or evidence of current varicosities. Suspect superficial venous thrombosis in a woman with varicose veins who reports tenderness and discomfort over the site of the thrombosis, most commonly in the calf area. The area appears reddened along the vein and is warm to the touch. The woman will report increased pain in the affected leg when she ambulates and bears weight.

Manifestations of deep venous thrombosis are often absent and diffuse. If they are present, they are caused by an inflammatory process and obstruction of venous return. Calf swelling, erythema, warmth, tenderness, and pedal edema may be noted. A positive Homans sign (pain in the calf upon dorsiflexion) is not a definitive diagnostic sign because pain can also be caused by a strained muscle or contusion (Engstrom, 2004).

Assess for signs and symptoms of pulmonary embolism, including unexplained sudden onset of shortness of breath, tachypnea, sudden chest pain, tachycardia, cardiac arrhythmias, apprehension, profuse sweating, hemoptysis, and sudden change in mental status as a result of hypoxemia (Lewis et al., 2004). Expect a lung scan to be done to confirm the diagnosis.

Nursing Interventions

For the woman with superficial venous thrombosis, care includes administering NSAIDs for analgesia, providing for rest and elevation of the affected leg, applying warm compresses to the affected area to promote healing, and using antiembolism stockings to promote circulation to the extremities.

Nursing interventions for a woman with deep vein thrombosis includes bed rest and elevation of the affected extremity to decrease interstitial swelling and promote venous return from that leg. Apply antiembolism stockings to both extremities as ordered. Fit the stockings correctly and urge the woman to wear them at all times. Sequential compression devices can also be used for women with varicose veins, a history of thrombophlebitis, or a surgical birth. Anticoagulant therapy using a continuous IV infusion of heparin is started to prolong blood clotting time and prevent extension of the thrombosis. Monitor the woman's coagulation studies closely; these might include activated partial thromboplastin time (APTT), whole blood partial thromboplastin time, and platelet levels. A therapeutic APTT values typically ranges from 35 to 45 seconds, depending on which standard values are used (Cavanaugh, 2003). Also apply warm moist compresses to the affected leg and administer analgesics as ordered to decrease the discomfort.

After several days of IV heparin therapy, expect to begin oral anticoagulant therapy with warfarin (Coumadin) as ordered. In most cases, the woman will continue to take this medication for several months after discharge. Provide teaching about the use of anticoagulant therapy and possible danger signs (Teaching Guidelines 22-1).

For the woman who develops a pulmonary embolism, institute emergency measures immediately. The objectives of treatment are to prevent further growth or multiplication of thrombi in the lower extremities, prevent further thrombi from traveling to the pulmonary vascular system, and provide cardiopulmonary support if needed. Interventions include administering oxygen via mask or cannula and continuous IV heparin titrated according to the laboratory results, maintaining the client on bed rest, and administering analgesics for pain relief. Thrombolytic agents, such as tPA, might be used to dissolve pulmonary emboli and the source of the thrombus in the pelvis or deep leg veins, thus reducing the potential for a recurrence.

Additional interventions would include anticipatory guidance, support, and education about anticoagulants and associated signs of complications and risks. Focus discharge teaching on the following issues:

- Elimination of modifiable risk factors for deep vein thrombosis (smoking, use of oral contraceptives, a sedentary lifestyle, and obesity)
- Importance of using compression stockings

 TEACHING GUIDELINES 22-1

Teaching to Prevent Bleeding Related to Anticoagulant Therapy

- Watch for possible signs of bleeding and notify your health care provider if any occur:
  - Nosebleeds
  - Bleeding from the gums or mouth
  - Black tarry stools
  - Brown "coffee ground" vomitus
  - Red to brown speckled mucus from a cough
  - Oozing at incision, episiotomy site, cut, or scrape
  - Pink, red, or brown-tinged urine
  - Bruises, "black and blue marks"
  - Increased lochia discharge (from present level)
- Practice measures to reduce your risk of bleeding:
  - Brush your teeth gently using a soft toothbrush.
  - Use an electric razor for shaving.
  - Avoid activities that could lead to injury, scrapes, bruising, or cuts.
  - Do not use any over-the-counter products containing aspirin or aspirin-like derivatives.
  - Avoid consuming alcohol.
  - Inform other health care providers about the use of anticoagulants, especially dentists.
- Be sure to comply with follow-up laboratory testing as scheduled.
- If you accidentally cut or scrape yourself, apply firm direct pressure to the site for 5 to 10 minutes. Do the same after receiving any injections or having blood specimens drawn.
- Wear an identification bracelet or band that indicates that you are taking an anticoagulant.

- Avoidance of constrictive clothing and prolonged standing or sitting in a motionless, leg-dependent position
- Danger signs and symptoms (sudden onset of chest pain, dyspnea, and tachypnea) to report to the health care provider

Postpartum Infection

Infection during the postpartum period is a common cause of maternal morbidity and mortality. Overall, postpartum infection is estimated to occur in up to 8% of all births. There is a higher occurrence in cesarean births than in vaginal births (Gibbs et al., 2004). The incidence of postpartum infections is expected to increase because of the earlier discharge of postpartum women from the hospital (Kennedy, 2005).

Postpartum infection is defined as a fever of 38°C or 100.4°F or higher after the first 24 hours after childbirth, occurring on at least 2 of the first 10 days after birth, exclusive of the first 24 hours (Olds et al., 2004). Infections can easily enter the female genital tract externally and ascend through the internal genital structures. In addition, the normal physiologic changes of childbirth increase the risk of infection by decreasing the vaginal acidity due to the presence of amniotic fluid, blood, and lochia, all of which are alkaline. An alkaline environment encourages the growth of bacteria. Because today women are commonly discharged 24 to 48 hours after giving birth, nurses must assess new mothers for risk factors and identify early subtle signs and symptoms of an infectious process. Common postpartum infections include metritis, wound infections, urinary tract infections, and mastitis.

Etiology

The common bacterial etiology of postpartum infections involves organisms that constitute the normal vaginal flora, typically a mix of aerobic and anaerobic species. Postpartum infections generally are polymicrobial and involve the following microorganisms: *Staphylococcus aureus, Escherichia coli, Klebsiella, Gardnerella vaginalis,* gonococci, coliform bacteria, group A or B hemolytic streptococci, *Chlamydia trachomatis,* and the anaerobes that are common to bacterial vaginosis (Higgins, 2004).

Factors that place a woman at risk for a postpartum infection are highlighted in Box 22-2.

Clinical Manifestations

A postpartum infection is associated with an elevation in temperature, as mentioned previously. Other generalized signs and symptoms may include chills, headache, malaise, restlessness, anxiety, and tachycardia. In addition, the woman may exhibit specific signs and symptoms based on the type and location of the infection (Table 22-1).

Metritis

Although usually referred to clinically as endometritis, postpartum uterine infections typically involve more than just the endometrial lining. **Metritis** is an infectious condition that involves the endometrium, decidua, and adjacent myometrium of the uterus. Extension of metritis can result in parametritis, which involves the broad ligament and possibly the ovaries and fallopian tubes, or septic pelvic thrombophlebitis, which results when the infection spreads along venous routes into the pelvis (Kennedy, 2005).

The uterine cavity is sterile until rupture of the amniotic sac. As a consequence of labor, birth, and associated manipulations, anaerobic and aerobic bacteria can contaminate the uterus. In most cases, the bacteria responsible for pelvic infections are those that normally reside in the bowel, vagina, perineum, and cervix, such as *E. coli, Klebsiella pneumoniae,* or *G. vaginalis.*

The risk of metritis increases dramatically after a cesarean birth; it complicates from 10% to 20% of cesarean births. This is typically an extension of chorioamnionitis that was present before birth (indeed, that may have been why the cesarean birth was performed). In addition, trauma to the tissues and a break in the skin (incision) provide entrances for bacteria to enter the body and multiply (Kennedy, 2005).

Primary prevention of metritis is key and focuses on reducing the risk factors and incidence of cesarean births. When metritis occurs, broad-spectrum antibiotics are used to treat the infection. Management also includes measures to restore and promote fluid and electrolyte balance, provide analgesia, and provide emotional support. In most treated women, reduction of fever and elimination of symptoms will occur within 48 to 72 hours after the start of antibiotic therapy.

Wound Infections

Any break in the skin or mucous membranes provides a portal for bacteria. In the postpartum woman, sites of wound infection include cesarean surgical incisions, the episiotomy site in the perineum, and genital tract lacerations (Fig. 22-2). Wound infections are usually not identified until the woman has been discharged from the hospital because symptoms may not show up until 24 to 48 hours after birth. Because some infections may not manifest until after discharge, instructions about signs and symptoms to look for should be included in all discharge teaching. When a low-grade fever (<100.4°F), poor appetite, and a low energy level persist for a few days, a wound infection should be suspected.

Management for wound infections involves recognition of the infection, followed by opening of the wound to allow drainage. Aseptic wound management with sterile gloves and frequent dressing changes if applicable, good handwashing, frequent perineal pad changes, hydration, and ambulation to prevent venous stasis and improve circulation are initiated to prevent development of a more serious infection or spread of the infection to adjacent structures. Parenteral antibiotics are the mainstay of treatment. Analgesics are also important, because women often experience discomfort at the wound site.

Urinary Tract Infections

Urinary tract infections are most commonly caused by bacteria often found in bowel flora, including *E. coli, Klebsiella, Proteus,* and *Enterobacter* species. Any form of invasive manipulation of the urethra, such as urinary catheterization, frequent vaginal examinations, and genital trauma increase the likelihood of a urinary tract infection. Treatment consists of administering fluids if dehydration exists and antibiotics if appropriate.

BOX 22-2

FACTORS PLACING A WOMAN AT RISK FOR POSTPARTUM INFECTION

- Prolonged (>6 hours) premature rupture of membranes (removes the barrier of amniotic fluid so bacteria can ascend)
- Cesarean birth (allows bacterial entry due to break in protective skin barrier)
- Urinary catheterization (could allow entry of bacteria into bladder due to break in aseptic technique)
- Regional anesthesia that decreases perception to void (causes urinary stasis and increases risk of urinary tract infection)
- Staff attending to woman are ill (promotes droplet infection from personnel)
- Compromised health status, such as anemia, obesity, smoking, drug abuse (reduces the body's immune system and decreases ability to fight infection)
- Preexisting colonization of lower genital tract with bacterial vaginosis, *Chlamydia trachomatis*, group B streptococci, *Staphylococcus aureus*, and *Escherichia coli* (allows microbes to ascend)
- Retained placental fragments (provides medium for bacterial growth)
- Manual removal of a retained placenta (causes trauma to the lining of the uterus and thus opens up sites for bacterial invasion)
- Insertion of fetal scalp electrode or intrauterine pressure catheters for internal fetal monitoring during labor (provides entry into uterine cavity)
- Instrument-assisted childbirth, such as forceps or vacuum extraction (increases risk of trauma to genital tract, which provides bacteria access to grow)
- Trauma to the genital tract, such as episiotomy or lacerations (provides a portal of entry for bacteria)
- Prolonged labor with frequent vaginal examinations to check progress (allows time for bacteria to multiply and increases potential exposure to microorganisms or trauma)
- Poor nutritional status (reduces body's ability to repair tissue)
- Gestational diabetes (decreases body's healing ability and provides higher glucose levels on skin and in urine, which encourages bacterial growth)
- Break in aseptic technique during surgery or birthing process by the birth attendant or nurses (allows entry of bacteria)

Table 22-1 Signs and Symptoms of Postpartum Infections

Postpartum Infection	Signs and Symptoms
Metritis	Lower abdominal tenderness or pain on one or both sides Temperature elevation (>38°C) Foul-smelling lochia Anorexia Nausea Fatigue and lethargy Leukocytosis and elevated sedimentation rate
Wound infection	Weeping serosanguineous or purulent drainage Separation of or unapproximated wound edges Edema Erythema Tenderness Discomfort at the site Maternal fever Elevated white blood cell count
Urinary tract infection	Urgency Frequency Dysuria Flank pain Low-grade fever Urinary retention Hematuria Urine positive for nitrates Cloudy urine with strong odor
Mastitis	Flulike symptoms, including malaise, fever, and chills Tender, hot, red, painful area on one breast Inflammation of breast area Breast tenderness Cracking of skin or around nipple or areola Breast distention with milk

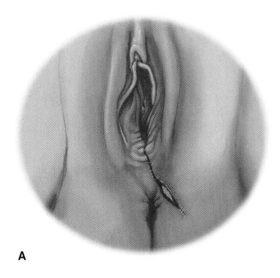

A

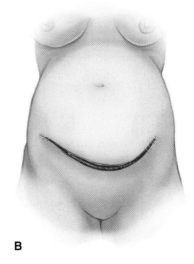

B

● Figure 22-2 Postpartum wound infections. (**A**) Infected episiotomy site. (**B**) Infected cesarean birth incision.

Mastitis

A common problem that may occur within the first 2 weeks postpartum is an inflammation of the breast termed **mastitis.** It can be caused by a missed infant feeding, a bra that is too tight, poor drainage of duct and alveolus, or an infection. The most common infecting organism is *S. aureus,* which comes from the breastfeeding infant's mouth or throat (Kennedy, 2005). Infection can be transmitted from the lactiferous ducts to a secreting lobule, from a nipple fissure to periductal lymphatics, or by circulation (Youngkin & Davis, 2004) (Fig. 22-3).

The diagnosis is usually made without a culture being taken. Unless mastitis is treated adequately, it may progress to a breast abscess. Treatment of mastitis focuses on two areas: emptying the breasts and controlling the infection. The breast can be emptied either by the infant sucking or by manual expression. Increasing the frequency of nursing is advised. Lactation need not be suppressed. Control of infection is achieved with antibiotics. In addition, ice or warm packs and analgesics may be needed.

Nursing Management

Perinatal nurses are primary caregivers for postpartum women and have the unique opportunity to identify subtle changes that place women at risk for infection. Nurses play a key role in identifying signs and symptoms that suggest a postpartum infection. Client teaching about danger signs and symptoms also is a priority due to today's short lengths of stay after delivery. (See Nursing Care Plan 22-1.)

Assessment

Review the client's history and physical examination and labor and birth record for factors that might increase her risk for developing an infection. Then complete the assessment (using the "BUBBLE-HE" parameters discussed in Chapter 16), paying particular attention to areas such as the abdomen and fundus, breasts, urinary tract, episiotomy, lacerations, or incisions, being alert for signs and symptoms of infection (see Table 22-1).

When assessing the episiotomy site, use the acronym "REEDA" (redness, erythema or ecchymosis, edema, drainage or discharge, and approximation of wound edges) to ensure complete evaluation of the site (Engstrom, 2004).

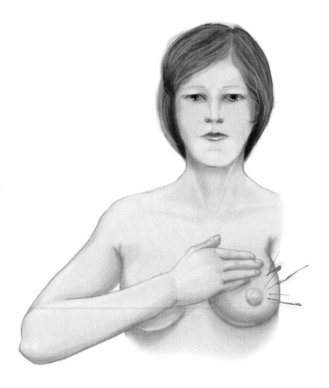

● Figure 22-3 Mastitis.

Nursing Care Plan 22-1

Overview of the Woman with a Postpartum Complication

Jennifer, a 16-year-old G1P1, gave birth to a boy by cesarean 3 days ago due to cephalopelvic disproportion following 25 hours of labor with ruptured membranes. Her temperature is 102.6°F (39.2°C). She is complaining of chills and malaise and severe pain at the incision site. The site is red and warm to the touch with purulent drainage. Jennifer's lochia is scant and dark red, with a strong odor. She tells the nurse to take her baby back to the nursery because she doesn't feel well enough to care for him.

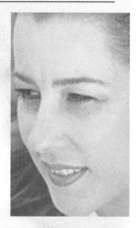

Nursing Diagnosis: Ineffective thermoregulation related to bacterial invasion

Outcome identification and *evaluation*	Interventions with *rationales*
Jennifer's body temperature decreases from current level and *remains within acceptable parameters for the next 24 hours*	Assess vital signs every 2 to 4 hours and record results *to monitor progress of infection.* Offer cool bed bath or shower *to reduce temperature.* Place cool cloth on forehead and/or back of neck *for comfort.* Change bed linen and gown when damp from diaphoresis *to provide comfort and hygiene.* Administer antipyretics as ordered *to reduce temperature.* Administer antibiotic therapy and wound care as ordered *to treat infection.* Use aseptic technique *to prevent spread of infection.* Force fluids to 2,000 mL per shift *to hydrate patient.* Document intake and output *to assess hydration status.*

Nursing Diagnosis: Acute pain related to infectious process

Patient reports decreased pain as evidenced by *pain rating of 0 or 1 on pain scale; client verbalizes no complaints and can rest comfortably.*	Place client in semi-Fowler's position *to facilitate drainage and relieve pressure.* Assess pain level on pain scale of 0 to 10 *to describe pain objectively.* Assess fundus gently *for appropriate involution changes.* Administer analgesics as needed and on time as ordered *to maintain pain relief.* Provide for rest periods *to allow for healing process.* Encourage good dietary intake *to promote healing.* Assist with positioning in bed with pillows *to promote comfort.* Offer a backrub *to ease aches and discomfort* if desired.

(continued)

Overview of the Woman with a Postpartum Complication (continued)

Nursing Diagnosis: Risk for impaired parental/infant attachment related to effects of postpartum infection

Outcome identification and *evaluation*	Interventions with *rationales*
Client begins to bond with newborn appropriately with each exposure; *expresses positive feelings toward newborn when holding him; demonstrates ability to care for newborn when feeling better; states that she has help and support at home so she can focus on newborn.*	Promote adequate rest and sleep *to promote healing.* Bring newborn to mother after she is rested and had an analgesic *to allow mother to focus her energies on the child.* Progressively allow the client to care for her infant or comfort him as her energy level and pain level improve *to promote self-confidence in caring for the newborn.* Offer praise and positive reinforcement for caretaking tasks; stress positive attributes of newborn to mother while caring for him *to facilitate bonding and attachment.* Contact family members to participate in care of the newborn *to allow mother to rest and recover from infection.* Encourage mother to care for herself first and then the newborn *to ensure adequate energy for newborn's care.* Arrange for assistance and support after discharge from hospital *to aid in providing necessary backup.* Refer to community health nurse *for follow-up care of mother and newborn at home.*

Monitor the woman's vital signs, especially her temperature, for changes that may signal an infection.

Nursing Interventions

Nursing care focuses on preventing postpartum infections. Use the following guidelines to help reduce the incidence of postpartum infections:

• Maintain aseptic technique when performing invasive procedures such as urinary catheterization, when changing dressings, and during all surgical procedures.
• Use good handwashing technique before, after, and in between each patient care activity.
• Reinforce measures for maintaining good perineal hygiene.
• Use adequate lighting and turn the client to side to assess the episiotomy site.
• Screen all visitors for any signs of active infections to reduce the client's risk of exposure.
• Review the client's history for preexisting infections or chronic conditions.

• Monitor vital signs and laboratory results for any abnormal values.
• Monitor the frequency of vaginal examinations and length of labor.
• Assess frequently for early signs of infection, especially fever and the appearance of lochia.
• Inspect wounds frequently for inflammation and drainage.
• Encourage rest, adequate hydration, and healthy eating habits.
• Reinforce preventive measures during any interaction with the client.

Client teaching is essential. Review the signs and symptoms of infection, emphasizing the danger signs and symptoms that need to be reported to the health care provider. Most importantly, stress proper handwashing, especially after perineal care and before and after breastfeeding. Also reinforce measures to promote breastfeeding, including proper breast care (see Chapter 16).

If the woman develops an infection, also review treatment measures, such as antibiotic therapy if ordered, and any special care measures, such as dressing changes. Teaching Guidelines 22-2 highlights the major teaching points for a woman with a postpartum infection.

Postpartum Emotional Disorders

The postpartum period involves extraordinary physiologic, psychological, and sociocultural changes in the life of a woman and her family. It is an exhilarating time for most women, but for others it may not be what they had expected. Women have varied reactions to their child-

 TEACHING GUIDELINES 22-2

Teaching for the Woman With a Postpartum Infection

- Continue your antibiotic therapy as prescribed.
  - Take the medication exactly as ordered and continue with the medication until it is finished.
  - Do not stop taking the medication even when you are feeling better.
- Check your temperature every day and call your health care provider if it is above 100.4°F (38°C).
- Watch for other signs and symptoms of infection, such as chills, increased abdominal pain, change in the color or odor of your lochia, or increased redness, warmth, swelling, or drainage from a wound site such as your cesarean incision or episiotomy. Report any of these to your health care provider immediately
- Practice good infection prevention:
  - Always wash your hands thoroughly before and after eating, using the bathroom, touching your perineal area, or providing care for your newborn.
  - Wipe from front to back after using the bathroom.
  - Remove your perineal pad using a front-to-back motion. Fold the pad in half so that the inner sides of the pad that were touching your body are against each other. Wrap in toilet tissue or place in a plastic bag and discard.
  - Wash your hands before applying a new pad.
  - Apply a new perineal pad using a front-to-back motion. Handle the pad by the edges (top and bottom or sides) and avoid touching the inner aspect of the pad that will be against your body.
  - When performing perineal care with the peri-bottle, angle the spray of water to that it flows from front to back.
  - Drink plenty of fluids each day and eat a variety of foods that are high in vitamins, iron, and protein.
  - Be sure to get adequate rest at night and periodically throughout the day.

bearing experiences, exhibiting a wide range of emotions. Typically, the delivery of a newborn is associated with positive feelings such as happiness, joy, and gratitude for the birth of a healthy infant. However, women may also feel weepy, overwhelmed, or unsure of what is happening to them. They may experience fear about loss of control; they may feel scared, alone, or guilty, or as if they have somehow failed.

Postpartum emotional disorders have been documented for years, but only recently have they received medical attention. Plummeting levels of estrogen and progesterone immediately after birth can contribute to postpartum mood disorders. It is believed that the greater the change in these hormone levels between pregnancy and postpartum, the greater the chance for developing a mood disorder (Elder, 2004).

Many types of emotional disorders occur in the postpartum period. Although their description and classification may be controversial, the disorders are commonly classified on the basis of their severity as postpartum or baby blues, postpartum depression, and postpartum psychosis.

Postpartum or Baby Blues

Many postpartum women (approximately 50% to 85%) experience the "baby blues" (Suri & Altshuler, 2004). The woman exhibits mild depressive symptoms of anxiety, irritability, mood swings, tearfulness, increased sensitivity, and fatigue (Clay & Seehusen, 2004). The "blues" typically peak on postpartum days 4 and 5 and usually resolve by postpartum day 10. Although the woman's symptoms may be distressing, they do not reflect psychopathology and usually do not affect the mother's ability to function and care for her infant. Baby blues are usually self-limiting and require no formal treatment other than reassurance and validation of the woman's experience, as well as assistance in caring for herself and the newborn. However, follow-up of women with postpartum blues is important, as up to 20% go on to develop postpartum depression (Henshaw et al., 2004).

Postpartum Depression

Depression is more prevalent in women than in men, which may be related to biological, hormonal, and psychosocial factors. If the symptoms of postpartum blues last beyond 6 weeks and seem to get worse, the mother may be experiencing **postpartum depression,** a major depressive episode associated with childbirth (MacQueen & Chokka, 2004). As many as 20% of all mothers develop postpartum depression (Vieira, 2003). It affects approximately 500,000 mothers in the United States each year, and about half of these women receive no mental health evaluation or treatment (Horowitz & Goodman, 2005).

As an assertive practicing attorney in her thirties, my first pregnancy was filled with nagging feelings of doubt about this upcoming event in my life. Throughout my pregnancy I was so busy with trial work that I never had time to really evaluate my feelings. I was always reading about the bodily changes that were taking place, and on one level I was feeling excited, but on another level I was emotionally drained. Shortly after the birth of my daughter, those suppressed nagging feelings of doubt surfaced big time and practically immobilized me. I felt exhausted all the time and was only too glad to have someone else care for my daughter. I didn't breastfeed because I thought it would tie me down too much. Although at the time I thought this "low mood" was normal for all new mothers, I have since found out it was postpartum depression. How could any woman be depressed about this wondrous event?

Thoughts: Now that postpartum depression has been "taken out of the closet" and recognized as a real emotional disorder, it can be treated. This woman showed tendencies during her pregnancy but was able to suppress the feelings and go forward. Her description of her depression is very typical of many women who suffer in silence, hoping to get over these feelings in time. What can nurses do to promote awareness of this disorder? Can it be prevented?

Unlike the postpartum blues, women with postpartum depression feel worse over time, and changes in mood and behavior do not go away on their own.

Several factors can increase a mother's risk of developing postpartum depression:

- History of previous depression
- History of postpartum depression
- Evidence of depressive symptoms during pregnancy
- Family history of depression
- Life stress
- Childcare stress
- Prenatal anxiety
- Lack of social support
- Relationship stress
- Difficult or complicated pregnancy
- Traumatic birth experience
- Birth of a high-risk or special-needs infant (Suri & Altshuler, 2004)

Postpartum depression affects not only the woman but also the entire family. Identifying depression early can substantially improve the client and family outcomes. Postpartum depression usually has a more gradual onset and becomes evident within the first 6 weeks postpartum. Some of the common manifestations are listed in Box 22-3.

Postpartum depression lends itself to prophylactic intervention because its onset is predictable, the risk period for illness is well defined, and women at high risk can be identified using a screening tool. Prophylaxis starts with a prenatal risk assessment and education. Based on the woman's history of prior depression, prophylactic antidepressant therapy may be needed during the third trimester or immediately after giving birth. Management mirrors that of any major depression—a combination of antidepressant medication, antianxiety medication, and psychotherapy in an outpatient or inpatient setting (Pavlovich-Danis, 2004). Marital counseling may be necessary when marital problems may be contributing to the woman's depressive symptoms.

Postpartum Psychosis

At the severe end of the continuum of postpartum emotional disorders is postpartum psychosis, which occurs in one or two women per 1,000 births (Elder, 2004). It generally surfaces within 3 weeks of giving birth. Symptoms of postpartum psychosis include sleep disturbances, fatigue, depression, and hypomania. The mother will be tearful, confused, and preoccupied with feelings of guilt and worthlessness. Early symptoms resemble those of depression, but they may escalate to delirium, hallucinations, anger toward herself and her infant, bizarre behavior, manifestations of mania, and thoughts of hurting herself and the infant. The mother frequently loses touch with reality and experiences a severe regressive breakdown, associated with a high risk of suicide or infanticide (MacQueen & Chokka, 2004).

Most women with postpartum psychosis are hospitalized for up to several months. Psychotropic drugs are almost always part of treatment, along with individual psychotherapy and support group therapy. The greatest hazard of postpartum psychosis is suicide. Infanticide and child abuse are also risks if the woman is left alone

---

BOX 22-3

COMMON MANIFESTATIONS OF POSTPARTUM DEPRESSION

- Loss of pleasure or interest in life
- Low mood, sadness, tearfulness
- Exhaustion that is not relieved by sleep
- Feelings of guilt
- Irritability
- Inability to concentrate
- Anxiety
- Despair
- Compulsive thoughts
- Loss of libido
- Loss of confidence
- Sleep difficulties (insomnia)
- Loss of appetite
- Feelings of failure as a mother (Horowitz & Goodman, 2005)

with her infant. Early recognition and prompt treatment of this disorder is imperative.

Nursing Management

Postpartum emotional disorders are often overlooked and go unrecognized despite the large percentage of women who experience them. The postpartum period is a time of increased vulnerability, but few women receive education about the possibility of depression after birth. In addition, many women may feel ashamed of having negative emotions at a time when they "should" be happy; thus, they don't seek professional help. Nurses can play a major role in providing provide guidance about postpartum emotional disorders, detecting manifestations, and assisting women to obtain appropriate care.

Assessment

Assessment should begin by reviewing the history to identify risk factors that could predispose them to depression:

- Poor coping skills
- Low self-esteem
- Numerous life stressors
- Mood swings and emotional stress
- Previous psychological problems or a family history of psychiatric disorders
- Substance abuse
- Limited social support networks

Be alert for possible physical findings. Assess the woman's activity level, including her level of fatigue. Ask about her sleeping habits, noting any problems with insomnia. When interacting with the woman, observe for verbal and nonverbal indicators of anxiety as well as her ability to concentrate during the interaction. Difficulty concentrating and anxious behaviors suggest a problem. Also assess her nutritional intake: weight loss due to poor food intake may be seen. Assessment can identify women with a high-risk profile for depression, and the nurse can educate them and make referrals for individual or family counseling if needed.

Nursing Interventions

Nursing interventions that are appropriate to assist any postpartum woman to cope with the changes of this period include:

- Encourage the client to verbalize her feelings of what she is going through.
- Recommend that the woman seek help for household chores and childcare.
- Stress the importance of good nutrition and adequate exercise and sleep.

- Encourage the client to develop a support system with other mothers.
- Assist the woman to structure her day to regain a sense of control.
- Emphasize the importance of keeping her expectations realistic.
- Discuss postponing major life changes, such as moving or changing jobs.
- Provide information about bodily changes (ICEA, 2003).

The nurse can play an important role in assisting women and their partners with postpartum adjustment. Providing facts about the enormous changes that can occur during the postpartum period is critical. Review the signs and symptoms of all three emotional disorders. This information is typically included as part of prenatal visits and childbirth education classes. Know the risk factors associated with these disorders and review the history of clients and their families. Use specific, nonthreatening questions to aid in early detection.

Discuss factors that may increase a woman's vulnerability to stress during the postpartum period, such as sleep deprivation and unrealistic expectations, so couples can understand and respond to those problems if they occur. Stress that many women need help after childbirth and that help is available from many sources, including people they already know. Assisting women to learn how to ask for help is important so they can gain the support they need. Also provide educational materials about postpartum emotional disorders. Have available referral sources for psychotherapy and support groups appropriate for women experiencing postpartum adjustment difficulties.

KEY CONCEPTS

- Postpartum hemorrhage is a potentially life-threatening complication of both vaginal and cesarean births. It is the leading cause of maternal mortality in the United States.
- A good way to remember the causes of postpartum hemorrhage is the "4 Ts": tone, tissue, trauma, and thrombosis.
- Uterine atony is the most common cause of early postpartum hemorrhage, which can lead to hypovolemic shock.
- Oxytocin (Pitocin), methylergonovine maleate (Methergine), ergonovine maleate (Ergotrate), and prostaglandin (PGF2a, Prostin/15m, Hemabate) are drugs used to manage postpartum hemorrhage.
- Failure of the placenta to separate completely and be expelled interferes with the ability of the uterus to contract fully, thereby leading to hemorrhage.
- Causes of subinvolution are retained placental fragments, distended bladder, uterine myoma, and infection.

- Lacerations should always be suspected when the uterus is contracted and bright-red blood continues to trickle out of the vagina.
- Conditions that cause coagulopathies may include idiopathic thrombocytopenic purpura (ITP), von Willebrand disease (vWD), and disseminated intravascular coagulation (DIC).
- Pulmonary embolism is a potentially fatal condition that occurs when the pulmonary artery is obstructed by a blood clot that has traveled from another vein into the lungs, causing obstruction and infarction.
- The major causes of a thrombus formation (blood clot) are venous stasis and hypercoagulation, both common in the postpartum period.
- Postpartum infection is defined as a fever of 38°C or 100.4°F or higher after the first 24 hours after childbirth, occurring on at least 2 of the first 10 days exclusive of the first 24 hours.
- Common postpartum infections include metritis, wound infections, urinary tract infections, and mastitis.
- Postpartum emotional disorders are commonly classified on the basis of their severity: "baby blues," postpartum depression, and postpartum psychosis.
- Management of postpartum depression mirrors the treatment of any major depression—a combination of antidepressant medication, antianxiety medication, and psychotherapy in an outpatient or inpatient setting.

References

Benedetti, T. J. (2002). Obstetric hemorrhage. In S. G. Gabbe, J. R. Niebyl, & J. L. Simpson (Eds.), *Obstetrics: normal and problem pregnancies* (4th ed., pp. 503–538). New York: Churchill Livingstone.

Bjoring, A., & Baxi, L. (2004). Use of DDAVP as prophylaxis against postpartum hemorrhage in women with von Willebrand's disease: a case series demonstrating safety and efficacy. *Journal of Women's Health, 13*(7), 845–847.

Blackwell, J., & Goolsby, M. J. (2003). Diagnosis and treatment of idiopathic thrombocytopenia purpura. *Journal of the American Academy of Nurse Practitioners, 15*(6), 244–245.

Cavanaugh, B. M. (2003). *Nurse's manual of laboratory and diagnostic tests.* Philadelphia: F. A. Davis.

Clay, E. C., & Seehusen, D. A. (2004). A review of postpartum depression for the primary care physician. *Southern Medical Journal, 97*(2), 157–161.

Cunningham, F. G., Gant, N. F., & Leveno, K. J. (2005). Conduct of normal labor and delivery. In: *Williams obstetrics* (22nd ed., pp. 320–325) New York: McGraw-Hill.

Elder, C. R. (2004). Beyond the baby blues: Postpartum depression. *Nursing Spectrum,* [Online] Available at: http://nsweb.nursingspectrum.com/ce/ce72.htm

Engstrom, J. (2004). *Maternal-neonatal nursing made incredibly easy.* Philadelphia: Lippincott Williams & Wilkins.

Geil, J. D. (2004). Von Willebrand disease. *eMedicine.* [Online] Available at: http://emedicine.com/ped/topic2419.htm

Gibbs, R. S., Sweet, R. L., & Duff, W. P. (2004). Maternal and fetal infectious disorders. In R. K. Creasy, R. Resnik, & J. D. Iams (Eds.), *Maternal-fetal medicine: principles and practice* (5th ed., pp. 741–801). Philadelphia: Saunders.

Gilbert, E. S., & Harmon, J. S. (2003). *Manual of high-risk pregnancy and delivery* (3rd ed.). St. Louis: Mosby.

Goldhaber, S. Z. (2003). Deep-vein thrombosis: advancing awareness to protect patient lives (White Paper). *Public Health Leadership Conference on Deep-Vein Thrombosis.* Washington, D.C.: American Public Health Association.

Green, C. J., & Wilkinson, J. M. (2004). *Maternal newborn nursing care plans.* St. Louis: Mosby, Inc.

Henshaw, C., Foreman, D., & Cox, J. (2004). Postnatal blues: a risk factor for postnatal depression. *Journal of Psychosomatic Obstetrics & Gynecology, 25,* 267–272.

Higgins, P. G. (2004). Postpartum complications. In S. Mattson & J. E. Smith, *Core curriculum for maternal-newborn nursing* (3rd ed., pp. 850–870). St. Louis: Elsevier Saunders.

Horowitz, J. A., & Goodman, J. H. (2005). Identifying and treating postpartum depression. *JOGNN, 34*(2), 264–273.

International Childbirth Education Association (ICEA) (2003). ICEA position statement and review of postpartum emotional disorders. *IJCE, 18*(3), 35–40.

Kennedy, E. (2005). Postpartum infections. *EMedicine.* [Online] Available at: http://www.emedicine.com/emerg/topic482.htm

Lewis, S. M., Heitkemper, M. M., & Dirksen, S. R. (2004). *Medical-surgical nursing* (6th ed.). St. Louis: Mosby.

London, M. L., Ladewig, P. W., Ball, J. W., & Bindler, R. C. (2003). *Maternal-newborn & child nursing: family-centered care.* Upper Saddle River, NJ: Prentice Hall.

Lowdermilk, D. L., & Perry, S. E. (2004). *Maternity & women's health care* (8th ed.). St. Louis: Mosby.

MacMullen, N. J., Dulski, L. A., & Meagher, B. (2005). Red alert: perinatal hemorrhage. *MCN, 30*(1), 46–51.

MacQueen, G., & Chokka, P. (2004). Special issues in the management of depression in women. *Canadian Journal of Psychiatry, 49*(1), 27–40.

McKinney, E. S., James, S. R., Murray, S. S., & Ashwill, J. W. (2005). *Maternal-child nursing* (2nd ed.). St. Louis: Elsevier Saunders.

Olds, S. B., London, M. L., Ladewig, P. W., & Davidson, M. R. (2004). *Maternal-newborn nursing & women's health care* (7th ed.). Upper Saddle River, NJ: Pearson Prentice Hall.

O'Toole, M. T. (2005). *Encyclopedia & dictionary of medicine, nursing & allied health* (7th ed.). Philadelphia: Saunders.

Paper, R. (2003). Can you recognize and respond to von Willebrand disease? *Nursing 2003, 33*(7), 54–56.

Pavlovich-Danis, S. J. (2004). When "can do" fades to "why bother": understanding depression in women. *Nursing Spectrum, 14*(11), 12–13.

Pope, C. S., & O'Grady, J. P. (2003). Malposition of the uterus. *eMedicine.* [Online] Available at: http://www.emedicine.com/med/topic3473.htm

Scott, J. R., Hamond, C., & Gordon, J. D. (Eds.) (2003). *Danforth's obstetrics and gynecology* (9th ed.). Philadelphia: Lippincott Williams & Wilkins.

Silverman, M. A. (2005). Idiopathic thrombocytopenic purpura. *eMedicine.* [Online] Available at: http://www.emedicine.com/emerg/topic282.htm

Smith, J. R., & Brennan, B. G. (2004). Postpartum hemorrhage. *eMedicine.* [Online] Available at: http://emedicine.com/med/topic3568.htm

Society of Obstetricians and Gynecologists of Canada (2002). *Advances in labor and risk management (ALARM) course manual* (9th ed.). Ottawa, Ontario, Canada: Society of Obstetricians and Gynecologists.

Suri, R., & Altshuler, L. L. (2004). Postpartum depression: risk factors and treatment options. *Psychiatric Times, 21*(11), 64–68.

Trizna, Z., & Goldman, M. P. (2005) Thrombophlebitis. *eMedicine.* [Online] Available at: http://www.emedicine.com/derm/topic808.htm

U.S. Department of Health and Human Services (USDHHS), Public Health Service. (2000). *Healthy people 2010* (conference edition, in two volumes). U.S. Department of Health and Human Services. Washington, D.C.: U.S. Government Printing Office.

Vieira, T. (2003). When joy becomes grief: screening tools for postpartum depression. *AWHONN Lifelines, 6*(6), 506–513.

Wainscott, M. P. (2004). Pregnancy, postpartum hemorrhage. *eMedicine.* [Online] Available at: http://emedicine.com/emerg/topic481.htm

Youngkin, E. Q., & Davis, M. S. (2004). *Women's health: a primary care clinical guide* (3rd ed.). Upper Saddle River, NJ: Pearson Prentice Hall.

Web Resources

A Place to Remember: **www.aplacetoremember.com**

Depression: **www.nimh.nih.gov/publicat/depwomenknows.cfm**

Depression After Delivery, Inc. (D.A.D.): **www.depressionafterdelivery.com**

International Childbirth Educator's Association: **www.icea.org**

LaLeche League & Breastfeeding Resource Center: **www.lalecheleague.org**

Learning about von Willebrand Disease: **www.allaboutbleeding.com**

National Hemophilia Foundation: **www.hemophilia.org**

National Institute of Mental Health: **www.nimh.nih.gov**

National Women's Health Information Center: **www.4women.gov**

Parents Helping Parents: **www.php.com**

Postpartum Support International: **www.postpartum.net**

World Federation of Hemophilia: **www.wfh.org**

ChapterWORKSHEET

● MULTIPLE CHOICE QUESTIONS

1. A postpartum mother appears very pale and states she is bleeding heavily. The nurse should *first:*

   a. Call the client's health care provider immediately.

   b. Immediately set up an intravenous infusion of magnesium sulfate.

   c. Assess the fundus and ask her about her voiding status.

   d. Reassure the mother that this is a normal finding after childbirth.

2. Hallucinations and expressions of suicide or infanticide are indicative of:

   a. Postpartum psychosis

   b. Postpartum anxiety disorder

   c. Postpartum depression

   d. Postpartum blues

3. The nurse assesses a woman closely in the first few hours after giving birth because which of the following could occur?

   a. Thrombophlebitis

   b. Breast engorgement

   c. Uterine infection

   d. Postpartum hemorrhage

4. Which of the following would the nurse expect to include in the plan of care for a woman with mastitis who is receiving antibiotic therapy?

   a. Stop breastfeeding and apply lanolin.

   b. Administer analgesics and bind both breasts.

   c. Apply warm or cold compresses and give analgesics.

   d. Remove the nursing bra and expose the breast to fresh air.

● CRITICAL THINKING EXERCISES

1. Mrs. Griffin had a 12-hour labor before a cesarean birth. Her membranes ruptured 6 hours before she came to the hospital. Her fetus showed signs of fetal distress, so internal electronic fetal monitoring was used. Her most recent test results indicate she is anemic.

   a. What postpartum complication is this new mother at highest risk for? Why?

   b. What assessments need to be done to detect this potential complication?

   c. What nursing measures will the nurse use to prevent this complication?

2. Tammy, a 32-year-old G9P9, had a spontaneous vaginal birth 2 hours ago. Tammy has been having a baby each year for the past 9 years. Tammy's lochia has been heavy, with some clots. She hasn't been up to void since she had epidural anesthesia and has decreased sensation to her legs.

   a. What factors place Tammy at risk for postpartum hemorrhage?

   b. What assessments are needed before planning interventions?

   c. What nursing actions are needed to prevent a postpartum hemorrhage?

3. Lucy, a 25-year-old G2P2, gave birth 2 days ago and is expected to be discharged today. She has a history of severe postpartum depression 2 years ago with her first child. Lucy has not been out of bed for the past 24 hours, is not eating, and provides no care for herself or her newborn. Lucy states she already has a boy at home and not having a girl this time is disappointing.

   a. What factors/behaviors place Lucy at risk for an emotional disorder?

   b. Which interventions might be appropriate at this time?

   c. What education does the family need prior to discharge?

● STUDY ACTIVITIES

1. Compare and contrast postpartum blues, postpartum depression, and postpartum psychosis in terms of their unique features and medical management.

2. Select a website from the ones listed at the end of the chapter. Critique it regarding its helpfulness to parents, the correctness of the information supplied, and when was it last updated.

3. Interview a woman who has given birth and ask about any complications she may have had and what was most helpful to her during the experience.

4. The number-one cause of postpartum hemorrhage is

   _____.

5. When giving report to the nurse who will be caring for a woman and her newborn in the postpartum period, what information should the labor nurse convey?

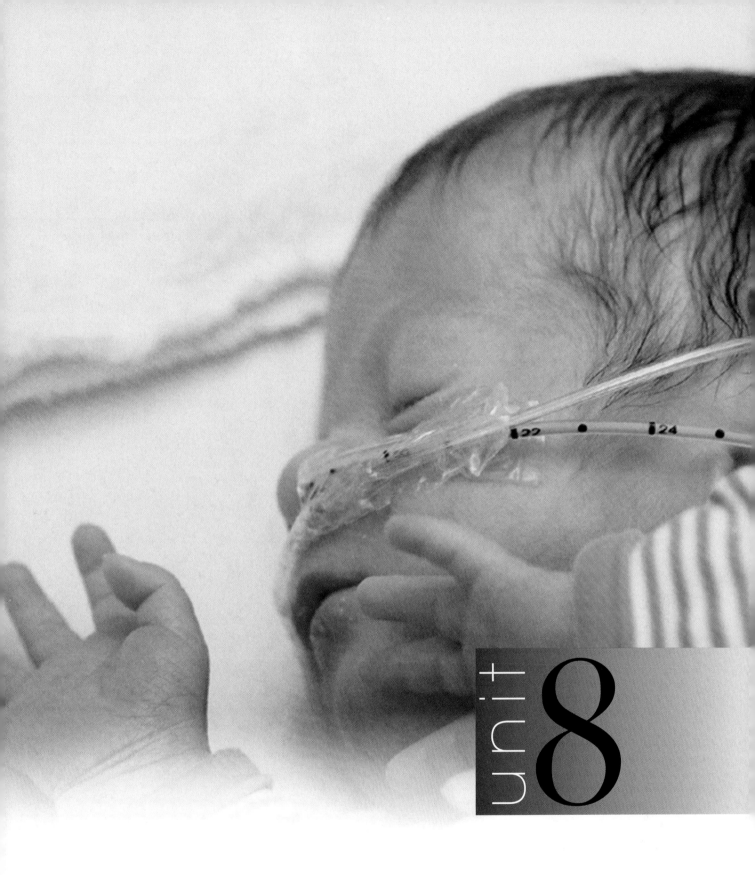

The Newborn at Risk

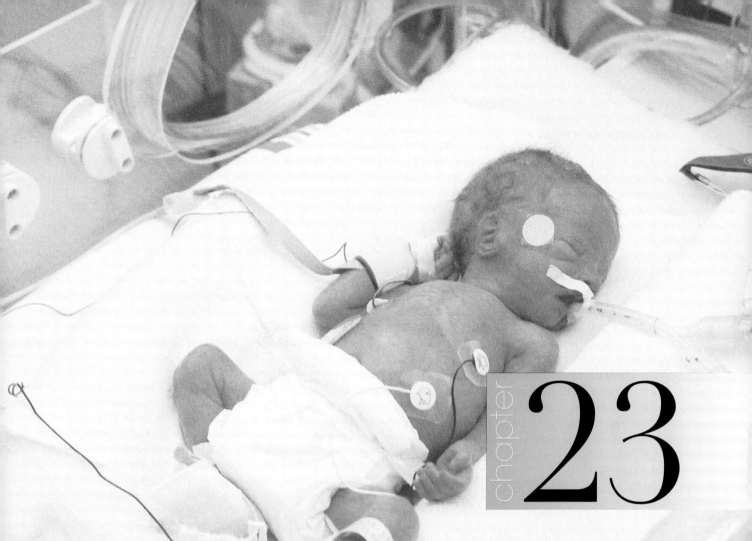

Nursing Management of the Newborn With Special Needs: Variations in Gestational Age and Birthweight

chapter 23

LearningOBJECTIVES

After studying the chapter content, the student should be able to accomplish the following:

1. Define the key terms.
2. Identify factors that assist in identifying a newborn at risk due to variations in gestational age and birthweight.
3. Describe contributing factors and common complications associated with dysmature infants and their management.
4. Discuss associated conditions and their management that affect the newborn with variations in gestational age and birthweight.
5. Outline the nurse's role in helping parents experiencing perinatal grief or loss.

WOW

Guiding a parent's hand to touch a frail or ill newborn demonstrates courage and compassion under very difficult circumstances, a powerful tool in helping to deal with the newborn's special needs.

Most newborns are born between 38 and 40 weeks' gestation and weigh 6 to 8 lb, but variations in gestational age and birthweight can occur, and infants with these variations have special needs. Gestational age at birth is inversely correlated with the risk that the infant will experience physical, neurologic, or developmental sequelae (Tufts, 2004). Some newborns are born very ill and need special advanced care to survive.

When a woman gives birth to a newborn with problems involving immaturity or birthweight, especially one who is considered high risk, she may go through a grieving process in which she mourns the loss of the healthy full-term newborn she had expected. Through this process she learns to come to terms with the experience she now faces.

The development of new technologies and regionalized care centers for the care of newborns with special needs has resulted in significant improvements and success. Nurses need to have a sound knowledge base to identify the newborn with special needs and to provide coordinated care.

The key to identifying a newborn with special needs related to gestational age or birthweight variation is an awareness of the factors that could place a newborn at risk. These factors are similar to those that would suggest a high-risk pregnancy:

• Maternal nutrition (malnutrition or overweight)
• Substandard living conditions
• Low socioeconomic status
• Maternal age of <20 or >35 years old
• Substance abuse
• Failure to seek prenatal care
• Smoking or exposure to passive smoke
• Periodontal disease
• Multiple gestation
• Extreme maternal stress
• Abuse and violence
• Placental complications (placenta previa or abruptio placentae)
• History of previous preterm birth
• Maternal disease (e.g., hypertension or diabetes)
• Maternal infection (e.g., urinary tract infection or chorioamnionitis)
• Exposure to occupational hazards (Gilbert & Harmon, 2003)

Being able to anticipate the birth of a newborn at risk allows the birth to take place at a health care facility equipped with the resources to meet the mother's and newborn's needs. This is important in reducing mortality and morbidity.

Healthy People 2010 has identified preterm births and low birthweight as important national health goals (Healthy People 2010).

This chapter discusses the nursing management of newborns with special needs related to variations in gestational age and birthweight. Selected associated conditions affecting these newborns are also described. Due to the frailty of these newborns, the care of the family experiencing perinatal loss and the role of the nurse in helping the family cope also are addressed.

Birthweight Variations

Fetal growth is influenced by maternal nutrition, genetics, placental function, environment, and a multitude of other

HEALTHY PEOPLE *2010*

National Health Goals Related to Newborns With Birthweight and Gestational Age Variations

Objective	Significance
Increase the proportion of very low birthweight (VLBW) infants born at level III hospitals or subspecialty perinatal centers	Will help to promote the delivery of high-risk infants in settings that have the technological capacity to care for them, ultimately reducing the morbidity and mortality rates for these infants
Reduce low birthweight (LBW) from a baseline of 7.6% to a target of 5%; reduce very low birthweight (VLBW) from a baseline of 1.4% to 0.9%	Will help to emphasize the issue of LBW as a risk factor associated with newborn death, helping to promote measures to reduce this risk factor and thus contributing to significant reductions in infant mortality
Reduce the total number of preterm births from a baseline of 11.6% to 7.6% Reduce the number of live births at 32 to 36 weeks' gestation from a baseline of 9.6% to 6.4% Reduce the number of live births at less than 32 weeks' gestation from a baseline of 2% to 1.1%	Will help to emphasize the role of preterm birth as the leading cause of newborn deaths unrelated to birth defects Will aid in promoting an overall reduction in infant illness, disability, and death

USDHHS, 2000.

638

factors. Assigning size to a newborn is a way to measure and monitor the growth and development of the newborn at birth. Newborns can be classified according to their weight and weeks of gestation, and knowing the group into which a newborn fits is important.

Appropriate for gestational age characterizes approximately 80% of newborns and describes a newborn with a normal height, weight, head circumference, and Body Mass Index (Venes, 2005). Being in the appropriate-for-gestational-age group confers the lowest risk for any problems. These infants have lower morbidity and mortality than other groups.

Small-for-gestational-age infants typically weigh less than 2,500 g (5 lb 8 oz) at term due to less growth in utero than expected. An infant is also classified as small for gestational age if his or her birthweight is at or below the 10th percentile as correlated with the number of weeks of gestation on a growth chart.

Large-for-gestational-age describes infants whose birthweight is above the 90th percentile on a growth chart and who weigh more than 4,000 g (8 lb 13 oz) at term due to accelerated growth for length of gestation (Cheffer & Rannalli, 2004).

The following terms describe other infants with marginal weights at birth and of any gestational age:

• **Low birthweight:** less than 2,500 g (5.5 lb) (Fig. 23-1)
• **Very low birthweight:** less than 1,500 g (3 lb 5 oz)
• **Extremely low birthweight:** less than 1,000 g (2 lb 3 oz)

Small-for-Gestational-Age Newborns

Newborns are considered small for gestational age (SGA) when they weigh less than two standard deviations for gestational age or fall below the 10th percentile on a growth chart for gestational age. These infants can be preterm, term, or postterm.

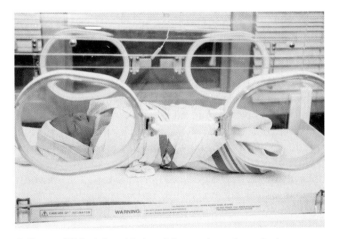

● Figure 23-1 A low-birthweight newborn in an isolette.

In some SGA newborns, the rate of growth does not meet the expected growth pattern. Termed intrauterine growth restriction (IUGR), these newborns also are considered at risk, with the perinatal morbidity and mortality rate increased substantially compared to that of the appropriate-for-age newborn (Cunningham et al., 2005). IUGR is the pathologic counterpart of SGA. However, an important distinction to make between SGA and IUGR newborns is that not all who are SGA have IUGR. The converse also is true: not all newborns who have IUGR are SGA. Some SGA infants are constitutionally small: they are statistically small but otherwise healthy.

Conditions altering fetal growth produce insults that affect all organ systems and are known to produce two patterns of growth that depend on the timing of the insult to the developing embryo or fetus. An early insult (typically <28 weeks) results in overall growth restriction, with all organs small. These SGA infants never catch up in size when compared with normal children. An insult later in gestation (>28 weeks) results in intrauterine malnutrition, but optimal postnatal nutrition generally restores normal growth potential and carries a better prognosis than earlier insults (Putman, 2004).

Historically, IUGR has been categorized as symmetric or asymmetric. Symmetric IUGR refers to fetuses with equally poor growth rate of the head, the abdomen, and the long bones. Asymmetric IUGR refers to infants whose head and long bones are spared compared to their abdomen and internal organs. It is now believed that most IUGR is a continuum from asymmetry (early stages) to symmetry (late stages) (Harper & Lam, 2005).

Fetal growth is dependent on genetic, placental, and maternal factors. Cognitive and motor development during infancy forms the basis for children's subsequent development. Newborns who experience nutritional deficiencies in utero and are born SGA are at risk for cognitive deficits that can undermine their academic performance throughout their lives (Black et al., 2004).

The fetus is thought to have an inherent growth potential that, under normal circumstances, yields a healthy newborn of appropriate size. The maternal-placental-fetal units act in harmony to provide for the needs of the fetus during gestation. However, growth potential in the fetus can be limited, and this is analogous to failure to thrive in the infant. The causes of both can be intrinsic or environmental. Factors that can contribute to the birth of an SGA newborn are highlighted in Box 23-1.

Characteristics of a Small-for-Gestational-Age Newborn

The typical appearance of the SGA newborn includes:

• Head disproportionately large compared to rest of body
• Wasted appearance of extremities

BOX 23-1

FACTORS CONTRIBUTING TO THE BIRTH OF SGA NEWBORNS

- Maternal causes
  - Chronic hypertension
  - Diabetes mellitus with vascular disease
  - Autoimmune diseases
  - Living at a high altitude (hypoxia)
  - Smoking
  - Substance abuse (heroin/cocaine/methamphetamines)
  - Hemoglobinopathies (sickle cell anemia)
  - Preeclampsia
  - Chronic renal disease
  - Malnutrition
  - "TORCH" group infections
- Placental factors
  - Abnormal cord insertion
  - Chronic abruption
  - Placenta previa
  - Placental insufficiency
- Fetal factors
  - Trisomy 13, 18, and 21
  - Turner's syndrome
  - Congenital anomalies
  - Multiple gestation

Sources: Harper & Lam, 2005; Thureen, Deacon, Hernandez, and Hall, 2005; Kenner & Lott, 2004; and Haws, 2004.

- Reduced subcutaneous fat stores
- Decreased amount of breast tissue
- Scaphoid abdomen (sunken appearance)
- Wide skull sutures secondary to inadequate bone growth
- Poor muscle tone over buttocks and cheeks
- Loose and dry skin that appears as if it is oversized
- Thin umbilical cord (Verklan & Walden, 2004)

Common Problems of Small-for-Gestational-Age Newborns

SGA newborns commonly face problems after birth because of the decrease in placental function during utero. These problems include perinatal asphyxia, hypothermia, hypoglycemia, polycythemia, and meconium aspiration.

Perinatal Asphyxia

Perinatal asphyxia is common in SGA infants because they tolerate the stress of labor poorly. As a result, they frequently develop acidosis and hypoxia. Typically they have low Apgar scores (Thureen et al., 2005).

The SGA newborn has lived in a hypoxic environment prior to birth and thus has little to no oxygen reserves available to withstand the stress of labor. Several alterations contribute to this hypoxic environment. Uterine contractions during labor increase hypoxic stress. Glycogen stores may be depleted secondary to the chronic hypoxic state,

leading to fetal distress as manifested by fetal bradycardia. In addition, impaired uteroplacental circulation secondary to maternal and uterine conditions predisposes them to perinatal depression. At birth, this compromised newborn experiences difficulty adjusting to the extrauterine environment. Care focuses on anticipating this problem and immediately initiating resuscitation measures at birth.

Hypothermia

Hypothermia frequently occurs in SGA newborns because they have less muscle mass, less brown fat, less heat-preserving subcutaneous fat, and limited ability to control skin capillaries (Lowdermilk & Perry, 2004). These physiologic conditions are associated with depleted glycogen stores, poor subcutaneous fat stores, and disturbances in central nervous system (CNS) thermoregulation mechanisms secondary to hypoxia (Kenner & Lott, 2004). Hypothermia stresses the SGA newborn metabolically, increasing the newborn's risk for acidosis and hypoglycemia (Thureen et al., 2005). Maintaining a neutral thermal environment is crucial to allow the newborn to stabilize his or her body temperature and to prevent cold stress, which could exacerbate the acidosis and thus the asphyxia.

Hypoglycemia

Hypoglycemia is prevalent in SGA newborns in the first few hours and days of life due to an increase in metabolic rate and lack of adequate glycogen stores to meet the newborn's metabolic demands. However, the symptoms of hypoglycemia can be easily overlooked because they are very subtle. Typically, the symptoms include lethargy, tachycardia, respiratory distress, jitteriness, poor feeding, hypothermia, diaphoresis, weak cry, seizures, and hypotonia. Blood glucose levels are below 40 mg/dL in term newborns and below 20 mg/dL in preterm newborns (Kenner & Lott, 2004).

Care focuses on monitoring glucose levels, maintaining fluid and electrolyte balance, observing for changes in the newborn's condition, such as increasing irritability or respiratory distress, and initiating early oral feedings if applicable. If oral feedings are not accepted, an intravenous infusion with 10% dextrose in water may be needed to maintain the glucose level above 40 mg/dL.

Polycythemia

Polycythemia is defined as a venous hematocrit of greater than 65%. Polycythemia exists because SGA fetuses experience chronic mild hypoxia secondary to placental insufficiency in utero. This hypoxic environment stimulates the release of erythropoietin, which leads to an increased rate of erythrocyte (red blood cell) production. The newborn exhibits a weak sucking reflex, ruddy appearance, tachypnea, jaundice, lethargy, jitteriness, hypotonia, and irritability. The goal of therapy is to reduce the viscosity of the blood via partial exchange transfusions of plasma, albumin, or normal saline to increase fluid volume to a hematocrit of approximately 60% (Lessaris, 2005).

Meconium Aspiration

Meconium aspiration occurs as a result of meconium being released into the amniotic fluid prior to birth. Historically, meconium contaminating amniotic fluid at birth was thought to be a sign of "fetal distress" in response to hypoxia. Currently, it is acknowledged as an indication of a normally maturing gastrointestinal tract, or the result of vagal stimulation from umbilical cord compression (Cunningham et al., 2005)

At times meconium-stained amniotic fluid may be a sign of fetal distress, especially if accompanied by diminished amniotic fluid and abnormal fetal heart rate patterns. Meconium-stained amniotic fluid is a signal indicating possible newborn depression at birth. If present, immediate resuscitation measures, including clearing the airway and supporting ventilation, are essential. (For more information on meconium aspiration syndrome, see Chapter 24.)

Large-for-Gestational-Age Newborns

A newborn whose weight is above the 90th percentile on growth charts or two standard deviations above the mean weight for gestational age is defined as large for gestational age (LGA). The range of weight is 4,000 to 5,000 g or more than 9 lb. LGA infants may be preterm, term, or postterm.

Maternal factors that increase the chance of bearing an LGA infant include maternal diabetes mellitus or glucose intolerance, multiparity, prior history of a macrosomic infant, postdates gestation, maternal obesity, male fetus, and genetics (Moses, 2004). Because of the infant's large size, vaginal birth may be difficult and occasionally results in birth injury. In addition, shoulder dystocia, clavicle fractures, and facial palsies are common. The incidence of cesarean births is very high with LGA infants to avoid arrested labor and birth trauma.

Characteristics of a Large-for-Gestational-Age Newborn

The typical LGA newborn has a large body and appears plump and full-faced. The increase in body size is proportional. However, the head circumference and body length are in the upper limits of intrauterine growth. These newborns have poor motor skills and have difficulty in regulating behavioral states. LGA infants are more difficult to arouse to a quiet alert state (Thureen et al., 2005).

Common Problems of Large-for-Gestational-Age Newborns

An LGA newborn can face several problems after birth: birth trauma due to fetopelvic disproportion, hypoglycemia, polycythemia, and jaundice secondary to hyperbilirubinemia.

Birth Trauma

Birth trauma secondary to the infant's large size is common. Because of their large size, LGA infants are more likely to be born by operative birth. If born vaginally, forceps or vacuum-assisted births may be necessary to overcome shoulder or body dystocia. Common birth traumas include depressed skull fracture, cephalhematoma, fracture of the clavicle or humerus, brachial plexus injuries, or facial palsy (Putman, 2004).

A thorough assessment of the LGA infant at birth is paramount to identify fractured clavicles, brachial palsy, facial paralysis, phrenic nerve palsy, skull fractures, or hematomas. Observation and documentation of any injuries discovered are essential for early intervention and improved outcomes.

Hypoglycemia

Hypoglycemia in the LGA infant is defined as a blood glucose level below 40 mg/dL. Like the SGA infant at risk for hypoglycemia, clinical signs are often subtle and include lethargy, apathy, irritability, tachypnea, weak cry, temperature instability, jitteriness, seizures, apnea, bradycardia, cyanosis or pallor, feeble suck and poor feeding, hypotonia, and coma. A similar presentation may be seen in several other disorders, including septicemia, severe respiratory distress, and congenital heart disease. Thus, the clinical signs of hypoglycemia are vague and a high index of suspicion is needed to identify it (Cloud & Haws, 2004).

Care of the LGA infant at risk for hypoglycemia includes checking the blood glucose on arrival at the nursery or within 2 hours of birth by reagent test strip (e.g., Dextrostix or Chemstrip BG). Repeat the screening every 2 to 3 hours or before feeds and also immediately in any infant suspected of having or showing clinical signs of hypoglycemia, regardless of age (Townsend, 2005).

Polycythemia

Polycythemia is defined as a venous hematocrit over 65%, resulting in the blood becoming increasingly hyperviscous and thus sluggish to circulate. Polycythemia in the LGA newborn can occur secondary to several events such as fetal hypoxia, trauma with bleeding, increase in fetal erythropoietin production, or delayed cord clamping (Mattson & Smith, 2004). Clinical manifestations include plethora (ruddy appearance), cyanosis, weak suck and feeding difficulties, lethargy, tachycardia, jitteriness, difficult to arouse, irritability, hypotonia, seizures, and jaundice.

Management focuses on decreasing blood viscosity by increasing the fluid volume. This is accomplished by partial exchange transfusion with plasma, normal saline, or albumin. The purpose of a partial exchange transfusion for polycythemia is to lower hematocrit and decrease blood viscosity. Polycythemia and hyperviscosity have been associated with fine and gross motor delays, speech delays, and neurologic sequelae (Gordon, 2003).

Hyperbilirubinemia

Hyperbilirubinemia in the LGA infant commonly accompanies polycythemia and erythrocyte breakdown. With increased numbers of red blood cells in circulation, their breakdown in large amounts predisposes the infant to hyperbilirubinemia and thus jaundice. In addition, many LGA infants cannot tolerate feedings in the first few days of life, thus increasing the enterohepatic circulation of bilirubin. Usually conjugated bilirubin, in the presence of intestinal flora initiated by feedings, is excreted via bile to the intestine and is not absorbed from the intestine back into the blood. In the absence of intestinal flora (due to limited or no feedings), unconjugated bilirubin can be reabsorbed across the intestinal mucosa into the portal circulation and return to the liver. This reabsorption path is referred to as the enterohepatic circulation (Thilo, 2005).

Measures to reduce bilirubin levels consist of hydration, early feedings, and phototherapy. (See Chapter 24 for a more detailed discussion of hyperbilirubinemia and phototherapy.)

Nursing Management of the Newborn With Birthweight Variations

Nursing management for the SGA or LGA infant involves keen observation skills and a solid knowledge base about the common problems each might develop. Since newborns cannot tell the nurse what is wrong, the nurse must maintain a high level of suspicion at all times to identify subtle newborn behaviors that might indicate a problem requiring immediate intervention to prevent a catastrophic event.

Assessment

Assessment of the SGA infant begins by reviewing the maternal history to identify possible risk factors, such as smoking, drug abuse, chronic maternal illness, hypertension, multiple gestation, or genetic disorders. This information allows the nurse to anticipate a possible problem and be prepared to intervene quickly should it occur. At birth, perform a thorough physical examination, closely observing for any congenital malformations, neurologic insults, or indications of infection. Anticipate the need for and provide resuscitation as indicated by the newborn's condition at birth.

Assessment of the LGA infant focuses on detecting any traumatic injuries, such as fractures of clavicle or humerus or facial nerve damage. Perform a neurologic examination to identify any nerve palsies, such as immobility of the upper arm. The maternal history can provide clues as to whether the woman has an increased risk of giving birth to a LGA infant. Also obtain frequent blood glucose levels as ordered to evaluate for hypoglycemia, and assess the LGA infant for subtle signs such as lethargy, jitteriness, seizures, hypotonia, or poor feeding.

Nursing Interventions

Interventions for the SGA infant may include obtaining weight, length, and head circumference, comparing them to standards, and documenting the findings. Perform frequent serial blood glucose measurements as ordered and monitor vital signs, being particularly alert for changes in respiratory status that might indicate respiratory distress. Institute measures to maintain a neutral thermal environment to prevent cold stress and acidosis.

Initiate early and frequent oral feedings unless contraindicated. Weigh the infant daily and ensure that the SGA infant has adequate rest periods to decrease metabolic requirements.

Observe for clinical signs of polycythemia and monitor blood results. If the infant is symptomatic, assist with the partial exchange transfusion procedure.

Provide anticipatory guidance to parents about any treatments and procedures that are being done. Emphasize the need for close follow-up and careful monitoring of the infant's growth in length, weight, and head circumference and feeding patterns throughout the first year of life to confirm any "catch-up" growth taking place.

For the LGA infant, assist in stabilizing the newborn. Monitor blood glucose levels and feeding during the first few hours of life to prevent hypoglycemia. Feedings can be formula or breast milk, with intravenous glucose supplementation as needed.

If the newborn's blood glucose level is below 25 mg/dL, institute immediate treatment with IV glucose, regardless of clinical symptoms (Thureen et al., 2005). Monitor and record intake and output and obtain daily weights to aid in evaluating nutritional intake. Also observe for signs and symptoms of polycythemia and hyperbilirubinemia and report any immediately to the health care provider so that early interventions can be taken to prevent poor long-term neurologic development outcomes. Provide parental guidance about the treatments and procedures being done and about the need for follow-up care for any abnormalities identified.

Gestational Age Variations

The mean duration of pregnancy calculated from the first day of the last normal menstrual period is approximately 280 days, or 40 weeks. Gestational age is typically measured in weeks: a newborn born before completion of 37 weeks is classified as preterm, and one born after completion of 42 weeks is classified as postterm. The infant born from the first day of 38th week through 42 weeks is classified as term. Precise knowledge of a newborn's gestational age is imperative for effective postnatal management. Determination of gestational age by the nurse assists in planning appropriate care for the newborn and provides important information regarding potential problems that need interventions. (See Chapter 18 for more information on assessing gestational age.)

Postterm Newborn

A pregnancy that extends beyond 42 weeks' gestation produces a **postterm newborn.** Other terms used to describe these late births include postmature, prolonged pregnancy, or postdates pregnancy. Postterm newborns may be LGA, SGA, or dysmature (newborn weighs less than established normal parameters for estimated gestational age [IUGR]), depending on placental function.

The reason why some pregnancies last longer than others is not completely understood. What is known is that women who experience one postterm pregnancy are at increased risk in subsequent pregnancies. The incidence of prolonged pregnancy is approximately 10% (Gilbert & Harmon, 2003).

The ability of the placenta to provide adequate oxygen and nutrients to the fetus after 42 weeks' gestation is thought to be compromised, leading to perinatal mortality and morbidity. As the placenta loses its ability to nourish the fetus, the fetus uses stored nutrients to stay alive, and wasting occurs. This wasted appearance at birth is secondary to the loss of muscle mass and subcutaneous fat.

Characteristics of a Postterm Newborn

Postterm newborns typically exhibit the following characteristics:

- Dry, cracked, wrinkled skin
- Long, thin extremities

Consider THIS!

I had been waiting for this baby my whole married life and now I was told to wait even longer. I was into my third week past my due date and was just told that if I didn't go into labor on my own, the doctor would induce me on Monday. As I waddled out of his office into the hot summer sun, I thought about all the comments that would await me at the office: "You're not still pregnant, are you?" "Weren't you due last month?" "You look as big as a house." "Are you sure you aren't expecting triplets?" I started to get into my car when I felt warm fluid slide down my legs. Although I was embarrassed at my wetness, I was thrilled I wouldn't have to go back to the office and drove myself to the hospital. Within hours my wait was finally over with the birth of my son, a postterm infant with peeling skin and a thick head of hair. He was certainly worth the wait!

Thoughts: Although most due dates are within plus or minus 2 weeks, we can't "go to the bank with it" because so many factors influence the start of labor. This woman was anxious about her overdue status, but nature prevailed. The old adage "when the fruit is ripe, it will fall" doesn't always bring a good outcome: many women need a little push to bring a healthy newborn forth. What happens when the fetus stays inside the uterus too long? What other features are typical of postterm infants?

- Creases that cover the entire soles of the feet
- Wide-eyed, alert expression
- Abundant hair on scalp
- Thin umbilical cord
- Limited vernix and lanugo
- Meconium-stained skin
- Long nails (Green & Wilkinson, 2004)

Complications in Postterm Newborns

The postern newborn is at risk for perinatal asphyxia, hypoglycemia, hypothermia, polycythemia, and meconium aspiration.

Perinatal Asphyxia

Perinatal asphyxia can be attributed to placental deprivation or oligohydramnios that leads to cord compression, thereby reducing perfusion to the fetus. Fetal distress will manifest as decelerations, bradycardia, or both on the fetal monitor during labor. Anticipating the need for newborn resuscitation is a priority. The newborn resuscitation team needs to be available in the birthing suite for immediate backup. The newborn may need to be transported to the neonatal intensive care unit (NICU) for continuous assessment, monitoring, and treatment, depending on the status after resuscitation.

Hypoglycemia

Hypoglycemia in the postterm infant is associated with hypoxia secondary to depleted glycogen reserves. In addition, placental insufficiency secondary to placental aging contributes to chronic fetal nutritional deficiency, further depleting glycogen stores. Since glucose is essential for cerebral metabolism, neurologic impairment, including intellectual and motor deficits, may result from hypoglycemia (Armentrout, 2004).

Care focuses on monitoring and maintaining blood glucose levels once stabilized. Intravenous dextrose 10% and/or early initiation of feedings will help stabilize the blood glucose levels to prevent CNS sequelae.

Hypothermia

Hypothermia results from loss of subcutaneous fat secondary to placental insufficiency. As the placenta loses its ability to nourish the growing fetus (placental insufficiency), the postterm fetus uses stored nutrients for nutrition, and wasting of subcutaneous fat, muscle, or both occurs (Putman, 2004). This loss of subcutaneous fat strips the infant of the natural insulation that would assist in temperature regulation.

Signs of hypothermia include bradycardia (<25 bpm), tachypnea (>60 bpm), tremors, irritability, wheezing, crackles, retractions, restlessness, lethargy, hypotonia, weak or high-pitched cry, hypothermia, temperature instability, seizures, poor feeding, and grunting (Green & Wilkinson, 2004).

Care focuses on assessing skin temperature, respiration characteristics, results of blood studies, such as arterial blood gases (ABGs), blood glucose levels, and serum bilirubin, and neurologic status. Measures to prevent or reduce the incidence of hypothermia involve eliminating sources of heat loss by thoroughly drying the newborn at birth, wrapping him or her in a warmed blanket, and placing a stockinet cap on the newborn's head. Providing environmental warmth via a radiant heat source will help stabilize the newborn's temperature.

Polycythemia

Polycythemia develops secondary to intrauterine hypoxia, which triggers increased red blood cell production to compensate for lower oxygen levels. Polycythemia leads to sluggish organ perfusion and hyperbilirubinemia from the red blood cell breakdown. The true incidence of this condition is not known, since the majority of infants are asymptomatic. Diagnosis is typically based on hematocrit values. Manifestations may be subtle and include respiratory distress, lethargy, seizures, hypoglycemia, tachypnea, plethora, tremors, hypotonia, irritability, feeding difficulties, vomiting, hepatomegaly, and jaundice (Lessaris, 2005).

Closely assess all postterm infants for polycythemia. Review the maternal history to aid in identifying the newborn at risk for this problem. Providing adequate hydration will help reduce the viscosity of the newborn's blood to prevent thrombosis. Be alert to the early, often subtle signs to promote early identification and prompt treatment to prevent any neurodevelopmental delays.

Meconium Aspiration

Meconium aspiration is a possible complication in postterm infants who have experienced chronic intrauterine hypoxia. Meconium-stained amniotic fluid is present in 25% to 30% of all postterm births (Clark & Clark, 2004). The presence of meconium in the amniotic fluid increases the risk for aspiration, and it may be associated with adverse fetal and newborn outcomes, including acute respiratory complications, and long-term pulmonary and neurologic abnormalities. Astute observation of the amniotic fluid color when membranes rupture as well as a meconium-stained umbilical cord and fingernails is essential to alert the healthcare professional in charge of the birth to the possibility of meconium aspiration. Careful suctioning at the time of birth and afterwards, if the condition dictates it, reduces the incidence of meconium aspiration.

Preterm Newborn

A **preterm newborn** is one who is born before the completion of 37 weeks of gestation. Although the national birth rate has been declining since the 1990s, the preterm birth rate has been climbing rapidly. Approximately one in eight babies, or 12%, are born before the 37th week of ges-

tation (Nelson, 2004). Prematurity is now the leading cause of death within the first month of life and the second leading cause of all infant deaths. While certain risk factors have been identified (e.g., a previous preterm delivery, low socioeconomic status, preeclampsia, hypertension, poor maternal nutrition, smoking, multiple gestation, infection, advanced maternal age, and substance abuse), the etiology of half of all preterm births is unknown (Damus, 2005).

Preterm births take an enormous financial toll, estimated to be in the billions of dollars. They also take an emotional toll on those involved.

Changes in perinatal care practices, including regional care, have reduced newborn mortality rates. Transporting high-risk pregnant women to a tertiary center for birth rather than transferring the neonate after birth is associated with a reduction in neonatal mortality and morbidity (Bakewell-Sachs & Blackburn, 2003). Despite increasing rates of survival, preterm infants continue to be at high risk for neurodevelopmental disorders such as cerebral palsy or mental retardation, intraventricular hemorrhage, congenital anomalies, neurosensory impairment, and chronic lung disease (Bakewell-Sachs & Blackburn, 2003). Prevention of preterm births is best accomplished by making sure all pregnant women receive quality prenatal care throughout their gestation.

Characteristics of a Preterm Newborn

Although there isn't a typical preterm newborn appearance, some common physical findings include:

- Birthweight of less than 5.5 lb
- Scrawny appearance
- Head disproportionately larger than chest circumference
- Poor muscle tone
- Minimal subcutaneous fat
- Undescended testes
- Plentiful lanugo (a soft downy hair), especially over the face and back
- Poorly formed ear pinna with soft, pliable cartilage
- Fused eyelids
- Soft and spongy skull bones, especially along suture lines
- Matted scalp hair, wooly in appearance
- Absent to a few creases in the soles and palms
- Minimal scrotal rugae in male infants; prominent labia and clitoris in female infants
- Thin, transparent skin with visible veins
- Breast and nipples not clearly delineated
- Abundant vernix caseosa (Engstrom, 2004) (Fig. 23-2)

Effects of Prematurity on Body Systems

Since the preterm neonate did not remain in utero long enough, every body system may be immature, affecting the newborn's transition from intrauterine to extrauterine life and placing him or her at risk for complications. Without full development, organ systems are not capable

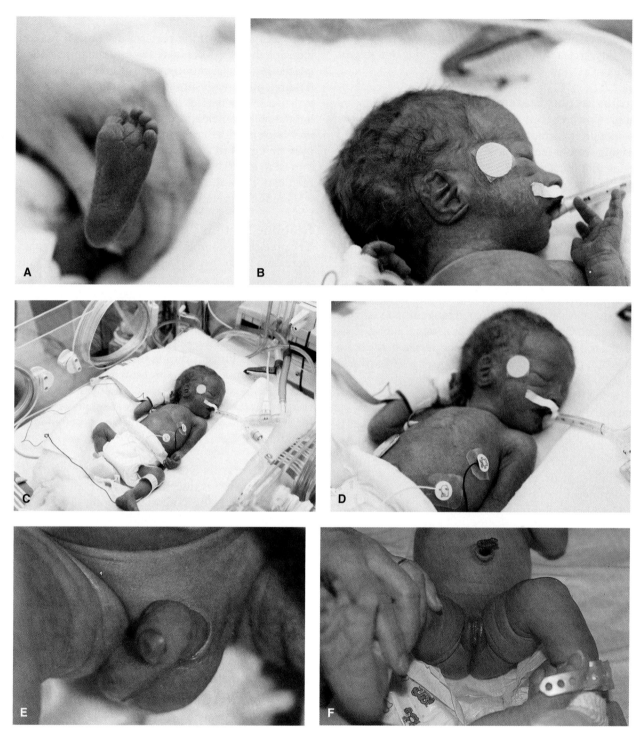

● Figure 23-2 Characteristics of a preterm newborn. (**A**) Few plantar creases. (**B**) Soft, pliable ear cartilage, matted hair, and fused eyelids. (**C**) Lax posture with poor muscle development. (**D**) Breast and nipple area barely noticeable. (**E**) Male genitalia. Note the minimal rugae on the scrotum. (**F**) Female genitalia. Note the prominent labia and clitoris.

of functioning at the level needed to maintain extra-uterine homeostasis (Mattson & Smith, 2004).

Respiratory System
Because the respiratory system is one of the last to mature, the preterm newborn is a great risk for respiratory compli-

cations. A few of the problems that affect the preterm baby's breathing ability and adjustment to extrauterine life include:

• Surfactant deficiency, leading to the development of respiratory distress syndrome
• Unstable chest wall, leading to atelectasis

- Immature respiratory control centers, leading to apnea
- Smaller respiratory passages, leading to obstruction
- Inability to clear fluid from passages, leading to transient tachypnea

Cardiovascular System

The preterm newborn has great difficulty in making the transition from intrauterine to extrauterine life in terms of changing from a fetal to a neonatal circulation pattern. Making that transition is prompted by higher oxygen levels in the circulation once air breathing begins. If the oxygen levels remain low secondary to perinatal asphyxia, the fetal pattern of circulation may persist, causing blood flow to bypass the lungs. Another problem affecting the cardiovascular system is the increased incidence of congenital anomalies associated with continued fetal circulation—patent ductus arteriosus and an open foramen ovale. In addition, impaired regulation of blood pressure in preterm newborns may cause fluctuations throughout the circulatory system. One of special note is cerebral blood flow, which may predispose the fragile blood vessels in the brain to rupture, causing intracranial hemorrhage (Mattson & Smith, 2004).

Gastrointestinal System

Preterm newborns usually lack the neuromuscular coordination to maintain the suck, swallow, and breathing regimen necessary for sufficient calorie and fluid intake to support growth. Perinatal hypoxia causes shunting of blood from the gut to more important organs such as the heart and brain. Subsequently, ischemia and damage to the intestinal wall can occur. This combination of shunting, ischemia, damage to the intestinal wall, and poor sucking ability places the preterm infant at risk for malnutrition and weight loss.

In addition, preterm infants have a small stomach capacity, weak abdominal muscles, compromised metabolic function, limited ability to digest proteins and absorb nutrients, and weak or absent suck and gag reflexes. All of these limitations place the preterm infant at risk for nutritional deficiency and subsequent growth and development delays (Gregory, 2005).

Currently, minimal enteral feeding is used to prepare the preterm newborn's gut to overcome the many feeding difficulties associated with gastrointestinal immaturity. It involves the introduction of small amounts, usually 0.5 to 1 mL/kg/h, of enteral feeding to induce surges in gut hormones that enhance maturation of the intestine. This minute amount of breast milk or formula given via gavage feeding prepares the gut to absorb future introduction of nutrients. It builds mucosal bulk, stimulates development of enzymes, enhances pancreatic function, stimulates maturation of gastrointestinal hormones, reduces gastrointestinal distention and malabsorption, and enhances transition to oral feedings (Blackburn, 2003).

Renal System

The renal system of the preterm newborn is immature, reducing the baby's ability to concentrate urine and slowing the glomerular filtration rate. As a result, the risk for fluid retention, with subsequent fluid and electrolyte disturbances, is increased. In addition, these newborns have limited ability to clear drugs from their systems, thereby increasing the risk of drug toxicity. Close monitoring of the preterm newborn's acid–base and electrolyte balance is critical to identify metabolic inconsistencies. Prescribed medications require strict evaluation to prevent overwhelming the preterm baby's immature renal system.

Immune System

The preterm newborn's immune system is very immature, increasing his or her susceptibility to infections. A deficiency of IgG may occur because transplacental transfer does not occur until after 34 weeks' gestation. This protection is lacking if the baby was born before this time. In addition, preterm newborns have an impaired ability to manufacture antibodies to fight infection if they were exposed to pathogens during the birth process. The preterm newborn's thin skin and fragile blood vessels provide a limited protective barrier, adding to the increased risk for infection. Thus, the focus of care is on anticipating and preventing infections, which has a better outcome than treating them.

Central Nervous System

The preterm baby is susceptible to injury and insult to the CNS, increasing the potential for long-term disability into adulthood. Like all newborns, preterm babies have difficulty in temperature regulation and maintaining stability. However, their risk for heat loss is compounded by inadequate amounts of insulating subcutaneous fat; lack of muscle tone and flexion to conserve heat; inadequate brown fat to generate heat; limited muscle mass activity, reducing the possibility of producing their own heat; inability to shiver to generate heat; and an immature temperature-regulating center in the brain (Lowdermilk & Perry, 2004). The major focus of care is preventing cold stress, which increases metabolic and oxygen needs. The goal is to create a neutral thermal environment in which oxygen consumption is minimal but body temperature is maintained (Kenner, 2003).

Nursing Management of the Newborn With Gestational Age Variations

The newborn with a gestational age variation often presents with multiple problems. Although preterm and postterm newborns may appear to be at opposite ends of the gestational age spectrum and are so different in appearance and size, both are at high risk and need special care. Postterm newborns are just as vulnerable as preterm ones.

When preterm labor develops and cannot be stopped by medical intervention, plans for appropriate management of the mother and the preterm newborn need to be made, such as transporting them to a regional center with facilities to care for preterm newborns or notifying the facility's NICU. Depending on the degree of prematurity, the preterm infant may be kept in the NICU for months.

The postterm infant poses the same high-risk situation as the preterm infant and needs special intensive monitoring and care to survive.

Assessment

A thorough assessment of the preterm or postterm newborn upon admission to the nursery provides a baseline from which to identify changes in clinical status. Nurses need to be aware of the common physical characteristics and must be able to identify any deviation from the expected. In addition, knowing the typical complications each is at risk for will assist in initiating early interventions.

Common assessments for preterm and postterm newborns might include:

- Review the maternal history to identify risk factors for pre- or postterm birth.
- Review antepartum and intrapartum records for maternal infections to anticipate treatment.
- Assess gestational age and assess for IUGR, if appropriate.
- Complete a physical examination to identify any abnormalities.
- Monitor skin condition to treat complications early.
- Screen for hypoglycemia upon admission and then every 1 to 2 hours, and observe for nonspecific signs of hypoglycemia such as lethargy, poor feeding, and seizures.
- Assess for complications such as respiratory distress syndrome in the preterm infant.
- Assess the baby's skin for color and perfusion (capillary refill).
- Assess respirations, including observations for periods of apnea lasting more than 20 seconds.
- Monitor vital signs, including temperature via skin probe to identify hypothermia or fever, and heart rate for tachycardia or bradycardia.
- Assess heart sounds for possible murmur, indicating presence of patent ductus arteriosus in a preterm newborn.
- Monitor oxygen saturation levels by pulse oximetry to validate perfusion status.
- Assess neurologic status through behavior (restlessness, hypotonia, weak cry or suck).
- Monitor laboratory studies such as hemoglobin and hematocrit for signs of polycythemia and bilirubin concentrations.
- Identify family strengths and coping mechanisms to establish a basis for intervention.

Nursing Interventions

The birth of a preterm or postterm infant creates a crisis for the mother and her family, as most have not anticipated having a newborn requiring special care. Preterm newborns present with immaturity of all organ systems, abundant physiologic challenges, and significant morbidity and mortality (Jotzo & Poets, 2005). Postterm infants are susceptible to several birth challenges secondary to placental dysfunction that place them at risk for asphyxia, hypoglycemia, and respiratory distress. The nurse must be vigilant for complications when managing both preterm and postterm infants (Nursing Care Plan 23-1).

Promoting Oxygenation

Newborns normally start to breathe without assistance and often cry after birth, stimulated by a change in pressure gradients and environmental temperature. The work of taking that first breath is primarily due to overcoming the surface tension of the walls of the terminal lung units at the gas–tissue interface. Subsequent breaths require less inspiratory pressure since there is an increase in functional capacity and air retained. By 1 minute of age, most newborns are breathing well. A newborn who fails to establish adequate, sustained respiration after birth is said to have **asphyxia.** On a physiologic level, it can be defined as impairment in gas exchange resulting in a decrease in oxygen in the blood (hypoxemia) and an excess of carbon dioxide or hypercapnia that leads to acidosis. Asphyxia is the most common clinical insult in the perinatal period that results in brain injury, which may lead to mental retardation, cerebral palsy, or seizures (Hernandez et al., 2005).

The preterm infant lacks surfactant, which lowers surface tension in the alveolus and stabilizes the alveoli to prevent their collapse. Even if they can initiate respirations, preterm infants have a limited ability to retain air due to insufficient surfactant. Therefore, preterm newborns develop atelectasis quickly without alveoli stabilization. Postterm infants experience respiratory distress secondary to placental insufficiency and intrauterine hypoxia. In either case, their inability to initiate and establish respirations leads to hypoxia (decreased oxygen), acidosis (decreased pH), and hypercarbia (increased carbon dioxide). This change in the newborn's biochemical environment may inhibit the transition to extrauterine circulation, and fetal circulation patterns may persist.

Failure to initiate extrauterine breathing or failure to breathe well after birth leads to hypoxia (too little oxygen in the cells of the body). As a result, the heart rate falls, cyanosis develops, and the newborn becomes hypotonic and unresponsive. Although this can happen with any newborn, the risk is increased in preterm and postterm newborns.

Prevention and early identification of newborns at risk are key. Be aware of the prenatal risk factors that can

(text continues on page 650)

Nursing Care Plan 23-1

Overview of the Care of a Preterm Newborn

Although Alice, an 18-year-old, felt she had done everything right during her first pregnancy, she didn't anticipate giving birth to a preterm infant at 32 weeks' gestation. When Mary Kaye was born, she had respiratory distress and hypoglycemia and couldn't stabilize her temperature. Assessment revealed the following: newborn described as scrawny in appearance; skin thin and transparent with prominent veins over abdomen; hypotonia with lax, extended positioning; weak sucking reflex when nipple offered; respiratory distress with tachypnea (70 breaths per minute), nasal flaring, and sternal retractions; low blood glucose level suggested by lethargy, tachycardia, jitteriness; temperature of 36°C (96.8°F) axillary despite warmed blanket; weight 2146 g (4.73 lb); length 45 cm (17.72 inches).

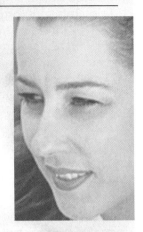

Nursing Diagnosis: Risk for imbalanced nutrition: less than body requirements related to poor sucking and lack of glycogen stores necessary to meet the newborn's increased metabolic demands

Outcome identification and *evaluation*	Interventions with *rationales*
Newborn will demonstrate adequate nutritional intake, remaining free of signs and symptoms of hypoglycemia *as evidenced by blood glucose levels being maintained above 45 mg/dL, enhanced sucking ability, and appropriate weight gain.*	Identify newborn at risk based on behavioral characteristics, body measurements, and gestational age *to establish a baseline and allow for early detection.*
	Assess blood glucose levels as ordered *to determine status and establish a baseline for interventions.*
	Obtain blood glucose measurements upon admission to nursery and every 1 to 2 hours as indicated *to evaluate for changes.*
	Observe behavior for clues of low blood glucose *to allow for early identification.*
	Initiate early oral feedings or gavage feedings *to maintain blood glucose levels.*
	If oral or gavage feedings aren't tolerated, initiate an IV glucose infusion *to aid in stabilizing blood glucose levels.*
	Assess skin for pallor and sweating *to identify signs of hypoglycemia.*
	Assess neurologic status for tremors, seizures, jitteriness, and lethargy *to identify further drops in blood glucose levels.*
	Monitor weights daily for changes *to determine effectiveness of feedings.*
	Maintain temperature using warmed blankets, radiant warmer, or warmed isolette *to prevent heat loss and possible cold stress.*
	Monitor temperature *to prevent cold stress resulting in decreased blood glucose levels.*
	Offer opportunities for nonnutritive sucking on premature-size pacifier *to satisfy sucking needs.*
	Monitor for tolerance of oral feedings, including intake and output, *to determine effectiveness.*
	Administer IV dextrose if newborn is symptomatic *to raise blood glucose levels quickly.*

Overview of the Care of a Preterm Newborn (continued)

Outcome identification and *evaluation*	Interventions with *rationales*
	Decrease energy requirements, including clustering care activities and providing for rest periods, *to conserve glucose and glycogen stores.* Inform parents about procedures and treatments, including rationale for frequent blood glucose levels, *to help reduce anxiety level.*

Nursing Diagnosis: Ineffective breathing pattern related to immature respiratory system and respiratory distress

Newborn's respiratory status returns to adequate level of functioning *as evidenced by rate remaining within 30 to 60 breaths per minute, maintenance of acceptable oxygen saturation levels, and minimal to absent signs of respiratory distress.*	Assess gestational age and risk factors for respiratory distress *to allow early detection.* Anticipate need for bag and mask setup and wall suction *to allow for prompt intervention should respiratory status continue to worsen.* Assess the respiratory effort (rate, character, effort) *to identify changes.* Assess heart rate for tachycardia and auscultate heart sounds *to determine worsening of condition.* Observe for cues (grunting, shallow respirations, tachypnea, apnea, tachycardia, central cyanosis, hypotonia, increased effort) *to identify newborn's need for additional oxygen.* Maintain slight head elevation *to prevent upper airway obstruction.* Assess skin color *to evaluate tissue perfusion.* Monitor oxygen saturation level via pulse oximetry *to provide objective indication of perfusion status.* Provide supplemental oxygen as indicated and ordered *to ensure adequate tissue oxygenation.* Assist with any ordered diagnostic tests, such as chest x-ray and arterial blood gases, *to determine effectiveness of treatments.* Cluster nursing activities *to reduce oxygen consumption.* Maintain a neutral thermal environment *to reduce oxygen consumption.* Monitor hydration status *to prevent fluid volume deficit or overload.* Explain all events and procedures to the parents *to help alleviate anxiety and promote understanding of the newborn's condition.*

Nursing Diagnosis: Ineffective thermoregulation related to lack of fat stores and hypotonia resulting in extended positioning

Newborn will demonstrate ability to regulate temperature *as evidenced by a temperature remaining in normal range (36.4° to 37.1°C), and absent signs of cold stress*	Assess the axillary temperature every hour or use a thermistor probe *to monitor for changes.* Review maternal history *to identify risk factors contributing to problem.*

(continued)

Overview of the Care of a Preterm Newborn (continued)

Outcome identification and *evaluation*	Interventions with *rationales*
	Monitor vital signs, including heart rate and respiratory rate, *to identify deviations.*
	Check radiant heat source or isolette *to ensure maintenance of appropriate temperature of the environment.*
	Assess environment for possible sources of heat loss or gain through evaporation, conduction, convection, or radiation *to minimize risk of heat loss.*
	Avoid bathing infant *to prevent cold stress.*
	Prewarm all blankets and equipment that come in contact with newborn; place warmed cap on the newborn's head and keep it on *to minimize heat loss.*
	Encourage kangaroo care (mother holds preterm infant underneath her clothing skin-to-skin and upright between her breasts) *to provide warmth.*
	Educate parents on how to maintain a neutral thermal environment, including importance of keeping the newborn warm with a cap and double-wrapping with blankets and changing them frequently to keep dry *to promote newborn's adjustment.*

help identify the newborn who may need resuscitation at birth secondary to asphyxia:

- History of substance abuse
- Gestational hypertension
- Fetal distress due to hypoxia before birth
- Chronic maternal diseases such as diabetes or a heart or renal condition
- Maternal or perinatal infection
- Placental problems (previa or abruptio)
- Umbilical cord problems (nuchal or prolapsed)
- Difficult or traumatic birth
- Multiple births
- Congenital heart disease
- Maternal anesthesia or recent analgesia
- Preterm or postterm birth (Woods, 2004)

Note the newborn's Apgar score at 1 and 5 minutes If the score is below 7 at either time, resuscitation efforts are needed. Several diagnostic studies may be done to identify possible underlying etiologies. For example, a chest x-ray helps to identify any structural abnormalities that might interfere with respirations. Blood studies may be done, such as cultures to rule out an infectious process, a toxicology screen to detect any maternal drugs in the newborn, and a metabolic screen to identify any metabolic conditions (Green & Wilkinson, 2004). In addition, monitor vital signs continuously, check blood glucose levels for hypoglycemia secondary to stress, and maintain a neutral environmental temperature to promote energy conservation and minimize oxygen consumption.

Resuscitation Measures

Resuscitation involves a series of actions taken to establish normal breathing in the preterm or postterm infant. These actions aim to improve heart rate, color, tone, and activity. Resuscitation is necessary for all newborns that do not breathe well after birth or have a low 1-minute Apgar score.

The newborn with asphyxia requires immediate resuscitation. Dry the newborn thoroughly with a warm towel and then place him or her under a radiant heater to prevent rapid heat loss through evaporation. At times, handling and rubbing the newborn with a dry towel may be all that is needed to stimulate respirations. However, if the newborn fails to respond to stimulation, then active resuscitation is needed.

Any newborn can be born with asphyxia without warning. It is essential, therefore, to be prepared to resuscitate any newborn and to have all basic equipment immediately available and in working order. The equipment should be evaluated daily, and its condition and any needed repairs should be documented. Equipment needed for basic newborn resuscitation includes:

- A wall vacuum suction apparatus
- A wall source or tank source of 100% oxygen with a flow meter
- A neonatal self-inflating ventilation bag with correct-sized face masks
- A selection of endotracheal tubes (2.5, 3.0, or 3.5 mm) with introducers
- A laryngoscope with a small, straight blade and spare batteries and bulbs
- Ampules of naloxone (Narcan) with syringes and needles
- A wall clock to document timing of activities and events
- A supply of disposable gloves in a variety of sizes for staff to use

The procedure for newborn resuscitation is easily remembered by "ABCD"—airway, breathing, circulation, and drugs. The steps are highlighted in Box 23-2.

Resuscitation measures are continued until the newborn has a pulse above 100 bpm, a good cry, or good breathing efforts and a pink tongue. This last sign indicates a good oxygen supply to the brain (Woods, 2004).

Throughout the resuscitation period, keep the parents informed of what is happening to their newborn and what is being done and why. Provide support through this initial crisis. Once the newborn is stabilized, encourage bonding with the newborn by stroking, touching, and when appropriate holding the newborn (Fig. 23-3).

Oxygen Administration

Oxygen administration is a common therapy in newborn nurseries. Despite its use in newborns for over 75 years, there is no universal agreement on the most appropriate range at which oxygen levels should be maintained for hypoxic newborns, nor is there a standard timeframe for oxygen to be administered (Cunningham et al., 2005). While this uncertainty continues, nurses will experience a wide variation in practice in terms of modes of administration, monitoring, blood levels, and target ranges for both short- and long-term oxygen therapy.

A guiding principle, though, is that oxygen therapy should be targeted to levels appropriate to the condition, gestational age, and postnatal age of the newborn. Oxygen therapy must be used judiciously to prevent **retinopathy of prematurity** (ROP), a major cause of blindness in preterm newborns in the past. ROP is a potentially blinding eye disorder that occurs when abnormal blood vessels grow and spread through the retina, eventually leading to retinal detachment. The incidence of ROP is inversely proportional to the preterm baby's birthweight. Approximately 500 to 700 children become blind because of ROP in the United States annually (Gerontis, 2004). Although the role of oxygen in the pathogenesis of ROP is unclear, current evidence suggests that it is linked to the duration of oxygen use rather than the concentration. Thus, the use of 100% oxygen to resuscitate a newborn should not pose a problem (National Eye Institute, 2004). However, an ophthalmology consult for follow-up after discharge is essential for preterm infants whom have received extensive oxygen therapy.

Respiratory distress in preterm or postterm newborns is commonly caused by a deficiency of surfactant, retained fluid in the lungs (wet lung syndrome), meconium aspiration, pneumonia, hypothermia, or anemia. The principles

---

BOX 23-2

ABCDs OF NEWBORN RESUSCITATION

- **Airway**
  - Open the airway by placing the newborn's head in neutral position.
  - Clear the throat via gentle suctioning with a bulb syringe or soft 10F catheter.
- **Breathing**
  - Hold mask ventilation (blow-by oxygen) over the newborn's nose and mouth.
  - If no improvement is noted in the newborn's respirations, then intubate.
  - Intubate with endotracheal (ET) tube and ventilate with positive-pressure ventilation bag.
- **Circulation**
  - Apply chest compressions at about 80 times a minute.
  - Place hand around infant's chest using thumb on lower sternum.
  - Compress the chest two times, then follow with one ventilation.
- **Drugs**
  - If depression is due to narcotics, expect to administer naloxone (Narcan).
  - If metabolic acidosis is present, expect to administer sodium bicarbonate.
  - To improve heart rate, expect to administer epinephrine via ET tube or IV rapidly.

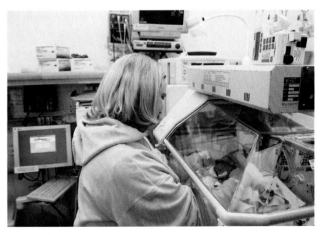

● Figure 23-3 Mother interacting with her preterm newborn in the isolette.

of care are the same regardless of the cause of respiratory distress. First, keep the newborn warm, preferably in a warmed isolette or with an overhead radiant warmer, to conserve the baby's energy and prevent cold stress. Handle the newborn as little as possible, because stimulation often increases the oxygen requirement. Provide energy through calories via intravenous dextrose or gavage or continuous tube feedings to prevent hypoglycemia. Treat cyanosis with an oxygen hood or blow-by oxygen placed near the newborn's face if respiratory distress is mild and short-term therapy is needed. Record the following important observations every hour, and document any deterioration or changes in respiratory status:

- Respiratory rate, quality of respirations, and respiratory effort
- Airway patency, including removal of secretions per hospital protocol
- Skin color, including any changes to duskiness, blueness, or pallor
- Lung sounds on auscultation to differentiate breath sounds in upper and lower fields
- Equipment required for oxygen delivery, such as:
  - Blow-by oxygen delivered via mask or tube for short-term therapy
  - Oxygen hood (oxygen is delivered via a plastic hood placed over the newborn's head)
  - Nasal cannula (oxygen is delivered directly through the nares) (Fig. 23-4A)
  - Continuous positive airway pressure (CPAP), which prevents collapse of unstable alveoli and delivers high inspired oxygen into the lungs
  - Mechanical ventilation, which delivers consistent assisted ventilation and oxygen therapy, reducing the work of breathing for the fatigued infant (see Fig. 23-4B)
- Correct placement of endotracheal tube (if present)

- Heart rate, including any changes
- Oxygen saturation levels via pulse oximetry to evaluate need for therapy modifications based on hemoglobin
- Maintenance of oxygen saturation level from 87% to 95% (Askin & Diehl-Jones, 2004)
- Nutritional intake, including calories provided, to prevent hypoglycemia and method of feeding, such as gavage, intravenous, or continuous enteral feedings
- Hydration status, including any signs and symptoms of fluid overload
- Laboratory tests, including ABGs, to determine effectiveness of oxygen therapy
- Administration of medication, such as exogenous surfactant

If the newborn shows worsening cyanosis or if oxygen saturation levels fall below 86%, prepare to give additional oxygen as ordered. Throughout care, strict asepsis, including handwashing, is vital to reduce the risks of infection.

Maintaining Thermal Regulation

Immediately after birth, dry the newborn with a warmed towel and then place him or her in a second warm, dry towel before performing the assessment. This drying prevents rapid heat loss secondary to evaporation. Newborns who are active, breathing well, and crying are stable and can be placed on their mother's chest ("kangaroo care") to promote warmth and prevent hypothermia. Preterm or postterm infants may not be stable enough to stay with their mother and thus need to be placed under a radiant warmer or in a warmed isolette after they are dried with a warmed towel.

Typically newborns use nonshivering thermogenesis for heat production by metabolizing their own brown adipose tissue. Neither the preterm nor the postterm newborn has an adequate supply of brown fat. The preterm newborn left the uterus before it was available; the postterm

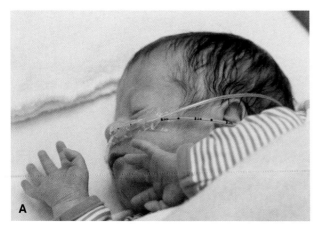
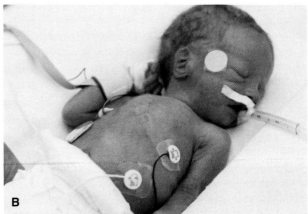

● Figure 23-4 (**A**) A preterm newborn receiving oxygen therapy via a nasal cannula. Note that the newborn also has an enteral feeding tube inserted for nutrition. (**B**) Preterm newborn receiving mechanical ventilation.

newborn used his or her supply for survival in a hypoxic environment. The preterm newborn has decreased muscle tone and thus cannot assume the flexed fetal position, which reduces the amount of skin exposed to a cooler environment. In addition, both preterm and postterm newborns have large body surface areas compared to their weight. This allows an increased transfer of heat from their bodies to the environment.

Typically, a preterm or postterm newborn who is having problems with thermal regulation will be cool to cold to the touch. The hands, feet, and tongue may appear cyanotic. Respirations will be shallow or slow, or the newborn will exhibit signs of respiratory distress. Lethargy, hypotonia, poor feeding, and feeble cry also may be noted. He or she is lethargic and hypotonic, feeds poorly, and has a feeble cry. Blood glucose levels most likely will be low, leading to hypoglycemia, due to the energy expended to keep warm.

When providing care for the preterm or postterm newborn to promote thermal regulation:

- Be knowledgeable about the four heat transfer mechanisms and how to prevent loss:
  - Convection: heat loss through air currents (avoid drafts near the newborn)
  - Conduction: heat loss through direct contact (warm everything the newborn comes in contact with, such as blankets, mattress, stethoscope)
  - Radiation: heat loss without direct contact (keep isolettes away from cold sources and provide insulation to prevent heat transfer)
  - Evaporation: heat loss by conversion of liquid into vapor (keep the newborn dry and delay the first bath until the baby's temperature is stable)
- Frequently assess the temperature of the isolette or radiant warmer, adjusting the temperature as necessary to prevent hypo- or hyperthermia.
- Assess the newborn's temperature every hour until stable.
- Observe for clinical signs of cold stress, such as respiratory distress, central cyanosis, hypoglycemia, lethargy, weak cry, abdominal distention, apnea, bradycardia, and acidosis.
- Be aware of the complications of hypothermia and frequently assess the newborn for signs and symptoms:
  - Metabolic acidosis secondary to anaerobic metabolism used for heat production, which results in the production of lactic acid
  - Hypoglycemia due to depleted glycogen stores
  - Pulmonary hypertension secondary to pulmonary vasoconstriction
- Monitor the newborn for signs of hyperthermia such as tachycardia, tachypnea, apnea, warm to touch, flushed skin, lethargy, weak or absent cry, and CNS depression; adjust the environmental temperature appropriately.
- Explain to the parents the need to maintain the newborn's temperature, including the measures used; demonstrate ways to safeguard warmth and prevent heat loss.

Promoting Nutrition and Fluid Balance

Providing nutrition is challenging for preterm and postterm newborns because their needs are great but their ability to take in optimal energy/calories is reduced due to their compromised health status. Individual nutritional needs are highly variable. Typically, adequate caloric intake for the preterm infant is 120 kcal/kg/day (Gregory, 2005).

Depending on their gestational age, preterm and postterm newborns receive nutrition orally, enterally, or parenterally, via an infusion. Several different methods can be used to provide nutrition for the preterm or postterm infant: parenteral feedings administered through a percutaneous central venous catheter for long-term venous access with delivery of total parenteral nutrition (TPN), or enteral feedings, which can include oral feedings (sucking on a nipple), continuous nasogastric tube feedings, or intermittent orogastric (gavage) tube feedings. Gavage feedings are commonly used for compromised newborns to allow them to rest during the feeding process. Many have a weak suck and become fatigued and thus cannot consume enough calories to meet their needs.

Most newborns born after 34 weeks' gestation without significant complications can feed orally. Those born before 34 weeks' gestation typically start with parenteral nutrition within the first 24 hours of life. Then, enteral nutrition is introduced and advanced based on the degree of maturity and clinical condition. Ultimately, enteral nutrition methods replace parenteral nutrition. Parenteral requirements are about 20% less than enteral requirements, or about 80 to 90 kcal/kg/day.

To promote nutrition and fluid balance in the preterm or postterm newborn:

- Measure daily weight and plot it on a growth curve.
- Monitor intake; calculate fluid and caloric intake daily.
- Assess fluid status by monitoring weight; urinary output; urine specific gravity; laboratory test results such as serum electrolyte levels, blood urea nitrogen, creatinine, and hematocrit; skin turgor; and fontanels (they will be sunken if the baby is dehydrated) (Kenner & Lott, 2004).
- Continually assess for enteral feeding intolerance; measure abdominal girth, auscultate bowel sounds, and measure gastric residuals before the next tube feeding.
- Assess for signs of dehydration, including a decrease in urinary output, sunken fontanels, temperature elevation, lethargy, and tachypnea.

Preventing Infection

Prevention of infection is critical when caring for preterm or postterm newborns. Infections are the most common cause of morbidity and mortality in the NICU population (Kenner & Lott, 2004). Nursing assessment and the ability to identify problems early are imperative for better newborn outcomes.

Preterm newborns are at risk for infection because their early birth deprived them of maternal antibodies needed for passive protection. Both preterm and postterm infants are susceptible to infection because of their limited ability to produce antibodies, asphyxia at birth, and thin, friable skin that is easily traumatized, leaving an entry for microorganisms.

Early detection is crucial. Be aware of the clinical manifestations, which can be nonspecific and subtle: apnea, diminished activity, poor feeding, temperature instability, respiratory distress, seizures, tachycardia, hypotonia, irritability, pallor, jaundice, and hypoglycemia. Report any of these to the primary care provider immediately so that treatment can be instituted.

Include the following interventions when caring for a preterm or postterm newborn to prevent infection:

- Assess for risk factors in maternal history that place the newborn at increased risk.
- Monitor for changes in vital signs such as temperature instability, tachycardia, or tachypnea.
- Assess oxygen saturation levels and initiate oxygen therapy as ordered if oxygen saturation levels fall below acceptable parameters.
- Assess feeding tolerance, typically an early sign of infection.
- Monitor laboratory test results for changes.
- Remove all jewelry on your hands prior to washing hands; wash hands upon entering the nursery and in between caring for newborns.
- Adhere to standard precautions; use clean gloves to handle dirty diapers and dispose of them properly.
- Avoid using tape on the newborn's skin to prevent tearing.
- Use sterile gloves when assisting with any invasive procedure; attempt to minimize the use of invasive procedures.
- Use equipment that can be thrown away after use.
- Avoid coming to work when ill, and screen all visitors for contagious infections.

Preventing Complications

Preterm or postterm newborns face a myriad of possible complications as a result of their fragile health status or the procedures and treatments used. Some of the more common complications in preterm newborns are respiratory distress syndrome, periventricular-intraventricular hemorrhage, bronchopulmonary dysplasia, ROP, hyperbilirubinemia, anemia, necrotizing enterocolitis, hypoglycemia, infection or septicemia, delayed growth and development, and mental or motor delays (March of Dimes, 2005). Several of these complications are described in Chapter 24.

Providing Appropriate Stimulation

Newborn stimulation involves a series of activities to encourage normal development in preterm and postterm infants. Research on developmental interventions has found that when preterm infants, in particular, receive sensorimotor interventions such as rocking, massaging, holding, or sleeping on waterbeds, they gain weight faster, progress in feeding abilities more quickly, and show improved interactive behavior compared to preterm newborns who were not stimulated (Dodd, 2005). Conversely, overstimulation may have negative effects by reducing oxygenation and causing stress in preterm infants. A newborn reacts to stress by flaying the hands or bringing an arm up to cover the face. When overstimulated, such as by noise, lights, excessive handling, alarms, and procedures, and stressed, heart and respiratory rates decrease and periods of apnea or bradycardia may follow (Bremmer et al., 2003).

Appropriate developmental stimulation that would not overtax the compromised newborn might include kangaroo (skin-to-skin) holding, rocking, singing softly, cuddling, soft music, stroking the infant's skin gently, colorful mobiles, gentle massage, waterbed mattresses, and nonnutritive sucking opportunities (Fig. 23-5) or using sucrose if tolerated.

The NICU environment can be altered to provide periods of calm and rest for the newborn by dimming the lights, lowering the volume and tone of conversations, closing doors gently, setting the telephone ringer at the lowest volume possible, clustering nursing activities, and covering the isolette with a blanket to act as a light shield to promote rest at night.

Encourage parents to hold and interact with their newborn. Doing so helps to acquaint the parents with their newborn, promotes self-confidence, and fosters parent–newborn attachment (Fig. 23-6).

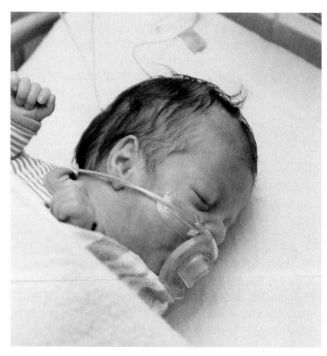

● Figure 23-5 A preterm newborn receiving non-nutritive sucking.

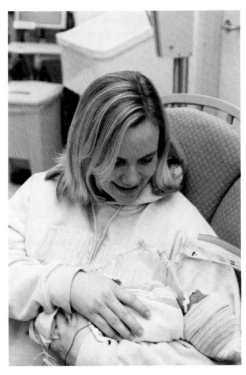

● Figure 23-6 A mother bonds with her preterm newborn.

Managing Pain

Pain is an unpleasant sensory and emotional experience felt by all humans. Newborns in the NICU are subjected to repeated procedures that cause them pain. Newborns, whether preterm, full term, or postterm, do experience pain, but the pain is difficult to validate with consistent behaviors. Considering that ill newborns undergo multiple noxious stimuli from invasive procedures, such as lumbar punctures, heel sticks, venipuncture, line insertions, chest tube placement, specimen collections, endotracheal intubation and suctioning, and mechanical ventilation, common sense would suggest that newborns experience pain from these many activities and interventions. However, pain management in infants was not addressed formally until various professional and accrediting organizations issued position statements and clinical recommendations in an effort to promote effective pain management (Verklan & Walden, 2004). An international consortium established principles of newborn pain prevention and management that all nurses should be familiar with and apply (Box 23-3).

Nurses play a key role in assessing a newborn's pain level. Assess the newborn frequently. Pain assessment is considered the "fifth vital sign" and should be done as frequently as the other four vital signs. Also, be able to differentiate pain from agitation by observing for changes in vital signs, behavior, facial expression, and body movement. Suspect pain if the newborn exhibits the following:

> BOX 23-3
>
> ### NEWBORN PAIN PREVENTION AND MANAGEMENT GUIDELINES
>
> - Newborn pain frequently goes unrecognized and undertreated.
> - Pain assessment is an essential activity prior to pain management.
> - Newborns experience pain, and analgesics should be given.
> - A procedure considered painful for an adult should also be considered painful for a newborn.
> - Developmental maturity and health status must be considered when assessing for pain in newborns.
> - Newborns may be more sensitive to pain than adults.
> - Pain behavior is frequently mistaken for irritability and agitation.
> - Newborns are more susceptible to the long-term effects of pain.
> - Adequate pain management may reduce complications and mortality.
> - Nonpharmacologic measures can prevent, reduce, or eliminate newborn pain.
> - Sedation does not provide pain relief and may mask pain responses.
> - A newborn's response to both pharmacologic and nonpharmacologic pain therapy should be assessed within 30 minutes of administration or intervention.
> - Health care professionals are responsible for pain assessment and treatment.
> - Written guidelines are needed on each newborn unit.

Anand, 2001; Spence et al., 2005; Walden, 2004; and Kenner & Lott, 2004.

- Sudden high-pitched cry
- Facial grimace with furrowing of brow and quivering chin
- Increased muscle tone
- Oxygen desaturation
- Body posturing, such as squirming, kicking, arching
- Limb withdrawal and thrashing movements
- Increase in heart rate, blood pressure, pulse, and respirations
- Fussiness and irritability (Littleton & Engebretson, 2005)

The goals of pain management are to minimize the amount, duration, and strength of pain and to assist the newborn in coping. Nonpharmacologic techniques to reduce pain may include:

- Gentle handling, rocking, caressing, cuddling, and massaging
- Rest periods before and after painful procedures
- Swaddling and positioning to establish physical boundaries
- Offering a pacifiers dipped in sucrose prior to procedure
- Use of minimal amount of tape, with gentle removal to avoid skin tears

- Use of warm blankets for wrapping to facilitate relaxation
- Reduction of environmental stimuli by removing or turning down noxious stimuli such as noise from alarms, beepers, loud conversations, and bright lights
- Use of distraction, such as colored objects or mobiles (Byers & Thornley, 2004)

Pain in the newborn is managed most effectively by preventing, limiting, or avoiding noxious stimuli and by administering pharmacologic agents when appropriate. The number of analgesics drugs available for preterm and postterm newborns is limited. Morphine and fentanyl, usually administered intravenously, are the most commonly used opioids to relieve moderate to severe pain. Mild pain relief is achieved with acetaminophen. Benzodiazepines are used as sedatives during painful procedures and can be combined with opioids for more effectiveness (AAP, 2000). Local or topical anesthetics (e.g., EMLA cream) also may be used before procedures (Walden & Franck, 2003).

Be vigilant for the potential adverse effects (respiratory depression or hypotension) when administering pharmacologic agents for pain management, especially in preterm newborns with neurologic impairment. These negative effects are usually dose- and route-related, so be knowledgeable about the pharmacokinetics and therapeutic dosing of any drug administered.

Promoting Growth and Development

In the late 1970s, researchers evaluated the NICU environment in terms of light and sound levels, caregiving activities, and handling of newborns. As a result of this research, many environmental modifications were made to reduce the stress and overstimulation of the NICU, and developmentally supportive care was introduced. Developmentally supportive care is defined as care of a newborn or infant to support positive growth and development. Developmental care focuses on what newborns or infants can do at that stage of development; it uses therapeutic interventions only to the point that they are beneficial; and it provides for the development of the newborn–family unit (Kenner & McGrath, 2004).

Developmental care is a philosophy of care that requires rethinking the relationships between newborns, families, and health care providers. It includes a variety of activities designed to manage the environment and individualize the care of the preterm or high-risk ill newborn based on behavioral observations. The goal is to promote a stable, well-organized newborn who can conserve energy for growth and development (Byers, 2003).

Developmental care includes these strategies:

- Clustering care to promote rest and conserve the infant's energy
- Flexed positioning to simulate the in utero positioning
- Environmental management to reduce noise and visual stimulation
- Kangaroo care to promote skin-to-skin sensation

- Placing twins in the same isolette or open crib to reduce stress
- Activities that promote self-regulation and state regulation:
  - Surrounding the newborn with nesting rolls/devices
  - Swaddling with a blanket to maintain the flexed position
  - Providing sheepskin or a waterbed to simulate the uterine environment
  - Providing nonnutritive sucking (calms the infant)
  - Providing objects to grasp (comforts the newborn)
- Promoting parent–infant bonding by making parents feel welcome in the NICU
- Providing open, honest communication with parents and staff
- Collaborating with the parents in planning the infant's care (Robison, 2003)

Developmental care can be fostered by clustering the lights in one area so that no lights are shining directly on newborns, installing visual alarm systems and limiting overhead pages to minimize noise, and monitoring continuous and peak noise levels. Nurses can play an active role by serving as members on committees that address these issues. In addition, nurses can provide direct developmentally supportive care. Doing so involves careful planning of nursing activities to provide the ideal environment for the newborn's development. For example, dim the lights and cover isolettes at night to simulate nighttime; support early extubation from mechanical ventilation; encourage early and consistent feedings with breast milk; administer prescribed antibiotics judiciously; position the newborn as if he or she was still in utero (a nesting fetal position); promote kangaroo care by encouraging parents to hold the newborn against the chest for extended periods each day; and coordinate care to respect sleep and awake states.

Throughout the newborn's stay, work with the parents, developing a collaborative partnership so they feel comfortable caring for their newborn. Be prepared to make referrals to community support groups to enhance coping (Carrier, 2004).

Promoting Parental Coping

Generally, pregnancy and the birth of a newborn are exciting times, with plans being made for the future. When the newborn has serious, perhaps life-threatening problems, the exciting experience suddenly changes to one of anxiety, fear, guilt, loss, and grief.

Anxiety Reduction

Parents who are typically unprepared for the birth of a preterm or postterm infant. They commonly experience an array of emotions, including disappointment, fear for the survival of the newborn, and anxiety due to the separation from their newborn immediately after birth (Jotzo & Poets, 2005). Early interruptions in the bonding process and concern about the newborn's survival can create extreme anxiety and interfere with attachment (Roller, 2005).

Nursing interventions aimed at reducing parental anxiety include:

- Review with them the events that have occurred since birth.
- Provide simple relaxation and calming techniques (visual imagery, breathing).
- Explore their perception of the newborn's condition, and offer explanations.
- Validate their anxiety and behaviors as normal reactions to stress and trauma.
- Provide a physical presence and support during emotional outbursts.
- Explore the coping strategies they used successfully in the past.
- Address their reactions to the NICU environment and explain all equipment used.
- Encourage frequent visits to the NICU.
- Identify family and community resources available to them.

Perinatal Loss

Nurses working in a NICU face a difficult situation when caring for newborns who may not survive. Newborn death is incomprehensible to most parents; this makes the grieving process more difficult because what is happening "can't be real." Deciding whether to see, touch, or hold the dying newborn is extremely difficult for many parents. Nurses play a major role in assisting parents to make their dying newborn "real" to them by providing them with as many memories as possible and encouraging them to see, hold, touch, dress, and take care of the infant and take photographs. These interventions help to validate the parents' sense of loss, to relive the experience, and to attach significance to the meaning of loss. A lock of hair, name card, and identification bracelet may serve as important mementoes that can ease the grieving process. The memories created by these interventions can be useful allies in the grieving process and in facilitating grief resolution (Cartwright & Read, 2004).

Parent–newborn interaction is vital to the normal processes of attachment and bonding. Equally important for parents is the detachment process involved in a newborn's death. Nurses can aid in this process by helping parents to see their newborn through the maze of equipment, explaining the various procedures and equipment, encouraging them to express their feelings about their fragile newborn's status, and providing time for them to be with their dying newborn (Lundquvist et al., 2002).

A common reaction by many people when learning that a newborn is not going to survive is one of avoidance. Nurses are no exception. It is difficult to initiate a conversation about such a sensitive issue without knowing how the parents are going to react and cope with the impending loss. One way to begin a conversation with the parents is to convey concern and acknowledge their loss. Active listening can provide parents a safe place to begin the healing process. The relationship that the nurse establishes with the parents is a unique one, providing an opportunity for both the nurse and the parents to share their feelings.

Be aware of personal feelings about loss and how these feelings are part of one's own life and personal belief system. Actively listen to the parents when they are talking about their experiences. Communicate empathy (understanding and feeling what another person is feeling), and respect their feelings and respond to them in helpful and supportive ways (Stevens, 2005).

When caring for the family experiencing a perinatal loss, include the following interventions:

- Help the family to accept the reality of death by using the word "died."
- Acknowledge their grief and the fact that their newborn has died.
- Help the family to work through their grief by validating and listening.
- Provide the family with realistic information about the causes of death.
- Offer condolences to the family in a sincere manner.
- Initiate spiritual comfort by calling the hospital clergy if needed.
- Acknowledge variations in spiritual needs and readiness.
- Encourage the parents to have a funeral or memorial service to bring closure.
- Encourage the parents to take photographs, make memory boxes, and record their thoughts in a journal.
- Suggest that the parents plant a tree or flowers to remember the infant.
- Explore with family members how they dealt with previous losses.
- Discuss meditation and relaxation techniques to reduce stress.
- Provide opportunities for the family to hold the newborn if they choose to do so.
- Assess the family's support network.
- Address attachment issues concerning subsequent pregnancies.
- Reassure the family that their feelings and grieving responses are normal.
- Provide information about local support groups.
- Provide anticipatory guidance regarding the grieving process.
- Recommend that family members maintain a healthy diet and get adequate rest and exercise to preserve their health.
- Present information about any impact on future childbearing, and refer the parents to appropriate specialists or genetic resources.
- Provide suggestions as to how friends can be helpful to the family.
- Offer to pray with the family if appropriate (Shuzman, 2004).

In a time of crisis or loss, individuals are often more sensitive to other people's reactions. For example, the parents may be extremely aware of the nurse's facial expressions, choice of words, and tone of voice. Talking quickly, in a businesslike fashion, or ignoring the loss may inhibit parents from discussing their pain or how they are coping with it. Parents may need to vent their frustrations and anger, and the nurse may become the target. Validate their feelings and attempt to reframe or refocus the anger toward the real issue of loss. An example would be to say, "I understand your frustration and anger about this situation. You have experienced a tremendous loss and it must be difficult not to have an explanation for it at this time." Doing so helps to defuse the anger while allowing them to vent.

When assisting bereaved parents, start where the parents are in the grief process to avoid imposing your own agenda on them. You may feel uncomfortable at not being able to change the situation or take the pain away. The nurse's role is to provide immediate emotional support and help facilitate the grieving process (Wallerstedt et al., 2003).

Preparing for Discharge

Discharge planning typically begins with evidence that recovery of the newborn is certain. However, the exact date of discharge may not be predictable. The goal of the discharge plan is to make a successful transition to home care. Essential elements for discharge are a physiologically stable infant, a family who can provide the necessary care with appropriate support services in place in the community, and a primary care physician available for ongoing care.

The care of each high-risk newborn after discharge requires careful coordination to provide ongoing multidisciplinary support for the family. The discharge planning team should include the parents, primary care physician, neonatologists, neonatal nurses, and a social worker. Other professionals, such as surgical specialists and pediatric subspecialists; occupational, physical, speech, and respiratory therapists; nutritionists; home health care nurses; and a case manager may be included as needed. Critical components of discharge planning are summarized in Box 23-4.

Nurses involved in the discharge process are instrumental in bridging the gap between the hospital and home. Interventions include:

- Assess the physical status of the mother and the newborn.
- Discuss the early signs of complications and what to do if they occur.
- Reinforce instructions for infant care and safety.
- Provide instructions for medication administration.
- Reinforce instructions for equipment operation, maintenance, and trouble-shooting.
- Teach infant cardiopulmonary resuscitation and emergency care.
- Demonstrate techniques for special care procedures such as dressings, ostomy care, artificial airway maintenance, chest physiotherapy, suctioning, and infant stimulation.

BOX 23-4

CRITICAL COMPONENTS OF DISCHARGE PLANNING

- Parental education—involvement and support in newborn care during NICU stay will ensure their readiness to care for the infant at home
- Evaluation of unresolved medical problems—review of the active problem list and determination of what home care and follow-up is needed
- Implementation of primary care—completion of newborn screening tests, immunizations, examinations such as funduscopic exam for ROP, and hematologic status evaluation
- Development of home care plan, including assessment of:
  - Equipment and supplies needed for care
  - In-home caregiver's preparation and ability to care for infant
  - Adequacy of the physical facilities in the home
  - An emergency care and transport plan if needed
  - Financial resources for home care costs
  - Family needs and coping skills
  - Community resources, including how they can be accessed

- Provide breastfeeding support or instruction on gavage feedings.
- Assist with defining roles in the adjustment period at home.
- Assess the parents' emotional stability and coping status.
- Provide support and reassurance to the family.
- Report abnormal findings to the health care team for intervention.
- Follow up with parents to assure them that they have a "lifeline."

KEY CONCEPTS

- Variations in birthweight and gestational age can place a newborn at risk for problems that require special care.
- Variations in birthweight include the following categories: small for gestational age, appropriate for gestational age, and large for gestational age. Newborns who are small or large for gestational age have special needs.
- The small-for-gestational-age newborn faces problems related to a decrease in placental function in utero; these problems may include perinatal asphyxia, hypothermia, hypoglycemia, polycythemia, and meconium aspiration.
- Risk factors for the birth of a large-for-gestational-age infant include maternal diabetes mellitus or glucose intolerance, multiparity, prior history of a macrosomic infant, postdates gestation, maternal obesity, male fetus, and genetics. Large-for-

gestational-age newborns face problems such as birth trauma due to cephalopelvic disproportion, hypoglycemia, polycythemia, and jaundice secondary to hyperbilirubinemia.

● Variations in gestational age include postterm and preterm newborns. Postterm newborns may be large or small for gestational age or dysmature, depending on placental function.

● The postterm newborn may develop several complications after birth, including fetal hypoxia, hypoglycemia, hypothermia, polycythemia, and meconium aspiration.

● Preterm birth is the leading cause of death within the first month of life and the second leading cause of all infant deaths.

● The preterm newborn is at risk for complications because his or her organ systems are immature, thereby impeding the transition from intrauterine life to extrauterine life.

● Newborns can experience pain, but their pain is difficult to validate with consistent behaviors.

● Newborns with gestational age variations, primarily preterm newborns, benefit from developmental care, which includes a variety of activities designed to manage the environment and individualize the care based on behavioral observations.

● Nurses play a key role in assisting the parents and family of a newborn with special needs to cope with this crisis situation, including dealing with the possibility that newborn may not survive. Nurses working with parents experiencing a perinatal loss can help by actively listening and understanding the parents' experiences and communicating empathy.

● The goal of discharge planning is to make a successful transition to home care.

References

American Academy of Pediatrics (AAP) (2000). Prevention and management of pain and stress in the neonate. *Pediatrics, 105*(2), 454–461.

Anand, K. J., & International Evidence-Based Group for Neonatal Pain (2001). Consensus statement for the prevention and management of pain in the newborn. *Archives of Pediatric and Adolescent Medicine, 155,* 173–180.

Armentrout, D. (2004). Glucose management. In M. T. Verklan & M. Walden (2004), *Core curriculum for neonatal intensive care nursing* (3rd ed., pp. 192–204). St. Louis: Elsevier Saunders.

Askin, D. F., & Diehl-Jones, W. (2004). Assisted ventilation. In M. T. Verklan & M. Walden, *Core curriculum for neonatal intensive care nursing* (3rd ed., pp. 536–568). St. Louis: Elsevier Saunders.

Black, M. M., Sazawal, S., Black, R. E., Khosla, S., Kumar, J., & Menon, V. (2004). Cognitive and motor development among small-for-gestational-age infants: impact of zinc supplementation, birth-weight, and care giving practices. *Pediatrics, 113*(5), 1297–1305.

Blackburn, S. (2003). *Maternal, fetal and neonatal physiology: a clinical perspective* (2nd ed.). Philadelphia: Saunders.

Bakewell-Sachs, S., & Blackburn, S. (2003) State of the science: achievements and challenges across the spectrum of care for preterm infants. *JOGNN, 32*(5), 683–695.

Bremmer, P., Byers, J. F., & Kiehl, E. (2003). Noise and the premature infant: physiological effects and practice implications. *JOGNN, 32*(4), 447–454.

Byers, J. F. (2003). Components of developmental care and the evidence for their use in the NICU. *MCN, 28*(3), 174–180.

Byers, J. F., & Thornley, K. (2004). Cueing into infant pain. *MCN, 29*(2), 84–91.

Carrier, C. T. (2004). Developmental support. In M. T. Verklan & M. Walden (Eds.), *Core curriculum for neonatal intensive care nursing.* St. Louis: Elsevier Saunders.

Cartwright, P., & Read, S. (2004). Perinatal loss: working with bereaved families. *Primary Health Care, 14*(2), 38–41.

Cheffer, N. D., & Rannalli, D. A. (2004). Newborn biologic/behavioral characteristics and psychosocial adaptations. In S. Mattson & J. E. Smith, *Core curriculum for maternal-newborn nursing* (3rd ed., pp. 437–464). St. Louis: Elsevier Saunders.

Clark, D. A., & Clark, M. B. (2004). Meconium aspiration syndrome. *eMedicine.* [Online] Available at: www.emedicine.com/ped/topic768.htm

Cloud, C. A., & Haws, P. (2004). Nutrition. In P. S. Haw, *Care of the sick neonate: a quick reference for health care providers* (p. 65). Philadelphia: Lippincott Williams & Wilkins.

Cunningham, F. G., Leveno, K. J., Bloom, S. L., Hauth, J. C., Gilstrap, L. C., & Wenstrom, K. D. (2005). *Williams obstetrics* (22nd ed.). New York: McGraw-Hill.

Damus, K. (2005). Prematurity. *March of Dimes.* [Online] Available at: www.marchofdimes.com/prematurity/5408_5576.asp

Dodd, V. L. (2005). Implications of kangaroo care for growth and development in preterm infants *JOGNN, 34*(2), 218–232.

Engstrom, J. (2004). *Maternal-neonatal nursing made incredibly easy.* Philadelphia: Lippincott Williams & Wilkins.

Gerontis, C. C. (2004). Retinopathy of prematurity. *eMedicine.* [Online] Available at: wwwemedicine.com/OPH/topic413.htm

Gilbert, E. S., & Harmon, J. S. (2003). *Manual of high-risk pregnancy and delivery* (3rd ed.). St. Louis: Mosby.

Gordon, E. A. (2003). Polycythemia and hyperviscosity of the newborn. *Journal of Perinatal and Neonatal Nursing, 17*(3), 209–221.

Gregory, J. (2005). Update on nutrition for preterm and full-term infants. *JOGNN, 34*(1), 98–108.

Green, C. J., & Wilkinson, J. M. (2004). *Maternal newborn nursing care plans.* St. Louis: Mosby.

Harper, T., & Lam, G. (2005). Fetal growth restriction. *eMedicine.* [Online] Available at: www.emedicine.com/med/topic3247.htm

Haws, P. S. (2004). *Care of the sick neonate: a quick reference for health care providers.* Philadelphia: Lippincott Williams & Wilkins.

Hernandez, J. A., Fashaw, L., & Evans, R. (2005). Adaptation to extrauterine life and management during normal and abnormal transition. In P. J. Thureen, J. Deacon, J. A. Hernandez, & D. M. Hall, *Assessment and care of the well newborn* (2nd ed., pp. 83–109). St. Louis: Elsevier Saunders.

Jotzo, M., & Poets, C. F. (2005). Helping parents cope with the trauma of premature birth: an evaluation of a trauma-preventive psychological intervention. *Pediatrics, 115*(4), 915–919.

Kenner, C. (2003). Resuscitation and stabilization of the newborn. In C. Kenner & J. Lott (Eds.), *Comprehensive neonatal nursing care: a physiologic perspective* (3rd ed.). St. Louis: Mosby.

Kenner, C., & Lott, J. W. (2004). *Neonatal nursing handbook.* St. Louis: Saunders.

Kenner, C., & McGrath, J. (2004). *Developmental care of newborns and infants: a guide for health professionals.* St. Louis: Mosby.

Lessaris, K. J. (2005). Polycythemia of the newborn. *eMedicine.* [Online] Available at: www.emedicine.com/ped/topic2479.htm

Littleton, L. Y., & Engebretson, J. C. (2005). *Maternity nursing care.* Clifton Park, NY: Thomson Delmar Learning.

Lowdermilk, D. L., & Perry, S. E. (2004). *Maternity & women's health care* (8th ed.). St. Louis: Mosby.

Lundquvist, A., Nilstun, T., & Dykes, A. K. (2002). Experiencing neonatal death: an ambivalent transition into motherhood. *Pediatric Nursing, 28*(6), 621–625.

March of Dimes (2005). Complications of preterm birth. March of Dimes Birth Defects Foundation. [Online] Available at: www. marchofdimes.com/prematurity/5512.asp

Mattson, S., & Smith, J. E. (2004). *Core curriculum for maternal-newborn nursing* (3rd ed.). St. Louis: Elsevier Saunders.

Moses, S. (2004). Fetal macrosomia: large for gestational age. *Family Practice Notebook.* [Online] Available at: www.fpnotebook.com/OB38.htm

National Eye Institute (2004). Retinopathy of prematurity (ROP). *U.S. National Institutes of Health Resource Guide.* [Online] Available at: http://nei.nih.gov/health/rop/index.asp

Nelson, R. (2004). Premature births on the rise. *AJN, 104*(6), 23–25.

Putman, M. A. (2004). Risks associated with gestational age and birthweight. In S. Mattson & J. E. Smith, *Core curriculum for maternal-newborn nursing* (3rd ed., pp. 465–496). St. Louis: Elsevier Saunders.

Robison, L. D. (2003). An organizational guide for an effective developmental program in the NICU. *JOGNN, 32*(3), 379–386.

Roller, C. G. (2005). Getting to know you: mothers' experiences of kangaroo care. *JOGNN, 34*(2), 210–217.

Shuzman, E. (2004). Facing stillbirth or neonatal death. *AWHONN Lifelines, 7*(6), 537–543.

Spence, K., Gillies, D., Harrison, D., Johnston, L., & Nagy, S. (2005). A reliable pain assessment tool for clinical assessment in the neonatal intensive care unit. *JOGNN, 33*(5), 80–86.

Stevens, S. (2005). The dark days of grief: how to lighten the load. *Advance for Nurse Practitioners, 13*(3), 31–33.

Thilo, E. H. (2005). Neonatal jaundice. In P. J. Thureen, J. Deacon, J. A. Hernandez, and D. M. Hall, *Assessment and care of the well newborn* (2nd ed., pp. 245–254). St. Louis: Elsevier Saunders.

Thureen, P. J., Deacon, J., Hernandez, J. A., & Hall, D. M. (2005). *Assessment and care of the well newborn* (2nd ed.). St. Louis: Elsevier Saunders.

Townsend, S. F. (2005). Approach to the infant at risk for hypoglycemia. In P. J. Thureen, J. Deacon, J. A. Hernandez, and D. M. Hall (2005), *Assessment and care of the well newborn* (2nd ed., pp. 261–266). St. Louis: Elsevier Saunders.

Tufts, G. (2004). Primary care of the premature infant. *American Journal for Nurse Practitioners, 8*(10), 25–41.

U.S. Department of Health and Human Services (USDHHS), Public Health Service. (2000). *Healthy people 2010* (conference edition, in two volumes). U.S. Department of Health and Human Services. Washington, D.C.: U.S. Government Printing Office.

Venes, D. (2005). *Taber's cyclopedic medical dictionary* (20th ed.). Philadelphia: F. A. Davis.

Verklan, M. T., & Walden, M. (2004). *Core curriculum for neonatal intensive care nursing* (3rd ed.). St. Louis: Elsevier Saunders.

Walden, M. (2004). Pain assessment and management. In M. T. Verklan & M. Walden, *Core curriculum for neonatal intensive care nursing* (3rd ed., pp. 375–391). St. Louis: Elsevier Saunders.

Walden, M., & Franck, L. (2003). Identification, management, and prevention of newborn/infant pain. In C. Kenner & J. Lott (Eds.), *Comprehensive neonatal nursing care: a physiologic perspective* (3rd ed.). St. Louis: Mosby.

Wallerstedt, C., Lilley, M., & Baldwin, K. (2003). Interconceptional counseling after perinatal and infant loss. *JOGNN, 32*(4), 533–542.

Woods, D. (2004). Neonatal resuscitation. *International Association for Maternal and Neonatal Health* (IAMANEH). [Online] Available at: www.gfmer.ch/Medical_education_En/PGC_RH_2004/Neonatal_asphyxia.htm

Web Resources

March of Dimes: **www.marchofdimes.com**

National Association of Neonatal Nurses: **www.nann.org**

Neonatal Network: **www.neonatalnetwork.com**

Parental Guide for Developmentally Supportive Care: **www.comeunity.com/premature/baby/supportive-care.html**

Physical and Developmental Environment of the High-Risk Infant: **www.med.usf.edu/-tsinger**

Premature Infant: **www.premature-infant.com**

ChapterWORKSHEET

● MULTIPLE CHOICE QUESTIONS

1. The nurse would classify a newborn as postterm if he was born after:

   a. 38 weeks' gestation

   b. 40 weeks' gestation

   c. 42 weeks' gestation

   d. 44 weeks' gestation

2. SGA and LGA newborns have an excessive number of red blood cells because of:

   a. Hypoxia

   b. Hypoglycemia

   c. Hypocalcemia

   d. Hypothermia

3. Because subcutaneous and brown fat stores were used for survival in utero, the nurse would be alert for which possible complication after birth in an SGA newborn?

   a. Hyperbilirubinemia

   b. Hypothermia

   c. Polycythemia

   d. Hypoglycemia

4. In dealing with parents experiencing a perinatal loss, which of the following nursing interventions would be most appropriate?

   a. Shelter them from the bad news.

   b. Make all the decisions regarding care.

   c. Encourage them to participate in care.

   d. Leave them alone to grieve.

5. In assessing a preterm newborn, which of the following findings would be of greatest concern?

   a. Milia over the bridge of the nose

   b. Thin transparent skin

   c. Poor muscle tone

   d. Heart murmur

● CRITICAL THINKING EXERCISES

1. After fetal distress was noted on the monitor, a postterm newborn was delivered via a difficult vacuum extraction. The newborn had low Apgar scores and had to be resuscitated before being transferred to the nursery. Once admitted, the nurse observed the following behavior: jitters, tremors, hypotonia, lethargy, and rapid respirations.

   a. What might these behaviors indicate?

   b. What other conditions is this neonate at high risk for?

   c. What intervention is needed to address this condition?

2. A preterm newborn was born at 35 weeks following an abruptio placentae due to a car accident. He was transported to the NICU at a nearby regional medical center. After being stabilized, he was placed in an isolette close to the door and placed on a heart monitor. A short time later, the nurse notices that he is cool to the touch and lethargic, has a weak cry, and has an axillary temperature of 36°C.

   a. What might have contributed to this infant's hypothermic condition?

   b. What transfer mechanism may have been a factor?

   c. What intervention would be appropriate for the nurse to initiate?

3. A term SGA newborn weighing 4 lb was brought to the nursery for admission a short time after birth. The labor and birth nurse reports the mother was a heavy smoker and a cocaine addict and experienced physical abuse throughout her pregnancy. After stabilizing the newborn and correcting the hypoglycemia with oral feedings, the nurse observes the following: acrocyanosis, ruddy color, poor circulation to the extremities, tachypnea, and irritability.

   a. What complication common to SGA infants might be manifested in this newborn?

   b. What factors may have contributed to this complication?

   c. What is the appropriate intervention to manage this condition?

● STUDY ACTIVITIES

1. At a community maternity center, secure permission to present a program about the effects of smoking during pregnancy and how it can be harmful to the infant. Start the session by asking about the women's perception of how smoking affects babies, and then after the session ask if any of their views have changed. Encourage them to take steps to quit smoking.

2. Visit the March of Dimes website and review this group's national campaign to reduce the incidence of prematurity. Are their strategies workable or not? Explain your reasoning.

3. A common metabolic disorder present in both SGA and LGA infants after birth is _____.

4. A 10-lb LGA newborn is brought to the nursery after a difficult vaginal birth. The nursery nurse should focus on detecting birth injuries such as _____.

5. Nursing care that is organized to require minimal infant energy expenditure will promote growth and development of newborns with variations in gestational age or birthweight. Nursing measures to facilitate energy conservation include:

(Select all that apply)

a. Minimal handling of the infant

b. Maintaining a neutral thermal environment

c. Decreasing environmental stimuli

d. Initiating early oral feedings

e. Using thermal warmers in all cribs

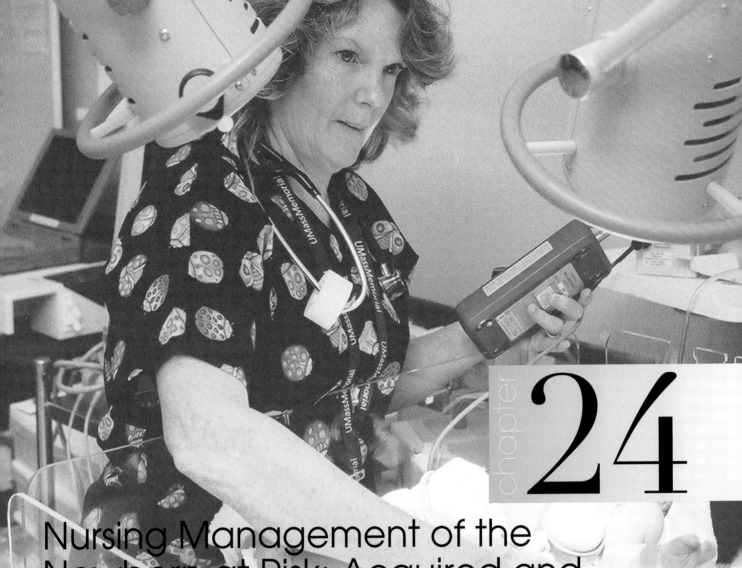

chapter24

Nursing Management of the Newborn at Risk: Acquired and Congenital Newborn Conditions

alcohol-related birth defects
anencephaly
asphyxia
congenital diaphragmatic
  hernia
congenital heart disease
developmental dysplasia
  of the hip
galactosemia
hydrocephalus
hyperbilirubinemia
hypospadias
infant of a diabetic mother

kernicterus
meconium aspiration
  syndrome
microcephaly
myelomeningocele
neonatal abstinence
  syndrome
neonatal sepsis
omphalocele
respiratory distress
  syndrome
spina bifida

Learning OBJECTIVES

After studying the chapter content, the student should be able to accomplish the following:

1. Define the key terms.
2. Identify the most common acquired conditions affecting the newborn.
3. Describe the nursing management of a newborn experiencing respiratory distress syndrome.
4. Outline the birthing room preparation and procedures necessary to prevent meconium aspiration syndrome in the newborn at birth.
5. Identify risk factors for the development of necrotizing enterocolitis.
6. Discuss parent education for follow-up care needed by newborns with retinopathy of prematurity.
7. Discuss the impact of maternal diabetes on the newborn and care needed.

(Continued)

LearningOBJECTIVES Continued

8. Describe the assessment and intervention for an infant experiencing drug withdrawal after birth.
9. Identify assessment and nursing management for newborns sustaining trauma and birth injuries.
10. Outline assessment, interventions, prevention, and management of hyperbilirubinemia in newborns.
11. Summarize the interventions appropriate for a newborn with neonatal sepsis.
12. Compare and contrast the four classifications of congenital heart disease.
13. Identify the major structural disorders affecting the gastrointestinal tract, nervous system, respiratory system, genitourinary tract, and skeletal system.
14. Describe three inborn errors of metabolism.
15. Formulate a plan of care for a newborn with an acquired or congenital condition.
16. Discuss the importance of parental participation in care of the newborn with a congenital or acquired condition, including the nurse's role in facilitating parental involvement.

Advances in prenatal and neonatal medical and nursing care throughout the industrialized world have led to a marked increase in the number of newborns who have survived a high-risk pregnancy but experience acquired or congenital conditions. These newborns are considered at risk: that is, they are susceptible to morbidity and mortality because of the acquired or congenital disorder. Several National Health Goals address the issues of acquired and congenital conditions in newborns (Healthy People 2010).

Technological and pharmacologic advances, in conjunction with standardized policies and procedures, over the past several decades have significantly improved survival rates for at-risk newborns. However, morbidity remains an important sequela. For example, some of these newborns are at risk for long-term health problems that require long-term technological support. Other newborns remain at risk for physical and developmental problems into the school years and beyond. Providing the complex care needed to maintain the child's health and well-being will have a tremendous emotional and economic impact on the family. Nurses are challenged to provide support to mothers and their families when neonatal well-being is threatened.

Acquired disorders typically occur at or soon after birth. They may result from problems or conditions experienced by the woman during her pregnancy or at birth, such as diabetes, maternal infection, or substance abuse, or conditions associated with labor and birth, such as prolonged rupture of membranes or fetal distress. There may be no identifiable cause for the disorder.

Congenital disorders are disorders present at birth, usually due to some type of malformation that occurred during the antepartal period. Congenital disorders, which typically involve a problem with inheritance, include structural anomalies (commonly referred to as birth defects), chromosomal disorders, and inborn errors of metabolism. Most congenital disorders have a complex etiology, involving many interacting genes, gene products, and social and environmental factors during organogenesis. Some alterations can be prevented or compensated for with pharmacologic, nutritional, or other types of interventions, while others cannot be changed. Only through a better understanding of the complex interplay of genetic, environmental, social, and cultural factors can these devastating and life-changing outcomes be prevented (Cleves & Hobbs, 2004).

This chapter addresses selected acquired and congenital newborn conditions. In addition, the nurse's role in assessment and intervention is discussed. Parental education and measures to help the parents cope are emphasized. Nurses play a key role in helping the parents deal with all aspects of the situation.

Acquired Disorders

Neonatal Asphyxia

Newborns normally start to breathe without assistance and often cry just after birth. By 1 minute of age, most newborns are breathing well. A newborn who fails to establish adequate, sustained respiration after birth is said to have **asphyxia.** On a physiologic level, asphyxia can be defined as impairment in gas exchange resulting in a decrease in blood oxygen levels (hypoxemia) and an excess of carbon dioxide or hypercapnia that leads to acidosis.

Incidence and Risk Factors

Asphyxia is the most common clinical insult in the perinatal period. As many as 10% of newborns require some degree of active resuscitation to stimulate breathing (Cunningham et al., 2005). According to the World Health Organization, 4 to 9 million cases of neonatal asphyxia occur annually worldwide, accounting for approximately 20% of all newborns deaths. More than a million newborns who survive asphyxia at birth develop long-term problems such as cerebral palsy, mental retardation, and speaking, hearing, visual, and learning disabilities (MNH, 2005).

National Health Goals Related to Acquired and Congenital Newborn Conditions

Objective	Significance
1. Reduce fetal and infant deaths Decrease the number of all infant deaths (within 1 year) from a baseline of 7.2/1,000 live births to 4.5/1,000 live births. Decrease the number of neonatal deaths (within the first 28 days of life) from a baseline of 4.8 to 2.9 deaths/1,000 live births. Decrease the number of post-neonatal deaths from a baseline of 2.4 to 1.2 deaths/1,000 live births. Reduce the number of deaths related to all birth defects from a baseline of 1.6 to 1.1 deaths/1,000 live births. Reduce the number of infant deaths related to congenital heart defects from a baseline of 0.53 to 0.38 deaths/1,000 live births. Reduce deaths from sudden infant death syndrome (SIDS) from a baseline of 0.72 to 0.25 deaths/1,000 live births.	Will foster early and consistent prenatal care, including education to place infants on their backs for naps and sleeping to prevent SIDS and avoidance of exposing the newborn to cigarette smoke
2. Reduce the occurrence of developmental disabilities Reduce the number of children with mental retardation from a baseline of 131 to 124 children/10,000. Reduce the number of children with cerebral palsy from a baseline of 32.2 to 31.5 children/10,000. Reduce the number of children with autism spectrum disorder.	Will promote measures for close antepartal and intrapartal monitoring of women at risk, subsequently reducing the incidence of disabilities, leading to a reduction in long-term effects and costs of care
3. Reduce the occurrence of spina bifida and other neural tube defects Reduce the number of new cases of spina bifida or other neural tube defects from a baseline of 6 to 3 new cases/10,000 live births.	Will increase awareness of the need for all women of childbearing age to take a multivitamin containing at least 400 mg of folic acid and consume foods high in folic acid
4. Reduce the occurrence of fetal alcohol syndrome	Will foster programs for at-risk groups, including adolescents, about the effects of substance abuse, especially alcohol, during pregnancy
5. Ensure appropriate newborn bloodspot screening, follow-up testing, and referral to services Ensure all newborns are screened at birth for conditions as mandated by their state-sponsored newborn screening programs. Ensure that follow-up diagnostic testing for screening positives is performed within an appropriate time period. Ensure that infants with diagnosed disorders are enrolled in appropriate service interventions within an appropriate time period	Will help in the development of protocols and procedures to ensure appropriate screening and follow-up for all newborns

DHHS, 2000; available on-line at: www.healthypeople.gov

Risk factors associated with newborn asphyxia include:

- History of maternal substance abuse
- Gestational hypertension
- Fetal distress due to hypoxia before birth
- Chronic maternal diseases such as diabetes or a heart or renal condition
- Maternal or perinatal infection
- Placental problems, such as placenta previa or abruptio placentae
- Umbilical cord problems, such as a nuchal or prolapsed cord
- Difficult or traumatic birth
- Multiple births
- Postterm newborn
- Congenital heart disease in newborn

• Maternal anesthesia or recent analgesia
• Abnormal fetal lie or presentation
• Preterm newborn (Woods, 2004)

Nursing Management

Newborn asphyxia is treatable if the perinatal team identifies and recognizes newborns who may be at risk and uses basic, effective resuscitation measures soon after birth. Prompt assessment of the newborn at birth, with immediate intervention, is essential for a newborn experiencing distress.

Assessment

The newborn with asphyxia may have hypothermia, apnea, or respiratory distress manifested by gasping respirations, grunting, nasal flaring, sternal retraction, tachypnea, hypotonia, pallor, and bradycardia (Verklan & Walden, 2004).

With failure to breathe well after birth, the newborn will develop hypoxia (too little oxygen in the cells of the body). As a result, the heart rate falls, cyanosis develops, and the newborn becomes hypotonic and unresponsive.

In addition to the clinical signs, the Apgar scores at 1 minute and 5 minutes provide valuable information. If the score is below 7 at either time, resuscitation is needed.

Several diagnostic studies also assist in identifying underlying etiologies to help plan appropriate interventions. A chest x-ray is helpful to identify any structural abnormalities that might interfere with respiration. Blood studies include cultures to rule out an infectious process, a toxicology screen to detect any maternal drugs in the newborn, and a metabolic screen to identify any metabolic conditions (Green & Wilkinson, 2004).

Nursing Interventions

Management of the newborn experiencing asphyxia includes immediate clinical assessment and resuscitation. Ensure that the equipment needed for resuscitation is readily available and in working order. Dry the newborn quickly with a warm towel and then place him or her under a radiant heater to prevent rapid heat loss through evaporation. Handling and rubbing the newborn with a dry towel is usually all that is needed to stimulate the onset of breathing. If the newborn fails to respond to stimulation, then active resuscitation is needed. Essential equipment includes a wall suction apparatus, an oxygen source, a newborn ventilation bag, endotracheal tubes (2 to 3 mm), laryngoscope, and ampules of naloxone (Narcan) with syringes and needles for administration.

The procedure for newborn resuscitation is easily remembered by the "ABCDs"—airway, breathing, circulation, and drugs (see Chapter 23, Box 23-2). Continue resuscitation until the newborn has a pulse above 100 bpm, a good cry, or good breathing efforts and a pink tongue. This last sign indicates a good oxygen supply to the brain (Woods, 2004).

Additional nursing measures for the newborn with asphyxia include the following:

• Monitor vital signs to assess the level of hypoxia.
• Check the blood glucose level and observe for signs of hypoglycemia.
• Maintain a neutral thermal environment to prevent hypothermia.
• Inform and reassure the parents about the resuscitation activities being performed.
• Offer ongoing explanations to the parents about the procedures or medications given.
• Support the parents physically and emotionally through the initial crisis and throughout the newborn's stay.
• Promote bonding by allowing the parents to hold the stimulated infant, if stable.
• Continue observation and assessment of the successfully resuscitated infant.

Transient Tachypnea of the Newborn

Most newborns make the transition from fetal to newborn life without incident. During fetal life, the lungs are filled with a serous fluid. During and after birth, this fluid must be removed and replaced with air. Passage through the birth canal during a vaginal birth compresses the thorax, which helps remove this fluid. Pulmonary circulation and the lymphatic drainage remove the remaining fluid shortly after birth. Transient tachypnea of the newborn occurs when the liquid in the lung is removed slowly or incompletely. The condition is self-limiting, usually resolving within days after birth.

Incidence and Risk Factors

Transient tachypnea of the newborn occurs in approximately 11 per 1,000 live births (Asenjo, 2003) and is commonly seen in newborns who are sedated or have been born via cesarean birth. Prolonged labor, macrosomia of the fetus, and maternal asthma and smoking have also been associated with a higher incidence of this condition (Kicklighter, 2003).

Nursing Management

Astute observation of the newborn with respiratory distress is important because transient tachypnea of the newborn is a diagnosis of exclusion. Initially it might be difficult to distinguish from respiratory distress syndrome or group B streptococcal pneumonia, since the clinical picture is similar. The symptoms of transient tachypnea rarely last more than 72 hours (Mattson & Smith, 2004). Nursing management focuses on providing adequate oxygen and determining whether these respiratory manifestations appear to be resolving or persisting.

Assessment

Newborns with transient tachypnea present within the first few hours of birth with tachypnea, expiratory grunting, retractions, labored breathing, nasal flaring, and mild cyanosis (Asenjo, 2003). Mild to moderate respiratory distress is present by 6 hours of age, with respiratory rates as high as 100 to 140 breaths per minute (Olds et al., 2004). Breath sounds might be slightly decreased secondary to reduced air entry. The chest may appear hyperextended or barrel-shaped.

A chest x-ray usually reveals mild symmetric lung overaeration and prominent perihilar interstitial markings and streaking, which correlates with lymphatic engorgement of retained fetal fluid (Asenjo, 2003).

Nursing Interventions

Care of the newborn with transient tachypnea is mainly supportive while the retained lung fluid is reabsorbed. Supportive care includes administration of IV fluids and gavage feedings until the respiratory rate decreases enough to allow oral feedings. Supplemental oxygen under an oxygen hood to maintain adequate oxygen saturation and maintenance of a neutral thermal environment with minimal stimulation are important to minimize oxygen demand. As transient tachypnea resolves, the newborn's respiratory rate declines to 60 breaths per minute or less, oxygen requirement decreases, and the x-ray shows resolution of the perihilar streaking. The condition usually resolves within 72 hours after birth. Reassurance and progress reports to the parents are paramount in helping them cope with this crisis.

Respiratory Distress Syndrome

Despite improved survival rates and advances in perinatal care, many high-risk newborns are at risk for respiratory problems, particularly **respiratory distress syndrome** (RDS), a breathing disorder caused by lack of alveolar surfactant, which leads to decreased pulmonary compliance and increased work of breathing. Since the link between RDS and surfactant deficiency was discovered more than 30 years ago, tremendous strides have been made in understanding the pathophysiology and treatment of this disorder. The introduction of prenatal steroids to accelerate lung maturity and the development of synthetic surfactant can be credited with the dramatic improvements in the outcome of neonates with RDS (Rodriguez, 2003).

Incidence and Risk Factors

RDS affects an estimated 25,000 infants born alive in the United States annually. The incidence declines with degree of maturity at birth. It occurs in 60% of preterm newborns of less than 28 weeks' gestation, 30% of those born at 28 to 34 weeks, and less than 5% of those born after 34 weeks (ALA, 2004). Common risk factors contributing to the development of RDS include low gestational age, perinatal asphyxia regardless of gestational age, cesarean birth in the absence of labor related to the lack of thoracic squeezing, male gender, and maternal diabetes.

RDS is decreased with prolonged rupture of membranes, intrauterine growth restriction (IUGR), gestational hypertension, maternal heroin addiction, and use of prenatal corticosteroids because of the physiologic stress imposed on the fetus. Chronic stress experienced by the fetus in utero accelerates the production of surfactant before the 35th week of gestation and thus reduces the incidence of RDS at birth.

Pathophysiology

The pathophysiology of RDS relates to surfactant deficiency. Surfactant is a complex mixture of phospholipids and proteins that adheres to the alveolar surface of the lungs. It forms a coating over the inner surface of the alveoli to reduce the surface tension, thereby preventing alveolar collapse at the end of expiration. In the affected newborn, lack of surfactant results in stiff lungs and alveoli that tend to collapse, leading to diffuse atelectasis. The x-ray findings validate the pathophysiology by showing hypoaeration, underexpansion, reticulogranular ("ground glass") pattern, and decreased lung volumes (Mattson & Smith, 2004). The diagnosis of RDS is based on the clinical symptoms and abnormal x-rays.

Nursing Management

Nursing management focuses on differentiating RDS from other respiratory conditions, such as transient tachypnea or group B pneumonia, and supporting respirations to ensure adequate oxygenation. RDS usually begins at or soon after birth and tends to escalate. Continual observation of the baby's respiratory status is important in determining the underlying respiratory condition to plan appropriate treatment.

Assessment

The newborn with RDS presents at birth or within a few hours of birth with expiratory grunting respirations, nasal flaring, chest wall retractions, see-saw respirations, tachypnea with rates above 60 breaths per minute, fine inspiratory crackles on auscultation, tachycardia with rates above 150 to 180 bpm, and generalized cyanosis secondary to hypoxemia. To help determine the degree of respiratory distress, use an assessment tool such as the Silverman-Anderson index. This tool involves observation of five features, each of which is scored as 0, 1, or 2 (Fig. 24-1). The higher the score, the greater the respiratory distress. A score over 7 suggests severe respiratory distress.

If untreated, RDS will worsen. It appears to be a self-limiting disease, though, with the respiratory symptoms declining after 72 hours. This decline parallels the production of surfactant in the alveoli (Haws, 2004). The newborn needs supportive care until surfactant is produced.

Nursing Interventions

Identification of newborns at high risk for RDS is crucial because the associated atelectasis increases the work of breathing. This results in hypoxemia and acidemia, leading to vasoconstriction of the pulmonary vasculature.

Score

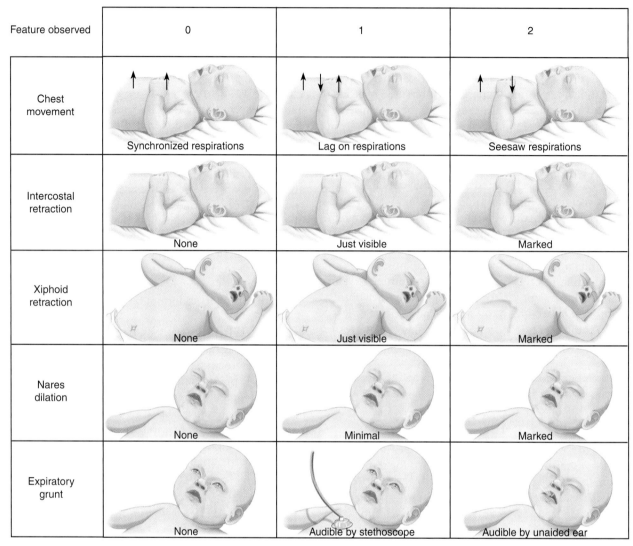

Feature observed	0	1	2
Chest movement	Synchronized respirations	Lag on respirations	Seesaw respirations
Intercostal retraction	None	Just visible	Marked
Xiphoid retraction	None	Just visible	Marked
Nares dilation	None	Minimal	Marked
Expiratory grunt	None	Audible by stethoscope	Audible by unaided ear

● Figure 24-1 Assessing the degree of respiratory distress. (Used with permission from Silverman, W. A. & Anderson, D. H. [1956]. A controlled clinical trial of effects of water mist on obstructive respiratory signs, death rate, and necroscopy findings among premature infants. *Pediatrics, 17*[4], 1–9.)

Subsequently, alveolar capillary circulation is limited, further inhibiting surfactant production. A vicious cycle is created, compounding the problem (Zukowsky, 2004).

Care of the newborn with RDS is primarily supportive and requires a multidisciplinary approach to obtain the best outcomes. Applying the basic principles of newborn care, such as thermoregulation, cardiovascular and nutritional support, and infection prevention, is crucial to achieve therapeutic goals, primarily reducing mortality and minimizing lung trauma. Effective therapies for established RDS include conventional mechanical ventilation, continuous positive airway pressure (CPAP), and surfactant therapy. The use of exogenous surfactant replacement therapy to stabilize the newborn's lungs until postnatal surfactant synthesis matures has become a life-saver.

Anticipate the administration of surfactant replacement therapy, prophylactically or as a rescue approach. With prophylactic administration, surfactant is given within minutes after birth through an endotracheal tube, thus providing replacement surfactant before severe RDS develops. Rescue treatment is indicated for newborns with established RDS who require mechanical ventilation and supplemental oxygen. The ideal timing of therapy has not been established: research is needed to determine which one affords better outcomes (Horbar et al., 2004).

Administer the prescribed oxygen concentration, via oxygen hood or nasal cannula. Anticipate the need for ventilator therapy, which has greatly improved in the past several years, with significant expansion of conventional and high-frequency ventilation therapies (Fig. 24-2). Recent

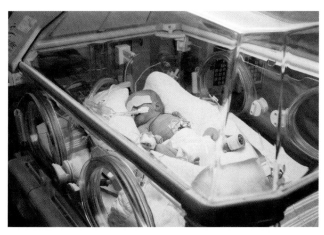

● Figure 24-2 A newborn with RDS receiving mechanical ventilation.

studies show no difference in outcomes for newborns who received early treatment with high-frequency oscillatory ventilation compared with those receiving conventional mechanical ventilation (Bakewell-Sachs & Blackburn, 2003). Although mechanical ventilation has improved survival rates, it is also a contributing factor to bronchopulmonary dysplasia, pulmonary hypertension, and retinopathy of prematurity (Cunningham et al., 2005).

Additional interventions to support the newborn with RDS include the following:

- Administer exogenous surfactant as ordered.
- Transfer the newborn to the neonatal intensive care unit (NICU) soon after birth.
- Continuously monitor the infant's cardiopulmonary status via invasive or noninvasive means (e.g., arterial lines or auscultation, respectively).
- Continuously monitor oxygen saturation levels.
- Closely monitor vital signs, acid–base status, and arterial blood gases.
- Administer broad-spectrum antibiotics if blood cultures are positive.
- Administer sodium bicarbonate or acetate as ordered to correct metabolic acidosis.
- Prevent or treat hypotension via fluids and pressor agents as needed.
- Prevent or treat hypoglycemia, including testing for blood glucose levels and administering dextrose as ordered.
- Cluster caretaking activities to avoid overtaxing and compromising the newborn.
- Place the newborn in the prone position to optimize respiratory status and reduce stress.
- Perform gentle suctioning to remove secretions and maintain a patent airway.
- Observe for signs and symptoms of respiratory complications such as pneumothorax.
- Assess level of consciousness to identify intraventricular hemorrhage.

- Provide sufficient calories via gavage and intravenous feedings.
- Maintain adequate hydration and assess for signs and symptoms of fluid overload.
- Provide information to the parents about treatment modalities; give thorough but simple explanations about the rationales for interventions.
- Encourage the parents to participate in care (Blackburn, 2003).

Meconium Aspiration Syndrome

Meconium is a viscous green substance composed primarily of water and other gastrointestinal secretions that can be noted in the fetal gastrointestinal tract as early as 10 to 16 weeks' gestation (Clark & Clark. 2004). It is expelled as the newborn's first stool after birth. **Meconium aspiration syndrome** occurs when the newborn inhales meconium mixed with amniotic fluid into the lungs while still in utero or on taking the first breath after birth. It is a common cause of newborn respiratory distress and can lead to severe illness. Aspiration induces airway obstruction, surfactant dysfunction, hypoxia, and chemical pneumonitis with inflammation of pulmonary tissues. In severe cases, it progresses to persistent pulmonary hypertension and death (Cunningham et al., 2005).

Incidence and Risk Factors

Meconium staining of the amniotic fluid, with the possibility of aspiration, occurs in approximately 20% of pregnancies at term (Cunningham et al., 2005). Meconium may be passed in utero secondary to hypoxic stress and aspirated in the presence of gasping or deep fetal breathing movements. Although the etiology is not well understood, the effects of meconium can be harmful to the fetus. Meconium alters the amniotic fluid by reducing antibacterial activity and subsequently increasing the risk of perinatal bacterial infection. Additionally, meconium is very irritating because it contains enzymes from the fetal pancreas.

Predisposing factors for meconium aspiration syndrome include postterm pregnancy; breech, forceps, or vacuum extraction births; prolonged or difficult labor associated with fetal distress in a term or postterm newborn; maternal hypertension or diabetes; oligohydramnios; IUGR; prolapsed cord; or acute or chronic placental insufficiency (Mattson & Smith, 2004).

Nursing Management

Nursing management focuses on ensuring adequate tissue perfusion and minimizing oxygen demand and energy expenditure. Observe for meconium-stained amniotic fluid when the maternal membranes rupture. Have a bulb syringe or suctioning equipment readily available. Proper oropharyngeal suctioning following the birth of the fetal head but before the birth of the chest can help reduce the incidence of meconium aspiration in newborns.

Assessment

Review prenatal and birth records to identify newborns who may be at high risk for meconium aspiration. Assess the amniotic fluid when the membranes rupture. Green-stained amniotic fluid suggests meconium aspiration syndrome and should be reported immediately. Also note any yellowish-green staining of the umbilical cord and nails and skin.

Other assessment findings include a barrel-shaped chest with an increased anterior-posterior (AP) chest diameter (similar to that found in a patient with chronic obstructive pulmonary disease), prolonged tachypnea, progression from mild to severe respiratory distress, intercostal retractions, end-expiratory grunting, and cyanosis (Clark & Clark, 2004). Chest x-rays show patchy, fluffy infiltrates unevenly distributed throughout the lungs, marked hyperaeration mixed with areas of atelectasis. Direct visualization of the vocal cords for meconium staining using a laryngoscope can confirm aspiration. Lung auscultation typically reveals coarse crackles and rhonchi. Arterial blood gas analysis will indicate metabolic acidosis with a low blood pH, decreased Pa_{O_2}, and increased Pa_{CO_2} (Engstrom, 2004).

Nursing Interventions

Caring for the newborn with meconium aspiration begins in the birthing unit when the birth attendant identifies meconium-stained amniotic fluid with membrane rupture during labor. Immediately, an amnioinfusion with sterile saline is administered to dilute the meconium. Upon delivery of the newborn's head, before the newborn takes the first breath, the posterior pharynx is gently suctioned to decrease the potential for aspiration. If the newborn is significantly depressed at birth, secondary clearing of the lower airways by direct tracheal suctioning may be necessary. Repeated suctioning is limited to prevent overstimulation and further depression (Hashim & Guillet, 2002). Usually the newborn is transferred to the NICU for close monitoring.

Other interventions include the following:

- Maintain a thermoneutral environment, including placing the newborn under a radiant warmer or in a warmed isolette, to prevent hypothermia.
- Minimize handling, to reduce energy expenditure and oxygen consumption that could lead to further hypoxemia and acidosis.
- Administer oxygen therapy as ordered via oxygen hood or with positive-pressure ventilation. Monitor oxygen saturation levels via pulse oximetry to evaluate the baby's response to treatment and to detect changes. Administer hyperoxygenation to dilate the pulmonary vasculature and close the ductus arteriosus or nitric oxide inhalation to decrease pulmonary vascular resistance, or use high-frequency oscillatory ventilation to increase the chance of air trapping (Haws, 2004).

- Monitor arterial blood gas results for changes and assist with measures to correct acid–base imbalances to facilitate perfusion of tissues and prevent pulmonary hypertension (Cunningham et al., 2005).
- Administer vasopressors and pulmonary vasodilators as prescribed.
- Cluster newborn care to minimize oxygen demand.
- Administer surfactant as ordered to counteract inactivation by meconium.
- Administer broad-spectrum antibiotics to treat bacterial pneumonia.
- Assist with the use of extracorporeal membrane oxygenation (ECMO), a modified type of heart–lung machine, if all else fails.
- Administer sedation to reduce oxygen consumption and energy expenditure.
- Continuously monitor the newborn's condition.
- Reassure and support the parents throughout the experience (Haws, 2004).

Persistent Pulmonary Hypertension of the Newborn

Persistent pulmonary hypertension of the newborn, previously referred to as persistent fetal circulation, is a cardiopulmonary disorder characterized by marked pulmonary hypertension that causes right-to-left extrapulmonary shunting of blood and hypoxemia. Pulmonary vascular resistance is elevated to the point that venous blood is diverted to some degree through fetal structures (i.e., the ductus arteriosus and foramen ovale) into the systemic circulation. This diversion of blood bypasses the lungs, resulting in systemic arterial hypoxemia.

Incidence and Risk Factors

Persistent pulmonary hypertension can occur idiopathically or it can be a complication of perinatal asphyxia, meconium aspiration syndrome, pneumonia, congenital heart defects, metabolic disorders such as hypoglycemia, hypothermia, hypovolemia, hyperviscosity, acute hypoxia with delayed resuscitation, sepsis, and RDS. It occurs in 2 to 6 newborns per 1,000 live births of term, near-term, or postterm infants (Steinhorn, 2004).

Nursing Management

The management of persistent pulmonary hypertension requires meticulous attention to detail, with continuous monitoring of the newborn's oxygenation and perfusion status and blood pressure. The goals of therapy include improving alveolar oxygenation, inducing metabolic alkalosis by administering sodium bicarbonate, correcting hypovolemia and hypotension with the administration of volume replacement and vasopressors, and anticipating use of ECMO when support has failed to maintain acceptable oxygenation (Steinhorn, 2004).

Assessment

A newborn with persistent pulmonary hypertension demonstrates tachypnea within 12 hours after birth. Additional findings include marked cyanosis, grunting, retractions, systolic ejection murmur, and hypotension resulting from both heart failure and persistent hypoxemia (Green & Wilkinson, 2004). An echocardiogram confirms the diagnosis.

Nursing Interventions

The condition can be prevented by instituting early and effective resuscitation and correcting acidosis and hypoxia in all compromised newborns. These compromised infants are treated in the NICU so that they can receive close monitoring and supervision and ventilatory assistance if needed.

Typically, immediate resuscitation is needed after birth and oxygen therapy is initiated. Monitor arterial blood gases frequently to evaluate the effectiveness of oxygen therapy. Respiratory support with mechanical ventilation is used frequently. Administer prescribed medications, monitor cardiopulmonary status, cluster care to reduce stimulation, and provide support and education to the parents.

Bronchopulmonary Dysplasia

Bronchopulmonary dysplasia is a chronic lung disorder of the newborn that follows a lung injury. The lung injury commonly occurs secondary to mechanical ventilation and oxygen toxicity. High inspired oxygen concentrations cause an inflammatory process in the lungs that leads to parenchymal damage (Zukowsky, 2004).

Although the etiology of the lung injury is multifactorial, it is associated with surfactant deficiency, pulmonary edema, lung immaturity, barotrauma from mechanical ventilation, and fluid overload. These newborns often need hospital care for several months after birth and home oxygen therapy after being discharged. The overall costs of treating bronchopulmonary dysplasia in the United States are estimated to be $2.4 billion annually (ALA, 2004).

Incidence and Risk Factors

Approximately 5,000 to 10,000 new cases of bronchopulmonary dysplasia occur each year. White male infants seem to be at greatest risk for developing bronchopulmonary dysplasia (ALA, 2004). Risk factors include male gender, preterm birth (<32 weeks), nutritional deficiencies, white race, excessive fluid intake during the first few days of life, presence of patent ductus arteriosus, severe RDS treated with mechanical ventilation for more than 1 week, and sepsis (Dugas et al., 2005).

Nursing Management

Bronchopulmonary dysplasia can be prevented by administering steroids to the mother in the antepartal period and exogenous surfactant to the newborn to aid in reducing the development of RDS and its severity. In addition, using high-frequency ventilation and nitric oxide helps reduce the need for respiratory support with mechanical ventilation (Lowdermilk & Perry, 2004).

Supplemental oxygen, antibiotics, and fluid restriction and diuretics to decrease fluid accumulation in the lungs are used. Intravenous feedings are given to meet the infant's nutrition needs, and physical therapy is used to improve muscle performance and to help the lungs expel mucus. Nursing management involves implementing all treatment modalities along with supporting and educating the parents throughout care.

Assessment

Although bronchopulmonary dysplasia is most common in preterm newborns, it can also occur in full-term ones who have respiratory problems during their first days of life. Thus, it is essential to assess the newborn's history related to the administration of supplemental oxygen, the length of exposure to oxygen therapy, and the use of ventilatory support.

Clinical signs and symptoms of bronchopulmonary dysplasia include tachypnea, poor weight gain related to the increased metabolic workload, tachycardia, sternal retractions, nasal flaring, and bronchospasm with abnormal breath sounds (crackles, rhonchi, and wheezes). Hypoxia, as evidenced by abnormal blood gas results, and acidosis and hypercapnia also are noted. Diagnosis is based on x-rays showing hyperinflation, infiltrates, and cardiomegaly and clinical signs.

Nursing Interventions

Nursing care includes providing continuous ventilatory and oxygen support and optimal nutrition to support growth, and administering bronchodilators, anti-inflammatory agents, and diuretics to control fluid retention. Continuously monitor the newborn's respiratory status to determine the need for continued ventilatory assistance. When the newborn is clinically stable and ready, expect to wean him or her slowly so that the baby can compensate for the changes. Supplemental oxygen may be needed after discharge from the hospital. Provide a high caloric intake to promote growth and to compensate for the calories expended due to the increased work of breathing.

Newborns with bronchopulmonary dysplasia may require continued care at home. When planning for discharge, educate the family caretaker about how to manage a chronically ill child that may be oxygen-dependent for an extended time. Also instruct the family about the safe use of oxygen in the home, including the need to notify emergency medical services and utility companies that a technology-dependent child is living in their district. In addition, initiate a social service referral to help the family access community resources (McKinney et al., 2005).

Retinopathy of Prematurity

The retina transmits visual information to the brain. Retinopathy of prematurity (ROP) is a developmental abnormality that affects the immature blood vessels of the retina. It develops in both eyes secondary to an injury such as hyperoxemia due to prolonged assistive ventilation and high oxygen exposure, acidosis, and shock. These events cause abnormal blood vessels to proliferate in the retina, resulting in scar tissue. ROP can lead to lifelong vision impairment (NEI, 2005). It can also lead to vitreous hemorrhage, retinal detachment, and blindness (Brooks, 2004).

Incidence and Risk Factors

The incidence of ROP in preterm newborns is inversely proportional to their birth weight. Of the approximately 4 million infants born in the United States annually, about 57,000 weigh 1,500 grams (2.75 lb) or less. About 14,000 to 16,000 of these infants are affected by some degree of ROP (NEI, 2005). Other risk factors include the duration of intubation and the use of oxygen therapy, intraventricular hemorrhage, multiple prenatal maternal risk factors (substance abuse, hypertension, preeclampsia, heavy smoker, or inadequate oxygen supply to placenta), and sepsis (Vision Channel, 2004).

The eye develops rapidly between 28 and 40 weeks' gestation. When the baby is born preterm, normal blood vessel development may cease. Exposure to high oxygen concentrations leads to severe retinal vasoconstriction with endothelial damage and vessel obliteration. Adhesions form, causing retinal detachment. Although the precise levels of hyperoxemia that can be sustained without causing retinopathy are not known, very immature newborns who develop respiratory distress often must be given high oxygen concentrations to maintain life (Cunningham et al., 2005).

Nursing Management

The incidence of ROP can be decreased by minimizing the risk of preterm birth through providing quality prenatal care and health counseling to all new mothers. When ROP does develop, care depends on the stage and degree of retinal findings. ROP is classified in five stages, ranging from mild (stage I) to severe (stage V). Typically, stages I and II resolve on their own and require only periodic evaluation by the ophthalmologist. For more advanced stages, surgical intervention such as laser photocoagulation and scleral buckling surgery and/or vitrectomy is performed.

Assessment

The newborn who develops ROP exhibits no signs or symptoms, so assessment involves identifying the newborn at risk. Any newborn with a birthweight of less than 1,500 g or born at less than 28 weeks' gestation should be examined by a pediatric ophthalmologist within 4 to 6 weeks after birth. Diagnosis is made by an ophthalmic examination (Kenner & Lott, 2004).

Nursing Interventions

Cautious, judicious use of oxygen is imperative in preventing this serious eye condition. Continuously assess and monitor the newborn who is receiving oxygen therapy. Cover the isolette with a blanket and dim the surrounding lights to protect the newborn's eyes.

Assist with scheduling an ophthalmic examination for the newborn and administer a mydriatic eye agent to dilate the newborn's pupils approximately 1 hour prior to the examination as ordered. During this time, take extra care to protect the newborn's eyes from bright light. If necessary, assist with the examination by holding the newborn's head. Follow-up eye examinations are scheduled every 2 to 3 weeks depending on the severity of the clinical findings at the first examination (Verklan & Walden, 2004).

Provide support to the parents. This is an extremely difficult time for them: in addition to learning to meet the needs of their preterm newborn, they must also deal with the possibility that their baby may have a condition that could lead to blindness. Consider the family's needs and provide individualized support and guidance. Provide information about the newborn's condition and treatment options. Stress the need for follow-up vision screenings, because ROP is considered a life-long disease with numerous late-onset problems.

Periventricular–Intraventricular Hemorrhage

Periventricular–intraventricular hemorrhage is defined as bleeding that usually originates in the subependymal germinal matrix region of the brain, with extension into the ventricular system (Haws, 2004). Each ventricular area contains a rich network of capillaries that are very thin and fragile and can easily rupture. It is a common problem of preterm infants, especially those born before 32 weeks. A significant number of these newborns will incur brain injury, leading to cerebral palsy, hydrocephalus, and behavioral, learning, auditory, or visual deficits in their early and later school-age years. Identifying preventive strategies to reduce the incidence of these brain insults is a national public health priority (Bloch, 2005).

Periventricular–intraventricular hemorrhage is classified according to a grading system of I to V (least severe to most severe) (Blackburn, 2003). The prognosis is guarded, depending on the grade and severity of the hemorrhage. Generally, newborns with mild hemorrhage (grades I and II) have a much better developmental outcome than those with severe hemorrhage (grades III and IV). Complications include obstructive hydrocephalus, developmental impairment, cerebral palsy, and seizure disorders (Haws, 2004).

Incidence and Risk Factors

The incidence of ventricular hemorrhage depends on the gestational age at birth. About 30% to 40% of newborns weighing 1,500 g or less or born at 30 weeks' gestation or less will have evidence of hemorrhage. Only about 4% of term newborns show evidence of ventricular hemorrhage. Very-low-birthweight infants have the earliest onset of hemorrhage and the highest mortality rate (Cunningham et al., 2005).

The preterm newborn is at greatest risk for periventricular–intraventricular hemorrhage because the immaturity of the brain makes it more vulnerable to injury. The more preterm the newborn is, the greater likelihood of brain damage. While all areas of the brain can be injured, the periventricular area is the most vulnerable.

With a preterm birth, the fetus is suddenly transported from a well-controlled uterine environment into a highly stimulating one. This tremendous physiologic stress and shock may contribute to the rupture of periventricular capillaries and subsequent hemorrhage. Other associated risk factors include acidosis, asphyxia, unstable blood pressure, meningitis, seizures, acute blood loss, hypovolemia, respiratory distress with mechanical ventilation, intubation, apnea, hypoxia, suctioning, hyperosmolar solutions, rapid volume expansion, as well as most nursing activities that involve handling. Most hemorrhages occur in the first 72 hours after birth (Cunningham et al., 2005).

Nursing Management

Nursing management focuses on identifying the risk factors leading to hemorrhage and interventions to decrease the risk of hemorrhage. Using a developmental care environment in the NICU is helpful to minimize the risk of hemorrhage. Support for the parents to cope with the diagnosis and potential long-term sequelae is essential. The long-term neurodevelopmental outcome is determined by the severity of the bleed.

Assessment

Assessment of a newborn with periventricular–intraventricular hemorrhage varies significantly. Some newborns have no signs; in others the findings are dramatic. Signs include a sudden unexplained drop in hematocrit, pallor, poor perfusion as evidenced by respiratory distress and oxygen desaturation, lethargy, sudden deterioration in vital signs associated with shock secondary to hemorrhage, changes in level of consciousness, seizures, metabolic acidosis, glucose instability and hypotonia, bradycardia, shock, and a tense anterior fontanel (Annibale & Hill, 2003). Frequently a bleed can progress rapidly and result in shock and death. Cranial ultrasonography is the diagnostic tool of choice to detect hemorrhage.

Nursing Interventions

Prevention of preterm birth is essential in preventing periventricular–intraventricular hemorrhage. In addition, the nurse plays a major role in preventing perinatal asphyxia and birth trauma. If a preterm birth is expected, having the mother deliver at a tertiary facility with a NICU would be most appropriate.

Nursing care for periventricular–intraventricular hemorrhage is primarily supportive and includes the following:

- Correct anemia, acidosis, and hypotension with fluids and medications.
- Prevent fluctuations in blood pressure by slowly administering fluids; avoid rapid volume expansion to minimize changes in cerebral blood flow.
- Limit stimulation in the newborn's environment to reduce stress.
- Minimize handling of the newborn by clustering nursing care; reduce the newborn's exposure to noxious stimuli to avoid a fluctuation in blood pressure and energy expenditure.
- Keep the newborn in a flexed, contained position with the head elevated to prevent or minimize fluctuations in intracranial pressure.
- Provide adequate oxygenation to promote adequate tissue profusion but controlled ventilation to decrease the risk of pneumothorax.
- Assess for signs of hemorrhage, such as changes in the level of consciousness, bulging fontanel, seizures, apnea, and reduced activity level.
- Provide education and emotional support for the parents throughout the newborn's stay.
- Discuss expectations for short-term and long-term care needs with the parents.
- Promote community awareness of factors that may contribute to periventricular–intraventricular hemorrhage, such as a lack of prenatal care, maternal infection, alcohol consumption, and smoking (Bloch, 2005).

Necrotizing Enterocolitis

Necrotizing enterocolitis (NEC) is a serious gastrointestinal disease of unknown etiology in newborns. Although it is more common in preterm newborns, it can be observed in term newborns. The precise pathogenesis is unclear, but four major factors have been proposed: the presence of a pathogenic organism, a hypoxic/ischemic event, the challenge of enteral feeding, and altered enteric mucosa integrity. Currently there are no effective prevention strategies (Lin et al., 2005).

Incidence and Risk Factors

NEC occurs in up to 10% of all admissions to the NICU; approximately 90% of cases are found in preterm newborns (Bell, 2005). Predisposing risk factors are highlighted in Box 24-1.

Pathophysiology

NEC is characterized by mucosal or transmucosal necrosis of part of the intestine (Wood, 2005). Although any region of the bowel can be affected, the distal ileum and proximal colon are the regions most commonly involved. NEC usually occurs between 3 and 10 days of life.

Several factors contribute to the development of newborn NEC, but three events are typically found: perinatal

**PREDISPOSING FACTORS FOR THE DEVELOPMENT
OF NECROTIZING ENTEROCOLITIS**

Prenatal Factors
• Preterm labor
• Prolonged rupture of membranes
• Preeclampsia
• Maternal sepsis
• Amnionitis
• Uterine hypoxia

Postnatal Factors
• Respiratory distress syndrome
• Patent ductus arteriosus
• Congenital heart disease
• Exchange transfusion
• Low birthweight
• Low Apgar scores
• Umbilical catheterization
• Hypothermia
• Gastrointestinal infection
• Hypoglycemia
• Asphyxia

hypoxia, bacterial invasion, and high-solute feedings. In perinatal hypoxia, blood is shunted from the gut to more important organs (heart and brain), resulting in ischemia and damage to the intestinal wall. Bacterial invasion follows, and high-solute feedings provide sustenance for bacteria to flourish. In an attempt to improve gastrointestinal function and reduce the risk of NEC, many neonatologists are trying enteral antibiotics, judicious administration of parenteral fluids, human milk feedings, antenatal corticosteroids, enteral probiotics (*Lactobacillus acidophilus*), and delayed or slow feedings (Bell, 2005).

Nursing Management

Nursing management focuses on being alert to the risk factors associated with NEC and meticulous observation for clinical manifestations of this potentially devastating condition. Frequently the infant has nonspecific symptoms that can be easily overlooked. The nurse schedules and assists with the various diagnostic tests ordered to evaluate the infant for this condition.

Assessment

Assessment of a newborn with NEC typically reveals abdominal distention and tenderness, bile-stained emesis, lethargy, feeding intolerance, decreased activity, respiratory distress, visible loops of bowel, metabolic acidosis, temperature instability, hypotension, grossly bloody stools, delayed gastric emptying, diarrhea, oliguria, hypoglycemia, and cyanosis (Verklan & Walden, 2004).

The diagnosis of NEC is based on clinical suspicion supported by x-rays and laboratory studies. Diagnostic findings typically indicate leukocytosis, thrombocytopenia, electrolyte imbalances, metabolic acidosis, hypoxemia, blood in stools, and disseminated intravascular coagulation (DIC). The x-rays show diffuse gaseous distention of the intestines, with air within the wall of the intestine (pneumatosis) and persistently dilated loops of bowel (Verklan & Walden, 2004).

Nursing Interventions

As soon as NEC is suspected, expect to stop oral feedings and withhold food and fluids, placing the newborn on NPO status. Institute gastric decompression as ordered with an orogastric tube attached to low intermittent suction. Administer antibiotics as ordered, because it is thought that NEC involves bacterial invasion. Give parenteral fluid therapy to replace formula or breast milk. Continue to monitor the newborn's condition via abdominal x-rays, blood tests, and arterial blood gases, as ordered.

Supportive treatment is continued as long as there is no evidence of intestinal necrosis or perforation (free air in the abdomen on x-ray). If necrosis or perforation occurs, surgery is indicated and may include laparotomy with resection of necrotic bowel and possibly creation of an ostomy (Kenner & Lott, 2004).

Key nursing interventions for the newborn with NEC include the following:

• Manage pain by administering analgesics as ordered.
• Stress infection control, with an emphasis on careful handwashing.
• Make continuous nursing assessments, including:
  ◦ Checking for guaiac-positive stools
  ◦ Measuring abdominal girth frequently
  ◦ Palpating the abdomen for tenderness and rigidity
  ◦ Auscultating bowels to assess for paralytic ileus
  ◦ Observing for abdominal redness or shininess, which indicates peritonitis
  ◦ Careful monitoring of intake and output
  ◦ Coordinating laboratory and x-ray studies to monitor the newborn's status
• Maintain fluid and electrolyte balance.
• Support the parents throughout medical and/or surgical interventions by:
  ◦ Listening to their worries and fears
  ◦ Answering their questions honestly and hopefully
  ◦ Teaching them about therapies and procedures
  ◦ Encouraging interaction with the newborn through gentle touching

Infants of Diabetic Mothers

An **infant of a diabetic mother** is one born to a woman with pregestational or gestational diabetes (see Chapter 20 for additional information). The newborn of a diabetic woman is at high risk for numerous health-related complications, especially hypoglycemia. In light of the increasing incidence of type 2 diabetes among women of childbearing age due to obesity, it is important to educate women about the potential impact of poor glycemic control on their offspring.

Impact of Diabetes on the Newborn

For more than a century, it has been known that diabetes during pregnancy can have severe adverse effects on fetal and newborn outcomes. Infants of diabetic mothers have an increased morbidity and mortality in the perinatal period. The incidence of major congenital anomalies is much greater for these newborns than for other newborns. Poor glycemic control in the first trimester, during organogenesis, is thought to be the major reason for congenital malformations. The most common types of malformations in infants of diabetic mothers involve the cardiovascular, skeletal, central nervous, gastrointestinal, and genitourinary systems; cardiac anomalies are the most common (Cleves & Hobbs, 2004).

Infants of diabetic mothers are longer and weigh more than newborns of similar gestational age. They also have increased organ weights (organomegaly) and excessive fat deposits on the shoulders and trunk, contributing to the increased overall body weight and predisposing them to shoulder dystocia. These newborns are macrosomic (an infant whose birthweight exceeds 4,500 g). These oversized newborns frequently require cesarean births for cephalofetal disproportion and are often hypoglycemic in the first few hours after birth.

Despite their increased size and weight, they may be remarkably feeble, showing behaviors similar to those of a preterm newborn. Thus, birthweight may not be a reliable criterion of maturity. Newborns of women with diabetes but without vascular complications often tend to be large for gestational age (LGA), whereas those of women with diabetes and vascular disease are usually small for gestational age (SGA).

The large size of the infant born to a diabetic mother is secondary to exposure to high levels of maternal glucose crossing the placenta into the fetal circulation. Maternal hyperglycemia acts as a fuel to stimulate increased production of fetal insulin, which in turn promotes somatic growth within the fetus. The fetus responds to these high levels by producing more insulin, which acts as a growth factor in the fetus (Olds et al., 2004). How the fetus will be affected depends on the severity, duration, and control of the diabetes in the mother.

Common Problems in Infants of Diabetic Mothers

Common problems include macrosomia, RDS, birth trauma, hypoglycemia, hypocalcemia and hypomagnesemia, polycythemia, hyperbilirubinemia, and congenital anomalies (Table 24-1).

Nursing Management

The focus of care for these infants is early detection and initiation of therapy to address potential problems (Nursing Care Plan 24-1). Care begins in the prenatal period by identifying women with diabetes and taking measures to control maternal glucose levels (see Chapter 20 for information on management of the pregnant woman with diabetes).

Treatment focuses on correcting hypoglycemia, hypocalcemia, hypomagnesemia, dehydration, and jaundice. Oxygenation and ventilation are supported as necessary.

Assessment

The infant of a diabetic mother has a characteristic appearance:

- Full rosy cheeks with a ruddy skin color
- Short neck (some describe "no-neck" appearance)
- Buffalo hump over the nape of the neck
- Massive shoulders with a full intrascapular area
- Distended upper abdomen due to organ overgrowth
- Excessive subcutaneous fat tissue, producing fat extremities (Fig. 24-3)

Be alert for hypoglycemia, which may occur immediately after birth or within an hour. Assess blood glucose levels, which should remain above 40 mg/dL. Closely assess the newborn for signs of hypoglycemia, including listlessness, hypotonia, apathy, poor feeding, apneic episodes with a drop in oxygen saturation, cyanosis, temperature instability, pallor and sweating, tremors, irritability, and seizures.

Determine baseline serum calcium, magnesium, and bilirubin levels and monitor frequently for changes (Table 24-2). Hypocalcemia is typically manifested in the first 2 to 3 days of life as a result of birth injury or a prolonged delay in parathyroid hormone production. Hypomagnesemia parallels calcium levels and is suspected only when hypocalcemia does not respond to calcium replacement therapy. Red blood cell breakdown leads to increased hematocrit and polycythemia. In addition, hyperbilirubinemia may be caused by slightly decreased extracellular fluid volume, hepatic immaturity, and birth trauma forming enclosed hemorrhages. It can appear within the first 24 hours of life (pathologic) or after 24 hours of life (physiologic).

Assess the newborn for signs of birth trauma involving the head (tense, bulging fontanels, cephalhematoma, skull fractures, and facial nerve paralysis), shoulders and extremities (posturing, paralysis), and skin (bruising). Inspect the newborn for compromised oxygenation by examining the skin for cyanosis, pallor, mottling, and sluggish capillary refill. Take the newborn's temperature frequently and provide a neutral thermal environment to prevent cold stress, which would increase the glucose utilization and contribute to the hypoglycemic state.

Table 24-1 Common Problems of Infants of Diabetic Mothers (IDMs)

Condition	Description	Effects
Macrosomia	– Newborn with an excessive birthweight; arbitrarily defined as a birthweight >4,000 g (8 lb 13 oz) to 4,500 g (9 lb 15 oz) or >90% for gestational age – Complication in 10% of all pregnancies in the United States	– Increased risk for shoulder dystocia, traumatic birth injury, birth asphyxia – Risks for newborn hypoglycemia and hypomagnesemia, polycythemia, and electrolyte disturbances – Increased maternal risk for surgical birth, postpartum hemorrhage and infection, and birth canal lacerations – Increased risk of developing type 2 diabetes later in life for both – Higher weight and accumulation of fat in childhood and a higher rate of obesity in adults
Respiratory distress syndrome (RDS)	– Cortisol-induced stimulation of lecithin/sphingomyelin (phospholipids) necessary for lung maturation is antagonized due to the high insulin environment within the fetus due to mother's hyperglycemia. – Less mature lung development than expected for gestational age – Decrease in the phospholipid phosphatidylglycerol (PG), which stabilizes surfactant, compounding risk	– Most commonly, breathing normally at birth but developing labored, grunting respiration with cough and a hoarse complaining cry within a few hours with chest retractions and varying degrees of cyanosis – IDMs with vascular disease seldom develop RDS because the chronic stress of poor intrauterine perfusion leads to increased production of steroids, which accelerates lung maturation.

Hypoglycemia	– Glucose is the major source of energy for organ function.
	– Typical characteristics:
	  – Poor feedings
	  – Jitteriness
	  – Lethargy
	  – High-pitched or weak cry
	  – Apnea
	  – Cyanosis and seizures
	  – Some newborns asymptomatic
		– Low blood glucose levels are problematic during early post-birth period due to abrupt cessation of high-glucose maternal blood supply and the continuation of insulin production by the newborn.
		– Limited ability to release glucagon and catecholamines, which normally stimulate glucagon breakdown and glucose release
		– Prolonged and untreated hypoglycemia leads to serious, long-term adverse neurologic sequelae such as learning disabilities and mental retardation.

Hypocalcemia and hypomagnesemia	Hypocalcemia (drop in calcium levels) manifested by tremors, hypotonia, apnea, high-pitched cry, and seizures due to abrupt cessation of maternal transfer of calcium to fetus primarily in third trimester and birth asphyxia Associated hypomagnesemia directly related to the maternal level before birth About half of IDMs affected	Newborn is at risk for a prolonged delay in parathyroid hormone production and cardiac dysrhythmias.

Table 24-1 Common Problems of Infants of Diabetic Mothers (IDMs) (continued)

Condition	Description	Effects
Polycythemia	– Venous hematocrit of >65% in the newborn – Increased oxygen consumption by IDM secondary to fetal hyperglycemia and hyperinsulinemia – Increased fetal erythropoiesis secondary to intrauterine hypoxia due to placental insufficiency from maternal diabetes – Hypoxic stimulation of increased red blood cell (RBC) production as compensatory mechanism	Increased viscosity, resulting in poor blood flow predisposing newborn to decreased tissue oxygenation and development of microthrombi
Hyperbilirubinemia	Usually seen within the first few days after birth, manifested by a yellow appearance of the sclera and skin Excessive red cell hemolysis necessary to break down increased RBCs in circulation due to polycythemia Resultant elevated bilirubin levels Excessive bruising secondary to birth trauma of macrosomic infants, further adding to high bilirubin levels	If untreated, high levels of unconjugated bilirubin may lead to kernicterus (neurologic syndrome that results in irreversible damage) with long-term sequelae that include cerebral palsy, sensorineural hearing loss, and mental retardation.
Congenital anomalies	– Occur in up to 10% of IDMs, accounting for 30% to 50% of perinatal deaths – Incidence is greatest among SGA newborns. – Overall, approximately three times the usual incidence of congenital anomalies compared to newborns from the non-diabetic general population	Most common anomalies: – Coarctation of the aorta – Atrial and ventricular septal defects – Transposition of the great vessels – Sacral agenesis – Hip and joint malformations – Anencephaly – Spina bifida – Caudal dysplasia – Hydrocephalus

Sources: Jazayeri & Contreras, 2005; Moore, 2004; Harris, 2004; Mattson & Smith, 2004; Lessaris, 2005; Barbour, 2003; Schaefer-Graf et al., 2003; and Johnson, 2003.

Nursing Interventions

Appropriate nursing interventions for infants of diabetic mothers include the following:

• Monitor blood glucose levels via heel stick every hour for the first 4 hours of life and then every 3 to 4 hours until stable. Document the results. Report unstable glucose values if oral feedings do not maintain and stabilize the newborn's blood glucose levels.

• Prevent hypoglycemia by providing early oral feedings with formula or breast milk at frequent intervals (every 2 to 3 hours). Feedings help to control glucose levels, reduce hematocrit, and promote bilirubin excretion.

• If glucose levels are not stabilized, initiate IV glucose infusions as ordered and monitor the infusions at the prescribed rate.

• Monitor serum calcium levels for needed supplementation (oral or IV calcium gluconate), and observe for signs and symptoms of hypocalcemia, such as tremors, jitteriness, twitching, seizures, and high-pitched cry.

• Monitor serum bilirubin levels and prepare to administer fluid therapy as ordered for needed hydration, and institute phototherapy if the newborn is over 24 hours old.

• Maintain a neutral thermal environment to avoid cold stress, which may stimulate the metabolic rate, thereby increasing the demand for glucose.

Nursing Care Plan 24-1

Overview of an Infant of a Diabetic Mother (IDM)

Jamie, a 38-year-old Hispanic woman, gave birth to a term LGA newborn weighing 10 lb. She had a history of gestational diabetes but had not received any prenatal care. She arrived at the hospital in active labor. Despite macrosomia, the newborn's Apgar scores were 8 and 9. No resuscitative measures were needed. The nursery nurse notices a quiet newborn with tremors of the extremities. A glucose level via a heel stick was 35 mg/dL. The newborn is now demonstrating signs of respiratory distress—grunting, nasal flaring, and tachypnea.

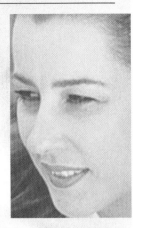

Nursing Diagnosis: Risk for injury related to hypoglycemia secondary to maternal gestational diabetes

Outcome identification and *evaluation*	Interventions with *rationales*
The newborn will exhibit adequate glucose control *as evidenced by blood glucose levels above 40 mg/dL and an absence of clinical signs of hypoglycemia.*	Monitor blood glucose levels *to detect hypoglycemia, which would be <40 mg/dL secondary to the infant's hyperinsulin state in utero.* Observe for manifestations of hypoglycemia such as pallor, tremors, jitteriness, lethargy, and poor feeding *to allow for early detection and prompt intervention to minimize the risk of complications associated with hypoglycemia.* Maintain a neutral thermal environment *to reduce heat loss through evaporation, convection, conduction, and radiation, which further depletes glycogen stores.* Monitor temperature *to prevent cold stress and use of glucose to maintain temperature.* Initiate early feedings or administer glucose supplements as ordered *to prevent hypoglycemia caused by the infant's hyperinsulin state.* Cluster infant care activities *to conserve energy to reduce use of glucose and glycogen stores.* Reduce environmental stimuli by dimming lights and speaking softly *to reduce energy needs and further utilization of glucose.*

Nursing Diagnosis: Risk for impaired gas exchange related to respiratory distress secondary to fetal hyperinsulinemia inhibiting pulmonary surfactant production and delaying lung maturation

Newborn will demonstrate signs of adequate oxygenation without respiratory distress *as evidenced by respiratory rate and vital signs within acceptable parameters, absence of nasal flaring and grunting, and oxygen saturation and arterial blood gas levels within acceptable parameters.*	Assess newborn's skin *to identify cyanosis, pallor, and mottling, which may indicate compromised oxygenation.* Monitor newborn's vital signs *to establish a baseline and evaluate for changes.* Assess airway patency and suction as ordered *to promote adequate oxygen intake and maintain patency.*

Overview of an Infant of a Diabetic Mother (IDM) (continued)

Outcome identification and *evaluation*	Interventions with *rationales*
	Assess lung sounds for changes *to allow for early detection of change in status.*
	Monitor oxygen saturation levels *to determine adequacy of tissue perfusion.*
	Assess arterial blood gases *to determine presence of acidosis, hypoxemia, or hypercarbia, which would indicate hypoxia.*
	Administer oxygen as ordered *to increase the availability of oxygen and reduce hypoxia.*
	Maintain normal blood glucose levels and a neutral thermal environment and reduce excessive stimuli *to decrease oxygen consumption.*

• Provide rest periods to decrease energy demand and expenditure.
• Closely monitor the baby's respiratory status to identify signs and symptoms of respiratory distress.
• Perform a head-to-toe physical assessment to identify congenital anomalies.
• Provide support and information to the parents and family. They may erroneously interpret the newborn's large size as an indication that the newborn is free of problems. Encourage open communication and listen with empathy to the family's fears and concerns.
• Offer frequent opportunities for the parents to interact with their newborn.
• Make appropriate referrals to social services and community resources as necessary to help the family cope.

Birth Trauma

Injuries to the newborn from the forces of labor and birth are categorized as birth trauma. In the past, numerous injuries were associated with difficult births requiring external or internal version or mid- or high forceps deliveries. Today, however, cesarean births have contributed to the decline in birth trauma.

Incidence and Risk Factors
The process of birth is a blend of compression, contractions, torques, and traction. When fetal size, presentation, or neurologic immunity complicates this process, the forces of labor and birth may lead to tissue damage, edema, hemorrhage, or fracture in the newborn. Significant birth

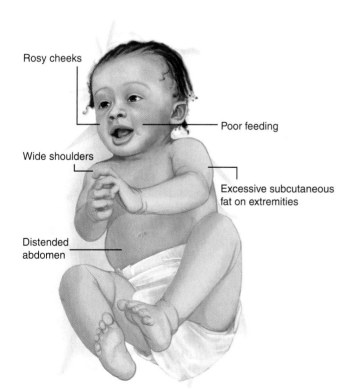

Rosy cheeks

Poor feeding

Wide shoulders

Excessive subcutaneous fat on extremities

Distended abdomen

● Figure 24-3 Characteristics of an infant of a diabetic mother.

Table 24-2 Critical Laboratory Values for Infants of Diabetic Mothers

Hypoglycemia	<40 mg/dL
Hypocalcemia	<7 mg/dL
Hypomagnesemia	<1.5 mg/dL
Hyperbilirubinemia	>12 mg/dL (term infant)
Polycythemia	>65% (venous hematocrit)

trauma accounts for fewer than 2% of neonatal deaths and stillbirths in the United States (Lynam & Verklan, 2004). Improved prenatal diagnosis and monitoring during labor have helped to reduce the incidence of birth injuries today.

Factors placing the newborn at risk for birth injury include cephalopelvic disproportion, maternal pelvic anomalies, oligohydramnios, prolonged or rapid labor, abnormal presentation (breech, face, brow), instrument-assisted extraction (vacuum or forceps), fetal prematurity, fetal macrosomia, and fetal abnormalities (Lynam & Verklan, 2004).

Types of Birth Trauma
Fractures
Fractures most often occur during breech births or shoulder dystocia in newborns with macrosomia. Midclavicular fractures are the most common type of fracture, secondary to shoulder dystocia. The newborn presents with irritability and does not move the arm on the affected side either spontaneously or when the Moro reflex is elicited. X-rays confirm the fracture. Typically, healing is rapid and uneventful. Arm motion may be limited by pinning the newborn's sleeve to the shirt. Explanation to the parents and reassurance are needed.

Loss of spontaneous arm or leg motion indicates a long-bone fracture of the humerus or femur, respectively. Usually swelling and pain accompany the limited movement. Femoral and humeral shaft fractures are usually mid-shaft and treated with splinting. Healing and complete recovery are expected within 2 to 4 weeks without incident (Laroia, 2004).

Brachial Plexus Injury
Brachial plexus injury occurs most often in large newborns, frequently with shoulder dystocia or in breech births. These injuries are relatively common, complicating between 1 in 500 and 1 in 1,000 term births (Cunningham et al., 2005). Most cases involve *Erb's palsy,* in which cervical nerves 5 and 6 are damaged, leading to paralysis of the upper portion of the arm. Injury to the upper plexus results from stretching or pulling the head away from the shoulder during a difficult birth. The involved extremity lies adducted, prone, and internally rotated. Shoulder movement is absent. Immobilization of the arm across the upper chest protects the shoulder from excessive motion. Gentle passive range-of-motion exercises are performed daily to prevent contractures.

Injury to the lower brachial plexus is less common, but *Klumpke's palsy* can occur, resulting in hand and wrist weakness. The grasp reflex is absent on assessment. The hand is placed in a neutral position and passive range-of-motion exercises are used.

Cranial Nerve Trauma
Pressure on the facial nerve before birth or from the use of obstetric forceps may cause a transient palsy to the face. It results in facial asymmetry, especially during crying. The mouth is drawn toward the unaffected side, wrinkles are deeper on the unaffected side, and the eye is persistently open on the affected side. Most newborns begin to recover within the first week, but full resolution may take several months. The open eye is protected with a patch and artificial tears are instilled frequently. Parents need instruction about how to feed the newborn, since he or she cannot close the lips around the nipple without having milk seep out. Parents also need reassurance that most facial trauma is self-limiting and resolves in a short time.

Head Trauma
Mild trauma can cause soft tissue injuries such as cephalhematoma and caput succedaneum. Greater trauma can cause depressed skull fractures. *Cephalhematoma* is a subperiosteal collection of blood secondary to the rupture of blood vessels between the skull and periosteum. The suture lines delineate its extent. Cephalhematoma typically is located on one side over the parietal bone. It occurs in 2.5% of all births and typically appears within hours after birth (Cunningham et al., 2005). Resolution occurs gradually over 2 to 3 weeks without treatment (see Chapter 18).

Caput succedaneum is a soft tissue swelling caused by edema of the head against the dilating cervix during the birth process. It is not limited by suture lines, extends across the midline, and is associated with head molding. It does not usually cause complications other than a misshaped head. The swelling from caput succedaneum is maximal at birth, rapidly decreases in size, and usually resolves over the first few days without treatment (see Chapter 18).

Subarachnoid hemorrhage is probably one of the most common types of intracranial trauma. Hypoxia/ischemia, variations in blood pressure, and the pressure exerted on the head during labor are major causes of this type of intracranial hemorrhage. Bleeding is of venous origin, and underlying contusions also may occur (Haws, 2004). Some red blood cells may appear in the cerebrospinal fluid of full-term newborns. Newborns with subarachnoid hemorrhage may present with apnea, seizures, lethargy, or abnormal findings on a neurologic examination (Becske & Jallo, 2004). Minimal handling to reduce stress is important.

Subdural hemorrhage (hematomas) occurs less often today because of improved obstetric techniques. Typically, tears of the major veins or venous sinuses overlying the cerebral hemispheres or cerebellum are the cause. Such tears are most common in newborns of primaparas, in large newborns, or after an instrumented birth. All of these conditions can produce increased pressure on the blood vessels inside the skull, leading to tears. The newborn with a subdural hemorrhage can be asymptomatic or can exhibit seizures, enlarging head size, decreased level of consciousness, or abnormal findings on a neurologic examination, with hypotonia, a poor Moro reflex, or extensive retinal hemorrhages (Lynam & Verklan, 2004). A subdural hematoma can be life-threatening if it is in an inaccessible location and cannot be aspirated (Whitby et al., 2003).

Depressed skull fractures, although rare, may result from the pressure of a forceps delivery but can also occur during spontaneous or cesarean births. They also may be associated with other head trauma causing subdural bleeding, subarachnoid hemorrhage, or brain trauma (Laroia, 2004). Depressed skull fractures can be observed and palpated as depressions. Confirmation via x-ray is necessary. Neurosurgical consultation is typically needed.

Nursing Management

Recognition of trauma and birth injuries is imperative so that early treatment can be initiated. The nurse needs to complete a careful physical and neurologic assessment of every newborn admitted to the nursery to establish whether injuries exist. Assess and document symmetry of structure and function thoroughly. Be prepared to assist with scheduling diagnostic studies to confirm trauma or injuries, which will be important in determining treatment modalities.

Provide parents with a realistic picture of the situation to gain their understanding and trust. Be readily available to answer questions and teach them how to care for the newborn, including any modifications that might be necessary. Allow parents adequate time to understand the implications of the birth trauma or injury and what treatment modalities are needed, if any. Spending time with the parents and providing them with support, information, and teaching are important to allow them to make decisions and care for their newborn. Anticipate the need for community referral for ongoing follow-up and care.

Newborns of Substance-Abusing Mothers

It is generally assumed that all pregnant women want to provide a healthy environment for their unborn child and know how to avoid harmful consequences. However, for women who use substances such as drugs or alcohol, this may not be the case. Substance use during pregnancy exposes the fetus to the possibility of IUGR, prematurity, neurobehavioral and neurophysiologic dysfunction, birth defects, infections, and long-term developmental sequelae (Verklan & Walden, 2004).

It is difficult to establish the true prevalence of substance use in pregnant women: many women deny taking any nonprescribed substance because of the associated social stigma and legal implications. The National Institute on Drug Abuse (NIDA) suggests that approximately 1 in 10 infants are exposed to one or more mood-altering drugs in utero (NIDA, 2005). Drug exposure may go unrecog-

Consider THIS!

I admit, I had led a reckless life since I was a teen. I rebelled against my mother's authority and started smoking and doing drugs just to "check out" of my painful world. It was one big blast after another with a high and then a low. I never considered the consequences of my behavior then and never thought it would hurt anyone until I learned I was about 4 months pregnant. I convinced myself that if I cut back, everything would be fine.

Now, as I stand here in the NICU watching my tiny son struggle for air and tremble all over, I am not so convinced that I didn't hurt anyone except myself. As I witness my son fight against MY nicotine and drug addiction, my heart is heavy with guilt. I wonder how I could have thought that my troubles wouldn't become another's plight sooner or later. What must I have been thinking to isolate my addiction and not consider the impact that it would have on my mother and my son?

Thoughts: This woman honestly regrets what her addiction has done to her son as she stands watching him go through withdrawal. Her lifestyle choices do affect others, despite her previous denial. One problem with addiction is the difficulty in getting help after deciding to finally quit. There aren't enough rehab centers to deal with the large numbers needing their services and it can be difficult to get into one. What can be offered to pregnant women who abuse substances? How can nurses increase community awareness about the impact of this problem, especially during pregnancy?

nized in these infants, and they may be discharged from the newborn nursery at risk for a complex of medical and social problems, including abuse and neglect.

Tobacco, alcohol, and marijuana are the most commonly abused substances during pregnancy; others are highlighted in Box 24-2.

Substance abuse during pregnancy is the subject of much controversy. The timing of drug ingestion usually determines the type and severity of damage to the fetus. Frequently, the woman uses more than one substance, which compounds the problem. Nurses must be knowledgeable about the issues of substance abuse and must be alert for opportunities to identify, prevent, manage, and educate women and families about this key public health issue.

Alcohol

The consumption of alcohol in the United States is pervasive and widely accepted. Alcohol use, abuse, and addiction affect all levels of our society. If a drug or substance is sold to the public without restrictions, there is a common misconception that it is safe. However, a "safe" level of alcohol consumption during pregnancy has yet to

BOX 24-2

SUBSTANCES OFTEN ABUSED DURING PREGNANCY

Opioids
- Morphine
- Codeine
- Methadone
- Meperidine (Demerol)
- Heroin

CNS Stimulants
- Amphetamines
- Cocaine

CNS Depressants
- Barbiturates
- Diazepam (Valium)
- Sedative–hypnotics

Hallucinogens
- LSD
- Inhalants
- Glue, paint thinner, nail polish remover
- Nitrous oxide (NIDA, 2005)

and hyperactivity. Box 24-3 summarizes the manifestations of fetal alcohol syndrome.

Worldwide, the incidence of fetal alcohol syndrome is 1 to 3 cases per 1,000 live births, and that of fetal alcohol effects is 3 to 5 per 1,000 live births (March of Dimes, 2005). Current estimates indicate that approximately 13% of women of childbearing age are either problem drinkers or alcoholics; therefore, the number of fetuses exposed to alcohol during utero increases dramatically (March of Dimes, 2005).

Fetal alcohol syndrome is one of the most common known causes of mental retardation, and it is the only cause that is entirely preventable. The effects last a lifetime. Children with this syndrome have varying degrees of psychological and behavioral problems and often find it difficult to hold a job and live independently (CDC, 2005).

Decreasing or eliminating alcohol consumption during pregnancy is the only way to prevent fetal alcohol syndrome and fetal alcohol effects. Unfortunately, few treatment programs address the needs of pregnant women, so many newborns are exposed to alcohol in utero.

Women who are pregnant or are planning to become pregnant need to be informed of the detrimental effects

be established. Therefore, the prudent choice for women who are or may become pregnant is to abstain from alcohol entirely.

The adverse effects of alcohol consumption have been recognized for centuries, but the associated pattern of fetal anomalies was not labeled until the early 1970s. The distinctive pattern identified three specific findings: growth restriction (prenatal and postnatal), craniofacial structural anomalies, and central nervous system (CNS) dysfunction. These distinctive findings were called fetal alcohol syndrome, characterized by physical and mental disorders that appear at birth and remain problematic throughout the child's life. However, there are also circumstances in which effects of prenatal alcohol exposure are apparent, but the newborn does not meet all of the criteria. In an attempt to include those who do not meet the strict criteria, the terms fetal alcohol effects, alcohol-related birth defects, and alcohol-related neurologic defects are used to describe children with a variety of problems thought to be related to alcohol consumption during pregnancy. The Institutes of Medicine coined the term fetal alcohol spectrum disorder as a way of describing the broader effects of prenatal alcohol exposure. Children with fetal alcohol syndrome are at the severe end of the spectrum (Weiner, 2005). Newborns with some but not all of the symptoms of fetal alcohol syndrome are described as having **alcohol-related birth defects.** Fetal alcohol effects may include such problems as low birthweight, developmental delays,

BOX 24-3

CLINICAL PICTURE OF FETAL ALCOHOL SYNDROME

- Microcephaly (head circumference <10th percentile)★
- Small palpebral (eyelid) fissures★
- Abnormally small eyes
- Maxillary hypoplasia (flattened or absent)
- Epicanthal folds (folds of skin of the upper eyelid over the eye)
- Thin upper lip★
- Missing vertical groove in median portion of upper lip★
- Short upturned nose
- Short birth length and low birthweight
- Joint and limb defects
- Altered palmar crease pattern
- Prenatal or postnatal growth ≤10th percentile★
- Congenital cardiac defects (septal defects)
- Delayed fine and gross motor development
- Poor eye–hand coordination
- Clinically significant brain abnormalities★
- Mental retardation
- Narrow forehead
- Performance substantially below expected level in cognitive or developmental functioning, executive or motor functioning, and attention or hyperactivity; social or language skills★
- Inadequate sucking reflex and poor appetite (March of Dimes, 2005)

★Diagnostic criteria for fetal alcohol syndrome.

of alcohol during pregnancy. Educate women using a nonjudgmental, culturally connected approach. There is little debate today about drinking and pregnancy—*there is no safe time to drink, nor is there a safe amount of alcohol to drink.*

Tobacco and Nicotine

The tobacco industry recently admitted that nicotine is addictive. In the United States, approximately one in four women smoke. Although the incidence of smoking in the United States is declining, more women than men now smoke. Currently, at least 11% of women in the United States smoke during pregnancy (March of Dimes, 2005). The risks of smoking, such as cancer and cardiovascular and pulmonary disease, are widely known, and smoking during pregnancy places the mother and fetus at additional risk.

Cigarette smoke contains more than 2,500 chemicals. The active constituents of cigarette smoke are nicotine, tar, carbon monoxide, and cyanide. It is not known for certain which of these chemicals are harmful to a developing fetus, but both nicotine and carbon monoxide are believed to play a role in causing adverse pregnancy outcomes. Nicotine crosses the placenta and carbon monoxide combines with hemoglobin, impairing oxygenation for the mother and the fetus. Nicotine is highly addictive and provides an almost immediate "kick" because it causes a discharge of epinephrine from the adrenal cortex. This stimulation is then followed by depression and fatigue, leading the abuser to seek more nicotine.

The fetus of a woman who smokes is at risk for low birthweight (the risk almost doubles), small-for-gestational-age status, and preterm birth. The risk for sudden infant death syndrome (SIDS) increases, as does the risk for chronic respiratory illness (MWH, 2005).

Women smoke for many reasons and are influenced by both external and internal factors. External factors include social and cultural norms and the smoking behavior of people with whom the woman lives and works. Internal factors include stress, addiction, boredom, weight control, and the need for a coping mechanism. Some groups of women are more likely than others to smoke: for example, women who are single, separated, or divorced and women with less education, lower incomes, and lower-status occupations than the norm have higher rates of smoking (CDC, 2004).

Smokers who are contemplating pregnancy are faced with a dilemma. On the one hand, they wish a healthy outcome for the fetus; however, smoking is an addiction that is difficult to break. Nurses play a major role in teaching women about healthy behaviors and providing support for smoking cessation. Assisting the woman in smoking cessation requires a thorough consideration of all the factors associated with the woman's smoking and the challenges she faces—for example, why she smokes, the stressors in her life, and her social support network. Options to explore include group smoking cessation programs, relaxation techniques, individual counseling, hypnosis, and partner-support counseling. The major motivation is the woman's desire to change.

Nurses can be instrumental in increasing the number of pregnant women who make a serious attempt to quit smoking by using the "5 A's" approach:

- *Ask:* Ask all women if they smoke and would like to quit.
- *Advise:* Encourage the use of clinically proven treatment plans.
- *Assess:* Provide motivation by discussing the 5 R's:
  - Relevance of quitting to the woman
  - Risk of continued smoking to the fetus
  - Rewards of quitting for both
  - Roadblocks to quitting
  - Repeat at every visit
- *Assist:* Help the woman to protect her fetus and newborn from the negative effects of smoking.
- *Arrange:* Schedule follow-up visits to reinforce the woman's commitment to quit.

Health-promotion activities for smoking cessation are also important, such as joining with other community organizations and private-sector partners to reduce tobacco use and improve the health of newborns (Murray & Wewers, 2004).

Marijuana

Marijuana remains the most widely used illicit psychoactive substance in the Western world and the most commonly used illicit drug in the United States (NIDA, 2005). Marijuana, derived from the *Cannabis sativa* plant, has not been shown to have a teratogenic effect on the fetus, and no consistent types of malformations have been identified. However, marijuana does have significant effects during pregnancy. Similar to tobacco smoking, the carbon monoxide in the smoke will be delivered to the fetus, and thus IUGR is common in heavy marijuana smokers (NIDA, 2005). Mothers who smoke marijuana during pregnancy risk having a smaller infant. Research has shown that infants born to mothers who smoked marijuana during their pregnancies have altered responses to visual stimuli, sleep-pattern abnormalities, photophobia, lack of motor control, hyperirritability, increased tremulousness, and a high-pitched cry, which may indicate neurologic problems in development. Long-term effects on childhood development have not been established; research continues (NIDA, 2005).

Methamphetamines

Methamphetamine is an addictive stimulant drug that releases high levels of the neurotransmitter dopamine, which stimulates brain cells, enhancing mood and body movement. Methamphetamine is made in illegal laboratories and has a high potential for abuse and addiction. Street methamphetamine is called by many names, such as "speed," "meth," "ice," and "chalk." It can be inhaled, injected, smoked, or taken orally (NIDA, 2005). Methamphetamines are used medically to treat obesity and narcolepsy in adults and hyperkinetic children.

Methamphetamines accelerate heart and respiratory rate, elevate blood pressure, and dilate the pupils of the eyes. A secondary effect, loss of appetite, has contributed to their use in the weight-loss industry. The illicit use of amphetamines during pregnancy has received relatively little research interest because it is less common than cocaine and narcotic use.

Fetal effects from methamphetamines are similar to the effects of cocaine (see below), suggesting vasoconstriction as a mechanism. Because they suppress appetite during pregnancy, maternal malnutrition may lead to problems with fetal growth and development. Infants born to mothers dependent on amphetamines have an increased risk of preterm births and low birthweight. Also, these infants may experience symptoms of withdrawal, as manifested by dysphoria, agitation, jitters, poor weight gain, abnormal sleep patterns, poor feeding, frantic fist sucking, high-pitched cry, respiratory distress soon after birth, frequent infections, and significant lassitude (Pitts, 2004). The long-term effects of methamphetamines have not been documented.

Cocaine

Cocaine is a strong CNS stimulant that interferes with the reabsorption of dopamine, a neurotransmitter associated with pleasure and movement. Physical effects of cocaine use include constricted blood vessels, dilated pupils, and increased temperature, heart rate, and blood pressure. It can be taken orally, sublingually, intranasally, intravenously, or by inhalation (Pitts, 2004).

The abuse of cocaine has become an alarming problem during the past decade. It is estimated that up to 8 million Americans use cocaine regularly, and 30% to 40% of cocaine addicts are women (NIDA, 2005). Maternal use of cocaine during pregnancy remains a significant public health problem, particularly in urban areas of the United States and among women of low socioeconomic status (March of Dimes, 2005). Cocaine exposure is associated with premature birth and lower birthweight, but its impact on later development is less clear. It is speculated that maternal cocaine use may interfere with the infant's cognitive development, resulting in learning and memory difficulties later in life (Messinger et al., 2004). Several congenital anomalies have also been associated with maternal cocaine use, including genitourinary anomalies, cardiac and CNS defects, and "prune belly syndrome" (absence of abdominal muscles at birth) (Cunningham et al., 2005).

Cocaine is a psychomotor stimulant and when used in low doses produces an increase in pleasure, alertness, and a sense of well-being. It lowers anxiety and social inhibitions. It can be ingested in several ways: intranasally by snorting, intravenously, and by smoking. Users soon discover that if they take more cocaine or "crack," the intensity of euphoria increases (NIDA, 2005).

It can be difficult to determine the effects of cocaine on the newborn due to the likelihood that the mother using cocaine also takes other drugs. Two major side effects of cocaine use—vasoconstriction and hypertension—are responsible for most of the fetal and newborn effects. Characteristics of cocaine-exposed newborns include:

- Prematurity
- Low birthweight
- Smaller head circumference
- A piercing cry (indicative of neurologic dysfunction)
- Genitourinary tract abnormalities
- Cardiac anomalies
- Limb defects
- Ambiguous genitalia
- Poor feeding
- Poor visual and auditory responses
- Poor sleep patterns
- Decreased impulse control
- Stiff, hyperextended positioning
- Irritability and hypersensitivity (hard to console when crying)
- Inability to respond to caretaker
- Higher incidence of SIDS (Pitts, 2004)

Cocaine-exposed newborns are typically fussy, irritable, and inconsolable at times. Techniques such as swaddling, gentle rocking, using a flexed position, and offering a pacifier can help manage CNS irritation. Keeping environmental stimuli to a minimum will also help. Cocaine-exposed infants demonstrate poor coordination of sucking and swallowing, making feeding time frustrating for the newborn and caregiver alike. A calm, gentle approach combined with proper positioning and handling will increase feeding success.

Heroin

Heroin is an illegal, highly addictive opiate derived from morphine. The white or brown powder can be sniffed, smoked, or injected. The medical and social consequences of its abuse, such as HIV infection, tuberculosis, fetal effects, crime, violence, and disruption of families, have a devastating impact on society, costing billions of dollars each year (NIDA Research Report, 2005). Heroin produces a sense of euphoria and readily crosses the placenta in the pregnant woman.

Heroin addiction during pregnancy poses serious health risks to the mother and the fetus. Heroin causes severe physical addiction. It is a CNS depressant that produces mental dullness and drowsiness. Although no teratogenic effects have been associated with its use, newborns of heroin-addicted mothers are born dependent on heroin. In addition, pregnant women who share needles are at risk for contracting hepatitis B and C and HIV, which can be transmitted to the newborn (Cunningham et al., 2005). The rates of stillbirth, IUGR, prematurity, and newborn mortality are three to seven times higher in heroin-addicted pregnant women than in women in the general population (NIDA, 2005).

The effects of heroin on the newborn include low birthweight, meconium aspiration secondary to hypoxia, a high incidence of SIDS, and delayed effects from subacute withdrawal, with symptoms such as restlessness, continual crying, agitation, sneezing, vomiting, fever, diarrhea, seizures, irritability, and poor socialization that may persist for 4 to 6 months (March of Dimes, 2005).

In general, abrupt cessation of the use of heroin or any opiate during pregnancy is not advised because intrauterine death or prematurity may result. Treatment for heroin-dependent mothers consists of methadone maintenance. Women who enroll in a methadone maintenance program often have a good outcome, including a longer gestation time and increased birthweight, compared to women who go untreated (March of Dimes, 2005). Most newborns of mothers who abuse heroin begin withdrawal within 24 to 72 hours as opposed to a week after birth for infants whose mothers have been maintained on methadone (Pitts, 2004). Treatment is supportive for the newborn experiencing heroin withdrawal.

Methadone

Methadone is a synthetic opiate narcotic that is used primarily as maintenance therapy for heroin addiction. It blocks the effects of heroin for about 24 hours. When combined with prenatal care and a comprehensive drug treatment program, many of the detrimental maternal and newborn outcomes associated with heroin abuse can improve. There is preliminary evidence that buprenorphine (Buprenex) also is safe and effective in treating heroin dependence during pregnancy, although infants exposed to methadone or buprenorphine during pregnancy typically require treatment for withdrawal symptoms (NIDA Research Report, 2005).

Although methadone poses some threat to the fetus, it is important to weigh the benefits of methadone in pregnancy against the risks associated with the continuing use of heroin. For this reason, methadone maintenance is often recommended for pregnant heroin-dependent women, and it remains the standard of care for treatment of women with narcotic addiction.

Methadone maintenance is advantageous because it provides the woman with an alternative to an illicit sub-

stance. This substance can be monitored by a medical team, which helps her to stay heroin-free. It also helps to promote compliance with prenatal care: the woman is given a prescribed dose and must return on a consistent basis to receive more. Other advantages include improved fetal and newborn growth, a reduced risk of fetal death (maternal opiate withdrawal can cause fetal death or pregnancy loss), and a reduced risk of HIV infection because the woman no longer needs to engage in the high-risk behaviors involved in obtaining illegal drugs. The woman on methadone maintenance also can breastfeed (Weiner, 2005).

Despite the significant advantages of methadone to a heroin-dependent pregnant woman, dangers to the fetus and newborn remain. In utero exposure to methadone may lead to low birthweight caused by symmetric fetal growth restriction involving weight, length, and head circumference. Withdrawal from methadone is more severe than from heroin and more prolonged, possibly lasting up to 3 weeks due to the much longer half-life of methadone. Also, seizures attributed to withdrawal are commonly severe and may not occur until 2 to 3 weeks of age, after the newborn has been discharged and is home without medical supervision. Finally, the rate of SIDS among opiate-exposed infants is three to four times higher than for the general population (Cunningham et al., 2005). Nurses play a major role in teaching mothers and caregivers to monitor the newborn for methadone withdrawal symptoms after returning home.

Neonatal Abstinence Syndrome

Newborns of women who abuse tobacco, illicit substances, caffeine, and alcohol can exhibit withdrawal behavior. Withdrawal symptoms occur in 60% of all newborns exposed to drugs (Wang, 2004). Drug dependency acquired in utero is manifested by a constellation of neurologic and physical behaviors and is known as **neonatal abstinence syndrome.** Although often treated as a single entity, neonatal abstinence syndrome is not a single pathologic condition. Manifestations of withdrawal are a function of the drug's half-life, the specific drug or combination of drugs used, dosage, route of administration, timing of drug exposure, and length of drug exposure (Engstrom, 2004). Neonatal abstinence syndrome has both medical and developmental consequences for the newborn.

The newborn's behavior often prompts the healthcare provider or nurse to suspect intrauterine drug exposure (Box 24-4). The newborn physical examination may also reveal low birthweight for gestational age or drug or alcohol-related birth defects and dysfunction.

To remember the symptoms of neonatal abstinence syndrome, use the acronym WITHDRAWAL:

W = Wakefulness: sleep duration less than 1 to 3 hours after feeding

BOX 24-4

MANIFESTATIONS OF NEONATAL ABSTINENCE SYNDROME

CNS Dysfunction
- Tremors
- Generalized seizures
- Hyperactive reflexes
- Restlessness
- Hypertonic muscle tone, constant movement
- Shrill, high-pitched cry
- Disturbed sleep patterns

Metabolic, Vasomotor, and Respiratory Disturbances
- Fever
- Frequent yawning
- Mottling of the skin
- Sweating
- Frequent sneezing
- Nasal flaring
- Tachypnea >60 bpm
- Apnea

Gastrointestinal Dysfunction
- Poor feeding
- Frantic sucking or rooting
- Loose or watery stools
- Regurgitation or projectile vomiting (Belik & Al-Hamad, 2004)

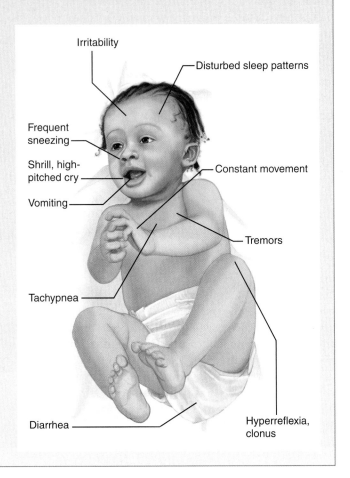

I = Irritability
T = Temperature variation, tachycardia, tremors
H = Hyperactivity, high-pitched persistent cry, hyperreflexia, hypertonus
D = Diarrhea, diaphoresis, disorganized suck
R = Respiratory distress, rub marks, rhinorrhea
A = Apneic attacks, autonomic dysfunction
W = Weight loss or failure to gain weight
A = Alkalosis (respiratory)
L = Lacrimation (AAP Committee on Substance Abuse, 2005)

Diagnostic studies to help identify the severity of withdrawal include various scoring systems to rate the infant's withdrawal behaviors. Toxicology screening of the newborn's blood, urine, and meconium helps to identify the substances to which the newborn has been exposed. In general, a urine screen signifies only recent use of drugs: it can detect marijuana use up to a month earlier, cocaine use up to 96 hours earlier, heroin use 24 to 48 hours earlier, and methadone use up to 10 days earlier (Wang, 2004).

Nursing Management

Management of the substance-exposed newborn remains a major challenge to health care professionals. The major goals include providing comfort to the newborn by relieving symptoms, improving feeding and weight gain, preventing seizures, promoting mother–newborn interactions, and reducing the incidence of newborn mortality and abnormal development (Belik & Al-Hamad, 2004).

Pharmacologic treatment is warranted if conservative measures, such as swaddling and decreased environmental stimulation, are not adequate. The AAP recommends that for newborns with confirmed drug exposure, drug therapy should be indicated if the newborn has seizures, diarrhea and vomiting resulting in excessive weight loss and dehydration, poor feeding, inability to sleep, and fever unrelated to infection (AAP Committee on Substance Abuse, 2005). Common medications used in the management of newborn withdrawal include morphine, paregoric, phenobarbital, tincture of opium, methadone clonidine, chlorpromazine, and diazepam (Wang, 2004).

For a substance-abusing mother, the birth of a drug-exposed newborn is both a crisis and an opportunity. The mother may feel guilty about the newborn's condition. Many of these newborns are unresponsive and disorganized in sleeping and feeding patterns. When awake, they can be easily overstimulated and irritated. Such characteristics make parent–newborn interaction difficult and frustrating, leading to possible detachment and avoidance (Pitts, 2004). The mother may be single and a victim of physical and sexual abuse and may have a limited support system. Many of these mothers had poor parenting themselves, lack information about characteristic infant behaviors, and have unrealistic expectations about the newborn's abilities (Ballard, 2002). On the other hand, the newborn may be a powerful motivator for the mother to undergo treatment and seek recovery. Nurses can play a pivotal role in assisting her to abstain from drug use and become a good mother to her newborn.

Assessment

Several assessment tools can be used to assess a drug-exposed newborn. Figure 24-4 shows an example. Key areas to assess include:

- Maternal history to identify risk behaviors for substance abuse:
  ○ Previous unexplained fetal demise
  ○ Lack of prenatal care
  ○ History of missed prenatal appointments
  ○ Severe mood swings
  ○ Precipitous labor
  ○ Poor nutritional status
  ○ Abruptio placentae
  ○ Hypertensive episodes
  ○ History of drug abuse
- Laboratory test results (toxicology) to identify substances in mother and newborn
- Signs of neonatal abstinence syndrome (use the "WITHDRAWAL" acronym)
- Evidence of seizure activity and need for protective environment

Nursing Interventions

Nursing interventions focus on promoting a calming, supportive environment. Decrease stimuli by dimming the lights in the nursery, and swaddle the newborn tightly to decrease irritability behaviors. Plan activities to allow for minimal stimulation of the newborn. Use a pacifier to satisfy needs for nonnutritive sucking.

When feeding the newborn, use small amounts and position the newborn upright to prevent aspiration and to facilitate rhythmic sucking and swallowing. Breastfeeding is encouraged unless the mother is still using drugs. Monitor the newborn's weight daily to evaluate success of food intake. Assess hydration; check skin turgor and fontanels. Monitor the newborn's fluid and electrolyte and acid–base status.

In addition, implement the following interventions:

- Assess the frequency and characteristics of bowel movements.
- Monitor for any changes in condition or signs.
- Protect the neonate's elbows and knees against friction and abrasions.
- Administer ordered medications and document behavioral changes.
- Teach the mother or caretaker how to care for the newborn at home (Teaching Guidelines 24-1).
- Refer the mother to community agencies to address addiction and the infant's developmental needs (Green & Wilkinson, 2004).

The needs of the substance-exposed newborn are multiple, complex, and costly, both to the healthcare system and to society. Substance abuse takes place among people of all colors, sizes, shapes, incomes, types, and conditions. Most pregnant women are unaware of the adverse impact their substance abuse can have on the newborn.

Nurses are in a unique position to help because they interact with high-risk mothers and newborns in many settings, including the community, healthcare facilities, and family agencies. It is the responsibility of all nurses to identify, educate, counsel, and refer pregnant women with substance-abusing problems. Early, supportive, ongoing nurse care is critical to the well-being of the mother and her newborn.

Hyperbilirubinemia

Hyperbilirubinemia is a total serum bilirubin level above 5 mg/dL resulting from unconjugated bilirubin being deposited in the skin and mucous membranes (Mattson & Smith, 2004). Hyperbilirubinemia is exhibited as jaundice. Newborn jaundice is one of the most common reasons for hospital readmission. It occurs in 60% to 80% of term newborns in the first week of life and in virtually all preterm newborns (Madan et al., 2004).

Pathophysiology

Newborn jaundice results from an imbalance in the rate of bilirubin production and bilirubin elimination. This relative imbalance determines the pattern and degree of newborn hyperbilirubinemia (Dixon, 2004).

During the newborn period, a rapid transition from the intrauterine to the extrauterine pattern of bilirubin physiology occurs. Fetal unconjugated bilirubin is normally cleared by the placenta and the mother's liver in utero, so total bilirubin at birth is low. After the umbilical cord is cut, the newborn must conjugate bilirubin (convert a lipid-soluble pigment into a water-soluble pigment) in the liver on his or her own. The rate and amount of bilirubin conjugation depend on the rate of red blood cell breakdown, the bilirubin load, the maturity of the liver, and the number of albumin-binding sites (Olds et al., 2004). Bilirubin production increases after birth mainly because of a shortened

CENTRAL NERVOUS SYSTEM DISTURBANCES

SIGNS AND SYMPTOMS	SCORE	AM						PM					
Excessive high-pitched cry	2												
Continuous high-pitched cry	3												
Sleeps <1 hour after feeding	3												
Sleeps <2 hours after feeding	2												
Sleeps <3 hours after feeding	1												
Hyperactive Moro reflex	2												
Markedly hyperactive Moro refex	3												
Mild tremors disturbed	1												
Moderate–severe tremors disturbed	2												
Mild tremors undisturbed	1												
Moderate–severe tremors undisturbed	4												
Increased muscle tone	2												
Excoloration (specify area)	1												
Myoclonic jerks	3												
Generalized convulsions	5												
METABOLIC / VASOMOTOR/RESPIRATORY DISTURBANCES													
Sweating													
Fever <101 (99–100.8°F/37.2–38.2°C)	1												
Fever <101 (38.2°C and higher)	2												
Frequent yawning (>3– 4 times/interval)	1												
Mottling	1												
Nasal stuffiness	1												
Sneezing (>3–4 times/interval)	1												
Nasal flaring	2												
Respiratory rate >60 / min	1												
Respiratory rate >60 / min, with retractions	2												
GASTROINTESTINAL DISTURBANCES													
Excessive sucking	1												
Poor feeding	2												
Regurgitation	2												
Projectile vomiting	3												
Loose stools	2												
Watery stools	3												
TOTAL SCORE													

● Figure 24-4 Neonatal abstinence scoring system. (From Cloherty, J. P. & Stark, A. R. [1998]. *Manual of neonatal care* [4th ed., pp. 26–27]. Boston: Little, Brown.)

TEACHING GUIDELINES 24-1

Caring for Your Newborn at Home

- Position your newborn with the head elevated to prevent choking.
- To aid your newborn's sucking and swallowing during feeding, position the chin downward and support it with your hand.
- Place your newborn on his or her back to sleep or nap, never on the stomach.
- Keep a bulb syringe close by to suction your newborn's mouth in case of choking.
- Cluster newborn care (bathing, feeding, dressing) to prevent overstimulation.
- If your newborn is fussy or crying, try these measures to help calm him or her:
  ○ Wrap your newborn snugly in a blanket and rock in rocking chair.
  ○ Take the baby for a ride in the car (using a newborn car seat).
  ○ Play soothing music and "dance" with the newborn.
  ○ Use a wind-up swing with music.
- To help your newborn get to sleep, try these measures:
  ○ Schedule a bath with a gentle massage prior to bedtime.
  ○ Change diaper and clothes to make the baby comfortable.
  ○ Feed the baby just prior to bedtime.
  ○ If the newborn cries when put in crib and all needs are met, allow him or her to cry.
  ○ Use a rocking chair to feed and sing a soft lullaby.
- Call your primary care provider if you observe withdrawal behaviors such as:
  ○ Slight tremors (shaking) of hands and legs
  ○ Stiff posture when held in your arms
  ○ Irritable and frequently fussy
  ○ High-pitched cry, excessive sucking motions
  ○ Erratic sleep pattern
  ○ Frequent yawning, nasal stuffiness, sweating
  ○ Prolonged feeding time needed
  ○ Frequent vomiting after feeding

red blood cell lifespan (70 days vs. 90 days in the adult) combined with an increased red blood cell mass. Therefore, the amount of bilirubin the newborn must deal with is large when compared to that of an adult. Additional risk factors contributing to newborn jaundice include:

- Polycythemia
- Significant bruising or cephalhematoma, which increases bilirubin production
- Infections such as TORCH (toxoplasmosis, hepatitis B, rubella, cytomegalovirus, herpes simplex virus)
- Use of drugs during labor and birth such as diazepam (Valium) or oxytocin (Pitocin)

- Prematurity
- Gestational age of 34 to 36 weeks
- Hemolysis due to ABO incompatibility or Rh iso-immunization
- Macrosomic infant of a diabetic mother
- Delayed cord clamping, which increases the erythrocyte volume
- Decreased albumin binding sites to transport unconjugated bilirubin to the liver because of acidosis
- Delayed meconium passage, which increases the amount of bilirubin that returns to the unconjugated state and can be absorbed by the intestinal mucosa
- Siblings who had significant jaundice
- Inadequate breastfeeding leading to dehydration, decreased caloric intake, weight loss, and delayed passage of meconium
- Ethnicity, such as Asian-American, Mediterranean, or Native American
- Male gender (AAP, 2004)

Bilirubin has two forms—unconjugated or indirect, which is fat-soluble and toxic to body tissues, and conjugated or direct, which is water-soluble and nontoxic. Elevated serum bilirubin levels are manifested as jaundice in the newborn. Typically the total serum bilirubin level rises over the first 3 to 5 days and then declines.

Physiologic Jaundice

Physiologic jaundice is the manifestation of the normal hyperbilirubinemia seen in newborns, appearing during the third to fourth days of life, due to the limitations and abnormalities of bilirubin metabolism. It occurs in 60% of term infants and up to 80% of preterm infants (Blackburn, 2003). Serum bilirubin levels reach up to 10 mg/dL and then decline rapidly over the first week after birth (Cunningham et al., 2005). Most newborns have been discharged by the time this jaundice peaks (at about 72 hours).

Factors that contribute to the development of physiologic jaundice include an increased bilirubin load because of relative polycythemia, a shortened red blood cell lifespan, immature hepatic uptake and conjugation process, and increased enterohepatic circulation (Holcomb, 2005).

Physiologic jaundice differs between breast-fed and bottle-fed newborns in relation to the onset of symptoms. Breast-fed newborns typically have peak bilirubin levels on the fourth day of life; levels for bottle-fed newborns usually peak on the third day of life. The rate of bilirubin decline is less rapid in breast-fed newborns compared to bottle-fed newborns (Cunningham et al., 2005).

Jaundice associated with breastfeeding presents in two distinct patterns: early-onset breastfeeding jaundice and late-onset breast milk jaundice. Early-onset breastfeeding jaundice is probably associated with ineffective breastfeeding practices because of relative caloric deprivation in the first few days of life. Decreased volume and frequency of feedings may result in mild dehydration and the delayed passage of meconium. This delayed defecation allows enterohepatic circulation reuptake of bilirubin and an increase in the serum level of unconjugated bilirubin. To prevent this, strategies to promote early effective breastfeeding are important. The AAP Work Group on Breastfeeding (2005) recommends early and frequent breastfeeding without supplemental water or dextrose-water unless medically indicated. Early frequent feedings can provide the newborn with adequate calories and fluid volume (via colostrum) to stimulate peristalsis and passage of meconium to eliminate bilirubin.

Late-onset breast milk jaundice occurs later in the newborn period, with the bilirubin level usually peaking in the 6th to 14th day of life. Total serum bilirubin levels may be 12 to 20 mg/dL, but the levels are not considered pathologic (Sarici et al., 2004). The specific cause of late-onset breast milk jaundice is not entirely understood, but it may be related to a change in the milk composition resulting in enhanced enterohepatic circulation. Additional research is needed to determine the cause. Interrupting breastfeeding is not recommended unless bilirubin levels reach dangerous levels; if this occurs, breastfeeding is stopped for only 1 or 2 days. Substituting formula during this short break usually results in a prompt decline of bilirubin levels.

Pathologic Jaundice

Pathologic jaundice is manifested within the first 24 hours of life when total bilirubin levels increase by more than 5 mg/dL/day and the total serum bilirubin level is higher than 17 mg/dL in a full-term infant (Ozen & Mukherjee, 2004). Conditions that alter the production, transport, uptake, metabolism, excretion, or reabsorption of bilirubin can cause pathologic jaundice in the newborn. A few conditions that contribute to red blood cell breakdown and thus higher bilirubin levels include polycythemia, blood incompatibilities, and systemic acidosis. These altered conditions can lead to high levels of unconjugated bilirubin, possibly reaching toxic levels and resulting in a severe condition called kernicterus.

Kernicterus (yellow nucleus) or bilirubin encephalopathy is a preventable neurologic disorder characterized by encephalopathy, motor abnormalities, hearing and vision loss, and death (Springer & Annibale, 2004). Neurotoxicity develops because unconjugated bilirubin has a high affinity for brain tissue, and bilirubin not bound to albumin is free to cross the blood–brain barrier and damage cells of the CNS.

In the acute stage, the newborn becomes lethargic, irritable, and hypotonic and sucks poorly. If the hyperbilirubinemia is not treated, the newborn becomes hypertonic, with arching and seizures. A high-pitched cry may be noted. These changes can occur rapidly, so all newborns must be assessed for jaundice and tested if indicated so that treatment can be initiated.

The most common condition associated with pathologic jaundice is hemolytic disease of the newborn secondary to incompatibility of blood groups of the mother and the newborn. The most frequent conditions are Rh factor and ABO incompatibilities. *Rh incompatibility* or isoimmunization develops when an Rh-negative woman who has experienced Rh isoimmunization subsequently becomes pregnant with an Rh-positive fetus. The maternal antibodies cross the placenta into the fetal circulation and begin to break down the red blood cells (Fig. 24-5). Destruction of the fetal red blood cells leads to fetal anemia and hemolytic disease of the newborn. The severity of the fetal hemolytic process depends on the level and effectiveness of anti-D antibodies and the capacity of the fetal system to remove antibody-coated cells.

Clinical manifestations of hemolytic disease of the newborn include ascites, congestive heart failure, edema, pallor, jaundice, hepatosplenomegaly, hydramnios, thick placenta, and dilation of the umbilical vein (Harrod et al., 2003). The jaundice typically manifests at birth or in the first 24 hours after birth with a rapidly rising unconjugated bilirubin level.

Subsequent Rh⊕fetus

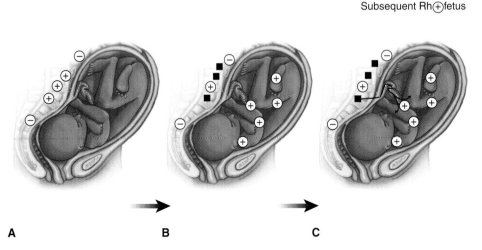

A   **B**   **C**

● Figure 24-5 Rh isoimmunization. (**A**) The Rh-negative mother is exposed to Rh-positive antigens. (**B**) Maternal antibodies form. (**C**) Rh antibodies are transferred to the fetus.

Immune hydrops, also called hydrops fetalis, is a severe form of hemolytic disease of the newborn that occurs when pathologic changes develop in the organs of the fetus secondary to severe anemia. Hydrops fetalis results from fetal hypoxia, anemia, congestive heart failure, and hypoproteinemia secondary to hepatic dysfunction. ABO and Rh incompatibilities can both cause hydrops fetalis, but Rh disease is the more common cause. Typically, hydrops is not observed until the hemoglobin drops below approximately 4 g/dL (hematocrit <15%) (Wagle & Deshpande, 2003). Fetuses with hydrops may die in utero from profound anemia and circulatory failure. The placenta is very enlarged and edematous. One sign of severe anemia and impending death is the sinusoidal fetal heart rate pattern (Cunningham et al., 2005). The newborn hydropic infant appears pale, edematous, and limp at birth and typically requires resuscitation.

The newborn with immune hydrops exhibits severe generalized edema, organ hypertrophy and enlargement, and effusion of fluid into body cavities. Intrauterine transfusions with Rh-negative, type O blood may be life-saving if done in time. The widespread administration of Rh immune globulin (RhoGAM), combined with aggressive fetal surveillance and transfusion, has reduced the incidence of hemolytic disease of the newborn.

ABO incompatibility is an immune reaction that occurs when the mother has type O blood and the fetus has type A, B, or AB blood. Although it occurs more frequently than Rh incompatibilities, it causes less severe problems and rarely results in hemolytic disease severe enough to be clinically diagnosed and treated. Enlargement of the spleen and liver may be found in newborns with ABO incompatibility, but hydrops fetalis is rare (Diehl-Jones & Askin, 2004).

Women with type O blood develop anti-A or anti-B antibodies throughout their life through foods they eat and exposure to infections. Most species of anti-A and anti-B antibodies are immunoglobin M (IgM), which cannot cross the placenta and thus cannot gain access to the fetal red blood cells. Some anti-A and anti-B antibodies from the mother may cross the placenta to the fetus during the first pregnancy and can cause hemolysis of fetal blood cells.

Clinically, the newborn may present with mild hemolysis, anemia, and hyperbilirubinemia. Very few newborns develop anemia or hepatosplenomegaly, and most often the elevated bilirubin levels respond to phototherapy after birth. Because the antibodies resulting in ABO incompatibility occur naturally, it is impossible to eliminate this type of incompatibility. Therefore, nurses need to be aware of this potential cause of hyperbilirubinemia.

Nursing Management

Nursing management of a newborn with hyperbilirubinemia requires a comprehensive approach. As members of the health care team, nurses share in the responsibility for early detection and identification, family education, proper management, and follow-up of the mother and newborn. It is important for nurses to obtain a complete, detailed history to identify factors that may place the infant at risk for hyperbilirubinemia. Nurses can help the mother to understand the diagnostic tests and treatment modalities by offering individualized teaching. Throughout the continuum of care, nurses can improve care by their presence and support.

Assessment

Review the medical record for factors that might predispose the newborn to hyperbilirubinemia. Identify maternal and fetal blood types, checking for possible incompatibilities (Table 24-3). Perform a complete physical examination.

Detect jaundice by observing the infant in a well-lit room and blanching the skin with digital pressure over a bony prominence. Inspect the eyes and mucous membranes for discoloration. Typically, jaundice begins on the head and gradually progresses to the abdomen and extremities. Jaundice in a term newborn fewer than 24 hours old is always pathologic and needs thorough investigation and prompt treatment to prevent kernicterus. Observe for pallor (anemia), excessive bruising (bleeding), and dehydration (sluggish circulation), which may

Table 24-3 Comparing Rh and ABO Incompatibility in the Newborn

Clinical Picture	Rh Incompatibility	ABO Incompatibility
First-born	Rare	Common
Later pregnancies	More severe	No increase in severity
Jaundice	Moderate to severe	Mild
Hydrops fetalis	Frequent	Rare
Anemia	Frequently severe	Rare
Ascites	Frequent	Rare
Hepatosplenomegaly	Frequent	Common

contribute to the development of jaundice and the risk for kernicterus.

Diagnostic tests that may be ordered to aid in diagnosing the condition include:

- Direct Coombs test—to identify hemolytic disease of the newborn; positive results indicate that the newborn's red blood cells have been coated with antibodies and thus are sensitized
- Blood type—to determine Rh status and any incompatibility of the newborn
- Total and direct bilirubin—establishes the diagnosis of hyperbilirubinemia
- Total serum protein—detects reduced binding capacity of albumin
- Reticulocyte count—an elevated level indicates increased hemolysis

Assist with obtaining blood specimens. Cord blood is used for hemoglobin concentration measurements; a heel stick is used for direct Coombs testing and bilirubin levels.

Nursing Interventions

For the newborn with jaundice, regardless of its etiology, phototherapy is used to convert unconjugated bilirubin to the less toxic water-soluble form that can be excreted. Phototherapy, via special lights placed above the newborn or a fiber-optic blanket placed under the newborn and wrapped around him or her, involves blue wavelengths of light to alter unconjugated bilirubin in the skin. The newborn is exposed to the lights continuously except for feeding. Only the newborn's eyes and genital area are covered to ensure exposure of the greatest surface area (Fig. 24-6).

If the total serum bilirubin level remains elevated after intensive phototherapy has been used, an exchange transfusion, the most rapid method for lowering serum bilirubin levels, may be necessary (Springer & Annibale, 2004). In the presence of hemolytic disease, severe anemia, or a rapid rise in the total serum bilirubin level, an exchange transfusion is recommended. Exchange transfusion removes the newborn's blood and replaces it with nonhemolyzed red blood cells from a donor. During the transfusion, the newborn cardiovascular status is continuously monitored because serious complications can arise, such as acid–base imbalances, infection, hypovolemia, and fluid and electrolyte imbalances. Therefore, exchange transfusion is used only as a second-line therapy after phototherapy has failed to yield results. Intensive nursing care is needed.

General nursing interventions for the newborn with jaundice related to hyperbilirubinemia include the following:

- Educate parents about jaundice and its potential risk by providing written and verbal material.
- Encourage the early initiation of feedings to prevent hypoglycemia and provide protein to maintain the albumin levels to transport bilirubin to the liver.

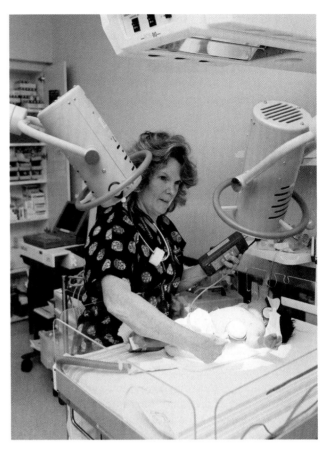

● Figure 24-6 Newborn receiving phototherapy.

- Ensure newborn feedings (breast or formula) every 2 to 3 hours to promote prompt emptying of bilirubin from the bowel.
- Encourage the mother to breastfeed (8 to 12 feedings per day) to prevent inadequate intake and thus dehydration.
- Supplement breast milk with formula to supply protein if bilirubin levels continue to increase with breastfeeding only.
- Show the parents how to identify newborn behaviors that might indicate rising bilirubin levels; urge them to seek treatment from their pediatrician:
  ○ Lethargic, sleepy, poor muscle tone, floppy
  ○ Poor suck, not interested in feeding
  ○ High-pitched cry
- Document the timing of onset of jaundice to differentiate between physiologic (>24 hours) and pathologic jaundice (<24 hours).
- Explore with the family their understanding of jaundice and treatment modalities to reduce anxiety and gain their cooperation in monitoring the infant.
- Monitor serum bilirubin levels to reduce the risk of developing severe hyperbilirubinemia.
- Emphasize appropriate follow-up with the primary care provider within 48 to 72 hours after discharge to assess jaundice status (AAP, 2004).

For the newborn receiving phototherapy, place the newborn under the lights or on the fiberoptic blanket, exposing as much skin as possible. Cover the newborn's genitals and shield the eyes to protect these areas from becoming irritated or burned. Assess the intensity of the light source to prevent burns and excoriation. Turn the newborn every 2 hours to maximize the area of exposure, removing the newborn from the lights only for feedings. Maintain a neutral thermal environment to decrease energy expenditure, and assess the newborn's neurologic status frequently.

Assess the newborn's temperature every 3 to 4 hours as indicated. Monitor fluid intake and output closely and assess daily weights for gains or losses. Check skin turgor for evidence of dehydration. With feedings, remove the newborn from the lights and remove the eye shields to allow interaction with the newborn. Encourage breast or bottle feedings every 2 to 3 hours. Follow agency policy about removing the eye shields periodically to assess the eyes for discharge or corneal irritation secondary to eye shield pressure. Typically, the eyes are assessed and eye shields removed once a shift.

Monitor stool characteristics for consistency and frequency. Unconjugated bilirubin excreted in the feces will produce a greenish appearance, and typically stools are loose. Lack of frequent green stools is a cause for concern.

Provide meticulous skin care. Assess skin surfaces and turgor frequently for dryness and irritation secondary to the dehydrating effects of phototherapy and irritation from highly acidic stool to prevent excoriation and skin breakdown (Green & Wilkinson, 2004).

The use of phototherapy can be anxiety-producing for the parents. Explain the rationale for the procedure and demonstrate techniques that the parents can use to interact with their newborn.

If an exchange transfusion is necessary, assist the physician with the procedure. Monitor the newborn's status closely before, during, and after the procedure for any changes, especially in vital signs and heart rate and rhythm.

Parents need instruction about how to assess their newborn for signs and symptoms of jaundice because physiologic jaundice may not occur until after the newborn is discharged. Additional education related to phototherapy may be necessary when home phototherapy is used (Teaching Guidelines 24-2).

Newborn Infections

Newborns are susceptible to infections because their immune system is immature and slow to react. The antibodies newborns received from their mother during pregnancy and from breast milk help protect them from invading organisms. However, these need time to reach optimal levels.

 TEACHING GUIDELINES 24-2

Caring for Your Newborn
Receiving Home Phototherapy

- Inspect your newborn's skin, eyes, and mucous membranes for a yellow color.
- Remember that a home health nurse will come to visit and help you set up the light system.
- Keep the lights about 12 to 30 inches above your newborn.
- Cover your newborn's eyes with patches or cotton balls and gauze to protect them.
- Keep the newborn undressed except for the diaper area; fold the diaper down below the newborn's navel in the front and as far as possible in the back to expose as much skin area as possible.
- Turn your newborn every 2 hours to make sure to expose all areas of the body.
- Remove the newborn from the lights only during feeding.
- Remove the eye patches during feedings so that you can interact with your newborn.
- Record your newborn's temperature, weight, and fluid intake daily.
- Document the frequency, color, and consistency of all stools; the stools should be loose and green as the bilirubin is broken down.
- Keep the skin clean and dry to prevent irritation.
- Feed your newborn frequently, including supplemental glucose water if allowed to provide added fluid, protein, and calories.
- Rock, cuddle, or hold the newborn to promote bonding when out of the lights.
- Contact your pediatrician or home health care agency with any questions or changes, including refusing feedings, fewer than five wet diapers in one day, vomiting of complete amounts of feeding, or elevated temperature.
- Keep appointments for follow-up laboratory testing to monitor bilirubin levels.

Pathophysiology

When a pathologic organism overcomes the newborn's defenses, infection and sepsis results. **Neonatal sepsis** is the presence of bacterial, fungal, or viral microorganisms or their toxins in blood or other tissues. Infections that have an onset within the first month of life are termed newborn infections. Exposure to a pathogenic organism, whether a virus, fungus, or bacteria, occurs and it enters the newborn's body and begins to multiply.

Etiologies and Risk Factors

Bacterial infections of the newborn affect approximately 4 out of every 1,000 live births (Stoll, 2004). Making the diagnosis of sepsis in newborns is difficult due to its non-specific symptoms. The mortality rate from newborn sepsis may be as high as 50% if untreated. Infection is a major cause of death during the first month of life, contributing to 13% to 15% of all neonatal deaths (Bellig & Ohning, 2004). An awareness of the myriad of risk factors associated with newborn sepsis prepares the nurse for early identification and treatment, thus reducing mortality and morbidity. Among the factors that contribute to the newborn's vulnerability to infection are poor skin integrity, invasive procedures, and exposure to numerous caregivers and an environment conducive to bacterial colonization (Aly et al., 2005).

Newborn infections are usually grouped into three classes according to their time of onset: congenital infection, acquired in utero by vertical transmission with onset before birth; early-onset infections, acquired by vertical transmission in the perinatal period, either shortly before or during birth; and late-onset infections, acquired by horizontal transmission in the nursery. As many as 80% to 90% of neonatal infections have their onset in the first 2 days of life (CDC, 2002).

Intrauterine infections occur when pathogenic organisms cross the placenta into the fetal circulatory system or ascend from the vagina and begin to multiply. The organism can reside in the amniotic fluid, as with cytomegalovirus, or can travel up from the vagina, infecting the membranes and causing them to rupture. This rupture can cause respiratory and gastrointestinal tract infections of the neonate.

Early-onset or intrapartum factors that increase the risk for infection include prolonged rupture of the membranes, urinary tract infections, preterm labor, prolonged or difficult labor, maternal fever, colonization with group B streptococci, and maternal infections. The most common organisms involved in early-onset newborn infections are *Escherichia coli*, group B streptococci, *Klebsiella pneumoniae*, *Listeria monocytogenes*, and other enteric gram-negative bacilli (Hoerst & Samson, 2002). Most infections during the birthing process occur when the newborn comes into contact with an infected birth canal, which can host bacteria against which the newborn cannot defend. The newborn's susceptibility to infection by exogenous organisms may be in part due to the inadequacy of physical barriers: the newborn has thin, friable skin with little subcutaneous tissue. Lack of gastric acidity may also result in easy colonization by environmental organisms. Newborns also may aspirate microorganisms during birth and develop pneumonia.

Risk factors for late-onset infection in the newborn include low birthweight, prematurity, meconium staining, need for resuscitation, birth asphyxia, and improper handwashing. Infections are more common in newborns undergoing invasive procedures such as endotracheal intubation or catheter insertion. Common pathogens implicated in causing late-onset infections include *Candida albicans*, coagulase-negative staphylococci, *Staphylococcus aureus*,

E. coli, Enterobacter, Klebsiella, Serratia, Pseudomonas, and group B streptococci (Merenstein et al., 2002).

Nursing Management

Nursing management requires keen assessment skills to identify a newborn with an infection because the signs and symptoms are often subtle, such as apnea, lethargy, poor feeding, temperature instability, respiratory distress, and poor color (Thureen et al., 2005). Obtaining specimens and coordinating therapies are paramount in treating the newborn with an infection.

Assessment

Manifestations of infections in the newborn usually are nonspecific. Few newborn infections are easy to recognize. Early symptoms can be vague because of the newborn's inability to mount an inflammatory response. Often the nursery nurse reports that the newborn does not "look right." Assess the newborn for common nonspecific signs of infection:

- Hypothermia
- Pallor or duskiness
- Hypotonia
- Cyanosis
- Poor weight gain
- Irritability
- Seizures
- Jaundice
- Grunting
- Nasal flaring
- Apnea and bradycardia
- Lethargy
- Hypoglycemia
- Poor feeding (lack of interest in feeding)
- Abdominal distention (Bellig & Ohning, 2004)

Since infection can be confused with other newborn conditions, laboratory and radiographic tests are needed to confirm the presence of infection. Be prepared to coordinate the timing of the various tests and assist as necessary.

Workups for sepsis may include a complete blood count with a differential to identify anemia, leukocytosis, or leukopenia. A C-reactive protein may also be ordered to validate inflammation. An elevated C-reactive protein level is associated with tissue injury and inflammation. It is not used as a sole indicator of neonatal sepsis but can be used along with other studies to evaluate the infectious process. X-rays of the chest and abdomen are also ordered to detect infectious processes located there. Blood, cerebrospinal fluid, and urine cultures are taken to identify the location and type of infection present. Positive cultures confirm that the newborn has an infection.

Nursing Interventions

To enhance the newborn's chance of survival, early recognition and diagnosis are key. Often the diagnosis of sepsis is based on suspicion of the presenting clinical picture. Antibiotic therapy is usually started before the laboratory results identify the infecting pathogen. Along with antibiotic therapy, circulatory, respiratory, nutritional, and developmental support is important. Antibiotic therapy is continued for 7 to 21 days if cultures are positive, or it is discontinued within 72 hours if cultures are negative. With the use of antibiotics along with early recognition and supportive care, mortality and morbidity rates have been reduced greatly.

Perinatal infections continue to be a public health problem, with severe consequences for those affected. By promoting a better understanding of newborn infections and appropriate use of therapies, nurses can lower the mortality rates associated with severe sepsis, especially with appropriate timing of interventions. The potential for nursing interventions to identify, prevent, and minimize the risk for sepsis is significant. Primary disease prevention must be a major focus for nurses. Family education plays a key role in the prevention of perinatal infections, in addition to following accepted practices in immunization.

Nurses possess the education and assessment tools to decrease the incidence of and reduce the impact of infections on women (see Chapter 20 for additional information) and their newborns by implementing measures for prevention and early recognition, including:

- Formulate a sepsis prevention plan that includes education of all members of the healthcare team on identification and treatment of sepsis.
- Screen all newborns daily for signs of sepsis.
- Monitor sepsis cases and outcomes to reinforce continued quality-improvement measures or modify current practices.
- Outline and carry out measures to prevent nosocomial infections:
  ◦ Thorough handwashing hygiene for all staff
  ◦ Frequent oral care and inspections of mucous membranes
  ◦ Proper positioning and turning to prevent skin breakdown
  ◦ Use of strict aseptic technique for all wound care
  ◦ Frequent monitoring of invasive catheter sites for signs of infection
- Identify newborns at risk for sepsis by reviewing risk factors.
- Monitor vital sign changes and observe for subtle signs of infection.
- Monitor for signs of organ system dysfunction:
  ◦ Cardiovascular compromise—tachycardia and hypotension
  ◦ Respiratory compromise—respiratory distress and tachypnea
  ◦ Renal compromise—oliguria or anuria
  ◦ Systemic compromise—abnormal blood values
- Provide comprehensive sepsis treatment:

  ◦ Provide circulatory support with fluids, vasopressors.
  ◦ Provide supplemental oxygen and mechanical ventilation.
  ◦ Obtain and assist with culture samples as requested.
  ◦ Administer antibiotics as ordered, observing for side effects.
  ◦ Provide for the newborn's comfort level.
  ◦ Assess the family's educational needs and provide information as needed.

Congenital Conditions

Congenital conditions can arise from many etiologies, including single-gene disorders, chromosome aberrations, exposure to teratogens, and many sporadic conditions of unknown cause. Congenital conditions may be inherited or sporadic, isolated or multiple, apparent or hidden, gross or microscopic. They cause nearly half of all deaths in term newborns and cause long-term sequelae for many. The incidence varies according to the type of defect. When a serious anomaly is identified prenatally, the parents can decide whether or not to continue the pregnancy. When an anomaly is identified at or after birth, parents need to be informed promptly and given a realistic appraisal of the severity of the condition, the prognosis, and treatment options so that they can participate in all decisions pertaining to their child.

Congenital Heart Disease

Congenital heart disease is a structural defect involving the heart, the great vessels, or both that is present at birth (O'Toole, 2005). It is a broad term that can describe a number of abnormalities affecting the heart. One in 100 newborns in North America has congenital heart disease—about 8 to 10 of every 1,000 live births (Rempel et al., 2004). It is responsible for more deaths in the first year of life than any other birth defects (Cheffer & Rannalli, 2004). The defect may be very mild and the newborn appears healthy at birth, or it may be so severe that the newborn's life is in immediate jeopardy. Severe congenital cardiac defects usually present in the first few days or weeks of life, while the newborn's circulation is continuing to adapt to the demands of extrauterine life. Advances in diagnosis and medical and surgical interventions have led to dramatic increases in survival rates for newborns with serious heart defects.

Etiology and Risk Factors

In most cases, the exact cause of congenital heart disease is unknown. Most congenital heart defects develop during the first 8 weeks of gestation and are usually the result of genetic and environmental forces, which might include:

- Maternal alcoholism
- Maternal diabetes mellitus

- Single-gene mutation or chromosomal disorders
- Maternal exposure to x-rays
- Maternal exposure to rubella infection
- Poor maternal nutrition during pregnancy
- Maternal age over 40
- Maternal use of amphetamines
- Genetic factors (family recurrence patterns)
- Maternal metabolic disorder of phenylketonuria
- Maternal use of anticonvulsants, estrogen, progesterone, lithium, warfarin (Coumadin), or isotretinoin (Accutane) (Littleton & Engebretson, 2005)

Classification

Typically, congenital heart disease is divided into four physiologic categories based on structural abnormalities and functional alterations (Table 24-4):

- Defects causing increased pulmonary blood flow, such as atrial septal defect and ventricular septal defect
- Defects causing obstructed blood flow out of the heart, such as pulmonary or aortic stenosis
- Defects causing decreased pulmonary blood flow, such as tetralogy of Fallot
- Defects with cyanosis and increased pulmonary blood flow or mixed defects, such as truncus arteriosus or transposition of the great arteries

These four categories are more descriptive than the system used previously, which classified the disorder only as cyanotic or acyanotic. This previous classification was imprecise because some newborns with "acyanotic" defects developed cyanosis, and delayed symptoms often become apparent during infancy and early childhood. With the hemodynamic classification, the clinical picture of each grouping is more uniform and predictable (Hockenberry, 2005).

Nursing Management

Ideally, nursing management begins prenatally by reviewing the maternal history for risk factors that might predispose the newborn to a congenital heart defect. While most congenital heart defects cannot be prevented, several key areas need to be addressed to ensure the optimal health status for the woman and her fetus. For example, ensure that all women are tested prior to pregnancy for immunity to rubella so that they can be immunized if necessary. Any chronic health problems, such as diabetes, hypertension, seizures, and phenylketonuria, should be controlled and any medication or dietary adjustments should be made before attempting conception. Once pregnant, the woman should be encouraged to avoid alcohol, smoking, and the use of unprescribed drugs. Refer the woman and her partner for genetic counseling if cardiac defects are present in the family to provide the parents with a risk assessment for future offspring.

Some defects can be discovered on routine prenatal ultrasound. Therefore, stress the importance of receiving prenatal care throughout pregnancy so that appropriate interventions can be initiated early if the need arises.

After birth, when the newborn is admitted to the nursery, carefully assess the cardiovascular and respiratory systems, looking for signs and symptoms of respiratory distress, cyanosis, or congestive heart failure that might indicate a cardiac anomaly. Assess rate, rhythm, and heart sounds, reporting any abnormalities immediately. Note any signs of heart failure, including edema, diminished peripheral pulses, hepatomegaly, tachycardia, diaphoresis, respiratory distress with tachypnea, peripheral pallor, and irritability (Kenner & Lott, 2004). Assist with diagnostic testing, such as:

- Arterial blood gases to determine oxygenation levels and to differentiate lung disease from heart disease as the cause of cyanosis
- Chest x-rays to identify cardiac size, shape, and position
- Magnetic resonance imaging (MRI) to evaluate for cardiac malformations
- Electrocardiogram to detect atrial or ventricular hypertrophy and dysrhythmias
- Echocardiogram to evaluate heart anatomy and flow defects
- Blood studies to assess anemia, blood glucose, and electrolyte levels
- Catheterization to obtain data for definitive diagnosis or in preparation for cardiac surgery (Montoya & Washington, 2002)

Provide continuous monitoring of the newborn's cardiac and respiratory status, administer medications as ordered, and provide comfort measures to the newborn who will be subjected to a variety of painful procedures. Be vigilant in ensuring the newborn's comfort, since he or she cannot report or describe pain. Assist in preventing pain as much as possible, interpreting the newborn's cues suggesting pain and managing it appropriately (Pasero, 2004). Make pain assessment part of routine newborn nursing care.

Include the parents in the plan of care. Parents want to make informed decisions based on their beliefs and values and desire to make them in the best interest of their infant (Rempel et al., 2004). Nurses can play a key role in meeting the parents' needs by doing the following:

- Assess their ability to cope with the diagnosis.
- Encourage them to verbalize their feelings about the newborn's condition and treatment.
- Instruct them about the medications prescribed, including side effects and doses, and how to observe for signs and symptoms indicating heart failure.
- Educate them about the specific cardiac defect; include written information and pictures to enhance understanding.

Table 24-4 Classifications of Congenital Heart Disease

Cardiac Defect	Examples	Pathophysiology	Clinical Picture
Increased pulmonary blood flow (left-to-right shunting)	Atrial septal defect (ASD) Ventricular septal defect (VSD) Patent ductus arteriosus (PDA)	Cardiac septum communication or abnormal connection between the great arteries permits blood to flow from higher pressure (left side of heart) to lower pressure (right side of heart).	Asymptomatic or murmur, fatigue with feedings, and symptoms of CHF: pallor, cyanosis, or gray coloring, diminished peripheral pulses, edema, diaphoresis, tachypnea, and tachycardia
Decreased pulmonary blood flow	Tetralogy of Fallot (TOF) Tricuspid atresia	Pulmonary blood flow obstruction accompanied by an anatomic defect such as ASD or VSD between the right and left sides of the heart, which allows desaturated blood to shunt right to left, causing desaturated blood to enter into the systemic circulation	Cyanosis, murmur, hypoxemia, dyspnea, increased cardiac workload, and marked exercise intolerance
Obstruction to blood flow out of the heart	Pulmonary stenosis Aortic stenosis Coarctation of the aorta	A narrowing or constriction of an opening causes pressure to rise in the area behind the obstruction and a decrease in blood available for systemic perfusion	CHF, decreased cardiac output, and pump failure
Cyanotic defects with increased pulmonary blood flow or mixed defects	Transposition of the great arteries Truncus arteriosus Hypoplastic left heart syndrome	Fully saturated systemic blood flow mixes with desaturated pulmonary blood flow, causing desaturation of the systemic circulation. This leads to pulmonary congestion and a decrease in cardiac output. To support life, intervention must bring about a mixing of arterial and venous blood.	Cyanosis, CHF, ruddiness, dusky or gray color, dyspnea

CHF, congestive heart failure

Sources: Hockenberry, 2005; Verklan & Walden, 2004; Mattson & Smith, 2004; McKinney et al., 2005.

- Present an overview of the prognosis and possible interventions.
- Assist them with making decisions about treatment, and support their decisions for the newborn's care.
- Orient them to the NICU prior to surgery.
- Provide emotional support throughout care.

The parents also need clear instructions about how to monitor the newborn at home, especially if the newborn will be discharged and then brought back later so the condition can be corrected. The parents also need instructions about caring for their newborn after the defect is corrected. Educate the parents about signs and symptoms that need to be reported, such as weight loss, poor feeding, cyanosis, breathing difficulties, irritability, increased respiratory rate, and fever. Referrals to local support groups, national organizations, and websites also are helpful. Emphasize the importance of close supervision and follow-up care.

Inborn Errors of Metabolism

Inborn errors of metabolism are genetic disorders that disrupt normal metabolic function. Most are due to a defect in an enzyme or transport protein, resulting in a blocked metabolic pathway. Clinical symptoms are manifested secondary to toxic accumulations of substances before the block. When viewed individually, inborn errors of metabolism are rare, but collectively they are responsible for significant levels of infant mortality and morbidity. Table 24-5 summarizes four common inborn errors.

A successful outcome for the affected newborn depends on early diagnosis and prompt intervention. Most inborn errors present in the newborn period with nonspecific and subtle manifestations—lethargy, hypotonia, respiratory distress, poor feeding and weight gain, vomiting, and seizures (Weiner, 2005). Identification of an inborn error of metabolism in a newborn depends largely on the awareness of the nurse and clues from the maternal history, laboratory work, and clinical examination.

Congenital CNS Structural Defects

Congenital CNS structural defects are serious malformations involving the spine (spina bifida) and brain (anencephaly). They are more commonly described as neural tube defects because they occur when the neural tube fails to close properly during early embryogenesis. The neural tube develops into the brain and spinal cord and normally closes between the 17th and 30th day of gestation. Neural tube defects develop during this first month, when most women are still unaware of their pregnancy and the embryo is estimated to be about the size of a grain of rice. In pregnancies in which the fetus has a neural tube defect, the level of alpha-fetoprotein in the amniotic fluid and maternal serum is elevated.

Neural tube defects involve abnormalities in the region-specific neural tube closure junctions with the cranial and caudal levels of the neural tube, often resulting in frank exposure of neural tissue. These defects vary in their severity, depending on the type and level of the lesion. Neural tube defects affect 0.6 per 1,000 live births in the United States, where there are approximately 3,000 pregnancies annually that are complicated by neural tube defects (Becske & Jallo, 2004). They are the second most common major congenital anomaly worldwide, behind cardiac malformations (CDC, 2004).

Neural tube defects may be either closed (covered by skin or a membrane) or open (neural tissue exposed). Some common defects are anencephaly, hydrocephalus, microcephaly, spina bifida, myelomeningocele, and meningo-

cele. Defects that will be discussed here are hydrocephalus, microcephaly, anencephaly, and spina bifida.

A worldwide decline in neural tube defects has occurred over the past few decades as a result of prevention (preconception folic acid supplementation and monitoring of maternal serum alpha-fetoprotein levels) and use of ultrasonography and amniocentesis to identify affected fetuses (Blackburn, 2003). Despite this decline, still more infants could be born free of these birth defects if all women consumed the necessary amount of folic acid (CDC, 2004). Early prenatal diagnosis can offer parents the option for elective termination if desired.

Hydrocephalus

Hydrocephalus is an increase in cerebrospinal fluid (CSF) in the ventricles of the brain due to overproduction or impaired circulation and absorption. The term stems from the Greek words *hydor* (water) and *cephalic* (head). Normal growth of the brain is altered secondary to the increase in intracranial pressure from the CSF. Congenital hydrocephalus usually arises as a result of a malformation in the brain or an intrauterine infection (toxoplasmosis or cytomegalovirus). It occurs in about 3 or 4 per 1,000 live births (Allen & Vessey, 2004).

Hydrocephalus rarely occurs as an isolated defect; it is usually associated with spina bifida or other neural tube anomalies. Clinical manifestations include large head, widened sutures, poor feeding, bulging and tense fontanels, "setting sun" eyes, vomiting, lethargy, visible scalp veins, and irritability (Haws, 2004). Diagnosis is by computed tomography (CT) scan or MRI (Fig. 24-7).

No treatment is available that can counteract the accumulation of CSF in the brain. Therefore, surgery with the insertion of a ventricular shunt is the mainstay of treatment to relieve pressure within the cranium. Shunts are designed to maintain normal intracranial pressure by draining off excess CSF. Shunting has dramatically improved the outcome of newborns with hydrocephalus (Sgouros, 2004).

A ventriculoperitoneal shunt is inserted from the ventricle in the brain and threaded down into the peritoneal cavity to allow drainage of excess CSF. The long-term prognosis for this condition varies and depends on the patency of the shunt, the presence of other CNS anomalies and their impact on the newborn, and the quality of care the newborn receives.

Prior to shunt insertion, nursing management focuses on daily documentation of the newborn's head circumference and associated neurologic behaviors that might indicate an increase in intracranial pressure: irritability, high-pitched cry, poor feeding and sucking, vomiting, or decrease in consciousness. Gently palpate the fontanels for signs of bulging and tenseness, and palpate the suture lines for increasing separation. Protect the enlarged head to prevent skin breakdown. Handle the head gently and use a sheepskin or a waterbed or egg-crate mattress. Change the newborn's position frequently to minimize pressure.

Table 24-5 Inborn Errors of Metabolism

Condition	Incidence and Etiology	Clinical Picture	Management
Phenylketonuria (PKU)	1:15,000 live births Autosomal recessive genetic disorder caused by a deficiency of the hepatic enzyme phenylalanine hydroxylase Enzyme deficiency with subsequent accumulation of amino acid phenylalanine	Newborns appear normal at birth but by 6 months of age signs of slow mental development evident Vomiting, poor feedings, failure to thrive, overactivity, irritability, musty-smelling urine If not treated, possible mental retardation	Screening of all newborns at about 48 hours after birth to ensure adequate intake of protein Dietary restriction of phenylalanine, with regular monitoring of serum phenylalanine levels (effective when started before the first month of age) Life-long dietary restriction of phenylalanine
Maple syrup urine disease (MSUR)	1:150,000 in general population; most prevalent among the Mennonite population in Lancaster, Pennsylvania Autosomal recessive inherited disorder Enzyme metabolism of certain amino acids is affected, with the buildup of acids causing ketoacidosis.	Lethargy, poor feeding, vomiting, weight loss, seizures, shrill cry, shallow respirations, loss of reflexes, coma, sweet maple syrup odor to urine	Dialysis to remove accumulated acids Life-long low-protein diet to prevent neurologic deficits of disease
Galactosemia	1:50,000 births Autosomal recessive inherited disorder in which an enzyme needed to convert galactose to glucose is missing and newborn cannot metabolize lactose	Vomiting, hypoglycemia, liver damage, hyperbilirubinemia, poor weight gain, cataracts, frequent infections	Routine newborn screening for galactosemia is performed in the majority of states. Life-long lactose-restricted diet to prevent mental retardation, liver disease, and cataracts.
Congenital hypothyroidism	1:4,000 live births Multiple causes—absent or underdeveloped thyroid gland or biochemical defects in thyroid hormone	Large protruding tongue, slow reflexes, distended abdomen, large, open posterior fontanel, constipation, hypothermia, poor feeding, hoarse cry, dry skin, coarse hair, goiter, and jaundice. If untreated, irreversible cognitive and motor impairment. Decreased levels of thyroid hormone (T4) and elevated levels of TSH.	Newborn screening program in all states Life-long thyroid replacement hormone therapy and continued monitoring of thyroid levels and clinical response to therapy

Sources: Weiner, 2005; Verklan & Walden, 2004; Lanting et al., 2005; Hockenberry, 2005; Littleton & Engebretson, 2005

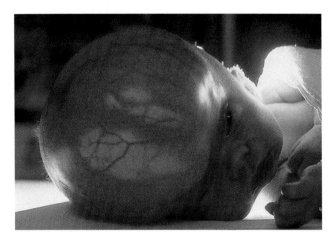

● Figure 24-7 Newborn with hydrocephalus.

Postoperatively, strictly monitor the newborn's neurologic status and behavior and report any changes that might indicate an increased intracranial pressure secondary to a blockage in the shunt. These finding may include papillary dilation (increased intracranial pressure places pressure on the oculomotor nerve, producing dilation), increasing head size, bulging fontanels, and change in level of consciousness. Assess the abdomen for distention because drainage of CSF into the abdomen can cause peritonitis. Paralytic ileus is another possible postoperative complication due to distal catheter placement (Hockenberry, 2005).

After surgery, continue to provide protective and comfort measures for the enlarged head. Position the newborn's head so that he or she does not lie on the shunt area. Educate the parents about caring for the shunt and signs and symptoms of infection or blockage. A referral for follow-up home care is appropriate.

Microcephaly

Microcephaly is a condition in which a small brain is located within a normal-sized cranium. This implies neurologic impairment. Risk factors for this anomaly include maternal viral infections (toxoplasmosis, rubella, cytomegalovirus, herpes, and syphilis), radiation exposure, diabetes, phenylketonuria, street drug exposure, and malnutrition (Verklan & Walden, 2004). Diagnosis is confirmed by a CT scan or MRI. Care is supportive since there is no known treatment to reverse the disorder. Parents need to be informed of potential cognitive impairment of their newborn. Ensure that appropriate community referrals are made to assist the parents and the child, who will have developmental delays.

Anencephaly

Anencephaly, the most severe neural tube defect, is the congenital absence of the cranial vault, with the cerebral hemispheres completely missing or reduced to small masses (O'Toole, 2003). It most commonly involves the forebrain and variable amounts of the upper brain stem, where there is no brain tissue above the brain stem. The incidence is approximately 0.2 per 1,000 live births, and both genetic and environmental insults appear to be responsible (Verklan & Walden, 2004). Anencephaly is apparent on visual inspection after birth, with exposed neural tissue without a cranium surrounding it. Prenatally, alpha-fetoprotein levels are elevated late in the first trimester. Most newborns with anencephaly are stillborn; those born alive die within a few days. Comfort measures for the newborn and support for the parents are needed as they grieve for the loss of their infant.

Spina Bifida

Spina bifida is a general category of caudal defects (below the level of T12) involving spinal cord tissue (Finnell et al., 2003). It is the most complex but treatable CNS abnormality that is visible at birth (Foster, 2004). Spina bifida is the leading cause of infantile paralysis in the world today; incidence rates are about 1 per 1,000 live births (Vachha & Adams, 2005). This classification includes two types of common defects: meningocele and myelomeningocele (Fig. 24-8).

A meningocele is an opening in the spine through a bony defect (spina bifida) where a herniation of the meninges and spinal fluid has protruded. The spinal cord and nerve roots do not herniate into this dorsal dural sac. Newborns with meningocele usually have normal examination findings and a covered (closed) dural sac. They typically do not have associated neurologic malformations. Surgical treatment to close the defect is usually warranted.

A **myelomeningocele** is a more severe form of spina bifida in which the spinal cord and nerve roots herniate into the sac through an opening in the spine, compromising the meninges. It is the most common form of spina bifida, accounting for 94% of cases (Foster, 2004). The incidence is 1 in 1,200 to 1,400 live births, affecting 6,000 to 11,000 newborns in the United States each year (Becske & Jallo, 2004).

This complex condition, resulting from a neurodevelopmental disruption early in gestation, affects not just the spine but also the CNS. Hydrocephalus frequently accompanies this anomaly (Ellenbogen, 2004). This protrusion is typically covered partially or completely by skin but is very fragile and may leak CSF if traumatized. Risk factors for myelomeningocele include both genetic and environmental factors:

- Celtic ancestry (highest incidence)
- Female sex (accounting for 60% to 70% of affected newborns)
- Low socioeconomic status
- Maternal diabetes
- Use of anticonvulsants (valproic acid and carbamazepine)
- Previous pregnancy with a newborn with a neural tube defect

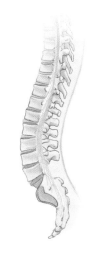 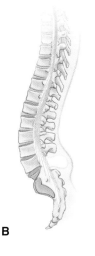 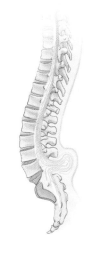

● Figure 24-8 Two common types of spina bifida. (**A**) Normal spinal cord. (**B**) Meningocele. (**C**) Myelomeningocele.

A

B

C

- Maternal obesity
- Maternal malnutrition
- Low folic acid intake (Cunningham et al., 2005)

Myelomeningoceles can arise at any point along the vertebral column, but they most commonly occur in the lower lumbar or sacral regions, causing neurologic deficits below the level of the defect. Paralysis, bladder and bowel incontinence, and hydrocephalus are the most common complications (Fig. 24-9). Surgical repair as soon as possible, usually within 72 hours after birth, helps prevent infection and preserve neurologic function (Ellenbogen, 2004).

Nursing management for a newborn with myelomeningocele involves the following actions:

- Use strict aseptic technique when caring for the defect to prevent infection.
- Avoid hypothermia: heat can be lost through the defect opening, placing the newborn at increased risk for cold stress.
- Avoid trauma to the sac (to prevent leakage of CSF or damage to the nerve tissue) through prone or side-lying positioning.

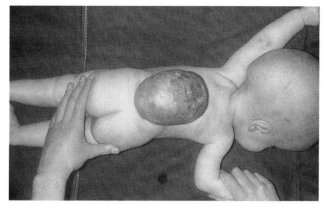

● Figure 24-9 Newborn with myelomeningocele and hydrocephalus.

- Apply a sterile dressing or protective covering over the sac to prevent rupture and drying, with frequent changes to prevent the dressing from adhering to the defect.
- Frequently monitor the sac for signs of oozing fluid or drainage.
- Meticulously clean the genital area to avoid contamination of the sac.
- Assess movement and sensation below the defect.
- Measure head circumference daily to observe for hydrocephalus.
- Provide support and information to help the parents cope.
- Allow the parents to vent their feelings.
- Make referrals to support groups.
- Encourage open discussions regarding the baby's prognosis and long-term care.
- Involve the parents in the newborn's care.

Respiratory System Structural Anomalies

Two structural anomalies of the respiratory system, choanal atresia and congenital diaphragmatic hernia, can be life-threatening.

Choanal Atresia

Choanal atresia is an uncommon congenital malformation of the upper airway involving a narrowing of the nasal airway by membranous or bony tissue. It typically presents with other anomalies involving the heart and CNS. It occurs in 1 in 8,000 live births, with a female preponderance (Dave, 2005). This structural anomaly can result in significant respiratory distress in the newborn. If the nasal airway is completely obstructed, death from asphyxia may occur at birth.

During attempted inspiration, the tongue is pulled to the palate and obstruction of the oral airway results. If the newborn cries and takes a breath through the mouth, the airway obstruction is momentarily relieved. When the crying stops, however, the mouth closes and the cycle of obstruction is repeated (Tewfik & Hagr, 2005).

The cause of this congenital defect is unknown, but it is thought to result from persistence of the membrane between the nasal and oral spaces during fetal development. This defect may be unilateral or bilateral and is often associated with other congenital anomalies.

Failure to pass a suction catheter through the nose into the pharynx is highly suggestive of choanal atresia. The diagnosis can be confirmed with a CT scan. Other signs include respiratory distress, cyanosis unless newborn is crying, and inability to suck and breathe simultaneously. Surgery to remove the obstruction and establish a patent airway is needed. Full recovery is the usual outcome.

Congenital Diaphragmatic Hernia

Congenital diaphragmatic hernia is a rare disorder (1 in 3,000 newborns) that frequently presents with significant respiratory distress in the immediate newborn period (Tesselaar et al., 2004). The abdominal contents are herniated into the thoracic cavity through a defect in the diaphragm. It is thought that the diaphragm failed to close properly during early embryonic development. The timing of the herniation and the amount of abdominal contents in the thoracic cavity greatly influence the clinical picture at birth and the survival rate (Cheffer & Rannalli, 2004).

Most hernias (85%) involve the left hemidiaphragm (Mattson & Smith, 2004). Prenatal diagnosis is possible through ultrasound. This diagnosis should be considered when hydramnios is present. The presence of the abdominal contents in the chest compresses the lung, leads to pulmonary hypoplasia, and promotes persistent pulmonary hypertension in the newborn (Haws, 2004).

Associated anomalies include congenital cardiac defects, genital or renal anomalies, neural tube defects, choanal atresia, or chromosomal anomalies, such as trisomy 13 and 18. The survival rate of newborns with a diaphragmatic hernia varies, but overall the rate has remained at about 50% for nearly half a century despite advances in neonatal intensive care, anesthesia, and surgery (Golombek, 2002) (Fig. 24-10).

Affected newborns present with profound respiratory distress because at least one of the lungs cannot expand or may not have fully developed, resulting in persistent pulmonary hypertension shortly after birth; aggressive resuscitation is needed. Other clinical features include absent breath sounds on the affected side of the chest, heart sounds displaced to the right, bowel sounds noted in the chest, barrel chest and a scaphoid-shaped abdomen, and cyanosis. Diagnosis is made by chest x-ray, which reveals an air-filled bowel in the chest cavity (Hockenberry, 2005). Surgery to correct the defect is needed.

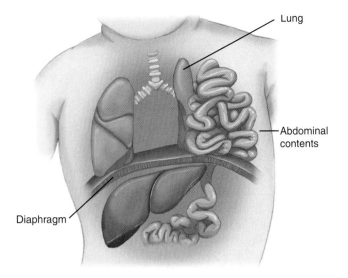

● Figure 24-10 Congenital diaphragmatic hernia. Note how some of the abdominal contents enters the thoracic cavity, subsequently compressing the lung.

Nursing care related to the care of the affected newborn includes the following:

- Assist with endotracheal intubation and positive-pressure ventilation to aid in lung expansion and improvement of ventilation.
- Position the newborn on the affected side with the head and chest elevated to promote normal lung expansion.
- Assist with placement of an orogastric tube for gastric decompression.
- Monitor ventilatory pressures to prevent pneumothorax.
- Monitor vital signs, weight, urinary output, and serum electrolytes to identify changes early.
- Maintain thermoregulation to prevent cold stress.
- Anticipate use of extracorporeal membrane oxygenation (ECMO) or high-frequency oscillatory ventilation if the newborn's condition does not stabilize.
- Maintain nothing by mouth (NPO) status to prevent aspiration.
- Administer inotropics to support systemic blood pressure.
- Administer surfactant, steroids, and inhaled nitric oxide as ordered to correct hypoxia and acid–base imbalance.
- Assist with insertion of a chest tube in the event of a pneumothorax.
- Monitor oxygen saturation levels to evaluate systemic perfusion status.
- Minimize environmental stimuli to reduce agitation and oxygen demand.
- Provide supportive positioning with a rolled blanket to promote comfort.

- Provide the parents with continuing updates about the newborn's condition.
- Encourage the parents to see and touch the infant frequently to promote bonding.
- Recognize and react to newborn clues (Mattson & Smith 2004).

Gastrointestinal System Structural Anomalies

Gastrointestinal anomalies that disrupt facial structures are found in about 1% (or 1 million) of the infants born worldwide each year. The most common of these is cleft lip and palate, a complex condition due to multiple genetic and environmental factors (Murray & Schuttem, 2004). Other gastrointestinal system anomalies include esophageal atresia, tracheoesophageal fistula, omphalocele, gastroschisis, and imperforate anus.

Cleft Lip and Palate

A cleft lip involves a congenital fissure or longitudinal opening in the lip; a cleft palate involves a congenital fissure or longitudinal opening in the roof of the mouth. The defect may be limited to the outer flesh of the upper lip or it may extend back through the midline of the upper jaw through the roof of the palate. It may occur as a single defect or part of a syndrome of anomalies. It can be unilateral or bilateral. Unilateral cleft lip occurs more commonly on the left side. Bilateral cleft lip is usually accompanied by a cleft palate (O'Toole, 2005). Cleft palate can range from a cleft in the uvula to a complete cleft in the soft and hard palates that can be unilateral, bilateral, or in the midline (Fig. 24-11).

Cleft lip and palate is the most common craniofacial birth defect. It is more common in white and Asian males. In addition to immediate feeding difficulties,

infants with cleft lip and palate may have problems with dentition, language acquisition, and hearing (Pelchat et al., 2004).

Risk factors for this anomaly include maternal use of phenytoin (Dilantin), alcohol, retinoic acid (Accutane), and cigarette smoking. In addition, a family history of cleft lip or palate increases the incidence (Mattson & Smith, 2004).

The diagnosis of cleft lip is readily apparent at birth. Treatment is surgical repair between the ages of 6 to 12 weeks. Successful surgery often leaves only a thin scar on the upper lip. The outcome of surgery depends on the severity of the defect: children with more severe cases will need additional surgery in stages (Lowdermilk & Perry, 2004).

Repairing the facial anomaly as soon as possible is important to facilitate bonding between the newborn and the parents and to improve nutritional status. Milk flow during feeding requires negative pressure and sucking pressure. Newborns with cleft lip and palate have feeding difficulties because they cannot generate a negative pressure in the mouth to facilitate sucking (Tolarova, 2004). Specialized nipples, bottles, and feeders are available to help meet the nutritional needs of infants with this anomaly.

Surgical correction for cleft palate is done around 6 to 18 months of age to allow for developmental growth to occur. A plastic palate guard to form a synthetic palate may need to be used to allow for introduction of solid foods and to prevent aspiration in the interim.

Caring for a newborn with a cleft lip and palate includes the following:

- Feed the infant in an upright position to prevent aspiration.
- Assess for adequate achievement of suction during feeding.
- Position the newborn on sides in an infant seat after feeding.
- Burp the infant frequently to reduce the risk for vomiting and aspiration; burp him or her in the sitting position on your lap to prevent trauma to the mouth on your shoulder.
- Limit feeding sessions to avoid poor weight gain due to fatigue.
- Use high-calorie formula to improve caloric intake.
- Be alert for bonding problems; encourage the parents to express their feelings about this visible anomaly.
- Encourage parental interaction and involvement with the newborn.
- Plan for discharge as soon as the parents feel comfortable with infant care.
- Show the family photos taken before and after surgical repair in other babies.

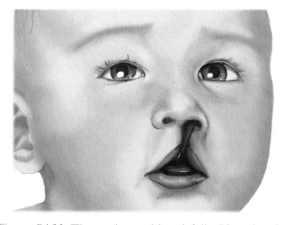

● Figure 24-11 The newborn with a cleft lip. Note that the defect may extend up through the roof of the palate.

- Allow the parents to vent their frustrations about feeding problems.
- Outline treatment modalities and explain the staging of surgical interventions.
- Model nurturing behaviors when interacting with the infant.
- Offer information and make appropriate referrals for community support and counseling as needed (Kenner & Lott, 2004).

Esophageal Atresia and Tracheoesophageal Fistula

Esophageal atresia and tracheoesophageal fistula are gastrointestinal anomalies in which the esophagus and trachea do not separate normally during embryonic development. Esophageal atresia refers to a congenitally interrupted esophagus where the proximal and distal ends do not communicate: the upper esophageal segment ends in a blind pouch and the lower segment ends a variable distance above the diaphragm (Fig. 24-12). Tracheoesophageal fistula is an abnormal communication between the trachea and esophagus. When associated with esophageal atresia, the fistula most commonly occurs between the distal esophageal segment and the trachea. The incidence of esophageal atresia is 1 per 3,000 to 4,500 live births (Blair & Konkin, 2004).

Several types of esophageal atresia exist, but the most common anomaly is a fistula between the distal esophagus and the trachea, which occurs in 86% of newborns with an esophageal defect. Esophageal atresia and tracheoesophageal fistula are thought to be the result of incomplete separation of the lung bed from the foregut during early fetal development. A large percentage of these newborns have other congenital anomalies involving the vertebra, renal, heart, musculoskeletal, and gastrointestinal systems (Haws, 2004); most have several anomalies.

The first sign of esophageal atresia may be hydramnios in the mother, because the fetus cannot swallow and absorb amniotic fluid in utero, leading to accumulation. The second sign soon after birth is copious, frothy bubbles of mucus in the mouth and nose accompanied by drooling. Abdominal distention develops as air builds up in the stomach. A gastric tube cannot be inserted beyond a certain point since the esophagus ends in a blind pouch. The newborn may have rattling respirations, excessive salivation and drooling, and "the three C's" (coughing, choking, and cyanosis) if feeding is attempted. The presence of a fistula increases the risk of respiratory complications such as pneumonitis and atelectasis due to aspiration of food and secretions (Kronemer & Snyder, 2004).

Diagnosis is made by x-ray: a gastric tube appears coiled in the upper esophageal pouch, and air in the gastrointestinal tract indicates the presence of a fistula (Verklan & Walden, 2004). Once a diagnosis of esophageal atresia is established, preparations for surgery are made if the newborn is stable.

Preoperative care focuses on the following:

- Prevent aspiration by elevating the head of the bed 30 to 45 degrees to prevent reflux.
- Maintain NPO status.
- Monitoring parenteral IV fluid infusions.
- Assess and maintain the patency of the orogastric tube; monitor the functioning of the tube, which is attached to low continuous suction; and avoid irrigation of the tube to prevent aspiration.
- Assist with diagnostic studies to rule out other anomalies.
- Use comfort measures to minimize crying and prevent respiratory distress.
- Inform the parents about the rationales for the aspiration prevention measures.
- Document frequent observations of the newborn's condition (Haws, 2004).

Surgery consists of closing the fistula and joining the two esophageal segments. Postoperative care involves close observation of all systems to identify any complications. Total parenteral nutrition and antibiotics are commonly used until the esophageal anastomosis is proven intact and patent. Then oral feedings are usually started within a week after surgery (Verklan & Walden, 2004). Keep the parents informed of their newborn's condition and progress. Demonstrate and reinforce all teaching prior to discharge.

Omphalocele and Gastroschisis

Omphalocele and gastroschisis are congenital anomalies of the anterior abdominal wall. An **omphalocele** is a defect of the umbilical ring that allows evisceration of abdominal contents into an external peritoneal sac. Defects vary in size; they may be limited to bowel loops or may include the entire gastrointestinal tract and liver (Fig. 24-13). Bowel malrotation is common, but the displaced organs are usually normal. Omphaloceles are associated with other anomalies in more than 70% of the cases. This anomaly is usually detected during routine prenatal ultrasound of the fetus or during investigation of an increased alpha-fetoprotein level (Khan & Thomas, 2004).

Gastroschisis is a herniation of abdominal contents through an abdominal wall defect, usually to the left or right of the umbilicus (Haws, 2004). Gastroschisis differs from omphalocele in that there is no peritoneal sac protecting the herniated organs, and thus exposure to amniotic fluid makes them thickened, edematous, and inflamed (Verklan & Walden, 2004). Gastroschisis is associated with significant newborn mortality and morbidity rates. Despite surgical correction, feeding intolerance, failure to thrive, and prolonged hospital stays occur in nearly all newborns with this anomaly (Laughon et al., 2003).

Factors associated with high-risk pregnancies, such as maternal illness and infection, drug use, smoking, and

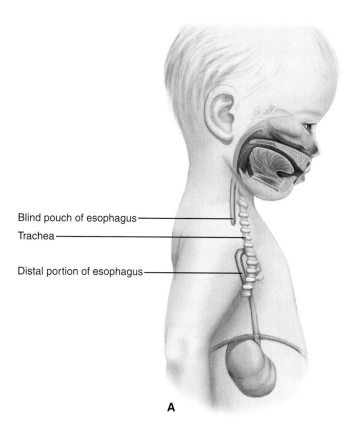

A

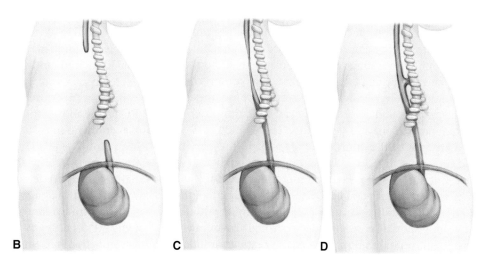

● Figure 24-12 Esophageal atresia and tracheoesophageal fistula. (**A**) The most common type of esophageal atresia, in which the esophagus ends in a blind pouch and a fistula connects the trachea with the distal portion of the esophagus. (**B**) The upper and distal portions of the esophagus end in a blind pouch. (**C**) The esophagus is one segment, but a portion of it is narrowed. (**D**) The upper portion of the esophagus connects to the trachea via a fistula.

Blind pouch of esophagus

Trachea

Distal portion of esophagus

B   C   D

genetic abnormalities, are also associated with omphalocele and gastroschisis. These factors contribute to placental insufficiency and the birth of a small-for-gestational-age or preterm newborn, the populations in which both of these abdominal defects most commonly occur. The combined incidence of both congenital abdominal wall anomalies is 1 in 2,000 births (Glasser, 2003).

Nursing care of newborns with omphalocele or gastroschisis focuses on preventing hypothermia, maintaining perfusion to the eviscerated abdominal contents by minimizing fluid loss, and protecting the exposed abdominal contents from trauma and infection. These objectives can be accomplished by placing the infant in a sterile drawstring bowel bag that maintains a sterile environment for the exposed contents, allows visualization, reduces heat and moisture loss, and allows heat from radiant warmers to reach the newborn. The newborn is placed feet-first into the bag and the drawstring is secured around the torso (Lockridge et al., 2002). Strict sterile technique is necessary to prevent contamination of the exposed abdominal

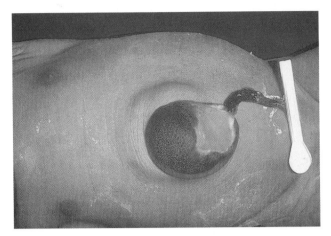

● Figure 24-13 Omphalocele in a newborn. Note the large, protruding sac.

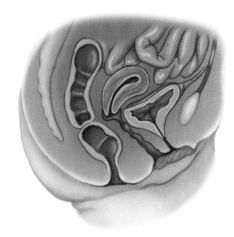

● Figure 24-14 Imperforate anus in which the rectum ends in a blind pouch.

contents. An orogastric tube attached to low suction is used to prevent intestinal distention. Intravenous therapy is administered to maintain fluid and electrolyte balance and provide a route for antibiotic therapy. Monitor the newborn's fluid status frequently. Closely observe the exposed bowel for vascular compromise, such as changes in color or a decrease in temperature, and report immediately.

Surgical repair of both defects occurs after initial stabilization and comprehensive evaluation for any other anomalies. It may have to occur in stages, depending on the defect. Postoperative care involves providing pain management, monitoring respiratory and cardiac status, monitoring intake and output, assessing for vascular compromise, maintaining the orogastric tube to suction, documenting the amount and color of drainage, and administering ordered medications and treatments (Haws, 2004).

Throughout the entire time after birth, the parents need continued support and progress reports on their newborn. Encourage the parents to touch the newborn and participate in care if possible. Because of the nature of this defect, bonding opportunities will be limited initially, but visiting should be permitted and strongly encouraged. Provide information about the defect, treatment modalities, prognosis, and home care instructions.

Imperforate Anus

An imperforate anus is a gastrointestinal system malformation of the anorectal area that may occur in several forms. The rectum may end in a blind pouch that does not connect to the colon or it may have fistulas (openings) between the rectum and the perineum, the vagina in girls or the urethra in boys (Fig. 24-14). The malformations occur during early fetal development and are associated with anomalies in other body systems.

Imperforate anus occurs in about 1 of every 5,000 live births (Hart, 2005). The defect can be further classified as a high or low type, depending on its level. The level significantly influences the outcome in terms of fecal continence as well as management (Molmenti, 2004).

Surgical intervention is needed for both high and low types of imperforate anus. Surgery for a high type of defect involves a colostomy in the newborn period, with corrective surgery performed in stages to allow for growth. Surgery for the low type of anomaly, which frequently includes a fistula, involves closure of the fistula, creation of an anal opening, and repositioning of the rectal pouch into the anal opening. A major challenge for either type of surgical repair is finding, using, or creating adequate nerve and muscle structures around the rectum to provide for normal evacuation.

Preoperatively, nursing care focuses on maintaining NPO status and gastric decompression and administering intravenous therapy and antibiotic therapy as ordered. Provide a full explanation of the defect, surgical options, potential complications, typical postoperative course, and long-term care needed to the parents. Make sure they are aware of the available treatment modalities.

Postoperative care includes providing pain relief, maintaining NPO status and gastric decompression until normal bowel function is restored, and providing colostomy care if applicable.

Genitourinary System Structural Anomalies

Although genitourinary structural anomalies typically are not life-threatening, they do pose problems. When a newborn has a structural anomaly involving the genitourinary system, parents begin to think about continence issues and the reproductive ability of their offspring. Discussing long-term outcomes immediately after the defect is diagnosed is often difficult. The nurse must provide continued support and teaching and give honest answers to the parents' questions. Developing a therapeutic relationship with the parents is important to allay their anxieties and fears during this stressful period.

Hypospadias

Hypospadias involves an abnormal positioning of the urinary meatus on the underside of the penis (Fig. 24-15A). The degree of hypospadias depends on the location of the opening. It is often accompanied by a downward bowing of the penis (chordee), which can lead to urination and erection problems in adulthood (CDC, 2004).

Hypospadias is a relatively common birth defect that occurs in approximately 1 of every 300 male births in the United States (Gatti & Kirsch, 2003). The malformation is the result of incomplete fusion of the urethral folds, which usually occurs between 9 and 12 weeks of gestation (Porter et al., 2005). The cause is unknown, but it is thought to be of multifactorial inheritance, because it occasionally occurs in more than one male in the same family.

Hypospadias can be corrected surgically. Depending on the severity, the correction can be completed in one or more procedures with good results. Surgical intervention should be completed during the first year of life to prevent any body image problems in the child.

Epispadias

Epispadias is a rare congenital genitourinary defect occurring in 1 of 117,000 male births and 1 of 484,000 female births (Gilbert, 2004). The condition is usually diagnosed at birth or shortly thereafter. In boys with epispadias, the urethra generally opens on the top or side rather than the tip of the penis. In females, the urinary meatus is located between the clitoris and the labia. This anomaly often occurs in conjunction with exstrophy of the bladder (McKinney et al., 2005). Surgical correction is necessary, and affected male newborns should not be circumcised (Lowdermilk & Perry 2004; see Fig. 24-15B).

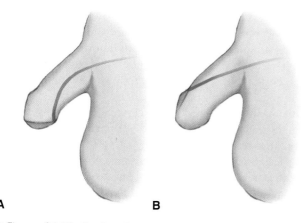

A   **B**

● Figure 24-15 Genitourinary tract structural anomalies. (**A**) Hypospadias. (**B**) Epispadias.

Bladder Exstrophy

In bladder exstrophy, the bladder protrudes onto the abdominal wall because the abdominal wall failed to close during embryonic development. Wide separation of the rectus muscles and the symphysis pubis accompanies this defect. Virtually all affected male infants have associated epispadias. The upper urinary tract is usually normal. The incidence is approximately 1 in 24,000 to 40,000 live births (Botwinski, 2004).

Treatment is surgical reconstruction performed in several stages. Goals of therapy include restoring urinary continence, preserving renal function, and reconstructing functional and cosmetically acceptable genitalia. Initial bladder closure is completed within 48 hours of birth, with epispadias repair taking place at the same time if possible. Surgery to reconstruct the bladder neck and reimplant the ureters is performed at about 2 to 3 years of age. Some children require permanent urinary diversion because a functional bladder cannot be reconstructed (Blaivas, 2004) (Fig. 24-16).

Nursing care for the newborn with bladder exstrophy includes the following activities:

- Identify the genitourinary defect at birth so that immediate treatment can be provided.
- Cover the exposed bladder with a sterile clear non adherent dressing to prevent hypothermia and infection.
- Irrigate the bladder surface with sterile saline after each diaper change to prevent infection.
- Assist with insertion and monitoring of a suprapubic catheter to drain the bladder and prevent obstruction.
- Administer antibiotic therapy as ordered to prevent infection.
- Schedule diagnostic tests to assess for additional anomalies.
- Assess the newborn frequently for any signs of infection.
- Maintain modified Bryant traction for immobilization after surgery.
- Administer antispasmodics, analgesics, and sedatives as ordered to prevent bladder spasm and provide comfort.
- Educate the parents about the care of the urinary catheter at home if applicable.
- Support the parents throughout.
- Promote bonding by encouraging the parents to visit and touch the newborn.
- Refer the parents to a support group to enhance their coping ability.
- Be a therapeutic listener to the family (Verklan & Walden, 2004).

Musculoskeletal System Structural Anomalies

Clubfoot and developmental dysplasia of the hip, two common congenital anomalies of the musculoskeletal system, can hamper the child's ability to become mobile.

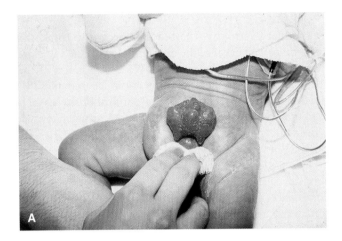

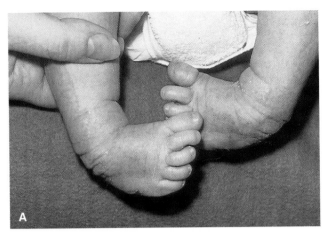

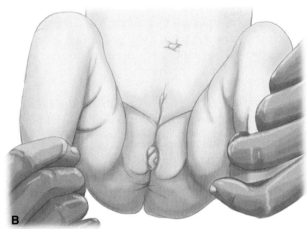

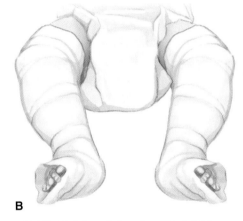

● Figure 24-16 Bladder exstrophy. (**A**) Before surgical correction. (**B**) After surgery.

● Figure 24-17 Clubfoot deformity. (**A**) Initial appearance. (**B**) Application of cast.

These anomalies can be identified with a careful examination at birth or soon after and need early intervention. Treatment is typically successful.

Congenital Clubfoot

Clubfoot, or talipes equinovarus, is a congenital deformity that typically has four components: inversion and adduction of the forefoot, inversion of the heel and hindfoot, limitation of extension of the ankle and subtalar joint, and internal rotation of the leg (Gore & Spencer, 2004). Reducing or eliminating all of the components of the deformity is the goal to ensure that the newborn has a functional, mobile, painless foot that does not require the use of special or modified shoes (Faulks & Luther, 2005).

The incidence of clubfoot is approximately 1 case per 1,000 live births in the United States. It is bilateral in about half of the cases and affects boys slightly more often than girls (Patel & Herzenberg, 2005) (Fig. 24-17). Clubfoot is a complex, multifactorial deformity with genetic and intrauterine factors. Heredity and race seem to factor into the incidence, but the means of transmission and the etiology are unknown. Most newborns who

have clubfoot have no identifiable genetic, syndromal, or extrinsic cause.

On examination, the foot appears "down and in." It is smaller, with a flexible, softer heel because of the hypoplastic calcaneus. The heel is internally rotated, making the soles of the feet face each other when the deformity occurs bilaterally.

Clubfoot can be classified into extrinsic (supple) type, which is essentially a severe positional or soft tissue deformity, or intrinsic (rigid) type, where manual reduction is not possible. The type of clubfoot deformity determines the treatment course. Treatment for the extrinsic (supple) type consists of serial casting, followed by maintenance splinting. Treatment for the intrinsic (rigid) type includes initial casting followed by surgery. It is generally agreed that the initial treatment should be nonsurgical and started soon after birth.

Treatment for either type starts with serial casting, which is needed due to the rapid growth of the newborn. Casts initially are changed weekly and are applied until the deformity responds and is fully corrected. If serial casting is not successful in correcting the deformity, surgical intervention is necessary between 4 and 9 months of age (Morcuenda et al., 2004).

Nursing management focuses on education, anticipatory guidance, and pain management. Educate the parents about their newborn's condition and the treatment protocol to reduce their anxiety, and provide reassurance that the clubfoot is not painful and will not hinder the child's development. Discuss challenges associated with sleep, play, and dressing. Inform them that slight modifications will be necessary to accommodate the plaster casts. Review positioning, bathing, and skin care along with pain management when new casts are applied. Stress the need to provide a calm, quiet environment to promote relaxation and sleep for their newborn.

Developmental Dysplasia of the Hip

Developmental dysplasia of the hip (DDH) involves abnormal growth or development of the hip that results in instability. This includes hips that are unstable, subluxated, or dislocated (luxated) or have a malformed acetabulum. This instability allows the femoral head to become easily displaced from the acetabulum. Typically, the newborn with DDH is otherwise healthy, usually without any other deformities.

The etiology of DDH is not clear, but associated factors include racial background (Native Americans), genetic transmission (runs in families), intrauterine positioning (breech), sex (female), oligohydramnios, birth order (first-born), and postnatal infant-carrying positions (swaddling, which forces the hips to be adducted). The incidence of hip instability is about 10 per 1,000 live births (McCarthy, 2005).

DDH is frequently not identified during the newborn examination. Newborns require careful evaluation for hip dysplasia at subsequent visits throughout the first year. Two maneuvers are used to assess hip instability in the newborn: Ortolani and Barlow (see Chapter 18 for more information on performing these maneuvers). Ortolani's maneuver elicits the sensation of the dislocated hip reducing; Barlow's maneuver detects the unstable hip dislocating from the acetabulum. Additional physical signs of DDH include an symmetric number of skin folds on the thigh or buttock, an apparent or true short leg, and limited hip abduction (Fig. 24-18; Hernandez & Glass, 2005).

Treatment is started as soon as DDH is identified to bring about a more favorable outcome. If a positive Ortolani or Barlow sign is found on the newborn examination, the newborn is referred to an orthopaedist. The goal of treatment is to relocate the femoral head in the acetabulum to facilitate normal growth and development. The Pavlik harness is the most widely used device; it prevents adduction while allowing flexion and abduction to accomplish the treatment goal (Fig. 24-19). The harness is worn continuously until the hip is stable, which make take several months. If harnessing is not successful, surgery is necessary.

Nursing care related to DDH starts with recognition of the disorder and early reporting to the health care provider. Early diagnosis is the crucial aspect; education also is key. Teach the parents how to care for their newborn while in the harness during treatment. Proper fit and adjustments for growth are essential for successful treatment. Frequent clinical assessment on an outpatient basis is needed to monitor progress. Through education, the nurse can be very effective in helping the parents to stay compliant with treatment.

KEY CONCEPTS

● Asphyxia, the most common clinical insult in the perinatal period, results in brain injury and may lead to mental retardation, cerebral palsy, or seizures.

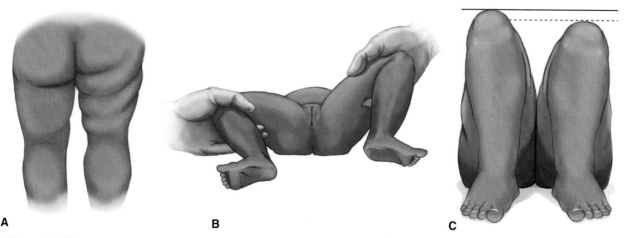

● Figure 24-18 Characteristics of developmental dysplasia of the hip. (**A**) Asymmetric number of skin folds on the thigh or buttock. (**B**) Limited hip abduction. (**C**) Appearance of short leg.

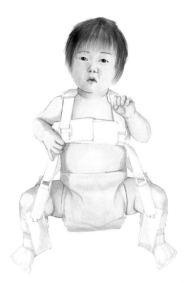

● Figure 24-19 The Pavlik harness to treat developmental dysplasia of the hip.

● Transient tachypnea of the newborn occurs when the liquid in the lung is removed slowly or incompletely.

● Common risk factors for respiratory distress syndrome (RDS) include young gestational age, perinatal asphyxia regardless of gestational age, cesarean birth in the absence of labor (related to the lack of thoracic squeeze), male gender, and maternal diabetes.

● Meconium aspiration has three major pulmonary effects: airway obstruction, surfactant dysfunction, and chemical pneumonitis.

● The management of persistent pulmonary hypertension of the newborn requires meticulous attention to detail, with continuous monitoring of oxygenation, blood pressure, and perfusion.

● Bronchopulmonary dysplasia is a newborn lung disease that follows a lung injury secondary to mechanical ventilation and oxygen toxicity.

● Retinopathy of prematurity (ROP) is a developmental abnormality that affects the immature vasculature of the retina: abnormal growth of blood vessels (neovascularization) takes place within the retina and vitreous.

● Periventricular/intraventricular hemorrhage is bleeding that usually originates in the subependymal germinal matrix region of the brain with extension into the ventricular system.

● Necrotizing enterocolitis (NEC) is a serious gastrointestinal disease of unknown etiology in newborns that can result in necrosis of a segment of the bowel.

● Infants of diabetic mothers are at risk for malformations most frequently involving the cardiovascular, skeletal, central nervous, gastrointestinal, and genitourinary systems; cardiac anomalies are the most common.

● Factors that place the newborn at risk for birth trauma include cephalopelvic disproportion, mater-

nal pelvic anomalies, oligohydramnios, prolonged or rapid labor, abnormal presentation, fetal prematurity, fetal macrosomia, and fetal abnormalities.

● Women who use drugs during their pregnancy expose their unborn child to the possibility of intrauterine growth restriction, prematurity, neurobehavioral and neurophysiologic dysfunction, birth defects, infections, and long-term developmental sequelae.

● Newborns of women who abuse tobacco, illicit substances, caffeine, and alcohol can exhibit withdrawal behavior.

● Physiologic jaundice is a common, normal newborn phenomenon that appears during the second or third day of life and then declines over the first week after birth. Pathologic jaundice is manifested within the first 24 hours of life when total bilirubin levels increase by more than 5 mg/dL/day and the total serum bilirubin level is higher than 17 mg/dL in a full-term infant.

● Newborn infections are usually classified according to the time of onset and grouped into three categories: congenital infection, acquired in utero by vertical transmission with onset before birth; early-onset neonatal infections, acquired by vertical transmission in the perinatal period, either shortly before or during birth; and late-onset neonatal infections, acquired by horizontal transmission in the nursery.

● There are several ways to classify pathogens that cause neonatal sepsis; typically three categories are used—bacterial, TORCH, and fungal.

● Congenital conditions, often referred to as birth defects, do not follow a recognized classical Mendelian inheritance pattern. Most have a complex etiology, involving many interacting genes, gene products, and social and environmental factors that may lead to structural malformations.

● Congenital heart disease is commonly classified physiologically as defects that result in increased pulmonary blood flow, defects that result in decreased pulmonary blood flow, defects that cause obstruction to blood flow out of the heart, and defects with cyanosis and increased pulmonary blood flow or mixed defects.

● Inborn errors of metabolism are genetic disorders that disrupt normal metabolic function. They are individually rare but collectively are responsible for significant levels of infant mortality and morbidity.

● Congenital structural anomalies may be inherited or sporadic, isolated or multiple, apparent or hidden, gross or microscopic. They cause nearly half of all deaths in term newborns and cause long-term sequelae for many.

● A worldwide decline in neural tube defects has occurred over the past few decades due to improved prevention secondary to preconception folic acid supplementation, maternal serum alpha-fetoprotein monitoring, and use of ultrasonography and amniocentesis.

- The birth of an infant who has a genetic condition, a syndrome, or a structural congenital anomaly is often a shocking and traumatic experience for the parents. Nurses play a primary role in setting the stage for the acceptance and adjustment process through their interaction with parents.

References

Allen, P. J., & Vessey, J. A. (2004). *Primary care of a child with a chronic condition* (4th ed.). St. Louis: Mosby.

Aly, H., Herson, V., Duncan, A., et al. (2005). Is bloodstream infection preventable among preterm infants? A tale of two cities. *Pediatrics, 115*(6), 1513–1518.

American Academy of Pediatrics (AAP) (2004). Management of hyperbilirubinemia in the newborn infant 35 or more weeks of gestation. *Pediatrics, 114*(1), 297–316.

American Academy of Pediatrics (AAP) (2003). Varicella-zoster infections. In L. K. Pickering (ed.), *Red book: report of the committee on infectious diseases* (26th ed., pp. 672–686). Elk Grove Village, IL: AAP.

American Academy of Pediatrics (AAP) (2000). Group B streptococcal infections. In L. K. Pickering (Ed.), *2000 red book: report of the Committee on Infectious Diseases* (25th ed., pp. 537–544). Elk Grove Village, IL: Author.

American Academy of Pediatrics (AAP) Committee on Substance Abuse (2005). Tobacco, alcohol, and other drugs: The role of the pediatrician in prevention, identification, and management of substance abuse. *Pediatrics, 115*(3), 816–821.

American Diabetes Association (ADA) (2005). Diabetic statistics for women. *American Diabetes Association.* [Online] Available at: http://www.diabetes.org/diabetes-statistics/women.jsp

American Diabetes Association (ADA) (2005). Gestational diabetes. *American Diabetes Association.* [Online] Available at: http://www.diabetes.org/gestational-diabetes.jsp

American Lung Association (ALA) (2004). Respiratory distress syndrome of the newborn fact sheet. *Lung Disease Data and Minority Lung Disease Data* [Online] Available at: http://www.lungusa.org/site/pp.asp?c=dvLUK9O0E&b=35693

American Lung Association (ALA) (2004). Bronchopulmonary dysplasia fact sheet. Search LungUSA [Online] Available at: http://www.lungusa.org/site/apps/s/content.asp?c=dvLUK9O0E&b=34706&ct=910851

Anadiotis, G. A., & Berry, G. T. (2003). Galactose-1-phosphate uridyltransferase deficiency (galactosemia). *eMedicine.* [Online] Available at: http://www.emdeicine.com/ped/topic818.htm

Annibale, D. J., & Hill, J. (2003). Periventricular hemorrhage-intraventricular hemorrhage. *eMedicine.* [Online] Available at: http://www.emedicine.com/ped/topic2595.htm

Asenjo, M. (2003). Transient tachypnea of the newborn. *eMedicine.* [Online] Available at: http://www.emedicine.com/radio/topic710.htm

Bakewell-Sachs, S., & Blackburn, S. (2003). State of the science: achievements and challenges across the spectrum of care for preterm infants. *JOGNN, 32*(5), 683–695.

Bale, J. F. (2002). Congenital infections. *Neurology Clinics, 20*(4), 1039–1060.

Ball, J. W., & Bindler, R. C. (2003). *Pediatric nursing: caring for children* (3rd ed.). Upper Saddle River, NJ: Prentice Hall.

Ballard, J. L. (2002). Treatment of neonatal abstinence syndrome with breast milk containing methadone. *Journal of Perinatal and Neonatal Nursing, 15*(4), 76–85.

Baltimore, R. S. (2003). Neonatal sepsis: epidemiology and management. *Pediatric Drugs, 5*(11), 723–740.

Barbour, L. A. (2003). New concepts: insulin resistance of pregnancy and gestational diabetes: long-term implications for mother and offspring. *Journal of Obstetrics and Gynecology, 23*(5), 545–549.

Bartlett, J. M., Wypij, D., Bellinger, D. C., et al. (2004). Effect of prenatal diagnosis on outcomes in D-transposition of the great arteries. *Pediatrics, 113*(4), 335–340.

Becske, T., & Jallo, G. (2004). Neural tube defects. *eMedicine.* [Online] Available at: http://www.emedicine.com/neuro/topic244.htm

Becske, T., & Jallo, G. (2004). Subarchnoid hemorrhage. *eMedicine.* [Online] Available at: http://www.emedicine.com/neuro/topic357.htm

Belik, J., & Al-Hamad, N. (2004). Neonatal abstinence syndrome. *eMedicine.* [Online] Available at: http://emedicine.com/ped/topic2760.htm

Bell, E. F. (2005). Preventing necrotizing enterocolitis: what works and how safe? *Pediatrics, 115*(1), 173–174.

Bellig, L. L., & Ohning, B. L. (2004). Neonatal sepsis. *eMedicine.* [Online] Available at: http://www.emedicine.com/PED/topic2630.htm

Blackburn, S. T. (2003). *Maternal, fetal and neonatal physiology: a clinical perspective* (2nd ed.). St. Louis: Saunders.

Blair, G., & Konkin, D. (2004). Esophageal atresia with or without tracheoesophageal fistula. *eMedicine.* [Online] Available at: http://emedicine.com/ped/topic2950.htm

Blaivas, A. J. (2004). Bladder exstrophy repair. *Medline Plus.* [Online] Available at: http://www.nlm.nih.gov/medlineplus/ency/article/002997.htm

Bloch, J. R. (2005). Antenatal events causing neonatal brain injury in premature infants. *JOGNN, 34*(3), 358–366.

Bodamer, O. A., & Lee, B. (2003). Maple syrup urine disease. *eMedicine.* [Online] Available at: www.emedicine.com/ped/topic1368.htm

Bosch, A. M., Grootenhuis, M. A., Bakker, H. D., Heijmans, H. S. A., Wijburg, F. A., & Last, B. F. (2004). Living with classic galactosemia: health-related quality of life consequences. *Pediatrics, 113*(5), 423–428.

Botwinski, C. (2004). Renal and genitourinary disorders. In M. T. Verklan & M. Walden, *Core curriculum for neonatal intensive care nursing* (3rd ed., pp. 794–820). St. Louis: Elsevier Saunders.

Bourgeois, M. J., & Varma, S. (2004). Congenital hypothyroidism. *eMedicine.* [Online] Available at: http://www.emedicine.com/ped/topic501.htm

Brooks, D. (2004). Retinopathy of prematurity. *Medline Plus.* [Online] Available at: http://www.nlm.nih.gov/medlineplus/ency/article/001618.htm

Cassio, A., Cacciari, E., Cicognani, A., et al. (2003). Treatment for congenital hypothyroidism: thyroxin alone or thyroxin plus triodothyronine? *Pediatrics, 111*(5), 1055–1061.

Centers for Disease Control and Prevention (CDC) (2000). Preventing congenital toxoplasmosis. *MMWR, 49*(RR-2): 57–75.

Centers for Disease Control and Prevention (CDC) (2002). Prevention of perinatal group B streptococcal disease: revised guidelines from the CDC. *MMWR, 51*(RR11), 1–12.

Centers for Disease Control and Prevention (CDC) (2004). *Surgeon General's report: women and smoking fact sheet: tobacco use and reproductive outcomes.* [Online] Available at: http://www.cdc.gov/tobacco/sgr/sgr_forwomen/factsheet_outcomes.htm

Centers for Disease Control and Prevention (CDC) (2005). Fetal alcohol syndrome: guidelines for referral and diagnosis. *National Task Force on FAS/FAE.* Atlanta: Centers for Disease Control and Prevention.

Centers for Disease Control and Prevention (CDC) (May 7, 2004). CDC report compares birth defect rates before and after folic acid mandate. *MMWR.*

Centers for Disease Control and Prevention (CDC) (2004). Use of vitamins containing folic acid among women of childbearing age, United States, 2004. *MMWR, 53*(36), 874–850.

Cheffer, N. D., & Rannalli, D. A. (2004). Newborn biologic/behavioral characteristics and psychosocial adaptations. In S. Mattson & J. E. Smith, *Core curriculum for maternal-newborn nursing* (3rd ed., pp. 437–464). St. Louis: Elsevier Saunders.

Clark, D. A., & Clark, M. B. (2004). Meconium aspiration syndrome. *eMedicine.* [Online] Available at: http://www.emedicine.com/ped/topic768.htm

Cleves, M. A., & Hobbs, C. A. (2004). Collaborative strategies for unraveling the complexity of birth defects. *Journal of Maternal-Fetal and Neonatal Medicine, 15*, 35–38.

Cowles, T., & Gonik, B. (2002). Perinatal infections. In A. Fanaroff & R. Martin (Eds.), *Neonatal-perinatal medicine: diseases of the fetus and infant* (7th ed.). St. Louis: Mosby.

Cunningham, F. G., Leveno, K. J., Bloom, S. L., Gilstrap, L. C., Hauth, J. C., & Wenstrom, K. D. (2005). *Williams's obstetrics* (22nd ed.). New York: McGraw-Hill.

Damato, E. G., & Winnen, C. W. (2002). Cytomegalovirus infection: perinatal implications. *JOGNN, 31*(1), 86–92.

Dave, A. (2005). Absent nasal flaring in a newborn with bilateral choanal stenosis. *Pediatrics, 109*(5), 989–990.

Diehl-Jones, W., & Askin, D. F. (2004). Hematologic disorders. In M. T. Verklan & M. Walden, *Core curriculum for neonatal intensive care nursing* (3rd ed., pp. 728–758). St. Louis: Elsevier Saunders.

Dixon, K. T. (2004). Newborn jaundice and kernicterus. *Advance for Nurse Practitioners, 12*(12), 43–63.

Dudek, S. G. (2006). *Nutrition essentials for nursing practice* (5th ed.). Philadelphia: Lippincott Williams & Wilkins.

Dugas, M. A., Nguyen, D., Frenette, L., et al. (2005). Fluticasone inhalation in moderate cases of bronchopulmonary dysplasia. *Pediatrics, 115*(5), 566–572.

Ellenbogen, R. G. (2004). Neural tube defects in the neonatal period. *eMedicine.* [Online] Available at: http://www.emedicine.com/ped/topic2805.htm

Engstrom, J. (2004). *Maternal-neonatal nursing made incredibly easy.* Philadelphia: Lippincott Williams & Wilkins.

Faulks, S., & Luther, B. (2005). Changing paradigm for the treatment of clubfeet. *Orthopedic Nursing, 24*(1), 25–31.

FDA/Center for Food Safety and Applied Nutrition (CFSAN) (2003). Reducing the risk of *Listeria monocytogenes: FDA/CDC 2003 Update of the Listeria Action Plan.* [Online] Available at: http://vm.cfsan.fda.gov/~dms/lmr2plan.html

Finnegan, L. P., & Kaltenbach, K. (1992). Neonatal abstinence syndrome. In Hoekelman & Nelson (Eds.), *Primary pediatric care* (2nd ed., pp. 1367–1378). St. Louis: Mosby Yearbook, Inc.

Finnell, R., Gould, A., & Spiegelstein, O. (2003). Pathology and genetics of neural tube defects. *Epilepsia* (Suppl. 3), 14–23.

Foster, M. R. (2004). Spina bifida. *eMedicine.* [Online] Available at: http://www.emedicine.com/orthoped/topic557.htm

Gatti, J. M., & Kirsch, A. J. (2003). Hypospadias. *eMedicine.* [Online] Available at: http://www.emedicine.com/ped/topic1136.htm

Gilbert, E. S., & Harmon, J. S. (2003). *Manual of high-risk pregnancy and delivery* (3rd ed.). St. Louis: Mosby.

Gilbert, S. M. (2004). Epispadias. *Medline Plus.* [Online] Available at: http://www.nlm.nih.gov/medlineplus/ency/article/001285.htm

Glasser, J. G. (2003). Omphalocele and gastroschisis. *eMedicine.* [Online] Available at: http://www.emedicine.com/ped/topic1642.htm

Goldenring, J. (2004). Congenital hypothyroidism. *Medline Plus.* [Online] Available at: http://www.nlm.nih.gov/medlineplus/print/ency/article/001193.htm

Golombek, S. G. (2002). The history of congenital diaphragmatic hernia from 1850s to the present. *Journal of Perinatology, 22,* 242–246.

Gore, A. L., & Spencer, J. P. (2004). The newborn foot. *American Family Physician, 69*(4), 865–872.

Green, C. J., & Wilkinson, J. M. (2004). *Maternal newborn nursing care plans.* St. Louis: Mosby, Inc.

Guttman, C. (Jan. 1, 2005). ROP: a lifelong disease that needs to be monitored. *Ophthalmology Times,* pp. 11–12.

Hadden, R. (2004). What nurses need to know: hepatitis C & pregnancy. *AWHONN Lifelines, 8*(3), 227–231.

Harris, T. (2004). Infant of the diabetic mother (IDM). [Online] Available at: http://www.ihs.gov/MedicalPrograms/MCH/M/MCHdownloads/Chap_E_34–41.pdf

Harrod, K. S., Hanson, L., VandeVusse, L., & Heywood, P. (2003). Rh-negative status and isoimmunization update: a case-based approach to care. *Journal of Perinatal and Neonatal Nursing, 17*(3), 166–178.

Hart, J. P. (2005). Imperforate anus. *Medline Plus.* [Online] Available at: http://www.nim.nih.gov/medlineplus/ency/article/001147.htm

Hashim, M. J., & Guillet, R. (2002). Common issues in the care of the sick neonate. *American Family Physician, 66*(9), 1685–1693.

Haws, P. S. (2004). *Care of the sick neonate: a quick reference for health care providers.* Philadelphia: Lippincott Williams & Wilkins.

Hernandez, J. A., & Glass, S. M. (2005). Physical assessment of the newborn. In P. J. Thureen, J. Deacon, J. A. Hernandez, & D. M. Hall, *Assessment and care of the well newborn* (2nd ed., pp. 119–172). St. Louis: Elsevier Saunders.

Hockenberry, M. J. (2005). *Wong's essentials of pediatric nursing* (7th ed.). St. Louis: Elsevier Mosby.

Hoerst, B., & Samson, L. (2002). Perinatal infections. *Nursing Spectrum.* [Online] Available at: http://nsweb.nursingspectrum.com/ce/m23b-2.htm

Holcomb, S. S. (2005). Managing jaundice in full-term infants. *The Nurse Practitioner, 30*(1), 6–12.

Horbar, J. D., Carpenter, J. H., Buzas, J., et al. (2004). Timing of initial surfactant treatment for infants 23 to 29 weeks gestation: is routine practice evidence based? *Pediatrics, 113*(6), 1593–1602.

Hupertz, V. F., & Wyllie, R. (2003). Perinatal hepatitis C infection. *Pediatric Infectious Diseases Journal, 22*(4), 369–371.

Jazayeri, A., & Contreras, D. (2005). Macrosomia. *EMedicine.* [Online] Available at: http://www.emedicine.com/med/topic3279.htm

Johnson, T. S. (2003). Hypoglycemia and the full-term newborn: how well does birth weight for gestational age predicts risk? *JOGNN, 32*(1), 48–57.

Jones, J., Lopez, A., & Wilson, M. (2003). Congenital toxoplasmosis. *American Family Physician, 67*(10), 2131–2138.

Kaul, A. J., & Balistreri, W. F. (2002). Part five: necrotizing enterocolitis. In A. A. Fanaroff & R. J. Martin (Eds.), *Neonatal-perinatal medicine: diseases of the fetus and infant* (7th ed.). St. Louis: Mosby.

Khan, A. N., & Thomas, N. (2004). Omphalocele. *eMedicine.* [Online] Available at: http://emedicine.com/radio/topic483.htm

Kenner, C., & Lott, J. W. (2004). *Neonatal nursing handbook.* St. Louis: Saunders.

Kicklighter, S. D. (2003). Transient tachypnea of the newborn. *eMedicine.* [Online] Available at: http://emedicine.com/ped/topic2597.htm

Kronemer, K., & Snyder, A. (2004). Esophageal atresia/tracheo-esophageal fistula. *eMedicine.* [Online] Available at: http://www.emedicine.com/radio/topic704.htm

Lanting, C. I., van Tijn, D. A., Loeber, J. G., et al. (2005). Clinical effectiveness and cost effectiveness of the use of thyroxine/thyroxine-binding globulin ratio to detect congenital hypothyroidism of thyroidal and central origin in a neonatal screening program. *Pediatrics, 116*(1), 168–173.

Laroia, N. (2004). Birth trauma. *eMedicine.* [Online] Available at: http://www.emedicine.com/ped/topic2836.htm

Laughon, M., Meyer, R., Bose, C., et al. (2003). Rising birth prevalence of gastroschisis. *Journal of Perinatology, 23,* 291–293.

Lessaris, K. J. (2005). Polycythemia of the newborn. *eMedicine.* [Online] Available at: http://www.emedicine.com/ped/topic2479.htm

Lin, H., Su, B., Chen, A., et al. (2005). Oral probiotics reduce the incidence and severity of necrotizing enterocolitis in very-low-birth-weight infants. *Pediatrics, 115*(1), 1–4.

Littleton, L. Y., & Engebretson, J. C. (2005). *Maternity nursing.* Clifton Park, NY: Thomson Delmar Learning.

Lockridge, T., Caldwell, A. D., & Jason, P. (2002). Neonatal surgical emergencies: stabilization and management. *JOGNN, 31*(3), 328–339.

Lowdermilk, D. L., & Perry, S. E. (2004). *Maternity & women's health care* (8th ed.). St. Louis: Mosby, Inc.

Lund, C. H. (2004). Extracorporeal membrane oxygenation. In M. T. Verklan & M. Walden, *Core curriculum for neonatal intensive care nursing* (3rd ed., pp. 569–583). St. Louis: Elsevier Saunders.

Lynam, L., & Verklan, M. T. (2004). Neurologic disorders. In M. T. Verklan & M. Walden, *Core curriculum for neonatal nursing* (3rd ed., pp. 821–857). St. Louis: Elsevier Saunders.

Madan, A., Huntsinger, K., Burgos, A., & Benitz, W. E. (2004). Readmission for newborn jaundice: the value of the Coombs' test in predicting the need for phototherapy. *Clinical Pediatrics, 43,* 63–68.

March of Dimes (MOD) (2005). Illicit drug use during pregnancy. *MOD Quick Reference: Fact Sheets.* [Online] Available at: http://www.marchofdimes.com/professionals/14332_1169.asp

March of Dimes (MOD) (2005). Medical References: Congenital heart defects. *March of Dimes Birth Defects Foundation* [Online] Available at: http://www.marchofdimes.com/printableArticles/681_1212.asp?printable=true

March of Dimes (MOD) (2005). Drinking alcohol during pregnancy. *March of Dimes Fact Sheets.* [Online] Available at: http://www.marchofdimes.com/professionals/681_1170.asp

March of Dimes (MOD) (2005). Smoking during pregnancy. *March of Dimes Fact Sheets.* [Online] Available at: http://www.marchofdimes.com/professionals/14332_1171.asp

Maternal & Neonatal Health (MNH) (2005). Best practices: detecting and treating newborn asphyxia. *MNH Program* [Online] Available at: http://www.mnh.jhpiego.org/best/detasphyxia.asp

Mattson, S., & Smith, J. E. (2004). *Core curriculum for maternal-newborn nursing* (3rd ed.). St. Louis: Elsevier Saunders.

McCarthy, J. (2005). Developmental dysplasia of the hip. *eMedicine.* [Online] Available at: http://www.emedicine.com/orthoped/topic456.htm

McKinney, E. S., James, S. R., Murray, S. S., & Ashwill, J. W. (2005). *Maternal-child nursing* (2nd ed.). St. Louis: Elsevier Saunders.

Meleski, M. E., & Damato, E. G. (2003). HIV exposure: neonatal considerations. *JOGNN, 32*(1), 109–116.

Merenstein, G., Adams, K., & Weisman, L. (2002). Infections in the neonate. In G. Merenstein & S. Gardner (Eds.), *Handbook of neonatal intensive care* (5th ed.). St. Louis: Mosby.

Messinger, D. S., Bauer, C. R., Das, A., et al. (2004). The maternal lifestyle study: cognitive and behavioral outcomes of cocaine-exposed and opiate-exposed infants through three years of age. *Pediatrics, 113*(6), 1677–1693.

Mijuskovic, Z. P., & Karadaglic, D. (2005). Phenylketonuria. *eMedicine.* [Online] Available at: http://www.emedicine.com/derm/topic712.htm

Minnesota Department of Health (MDH) (2004). Tobacco and pregnancy tip sheet. [Online] Available at: http://wwwhealth.state.mn.us/divs/fh/mch/mortality/tobacco-tipsheet.pdf

Molmenti, H. (2004). Imperforate anus repair. *Medline Plus.* [Online] Available at: http://nlm.nih.gov/medlineplus/ency/article/002926.htm

Morcuenda, J. A., Dolan, L. A., Dietz, F. R., & Ponseti, I. V. (2004). Radical reduction in the rate of extensive corrective surgery for clubfoot using the Ponseti method. *Pediatrics, 113*(2), 376–380.

Montoya, K. D., & Washington, R. L. (2002). Cardiovascular disease and surgical interventions. In G. B. Merenstein & S. L. Gardner (Eds.), *Handbook of neonatal intensive care* (5th ed.). St. Louis: Mosby.

Moore, T. R. (2004). Diabetes mellitus and pregnancy. *eMedicine.* [Online] Available at: http://www.emedicine.com/med/topic3249.htm

Mullaney, D. M. (2001). Group B streptococcal infections in newborns. *JOGNN, 30*(6), 649–658.

Murray, E., & Wewers, M. E. (2004). Nurses can play a significant role in reducing tobacco use in the U.S. *AWHONN Lifelines, 8*(3), 200–206.

Murray, J. C., & Schutte, B. C. (2004). Cleft palate: players, pathways, and pursuits. *Journal of Clinical Investigation, 113*(12), 1676–1678.

National Eye Institute (NEI) (2005). Retinopathy of prematurity. *NEI Health Information,* [Online] Available at: http://www.nei.nih.gov/health/rop/index.asp

National Institute on Drug Abuse (NIDA) (2005). NIDA InfoFacts: crack and cocaine. *National Institutes of Health.* [Online] Available at: http://www.drugabuse.gov/infofacts/cocaine.html

National Institute on Drug Abuse (NIDA) (2005). NIDA InfoFacts: heroin. *National Institutes of Health.* [Online] Available at: http://www.nida.nih.gov/Infofacts/heroin.html

National Institute on Drug Abuse (NIDA) (2005). NIDA InfoFacts: pregnancy and drug use trends. *National Institutes of Health.* [Online] Available at: http://www.drugabuse.gov/Infofacts/pregnancytrends.html

National Institute on Drug Abuse (NIDA) (2005). NIDA InfoFacts: marijuana. *National Institutes of Health.* [Online] Available at: http://www.nida.nih.gov/Infofacts/marijuana.html

National Institute on Drug Abuse (NIDA) (2005). NIDA InfoFacts: methamphetamine. *National Institutes of Health.* [Online] Available at: http://www.drugabuse.gov/infofacts/methamphetamine.html

National Institute on Drug Abuse (NIDA) (2005). NIDA Research Report: heroin abuse and addiction. *NIH Publication Number*

05–4165. [Online] Available at: http://www.drugabuse.gov/ResearchReports/Heroin/heroin4.html

National Institutes of Health (NIH) Consensus Development Conference Statement (2002). Management of hepatitis C. *Hepatology, 36*(5, Suppl.1), S3–S20.

Olds, S. B., London, M. L., Ladewig, P. W., & Davidson, M. R. (2004). *Maternal-newborn nursing & women's health care* (7th ed.). Upper Saddle River, NJ: Pearson Prentice Hall.

O'Toole, M. T. (2005). *Encyclopedia & dictionary of medicine, nursing and allied health* (7th ed.). Philadelphia: Elsevier Saunders.

Ozen, N., & Mukherjee, S. (2004). Hyperbilirubinemia, unconjugated. *eMedicine.* [Online] Available at: http://www.emedicine.com/med/topic1066.htm

Pasero, C. (2004). Pain relief for neonates. *AJN, 104*(5), 44–47.

Patel, M., & Herzenberg, J. (2005). Clubfoot. *eMedicine.* [Online] Available at: http://www.emedicine.com/orthoped/topic598.htm

Pelchat, D., Lefebvre, H., Proulx, M., & Reidy, M. (2004). Parental satisfaction with an early family intervention program. *Journal of Perinatal and Neonatal Nursing, 18*(2), 128–144.

Pitts, K. (2004). Perinatal substance abuse. In M. T. Verklan & M. Walden, *Core curriculum for neonatal intensive care nursing* (3rd ed., pp. 487–523). St. Louis: Elsevier Saunders.

Porter, M. L., & Dennis, B. L. (2002). Hyperbilirubinemia in the term newborn. *American Family Physician, 65*(4), 599–606.

Porter, M. P., Faizan, M. K., Grady, R. W., & Mueller, B. A. (2005) Hypospadias in Washington state: maternal risk factors and prevalence trends. *Pediatrics, 115*(4), 495–499.

Rawlins, S. (2001). Nonviral sexually transmitted infections. *JOGNN, 30*(3), 324–331.

Rempel, G. R., Cender, L. M., Lynam, M. J., Sandor, G. G., & Farquharson, D. (2004). Parents' perspectives on decision making after antenatal diagnosis of congenital heart disease. *JOGNN, 33*(1), 64–70.

Rodriguez, R. J. (2003). Management of respiratory distress syndrome: an update. *Respiratory Care, 48*(3), 279–287.

Sarici, S. U., Serdar, M. A., Korkmaz, A., et al. (2004). Incidence, course, and prediction of hyperbilirubinemia in near-term and term newborns. *Pediatrics, 113*(4), 775–780.

Schaefer, U. M., Kjos, S. L., Kilavuz, O., et al. (2003). Determinants of fetal growth at different periods of pregnancies complicated by gestational diabetes mellitus or impaired glucose tolerance. *Diabetes Care, 26*(1), 193–198.

Schleiss, M. R. (2005). Cytomegalovirus infection. *eMedicine.* [Online] Available at: http://www.emedicine.com/PED/topic544.htm

Sgouros, S. (2004). Management of spina bifida, hydrocephalus and shunts. *eMedicine.* [Online] Available at: http://www.emedicine.com/ped/topic2976.htm

Shaffer, T. H., Wolfson, M. R., & Panitch, H. B. (2004). Airway structure, function and development in health and disease. *Pediatric Anesthesia, 14*, 3–14.

Smith, A., & McHugh, M. (May 17, 2004). Atrial septal defect repair: a new device bypasses surgery. *Nursing Spectrum*, pp. 12–14.

Springer, S. C., & Annibale, D. J. (2002). Necrotizing enterocolitis. *eMedicine.* [Online] Available at: http://www.emedicine.com/ped/topic2601.htm

Springer, S. C., & Annibale, D. J. (2004). Kernicterus. *eMedicine.* [Online] Available at: http://www.emedicine.com/ped/topic1247.htm

Steinhorn, R. H. (2004). Pulmonary hypertension, persistent-newborn. *eMedicine.* [Online] Available at: http://www.emedicine.com/ped/topic2530.htm

Stewart, D. R. (2004). Galactosemia. *Medline Plus.* [Online] Available at: http://www.nlm.nih.gov/medlineplus/print/ency/article/000366.htm

Stoll, B. J. (2004). Infections of the neonatal infant. In R. E. Behrman, R. M. Kliegman, & H. B. Jenson (Eds.), *Nelson textbook of pediatrics* (17th ed., pp. 623–640). Philadelphia: Saunders.

Swearingen, P. L. (2004). *All-in-one care planning resource: medical-surgical, pediatric, maternity, and psychiatric nursing care plans.* St. Louis: Mosby, Inc.

Tesselaar, C. D., Postema, R. R., van Dooren, M. F., Allegaert, K., & Tibboel, D. (2004). Congenital diaphragmatic hernia and situs inversus totalis. *Pediatrics, 113*(5), 256–258.

Tewfik, T. L., & Hagr, A. A. (2005) Choanal atresia. *eMedicine.* [Online]. Available at: http://www.emedicine.com/ent/topic330.htm

Thureen, P. J., Deacon, J., Hernandez, J. A., & Hall, D. M. (2005). *Assessment and care of the well newborn* (2nd Ed.). St. Louis: Elsevier Saunders.

Tiller, C. M. (2002). Chlamydia during pregnancy: implications and impact on perinatal and neonatal outcomes. *JOGNN, 31*(1), 93–98.

Tolarova, M. M. (2004). Cleft lip and palate. *eMedicine.* [Online] Available at: http://www.emedicine.com/ped/topic2679.htm

U.S. Department of Health and Human Services (USDHHS) (2000). *Healthy people 2010:* Volumes 1 and 2 (Conference ed.) Washington, D.C: U.S. Government Printing Office.

Vachha, B., & Adams, R. (2005). Myelomeningocele, temperament patterns, and parental perceptions. *Pediatrics, 115*(1), 58–63.

Verklan, M. T., & Walden, M. (2004). *Core curriculum for neonatal intensive care nursing* (3rd ed.). St. Louis: Elsevier Saunders.

Vision Channel (2004). Retinopathy of prematurity. *Vision Channel* [Online] Available at: http://visionchannel.net/retinopathy

Wagle, S., & Deshpande, P. G. (2003). Hemolytic disease of the newborn. *eMedicine.* [Online] Available at: http://www.emedicine.com/ped/topic959.htm

Wang, M. (2004). Perinatal drug abuse and neonatal drug withdrawal. *eMedicine.* [Online] Available at: http://emedicine.com/ped/topic2631.htm

Weiner, D. L. (2005). Pediatrics, inborn errors of metabolism. *eMedicine.* [Online] Available at: http://emedicine.com/emerg/topic768.htm

Weiner, S. M. (2005). Perinatal substance abuse. *Advance for Nurses,* 6(13), 17–20.

Whitby, E. H., Griffiths, P. D., Rutter, S., et al. (2003). Frequency and natural history of subdural hemorrhages in babies and relation to obstetric factors. *Lancet, 362,* 846–851.

Wood, B. P. (2005). Necrotizing enterocolitis. *eMedicine.* [Online] Available at: http://www.emedicine.com/radio/topic469.htm

Woods, D. (2004). Neonatal resuscitation. *International Association for Maternal and Neonatal Health* (IAMANEH) [Online] Available at: http://www.gfmer.ch/Medical_education_En/PGC_RH_2004/Neonatal_asphyxia.htm

Wu, L., & Garcia, R. A. (2005). Toxoplasmosis. *eMedicine.* [Online] Available at: http://www.emedicine.com/oph/topic707.htm

Yerkes, E. B., & Rink, R. C. (2002). Exstrophy and epispadias. *eMedicine.* [Online] Available at: http://emedicine.com/ped/topic704.htm

Zukowsky, K. (2004). Respiratory distress. In M. T. Verklan & M. Walden, *Core curriculum for neonatal intensive care nursing* (3rd ed., pp. 487–523). St. Louis: Elsevier Saunders.

Web Resources

AHRQ's Tobacco Pathfinder: **www.ahrq.gov**
American Cleft Palate Association: **www.cleftline.org**
American Diabetes Association: **www.diabetes.org**
American Society of Plastic Surgeons: **www.plasticsurgery.org**
Anencephaly Support Foundation: **www.asfhelp.com**
Association for Bladder Exstrophy Community:
     www.bladderexstrophy.com
Association of Retinopathy of Prematurity: **www.ropard.org**
Birth Defects for Children: **www.birthdefects.org**
Centers for Disease Control and Prevention: **www.cdc.gov**
Congenital Heart Defects: **www.congenitalheartdefects.com**
Esophageal Atresia/Tracheoesophageal Fistula Family Support
     Connection: **www.eatef.org**
Maple Syrup Urine Disease Family Support Group:
     www.msud-support.org
March of Dimes Birth Defects Foundation:
     www.marchofdimes.com
Narcotics Anonymous: **www.na.org**
National Association for Continence: **www.nafc.org**
National Center on Birth Defects and Developmental Disabilities:
     www.cdc.gov/ncbddd/fas
National Clearinghouse for Alcohol and Drug Abuse Information:
     www.health.org
National Eye Institute: **www.nei.nih.gov**
National Institute on Alcohol Abuse and Alcoholism:
     www.niaaa.nih.gov
National Organization for Rare Disorders (NORD):
     www.rarediseases.org
National Organization on Fetal Alcohol Syndrome: **www.nofas.org**
National Women's Health Information Center: **www.4woman.gov**
Neonatal Network: **www.neonatalnetwork.com**
Parental Guide for Developmentally Supportive Care:
     www.comeunity.com/premature/baby/supportive-care.html
Parents of Galactosemic Children, Inc.: **www.galactosemia.org**
Partnership for a Drug-Free America: **www.drugfreeamerica.org**
Physical and Developmental Environment of the High-Risk Infant:
     www.med.usf.edu/-tsinger
Safe Motherhood Initiative: **www.safemotherhood.org**
SHARE Pregnancy & Infant Loss Support, Inc.:
     www.nationalshareoffice.com
Spina Bifida Association of America: **www.sbaa.org**
Substance Abuse & Mental Health Services:
     www.findtreatment.samhsa.gov

ChapterWORKSHEET

● MULTIPLE CHOICE QUESTIONS

1. Which findings would lead the nurse to suspect newborn respiratory distress?

   a. Abdominal distention

   b. Acrocyanosis

   c. Depressed fontanels

   d. Nasal flaring

2. When assessing the substance-exposed newborn, the nurse would expect to find:

   a. Calm facial appearance

   b. Daily weight gain

   c. Increasing irritability

   d. Feeding and sleeping well

3. Which newborn condition might be overlooked if there is inadequate ingestion of protein prior to screening?

   a. Congenital hypothyroidism

   b. Sickle cell anemia

   c. Cystic fibrosis

   d. Phenylketonuria (PKU)

4. A newborn with tracheoesophageal fistula is likely to present with which assessment finding?

   a. Subnormal temperature

   b. Absent Moro reflex

   c. Inability to swallow

   d. Foamy bubbles or drooling from mouth

● CRITICAL THINKING EXERCISES

1. As the nursery nurse, you receive a newborn from the labor and birth suite and place him under the radiant warmer. The nurse who gives you report states that the mother couldn't remember when her membranes broke before labor and that she ran a fever during labor for the past few hours. The Apgar scores were good, but the newborn seemed lethargic. As you begin your assessment, you note that she is pale and floppy and has a subnormal temperature; heart rate is 180 bpm and respiratory rate is 70 breaths per minute.

   a. What in the mother's history should raise a red flag to the nurse?

   b. What condition is this neonate at high risk for?

   c. What interventions are appropriate for this condition?

2. Terry, a day-old baby girl, is very fretful, and calming measures don't seem to work. As the nursery nurse you notice that she is losing weight and her formula intake is poor, even though she is manifesting hungry behavior. The mother received no prenatal care and denied drug use, but her drug screen was positive for heroin.

   a. What additional information do you need to obtain from the mother?

   b. What additional laboratory work might be needed for Terry?

   c. What specific measures need to be made for her ongoing care?

3. A baby girl weighing 7.5 pounds was born after a gestation of 41 weeks by cesarean section. She is brought to the nursery. On your initial assessment you find a floppy infant with short stature, dry, brittle hair, a short, thick neck, dull-appearing facial features, a thick, protruding tongue, and a hoarse-sounding cry.

   a. What is your impression of this newborn?

   b. What laboratory studies and results would you anticipate?

   c. What explanation could be offered to the parents concerning this condition?

● STUDY ACTIVITIES

1. Arrange for a tour of a regional NICU to see the nurse's role in caring for sick neonates. Ask the nurse to give a quick history of each newborn's condition. Was the nurse's role like you imagined? What was your impression of the NICU, and how would you describe it to expectant parents?

2. Select a website from the list at the end of the chapter. What kind of information is given? How helpful would it be for parents with an infant diagnosed with a specific condition?

3. Contact a local childbirth educator and ask permission to present a brief informational session to expectant parents at a natural childbirth class on the importance of newborn screening tests. What should be your "take-home message" to them?

4. A herniation of a newborn's abdominal contents present at birth describes _____.

5. An abnormal opening between the ventricles of the heart, a common cardiac defect found in infants of diabetic mothers, is _____.

Glossary

A

Abdominal effleurage: soft massage of the abdomen

Abortion: removal of products of conception from the uterus before viable fetal life

Abruptio placentae: separation of a normally implanted placenta from the uterine wall before birth

Abstinence: voluntary self-deprivation of potential pleasures (e.g., certain foods, alcohol, or sexual activity)

Acceleration: rise in baseline fetal heart rate for a period of time

Acme: peak intensity of a uterine contraction

Acquired disorder: bodily condition not inherited genetically

Acquired immunodeficiency syndrome (AIDS): serious impairment of cell immunologic functions occurring after a long incubation time, followed by prolonged debilitating body conditions that usually result in death

Acrocyanosis: bluish color of hands or feet caused by poor peripheral circulation

Active acquired immunity: antibody responses to illness or immunization

Active phase: the second phase of labor in which the cervix dilates from 3 or 4 cm to full dilation

Afterpains: abdominal cramp-like pains caused by uterine contractions after birth; they may last for a few days and tend to be more severe during breast-feeding

Alpha-fetoprotein (AFP): glycoprotein produced by the fetal development process that crosses the placenta and can be detected in the maternal blood; can be used as a marker for Down syndrome (decreased AFP) and neural tube defects (increased AFP)

Amnion: the innermost fetal membrane that forms the sac holding the embryo/fetus and amniotic fluid

Amniotic fluid embolism: leakage of amniotic and fetal matter into the maternal circulation; blocks pulmonary circulation and causes a life-threatening situation

Amniotomy: mechanical rupturing of fetal membranes using an instrument

Ampulla: outer area of the fallopian tube where fertilization of the ovum occurs

Androgen: substance that produces testosterone and other male characteristics

Anencephaly: lack of cerebral hemispheres and skull encasing the brain due to a congenital deformation

Anovulatory cycle: menstrual cycle in which an ovum is not released

Anovulatory: absence of ovulation

Anterior fontanel: diamond-shaped area above the newborn's forehead that is formed by two frontal and two parietal bones; it typically closes between 12 and 18 months

Antiretroviral therapy: drug regimen used to destroy or suppress viruses

Apgar score: numerical assessment system for infant heart rate, respiratory effect, muscle tone, reflex irritability, and color; it is taken at 1 and 5 minutes after birth

Apnea: cessation of respirations for 15 to 20 seconds, or long enough to cause cyanosis; it is of unknown cause and occurs 24 to 48 hours after birth; it resolves spontaneously in a few days with no special treatment

Asphyxia: decrease in oxygen and accumulation of carbon dioxide due to gas exchange problems; creates a life-threatening condition

Asymmetric intrauterine growth restriction: higher percentile growth rate of fetal length to head circumference than standardized weight-based rates

Atony: absence of uterine muscle tone

Attachment: affection-forming relationship and feeling of bonding between humans that occurs over time

Augmentation of labor: pharmacologic or physical methods of labor stimulation and uterine contractions after natural labor has begun

Autosome: chromosome included in the 22 pairs that is identical in males and females

B

Babinski reflex: a normal infant response characterized by hyperextension of the toes and dorsiflexion of the great toe upon stroking of the sole of the foot

Bacterial vaginosis: a vaginal bacteria infection characterized by a grayish discharge and a foul fishy odor

Ballottement: examination technique involving finger tapping to detect a floating fetus during pregnancy; the fetus is pushed away and rebounds against the examiner's fingers

Baseline fetal heart rate: average fetal heart rate between contractions and accelerations of labor

Beat-to-beat variability: variations in fetal heart rate between one beat and the next over a short interval

Bilirubin: a yellow bile pigment associated with jaundice that is produced during the destruction of red blood cells

Biophysical profile (BPP): noninvasive fetal risk assessment based on breathing, body movement, volume of amniotic fluid, fetal heart rate, and tone

Birth rate: calculation of annual rate of births per 1,000 people

Blastocyst: inner cell mass of the morula occurring approximately 3 days after fertilization; it develops into the embryo

Bloody show: secretion of blood-tinged vaginal discharge resulting from rupture of small capillaries in the cervix as it begins to dilate about 24 to 48 hours before labor

Boggy: adjective used to describe softening of the uterus that occurs due to a lack of muscle tissue contraction; carries a risk for postpartum hemorrhage

Brachial palsy: partial or complete paralysis of arm parts resulting from prolonged labor or difficult birth

Braxton Hicks contractions: intermittent, painless uterine contractions occurring during pregnancy without cervical dilation; they are not associated with true labor but are sometimes mistaken as such and referred to as "false labor"

Breast self-examination (BSE): touching and visual inspection of the breasts to detect abnormalities such as masses, nipple discharge, or changes that could indicate malignancy or conditions needing assessment

Breech presentation: the fetal buttocks or feet appear in the maternal pelvis first instead of the head

Bronchopulmonary dysplasia (BPD): chronic pulmonary disease that occurs from the use of mechanical ventilation and high levels of oxygen in the weeks after birth

Brown adipose tissue: fetal and neonate fat deposits around the kidneys and adrenals, in the neck, between the scapulae, and behind the sternum

C

Caput succedaneum: soft tissue swelling or edema in or under the fetal scalp due to birth trauma

Carcinoma in situ: cancer contained only in the cells of an organ in which it originated without spreading to other tissue

Cardinal movements of labor: natural fetal position changes and movements that are accommodated by the maternal pelvis as the fetus moves from the abdominal region through the birth canal to delivery

Cephalhematoma: subperiosteal collection of blood in the infant's skull due to blood vessel rupture during labor and birth; lasts for a few weeks to 2 months

Cephalofetal disproportion: abnormal condition of fetal head size, shape, or position preventing descent through the maternal pelvis for delivery

Cerclage: suturing used to close a recurrent premature dilation of the cervix, which usually occurs between 14 and 20 weeks of gestation

Cervical cap: cup-shaped mechanical barrier contraceptive that is held in place over the cervix by suction

Cervical dilation: gradual widening of the cervical opening from less than 1 cm to nearly 10 cm to accommodate passage of the fetal head

Cervical funneling: recess in the cervix that is commonly associated with recurrent premature dilation of the cervix

Cervical ripening: softening and thinning of the cervix through the normal physiologic labor process or through induction of labor

Cesarean section: fetal delivery through a surgical incision in the abdominal wall and uterus

Chadwick's sign: violet or blue discoloration in the vaginal mucous membranes visible during pregnancy around the fourth week; due to vasocongestion

Childbirth education: prenatal courses that focus on breathing, relaxation, and position techniques during labor; the goal is to minimize the need for medication and medical procedures

Chlamydia **infection:** the most common sexually transmitted bacterial infection in the United States; caused by *Chlamydia trachomatis;* a frequent cause of sterility

Chloasma: a brown or darker pigmentation of the nose, forehead, and cheeks during pregnancy or from ingesting oral contraceptives; referred to as a "mask of pregnancy"

Chorioamnionitis: infection of the chorion, amnion, and amniotic fluid caused by organisms that can be transferred to the fetus; potentially life-threatening to the infant

Chorion: outer fetal membrane closest to the uterine wall that is lined by the trophoblast and mesoderm surrounding the amnion; forms the fetal area of the placenta

Chorionic villi: hair-like projections that carry vascular circulation to the fetus

Chorionic villus sampling: procedure to obtain fetal cells during the first trimester in order to diagnose chromosomal and congenital disorders

Chromosome: hair-like chromatin structures of the cell nucleus that contain genetic information as codes in DNA

Chronic hypertension: maternal hypertension occurring prior to week 20 of gestation, or hypertension that continues 42 days past childbirth

Circumcision: surgical removal of foreskin from the penis

Circumoral cyanosis: bluish coloration around the mouth

Clitoris: small oval-shaped area comprising erectile tissue at the anterior junction of the female vulva; homologous to the penis

Coitus interruptus: contraceptive technique in which the man withdraws his penis from the woman's vagina prior to ejaculation

Cold stress: excessive loss of body heat resulting in a compensatory mechanism such as increased respirations to maintain the core body temperature

Colostrum: yellowish breast secretion of serum and white blood cells that precedes mature breast milk; has a high level of protein and some immune and cleansing properties for the newborn's intestinal tract

Colposcopy: procedure in which a magnifying lens is inserted into the vagina for cervical and vaginal tissue examination

Conception: process in which the ovum is fertilized by union with sperm

Condom: mechanical contraceptive device that blocks sperm from entering the vagina; it is worn over the erect penis or in the female vagina; also helps prevent sexually transmitted infections

Conduction: heat transfer to a cooler area or surface through direct skin contact

Contraction stress test: method used to assess fetal reaction to natural or induced contractions

Contraction: regular or periodic tightening and shortening of the uterine muscles during natural or artificially induced labor, causing effacement and dilation of the cervix

Convection: heat transfer to cooler air from a warm body surface

Coombs test: test to check for either Rh-positive antibodies in maternal red blood cells or Rh-positive antibodies in fetal cord red blood cells

Corpus luteum: small yellow glandular mass that develops within a ruptured ovarian follicle after it has matured and discharged its ovum

Corpus: the upper two thirds of the uterus

Cotyledons: subdivisions composed of villi that are located along the uterine surface of the placenta

Crowning: appearance of the fetal head at the vulvar opening during labor

Cyanosis: blue coloration of the infant's chest, face, fingers, toes, or mucous membranes as a result of the circulatory system's inability to oxygenate the tissues fully

Cystocele: a bulge in the anterior vaginal wall as a result of downward displacement of the bladder

D

Deceleration: periodic slowing of the fetal heart rate below baseline

Decidua: nourishing cell membrane surrounding the fetus in the uterus that is shed after childbirth

Depo-Provera: progestin contraceptive that can be injected for long-term use

Descent: start of the downward movement of the fetal presenting position into the pelvis

Dilatation and curettage (D&C): dilation of the cervix and passage of a curet to scrape the endometrium; performed to eliminate the uterine contents and end pregnancy, or to obtain tissue for examination

Dilation: gradual expansion of the external os of the cervix from a few millimeters to 10 cm so that the fetus can be born

Disseminated intravascular coagulation (DIC): complex hemorrhagic disorder resulting in tissue necrosis and bleeding; possibly caused by sepsis, fetal demise, or abruptio placentae

Dizygotic: fetuses derived from two separate zygotes; referred to as fraternal twins

Doula: a companion, possibly paid, who attends to the needs of a pregnant woman through labor

Down syndrome: a genetic birth defect resulting from an extra chromosome (number 21)

Ductus arteriosus: a shunt between the pulmonary artery and the descending aorta of the fetus

Ductus venosus: a fetal shunt passing through the liver and carrying oxygenated blood between the umbilical vein and the inferior vena cava

Duration: the length of time a contraction lasts

Dysfunctional labor pattern: labor that does not exhibit normal processes

Dysfunctional uterine bleeding (DUB): any deviation from usual uterine bleeding

Dysmenorrhea: painful side effects of menstruation, including cramping in the lower abdomen, nausea, vomiting, diarrhea, and headache

Dyspareunia: pain associated with sexual intercourse

Dystocia: failed or difficult progression of labor due to physical problems between the fetus and the maternal pelvis, or from uterine or other muscular problems

E

Early-onset deceleration: fetal heart rate slowing in which the head compresses at the onset of a uterine contraction; as the contraction ends, the fetal heart rate slowly returns to baseline

Eclampsia: a major seizure complication of unknown causes that sometimes occurs after 20 weeks of gestation or within 48 hours postpartum

Ectopic pregnancy: implantation of a fertilized ovum in the fallopian tubes, ovaries, or abdomen instead of the usual location (the lining of the uterus)

EDB: estimated date of birth

EDC: estimated date of confinement or fetal due date

Effacement: process of thinning, shortening, and flattening of the cervix that occurs late in pregnancy or during labor

Ejaculation: release of seminal fluids due to stimulation of the penis

Electronic fetal monitoring: monitoring device placed on the fetus for continuous tracking and assessment of fetal heart rate characteristics

Embryo: name for the developing organism between 2 and 8 weeks of gestation

Emergency contraception: postcoital pregnancy-prevention methods

Endometrial biopsy: procedure used during a fertility workup to obtain information about the effects on the uterus of progesterone produced by the corpus luteum after ovulation and endometrial receptivity

Endometriosis: chronic condition in which endometrial tissue grows outside the uterus in the pelvic cavity; often associated with infertility

Endometritis: infection of the inner uterus lining

Endometrium: inner cellular lining of the uterus that is shed during menses

En-face positioning: parent and newborn maintain the same face-to-face vertical plane of vision

Engorgement: swelling of breast tissue from congestion due to increased blood supply and lymph supply after childbirth and before true lactation starts

Engrossment: parental (particularly paternal) sense of intense interest during early contact with the newborn

Epidural: technique used to provide local anesthesia to the lower body in which the anesthetic is instilled into the epidural space and transfers to the nerve roots exiting the dura

Episiotomy: surgical incision of the perineum to enlarge the vaginal opening to facilitate birth

Epispadias: condition in which the urethral meatus is located on the top surface of the penis

Erythema toxicum: temporary, pink, irregular, papular rash with superimposed vesicles

Erythroblastosis fetalis: hemolytic disease of the newborn caused by maternal antibodies; results in anemia, jaundice, enlarged liver and spleen, and generalized edema

Esophageal atresia: condition in which the esophagus ends in a pouch or narrows to a thin cord unconnected to the stomach

Estrogen: female sex hormone that is produced by the ovary and stored in fat cells; it influences reproduction

Evaporation: loss of heat resulting from water on the skin surface being converted to vapor

Evidence-based practice: medical decisions that are made based on conscientious problem-solving approaches from explicit, judicious use of research data, statistical analysis, and other reliable information sources

Exchange transfusion: replacement of circulating blood by withdrawal of the recipient's blood and injection of an equal amount of donor blood; done to prevent accumulation of bilirubin or other byproducts of hemolysis in the blood

External os: portion of the cervix opening into the vagina

Extremely low birthweight: neonate birth weight of 1,000 g or less

F

Face presentation: descent of fetus with hyperextension of head and neck, allowing the fetal face to descend into the maternal pelvis first

False labor: regular or irregular uterine contractions that are strong enough to be interpreted as real labor; however, they do not dilate the cervix

Female condom: thin, flexible, polyurethane contraceptive sheath placed inside the vagina to block sperm from entering the cervix

Fern test: procedure to determine the presence of amniotic fluid

Fertility awareness methods: natural family planning based on tracking the woman's ovulatory cycle; requires careful record keeping and sexual abstinence during the fertile part of the month

Fertility rate: number of annual births per 1,000 in women aged 15 to 44

Fertilization: the uniting of sperm with the outer layer of the female ovum that begins the development of a human embryo

Fetal acoustic stimulation test: process used to accelerate the fetal heart rate through use of a speaker, bell, or artificial larynx

Fetal alcohol syndrome (FAS): various fetal physical deformities and cognitive disabilities resulting from excessive alcohol consumption by the mother during pregnancy

Fetal attitude: relationship of fetal body parts to one another, characterized by normal flexion of the arms onto the chest and the legs onto the abdomen

Fetal circulation: path of fetal blood circulation

Fetal distress: problem involving the fetal heart rate or activity in response to the intrauterine environment

Fetal fibronectin testing: screening process used to predict preterm labor

Fetal heart rate (FHR): number of fetal heartbeats per minute; normal range is 110 to 160

Fetal lie: relationship of the fetal spine to the maternal spine; designated as longitudinal or transverse

Fetal movement counting: daily maternal record of fetal movements and activity within a set time period

Fetal position: presenting fetal part in relation to the left, right, front, or back of the maternal pelvis

Fetal presentation: fetal part that first enters the maternal pelvis; known as a cephalic, shoulder, or breech presentation

Fetus: unborn child from about 8 weeks of gestation until birth

Fibroadenoma: painless breast tumor or solid mass

Fibrocystic changes: age-related hormonal changes that commonly include breast tissue thickening and cyst formation

Fibroid tumor: benign tumor growing within the myometrium that can protrude into the uterine cavity and bulge through the outer uterine layer

First stage of labor: period that begins with regular uterine contractions and ends with complete dilation and effacement of the cervix; divided into latent, active, and transition phases

Flexion: position in which the fetal head is bent with chin on chest when resistance is met at the pelvic inlet and floor

Follicle-stimulating hormone: hormone produced by the anterior pituitary during the first half of the menstrual cycle; stimulates the ovary to prepare a mature ovum for release

Follicular phase: ovarian cycle phase that occurs when a follicle becomes mature and is prepared for ovulation

Fontanel: fetal membrane-filled area of strong, soft, connective tissue between the cranial bones of the skull that allows molding of the head during birth

Foramen ovale: opening between the right and left atria of the fetal heart

Forceps: obstetric instruments sometimes used on the presenting part of the fetus to aid in childbirth

Forth stage of labor: period that occurs during the first 2 to 4 hours after delivery of the placenta

Frequency: time from the beginning of one contraction to the beginning of the next

Fundus: upper section of the uterus between the fallopian tubes

G

Gavage feeding: nourishment supplied through a tube inserted into the nose or mouth and emptying into the stomach

Genetic counseling: information discussed with clients and families concerning genes and heredity

Genetic disorder: inherited gene defect passed from one generation to its offspring

Gestational diabetes: diabetes occurring with the onset of pregnancy or first diagnosed during pregnancy

Gestational trophoblastic disease: a malignant or benign (hydatidiform mole) disorder

Gonadotropin-releasing hormone (GnRH): neurohormone secreted by the hypothalamus that stimulates the pituitary to release prolactin and other hormones

Goodell's sign: softening of the cervix during the second month of pregnancy that usually indicates pregnancy

Graafian follicle: fully ripe ovum that secretes estrogen

Gravida: any pregnancy, regardless of outcome

Gravidity: state of pregnancy and number of times pregnant

Gynecoid pelvis: characteristic female pelvis with oval inlet slightly wider than it is high

H

Hegar's sign: softening and widening of the isthmus of the uterus; usually occurs in the second or third month of pregnancy and is detectable by palpitation

HELLP syndrome: changes associated with severe preeclampsia, including elevated liver enzyme levels, hemolysis, and a low platelet count

Hemolytic disease of the newborn: condition in which maternal antibodies cross the placenta and destroy fetal red blood cells due to isoimmunization; examples are ABO and Rh incompatibility, or inadequate vitamin K, leading to a lack of clotting factors and risk of hemorrhage

Hormone replacement therapy (HRT): supplemental use of hormones such as estrogen and progestin to ease menopausal symptoms

Human chorionic gonadotropin (hCG): hormone produced by the chorionic villi and secreted by the corpus luteum of the ovary after conception; detectable in the urine of pregnant women

Human immunodeficiency syndrome (HIV): a retrovirus that causes severe inability of the body to fight infection; leads to AIDS

Human placental lactogen: hormone produced by the syncytiotrophoblast cell around 3 weeks of ovulation; promotes lipolysis to increase free fatty acids during maternal metabolism; detectable in maternal serum around the first month after fertilization

Hydramnios: excess of amniotic fluid often found in pregnant diabetics; may occur even without fetal problems

Hydrocele: accumulated serous fluid in the scrotum

Hydrocephalus: excessive cerebrospinal fluid circulating in the cerebral ventricles, resulting in enlarged fetal head size

Hyperbilirubinemia: abnormally high level of bilirubin in the blood

Hyperemesis gravidarum: severe and excessive vomiting during pregnancy that may begin in the first trimester of pregnancy; can lead to dehydration and starvation

Hyperglycemia: abnormally high blood glucose level

Hypertonic contractions: uterine resting contractions of elevated strength or intensity, or occurring more than five times within 10 minutes

Hypertonic labor: condition characterized by a poor resting rate of contractions and contractions occurring too frequently during labor

Hypocalcemia: abnormally low calcium level in the blood

Hypoglycemia: abnormally low blood glucose level

Hypospadias: congenital abnormality of the penis in which the urethral meatus is on the ventral area or the shaft rather than at the end

Hypothermia: human body temperature of 97°F (37 °C) or less

Hypotonic labor: uterine contractions of insufficient intensity, frequency, or duration during labor

I

Implantation: embedding of the blastocyst into the endometrium, usually 7 to 9 days after fertilization

Infant mortality rate: annual number of infant deaths under age 1 per 1,000 live births of an identified population

Infant of a diabetic mother: at-risk infant born to a diabetic mother

Infertility: inability to conceive or produce viable offspring after regular unprotected intercourse for at least 1 year

Intensity: strength of a uterine contraction at its peak

Internal os: area of the cervix opening into the uterus that divides the cervical canal from the uterine cavity

Intrapartum: time beginning at true labor and lasting birth, until expulsion of the placenta

Intrauterine growth restriction (IUGR): fetal growth below the 10th percentile in terms of weight, length, or head circumference based on standardized gestational rates; may be due to many causes, including deficient nutrient supply, congenital malformation, or intrauterine infection

Intrauterine pressure catheter: tube placed through the cervix to monitor uterine pressure during contractions or to add warm saline to the intrauterine fluid if indicated

Intraventricular hemorrhage: bleeding into cerebral ventricles; common in preterm infants

Inversion of the uterus: condition in which the uterus turns inside out, resulting in serious hemorrhage and shock

Involution: return of the uterus to prepregnancy size and function after childbirth

J

Jaundice: yellow color of a newborn's skin, mucous membranes, and sclera caused by accumulated bilirubin

K

Kangaroo care: skin-to-skin contact between the parent and the newborn

Karyotype: set of an individual's chromosomes arranged in numeric order to assess genetic alterations

Kegel exercises: internal exercises that tighten and strengthen the perineal floor muscles

Kernicterus: a condition resulting from the deposit of excessive unconjugated bilirubin in the brain tissue; may result in impaired neurologic function or death

L

LaLeche League: an international organization that promotes breastfeeding through education and support to breastfeeding mothers

Labor induction: stimulating uterine contractions by physically rupturing the membranes or using medications

Labor: involuntary uterine contractions in which the fetus and placenta are expelled from the uterus to the external world

Laceration: a tear in the perineum or birth canal that occurs during childbirth

Lamaze childbirth: a psychoprophylactic method of childbirth

Lanugo: fine, downy hair on the fetus that develops after the fourth month of gestation

Large for gestational age (LGA): an infant whose birthweight exceeds the 90th percentile for gestational age on a growth chart; typically the weight exceeds 9 lb

Latching-on: proper position for the infant to attach to the breast during breastfeeding

Late-onset deceleration: slowing of the fetal heart rate that begins at the peak of a contraction and returns to baseline at the end of the contraction; caused by uteroplacental insufficiency and potentially inadequate oxygenation of the fetus

Latent phase: labor phase that begins with the onset of true labor and ends with cervical dilatation of 3 cm

Lecithin-sphingomyelin (L/S) ratio: amniotic fluid ratio of lecithin to sphingomyelin that changes during gestation; used to assess fetal lung maturity; an L/S ratio of 2:1 or greater indicates mature lungs and a low risk of respiratory distress syndrome if born at that time

Leopold's maneuvers: series of abdominal palpitation methods to determine presentation, position, lie, and engagement of the fetus

Let-down reflex: breast milk ejection reflex caused by emotional response to the infant or from stimulation of the breast nipple

Letting-go phase: adjustment to the maternal role

Lightening: downward movement of the fetus and uterus into the pelvic cavity

Linea nigra: a dark line of pigment sometimes appearing along the symphysis pubis during later months of pregnancy

LNMP: last normal menstrual period

Lochia alba: creamy white vaginal discharge that occurs after lochia serosa starting from 10 days postpartum to about 21 days postpartum

Lochia rubra: blood-tinged vaginal discharge that occurs for 2 to 4 days postpartum

Lochia serosa: pink, serous, vaginal discharge following lochia rubra that occurs from about 3 days postpartum to about 10 days postpartum

Lochia: normal vaginal discharge of uterine blood, mucus, and tissue after childbirth

Long-term variability: large rhythmic wave variations of the fetal heart rate occurring 2 to 6 times per minute as tracked with a monitor

Low birthweight (LBW): neonate birthweight of 2,500 g or less

Low-lying placenta: condition of an undetermined location of the placenta in relation to the cervical os, or apparent placenta previa occurring prior to the third trimester

Luteal phase: part of the ovarian cycle

Luteinizing hormone (LH): hormone secreted from the anterior pituitary to stimulate ovulation

M

Macrosomia: large newborn weighing more than 4 kg (8 lb 13 oz), or a newborn falling above the 90th percentile for gestational age and birthweight

Malposition: fetal position other than occiput anterior

Malpresentation: abnormal presenting part of the fetus into the birth canal; presentation other than the normal completely flexed head

Mastitis: breast inflammation caused by infection, usually in the milk duct

Maternal mortality rate: number of maternal deaths from any reproductive cause per 100,000 live births

Maternal role attainment: process of learning and applying maternal behaviors to gain a comfortable identity as a mother

Maternal serum alpha-fetoprotein: test of maternal blood at 16 to 22 weeks' gestation for the presence of alpha-fetoprotein to screen for neural tube disorders and genetic trisomies

Meconium aspiration syndrome: newborn respiratory distress caused when the fetus breathes meconium in the amniotic fluid into the lungs or trachea

Meconium: fecal matter present in the large intestine and passed as first the stools of newborn

Menarche: initiation of menstruation

Menopause: permanent cessation of menses for 12 consecutive months

Menorrhagia: profuse or excessive menstrual flow

Menses: vaginal bleeding that occurs approximately every 28 days in nonpregnant females in which the uterine lining is discharged

Metrorrhagia: menstrual periods that occur at irregular intervals

Milia: small, white papules appearing on the newborn's face and upper torso; caused by unopened or plugged sebaceous glands; normally disappear without treatment in a few weeks

Mittelschmerz: abdominal pain at the time of ovulation

Molding: overlapping capability of the fetal cranial bones to allow shape and size changes of the head so that it can pass through the maternal pelvis during labor

Mongolian spots: irregular dark coloration of no medical significance appearing on the lower back or buttocks of the newborn; may last until age 2

Monozygotic: originating from one zygote; identical twins

Morbidity rate: ratio of the number of cases of a given illness, disease, abnormal human quality, or condition to a given population

Mortality rate: ratio of the number of deaths from various causes to a given population

Morula: solid cell mass formed by the fertilized ovum in very early development

Mottling: temporary skin discoloration on irregular areas of the infant's body that appears as a blue or red blood vessel framework; found in combination with chills, hypoxia, or poor perfusion

Multipara: a woman having two or more pregnancies with viable fetuses of 20 weeks' gestation or more in each pregnancy

Multiple gestation: having more than one fetus in the uterus during the same pregnancy

Mutation: sudden genetic change that occurs in an individual and continues to occur in the offspring

N

Nagele's rule: a method for estimating the delivery date by determining the first day of the last menstrual period, subtracting 3 months, and adding 7 days

Necrotizing enterocolitis (NEC): acquired acute gastrointestinal disease that can be life-threatening to a newborn

Neonatal abstinence syndrome: newborn withdrawal symptoms resulting from the use of narcotics by the mother during fetal development; symptoms may include vomiting, irritability, sneezing, diarrhea, and seizures

Neonatal death: infant death at any gestational age within the first 28 days of life

Neonate: infant in the first 28 days of life

Neutral thermal environment: external conditions that sustain normal internal body temperature with minimal oxygen consumption and metabolism

Nitrazine test: indicates the presence of amniotic fluid based on alkaline content

Nonstress test: assessment of fetal heart rate in response to natural or stimulated fetal movement

O

Obstetrical conjugate: anteroposterior diameter of the pelvic inlet

Oligohydramnios: less-than-normal amount of amniotic fluid in the third trimester; may indicate a fetal urinary tract problem

Ophthalmia neonatorum: newborn eye infection usually caused by gonococci

Orgasmic phase: phase of the human sexual arousal and response process experienced as a release of intense sexual tension

Ortolani maneuver: manual procedure used to diagnose developmental dysplasia of the hip

Osteoporosis: progressively decreased bone mass that results in weak and brittle bones; common in postmenopausal women; associated with lower estrogen and androgen levels

Ovulation: normal release of a mature, unfertilized ovum by the ovary approximately 14 days before the beginning of the menstrual period

Oxytocin: hormone produced by the posterior pituitary that stimulates uterine contractions and the release of milk into the lactiferous ducts

P

Papanicolaou (Pap) smear: procedure to detect cervical cancer

Para: number of live births or stillbirths in a woman following 28 weeks' gestation

Parity: number of past pregnancies that have reached viability

Partial previa: category of placenta previa in which the cervical os is not completely covered by the placenta

Patent ductus arteriosus (PDA): newborn condition in which the ductus arteriosus does not close spontaneously after the first 24 hours of life

Pathologic jaundice: newborn condition characterized by an excessive breakdown of red blood cells, resulting from hematologic incompatibility

Pelvic inflammatory disease (PID): infection of the fallopian tubes, uterus, or ovaries due to vaginal bacteria; may cause pelvic abscess

Pelvic inlet: upper border of the true pelvis and entrance to the first of three pelvic planes through which the fetal head passes during delivery

Pelvic outlet: lower border of the true pelvis and opening of the third pelvic plane through which the fetal head passes during delivery

Pelvic relaxation: decline of muscle support in the pelvic region

Percutaneous umbilical blood sampling (PUB): an evaluation technique involving the direct aspiration of fetal blood from the umbilical cord in the uterus by a needle inserted through the mother's abdominal wall

Perimenopause: phase prior to menopause during which menstrual periods begin to cease

Perineum: area between the vagina and anus in women, or between the scrotum and anus in men

Phototherapy: treatment of newborn jaundice by exposure to a special ultraviolet light

Physiologic anemia of pregnancy: increased plasma volume disproportionate to red blood cells during pregnancy; results in subnormal hemoglobin and hematocrit levels

Physiologic jaundice: harmless normal breakdown and reduction of red blood cells occurring between 2 to 3 days after birth and resolving in 7 to 10 days

Pica: ingestion during pregnancy of non-food substances, such as clay, laundry starch, or ice

Placenta previa: abnormal implantation of the placenta in the lower uterus near or covering the cervical os

Plethora: red color of skin associated with hyperoxia, overheating, or polycythemia

Polycystic ovary syndrome: endocrine disorder of the ovary characterized by the failure to release an ovum for extended periods; due to excess androgens in the blood and cysts in the ovaries

Polycythemia: excessive red blood cells in the circulation

Polydactyly: development of extra digits on hands or feet

Postpartal hemorrhage: loss of more than 500 mL of blood from the birth canal within the first 24 hours of delivery ("early") or after the first 24 hours ("late")

Postpartum blues: maternal feelings of being "out of sorts" during first few days after giving birth

Postpartum depression: maternal feelings of severe depression during the first year after giving birth, with increased occurrence prior to resumed menses

Postpartum psychosis: severe maternal psychiatric condition occurring within first few months after childbirth

Postterm infant: any newborn assessed to be of more than 42 weeks' gestation

Postterm pregnancy: pregnancy that continues beyond 42 weeks of gestation

Precipitous birth: rapid labor and birth process, usually less than 3 hours in duration

Preconception care: medical information and counseling provided to a woman before she becomes pregnant; can promote optimal outcomes for the mother and infant

Pre-eclampsia: syndrome of pregnancy characterized by proteinuria, hypertension, and edema

Premature rupture of membranes (PROM): spontaneous or artificial tearing of the amniotic membranes prior to labor

Prematurity: childbirth prior to the end of 37 weeks' gestation

Premenstrual syndrome (PMS): emotional, behavioral, or physical symptoms that some women experience during the luteal phase of the menstrual cycle

Presenting part: fetal part closest to the internal os of the cervix

Preterm birth: childbirth before 37 weeks of gestation

Preterm infant: birth of an infant determined to be less than 37 weeks' gestational age

Preterm labor: any true labor occurring during 20 and 38 completed weeks of gestation

Preterm premature rupture of membranes (PPROM): spontaneous or artificial tearing of the amniotic membranes prior to labor, occurring before 37 completed weeks of gestation

Primigravida: woman in her first pregnancy

Primipara: woman in her first pregnancy who has given birth past 20 weeks of gestation

Progesterone: hormone produced by the corpus luteum of the ovary and the adrenal cortex to prepare the uterus for implantation of the fertilized ovum

Prolactin: hormone secreted by the pituitary gland that triggers and sustains milk production in response to tactile breast stimulation

Proliferative phase: time in the menstrual cycle when the uterine lining becomes prepared for reception and implantation of the fertilized ovum

Prostaglandins: hormones synthesized by many body cells that affect uterine smooth muscle, vasodilatation, and constriction

Q

Quickening: mother's experience of first fetal movements, usually between 17 and 20 weeks' gestation

R

Radiation: transfer and loss of human body heat to cooler objects and surfaces not in direct contact

Reactive nonstress test: detection of two or more fetal heart rate changes of 15 beats or more per minute for 15 seconds or more each within a 10-minute period

Recovery stage: first 4 hours after delivery of the placenta in the fourth stage of labor

Reference daily intakes (RDIs): food content standards for vitamins and minerals

Regional anesthesia: injection of an anesthetic affecting nerve tissue by blocking neural impulses in order to obtain the loss of sensation to an area of the body

Respiratory distress syndrome (RDS): pulmonary membrane disease that causes breathing difficulty and occurs most often in preterm neonates; also known as hyaline membrane disease

Resting tone: level of uterine firmness between contractions during labor

Resuscitation: emergency procedure involving control of the airway opening, positive-pressure ventilation, chest compressions, medication, and body temperature

Retinopathy of prematurity (ROP): fibrotic disease in the blood vessels of the retina in newborns; can cause blindness

Rh incompatibility: hemolytic disease resulting from incompatibility of Rh factors of maternal and fetal blood that causes an antigen–antibody reaction; also known as isoimmunization

RhoGAM: anti-Rh (D) gamma globulin given to an Rh-negative mother after the birth of an Rh-positive child to prevent development of permanent active immunity to the Rh antigen

Rooting reflex: an infant's natural response of turning the head toward a physical stimulus of the cheek or mouth area

Rugae: transverse mucous membrane ridges lining the vagina that expand to accommodate descent of the fetal head during birth

S

Screening: a test or examination to detect a bodily condition, disorder, or disease warranting medical investigation

Second stage of labor: period from the time the cervix is completely dilated and effaced until the birth of the fetus

Secretory phase: period during the menstrual cycle following ovulation and preceding menstruation

Semen: white fluid containing sperm and their nutrient secretions ejaculated from the erect penis during orgasm

Seminiferous tubules: structures that carry sperm from the testes

Sepsis: systemic infection in the blood due to virus, parasites, or bacteria

Sexually transmitted infection (STI): disease transmitted through unprotected sexual contact with an infected individual

Short-term variability: normal changes detected between successive fetal heartbeats

Shoulder dystocia: condition during labor in which the fetal shoulder cannot freely pass beneath the maternal symphysis pubis due to either a large fetus or a small maternal pelvis

Small for gestational age (SGA): infant whose birthweight is below the 10th percentile for gestational age

Spermatogenesis: process by which mature sperm (spermatozoa) develop from spermatogonia (sperm cells)

Spermicide: chemical contraception that either destroys sperm or neutralizes vaginal secretions to immobilize sperm

Station: relationship between the presenting fetal part and an imaginary line of the pelvic ischial spines

Sterilization: surgical procedure performed on males or females to prevent reproduction

Stress incontinence: involuntary discharge of urine during exercise, sneezing, laughing, or coughing; due to loss of muscle tone at the neck of the urethra

Striae gravidarum: reddish or darkened streaks on the stretched skin of the abdomen, hips, or breasts caused by pregnancy

Subinvolution: failure of the uterus to return to normal size after pregnancy due to prolonged involution from infection, hemorrhage, or retained parts of the placenta

Sudden infant death syndrome (SIDS): the death of a healthy, properly cared for infant from unexplained causes

Surfactant: a lipoprotein that stabilizes and lowers the alveolar surface tension of fluids in the lungs, allowing gases to be exchanged in the alveoli

T

Tachycardia: rapid heart rate; in a neonate, above 160 bpm; in an adult, above 100 bpm

Tachypnea: rapid respiratory rate; in a neonate, above 70 respirations/minute

Taking-hold phase: second phase of maternal adjustment, marking maternal readiness for newborn involvement

Taking-in phase: first phase of maternal adjustment, marking maternal need for care, food, and comfort

Teratogen: nongenetic factors or environmental substances that cause physical or functional malformations of the embryo and fetus

Term infant: newborn determined by examination to be 37 to 42 weeks' gestational age

Testes: male gonads; two oval organs in the scrotum in which sperm and testosterone are produced

Testosterone: androgen (male) hormone produced in the testes, adrenal cortex, and ovary; responsible for development of secondary male characteristics

Thelarche: beginning breast development of glandular tissue behind the nipples; occurs at puberty

Thermoregulation: control of body heat production and loss through physiologic changes activated by the hypothalamus

Third stage of labor: period of labor from birth until the expulsion of the placenta

Thrush: fungal infection caused by *Candida albicans*, most common in infants; marked by white plaque patches in the mouth and on the tongue

TORCH: acronym for a pregnancy syndrome of infections (toxoplasmosis, rubella, cytomegalovirus, and herpesvirus or hepatitis); linked to potentially severe fetal or neonatal problems

Transient tachypnea of the newborn: fetal respiratory disorder characterized by mild cyanosis and increased respiratory rate, possibly caused by delayed resorption of lung fluid

Transition: third phase of the first stage of labor, in which dilation of the cervix increases from 8 to 10 cm

Transvaginal ultrasound: procedure used to monitor early pregnancy, to treat women undergoing induction cycles, and to retrieve oocytes for in vitro fertilization

Transverse lie: crosswise or horizontally positioned fetus

Trimester: one third of a normal pregnancy; pregnancy is divided into three trimesters of 3 months each

Trisomy: abnormal presence of an extra, or third, homologous chromosome rather than the normal two, resulting in 47 chromosomes per cell; Down syndrome is the most common human manifestation of this condition

True labor: regular contraction and relaxation intervals of the uterus with progressive shortening, thinning, and dilation of the cervix

Tubal ligation: method of female sterilization that involves surgical severing and tying of the fallopian tubes

U

Ultrasonography: use of high-frequency (>20,000 Hz) sound waves directed into the maternal abdomen to reflect tissue densities and outlines for visualization and diagnosis of the fetus, gestational structures, bones, and fluids

Umbilical cord compression: in utero pressure on the umbilical cord by the fetus or the uterine wall that decreases blood circulation and oxygenation of the fetus

Umbilical cord prolapse: condition in which the umbilical cord precedes the presenting fetal part through the cervix and birth canal

Urge incontinence: involuntary loss of urine associated with a sudden, strong desire to urinate

Uterine atony: inability of uterine muscle to contract after childbirth

Uterine rupture: uterine wall separation that could allow penetration of fetal parts into the abdomen

Uteroplacental insufficiency: decrease in placental function of exchange of gases, wastes, and nutrients, leading to fetal hypoxia and acidosis; evidenced by late fetal heart rate decelerations

V

Vacuum extraction: use of a vacuum suction cup applied to the fetal head to assist in birth

Vaginal birth after cesarean (VBAC): vaginal birth of an infant by a woman who has had at least one previous cesarean birth

Vaginal ring: contraceptive device used to deliver steroids through the vaginal mucosa

Variable deceleration: periodic slowing of fetal heart rate due to umbilical cord compression, and possibly unrelated to normal uterine contractions

Varicocele: varicose veins in the spermatic cord

Vasectomy: male sterilization procedure that involves removing a section of the vas deferens

Vernix caseosa: fatty, white, cheese-like substance secreted by fetal sebaceous glands and epidermal cells that covers and protects fetal skin from abrasions in utero

Vertex: crown or top of the fetal head

Vertical transmission: passing of an infection to the fetus or neonate by the mother during pregnancy, delivery, or breastfeeding

Very low birthweight: birthweight of less than 1,500 g

W

Weaning: transition from breast- or bottle-feeding to a cup

ANSWERS TO WORKSHEET QUESTIONS

Chapter 1

● MULTIPLE CHOICE QUESTIONS

1. The correct response is B. Analgesia was only available in the hospital setting and women wanted to have the pain of laboring reduced; thus, they sought hospital care over home births. A is an incorrect response due to the fact that more infections occurred in the hospital setting than in the home setting after giving birth. C is an incorrect response since the home setting afforded greater privacy than in a public hospital. The woman could have her family present in the home birth, but not so in the hospital setting. D is an incorrect response since midwives were very well trained to perform births, and the gender of the birth attendant had no bearing on birthing experience.

2. The correct response is A. Infant mortality rates are compared to 1000 live births and maternal mortality rates are compared to 100,000 live births since they are much rarer than infant mortality. B is an incorrect response since both statistical rates are gathered in the same manner, but the comparison of maternal deaths is based on higher rates than the infant mortality ones. C is an incorrect response since both rates are compiled annually worldwide. D is an incorrect response since both maternal and infant mortality rates would be included in the health index of countries. The health index of a country examines many statistics to give an overall view of its health status.

3. The correct response is D. Over 500,000 women die from cardiovascular disease annually in the United States. This number is higher than that for men, but heart disease remains in the minds of many a "man's disease." A is an incorrect response in comparison to CVD, although most women believe this is their number one health concern. The breast cancer mortality rate pales when compared to cardiovascular deaths. B is an incorrect response since annually in the United States, approximately 350 deaths occur secondary to childbirth complications. C is an incorrect response since this statistic would be much less than when compared to the half million deaths from CVD.

4. The correct response is C. 43 million Americans have no health insurance, with the majority of them being women. Without health insurance, many have limited options to procure prenatal care. A is an incorrect response since statistics will demonstrate the better outcomes with prenatal care and most women do want to have medical supervision for a better outcome. B is an incorrect response because most women seek care early in the pregnancy, with the exception of teenagers hiding or not aware of their pregnancy. D is an incorrect response since the majority of women receive quality prenatal care and the outcome is positive. This mistrust of traditional medical practices may play a role in some women from different cultures since they differ from their own cultural health practices.

● CRITICAL THINKING EXERCISES

1.

a. **What changes in the clinic service hours might address this situation?**
Many of the clients may have employment based on an hourly wage. If they don't work, they don't get paid, and therefore can't attend the clinic during their normal work hours. Offer evening and Saturday hours to improve their attendance at clinic appointments.

b. **Outline what you might say at your next staff meeting to address the issue of clients making one clinic visit and then never returning.**
Acceptance and a supportive tone are frequently set at the initial meeting, and one may need to examine how this is communicated to the client at their first encounter with the clinic staff. Offer suggestions of how the staff can set a positive, welcoming tone so clients will return for additional care.

c. **What strategies might you use to improve attendance and notification?**
Have a staff person call each client to remind her of her appointment the next day and offer any needed assistance to get her there. Assign a staff member to be an "outreach" person to make home visits to follow up on clients who habitually miss appointments.

d. **Describe what cultural and customer service techniques might be needed.**
Educate staff concerning cultural norms regarding the clientele served. Based on the culture served, devise culturally appropriate policies and procedures.

● **STUDY ACTIVITIES**

1. Depending on the student's frame of reference, some will think it is a right and the government should provide it for all citizens. Others will think it should be a privilege and should be paid for by the person and not the government. There is no right or wrong answer, but this topic can provide for a lively classroom discussion.

2. Women lack insurance to pay for services, no transportation available to get to services, language or cultural barriers, health care agency hours are in conflict with their work hours, and negative health staff attitudes.

3. Depending on which article they select on which Web site, these answers will vary.

Chapter 2

● **MULTIPLE CHOICE QUESTIONS**

1. The correct response is C. Having a knowledge of the various cultural variations in health care practices helps the nurse to utilize them in his or her everyday practice settings. This cultural sensitivity and application of it makes a culturally competent nurse. A is an incorrect response because knowing your own culture doesn't foster tolerance and acceptance of people from different ones. Only when the nurse gains knowledge about other cultures will she or he become culturally competent. B is an incorrect response because being open to different cultural customs and beliefs is only the beginning of becoming culturally competent; application of this knowledge is critical too. D is an incorrect response because working on policies without seeing them applied in the health setting is not going to break down barriers to care. What is written policy may not be utilized in the real world; thus, everyone can refer to the policy, but attitudes and actions haven't changed.

2. The correct response is B. Secondary prevention includes early diagnosis, screening for disease, and treating it early to prevent spread or exacerbation. A is an incorrect answer because primary prevention would be carried out on people to prevent early symptoms of any disease or condition. Examples would include daily exercise, eating low-fat meals, getting adequate sleep, and maintaining ideal weight. These preventive measures would reduce risk of disease before it started. C is an incorrect answer due to the fact that tertiary prevention focuses on disease progression after the person already has acquired the disease. Going to rehabilitation after suffering a stroke will help prevent a worsening of the existing condition or extension of it. D is an incorrect response because the community can band together to reduce a particular disease or condition, but it is up to every individual to prevent it within himself or herself. Community

education can only go so far without individual action.

3. The correct response is A. Americans place great value on youth, technology, and their time. The wisdom and advice of the elders from past generations is not valued and respected in many cases. The use of technology has exploded in the last century, and much time and resources are being spent on its improvement. Time is very precious to Americans, and there never seems to be much of it to accomplish our goals. B is an incorrect response since elders of our society are not respected for their opinion or ideas in many families. As one ages in this society, their value becomes lessened. Americans believe in what can be scientifically proven through research and are skeptical about fate and spiritual phenomena. C is an incorrect response since many Americans live by the clock and can't be flexible or accept lateness in others. Family focus is important to some extent, but other cultures hold the family in higher regard. D is an incorrect response in two respects: extended families are not in the majority in our culture, and folk medicine is not practiced by the majority of the population. Traditional medicine with scientific proof is the norm within our society.

4. The correct response is A. Not enough studies have been done on natural herbs to validate their effectiveness or rule out their teratogenic properties. It is best to avoid them during any pregnancy to prevent any fetal or maternal complications. B is an incorrect response for the above reasons and because safety has not been established for pregnant women. C is an incorrect response since harm could be brought to the growing fetus, and the nurse should warn her not to take unproven remedies during pregnancy. D is an incorrect response since increasing her prenatal vitamins will not necessarily improve her energy level, but may harm the fetus by introducing mega doses of vitamins.

5. The correct response is C. The question doesn't imply any judgment on the nurse's part and it invites the patient to describe the nontraditional therapies that are used. A is an incorrect response because it may imply judgment, depending on the tone in which it was asked. B is similar to A since the negative attitude can be realized by the man- ner in which the question is asked. The patient may pick up a "disapproving attitude" and not admit to any non-traditional therapies. D is an incorrect response because it places a judgment on herbs in the question itself. It doesn't allow the patient the freedom of response without prejudice.

● CRITICAL THINKING EXERCISE

1.

a. What resources would you use to research this topic prior to the meeting?

Community leaders from diverse cultures, library resources, and the Internet

b. What information will you present to address the nursing staff's attitudes toward their culturally diverse clientele?

Give out a survey to ascertain the staff's feelings about working with people from different cultures and use these data to open the discussion up to bring about awareness of various attitudes, beliefs, and values. Discussion about prejudice, stereotyping, and ethno- centricity will be explained and explored.

c. What steps would you take to help the nursing staff to become culturally competent?

Set up weekly cultural awareness/educational meetings and invite speakers from various cultures that the com- munity-based clinic serves to help the staff learn and become more open-minded about different points of view. Also, send staff to culturally oriented conferences to bring back information to other staff members.

● STUDY ACTIVITIES

1. The discussion will vary depending on which cultures are represented on the panel. It will be an eye-open- ing experience for many nursing students to hear the various members describe the differences.

2. Cultural competence or cultural competency

3. Depending on the Web site selected, answers will vary, but most of them offer a variety of resources to learn about different cultures and could be helpful to nurses seeking information.

4. This visit would be very educational for nursing stu- dents to "see" what is happening in the real world when faced with cultural barriers in the health care setting. Hopefully, the community health center staff will be open to these students and will share their strategies. These strategies can be used by the stu- dent later in their practice.

Chapter 3

● MULTIPLE CHOICE QUESTIONS

1. The correct response is B. FSH is secreted from the anterior pituitary gland to initiate the devel- opment of the ovarian follicles and the secretion of estrogen by them within the ovarian cycle. A is incorrect: TSH stimulates the thyroid gland and plays a limited role in the menstrual cycle. C is incorrect: CRH is released from the hypothala- mus, not the anterior pituitary gland. D is incor- rect: GnRH is released from the hypothalamus to stimulate the release of FSH and LH from the anterior pituitary gland.

2. The correct response is C. Skene's glands since they are located close to the urethral opening and secrete mucus and lubricate during urina- tion and sexual intercourse. A is incorrect: Cowper's glands are located on either side of the male urethra, not the female urethra. B is incor- rect: Bartholin's glands are located on either side of the vaginal opening and secrete alkaline mucus that enhances the viability of the male sperm. D is incorrect: seminal glands are pouch- like structures at the base of the male urinary bladder that secrete an alkaline fluid to enhance the viability of the male sperm.

3. The correct response is A. The secretory phase is the second part of the endometrial cycle after ovulation, *not* a phase of the ovarian cycle. B, the follicular phase, is the first phase of the ovarian cycle, when the immature ovum begins to mature inside the follicle. C, ovulation, is the second phase of the ovarian cycle, when the rupture of the graafian follicle occurs with the release of the mature ovum. D, the luteal phase, is the final or postovulation phase of the ovarian cycle, when the corpus luteum degenerates and the levels of estrogen and progesterone decline if fertilization did not take place.

4. The correct response is D. Progesterone is the dominant hormone after ovulation to prepare the endometrium for implantation. A is incorrect: estrogen levels decline after ovulation, since it assists in the maturation of the ovarian follicles before ovulation. Estrogen levels are highest during the proliferative phase of the menstrual cycle. B is incorrect: prostaglandin production increases during the follicular maturation and is essential during ovulation but not after ovulation. C is incorrect: prolactin is inhibited by the high levels of estrogen and progesterone during pregnancy; when their levels decline at birth, an increase in prolactin takes place to promote lactation.

5. The correct response is C. The function of the epididymis is to store and mature sperm until ejaculation occurs. A is incorrect: the testes manufacture sperm and send them to the epididymis for storage and continued maturation. B is incorrect: the main function of the vas deferens is to rapidly squeeze the sperm from their storage site (epididymis) into the urethra. D is incorrect: the function of the seminal vesicles is to secrete an alkaline fluid rich in fructose and prostaglandins to help provide an environment favorable to sperm motility and metabolism.

● CRITICAL THINKING EXERCISES

1.

a. **How should the nurse respond to this question?**
The nurse should respond by explaining to the student that conception is achieved only during the time of ovulation, which occurs at midcycle and not during menstruation. Further explanation might outline the phases of the menstrual cycle and how each phase contributes to the preparation of the endometrial lining if conception were to take place. If conception does not occur, sloughing of the prepared endometrial lining takes place, and this is what is shed during menstruation.

b. **What factor regarding the menstrual cycle was not clarified?**
The student apparently did not understand the concept of ovulation and the potential uniting of sperm and ovum. At ovulation, bodily changes occur that assist the sperm to impregnate the ovum that was released from the ovary. It is only during this midcycle period that the sperm can find the ovum and begin a pregnancy.

c. **What additional topics might this question lead into that might be discussed?**
Sexually transmitted infections and barrier protection; abstinence until marriage and personal responsibility; responsibilities and outcomes of becoming a young parent; self-esteem and taking pride in their bodies; future educational and career goals

---

● STUDY ACTIVITIES

1. This answer will vary depending on which web site the student selects and which topic of interest he or she researches. With luck, a variety of topics will be presented and lend itself to a lively class discussion.

2. The predominant hormones involved in the menstrual cycle are gonadotropin-releasing hormone (GnRH), which is responsible for reproductive hormone control and timing of the cycle; follicle-stimulating hormone (FSH), which stimulates the ovary to produce estrogen and follicles in the ovary that will mature; luteinizing hormone (LH), which induces the mature ovum to burst from the ovary and stimulate production of corpus luteum; estrogen, which induces growth and thickening of the endometrial lining; progesterone, which prepares the endometrial lining for implantation; and prostaglandins, which help to free the mature ovum inside the graafian follicle.

3. Ovum or ova

4. The correct responses are F (testes) and G (seminiferous tubules). Sperm is produced in the seminiferous tubules of the testes. A is incorrect: the vas deferens is a cordlike duct that transports sperm from the epididymis and has no role in making sperm cells. B is incorrect: the penis is the organ for copulation and serves as the outlet for sperm, but it plays no role in the manufacture of sperm cells or testosterone. C is incorrect: the scrotum serves as the climate-control

system for the testes to allow for normal sperm development, but it plays no direct role in their manufacture. D is incorrect: the ejaculatory ducts secrete fluids to help nourish the sperm but do not play a part in their development. E is incorrect: the prostate gland produces fluid that nourishes the sperm but does not participate in the production of sperm cells. H is incorrect: the bulbourethral glands (Cowper's glands) secrete a mucus-like fluid that provides lubrication during the sex act.

Chapter 4

● MULTIPLE CHOICE QUESTIONS

1. The correct response is B. The definition of infertility is the inability of a couple to conceive after 12 months of unprotected sexual intercourse. A is incorrect: 6 months isn't long enough to diagnose infertility in a couple not using birth control. C is incorrect: 18 months is 6 months beyond the time needed to diagnose infertility based on the definition. D is incorrect: 24 months is double the time needed to diagnose infertility.

2. The correct response is B. If EC is taken within 72 hours after unprotected sexual intercourse, pregnancy will be prevented by inhibiting implantation. The next morning would still afford time to take EC and not become pregnant. A is incorrect: it would be too late to use a spermicidal agent to prevent pregnancy, since the sperm have already traveled up into the female reproductive tract. C is incorrect: douching with vinegar and hot water 24 hours after unprotected sexual intercourse will not change the course of events; by then it is too late to prevent a pregnancy, and this combination would not be effective anyway. D is incorrect: a laxative will stimulate the gastrointestinal tract to produce defecation but will not disturb the reproductive tract, where fertilization takes place.

3. The correct response is A. Seasonale is the only FDA-approved oral contraceptive that is packaged to provide 84 days of continuous protection. Although any oral contraceptive can be taken continuously, the FDA has not approved this, and it would be considered an "off-label" use. B is incorrect: this product has not gained FDA approval for continuous use; it is to be left in 3 weeks and then removed for 1 week to create monthly cycles. C is incorrect response: the FDA has not given approval to use this transdermal patch on a continuous basis; it is placed on the skin for 3 weeks and removed for 1 week. D is incorrect: this implantable device is protective for 5 years, but it is not a combination contraceptive; it releases synthetic progesterone only, not estrogen.

4. The correct response is D. Weight-bearing exercise is an excellent preventive measure to preserve bone integrity, especially the vertebral column and hips. Walking strengthens the skeletal system and prevents breakdown that leads to osteoporosis. A is incorrect: iron does not prevent bone breakdown; while iron supplementation will build up blood and prevent anemia, it has a limited effect on bones. B is incorrect: being in the horizontal position while sleeping is not helpful to build bone. Weight-bearing on long bones helps to maintain their density, which prevents loss of bone matrix. C is incorrect: protein gained from eating lean meats helps the body to build tissue and muscles but has a limited effect on maintaining bone integrity or preventing loss of bone density.

5. The correct response is B. Smoking cigarettes causes vasoconstriction of the blood vessels, increasing peripheral vascular resistance and thus elevating blood pressure. These vascular changes increase the chances of CVD by placing additional pressure on the heart to pump blood with increasing vessel resistance. A is an incorrect answer since fiber would be a positive diet addition and assist with elimination patterns and prevent straining, which stresses the heart. C is an incorrect response because vitamins do not cause narrowing of the vessel lumen, which places an additional burden on the heart. D is an incorrect response since alcohol produces vasodilation and reduces blood pressure. Alcohol in moderation is said to be good for the heart.

6. The correct response is C. Vasomotor instability, which causes hot flashes, is directly related to declining estrogen levels. Increasing the estrogen levels by hormone replacement therapy reduces vasomotor instability and thus hot flashes. A is an incorrect response since weight gain or loss is associated with calorie intake and metabolic output in the form of energy expended through exercise. Although many women report a weight gain associated with HRT, when question closely they admit to a reduction in activity level. B is incorrect since estrogen has the opposite effect on bone density—it increases and/or maintains it. HRT is prescribed for post-menopausal women to prevent osteoporosis, or loss of bone density. D is incorrect since the incidence of heart disease (myocardial infarction and

strokes) was found to increase in women taking HRT in the WHI research study, if hormones were taken in high doses over a long period. Based on that landmark study, women on HRT should take the lowest dose possible to relieve symptoms and should not take HRT for more than 5 years.

7. The correct response is A. Exercise is heart-healthy, weight-healthy, and emotionally healthy. The motto "Keep moving" is the basis for a healthy lifestyle, since it will help maintain an ideal weight, improve circulation, and improve moods. B is incorrect: socialization does not necessarily involve physical activity and would not be proactive in preserving health. C is incorrect: quiet time alone, although needed to reduce stress, reduces movement and may result in depression and weight gain. D is incorrect: water, although needed to hydrate the body, will not maintain circulation, prevent weight gain, or improve one's emotional mindset. Exercise will accomplish all three.

● CRITICAL THINKING EXERCISE

1.

a. Is an IUD the most appropriate method for her? Why or why not?

In this case, based on her history of STIs, PID, and multiple partners, she is not a candidate for an IUD. This method would increase her risk of further ascending infections, which could hinder her future fertility. Unless her lifestyle choices change dramatically, she is placing herself at risk. She should be encouraged to use barrier methods for contraception.

b. What myths/misperceptions will you address in your counseling session?

This client states she isn't interested in using birth control pills because they cause cancer. That is not true, and an explanation of risk factors for cancer needs to be given, along with a discussion of the lower doses of estrogen in the birth control pills prescribed today. Positive noncontraceptive impacts such as a reduction in ovarian and colorectal cancers should also be addressed.

c. Outline the safer sex discussion you plan to have with her.

• Having a monogamous relation reduces the incidence of STIs.
• Using barrier methods (condom, cap, diaphragm) protects against both pregnancy and STIs.
• Oral sex using a dental dam reduces the risk of STIs.
• Dry kissing with no sores or broken skin reduces the risk of STIs.
• Inform client of relationship between PID and infertility.
• Encourage prompt treatment of any vaginal discharge.

● STUDY ACTIVITIES

1. Typically, the family planning nurse will ask the woman about any sociocultural, spiritual, and religious beliefs that will influence the decision. Lifestyle and economics also play a big role in the choice of a family planning method. Ideally this should be a decision made by both partners, but rarely is the partner involved. Important teaching involves the risks, benefits, side effects, and efficacy of each method, along with instructions on how to use it correctly. Information regarding follow-up care should be stressed.

2. Numerous web sites are available, many of them sponsored by infertility healthcare agencies.

3. Prices will be higher in metropolitan versus rural areas of the county. Students will discover that the risk is higher for a woman undergoing a tubal ligation than a man undergoing a vasectomy. The costs will vary, but male sterilization is generally both less risky and less expensive.

4. The students will find numerous brands of male condoms and only one brand of female condom. Male condoms prices can range from 35 cents each to over $4, depending on the manufacturer. Most female condoms are priced around $2.50 to $3.50 each.

5. A, B, D, E, and G are correct responses: research studies have validated a reduced incidence of these cancers and conditions. C and F are incorrect: research has not shown a reduction, and some studies have actually found an increase in the incidence of breast cancer and deep vein thrombosis.

Chapter 5

● MULTIPLE CHOICE QUESTIONS

1. The correct response is C. It creates a mechanical barrier so that bacteria and viruses cannot gain access to the internal reproductive tract and proliferate. A is incorrect: there is no barrier or protection offered by taking an oral pill. Oral contraceptives offer protection against pregnancy by preventing ovulation, but none against STIs. B is incorrect: since an infected partner can still transmit the infection through preejaculate fluids, which may contain an active STI. D is incorrect: an IUD offers no barrier to prevent entrance of bacteria or viruses into the internal reproductive tract. Because it is an internal device, the string emerging from the external uterine os can actually enhance STI infiltration into the uterus in susceptible women.

2. The correct response is A. The HIV virus is not spread through casual contact between individuals. HIV is spread through unprotected sexual intercourse, breastfeeding, blood contact, or shared needles or sex toys. B is incorrect: HIV can be spread by sharing injection equipment because the user can come into contact with HIV-positive blood. C is incorrect: sexual intercourse (unprotected vaginal, anal, or oral) poses the highest risk of HIV transmission. D is incorrect: the newborn can receive the HIV virus through infected breast milk. HIV-positive women are advised not to breastfeed to protect their offspring from getting a HIV infection.

3. The correct response is B. The human papillomavirus (HPV) causes warts in the genital region. HPV is a slow-growing DNA virus belonging to the papilloma group. Types 6 and 11 usually cause visible genital warts. Other HPV types in the genital region (16, 18, 31, 33, and 35) are associated with vaginal, anal, and cervical dysplasia. A is incorrect: a pus-filled discharge is not typical of an HPV infection, but rather a chlamydial or gonococcal STI. C is incorrect: a single painless ulcer would be indicative of primary syphilis rather than an HPV infection. D is incorrect: multiple vesicles would indicate a herpes outbreak, not an HPV infection. The woman would also experience tingling, itching, and pain in the affected area.

4. The correct response is D. A ruptured tubal pregnancy secondary to an ectopic pregnancy can cause life-threatening hypovolemic shock. Without immediate surgical intervention, death can result. A is incorrect: involuntary infertility may be emotionally traumatic, but it is not life-threatening. B is incorrect: chronic pelvic pain secondary to adhesions is unpleasant but typically isn't life-threatening. C is incorrect: depression may be caused by the chronic pain or involuntary infertility but is not life-threatening.

5. The correct response is C. The classic chancre in primary syphilis can be described as a painless, indurated ulcer-like lesion at the site of exposure. A is incorrect: a highly variable rash is characteristic of secondary syphilis, not primary. B is incorrect: this is more descriptive of a trichomoniasis vaginal infection rather than primary syphilis, which manifests with a chancre on the external genitalia. D is incorrect: a localized gumma formation on the mucous membranes, such as the lips or nose, is characteristic of late syphilis, along with neurosyphilis and cardiovascular syphilis.

● CRITICAL THINKING EXERCISE

1.

a. What STI would the nurse suspect?
Based on the description of the genital lesions, the nurse would suspect genital herpes. Typically the herpetic lesions begin as erythematous papules that then develop into vesicles. The vesicles rupture and leave ulcerated lesions and then crust over. This is essentially what Sally described in her history.

b. The nurse should give immediate consideration to which of Sally's complaints?
As with any STI, treatment should aim at promoting comfort, promoting healing, preventing secondary infection, and decreasing transmission of the disease. A sample from a genital lesion should be obtained for a definitive diagnosis. A urine sample should be checked for bacteria to rule out a bladder infection. Giving information about the specific STI is important to promote understanding. Information concerning her antiviral medication therapy is paramount to reduce the viral shedding. Sitz baths and mild analgesics may be needed for pain relief.

c. What should be the goals of the nurse in teaching Sally about this STI?
Although acyclovir or another antiviral medication can reduce the symptoms of herpes, the nurse needs to point out that it is not a cure for herpes. Antiviral drugs act to suppress viral replication but do not rid the body of them. This STI is a lifetime one, and she may experience numerous episodes. The nurse should teach Sally that this condition is manageable, but she will need to be able to identify stress factors that may trigger a

recurrence and reduce them. Common triggers may include hormonal changes, such as ovulation during the menstrual cycle; prolonged exposure to sunlight; emotional distress; lack of sleep; and overwork. The

final goal is to make sure Sally understands how to prevent transmission of herpes and what changes in her behaviors need to take place immediately to protect her health.

● STUDY ACTIVITIES

1. Depending on which web site the students select and which STI they choose to learn educated, discussions will vary. We hope that each student will bring additional information to the discussion and will share interesting "finds" with his or her peers.

2. Statistics will vary depending on the student's location. This research will help students learn what is happening in their area and what preventive measures are being used to reduce the incidence of STIs.

3. The counseling role of the STI nurse should be one of patience and sensitivity. The nurse should be non-judgmental and should see the client as someone who needs both treatment and education. The nurse should counsel the patient about high-risk behaviors and prevention of disease transmission.

4. *Chlamydia* and *gonorrhea*

5. The correct responses are B, C, and D: all three therapies assist in reducing the viral load in the warty lesion. Treatment may reduce but does not necessarily eradicate infection. A is incorrect: penicillin is a bacteriostatic agent and is not effective against viruses. E is incorrect: antiretroviral therapy is used for HIV infections. F is incorrect: acyclovir is typically used to treat herpes infections.

Chapter 6
● MULTIPLE CHOICE QUESTIONS

1. The correct response is C. Visible changes to the skin of the breast takes place and can be seen if inspected in front of a mirror (dimpling, contour changes, nipple discharge). A is incorrect: breast cancer first spreads to the axillary lymph nodes, not the cervical nodes. Palpation of the axillary lymph nodes is warranted, not the cervical ones. B is incorrect: spontaneous nipple discharge is more indicative of breast cancer than discharged produced by squeezing the nipple. D is incorrect: a mammogram is not part of a breast self-examination, which the woman does in the privacy of her home.

2. The correct response is A. The incidence of breast cancer increases with aging, especially over age 50. Only 1% of breast cancers occur in men. B is incorrect: bearing children interrupts the menstrual cycle and decreases a woman's risk of breast cancer. C is incorrect: only 7% of women have a genetic mutation resulting in breast cancer, whereas in the remaining 93% it is a sporadic occurrence. D is incorrect: colon cancer is not a risk factor for breast cancer.

3. The correct response is B. This describes the procedure for performing a sentinel node biopsy. A is incorrect: there is no dye used and a biopsy is taken of the breast mass, not the node. C is incorrect: this is an actual surgical removal of the axillary nodes and not just a biopsy, and no dye is used in this procedure. D is incorrect: an advanced breast biopsy doesn't use dye and involves taking a tissue sample of the breast mass, not the nodes in the axillary area.

4. The correct response is D. When the bone marrow is suppressed secondary to chemotherapy, the woman experiences bleeding tendencies (low platelets), limited immunity (low white blood cells), and anemia (low red blood cells). This myelosuppression can become life-threatening. A is incorrect: a decrease in the number of platelets in the circulating blood may cause bleeding tendencies if the body is traumatized, but it is not as life-threatening as having all bone marrow cells depressed. B is incorrect: having blood clots in deep veins is typically not a frequent response to chemotherapy, whereas myelosuppression is very common. C is incorrect: losing one's hair, while emotionally and aesthetically traumatizing, it is not a life-threatening event, and the hair will grow back after therapy ends.

5. The correct response is B. The discomfort is usually mild and analgesics will relieve it in most cases. A is incorrect: women are advised to reduce caffeine to reduce the stimulation of breast tissue, not increase it. C is incorrect: women are advised to increase their intake of leafy vegetables, not reduce them, since this would be a part of a balanced healthy diet. D is incorrect: women are advised to wear a firm supportive bra to reduce the strain on the breast tissue, not a bra that offers no support.

6. The correct response is D. This volunteer organization offers support and practical advice to women with breast cancer; all the volunteers have had breast cancer themselves. A is incorrect: NOW doesn't focus on breast cancer per se, but all women's issues, especially equality ones.

B is incorrect: the FDA is concerned with the regulation, security, and safety of all foods and drugs in the United States, not breast cancer issues. C is incorrect: the March of Dimes focuses on prevention of preterm births and reduction of birth defects, not breast cancer.

● CRITICAL THINKING EXERCISE

1.
a. What specific questions would you ask this client to get a clearer picture?
The nurse needs to assess this client's risk factors for breast cancer by asking about:
• Her family history of breast or ovarian cancer
• Her own health history
• Her gynecologic history (menarche, parity, family planning)
• Her history of breast problems (previous benign disorders)
• Her lifestyle habits, which may be associated with cancer (i.e., smoking, high intake of fat, alcohol intake)

b. What education is needed for this client regarding breast health?
The nurse needs to reassure the client that most breast lesions are benign, but this problem will need to be

explored. The fact she experiences cyclic pain suggests this problem may be fibrocystic breast changes and not cancer, but she should undergo a further workup. Stress the importance of the performing monthly breast self-examinations, receiving yearly mammograms, and scheduling annual clinical breast examinations with her healthcare provider to assist in taking control of her health.

c. What community referrals are needed to meet this client's future needs?
During October of each year, many healthcare agencies honor National Breast Cancer month by offering free or reduced-cost mammograms. The nurse needs to make this client aware of this and urge her to receive a mammogram to maintain her health.

● STUDY ACTIVITIES

1. A woman's breasts have a variety of meanings and symbolize various things to women. To some women, her breasts symbolize her female self and her ability to suckle her newborn, and separate her biologically from a man. To society, a woman's breasts can be viewed as a sex symbol and denote sexiness. Different cultures view a woman's breasts differently, dictating whether if she is welcome to expose them for breast-feeding or not.

2. Feelings might include fear of cancer, anxiety, helplessness, embarrassment, denial, or depression. A

nurse can help her cope with these feelings by giving her the facts and reassuring her that most breast disorders are benign. Guide the woman through the diagnostic tests needed to validate her condition.

3. Lifestyle modifications that can reduce the discomfort of fibrocystic breast changes might include taking oral contraceptives, eating a low-fat diet rich in fruits and vegetables, avoiding caffeine intake, reducing salt intake, wearing a well-fitting, supportive bra most of the time, and taking over-the-counter analgesics to reduce mild discomfort.

4. Mastitis

Chapter 7
● MULTIPLE CHOICE QUESTIONS

1. The correct response is C. Pressure against adjacent structures and stretching of the uterine muscle with increasing growth of the fibroid creates pain. A is incorrect: migraines are not caused by growing fibroids, but rather a change within the vasculature in the cranium. B is incorrect: bladder pressure to cause urinary urgency would be secondary to pelvic structure relaxation, not uterine fibroids. D is incorrect: constipation would be more common in a

woman experiencing pelvic organ prolapse rather than one with fibroids, since fibroids usually involve the uterus, not the rectum.

2. The correct response is A. Both pessaries and Kegel exercises help hold up and strengthen the pelvic floor to restore the pelvic organs to their correct anatomic position. B is incorrect: an external fixation device would not be a tolerable long-term solution; it would also be invasive and would place the woman at risk for infection. C is incorrect: weight gain is not usually a healthy intervention for women as they age. Additional weight would increase the pressure on pelvic organs and exacerbate the problem. Yoga is relaxing and could reduce the woman's stress level, but it would not be therapeutic for pelvic organ prolapse. D is incorrect: wearing firm support garments might increase intra-abdominal pressure and cause further downward descent of the pelvic organs.

3. The correct response is A. Preventing constipation and straining with defecation would lessen the strain on pelvic organs. B is incorrect: sitting for long periods will not affect pelvic organ movement. Gravity will create a downward pull on all organs regardless of the position, sitting or standing. C is incorrect: exercise will help to tone muscles within the body and strengthen the pelvic floor. D is incorrect: frequent childbirth contributes to pelvic organ prolapse rather than preventing it. Spacing children only a year apart would negatively influence the pelvic-floor musculature and would be a contributing factor for prolapse.

4. The correct response is C. Insulin resistance is characterized by failure of insulin to enter cells appropriately, resulting in hyperinsulinemia, a characteristic of PCOS. Factors that contribute to this include obesity, physical inactivity, and poor dietary habits. This person is at risk for developing type 2 diabetes secondary to insulin resistance. A is incorrect: osteoporosis develops in aging women because of declining estrogen and calcium levels, not due to PCOS. B is incorrect: lupus is an autoimmune condition and is not related to PCOS. D is incorrect: migraine headaches are not associated with PCOS but rather changes in cranium vessels.

5. The correct response is D. GnRH agonists block the production of estrogen, which produces menopausal symptoms. A is incorrect: osteoporosis would be a long-term result of estrogen deprivation and calcium, and typically women do not stay on GnRH agonists for long-term therapy. B is incorrect: the blocking of estrogen would not contribute to the development of arthritis. C is incorrect: inhibiting estrogen is not a cause of depression; a change in serotonin levels in the brain is a cause of depression.

● CRITICAL THINKING EXERCISE

1.
a. What condition might Faith have based on her symptoms?
The symptoms are suggestive of uterine fibroids. She presents with a typical profile.

b. What treatment options are available to address this condition?
If Faith desires to preserve her childbearing ability, she can be treated medically with oral contraceptives, gonadotropin-releasing hormones, mifepristone, or a myomectomy. If she is finished with childbearing, a vaginal hysterectomy would be advised.

c. What educational interventions should the nurse discuss with Faith?
The nurse needs to make sure that Faith understands what the disorder is and how it can be treated and should provide information to assist her in making a decision about treatment. In addition to the treatment modalities for fibroids, her iron deficiency anemia needs attention with iron preparations and dietary changes to increase her iron and vitamin C intake.

● STUDY ACTIVITIES

1. Offer an explanation of how this inconspicuous exercise can help build muscle volume. Show a picture of where this pelvic floor muscle is located. Pelvic floor relaxation comes with the aging process in women secondary to childbirth, weight gain, and the force of gravity. The easiest way to instruct a woman how to do Kegel exercises is to have her practice using the pubococcygeus muscle by starting and stopping the flow of urine. Have her tighten the pubococcygeus muscle for a count of three, then relax it. This maneuver should be done at least 10 times each day.

2. The symptoms that accompany pelvic organ prolapse might include stress incontinence, urinary frequency and urgency, a feeling of bladder fullness after voiding, constipation, rectal fullness, painful intercourse, and pelvic pressure. All of the symptoms combined would tend to keep a woman isolated from society and her partner because of the embarrassment of odor, discomfort, and accidents. A woman would not feel in control of her body functions and would thus feel vulnerable in most social or intimate circumstances. Joining a support group of women experiencing similar problems would allow her to express her feelings and find support through others. Suggestions about what

works and what doesn't work and how to cope with this situation would be very helpful.

3. Symptoms common in women with uterine fibroids include low back pain, menorrhagia, anemia, dyspareunia, dysmenorrhea, bloating, and feelings of heaviness in the pelvic region. A woman might delay seeking treatment because she fears she has cancer and thus might be in denial as a protective mechanism. Many women associate irregular bleeding and pain with the diagnosis of cancer.

4. *cystocele*

5. *rectocele*

Chapter 8

● MULTIPLE CHOICE QUESTIONS

1. The correct answer is B. Typically, there are no glaring features of ovarian cancer. Many of the symptoms are nonspecific and can easily be explained away and rationalized as changes related to the aging process. A is incorrect: ovarian cancer is aggressive and spreads early. C is incorrect: women do not have to die to be diagnosed with ovarian cancer. D is incorrect: most women with acute pain bring it to the attention of their health care provider, but acute pain is a late symptom of cancer.

2. The correct response is D. Any postmenopausal bleeding is suspicious for endometrial cancer. This event warrants immediate evaluation, which would include an endometrial biopsy. A is incorrect: postmenopausal women do not have menstrual periods unless they are taking hormone replacement therapy. B is incorrect: any postmenopausal bleeding is abnormal and needs evaluation to determine its cause. The exception would be for a woman taking hormone replacement therapy and still experiencing monthly cycles. C is incorrect: warm-water douches would not be advised for a woman experiencing postmenopausal bleeding, since it would not be therapeutic or warranted. Determining the etiology of the spotting or bleeding is imperative.

3. The correct response is A. Women need clear information to make informed choices about treatment and aftercare. This information will help reduce her anxiety and chose the best course of action for her. B is incorrect: hand-holding is important if used appropriately, but having clear information about what to expect and treatment options will go a longer way to meet her psychosocial needs. C is incorrect: cheerfulness is not necessarily therapeutic in the face of a grave prognosis. D is incorrect: instilling hope is important, but giving clear information would be more of a priority.

4. The correct response is C. Pap smears are done specifically to detect abnormal cells of the cervix that might be cancerous. A is incorrect: a fecal occult blood test would be useful in detecting blood in the gastrointestinal tract and might be diagnostic of colorectal cancer, not cervical cancer. B is incorrect: this glycoprotein is not specific for cervical cancer, but levels may rise in pancreatic, liver, colon, breast, and lung cancers. D is incorrect: a sigmoidoscopy is used to visualize the sigmoid colon to identify cancer, polyps, or blockages. It is not diagnostic of cervical cancer.

5. The correct response is B. Typically, ovarian cancer is not diagnosed until it is in advanced stages, when the prognosis and survival rates are poor. A is incorrect: vulvar cancer is usually recognized earlier, and treatment when it is in its early stages is curable. C is incorrect: endometrial cancer can usually be detected secondary to postmenopausal bleeding and can be treated if detected early by surgery to remove the uterus or source of cancer. D is incorrect: cervical cancer, if detected early and treated, can be eliminated. With early treatment, it does not carry a high mortality rate.

● CRITICAL THINKING EXERCISES

1.
a. Based on her history, which risk factors for cervical cancer are present?
This client is at high risk for several conditions, including sexually transmitted infections as well as cervical cancer: smoking, early onset of sexual activity, multiple partners, and no previous Pap smears.

b. What recommendations would you make for her and why?
Schedule an appointment for a Pap smear and instruct her to keep it. It may save her life. The ACS strongly recommends cervical cancer screening for all women who are sexually active within 3 years of the start of sexual activity or at the age of 21. This client hasn't undergone any assessment and engages in high-risk behavior.

c. **What are this client's educational needs concerning health maintenance?**
Cigarette smoking and multiple sexual partners from an early age strongly correlate with cervical dysplasia and cancer and increase risk. This client needs to undergo a Pap smear annually, stop smoking, use barrier methods for protection, and reduce the number of sexual partners. The nurse should refer her to community social services to obtain employment and thus health insurance to continue health maintenance activities. The nurse should stress the importance of lifestyle behavioral changes that she needs to make to preserve her health.

d. **Is Jennifer typical for a woman with this diagnosis?**
Yes, Jennifer represents the typical presentation of a woman with epithelial ovarian cancer. She was diagnosed with advanced ovarian cancer that had spread to other abdominal organs and the lymph nodes by the time she was diagnosed. She essentially experienced no symptoms of concern prior to her diagnosis. Her 5-year survival rate is poor because of her advanced cancer state.

e. **What in her history might have increased her risk for ovarian cancer?**
Jennifer already had been diagnosed with breast cancer, which places her at an increased risk for ovarian cancer. In addition, she had no prior pregnancies to interrupt her menstrual cycles, which would be helpful in lowering her risk of developing ovarian cancer. Finally, Jennifer has a history of perineal talc exposure, which increases her risk because of its similarity to asbestos.

f. **What can this nurse do to increase awareness of this cancer for all women?**
Community education can be very effective in increasing awareness of this condition. Education should focus on pertinent information about risk-reduction measures, screening options for women at high risk, and the importance of annual examinations. In addition, nurses should keep current on research concerning ovarian cancer and should be able to disseminate this information at health fairs and women's support groups.

● STUDY ACTIVITIES

1. Depending on the type of reproductive cancer the student selects, the responses will vary. Typically the symptoms described are vague, and the woman may have delayed seeking help from her healthcare provider. Her preoperative emotions are usually fear, denial, and anxiety regarding the unknown. Her postoperative feelings can include relief, worry, depression, and anxiety again. Her future may seem bright if the cancer was detected early, but it may be bleak if it is advanced.

2. Depending on where the student lives and what community resources are available, their responses will vary. The purpose of this field trip to acquaint the students with their community resources and to visualize the equipment used in cancer treatment. Cancer treatment centers are very specialized and most offer numerous modalities of care. It is important that students know what is available in their communities and be informed referral agents.

3. Most web sites address the lay public and offer education about each type of cancer. Most urge clients to seek specific information concerning their symptoms or situation from their healthcare practitioner.

4. *Ovarian*

5. *Breast* and *ovarian*

Chapter 9
● MULTIPLE CHOICE QUESTIONS

1. The correct response is D. Giving women the ability to gain control over their lives allows them to make the changes needed to protect themselves and their children. As long as they feel victimized, they will take little action to make change. A is incorrect: being the victim of abuse is not a mental illness, but involves being in circumstances where her courage and self-esteem may be hindered. B is incorrect: leaving the abuser is a process, not an abrupt action, and a great deal of preparation is needed before making this move. C is incorrect: nurses don't have the resources to provide financial support to abused women, but they can make referrals to community agencies that could help with job training.

2. The correct response is B. Tension builds within the abuser and he demonstrates increased anger and violent behavior without any provocation from the woman. This tension-building phase starts the cycle of violence. A is incorrect: typically the woman doesn't provoke the abuser's violent behavior, but he blames her for his lack of anger control. C is incorrect: in the honeymoon phase, the final phase in the cycle of violence, the abuser says he is sorry, he loves her, and it will never happen again. D is incorrect: in the explosion stage of the cycle of violence, the abuser physically harms the woman. This stage follows the tension-building phase.

3. The correct response is C. Women with low self-esteem and limited communication skills

seem more likely to become victims of abuse than those with good communication skills and assertiveness. Women possessing these skills would be able to make changes in their life and would not fall victim to abuse. A is incorrect: cooking skills have a limited impact on abusive relationships. The woman's ability to communicate and feel strong within herself will provide her with better preventive tools than her cooking skills. B is incorrect: being a good decorator will not prevent abuse. Good self-esteem and work skills will go further to help her recover from an abusive relationship than being a good homemaker. D is incorrect: improving her appearance would not prevent her from becoming a victim again if her self-esteem remains low. Improving her appearance through weight loss and exercise would, however, improve her overall health status and ability to survive her abusive past.

4. The correct response is A. This statement promotes a sense of self-worth, which may have been destroyed by her abuser in the relationship. This statement indicates to the woman that she has a lot to offer and that she shouldn't put up with this abusive behavior. The victim may not have heard this message before: her abuser may have convinced her that she did deserve the violence. B is incorrect: many children living in violent homes are abused themselves and extremely stressed. No children should live under such stressful circumstances; a two-parent household is not healthy if one is an abuser. C is incorrect: in most cases the woman doesn't trigger the abuse; rather, the abuser has limited control over his anger and does not need to be provoked before lashing out. There is not necessarily a cause-and-effect relationship between the woman's behavior and the violence. D is incorrect: over time the abuse typically escalates rather than lessens; thus, giving the partner more time will not bring him to his senses.

● CRITICAL THINKING EXERCISE

1.
a. Outline your conversation when you broach the subject of abuse with Mrs. Boggs.

Since you suspect abuse, asking a direct question about whether she feels safe in her own home might open up the conversation and allow Mrs. Boggs to talk about the situation. If she denies that there is a problem, reassure her that you care, that you are afraid for her safety, and that she deserves better. Opening the door for discussion is the first step toward change.

b. What is your role as a nurse in caring for this family in which you suspect abuse?

Allow Mrs. Boggs to know that you are there for her when she is ready to talk about her situation and that she

deserves better than this. If she is unwilling to do so at this time, continue to ask screening questions about abuse on each subsequent visit. Providing her with the National Domestic Violence Hotline number might be helpful.

c. What ethical/legal considerations are important in planning care for this family?

If you notice that Mrs. Boggs has suffered acute abuse, by law you must report it. You also need to document any injuries to strengthen this case if it were to go to trial. Accurate documentation can also be used as justification for a variety of other actions, such as restraining orders, compensation, and insurance and welfare payments. You have an ethical and legal responsibility to report the abuse and assist the woman; do not ignore it and pass it off as "a private family dispute."

● STUDY ACTIVITIES

1. This web site includes postings from women in abusive relationships. It may help the students grasp the extent of violence in our society and may prompt them to lobby legislators to pass stricter laws to protect the victims of abuse.

2. This exercise may help the students put the issue of domestic violence into perspective and determine whether they live in a safe state. They may also discover what interventions might help to reduce domestic violence.

3. Campus security personnel often present safety programs for women about how to protect themselves against date rape and sexual assault. This information will serve any woman well whether she lives on the campus or not.

4. This activity should provide an eye-opening experience about the frequency of calls related to domestic violence and how much time police officers spend dealing with it.

Chapter 10

● MULTIPLE CHOICE QUESTIONS

1. The correct response is C. Scientists have determined that conception/fertilization occurs in the upper portion of the fallopian tube. A is an incorrect response because this is where implantation takes place after fertilization has occurred. B is an incorrect response because this describes the inner lining of the uterus, where implantation takes place; not where fertilization of the ovum and sperm occur. D is an incorrect response because the sperm does not travel outside the fallopian tube to the ovary, but rather meets the ovum for purposes of fertilization in the fallopian tube.

2. The correct response is B. hCG is secreted by the formation of the zygote after fertilization has taken place. Its presence in the maternal urine or serum signals a pregnancy has started. Its absence denotes no pregnancy. A is an incorrect response because it is not detected until weeks later, after fertilization has taken place. It is secreted by the placenta after it is formed. C is an incorrect response because FSH stimulates ovulation, but bows out once ovulation is accomplished. D is an incorrect response because TSH, although needed to support a pregnancy, has a limited affect on fertilization and its aftermath.

3. The correct response is A. Alpha-fetoprotein is produced by the fetal liver, and increasing levels are detectable in the serum of pregnant women from 14 to 34 weeks. Through scientific studies, a lower than normal level of alpha-fetoprotein is associated with Down syndrome, and elevated levels are associated with neural tube defects such as spina bifida or anencephaly. B is an incorrect response because fetoscopy, once popular in the 1970s and 1980s, has been replaced by amniocentesis and serum marker tests to detect neural tube defects. C is an incorrect response because CT scans are rarely used on pregnant women except in trauma cases, because it would expose the fetus to ionizing radiation, which might be harmful to the developing fetus. D is an incorrect response because Coombs tests are used to detect RBCs coated with antibody such as what would occur in Rh incompatibility.

4. The correct response is D. Many common congenital malformations are caused by the interaction of many genes and environmental factors, such as health status, age, and potential exposure to pollutants and viruses. A is an incorrect response to this question because human genetics plays a major role in fetal development from conception on. B is an incorrect response because there is an understanding of cause-and-effect relationships of most health conditions. C is an incorrect response because although poor lifestyles can have a major impact on fetal development, genetics must also be factored into the equation. Poor outcomes secondary to poor nutrition and health status can negatively influence any pregnancy, but they are not necessarily the sole factor.

5. The correct response is C. Uncovering an individual's family history can identify previous genetic disorders that have a high risk for recurrence in subsequent generations. A is an incorrect response to this question because observing a patient and their family would be costly and unproductive to diagnose a genetic disorder. This observation would have to take place over several generations to yield results. B is an incorrect response because psychological testing might not uncover genetic predispositions to disorders. D is an incorrect response because excluding the numerous genetic conditions would be a time-consuming and tedious task.

6. The correct response is D. The risk of having a Down syndrome offspring or other chromosomal disorder increases with advancing age in women. It is thought that the woman's ovum become aged and malformations can result. A is an incorrect response because multiple pregnancies do not carry any higher risk of chromosomal abnormalities than a singleton gestation. B is an incorrect response because emotions, although they play a big role in accepting the pregnancy, have limited impact on causing chromosomal abnormalities. C is an incorrect response because primigravidas run no higher risk of producing genetic mutations than multigravidas, unless maternal age is advanced.

7. The correct response is D. Down syndrome offspring will receive the abnormal chromosome from one parent, plus a normal 21 chromosome from the carrier parent, which will result in an extra amount of chromosomal material on the 21st gene pair. A is an incorrect response because a Down syndrome infant has 47 chromosomes (47,XX+21 or 47,XY+21). B is an incorrect response because not only male offspring are affected by this genetic abnormality. C is an incorrect response because the genetic mutation occurs on gene pairing 21 and not on the sex chromosome determining the sex.

● CRITICAL THINKING EXERCISES

1.

a. What information/education is needed for this couple to consider before deciding whether to have the test? The nurse needs to outline the facts about the genetic inheritance:

- CF is a recessive disorder that affects 1 in every 2500 babies.
- It predominately is seen in white infants and is less common in other races.
- Because it is a recessive disorder, Mrs. Martin must also be a carrier to pass it on to their offspring.
- If Mrs. Martin is a carrier, their chance of having a child with CF is one in four.
- The risk is the same each time they have a child.
- The nurse should provide general information about cystic fibrosis.

b. How can you assist this couple in their decision-making process?

Start by providing all the facts about the nature of the inheritance risk. Also, outline all options so the couple can make an informed decision. Options include the following:

- The couple does not receive genetic testing and takes their chances.

- If Mrs. Martin is a CF carrier, then they could choose not to have children or adopt a baby.
- Prenatal testing could be done on the fetus to determine whether both its genes carry a CF mutation. If so, the couple could elect to abort the pregnancy.
- Use an ovum or sperm from a donor who does not carry CF.
- Make a referral to a reproductive technology health facility for the couple to become educated regarding alternatives to maximize their outcome.
- Be realistic with this couple about not having any guarantees that another genetic disorder might not occur.
- Discuss the expense involved in genetic testing and in vitro fertilization that probably will not be covered by health insurance.

c. What is your role in this situation if you do not agree with their decision?

As a nurse, your role is to provide the facts and allow the couple to make their own decision about what they wish to do. They must live with their decision, not the nurse. As a nurse, your role would be to respect and support whatever this couple decides to do.

● STUDY ACTIVITIES

1. The video entitled *Miracle of Life* is a wonderful visualization of conception through fetal development and birth. A photographer was able to photograph sperm swimming and ovum being released from the ovary. He then photographed the developing embryo and fetal development through birth. It is realistic and a true wonder of life. The title depicts the images.

2. Most large hospitals have obstetric ultrasound departments that schedule pregnant women throughout the day for a variety of ultrasounds for diagnostic purposes. Some departments offer level II and three-dimensional ultrasounds, which demonstrate facial features of the fetus. It would provide a tremendous learning experience for a nursing student to see the developing fetus via ultrasound. This field trip would enhance the student's understanding of fetal growth and development.

3. Depending on which Web site the student selects, the critique will vary. Most sites are very user friendly and are geared to the lay public's understanding. Student will choose their own area of

interest, depending on their frame of reference. Their information would make for an educational discussion in class.

4. Students should draw their own family pedigree to identify their past health history. This information is important to determine genetic conditions and inheritable diseases. By identifying their past health ancestry, perhaps motivation for wiser lifestyle choices might surface.

5. Results will vary depending on which fetal screening test is chosen. An example might be the fetal nuchal translucency screening test. The *purpose* of the test is to identify genetic disorders and/or physical anomalies. The *procedure* involves ultrasound measurement of fluid in the nape of the neck between 10 and 14 weeks' gestation. A nuchal translucency measurement of 3 mm or more is highly suggestive of fetal abnormalities and diagnostic genetic testing is indicated. The student playing the role of the nurse discussing this test should be very supportive, but factual to the expectant couple. They can reverse roles with a different fetal screening test to discuss.

Chapter 11

● MULTIPLE CHOICE QUESTIONS

1. The correct response is B. Progesterone is the relaxation hormone throughout pregnancy because it relaxes smooth muscles, including the uterus. Estrogen is responsible for vascularization of the reproductive organs and preparing the breasts for lactation, and does not cause the uterine muscle to relax to prevent contractions. Oxytocin is secreted by the posterior pituitary gland and is responsible for stimulating uterine contractions and initiating the milk let-down reflex for lactating mothers. Prolactin promotes lactation but has no influence on calming the uterus.

2. The correct response is C. Urinary frequency occurs during early pregnancy secondary to pressure on the bladder by the expanding uterus. This is one of the presumptive signs of pregnancy. Restlessness or elevated mood is not a sign of pregnancy. As hormones increase during pregnancy, the mood might change, but it is not indicative of pregnancy. Low backache is frequently experienced by many women during the third trimester of pregnancy secondary to the change in their center of gravity, but it is not a presumptive sign of pregnancy.

3. The correct response is A. The corpus luteum secretes hCG early after conception to signal that fertilization has taken place. Without fertilization, hCG is not detected. Thus, it is the basis for pregnancy tests. hPL is the hormone secreted by the placenta to prepare the breasts for lactation. It is also an antagonist to insulin, competing for receptor sites that force insulin secretion to increase to meet the body's demands. FSH is secreted by the anterior pituitary gland to stimulate the ovary to mature an ovum for ovulation. It is not detected during pregnancy tests. LH is secreted by the pituitary gland. An increase in LH occurs immediately before ovulation and is responsible for release of the ovum. It is not the basis for pregnancy tests.

4. The correct response is D. The feeling of ambivalence is experienced by most women when they question their ability to become a mother. Feelings fluctuate between happiness about the pregnancy, and anxiety and fear about the prospect of new responsibilities and a new family member. Acceptance usually develops during the second trimester after fetal movement is felt by the mother and the infant becomes real to her. Depression is not a universal feeling experienced by most women unless there has been past history of underlying depression experienced by the woman. Jealousy is not a universal feeling of pregnant women. It can occur in partners, because attention is being diverted from them to the pregnancy and the newborn.

5. The correct response is C. Seeking acceptance of self to the infant is the basis for establishing a mutually gratifying relationship between mother and infant. This "binding in" is a process that changes throughout the pregnancy, starting with the mother's acceptance of the pregnancy and then the infant as a separate entity. Ensuring safe passage through pregnancy, labor, and birth focuses on the mother initially and her concern for herself. As the pregnancy progresses, the fetus is recognized and concern for its safety becomes a priority. The mother–infant relationship is not the mother's concern yet. Seeking acceptance of this infant by others includes the world around the mother and how they will integrate this new infant into their world. The infant–maternal relationship is not the focus in this task. Learning to give of one's self on behalf of one's infant focuses on delaying maternal gratification, focusing on the infant's needs before the mother's needs.

● CRITICAL THINKING EXERCISES

1.
a. How should the nurse answer her question?
The feelings that the woman is describing are those of ambivalence and they are very common in women when they first learn they are pregnant. The nurse needs to explain this to the woman, emphasizing that it is common for women to question themselves in relation to the pregnancy because it is "unreal" to them during this early period. Fetal movement helps to make the pregnancy a reality.

b. What specific information is needed to support the client during this pregnancy?
The nurse can be supportive to this woman during this time by providing emotional support and validating the various ambivalent feelings she is experiencing. Including her husband and/or family members might also provide support for her.

2.
a. What explanation can the nurse offer Sally regarding her fatigue?
The nurse can explain in simple terms that the new embryo needs a great deal of her glucose and nutrients

to grow, and thus her energy level will be affected during early pregnancy, and this is why she is feeling tired frequently. The nurse can also inform her that her energy level will increase by the second trimester and she should not feel as drained.

b. **What interventions can the nurse offer to Sally?**
Interventions to help Sally cope with her fatigue during her early pregnancy would be for her to plan rest periods throughout the day and make sure she gets a good night's sleep daily. Taking naps on weekends to refresh her may also help her. Also, help with meal preparation would be beneficial.

3.
a. **What strategies can a nurse discuss with a concerned mother when she asks how to deal with this?**
Strategies to integrate a new infant into the family unit would include involving the sibling in planning the nursery for their new brother or sister, answering their questions about the new infant during the pregnancy, using age-specific books to inform the sibling of the fetus' growth and development, and providing special time set aside to be with that sibling before and after the new infant arrives into the home.

● STUDY ACTIVITIES

1. Depending on the information obtained by the interview, each symptom and/or feeling can be placed on a list and matched to the appropriate trimester. For example: fatigue, breast tenderness, urinary frequency, ambivalence = first trimester. Increased energy level, less urinary frequency, fetal movement = second trimester. Backache, frequency, introspection = third trimester.

2. The student should select about three Web sites and present the URLs during a post conference or in a group with a thorough description of what each site has to offer.

3. Physiologic anemia of pregnancy

4. Compression of the vena cava by the heavy gravid uterus

Chapter 12

● MULTIPLE CHOICE QUESTIONS

1. The correct response is A. Research has linked a deficiency of folic acid to an increased incidence of neural tube defects. Pregnant women are given a folic acid supplement to prevent this fetal deformity. Vitamin A is not linked to neural tube defects. Vitamin C is not responsible for preventing neural tube defects. Vitamin K helps with blood clotting and is not linked to neural tube defects in newborns.

2. The correct response is C. Kegel exercises help to tighten and strength pelvic floor muscles to improve tone. They can help prevent stress incontinence in women after childbirth. These exercises don't strengthen the perineal area on the outside to prevent lacerations, but rather the internal pelvic floor muscles. Kegel exercises have nothing to do with the start of labor for postdates infants. A drop in progesterone levels and an increase in prostaglandins augment labor, not exercise. Kegel exercises don't burn calories.

3. The correct response is D. The uterus is constantly contracting throughout pregnancy, but the contractions are irregular and not usually felt by the woman, nor do they cause dilation of the cervix. Braxton Hicks contractions are not the start of early labor, since there aren't any measurable cervical changes. They are normal throughout the pregnancy, not an ominous sign of an impending abortion. A woman's hydration status is not related to Braxton Hicks contractions; they occur regardless of her fluid status.

4. The correct response is C. The underwater pressure incurred during scuba diving may cause oxygenation changes and a decrease in perfusion to the placenta. There is also a risk of trauma from coral reefs and boating. Swimming is an appropriate sport if the woman does not swim alone or after a heavy meal. Walking is an appropriate exercise to promote well-being. Bike riding provides good leg exercise and is appropriate if safety precautions are observed.

5. The correct response is D. In using Nagele's rule, 3 months are subtracted and 7 days are added, plus 1 year from the date of the last menstrual period.

● CRITICAL THINKING EXERCISES

1.

a. What subjective and objective data do you have to make your assessment?

Subjective data: reports feeling extreme fatigue; sleeps 8 to 9 hours each night; eats poorly

Objective data: pale and tired appearance; pale mucous membranes, low H & H

b. What is your impression of this woman?

She is in her first trimester of pregnancy, when fatigue is a normal complaint due to the diversion of the maternal glucose to the developing fetus. In addition, she is anemic (low H & H) due to eating habits or perhaps pica. It is important for the nurse to report this finding to the health care professional for further investigation of the cause.

c. What nursing interventions would be appropriate for this client?

Reassure her that the fatigue is a common complaint of pregnancy in the first trimester, but her poor dietary habits are contributing to her fatigue. She is anemic and needs to improve her diet and increase the amount of iron and vitamin C she takes. She also needs to increase her fiber intake to prevent constipation. An iron supplement might be advised by the healthcare provider to address her anemia. Request that the client keep a food log to bring with her to the next visit to review. A referral for nutritional counseling would be appropriate.

d. How will you evaluate the effectiveness of your interventions?

To assess compliance with the iron supplement, ask her what color her stools are. If they are dark, then she is taking the iron; if not, she probably isn't. Ask what dietary changes she has made to improve her nutrition by reviewing her food log and making suggestions to increase her iron consumption. Also review the importance of good nutrition for the positive outcome of this pregnancy. Do another H & H level to monitor her anemia.

2.

a. In addition to the routine obstetric assessments, which additional ones might be warranted for this teenager?

Calculate Monica's body mass index (BMI) based on height and weight (BMI = 17.8, which places her at high risk for not gaining enough weight during pregnancy).

Ask Monica if she takes drugs or alcohol, which might have a negative impact on the pregnancy.

Request a 24-hour diet recall, which might reveal low calorie and calcium intake.

Ascertain who does the cooking and food purchasing in her house; ask that the person accompany her to the clinic for her next visit for dietary teaching.

Explore reasons why she won't drink milk, and provide her with information about other sources of calcium that she might substitute for milk, such as yogurt.

b. What dietary instruction should be provided to this teenager based on her history?

Stress the importance of gaining weight for the baby's health.

Encourage she eat three meals each day plus three high-fiber snacks.

Go over the Food Guide Pyramid with her to show her selections from each group that she needs to consume daily.

Request that she take a peanut butter and jelly sandwich on whole-wheat bread to school to make sure she eats a good lunch each day.

Instruct her on limiting her intake of sodas and caffeinated drinks.

Encourage her to drink calcium-fortified orange juice for breakfast daily.

Reinforce the importance of taking her prenatal vitamin daily.

Send her home with printed materials for review.

c. What follow-up monitoring should be included in subsequent prenatal visits?

Increase the frequency of prenatal visits to every 2 weeks to monitor weight gain for the next few months.

Refer Monica and her mother to the nutritionist in the WIC program for a more thorough dietary instruction.

Request a 24-hour dietary recall at each prenatal visit to provide a basis for instruction and reinforcement.

3.

a. What additional information would the nurse need to assess her complaint?

Ask Maria for a 24-hour food intake recall to assess what other food she eats.

Ask Maria if she had this problem before becoming pregnant.

Ask Maria if she takes iron supplementation in addition to her prenatal vitamin.

Ask Maria how much and what kind of fluid intake she has in 24 hours.

Ask Maria whether she engages in any exercise consistently.

b. What advice would be appropriate for the nurse to give Maria?

The nurse needs to discuss with her the reasons why she is constipated: heavy gravid uterus compressing the intestines, reduced peristalsis and smooth muscle relaxation secondary to progesterone, low fiber and fluid intake, and limited exercise. To reduce the problem, Maria will need to make changes in the areas of food, fluid, and exercise.

c. What lifestyle adaptations will Maria need to make to alter her constipation?

Maria will need to consume high-fiber foods (fruits and vegetables) and increase her fluid intake to 2,000 mL daily to overcome the constipation. In addition, she will need to get off the couch and get some exercise, perhaps walking. Finally, she will need to stop taking stimulant laxatives and change to bulk-forming ones if the increase in high-fiber foods and fluids doesn't work for her.

● STUDY ACTIVITIES

1–4. The answers to activities 1 to 4 are highly individualized.

5. Doula

Chapter 13

● MULTIPLE CHOICE QUESTIONS

1. The correct response is A. Frequency is measured from the start of one contraction to the start of the next contraction. The duration of a contraction is measured from the beginning of one contraction to the end of that same contraction. The intensity of two contractions is measured by comparing the peak of one contraction with the peak of the next contraction. The resting interval is measured from the end of one contraction to the beginning of the next contraction.

2. The correct response is B. A longitudinal lie places the fetus in a vertical position, which would be the most conducive for a spontaneous vaginal birth. A transverse lie would not allow for a vaginal birth because the fetus would be lying perpendicular to the maternal spine. A perpendicular lie describes the transverse lie, which would not be conducive for a spontaneous birth. An oblique lie would not allow for a spontaneous vaginal birth because the fetus would not fit through the maternal pelvis in this side-lying position.

3. The correct response is C. After the placenta separates from the uterine wall, the shape of the uterus changes from discord to globular. The uterus continues to contract throughout the placental separation process and the umbilical cord continues to pulsate for several minutes after placental separation occurs. Maternal blood pressure is not affected by placental separation because the maternal blood volume has increased dramatically during pregnancy to compensate for blood loss during birth.

4. The correct response is A. The release of amniotic fluid through an amniotomy stimulates uterine contractions and is used to augment labor by reducing the distention of the uterus. Rupturing the amniotic sac will increase the risk of an ascending infection by removing the protection of a closed system. An amniotomy allows an increase in fetal head compressions; thus, fetal heart decelerations, not accelerations, might result. With less fluid to absorb the impact of muscular contractions, contraction intensity increases and discomfort increases.

5. The correct response is C. The transitional phase of the first stage of labor occurs when the contractions are 1 to 2 minutes apart and the final dilation is taking place. The transition phase is the most difficult and, fortunately, the shortest phase for the woman, lasting approximately 1 hour in the first birth and perhaps 15 to 30 minutes in successive births. Many women are not able to cope well with the intensity of this short period, become restless, and request pain medications. During the latent phase, contractions are mild. The women is in early labor and able to cope with the infrequent contractions. This phase can last hours. The active phase involves moderate contractions that allow for a brief rest period in between, helping the woman to be able to cope with the next contraction. This phase can last hours. The placental expulsion phase occurs during the third stage of labor. After separation of the placenta from the uterine wall, continued uterine contractions cause the placenta to be expelled. Although this phase can last 5 to 30 minutes, the contraction intensity is less than that of the transition phase.

● CRITICAL THINKING EXERCISES

1.

a. What additional information do you need to respond appropriately?

• Ask about the frequency and duration of her contractions.
• Ask about how long she has experienced "labor pains."
• Ask about any other signs she may have experienced such as bloody show, lightening, backache, ruptured membranes, and so forth.
• Ask if walking tends to increase or decrease the intensity of contractions.
• Ask her when she last felt fetal movement.
• Ask her how far away (distance) she is from the birthing center.
• Ask her if she has a support person in the home with her.

b. What suggestions/recommendations would you make to her?

• Stay in the comfort of her home environment as long as possible.
• Advise her to walk as much as possible to see what effect it has on the contractions. Also, tell her to drink fluids to hydrate herself.
• Review nonpharmacologic comfort measures she can try at home.
• Tell her to keep in contact with the birthing center staff regarding her experience.

c. What instructions need to be given to guide her decision making?

• Instruct her on how to time frequency and duration of contractions.
• Wait until contractions are 5 minutes apart or her membranes rupture to come to the birthing center.
• Tell her to come to the birthing center when she cannot talk during a contraction.
• Reinforce all instructions with her support partner.

2.

a. What other premonitory signs of labor might the nurse ask about?

• Has she experienced the feeling of the fetus dropping (lightening) lower down?
• Has her energy level changed (increased) in the last day or so?
• Has she noticed any reddish discharge (bloody show) from her vagina?
• Has she had any episodes of diarrhea within the last 48 hours?
• Has her "bag of waters" broken or does she feel any leakage?

b. What manifestations would be found if Cindy is experiencing true labor?

There would be progressive dilation and effacement of her cervix if true labor is occurring. Contraction pain also would not be relieved with walking, and the pain would start in the back and radiate around toward the front of the abdomen. Contractions also would occur regularly, becoming closer together, usually 4 to 6 minutes apart, and last 30 to 60 seconds. If she is experiencing false labor, slight effacement might be present, but not dilation.

3.

a. Topics to address in the community education program would include

• Information about the stages of labor, including what to expect
• Explanation of risks and benefits about any interventional procedures that might be performed during the labor process
• Information about the available pain relief measures
• Methods of involvement and participation during the labor and birthing process by partner/doula/family member
• Information about variables that may alter or influence the course of labor and include preoperative teaching for cesarean birth

● STUDY ACTIVITIES

1. This discussion should involve the passenger, powers, passageway, position, and psychological response of the student's assigned women going through labor and how each affected the length and stages of labor.

2. Answers A, B, and E are correct. The cardinal movements of labor by the fetus include engagement, descent, flexion, international rotation, extension, external rotation, and expulsion only. The other choices describe the various fetal positions.

3. This discussion will vary depending on the women's labor and birth experience. Psychological factors that could be addressed might include previous birth experiences, age, pregnancy discomforts, cultural beliefs, expectations for this birth experience, preparation for birth, and effectiveness and participation of support system.

4. See the following figure. For duration, the "X" is placed at the start of one contraction and at the end of it.

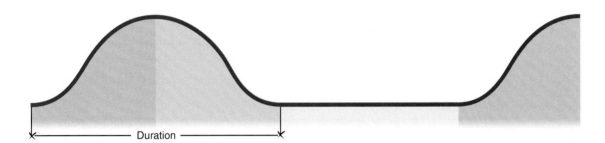

Duration

Chapter 14

● MULTIPLE CHOICE QUESTIONS

1. The correct response is D. Intermittent pushing with each contraction is more effective than continuous pushing, which reduces perfusion to the placenta. Holding the breath and pushing through the entire contraction is incorrect because this action reduces blood flow and oxygenation to the uterus and to the fetus. Chest breathing is not an effective breathing pattern to increase intra-abdominal pressure, which assists the contraction to expel the fetus. Panting and blowing is used between contractions to abstain from pushing.

2. The correct response is B. A full bladder causes displacement of the uterus above it, and increased bleeding results secondary to the uncontracted status of the uterus. Massaging the uterus will help to make it firm but will not help to bring it back into the midline, since the full bladder is occupying the space it would normally assume. Notifying the primary healthcare provider is not necessary unless the woman continues to have difficulty voiding and the uterus remains displaced. The normal location of the uterus in the fourth stage of labor is in the midline. Displacement suggests a full bladder, which is not considered a normal finding.

3. The correct response is C. The entire focus of the labor and birth experience is for the family to make decisions, not the caretakers. The nurse's role is to respect and support those decisions.

Decisions about pain management are not based on length of the various stages of labor, but rather on what provides effective pain relief for the laboring woman. Pain-relief measures differ. Each individual responds differently and uniquely to various pain-relief measures. Not recommending nonpharmacologic measures demonstrates bias on the nurse's part; it is not the nurse's decision to make, but rather the client's decision.

4. The correct response is A. Several professional women's health organizations have published guidelines concerning the timing of intermittent FHR assessments during the active stage of labor. The current recommendation is that intermittent FHR is assessed every 15 minutes during the active phase of labor.

5. The correct response is C. Fetal accelerations denote an intact central nervous system and appropriate oxygenation levels demonstrated by an increase in heart rate associated with fetal movement. Accelerations are a reassuring pattern, so no intervention is needed. Turning the woman on her left side would be an appropriate intervention for a late deceleration pattern. Administering 100% oxygen via face mask would be appropriate for a late or variable deceleration pattern. Since fetal accelerations are a reassuring pattern, no orders are needed from the healthcare provider, nor does the healthcare provider need to be notified of this reassuring pattern.

● CRITICAL THINKING EXERCISE

1.

a. Based on your assessment data and the woman's request not to have medication, what nonpharmacologic interventions could the nurse offer her?

• Progressive relaxation techniques of locating, then releasing tension from one muscle group at a time until the entire body is relaxed
• Visual imagery such as taking a journey in the woman's mind to a relaxing place that is far away from the discomfort of labor
• Music to bring about a calming effect as well as a distraction or attention focusing to divert attention away from the laboring process; focusing on sound or rhythm helps release tension and promote relaxation.
• Massage/acupressure to enhance relaxation, improve circulation, and reduce pain in labor; counterpressure on the lower back to help relieve back pain
• Breathing techniques for effective attention-focusing strategies to enhance coping mechanisms during labor

b. What positions might be suggested to help facilitate fetal descent?

• Upright positions such as walking, swaying, slow-dancing with her partner, or leaning over a birthing ball will all enhance comfort and use the force of gravity to facilitate fetal descent.
• Kneeling and leaning forward will help relieve back pain.
• Pelvic rocking on hands and knees and lunging with one foot elevated on a chair may help with internal fetal rotation and speed a slow labor.

2.

a. What assessment needs to be done to determine what is happening?

The nurse should perform a vaginal examination to validate that she is in the transition phase (8 to 10 cm dilated).

b. What explanation can you offer Carrie's partner regarding her change in behavior?

Explain to her partner that she is in the transition phase of the first stage of labor and that her behavior is typical, since she is having hard contractions frequently. Reassure him not to take Carrie's comments personally, but to stay and be supportive to her.

● STUDY ACTIVITIES

1. This information will vary depending on what the woman reports to the student. Unrealistic pain-management plans need to be identified and valid evidence-based ones presented to the woman. Misconceptions can be cleared up also.

2. *Acceleration*—elevation of FHR above the baseline; a reassuring pattern

3. The findings will vary from facility to facility, but the student might find a more liberal use of non-pharmacologic techniques in the birthing center compared to the hospital setting and more frequent use of hydrotherapy and ambulation to relieve discomfort. Also, intermittent assessment using a hand-held Doppler is probably used more frequently in the birthing center compared to the hospital, where continuous electronic fetal monitoring is prevalent.

4. Many childbirth web sites present very basic information about childbirth and attempt to target a wide audience of educational levels. Many of the childbirth web sites promote various pregnancy and infant products.

Chapter 15

● MULTIPLE CHOICE QUESTIONS

1. The correct response is A. Engorgement refers to the swelling of the breast tissue as a result of an increase in blood and lymph supply to produce milk for the newborn. Estrogen and progesterone levels decrease considerably and are not restored until the first menses returns several weeks or months later, depending on the lactation status of the mother. Colostrum can be secreted as early as 16 weeks' gestation. The mother's body is going through profuse diuresis to restore prepregnant fluid levels to her body and therefore would not be retaining fluid in the breasts.

2. The correct response is C. According to Reba Rubin, the mother is very passive and is dependent on others to care for herself for the first 24 to 48 hours after giving birth. Gaining self-confidence would characterize a mother in the taking-hold phase, during which the mother demonstrates mastery over her own body's functioning and feels more confident in caring for her newborn. Adjustment to relationships does not occur until the third phase—letting go, when the mother begins to separate from the symbiotic relationship she and her newborn enjoyed during pregnancy and birth. Resuming control over her life would denote the second phase of

taking hold, during which the mother does resume control over her life and gains self-confidence in her newborn care.

3. The correct response is D. The direct cause of afterpains is uterine contractions. Mothers experience abdominal pain secondary to contractions, especially when breast-feeding because sucking stimulates the release of oxytocin from the posterior pituitary gland, which causes uterine contractions. Manipulation of the uterus during labor would only occur during a surgical birth and this discomfort would not be sustained weeks later. The size of the infant might cause additional stretching of the uterus, but it is not the underlying cause of the afterpains. Pregnancies spaced too close together can contribute to frequent stretching of the uterus, but this is not the cause of afterpains.

4. The correct response is B. Lochia discharge from the uterus proceeds in an orderly fashion, regardless of a surgical or vaginal birth. Its color changes from red to pink to whitish cream consistently, unless there is a complication. The correct sequence is rubra (red), then serosa (pink), and then alba (white, creamy).

5. The correct response is C. The body attempts to rid the woman's body of excess fluids retained during pregnancy after giving childbirth. This is accomplished in two ways: an increase in urinary output and profuse diaphoresis. There is no relationship between lactation and profuse diaphoresis. The body increases blood and lymph fluid to the breasts in preparation for lactation. Pain medications used during labor and birth are metabolized in the liver and excreted in the urine, not through profuse sweating. Fever would accompany an infectious process and there is no mention of an elevated temperature in the mother.

● CRITICAL THINKING EXERCISES

1.

a. Is there something "wrong" with Ms Griffin's behavior?

No, this is typical behavior for a new mother within the first 2 days after giving birth.

b. What maternal role phase is being described by the new nurse?

This behavior is characteristic of Reba Rubin's taking-in phase, which covers the first 48 hours after childbirth. The new mother is typically focused on her own needs for rest, food, and comfort. New mothers in this phase tend to be passive and take directions/suggestions well from staff. Preoccupation with themselves rather than their newborns is normal during this phase. Their needs must be met before they can begin to care for others.

c. What role can the nurse play to support the mother through this phase?

The nurse can be supportive through this early phase by providing a restful, quiet environment to facilitate her recovery from childbirth. Providing her with simple guidance and suggestions of how she can care for herself and her newborn will assist the new mother in expanding her focus. Praising her for her accomplishments in care will reinforce it.

2.

a. Would you consider Mr. Lenhart's paternal behavior to be normal at this time?

Yes, inexperienced first-time fathers are anxious around their newborns because this is a new experience for them and many do not know how to handle or care for their newborns yet. Paternal attachment is a gradual process that occurs over weeks and months.

b. What might Mr. Lenhart be feeling at this time?

He is probably feeling overwhelmed with this tiny baby and, although he probably wants to help, he is anxious about how or what to do without appearing awkward.

c. How can the nurse help this new father adjust to their new role?

The nurse can help new fathers adjust to their role by taking time to listen to their concerns and demonstrating how they can become involved in the care of their newborn. Staying in the room and physically supporting the father as he tries out his new role will provide encouragement for him to become involved. The nurse can slowly introduce fathers to the care needs of their newborn and encourage their participation. This supportive role by the nurse can help reduce role strain and enhance family adjustment.

● STUDY ACTIVITIES

1. Possible Internet resources helpful to parents after childbirth would be
   • The Center for Postpartum Health, www.postpartumhealth.com
   • Postpartum Support International, www.chss.iup.edu/postpartum

2. The teaching plan might include the following topics:
   • Involution of uterus
   • Stages and color of lochia
   • Diaphoresis
   • Breast changes (lactating and nonlactating)
   • Discomforts after birth, such as perineal healing (ice packs, sitz baths), afterpains (analgesics), breast engorgement (supportive bra)
   • Follow-up care for mother

3. Involution

4. Full bladder

Chapter 16

● MULTIPLE CHOICE QUESTIONS

1. The correct response is C. Periodic crying and insomnia are characteristic of postpartum blues, in addition to mood changes, irritability, and increased sensitivity. Panic attacks and suicidal thoughts or anger toward self and the infant would be descriptive of postpartum psychosis, when some women turn this anger toward themselves and have committed suicide or infanticide. Women experiencing postpartum blues do not lose touch with reality. Obsessive thoughts and hallucinations would be more descriptive of postpartum psychosis.

2. The correct response is D. Nurses need first to become educated about various cultural practices to incorporate them into their care delivery. By gaining an understanding of diverse cultures different from their own, nurses can become sensitive to these different practices and not violate them. Attending a transcultural course might be beneficial, but this would take several weeks to complete and the information is needed much sooner to provide culturally sensitive care for an admitted patient and her family. Caring for only families of the nurse's cultural origin would not be possible or realistic in our global, culturally diverse population within the United States. Nurses need to care for every person regardless of their color, creed, or nationality with respect and competence. Teaching diverse cultural families Western beliefs would demonstrate ethnocentric behavior and would not be professional. Each culture needs to be respected and learned about with tolerance and understanding.

3. The correct response is B. Because weight loss is based on the principle of intake of calories and output of energy, instructing this woman to avoid high-calorie foods that yield no nutritive value and expending more energy through active exercise would result in weight loss for her. Acid-producing foods (plums, cranberries, and prunes) are typically recommended for women to prevent urinary tract infections to acidify the urine and not for weight loss purposes. Increasing fluid intake (water) would be good for weight loss because it fills the stomach and reduces hunger sensations; however, this option does not identify which fluids should be increased. Increasing high-calorie juice and soda drinks would be counterproductive to weight loss measures. Fluid restriction combined with a high-protein diet would increase the risk of gout and formation of kidney stones. Carbohydrates are needed by the body to make ATP and convert it to energy for cellular processes. Limiting snacks might be a good suggestion depending on which ones are selected. Raw fruits and vegetables are excellent high-fiber snacks that will help in an overall weight loss program.

4. The correct response is C. Lactating mothers need an extra 500 cal to sustain breast-feeding. An additional 20 g of protein is also needed to help build and regenerate body cells for the lactating woman. Additional intake of carbohydrates or fiber is not suggested for lactation. An increase in fats is not recommended nor is it needed for breast-feeding. To obtain adequate amounts of vitamins during lactation, women are encouraged to choose a varied diet that includes enriched and fortified grains and cereals, fresh fruits and vegetables, and lean meats and dairy products. An increase in vitamins via supplements is not recommended. Choosing a variety of foods from the food pyramid will provide the lactating women with adequate iron and minerals.

5. The correct response is D. A swollen, tender area on the breast would indicate mastitis, which would need medical intervention. Fatigue and irritability are not complications of childbearing, but rather the norm during the early postpartum period secondary to infant care demands and lack of sleep on the caretaker's part. Perineal dis-

comfort and lochia serosa are normal physiologic events after childbirth and indicate normal uterine involution. Bradycardia is a normal vital sign for several days after childbirth because or the dramatic circulatory changes that take place with the loss of the placenta at birth and the return of blood back to the central circulation.

6. The correct response is A. Desiring to be in close proximity to another human being is all part of the bonding process. Bonding cannot take place with separation of individuals. Closeness is needed by the two people bonding, and not having others hold the infant. Buying or wearing expensive clothes has no emotional effect on a bonding relationship. Requesting that nurses provide care separates the parent from the infant and suggests that the parents lack the desire for closeness with their infant.

7. The correct response is C. Older sibling needs to feel they are still loved and not upstaged by the newest family member. Allowing special time for that sibling reinforces the parent's love for them also. Regression behavior is common when there is stress in that sibling's life, and punishing him brings attention to negative behavior, possibly reinforcing it. The older sibling might feel he/she is being replaced and is not wanted by the parents when he/she is sent away. Including the older sibling in the care of the newborn is a better way to incorporate the newest member into the family unit. Sharing a room with the infant could lead to feelings of displacement in the sibling. In addition, frequent interruptions during the day and night will awaken the sibling and not allow a full night's sleep or undisturbed nap.

● CRITICAL THINKING EXERCISES

1.

a. What is your nursing assessment of this encounter?

Nursing observations would indicate poor bonding/attachment behaviors between mother and infant based on
• Disinterest in holding or being close to infant
• Lack of concern for infant's needs
• More concerned about phone conversation
• Negative comment about newborn ("monkey")

b. What nursing interventions would be appropriate?

Assess for risk factors in client—age, outside family support, multiple life stressors, unrealistic expectations of newborn behaviors, level of education, family support system—and determine the client's perception of newborn behaviors and educate her about normal newborn behaviors and mothering activities needed. In addition, model parent care behaviors in caring for a newborn and ascertain the availability of any family support—extended family, neighbors, and community resources.

c. What specific discharge interventions may be needed?

Based on observations and assessment data, this client would need a referral to the discharge planner, social services department, or local health department for home visit follow-up care. Bonding/attachment behaviors are lacking, possibly placing the newborn at risk for neglect or abuse.

2.

a. Which of these assessment findings warrants further investigation?

• Tearful client pacing the floor holding her crying son
• Distended bladder upon palpation; reporting frequency
• Fundus firm and displaced to right of midline

b. What interventions are appropriate at this time and why?

It is apparent that Jennifer is overwhelmed and does not seem to be coping well with her new parenting role. She may be experiencing postpartum blues as well. She needs support during this critical period. The home care nurse needs to ascertain what family or support systems are available and make contact with them for help. Questioning Jennifer about previous crying episodes or feeling "down" recently is in order to ascertain whether she is feeling the "blues" in addition to being overwhelmed. If limited resources are available, assigning a home health aide to come daily to assist Jennifer might be needed. Counseling and active listening will be helpful during the home care visit.

The uterine fundus is displaced out of the midline as a result of a distended bladder. The bladder needs to be emptied for the uterus to assume midline positioning. Jennifer's urinary frequency may be the result of distention secondary to poor bladder tone or a developing urinary tract infection. The nurse should attempt to get Jennifer to void on her own and obtain a clean-catch urine specimen. Checking for bacteria with a chemical reagent strip ("dipstick") is appropriate. Instituting measures to promote voiding—tap water running, forcing fluids, and cranberry juice—also would be appropriate interventions. If a bacterium is found in the clean-catch urine specimen, calling Jennifer's health care provider to obtain an order for medication would be necessary. Otherwise, advising Jennifer to increase her fluid intake and voiding frequently to empty her bladder would be in order.

c. **What health teaching is needed before you leave this home?**

Information about postpartum blues should be discussed, emphasizing that it is benign and self-limiting. Assuring Jennifer that this is very common and allowing time for Jennifer to vent her frustrations and to express her feelings can be very therapeutic. Increasing awareness about postpartum blues can bring it into focus and help her understand this event in her life. In addition, review of self-care and newborn care measures that allow Jennifer to rest need to be outlined. Suggesting that Jennifer nap when the baby sleeps throughout the day is a start. Attempting to cluster baby care (bathing, feeding, and dressing) might give her additional time for herself. Calling on friends and family to help out should be stressed. Other interventions would include

• Reassurance that her mothering ability is fine and the newborn is healthy
• Referral to community home health agency to gain home health aide assistance
• Discussions concerning accepting help and support from others
• Times and dates of follow-up care appointments
• Community resources available to assist her through this time

● STUDY ACTIVITIES

1. How have you been feeling recently? How has your sleep been? Have you felt low in spirits and/or able to enjoy the things you usually enjoy?

2. A possible Internet site might be La Leche League International (www.lalecheleague.org)

3.
   • Wash your hands with soap and water, and dry them.
   • Fill your peribottle with warm tap water and replace the top.

3.
a. **What response by the nurse would be appropriate at this time?**
Reply in a sensitive, nonjudgmental manner that this bottle of formula has been sitting out for 3 hours since the last feeding and has not been refrigerated. It may be contaminated and would not be appropriate to feed her baby with now.

b. **What action by the nurse should take place?**
Take the old bottle of formula and tell Lisa that you will get her a fresh bottle for this feeding. Leave the room with the formula bottle and replace it with another one.

c. **What health teaching is needed for Lisa prior to discharge?**
A thorough explanation is needed about feeding practices, emphasizing that formula is milk and needs to be refrigerated when not being used for feeding at that time. Leaving formula sit at room temperature for long periods increases the risk of bacterial contamination and may give her infant gastroenteritis. In addition, as the infant grows, more formula will be consumed at each feeding, and making up an approximate amount that will consumed will become easier for her to avoid waste.

• Straddle the toilet and spray all the water from the peribottle over your perineal area.
• Pat the area dry with a clean towel and replace your peripad from front to back.
• Place the empty peribottle on the sink for the next time.
• Wash your hands with soap and water before leaving the bathroom.

4. Engorgement

Chapter 17
● MULTIPLE CHOICE QUESTIONS

1. The correct response is B. The behaviors demonstrated by the newborn, such as alertness, stabilized heart and respiratory rates, and passage of meconium are associated with the second period of reactivity. The first period of reactivity starts with a period of quiet alertness followed by an active alertness with frequent bursts of movement and crying. During the decreased responsiveness period, also called the *sleep period,* the newborn is relatively unresponsive and difficult to waken.

2. The correct response is C. Convection is loss of heat from an object to the environment. Using the portholes instead of opening the isolette door

prevents rapid heat loss from the inside of the isolette. This action also protects the newborn from drafts. Evaporation is the loss of heat as water is lost from the skin to the environment. Keeping the newborn dry will prevent this type of heat loss. Conduction is the transfer of heat from one object to another when in direct contact, such as placing a newborn onto a cold scale to be weighed. Radiation is the loss of heat between objects that are not in direct contact, such as a cold window near the newborn's isolette.

3. The correct response is D. Evaporation is the loss of heat as water is lost from the skin to the environment. Drying the newborn at birth and after bathing, keeping linens dry, and using plastic wrap blankets and heat shields will all prevent

heat loss through evaporation. Placing the newborn on a warmed surface will prevent heat loss via conduction. Maintaining a warm room temperature will prevent heat loss via convection. Transporting the newborn in an isolette will prevent heat loss via radiation.

4. The correct response is A. The foramen ovale is the fetal structure within the heart that allows blood to cross immediately to the left side and bypass the pulmonary circuit. When left-side pressure gradients increase at birth, this opening closes, thereby establishing an extrauterine circulation pattern. The ductus venosus is not located in the heart; it is located between the umbilical vein and the inferior vena cava, and it shunts blood away from the liver during fetal life. The ductus arteriosus connects the pulmonary artery to the aorta to bypass the pulmonary circuit. It begins to constrict as pulmonary circulation increases and arterial oxygen tension increases. The umbilical vein, along with two umbilical arteries, is part of the umbilical cord that is cut at birth.

● CRITICAL THINKING EXERCISE

1.
a. What is your impression of this observation?
It is evident the new nurse's behaviors demonstrate a lack of awareness or knowledge about thermoregulation in newborns. Reinforcement of these principles is needed. Perhaps she needs to be reminded of newborns' inability to keep themselves warm as a result of a variety of factors. Or perhaps she may feel overwhelmed with caring for more than one newborn at a time. An in-service for all nursery personnel might be a good reinforcement of this concept.

b. What principles concerning thermoregulation need to be reinforced?
All four. The nurse is subjecting the newborn to heat loss by all four methods—evaporation (bathing), radiation (leaving door open), convection (cap off), and conduction (weighing). Newborns have an inability to conserve body heat and experience heat loss through four mechanisms: conduction, convection, evaporation, and radiation. Placing newborns on cold surfaces without any protection (such as a blanket or cover), will cause them to lose body heat via conduction. By exposing them while wet, such as during bathing, heat is lost through evaporation. Leaving the storage room open permits cool air flow over the newborn, allowing heat loss by convection. Placing the infant transporter near cold rooms allows for transfer of neonatal body heat via radiation.

c. How will you evaluate your instruction after the in-service is presented?
The effectiveness of the in-service can be evaluated by observing the behavior of the staff while caring for the newborns. Hopefully, the principles reinforced during the discussion will be applied in the handling of the newborns. For the new nurse, it would be important to observe the nurse covering the newborn when bathing, placing a warmed blanket on the scale prior to weighing, closing hallway doors to prevent drafts, and keeping a cap on the newborn's head when showing him or her to his or her parents. In addition, the nurse should verbalize why she is performing all these actions.

● STUDY ACTIVITIES

1. First period of reactivity behavior: burst of rapid, jerky movements of the extremities; sucking activity; smacking and rooting; and fine tremors of the extremities. Second period behavior: newborn's alertness gradually declines and they sleep. Third period: newborns awaken and become more interactive with the environment. Movement is smoother compared with the first period of reactivity. Meconium may be passed during this period.

2. Initially the heart rate immediately on admission to the nursery would be high (120–180 bpm), but after several hours it typically will decline (120–140 bpm). The respiratory rate will be rapid (60–80 bpm), with periods of apnea lasting 5 seconds or less. After several hours, the respiratory rate will decline (30–50 bpm) and periods of apnea will become less frequent. The temperature of the newly admitted newborn may be on the low end of normal (36.5–37°C) if there has been no hypothermia while transporting the newborn from the birthing area. After being under a radiant heat source for several hours and not exposed to drafts or moisture, the temperature should be in the mid range of temperature norms. If the temperature remains stabilized, a bath can be given.

3. American Academy of Pediatrics, www.aap.org; Neonatal Network, www.neonatalwork.com

4. Evaporation

Chapter 18

● MULTIPLE CHOICE QUESTIONS

1. The correct response is D. One point would be subtracted for color (acrocyanosis) and 1 point for fair flexion of extremities. All the assessment parameters should rate 2 points, except for color and flexion. Therefore, any score except 8 points would be incorrect.

2. The correct response is D. Phototherapy reduces the bilirubin on the newborn's skin via oxidation. Phototherapy does not affect surfactant levels in the newborn's lungs nor does it help to stabilize temperatures in the newborn. In fact, it might cause hyperthermia at times if not monitored closely. Phototherapy cannot destroy Rh antibodies attached to RBCs within the circulation.

3. The correct response is B. Vitamin K is needed for blood clotting and is a vital component of the blood-clotting cascade. The newborn's gut is sterile at birth and unable to manufacture vitamin K on its own without an outside source initially. Vitamin K has no impact on bilirubin conjugation, transport, or excretion. It is not involved in closing the foreman ovale; cutting the cord and changing gradient vascular pressures are responsible for this closure. Vitamin K has no influence over the digestive process of complex proteins.

4. The correct response is A. The eyes of newborns can be exposed to gonorrhea and/or chlamydial organisms if present in the mother's vagina during the birth process, possibly resulting in a severe infection and blindness. Therefore, eye prophylaxis is administered. Thrush and *Enterobacter* typically do not affect the eyes. Thrush develops in the newborn's mouth after exposure to maternal vaginal yeast infections during the birth process. Infections with *Staphylococcus* and syphilis are contracted through blood stream exposure or via the placenta and not by contact with the maternal vagina during birth. Eye treatment would not impact/treat either infectious process. Hepatitis B and herpes are not treatable with eye ointment.

5. The correct response is C. Research has identified sleeping position and its link to SIDS. Since 1992, the AAP has recommended all newborns be placed on their backs to sleep. This recommendation has reduced the incidence of SIDS dramatically. Respiratory distress syndrome involves a lack of surfactant in the lungs, not sleeping position. The intake of formula or juice (high lactose exposure) being allowed to sit in the infant's mouth while sleeping is the cause of bottle mouth syndrome. Positioning on the back might aggravate the GI regurgitation syndrome rather than help it.

6. The correct response is D. Most newborns are started on the hepatitis B series before discharge from the hospital and receive the remaining two immunizations at 1 month and at 4 to 6 months of age. The pneumococcal vaccine is given between 2 to 23 months of age, not at birth. Varicella immunization is not given until 12 to 18 months of age. Hepatitis A immunization is recommended for children and adolescents in selected states and regions, and for high-risk groups. It is not a universal vaccine for all children.

7. The correct response is C. Ingestion of certain amino acids found in breast milk or formula must be accumulated in the newborn to identify a deficiency in an enzyme that cannot metabolism them. If the PKU test is done prior to 24 to 48 hours after feeding, it must be repeated after the infant has tolerated feedings for at least that length of time. Identifying hypothyroidism is not linked to ingesting protein feedings. Cystic fibrosis is a genetic inherited condition not related to protein intake. Sickle cell disease is a genetically inherited condition unrelated to protein ingestion in the newborn.

● CRITICAL THINKING EXERCISES

1.

a. How should the nurse respond to Ms. Scott's questions?

In a calm manner, explain to Ms. Scott that all her observations are normal variations and address each one separately:

• "Banana-shaped head"—is molding where the newborn had a slight overriding of the skull bones to navigate the bony pelvis and birth canal during the birth process

• "Mushy" feel to head—caput succedaneum, which is an edematous area of the scalp as a result of sustained pressure of the occiput against the cervix during labor and birth process

• "White spots on nose"—milia, which are plugged, distended, small, white sebaceous glands that are present in most newborns and should not be squeezed by the mother

• "Blue bruises on buttocks"—Mongolian spots, which are bluish black areas of pigmentation that are common in African-Americans and have no clinical significance, but can be mistaken for bruises

b. **What additional newborn instruction might be appropriate at this time?**

At this time, it might be appropriate for the nurse to unwrap the newborn and complete a thorough bedside assessment, pointing out any minor deviations to the mother and explaining their significance. This will allay any future anxiety about her newborn and will afford the opportunity to instruct Ms. Scott on various physiologic and behavioral adaptations present in her daughter.

c. **What reassurance can be given to Ms. Scott regarding her daughter's appearance?**

One can assume that Ms. Scott's concern about these various normal deviations might be permanent. The nurse can identify each and provide reassurance about their approximate time of disappearance:
• Molding—transient in nature and should disappear within 72 hours
• Caput succedaneum—disappears spontaneously within 3 to 4 days
• Milia—will clear up spontaneously within the first month
• Mongolian spots—will gradually fade during the first or second year

2.
a. **What impact does an infant abduction have on family and the hospital?**

The abduction of an infant is a devastating event that poses significant emotional, legal, and financial risks to both the family and the hospital. The sudden, unexpected loss of an infant followed by an infinite period of uncertainty concerning the child's well-being places the traumatized family in crisis. The hospital typically will change their security systems, policies, and procedures; heighten supervision; and increase accountability for all staff.

b. **What security measure was the weak link in the chain of security here?**

The nurse was able to pass into the hospital via the emergency room posing as a "nurse" without anyone checking her name tag. The security cameras were not working at the time of the abduction. This allowed the abductor to pass down the hall with the infant unnoticed and unrecorded. The nurses on the unit were unaware of this woman on their unit, which should not happen. There should be an alarm on the doors leading into the unit and the doors should remain locked and only be opened electronically by a staff member on the unit after the person has been identified. There was truly a breakdown of several security measures in this scenario.

c. **What can hospitals do to prevent infant abduction from happening?**

Keys to infant security are awareness and education. The hospital staff should attend annual in-services on these measures and participate in a mock infant abduction drill to heighten awareness of infant security. Specially color-coded staff badges should be worn by all obstetrics staff, and parents should be instructed not to give their newborn to any one without that specific color badge. Parents' wristbands should match the infant's ankle and wrist bands. Everyone must work together to keep all infants safe.

● **STUDY ACTIVITIES**

1. The discussion of newborn changes noticed will vary from student to student, depending on the interview information obtained from the new mother.

2. This discussion will vary depending on questions asked during the bath demonstration as well as each individual mother's response to it.

3. The La Leche Web site is filled with helpful information with pictures to assist new mothers with breastfeeding. Each student will have their own opinion about how helpful and what educational level the Web site addresses.

4. The risks of neonatal circumcision include hemorrhage, infection, adhesions, dehiscence, urethral fistula, meatal stenosis, and pain. The benefits of neonatal circumcision include prevention of penile cancer, decreased incidence of UTIs and STIs, and preservation of male body consistent with father and peers where the procedure is common. Students will express their own opinion about their thoughts based on their value system and cultural background.

Chapter 19

● **MULTIPLE CHOICE QUESTIONS**

1. The correct response is A. Magnesium sulfate is a central nervous system depressant that interferes with calcium uptake in the cells of the myometrium, thus reducing the muscular ability to contract. Magnesium sulfate is not used as supplementation during pregnancy because most pregnant women do not have a deficiency of this mineral. Magnesium sulfate would not be effective against constipation in pregnant women. Magnesium sulfate does not stimulate musculoskeletal tone to augment labor contractions; rather, it has the opposite effect.

2. The correct response is D. Women with a history of preterm birth are at highest risk for the same in subsequent pregnancies. Because there is not a

complete understanding of causes of preterm labor, whatever situation existed in a previous pregnancy to initiate early labor may still be present for this pregnancy. Having had twins previously would have no bearing on this singleton pregnancy to influence a preterm labor. Location of residence is not a risk factor for preterm labor. The woman's occupation as a computer programmer and sitting at a computer all day would not increase her risk for preterm labor. However, standing for long periods in a work environment might increase her risk.

3. The correct response is B. When the placenta separates from the uterine wall, it causes irritation and bleeding into the muscle fibers, which causes pain. Painless, bright-red bleeding indicates placenta previa symptomatology. Excessive nausea and vomiting would be characteristic of hyperemesis gravidarum. Hypertension and headache would be associated with gestational hypertension.

4. The correct response is C. Calcium channel blockers, such as nifedipine (Procardia), inhibit calcium from entering smooth muscle cells, thus reducing uterine contractions. This type of drug would help in slowing down contractions associated with preterm labor. Diazepam (Valium) has little or no effect on uterine muscles. It was used in the past to inhibit seizure activity, but fetal side effects were great. Phenobarbital, although a central nervous system depressant, has little effect on calming uterine muscles. It was previously used to control maternal anxiety and prevent seizures. Butorphanol (Stadol) is an analgesic to decrease pain and has no effect on uterine muscles to stop contractions.

5. The correct response is A. Any time there is a pregnancy with the chance of maternal and fetal blood mixing, RhoGAM is needed to prevent sensitization or antibody production. Head injury resulting from a car crash is not a situation in which there would be mixing of fetal or maternal blood. The trauma would cause hemorrhage, but not a sensitization reaction. A blood transfusion after hemorrhage would require typing and cross-matching of the client's blood; thus, she would receive blood with her own Rh factor, not one with Rh-positive blood. Because the artificial insemination procedure was unsuccessful, no pregnancy occurred and RhoGAM would not be necessary.

● CRITICAL THINKING EXERCISES

1.
a. What is your impression of this condition?
From her history, it appears she has hyperemesis gravidarum, because she is beyond the morning sickness time frame (6–12 weeks) and her symptoms are continual.

b. What risk factors does Suzanne have for this condition?
Her risk factors include young age and primigravida status.

c. What intervention is appropriate for this woman?
• Question Suzanne further concerning previous eating patterns and food intake.
• Ask what measures has she used at home to stop the nausea and vomiting.
• Consult the healthcare provider concerning hospitalization of Suzanne for IV therapy to correct hypovolemia and electrolyte imbalances.
• If home care is in order, advise her to avoid the intake of greasy or highly seasoned foods and to separate food from fluid intake, instruct her on antiemetic medication ordered and possible side effects, and instruct her to return to the clinic if symptoms do not subside within 48 hours.

2.
a. Based on her history, what might this client be at risk for? Why?
This client is at high risk for preterm labor and birth because of the following risk factors in her history: African-American race, smoker, poor nutrition, anemia, history of UTIs, and low socioeconomic and educational status.

b. What client education is needed at this visit?
A frank discussion of risk factors associated with preterm labor and birth and how they can be changed to reduce her risk is needed. Signs and symptoms of preterm labor need to be stressed. Education should address diet, working conditions, taking prenatal vitamins, hydration, and goals for her future.

c. What specific nursing interventions might reduce her risk?
A smoking cessation program and a referral to a nutritionist and enrollment in the WIC program should be made. A Healthy Start referral would allow closer supervision of this client throughout the pregnancy. Increasing the frequency of her visits would be helpful in monitoring her closely. Reinforcing the signs and symptoms of preterm labor at each visit would help her identify it early. A referral to a social worker to assess her home environment would also be beneficial.

● STUDY ACTIVITIES

1. The answers will vary, but a common theme would probably be more diversional activities to combat the boredom and additional information regarding the health status of the fetus. Additional attention/participation in the treatment plan might also be discussed as a possible problematic area.

2. Hopefully the signs and symptoms would be taught to woman during their first trimester, and written material would be handed out too. During each prenatal visit, the information should be reinforced to make sure the woman understands what they are and what to do about them if they should occur.

3. Appropriate Internet sites might include Sidelines High Risk Pregnancy Support Office (www.sidelines.org) and Resolve through Sharing (http://www.ectopicpregnancy.com).

4. Ectopic

5. Choriocarcinoma

6. Various activities for the woman on prolonged bed rest at home could in include watching TV, reading, visiting computer sites with chat rooms, talking on the telephone, playing cards or engaging in crafts, having visitors in frequently, and completing educational courses online. The woman could also use the bed rest time to develop lists for managing the house while on bed rest, read or play games with her other children, and expand her knowledge related to the upcoming birth of her babies.

7. Tocolytics

Chapter 20

● MULTIPLE CHOICE QUESTIONS

1. The correct response is B. Levels of the hormone hPL (insulin antagonist) progressively rise throughout pregnancy, and additional insulin is needed to overcome its resistance. Having a carbohydrate craving is not associated with gestational diabetes. Hyperinsulinemia in the fetus develops in response to the mother's high blood glucose levels. Glucose levels are diverted across the placenta for fetal use, and thus maternal levels are reduced in the first trimester. This lower glucose level doesn't last throughout the gestation, just the first trimester. For the remaining two trimesters, the maternal glucose levels are high because of the insulin resistance caused by hPL.

2. The correct response is D. A pregnant woman with asthma who is having an acute exacerbation will be poorly oxygenated, and thus perfusion to the placenta is compromised. Immediate treatment is needed for her well-being as well as that of the fetus. Corticosteroids are used as a first-line drug therapy for asthma treatment and management because of their anti-inflammatory properties. Having asthma has no influence on the woman's glucose levels, unless she also had diabetes. Bronchodilators usually are inhaled, not given subcutaneously, so instruction about this route of administration would not be necessary.

3. The correct response is B. Extreme nausea and vomiting as part of hyperemesis gravidarum would cause fluid and electrolyte imbalances and would alter blood glucose levels tremendously. With placenta previa, the placenta is dislocated, not malfunctioning; it would not have as much of an impact on the pregnancy as would an imbalance of fluids and electrolytes. Abruptio placentae would place the mother at risk for hemorrhage, but the placenta does not govern the blood glucose levels of the mother. Rh incompatibility affects the fetus, not the mother, by causing hemolysis of the red blood cells in the fetus. This process would not influence the mother's glucose levels.

4. The correct response is C. Alcohol ingested by the woman during pregnancy is teratogenic to the fetus, and the newborn can be born with fetal alcohol spectrum disorder. Drinking alcohol would decrease production of dehydrogenase, an enzyme that mobilizes the hydrogen of a substrate so that it can pass it to a hydrogen acceptor. Becoming intoxicated faster during pregnancy is not the underlying problem associated with alcohol ingestion and pregnancy. The woman's genetic makeup, how much alcohol is ingested, her amount of body fat, metabolic rate, and ingestion of food are a few of the factors that determine the metabolism of alcohol. Alcohol contains calories and if enough is ingested along with food, weight gain would occur, not weight loss.

5. The correct response is B. The highest percentage of HIV transmission results from sexual activity, followed by intravenous drug use. Transmission can occur despite a low viral load in the blood of the infected person. Pregnant women who take antiretroviral therapy during their gestation significantly reduce the chances of transmitting HIV to their newborn. The use of standard precautions will minimize the risk of transmission of HIV to healthcare workers. A very small percentage of nurses contract HIV through needlesticks if using appropriate precautions.

● CRITICAL THINKING EXERCISES

1.

a. What additional information will you need to provide care for her?
- Explore her typical daily dietary intake.
- Ask her if there is a family history of diabetes mellitus.
- Take her vital signs, weight, and fetal heart rate.
- Assess her coping abilities and capacity for managing diabetes.
- Assess her knowledge of the disease process and lifestyle changes needed.
- Ask her about symptoms of fatigue, polyuria, polyphagia, and polydipsia.
- Ask about previous pregnancy outcomes and the weight of infants.

b. What education will she need to address this new diagnosis?
- Dietary modifications to reduce the amount of simple sugars and carbohydrates
- Thorough explanation of potential complications of diabetes in pregnancy:
  - Infection: urinary tract infections and monilial vaginitis
  - Difficult labor and birth: shoulder dystocia, birth trauma, cesarean section
  - Congenital anomalies: cardiac, CNS, and skeletal anomalies
- Literature describing diet, exercise, and glucose monitoring
- Outline of hypoglycemia and hyperglycemia symptoms
- Referral to nutritionist for diet planning

c. How will you evaluate the effectiveness of your interventions?
- Schedule more frequent prenatal visits to evaluate her health status.
- Evaluate glucose values at each visit to validate that they are in the normal range.
- Monitor HbA1C to determine past glucose levels.

2.

a. What is your first approach with the client to gain her trust?
Open the conversation by asking questions about school activities and her friends. Remain nonjudgmental, and bring the discussion to general questions about her monthly cycles. Finally work toward questions about when she last had her period, and assess how many months pregnant she is. Adolescents usually deny a pregnancy for several months, so she may be well into her second trimester.

b. List the client's educational needs during this pregnancy.
- Signs and symptoms of preterm labor
- Nutritional needs during pregnancy
- Need for prenatal care throughout pregnancy
- Importance of early detection of complications
- Decision about whether to involve her partner
- Reasons for the frequency of prenatal visits and importance of keeping them
- Symptoms of sexually transmitted infections
- Impact of substance abuse on fetal growth and development
- Childbearing and parenting classes
- Infant growth and development and newborn care

c. What prevention strategies are needed to prevent a second pregnancy?
- Ask about her educational goals and encourage her to complete school; perhaps refer her for vocational counseling.
- Identify her personal strengths and reinforce positive self-esteem.
- Actively involve her in her care at each visit and praise her for her efforts.
- Discuss family planning methods appropriate for her and let her decide.
- Enhance a positive perception of her ability to succeed in life.

3.

a. What aspects of this woman's history make you concerned that this infant is at risk for fetal alcohol spectrum disorder?
- Lack of prenatal care
- History of substance abuse (alcohol) during previous pregnancies
- Children placed in foster care from birth due to poor mothering ability
- Appearance on arrival and evidence of being malnourished
- Statement about not having any "recent" use of alcohol
- Delivery of newborn weighing 4 lb

b. What additional screening or laboratory tests might validate your suspicion?
Screening questionnaires can be used to diagnose problem drinking, along with a drug screen (urine or blood) on both her and the newborn to identify specific substances present. The social service agency can also be called to do a more thorough history on this woman.

c. What physical and neurodevelopmental deficits might present later in life if the infant has fetal alcohol spectrum disorder?
The infant might have attention-deficit/hyperactivity disorder (ADHD), poor impulse control, learning disabilities, communication problems, as well as growth restriction/developmental problems. It is important to address this woman's alcohol dependence by offering care options such as addiction treatment, mental health therapy, and support. As a nurse, it is important to be sensitive to the client's cultural, spiritual, religious, and emotional needs during this time. Discussion of effective contraception while she is struggling with her addiction is important to prevent fetal alcohol spectrum disorder.

● STUDY ACTIVITIES

1. Responses will vary based on the woman's preexisting condition. Common themes might be changes in activity level if the woman interviewed has one of the anemias or hypertension and dietary modifications if she is diabetic; all might express concern about the pregnancy outcome.

2. This study activity is one to which many college students can relate. Confronting the friend who is in denial is the most effective way to bring the issue up. Back it up with observed behaviors that demonstrate the friend's drug or alcohol dependency. Telling the person that you care about her and her well-being can go a long way toward modifying her behavior.

3. The answers will vary depending on which side the student takes. Some of the common themes might center on civil rights and the positive aspects marijuana has had on nausea and vomiting for cancer patients and controlling glaucoma pressure. On the other side of the debate, allowing this drug to be legalized might afford many pregnant women access to it, without long-term research studies to document effects on offspring.

4. The nurse should present the facts that taking the medications will reduce the risk of transmission of HIV and should discuss how the woman and her newborn will benefit from them. Stressing the importance of lowering her viral load throughout her pregnancy and relating it to her well-being might help. Presenting her with the facts is all that the nurse can do, since the final decision will be hers.

5. A, B, C, E, and F. Women with all the infections listed except HIV can choose to breastfeed. An HIV-positive woman can pass the virus to her newborn through breast milk and should be discouraged from breastfeeding.

Chapter 21

● MULTIPLE CHOICE QUESTIONS

1. The correct response is D. Fetopelvic disproportion is defined as a condition in which the fetus is too large to pass through the maternal pelvis. Cervical insufficiency would lead to an abortion, typically in the second trimester, when the heavy gravid uterus would cause pressure on the weakened cervix. A contracted pelvis might cause passageway problems, but if the fetus was small, no problem might occur. Maternal disproportion doesn't indicate where the disproportion is located.

2. The correct response is B. Herpes exposure during the birth process poses a high risk for mortality to the neonate. If the woman has active herpetic lesions in the genital tract, a surgical birth is planned to avoid this exposure. Hepatitis is a chronic liver disorder, and the fetus if exposed would at most become a carrier; a surgical birth would not be expected for this woman. Toxoplasmosis is passed through the placenta to the fetus prior to birth, so a cesarean birth would not prevent exposure. HPV would be manifest clinically by genital warts on the woman, and a surgical birth would not be anticipated to prevent exposure unless the warts caused an obstruction.

3. The correct response is A. Having a fetus in a posterior position would cause intense back pain secondary to the fetal head facing the maternal vertebra and causing pressure. Leg cramps are common during pregnancy and not caused by an occiput posterior position, but rather pressure from the heavy gravid uterus toward term. Fetal position would not contribute to nausea and vomiting. Going through transition in labor might cause nausea and vomiting, not the fetal position. A precipitous birth occurs rapidly and is not associated with intense back pain.

4. The correct response is D. Prostaglandins soften and thin out the cervix in preparation for labor induction. Although they do irritate the uterus, they aren't as effective as oxytocin in stimulating contractions. Prostaglandin gel would stimulate cervical nerve receptors rather than numb them. Prostaglandins have no power to prevent cervical lacerations, only to soften and thin the cervix.

5. The correct response is C. Hypotonic labor typically occurs in the active phase; it involves ineffective contractions to evoke cervical dilation and causes secondary inertia. Hypertonic labor is characterized by painful, high-intensity contractions that usually occur in the latent phase. A precipitous labor occurs within 3 hours and cervical dilation is very fast secondary to effective, high-intensity contractions. Dysfunctional labor describes any pattern that doesn't produce dilation and effacement in a timely manner.

● CRITICAL THINKING EXERCISES

1.

a. Based on the nurse's findings, what might you suspect is going on?
Since Marsha is multiparous and is in the active phase of labor without progression and the contraction pattern has become less intense, a hypotonic uterine dysfunction should be suspected.

b. How can the nurse address Marsha's anxiety?
Give her, in an easily understood manner, facts about dysfunctional labor. Outline expected treatment and outcome. Encourage questions and expression of feelings. Identify how this dysfunctional labor pattern may alter her labor plan. Reassure Marsha about the status of her fetus. Maintain a positive attitude about her ability to cope with this situation.

c. What are the appropriate interventions to change this labor pattern?
Typically some form of labor augmentation is initiated to produce more effective contractions to facilitate cervical dilatation—rupture of membranes or use of IV oxytocin to stimulate the intensity of contractions. If neither one of these interventions changes the hypotonic pattern, a surgical birth is in order.

2.

a. What new development might be occurring?
Based on Marsha's description, the nurse might suspect spontaneous rupture of membranes.

b. How will the nurse confirm her suspicion?
Depending on the agency protocol, the nurse may perform or assist with a sterile speculum examination to observe for evidence of fluid pooling in the posterior vagina, any discharge present, inflammation or lesions, or protrusion of the membranes through the cervix. The nurse should also document the amount, color, and consistency of any fluid found during the examination.

c. What interventions are appropriate for this finding?
• Obtain a baseline set of vital signs to assess FHR patterns for changes possibly indicating a prolapsed umbilical cord.
• Use Nitrazine paper to test for the presence of amniotic fluid: it will turn blue in the presence of amniotic fluid because it is alkaline.
• Examine a sample of fluid from the vagina under the microscope for a fern pattern once it dries.

● STUDY ACTIVITIES

1. This international web site offers numerous educational and personal testimonies to assist parents who have suffered a perinatal loss. There are listings of local support groups in which they can participate.

2. Maternal/fetal risks associated with a prolonged pregnancy include maternal exhaustion, psychological depression, macrosomia, dysmaturity syndrome, fetal hypoxia, meconium aspiration syndrome, hypoglycemia, and stillbirth.

3. Dystocia

Chapter 22

● MULTIPLE CHOICE QUESTIONS

1. The correct response is C. It is important to assess the situation before intervening. In addition, checking the bladder status and emptying a full bladder will correct uterine displacement so that effective contractions to stop bleeding can occur. Assessment of the situation is needed before the nurse can notify the healthcare provider. At this point, the nurse has no facts to report about the client's condition. Magnesium sulfate would relax the uterus and increase bleeding. Pallor and heavy bleeding are not normal findings during the postpartum period.

2. The correct response is A. Psychotic persons tend to lose touch with reality and frequently attempt to harm themselves or others. This behavior may occur when a woman experiences postpartum psychosis. Anxiety typically does not induce hallucinations or cause a person to want to harm herself or others. Depression involves feelings of sadness rather than hallucinations or thoughts of harming herself or others. Feeling "down," but not to the extreme of wanting to harm herself or her newborn, is suggestive of postpartum blues.

3. The correct response is D. Hemorrhage is possible if the uterus cannot contract and clamp down on the vessels to reduce bleeding. When the placenta is expelled, open vessels are then exposed and the risk of hemorrhage is great. Thrombophlebitis typically is manifested later in the postpartum period rather than within the first few hours after birth. Breast engorgement usually occurs on postpartum day 3 or later when the milk comes in, not within hours after birth. Infection usually is manifested 24 to 48 hours after birth, not within the first few hours.

4. The correct response is C. Applying compresses and giving analgesics would be helpful in provid-

ing comfort to the woman with painful breasts. Treatment for mastitis encourages frequent breastfeeding to empty the breasts. Lanolin applied to the breasts will have little impact on mastitis other than to keep them moist. Binding both breasts will not bring relief; in fact, it could

cause additional discomfort. Emptying the breasts frequently through breastfeeding would be helpful. Although wearing a nursing bra will help support the heavy breasts and fresh air is helpful to prevent cracked nipples, these are ineffective once mastitis develops.

● CRITICAL THINKING EXERCISES

1.
a. What postpartum complication is this mother at highest risk for? Why?
Postpartum infection would be the highest risk for this client because of the risk factors present: anemia, prolonged ruptured membranes, prolonged labor before a surgical birth with an incision, the likelihood of frequent vaginal examinations during the prolonged labor, and the use of internal fetal monitoring devices.

b. What assessments need to be done to detect this potential complication?
Monitor the client for signs of early infection: fever, malaise, abdominal pain, foul-smelling lochia, boggy uterus, tachycardia, and anorexia. Test results would indicate an elevated white blood cell count and sedimentation rate. Assessment of her incision for drainage and approximation of edges should be done frequently.

c. What nursing measures will the nurse use to prevent this complication?
• Adhere to strict aseptic technique in providing nursing care to the incision.
• Instruct the client about self-care measures to help prevent infection such as handwashing, perineal hygiene, wiping from front to back, and hydration.
• Complete a thorough "BUBBLE=HE" assessment and record findings.
• Urge the client to change her peripads frequently and use the peri-bottle.
• Reinforce home care instructions to continue infection prevention.

2.
a. What factors place Tammy at risk for postpartum hemorrhage?
Tammy is a grand multipara with nine previous pregnancies, and thus her uterus has been stretched repeatedly with close pregnancies. She also had an epidural during labor and therefore has limited sensation to her bladder.

b. What assessments are needed before planning interventions?
If Tammy's fundus is boggy (uterine atony) and her bladder is full, intervention is needed to promote voiding. If the fundus is firm and her bladder is

empty, additional evaluation is needed to rule out lacerations or retained placental fragments as a causative factor contributing to her heavy vaginal bleeding.

c. What nursing actions are needed to prevent a postpartum hemorrhage?
After the assessment is completed and the uterus is found to be boggy and bladder is full, the next step is to get the client up to void. After Tammy empties her bladder, reassess the fundus for firmness and location. With a full bladder, the uterus is typically displaced to the right of the midline. After emptying the bladder, the fundus should return to the midline and be firm. As a result, bleeding should decrease.

3.
a. What factors/behaviors place Lucy at risk for an emotional disorder?
Lucy had a previous episode of postpartum depression. Her behavior indicates limited interest in her newborn and herself by not providing care. She reports she is disappointed in the sex of this child. Lucy's inactivity and lack of appetite are also problematic since she will be going home and needs to care for herself and her newborn.

b. Which interventions might be appropriate at this time?
In a sensitive, caring manner, the nurse should approach Lucy and ask her questions to get a complete picture of her emotional status. Demonstrating concern and care might encourage Lucy to express her feelings about her situation and the newborn. Using therapeutic communication through open-ended questions might assist in gathering data. Notifying the healthcare provider of the findings is also crucial.

c. What education does the family need prior to discharge?
The family needs information on postpartum emotional disorders and referrals to community counseling centers to assist Lucy through this time. Providing the family with the addresses of web sites that offer assistance and information about emotional disorders might also be helpful. A good social support network of family and friends will be needed to care for both Lucy and her newborn initially when she is discharged.

● STUDY ACTIVITIES

1. *Baby blues* are usually self-limiting and benign, occurring a few days after childbirth and ending within 2 weeks. The woman cries easily, is irritable, and is more emotionally labile than normal. This emotional disorder usually resolves without specific treatment other than reassurance and support from the family. *Postpartum depression* occurs within 6 months after childbirth and is similar to other depressive disorders. The woman feels inadequate as a parent and has disturbances in appetite, mood, sleep, concentration, and energy. Psychotherapy and antidepressants are helpful to address this disorder, which may take months to resolve. Family patience and support are very important for her. *Postpartum psychosis* may result in suicidal or homicidal behavior and requires immediate medical and psychiatric intervention. Clinical manifestations include hallucinations, delusions, or both within 3 weeks after giving birth. Inpatient psychiatric services may be needed for this severe emotional disorder.

2. Students will offer varying opinions based on the web site they select.

3. The information obtained from this interview will vary depending on the woman's experience. It is hoped that some of the comments about helpfulness will center on a nurse who was present and provided assistance to her.

4. Uterine atony

5. Information the nurse needs to care for this mother and her newborn should include vital signs, fundal assessment (firm or boggy and location), lochia characteristics (color, amount, smell, consistency), appearance of perineum (episiotomy site, lacerations, swelling, bruising), breast status (wearing a soft, supportive bra; any nipple problems), and elimination status (empty or not voiding).

Chapter 23

● MULTIPLE CHOICE QUESTIONS

1. The correct response is C. A postterm infant is one born after the 42nd week of gestation. Birth between 38 and 41 weeks is considered within a normal range for a term newborn. A gestation of 44 weeks would be considered extremely long if the dates were calculated correctly.

2. The correct response is A. The fetus's body, in an attempt to compensate for the low oxygen level, produces more red blood cells to carry the limited amount of oxygen available. Thus, polycythemia will be present at birth in a fetus experiencing hypoxia in utero. Hypoglycemia is typically caused by inadequate stores of glycogen and overuse while living in a hostile environment. Low serum calcium levels are associated with perinatal asphyxia and not an increase in red blood cells. Hypothermia is associated with a decrease in body fat, particularly brown fat stores, and is not linked to increased production of red blood cells.

3. The correct response is B. Subcutaneous and brown fat stores may be used by the stressed fetus to survive in utero and thus will not be available to provide extrauterine warmth. Excessive red blood cell breakdown is responsible for hyperbilirubinemia, not the breakdown of brown fat stores. Polycythemia is caused by a buildup of red blood cells in response to a hypoxic state in utero; it is not linked to loss of subcutaneous and brown fat stores. Glycogen stores are used for survival in an environment with depleted glycogen and are unrelated to brown fat stores.

4. The correct response is C. The parents need to validate the experience of loss. The best way to do this is to encourage them to participate in their newborn's care so that the grieving process can take place. Avoiding the experience of loss inhibits the grieving process. Avoidance prolongs the experience of loss and does not allow the parents to vent their feelings so that they can progress through their grief. It is not the nurse's responsibility, nor is it healthy for the family, to take over decisions for a family. Family members need to support each other and need to decide what is best for their situation. Leaving the family alone can be viewed as abandonment; privacy is important, but leaving them totally alone is not therapeutic.

5. The correct response is D. The ductus arteriosus and foramen ovale may remain open if pulmonary vascular resistance remains high and oxygen levels remain low. When a newborn is born too soon, fetal circulation may persist in extrauterine life; this would be manifested by a heart murmur. Milia (clogged sebaceous glands) are present in most newborns and are not a pathologic sign. The preterm newborn has not been able to store subcutaneous fat, which does not occur until the eighth month of gestation. Poor muscle tone is apparent in most preterm newborns due to poor development secondary to the premature birth.

● CRITICAL THINKING EXERCISES

1.
a. What might these behaviors indicate?
These behaviors are clinical signs of hypoglycemia, which is common in a postterm infant after a difficult birth; glycogen stores are depleted secondary to chronic placental insufficiency.

b. For what other conditions is this newborn at high risk?
Besides hypoglycemia, hypothermia, polycythemia, meconium aspiration, and hyperbilirubinemia are common in the postterm infant.

c. What intervention is needed to address this condition?
Feed the newborn as early as possible, or administer glucose/glucagon to counter the low blood glucose level. Decrease energy requirements to conserve glucose and glycogen stores. Maintain a neutral thermal environment to prevent cold stress, which can exacerbate the hypoglycemia.

2.
a. What might have contributed to this newborn's hypothermic condition?
The simple fact that the newborn was premature predisposes him to thermal instability because of his larger surface-to-weight ratio, immature muscle tone and decreased muscular activity to generate heat, diminished stores of subcutaneous and brown fat, and poor nutritional intake, which makes him unable to meet energy requirements for growth and development. In addition, placing the isolette close to the door might produce cold drafts, causing hypothermia.

b. What transfer mechanism may have been a factor?
This preterm newborn could experience loss of heat by convection (heat transfer via air currents).

c. What intervention would be appropriate for the nurse to initiate?
Bundle or nest the preterm newborn with warmed blankets and move the isolette away from the door to prevent heat loss by convection. Place a knitted cap on the newborn's head and monitor his temperature frequently.

3.
a. What complication common to SGA newborns might be manifested in this newborn?
The signs indicate polycythemia, which is common in SGA infants.

b. What factors may have contributed to this complication?
In SGA infants, polycythemia is thought to be secondary to chronic hypoxia in utero, with resulting erythropoietin production. Complications of polycythemia are related to the increased viscosity of blood, which interferes with organ circulation.

c. What is the appropriate intervention to manage this condition?
Obtain a venous hematocrit measurement within 4 to 6 hours after birth to validate this condition, since its manifestations are very similar to those of hypoglycemia. Hematocrit values over 65% should be brought to the healthcare provider's attention. Typically it is treated by a dilutional exchange transfusion.

● STUDY ACTIVITIES

1. This program could be very effective to get the pregnant women to think about the harmful effects smoking has on a growing fetus. The emphasis should be on the vasoconstriction of the blood vessels and how this reduces nutritional and blood supplies to the fetus. Pictures of a narrowed blood vessel could be used to demonstrate this problem. Although each group will react in different ways to a presentation on smoking and pregnancy, ideally the seed will be planted for some to curtail or stop smoking.

2. The March of Dimes web site is full of ideas on how to prevent preterm births, which include early prenatal care for all women, diagnostic tests to detect changes in the cervix, and prevention of maternal infections. The students' comments may center on the inaccessibility of health care, which precludes some pregnant women from receiving early prenatal care, and the lack of insurance to cover the cost of diagnostic tests or prescriptions for treatment of infections.

3. hypoglycemia

4. Common birth injuries include clavicle fractures, facial palsies, and brachial plexus injuries.

5. Nursing measures to promote energy conservation would include a, b, and c.

Feeding and digestion will increase energy demands; thermal warmers might produce hyperthermia and thus increase energy demands; and preventing parents from visiting their infant is not a plan to reduce energy expenditure and could increase stress for both the parents and the baby.

Chapter 24

● MULTIPLE CHOICE QUESTIONS

1. The correct response is D. Nasal flaring is a cardinal sign of air hunger in respiratory distress syndrome. When an infant becomes hypoxic due to poor lung expansion, the nares expand to "search" for more oxygen to relieve the low oxygen concentration. Abdominal distention denotes air in the intestines, not hypoxia. Acrocyanosis is present only in the extremities and might indicate sluggish circulation. An infant with respiratory distress syndrome would demonstrate generalized cyanosis secondary to hypoxemia. Depressed fontanels would indicate dehydration, not respiratory distress syndrome.

2. The correct response is C. Irritability is a prime symptom of drug withdrawal in newborns. As they experience physiologic withdrawal from the addictive substance, irritability with crying and the inability to be consoled are prevalent behaviors. Newborns exposed to substances are anything but calm when withdrawing from an addictive substance. They are extremely distressed, and their faces commonly exhibit that distress. Weight loss, not weight gain, is typical of the newborn exposed to substances. Although they show signs of hunger, vomiting is common and thus weight loss follows. These newborns are extremely distressed and agitated. Their feeding and sleeping patterns are disrupted and would not be described as normal.

3. The correct response is D. Detection of PKU depends on an accumulation of phenylalanine, which is found in protein. Protein is ingested with breast milk or formula, so newborns need at least 48 hours of protein ingestion via milk before they can be screened for PKU. The ingestion of protein is not related to thyroid hormone levels and thus is not necessary to screen for hypothyroidism. A heel stick blood sample can be taken prior to 48 hours of age to diagnose sickle cell anemia. This newborn screening test is not dependent on protein intake since it is a genetic disease. Cystic fibrosis is an inherited disorder and present at birth, not 48 hours later.

4. The correct response is D. The newborn with this anomaly cannot handle oral secretions since the esophagus ends in a blind pouch. The secretions typically foam out of the mouth, and this becomes a clue that a fistula exists. A tracheoesophageal fistula alone doesn't affect the newborn's temperature unless an infection is present. This defect is structural, not neurologic. The newborn's ability to swallow is not related to this structural defect. There would have to be an insult to the CNS for swallowing to be affected as well as a structural defect in the pharynx.

● CRITICAL THINKING EXERCISES

1.

a. What in the mother's history might have raised a red flag to the nurse?

Prolonged rupture of the membranes provides an avenue for bacteria to ascend into the mother's genital tract. The fact she had a fever during labor is a key sign.

b. For what condition is this newborn at high risk?

Neonatal sepsis would be a likely diagnosis based on the mother's history and the nonspecific clinical manifestations in the newborn.

c. What interventions are appropriate for this condition?

The nurse should document the assessment findings and report them to the pediatrician so that cultures and blood work can be started to identify the offending organism. General antibiotic therapy is typically started until the offending organism is identified.

2.

a. What additional information do you need to obtain from her mother?

It is important to understand the extent and type of her drug use during pregnancy. Ask specific questions about her drug use so that you can plan care for her as well as her newborn. Place her at ease and ask direct, nonjudgmental questions.

b. What additional laboratory work might be needed for Terry?

Due to an increased risk of HIV in injection drug users, an HIV test along with a polydrug screen is needed. The mother's consent must be obtained prior to the HIV testing.

c. What specific referrals need to be made for her ongoing care?

After extensive counseling regarding the perinatal risks due to her heroin use, referral to a drug detoxification center and possibly methadone maintenance may be necessary. Depending on her commitment to stop taking drugs to reduce harm to her newborn, additional social services need to be explored. Although the decision to change her lifestyle is her choice, the nurse can play a vital role in guiding the care to achieve a better outcome for the mother and her infant. Terry also will need to undergo detoxification and will require close supervision until withdrawal has been achieved. Tight wrapping, calming techniques, and reduced stimuli will help decrease the newborn's irritability.

3.

a. What is your impression of this newborn?
Based on the newborn's characteristics documented during the nurse's assessment, congenital hypothyroidism should be suspected.

b. What laboratory studies and results would you anticipate?
Elevated thyroid stimulating hormone (TSH) levels and low thyroxine (T4) levels

c. What explanation could be offered to the parents concerning this condition?
Discuss the condition and stress that the mainstay of treatment for congenital hypothyroidism is early diagnosis and thyroid hormone supplementation. Parents should be provided with the hormone supplementation and taught proper administration. Reinforce that this is a lifetime supplementation.

● STUDY ACTIVITIES

1. This answer will vary depending on each student's perceptions, but common impressions of the role of NICU nurses would be their autonomy and the numerous types of technical equipment needed for each newborn. The students will probably note that the new parents seem overwhelmed because of the amount of equipment being used. Pointing out to expectant parents how capable and competent the nurses are will help in reducing their anxiety.

2. The students will find thorough descriptions of the specific congenital condition aimed at the level of laypeople. Many sites provide information about local support groups that parents can join.

3. The "take-home message" to all expectant parents concerning newborn screening tests is that they must actively participate in the follow-up testing to ensure that their newborn does not have an inborn error of metabolism or disease. It is critical for them to take their newborn back to the clinic or community laboratory after they are discharged from the hospital.

4. Gastroschisis

5. Ventricular septal defect

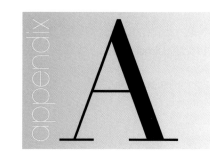

Standard Laboratory Values

Pregnant and Nonpregnant Women

Values	Nonpregnant	Pregnant
Hematologic		
Complete Blood Count (CBC)		
Hemoglobin, g/dL	12–16*	11.5–14*
Hematocrit, PCV, %	37–47	32–42
Red cell volume, mL	1600	1900
Plasma volume, mL	2400	3700
Red blood cell count, million/mm³	4–5.5	3.75–5.0
White blood cells, total per mm³	4500–10,000	5000–15,000
Polymorphonuclear cells, %	54–62	60–85
Lymphocytes, %	38–46	15–40
Erythrocyte sedimentation rate, mm/h	≤	30–90
MCHC, g/dL packed RBCs (mean corpuscular hemoglobin concentration)	30–36	No change
MCH (mean corpuscular hemoglobin per picogram)	29–32	No change
MCV/μm³ (mean corpuscular volume per cubic micrometer)	82–96	No change
Blood Coagulation and Fibrinolytic Activity†		
Factors VII, VIII, IX, X		Increase in pregnancy, return to normal in early puerperium; factor VIII increases during and immediately after delivery
Factors XI, XIII		Decrease in pregnancy
Prothrombin time (protime)	60–70 sec	Slight decrease in pregnancy
Partial thromboplastin time (PTT)	12–14 sec	Slight decrease in pregnancy and again decrease during second and third stage of labor (indicates clotting at placental site)

(continued)

Values	Nonpregnant	Pregnant
Bleeding time	1–3 min (Duke) 2–4 min (Ivy)	No appreciable change
Coagulation time	6–10 min (Lee/White)	No appreciable change
Platelets	150,000 to 350,000/mm^3	No significant change until 3–5 days after delivery, then marked increase (may predispose woman to thrombosis) and gradual return to normal
Fibrinolytic activity		Decreases in pregnancy, then abrupt return to normal (protection against thromboembolism)
Fibrinogen	250 mg/dL	400 mg/dL
Mineral and Vitamin Concentrations		
Serum iron, μg	75–150	65–120
Total iron-binding capacity, μg	250–450	300–500
Iron saturation, %	30–40	15–30
Vitamin B$_{12}$, folic acid, ascorbic acid	Normal	Moderate decrease
Serum protein		
Total, g/dL	6.7–8.3	5.5–7.5
Albumin, g/dL	3.5–5.5	3.0–5.0
Globulin, total, g/dL	2.3–3.5	3.0–4.0
Blood sugar		
Fasting, mg/dL	70–80	65
2-hour postprandial, mg/dL	60–110	Under 140 after a 100-g carbohydrate meal is considered normal
Cardiovascular		
Blood pressure, mm Hg	120/80†	114/65
Peripheral resistance, dyne/s · cm^{-5}	120	100
Venous pressure, cm H$_2$O		
Femoral	9	24
Antecubital	8	8
Pulse, rate/min	70	80
Stroke volume, mL	65	75
Cardiac output, L/min	4.5	6
Circulation time (arm-tongue), sec	15–16	12–14
Blood volume, mL		
Whole blood	4000	5600
Plasma	2400	3700
Red blood cells	1600	1900
Plasma renin, units/L	3–10	10–80
Chest x-ray studies		
Transverse diameter of heart	—	1–2 cm increase
Left border of heart	—	Straightened
Cardiac volume	—	70-mL increase
Electrocardiogram	—	15° left axis deviation
V$_1$ and V$_2$	—	Inverted T-wave
kV$_4$	—	Low T
III	—	Q + inverted T
aVr	—	Small Q

Values	Nonpregnant	Pregnant
Hepatic		
Bilirubin total	Not more than 1 mg/dL	Unchanged
Cephalin flocculation	Up to 2+ in 48 h	Positive in 10%
Serum cholesterol	110–300 mg/dL	↑ 60% from 16–32 weeks of pregnancy; remains at this level until after delivery
Thymol turbidity	0–4 units	Positive in 15%
Serum alkaline phosphatase	2–4.5 units (Bodansky)	↑ from week 12 of pregnancy to 6 weeks after delivery
Serum lactate dehydrogenase		Unchanged
Serum glutamic-oxaloacetic transaminase		Unchanged
Serum globulin albumin	1.5–3.0 g/dL 4.5–5.3 g/dL	↑ slight ↓ 3.0 g by late pregnancy
A/G ratio		Decreased
α_2-globulin		Increased
β-globulin		Increased
Serum cholinesterase		Decreased
Leucine aminopeptidase		Increased
Sulfobromophthalein (5 mg/kg)	5% dye or less in 45 min	Somewhat decreased
Renal		
Bladder capacity	1300 mL	1500 mL
Renal plasma flow (RPF), mL/min	490–700	Increase by 25%, to 612–875
Glomerular filtration rate (GFR), mL/min	105–132	Increase by 50%, to 160–198
Nonprotein nitrogen (NPN), mg/dL	25–40	Decreases
Blood urea nitrogen (BUN), mg/dL	20–25	Decreases
Serum creatinine, mg/kg/24 hr	20–22	Decreases
Serum uric acid, mg/kg/24 hr	257–750	Decreases
Urine glucose	Negative	Present in 20% of gravidas
Intravenous pyelogram (IVP)	Normal	Slight to moderate hydroureter and hydronephrosis; right kidney larger than left kidney
Miscellaneous		
Total thyroxine concentration	5–12 µg/dL thyroxine	↑ 9–16 µg/dL thyroxine (however, unbound thyroxine not greatly increased)
Ionized calcium		Relatively unchanged
Aldosterone		↑ 1 mg/24 hr by third trimester
Dehydroisoandrosterone	Plasma clearance 6–8 L/24 hr	↑ plasma clearance tenfold to twentyfold

* At sea level. Permanent residents of higher levels (e.g., Denver) require higher levels of hemoglobin.

From Scott, J. R., et al. (2000). *Obstetrics and gynecology*. Philadelphia: Lippincott Williams & Wilkins.

† Pregnancy represents a hypercoagulable state.

† For the woman about 20 years of age.

10 years of age: 103/70.

30 years of age: 123/82.

40 years of age: 126/84.

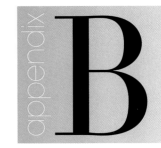

Clinical Paths

Labor and Delivery Clinical Path—Labor: Expected Outcomes

	Active Phase	Expulsion/Pushing	Recovery 1st Hour Post Partum
PATIENT EDUCATION	Patient coping with labor support Patient utilizing appropriate labor options Patient verbalizes satisfaction with plan Management interventions	Patient demonstrates effective pushing technique. Patient coping effectively with pushing. Support person coping effectively with labor	Bonding appropriately with baby
PATIENT STATUS	Cervix dilated 5 cms-complete Contraction regularly with progressive cervical change. Maternal/fetal well being maintained. Hydration maintained. If indicated: FSE and/or IUPC placed IV Pitocin started Epidural placed/WE encouraged Medicate with Prn pain meds	Vaginal birth	Placenta delivered Fundus firm Lochia small–moderate Without clots Perineum intact/repaired Hemodynamically stable EBL <500 cc
CONTINUUM OF CARE	Prenatal record available after 32 weeks Prenatal labs WNL Pre-registered to hospital Pediatrician identified Support after hospitalization identified Discharge plan discussed with patient/family. Communicates understanding of hospital and community resources		

	Interventions		
ASSESSMENT/ TREATMENT	Assess: Continuous EFM or auscultation Q 15 of 30 minutes as indicated. Vital signs hourly/Temp Q4 hours if intact membranes/Q 2 hrs if membranes ruptured Uterine by monitor or palpation Bladder for distention Hydration status Cervical dilation, effacement, station	Assess: Q 15 minutes monitoring of fetal well being (Low-Risk) and Q 5 minutes (High-Risk) Vital signs hourly Temp. Q 2–4 hrs. depending on membrane status Bladder for distention Hydration status Pushing effectiveness Descent of presenting part Caput	Assess: Uterus—fundus Vital signs Lochia Bladder Perineum Placenta
PATIENT EDUCATION	Reinforce comfort measures Encourage use of labor options Inform patient/support person of plan of care	Teaching of upright pushing positions Discourage prolonged maternal breath holding Encourage to assume position of choice Inform patient of progress	Baby status Breast feeding
TESTS/ PROCEDURES	Hgb or Hct (if not done recently) T & S (if ordered) VE as indicated IV therapy AROM by M.D. or CNM: assess for color, amount and odor, as appropriate FSE/IUPC placement if indicated	AROM: assess for color, amount and odor, as appropriate	Cord blood or Rhogam workup if appropriate Cord blood if O+ Mom
THERAPIES	Comfort measures/Birthing ball/ambulate/telemetry/ shower IV therapy Amnio Infusion for Variable decelerations If appropriate, Pain Mgmt. reviewed.	Perineal massage Warm soaks to perineal area Allow to rest until feels urge to push Frequent position changes Cool cloth/Ice chips	Ice pack to perineum Warm blankets
MEDS	Antibiotics as indicated for + GBS Pitocin if indicated PRN pain medication (Encourage WE if requesting this).	Pitocin if indicated	Pitocin IV
ACTIVITY/ SAFETY	Labor option usage Position changes	Provide wedge if supine Promote effective position for pushing: ie: squatting, side lying, upright Breathing technique patient/support person most comfortable with	Assist with ambulate to bathroom Infant care Assist with positioning for breast feeding Infant ID bands present

(continued)

Labor and Delivery Clinical Path—Labor: Expected Outcomes (continued)

	Interventions		
NUTRITION	Clear liquids Ice chips OTHER	Clear liquids Ice chips	Return to previous diet
UNIQUE PATIENT NEEDS			

Integrated Plan of Care for Cesarean Delivery

	Expected Patient Outcomes			
	Phase 1 Preadmission (Cesarean Delivery)	**Phase 2 Surgery/ Immediate Postop/ Day of Surgery**	**Phase 3 Post Op Day 1**	
Usual time in Phase	**N/A Date Started:**	Up to 23 hours	1 day	1–2 days
Assessment / Potential Complications	VS WNL for patient Hgb or Hct/values within normal SLH antepartum range	VS WNL for patient Systems assessment: Skin warm, dry, Clear → Alert & oriented → Neg. Homan's sign → Breast soft/nipples intact → Lungs clear → Bowel sounds present → Fundus firm u/u or u 1–2 (−/+) Lochia sm—mod Dsg dry and intact No signs infiltration IV site Verbalizes comfort using pain rating scale 0–10	VS. WNL for patient Afebrile Voiding without foley → Passing flatus Incision without redness or drainage Lochia small amount Fundus firm u/1–2 Verbalizes comfort using pain scale 0–10 on oral pain meds	Incision well approximated, without drainage or redness Passing flatus Lochia sm/mod amt Fundus firm u/1–2 Verbalizes comfort using pain medication as described

Expected Patient Outcomes

	Phase 1 Preadmission (Cesarean Delivery)	Phase 2 Surgery/ Immediate Postop/ Day of Surgery	Phase 3 Post Op Day 1	
Patient / Family Knowledge	**Date All Above Met** Verbalizes understanding of condition and need for surgery Verbalizes understanding of all pre-op teaching	**Date All Above Met** verbalizes correct use of PCA/ Fentanyl pump and when to request pain medication Turn, Cough & deep breath appropriately	**Date All Above Met** can state criteria for when to call doctor for problems post discharge → ↑ bleeding ↑ Temperature → incision redness, odor or drainage →	**Date All Above Met** Verbalizes follow-up appointment date and time Verbalizes proper dosing of pain medication
ADL's / Activity	**Date All Above Met** Verbalizes understanding of NPO status	**Date All Above Met** Able to ambulate with minimal assistance Tolerating clear/full liquid diet Bonding observed with newborn— Taking-in phase →	**Date All Above Met** Ambulating without assistance Tolerating soft to regular diet	**Date All Above Met** Ambulating in hall
Unique Patient Needs	**Date All Above Met**	**Date All Above Met**	**Date All Above Met**	**Date All Above Met**
	Date All Above Met **Entire Phase Outcomes Met; Progress patient to next phase**	**Date All Above Met** **Entire Phase Outcomes Met; Progress patient to next phase**	**Date All Above Met** **Entire Phase Outcomes Met; Progress patient to next phase**	**Date All Above Met** **Entire Phase Outcomes Met; Progress patient to next phase**

Plan of Care

	#1 Preadmission	# 2 Surgery/ Immediate Postop/ Day of Surgery	#3 Post Op Day 1	#4 Post Op Day 2- Discharge
Assessments	Vital Signs Fetal status immediately prior to surgery	VS per PACU then q 4 hr Systems assessment: *Skin, LOC, FROM, Homan's sign, *Breasts, Lungs, Fundus, Incision, *Lochia, bladder, bowel sounds, IV & site	VS q 6 hr Assess pain control 0–10 scale Incision Foley-volding Fundus/lochia Homan's sign IV site Breasts ID band on mother Activity	Assess pain control 0–10 scale Incision Volding Fundus lochia Homan's sign IV site as needed ID band on mother Activity

(continued)

Integrated Plan of Care for Cesarean Delivery (continued)

		Plan of Care		
	#1 Preadmission	# 2 Surgery/ Immediate Postop/ Day of Surgery	#3 Post Op Day 1	#4 Post Op Day 2-Discharge
		*I & O q shift *Assess pain control 0–10 scale *Assess Rhogam status *Assess Rubella titer status *ID band on mother		
Consults	Anesthesia	Social Work as needed, Anesthesia, Lactation, Dietitian as needed	Social Work, Lactation, Dietitian as needed	Social Work, Lactation, Dietitian as needed

Patient / Family Education Discharge Planning	— Need for surgery
	— Review Cesarean Delivery
	— Review procedure, postop expectations
	— Demonstrate/ Discuss equipment— PCA, Fentanyl pump
	— Tour of OR area & Nsy
		Review post-op expectations
		Review equipment us prn
		Instruct pt on:
		  Hospital/Infant security systems
		  Unity orientation
		  Newborn orientation/care /feeding (if breastfeeding problems see decision trees)
			Review dietary needs post surgery
			Review Bleeding/ Lochia
			Precautions post cesarean delivery
			Review follow-up care and doctor Appointments
			Review incision care, peri care
			Infant care
			Infant feeding
				Verify follow-up appointment date and time
				Activity restrictions
				Follow-up for staple removal as needed
				Offer Home follow-up care
				Discuss birth control

Tests and Procedures	PAT; Hgb or Hct (if not done recently—within one month) T & S (if ordered)			
Pharmacologic Needs		IV fluids as ordered Pain control: PCA, Fentanyl pump, IM to PO	IV lock PO pain meds Give Rhogam if indicated Give Rubella if indicated	DC IV lock as ordered

Plan of Care				
	#1 Preadmission	# 2 Surgery/ Immediate Postop/ Day of Surgery	#3 Post Op Day 1	#4 Post Op Day 2- Discharge
Activity / Rehabilitation	Patients usual	Change position q 2 hr while in bed, OOB stand at bedside post-op night/dangle and transfer to chair Progress to pt. endurance Observe bonding with infant Observe family support system (if inadequate consult SW)	Progress endurance/ begin Ambulation in hall OOB in AM May shower	Ambulate in halls without assistance
Nutrition / Elimination		NPO then clear liquids to DAT Foley empty q shift	DAT to regular or previous diet at home FOLEY DC'd	
Miscellaneous Interventions		TCDB q 2 hr while awake	Dressing removed by MD or RN with MD request	
Unique Patient Needs				

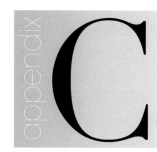

Cervical Dilation Chart

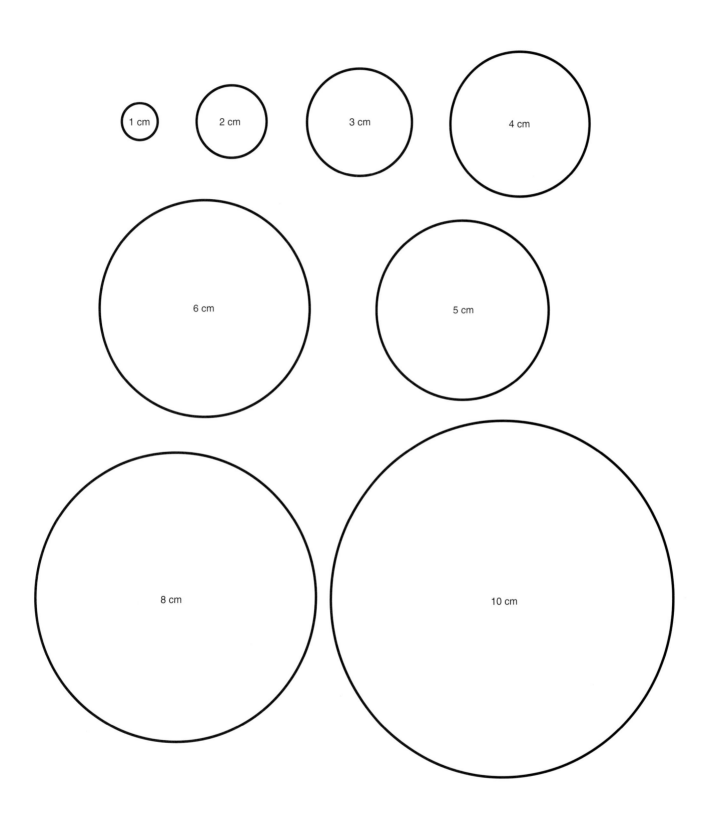

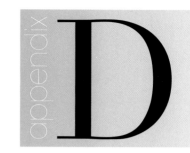

Weight Conversion Charts

Conversion of Pounds to Kilograms

Pounds	0	1	2	3	4	5	6	7	8	9
0	—	0.45	0.90	1.36	1.81	2.26	2.72	3.17	3.62	4.08
10	4.53	4.98	5.44	5.89	6.35	6.80	7.25	7.71	8.16	8.61
20	9.07	9.52	9.97	10.43	10.88	11.34	11.79	12.24	12.70	13.15
30	13.60	14.06	14.51	14.96	15.42	15.87	16.32	16.78	17.23	17.69
40	18.14	18.59	19.05	19.50	19.95	20.41	20.86	21.31	21.77	22.22
50	22.68	23.13	23.58	24.04	24.49	24.94	25.40	25.85	26.30	26.76
60	27.21	27.66	28.12	28.57	29.03	29.48	29.93	30.39	30.84	31.29
70	31.75	32.20	32.65	33.11	33.56	34.02	34.47	34.92	35.38	35.83
80	36.28	36.74	37.19	37.64	38.10	38.55	39.00	39.46	39.91	40.37
90	40.82	41.27	41.73	42.18	42.63	43.09	43.54	43.99	44.45	44.90
100	45.36	45.81	46.26	46.72	47.17	47.62	48.08	48.53	48.98	49.44
110	49.89	50.34	50.80	51.25	51.71	52.16	52.61	53.07	53.52	53.97
120	54.43	54.88	55.33	55.79	56.24	56.70	57.15	57.60	58.06	58.51
130	58.96	59.42	59.87	60.32	60.78	61.23	61.68	62.14	62.59	63.05
140	63.50	63.95	64.41	64.86	65.31	65.77	66.22	66.67	67.13	67.58
150	68.04	68.49	68.94	69.40	69.85	70.30	70.76	71.21	71.66	72.12
160	72.57	73.02	73.48	73.93	74.39	74.84	75.29	75.75	76.20	76.65
170	77.11	77.56	78.01	78.47	78.92	79.38	79.83	80.28	80.74	81.19
180	81.64	82.10	82.55	83.00	83.46	83.91	84.36	84.82	85.27	85.73
190	86.18	86.68	87.09	87.54	87.99	88.45	88.90	89.35	89.81	90.26
200	90.72	91.17	91.62	92.08	92.53	92.98	93.44	93.89	94.34	94.80

Conversion of Pounds and Ounces to Grams for Newborn Weights

Pounds	Ounces															
	0	1	2	3	4	5	6	7	8	9	10	11	12	13	14	15
0	—	28	57	85	113	142	170	198	227	255	283	312	430	369	397	425
1	454	482	510	539	567	595	624	652	680	709	737	765	794	822	850	879
2	907	936	964	992	1021	1049	1077	1106	1134	1162	1191	1219	1247	1276	1304	1332
3	1361	1389	1417	1446	1474	1503	1531	1559	1588	1616	1644	1673	1701	1729	1758	1786
4	1814	1843	1871	1899	1928	1956	1984	2013	2041	2070	2098	2126	2155	2183	2211	2240
5	2268	2296	2325	2353	2381	2410	2438	2466	2495	2523	2551	2580	2608	2637	2665	2693
6	2722	2750	2778	2807	2835	2863	2892	2920	2948	2977	3005	3033	3062	3090	3118	3147
7	3175	3203	3232	3260	3289	3317	3345	3374	3402	3430	3459	3487	3515	3544	3572	3600
8	3629	3657	3685	3714	3742	3770	3799	3827	3856	3884	3912	3941	3969	3997	4026	4054
9	4082	4111	4139	4167	4196	4224	4252	4281	4309	4337	4366	4394	4423	4451	4479	4508
10	4536	4564	4593	4621	4649	4678	4706	4734	4763	4791	4819	4848	4876	4904	4933	4961
11	4990	5018	5046	5075	5103	5131	5160	5188	5216	5245	5273	5301	5330	5358	5386	5415
12	5443	5471	5500	5528	5557	5585	5613	5642	5670	5698	5727	5755	5783	5812	5840	5868
13	5897	5925	5953	5982	6010	6038	6067	6095	6123	6152	6180	6209	6237	6265	6294	6322
14	6350	6379	6407	6435	6464	6492	6520	6549	6577	6605	6634	6662	6690	6719	6747	6776
15	6804	6832	6860	6889	6917	6945	6973	7002	7030	7059	7087	7115	7144	7172	7201	7228

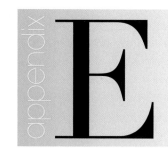

Breast-Feeding and Medication Use

General Considerations

- Most medications are safe to use while breast-feeding; however, the woman should always check with the pediatrician, physician, or lactation specialist before taking any medications, including over-the-counter and herbal products.
- Inform the woman that she has the right to seek a second opinion if the physician does not perform a thoughtful risk-versus-benefit assessment before prescribing medications or advising against breast-feeding.
- Most medications pass from the woman's bloodstream into the breast milk. However, the amount is usually very small and unlikely to harm the baby.
- A preterm or other special needs neonate is more susceptible to the adverse effects of medications in breast milk. A woman who is taking medications and whose baby is in the neonatal intensive care unit or special care nursery should consult with the pediatrician or neonatologist before feeding her breast milk to the baby.
- If the woman is taking a prescribed medication, she should take the medication just after breast-feeding. This practice helps ensure that the lowest possible dose of medication reaches the baby through the breast milk.
- Some medications can cause changes in the amount of milk the woman produces. Teach the woman to report any changes in milk production.

Lactation Risk Categories (LRC)

Lactation Category	Risk	Rationale
L1	Safest	Clinical research or long-term observation of use in many breast-feeding women has not demonstrated risk to the infant.
L2	Safer	Limited clinical research has not demonstrated an increase in adverse effects in the infant.
L3	Moderately safe	There is possible risk to the infant; however, the risks are minimal or nonthreatening in nature. These medications should be given only when the potential benefit outweighs the risk to the infant.

(continued)

Lactation Category	Risk	Rationale
L4	Possibly hazardous	There is positive evidence of risk to the infant; however, in life-threatening situations or for serious diseases, the benefit might outweigh the risk.
L5	Contraindicated	The risk of using the medication clearly outweighs any possible benefit from breast-feeding.

Potential Effects of Selected Medication Categories on the Breast-Fed Infant

Narcotic Analgesics

- Codeine and hydrocodone appear to be safe in moderate doses. Rarely the neonate may experience sedation and/or apnea. (LRC: L3)
- Meperidine (Demerol) can lead to sedation of the neonate. (LRC: L3)
- Low to moderate doses of morphine appear to be safe. (LRC: L2)
- Trace-to-negligible amounts of fentanyl are found in human milk. (LRC: L2)

Non-narcotic Analgesics and NSAIDs

- Acetaminophen and ibuprofen are approved for use. (LRC: L1)
- Naproxen may cause neonatal hemorrhage and anemia if used for prolonged periods. (LRC: L3 for short-term use and L4 for long-term use)
- The newer COX2 inhibitors, such as celecoxib (Celebrex), appear to be safe for use. (LRC: L2)

Antibiotics

- Levels in breast milk are usually very low.
- The penicillins and cephalosporins are generally considered safe to use. (LRC: L1 and L2)
- Tetracyclines can be safely used for short periods but are not suitable for long-term therapy (e.g., for treatment of acne). (LRC: L2)

- Sulfonamides should not be used during the neonatal stage (the first month of life). (LRC: L3)

Antihypertensives

- A high degree of caution is advised when antihypertensives are used during breast-feeding.
- Some beta blockers can be used.
- Hydralazine and methyldopa are considered to be safe. (LRC: L2)
- ACE inhibitors are not recommended in the early postpartum period.

Sedatives and Hypnotics

- Neonatal withdrawal can occur when antianxiety medications, such as lorazepam, are taken. Fortunately withdrawal is generally mild.
- Phenothiazines, such as Phenergan and Thorazine, may lead to sleep apnea and increase the risk for sudden infant death syndrome.

Antidepressants

- The risk to the baby often is higher if the woman is depressed and remains untreated, rather than taking the medication.
- The older tricyclics are considered to be safe; however they cause many bothersome side effects, such as weight gain and dry mouth, which may lead to noncompliance on the part of the woman.
- The selective serotonin uptake inhibitors (SSRIs) also are considered to be safe and have a lower side effect profile, which makes them more palatable to the woman. (LRC: L2 and L3)

Mood Stabilizers (Antimanic Medication)

- Lithium is found in breast milk and is best not used in the breast-feeding woman. (LRC: L4)
- Valproic acid (Depakote) seems to be a more appropriate choice for the woman with bipolar disorder. The infant will need periodic lab studies to check platelets and liver function.

Corticosteroids

- Corticosteroids do not pass into the milk in large quantities.
- Inhaled steroids are safe to use because they don't accumulate in the bloodstream.

Thyroid Medication

- Thyroid medications, such as levothyroxine (Synthroid), can be taken while breast-feeding.
- Most are in LRC category L1.

Medications That Usually Are Contraindicated for the Breast-Feeding Woman

- Amiodarone
- Antineoplastic agents
- Chloramphenicol
- Doxepin
- Ergotamine and other ergot derivatives
- Iodides
- Methotrexate and immunosuppressants
- Lithium
- Radiopharmaceuticals
- Ribavirin
- Tetracycline (prolonged use—more than 3 weeks)
- Pseudoephedrine (found in many over-the-counter medications)

Material in this Appendix was adapted from information found on the American Academy of Pediatrics website (www.aap.org) and from Riordan, J. (2005). *Breastfeeding and human lactation* (3rd ed.). Boston: Jones and Bartlett Publishers; Hale, T. W. (2004). *Medications and mother's milk* (11th ed.). Amarillo, TX: Pharmasoft Publishing.

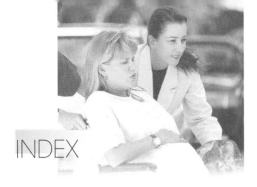

INDEX

Page numbers followed by *t* indicate tables; those followed by *f* indicate figures; those followed by *b* indicate boxes.